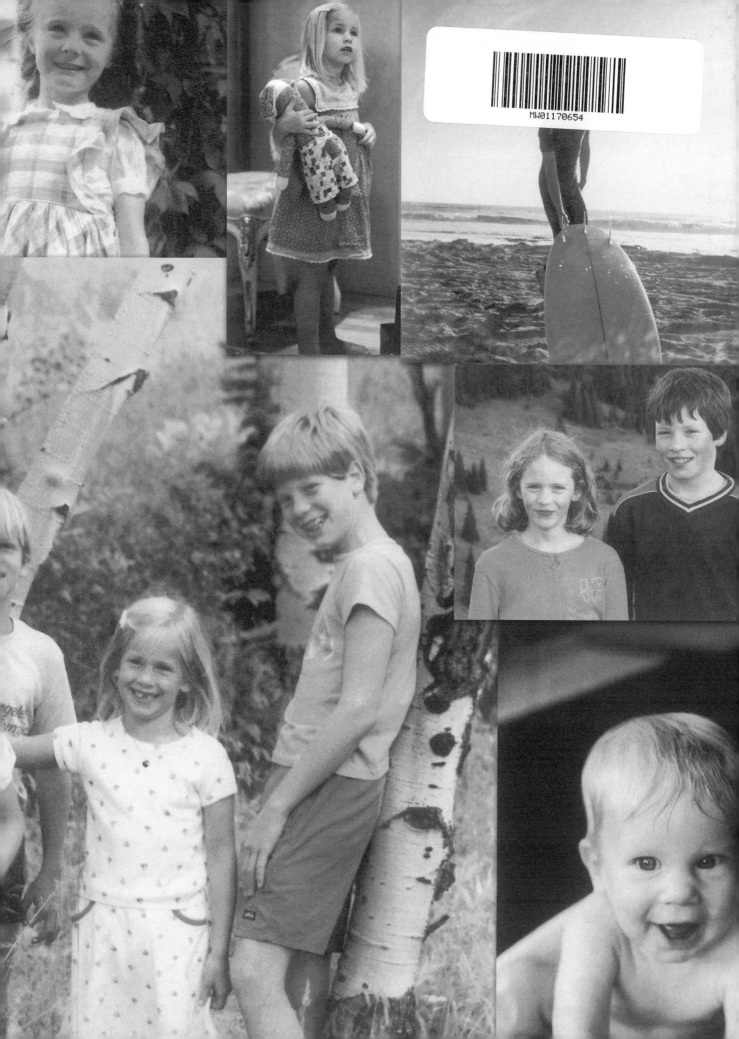

PRACTICAL
PEDIATRIC
RADIOLOGY

PRACTICAL PEDIATRIC RADIOLOGY

SASKIA V.W. HILTON, M.D.

DAVID K. EDWARDS, III, M.D.

Third Edition

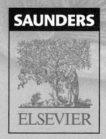

SAUNDERS

ELSEVIER

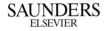

1600 John F. Kennedy Blvd.
Ste 1800
Philadelphia, PA 19103-2899

PRACTICAL PEDIATRIC RADIOLOGY, Third Edition

ISBN-13: 978-0-7216-9266-1
ISBN-10: 0-7216-9266-4

Library of Congress Cataloging-in-Publication Data

Practical pediatric radiology/[edited by] Saskia von Waldenburg Hilton, David K.
   Edwards III.–3rd ed.
      p.;cm
   Includes bibliographical references and index.
   ISBN 0-7216-9266-4
   1. Pediatric radiology. I. Hilton, Saskia von Waldenburg. II Edwards, David K.
   [DNLM: 1. Radiography–Child. 2. Radiography–Infant. WN 240 P895 2006]
RJ51.R3H54 2006
618.92′007572—dc22

2005051714

ISBN-13: 978-0-7216-9266-1
ISBN-10: 0-7216-9266-4

Acquisitions Editor: Meghan McAteer
Editorial Assistant: Elizabeth Schweizer
Publishing Services Manager: Joan Sinclair
Project Manager: Mary B. Stermel
Marketing Manager: Emily Christie

Chapter 1 images and illustrations courtesy of Dr. Ernst Richter; from Richter E., Oestreich, AE: Imaging Anatomy of the Newborn. Vienna, Urban & Schwarzenberg, 1990.

Printed in the United States of America

Last digit is the print number: 9   8   7   6   5   4   3   2   1

PREFACE

This third edition of our text retains the primary goals of the prior two editions. The first of these goals is to assist radiologists who deal only intermittently with infants and children and who thus regard pediatric radiology with some uncertainty and even trepidation. It is undeniable that pediatric radiology differs notably from adult radiology and typically is practiced primarily in tertiary medical centers. In such centers, pediatric radiology exists as a vibrant, growing specialty, but outside such centers the specialty becomes relatively arcane, so that general radiologists risk losing touch with its techniques and advances. We hope that this text is a valued resource for radiologists whose orientation is not primarily pediatric. Additionally, we intend the book to be of immediate, practical utility to emergency physicians, general pediatricians, and family medicine practitioners.

Another goal involves radiology teaching. Radiology residents, usually trained in tertiary centers, may face challenges that paradoxically are engendered by the nature of such centers. Tertiary centers and teaching facilities commonly treat children who are critically ill, often with uncommon disorders, as well as extraordinary populations such as infants in neonatal intensive care units. Although radiology residents thus trained are usually comfortable with new imaging modalities, contemporary techniques, and an assortment of unusual pediatric diseases, they risk unfamiliarity with the more mundane and commonplace aspects of general pediatric radiology. It is our hope and belief that a radiology resident familiar with the content of this book will not merely pass the pediatric portions of the Radiology Board examinations but will also be able to approach sick children professionally with skill and confidence.

A sick child usually presents at a primary care facility with a fairly well-defined symptom (or symptoms). The symptom suggests a limited differential diagnosis that is specific to the child's age. Diagnostic possibilities are best explored according to the likelihood of specific diseases, and the nature of the likely diseases focuses the diagnostic approach. Thus, the presenting symptom forms the practical basis of pediatric radiology. All three editions of this text are organized according to symptoms, which were chosen from the presenting symptoms of outpatient pediatric patients at the largest primary care facility in San Diego.

The first edition of this text, published more than 22 years ago, was gratifyingly well received because of this unique, symptom-oriented approach, which both radiologists and pediatricians found helpful in daily practice. The approach may be summarized as, "Given the child's major symptom, here is the most expeditious path to the diagnosis." This approach provides an effective and cost-containing evaluation in a medical environment beset with financial constraints and unfamiliar imaging modalities. For this reason, the text is additionally and especially suited to physicians practicing primary care pediatrics, emergency room medicine, and family practice.

The essential style and format have been retained in the successive editions of this text. Changes are intended to increase quality rather than size, and new chapters have selectively replaced those rendered less important by changing health care patterns. We have tried to limit all changes to those that are truly significant in a practical sense, rather than change for the sake of change.

This third edition's first chapter, an atlas of normal and preterm infant anatomy, is a new addition that greatly enriches the book. Its unique drawings by Roland Helmus and Marianne Lück are immensely helpful in understanding the radiographic findings of infants; additionally, many of these drawings exhibit artistic merit beyond their medical value, and one of them embellishes the cover.

We hope that this book meets and perhaps sometimes even exceeds our goals, and we remain grateful for any comments or criticisms that our readers may wish to offer.

SASKIA v.W. HILTON, M.D.

DAVID K. EDWARDS, III, M.D.

ACKNOWLEDGMENTS

The editors express their sincere appreciation to the contributors of this text for working successfully within a tightly confined framework that we believed necessary to produce a textbook of uniform style and format. We also thank them for accepting graciously and peacefully our often extensive and occasionally arbitrary revisions. We wished to produce a book that contained the wisdom, expertise, and experience of many scholars, which, for the reader's sake, suggested a single author.

Many colleagues contributed their time, effort, and material for this book. Experts in their specific fields reviewed several chapters, including Drs. Robert A. Kaufman, Paul K. Kleinman, Marilyn J. Siegel, Robert L. Lebowitz, John A. Kirkpatrick, N. Thorne Griscom, Martin Stein, and the Honorable Barbara Gamer. We are also notably grateful to our previous contributors from all editions of this book: Joel Blumhagen, M.D.; Calvin Colarusso, M.D.; Edmund A. Franken Jr., M.D.; Charles B. Higgins, M.D.; John W. Hilton, M.D.; Alan D. Hoffman, M.D.; Simon C. S. Kao, M.D.; Aryampur Kashani, M.D.; Kenneth Miller, M.D.; Lee H. Prewitt Jr., M.D.; Joanna Seibert, M.D.; Marilyn J. Siegel, M.D.; Philip Stanley, M.D.; Richard L. Wesenberg, M.D.; and Sandra Wooton-Gorges, M.D.

Dr. Judy A. Estroff provided the prenatal sonography. This material was widely employed throughout the text to demonstrate the utility of prenatal diagnosis.

Many individuals graciously provided us with superb images when our own files were lacking. A special word of gratitude is owed to Ron Cohen, who provided numerous illustrations. Many other colleagues provided us with valuable case material, including: Deborah S. Ablin, Bennett A. Alford, Richard D. Bellah, Gayle H. Bickers, George S. Bisset III, Joel D. Blumhagen, Robert C. Brasch, David Cranefield, James S. Donaldson, Paul Dukes, Judy A. Estroff, Sandra K. Fernbach, Lawrence E. Goldberger, Charles A. Gooding, Rick Greaney, N. Thorne Griscom, H. Theodore Harcke Jr., Deborah Harris, Alan D. Hoffman, George W. Kaplan, Robert A. Kaufman, Robert L. Lebowitz, Philippe L'Heureux, Massoud Majd, Kenneth E. Miller, Jenny Mitchell, Sheila G. Moore, David D. Payne, Paul S. Schulman, Joanna J. Seibert, Gary D. Shackelford, John R. Sty, Ina L. D. Tonkin, and Ulrich Willi.

We are especially grateful for the secretarial help of Gale Hurley, Tony McAfee, and Brenda Moreno. Marcia L. Earnshaw was responsible for the photography of the second edition. Ian Hilton provided the graphic art for this edition.

We are profoundly indebted to the staff at Elsevier Science, whose high standards of excellence produced the best possible book from our manuscript, photographs, and drawings. We are especially grateful to Meghan McAteer for her editorial assistance; her skill, advice, and patience made our interactions with the publisher a rewarding pleasure. Also invaluable were the seemingly tireless efforts of Bruce Siebert, Elizabeth Schweizer, and Mary B. Stermel.

A final word of love from Dr. Hilton is offered in memory of Reine Schofield whose presence enriched my life and the lives of my children and without whom this book would never have been written.

SASKIA v.W. HILTON, M.D.

DAVID K. EDWARDS, III, M.D.

DEDICATION

This book is most gratefully dedicated to my husband, Warren Gross, for his unfailing humor, and to our five children: Tiffany, Ian, Keith, Avery, and Megan.

SASKIA v.W. HILTON, M.D.

TABLE OF CONTENTS

CHAPTER 1

INTRODUCTION: ATLAS OF NORMAL ANATOMY OF THE PREMATURE AND TERM INFANT

Ernst Richter, MD

INTRODUCTION: ATLAS OF NORMAL ANATOMY OF THE PREMATURE AND TERM INFANT

Anatomy provides the foundation upon which diagnostic imaging is based. The anatomic relationships of the newborn child differ considerably from those of later childhood and adulthood. The statement "the child is not merely a small adult" is especially true for the newborn child. The topographic relationships and relative proportions are different and indeed to some extent so is nomenclature. Therefore, there are definite limitations to applying to the newborn an atlas that correlates anatomy and diagnostic imaging in the adult. Studies of the roentgenologic anatomy of the newborn were produced soon after the discovery of the x-ray. However, to date there have not been many atlases or monographs published concerning anatomy of the fetus and newborn, and most of these have been devoted to specific organ systems. In these sources one finds only isolated references to radiographic diagnosis, ultrasound imaging, and other forms of diagnostic imaging.

In this chapter we will touch upon all aspects of anatomy of the premature and term newborn, although we are not aiming for the completeness of a formal system of anatomy. Our emphasis will be on points of practical clinical application.

The material is intended principally for pediatricians and radiologists involved in the clinical care and diagnostic imaging of the newborn, especially during the period of intensive care. For that reason the book is divided into regions of clinical interest. Some anatomic preparations and sections are arranged to correspond to clinical images (e.g., obliquely oriented sections of brain for obliquely oriented sonographic images). Because of their clinical importance in the newborn period, sonography and conventional radiology will be emphasized.

The organs of premature newborns, as well as those of the term baby, develop rapidly. Birth is a variable point of time in terms of these processes of development. The illustrations offered from our investigations of premature and term newborns are like individual still frames from a rapidly projected, highly suspenseful movie. Development certainly does not cease with birth, but proceeds further in the extrauterine phase. To explain both this development and the varied possibilities for maldevelopment, it will be useful to review pertinent events in embryonic and fetal development.

Increasingly, immature premature infants are being cared for in modern high-level neonatal intensive care units; diagnosis and surveillance using radiology and sonography are essential to this process. This book is also intended as a guide for these situations.

The drawings and schematic diagrams in this chapter are based on anatomic preparations and sections of the human fetus and newborns (taken with the permission of the parents). Postmortem arteriograms and venograms permit vivid demonstration of the vascular system. Postmortem direct application of contrast material permits various structures to become radiographically visible (e.g., serous cavities such as the pleural space, pericardium, and peritoneum; joint cavities; the pharynx and esophagus; the tracheobronchial tree; and endocranial surfaces of the skull base). Because of concerns about radiation exposure, these radiographic anatomic illustrations are practical only as a postmortem endeavor.

Diagnostic imaging procedures will develop further with time, and both their nature and their indications will change. Newer methods will provide more precise information about the anatomy, pathology, and function of the organs of the living human. In the context of this process of development of diagnostic possibilities, we hope our work will provide a foundation for knowledge of the newborn period and that it will provide stimulation for our younger colleagues who will lead the future development of pediatric radiology.

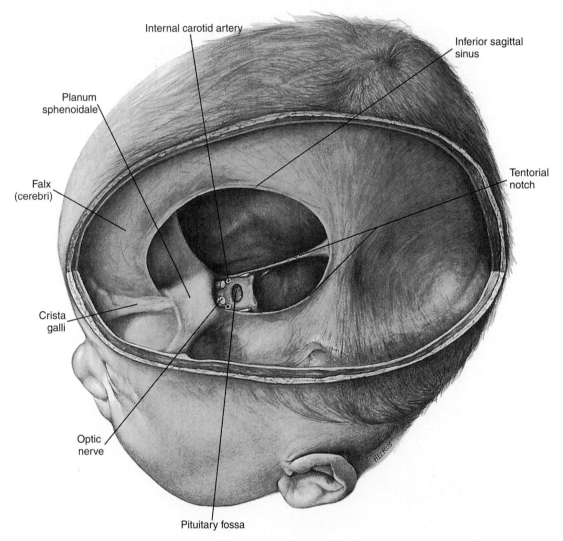

Internal carotid artery

Inferior sagittal sinus

Planum sphenoidale\

Tentorial notch

Falx (cerebri)

Crista galli

Optic nerve

Pituitary fossa

Figure 1–1
Cranial cavity of a nearly full-term newborn. The cranium has been opened from the left and the brain has been removed. The tentorial notch extends considerably upward. The cartilaginous dorsum sellae is well-developed.

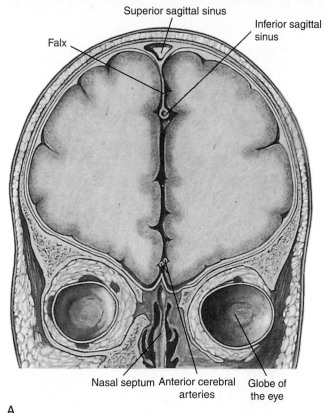

Superior sagittal sinus

Inferior sagittal sinus

Falx

Nasal septum   Anterior cerebral   Globe of
arteries   the eye

A

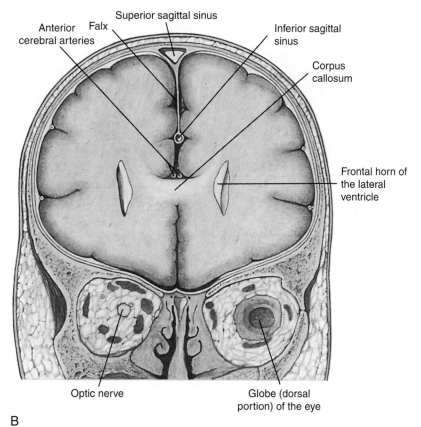

Anterior   Falx   Superior sagittal sinus
cerebral arteries

Inferior sagittal sinus

Corpus callosum

Frontal horn of the lateral ventricle

Optic nerve   Globe (dorsal portion) of the eye

B

Figure 1–2

A, Coronal section anterior to the frontal horns of the lateral ventricles.
B, Coronal section through the frontal horns of the lateral ventricles, as well as
the genu of the corpus callosum.   *Continued*

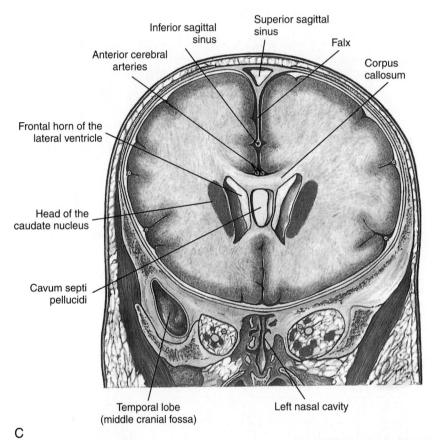

Inferior sagittal
sinus

Superior sagittal
sinus

Falx

Anterior cerebral
arteries

Corpus
callosum

Frontal horn of the
lateral ventricle

Head of the
caudate nucleus

Cavum septi
pellucidi

Temporal lobe
(middle cranial fossa)

Left nasal cavity

C

Figure 1–2—cont'd

C, Coronal section anterior to the foramina of Monro. Included are the cavum septi pallucidi, the midportions of the frontal horns of the lateral ventricles, and the heads of the caudate nuclei.

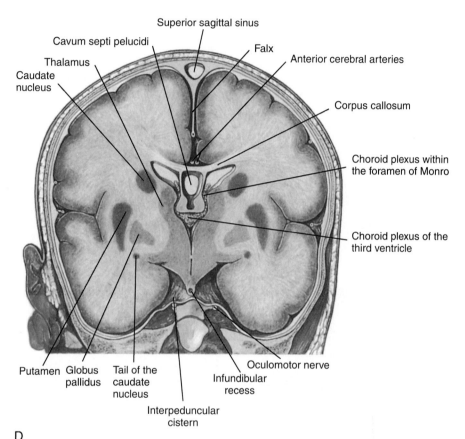

Superior sagittal sinus

Cavum septi pelucidi

Falx

Thalamus

Anterior cerebral arteries

Caudate
nucleus

Corpus callosum

Choroid plexus within
the foramen of Monro

Choroid plexus of the
third ventricle

Putamen Globus
pallidus

Tail of the
caudate
nucleus

Oculomotor nerve

Infundibular
recess

Interpeduncular
cistern

D

Figure 1–2—cont'd

D, Coronal section through the foramina of Monro. The body of the corpus callosum is still thin at this early stage of development. The tela choroidea and the choroid plexus of both lateral and third ventricles are encountered. *Continued*

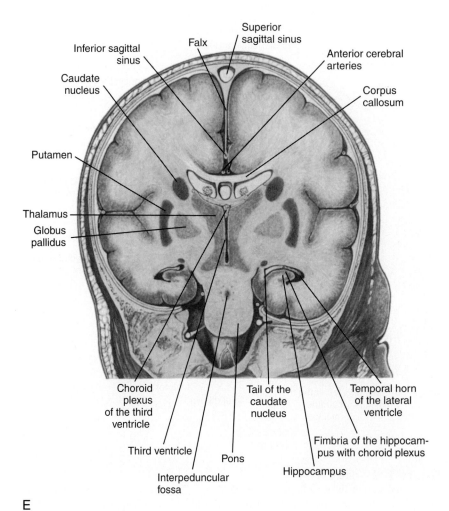

E

Figure 1–2—cont'd

E, Coronal section just posterior to the foramen of Monro.

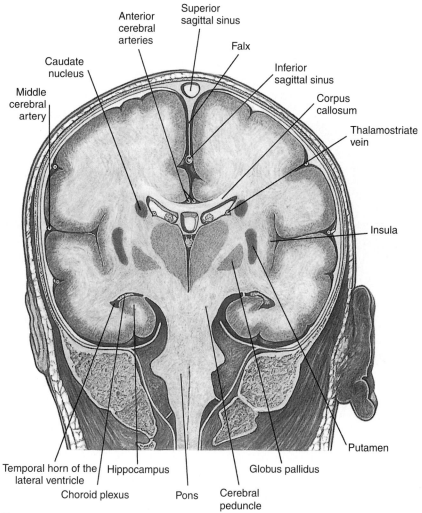

F

Figure 1–2—cont'd

F, Coronal section containing the junction of the brain stem, directed somewhat occipitally from the anterior fontanelle.

Continued

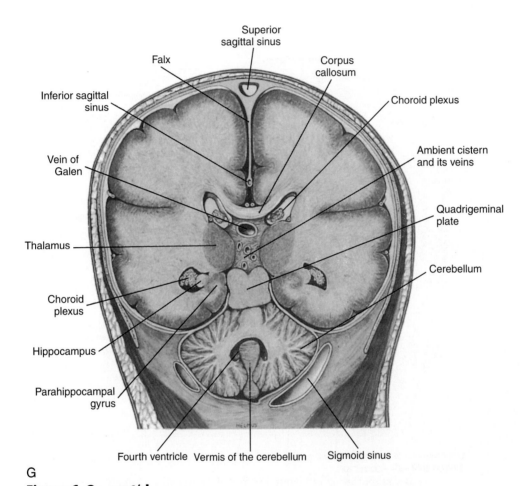

G

Figure 1–2—cont'd

G, Coronal section directed more occipitally through the pulvinar and cerebellum. The roof of the midbrain is sectioned just dorsal to the aqueduct. The fourth ventricle is exposed. In the large ambient cistern lies the relatively prominent great vein of Galen.

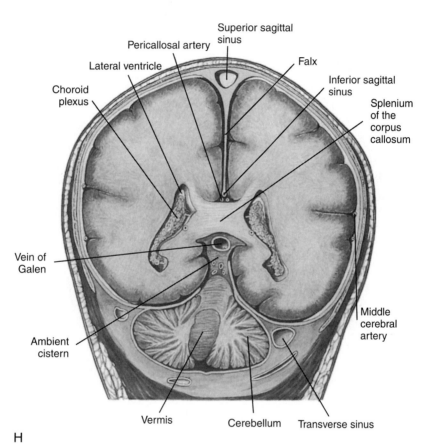

H

Figure 1–2—cont'd
H, Coronal section through the anterior fontanelle tipped occipitally to pass through the splenium of the corpus callosum, dorsal to the midbrain and fourth ventricle. Voluminous portions of choroid plexus (i.e., glomus) in the trigone of the lateral ventricle bilaterally.

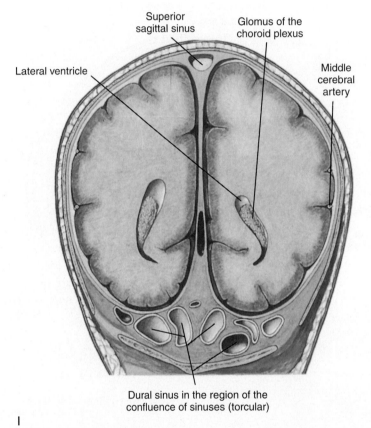

Superior
sagittal sinus

Glomus of the
choroid plexus

Lateral ventricle

Middle
cerebral
artery

Dural sinus in the region of the
confluence of sinuses (torcular)

Figure 1–2—cont'd
I, The most posteriorly tilted coronal section through the occipital
horns of the lateral ventricles. The occipital portions of the dural
sinuses are particularly spacious at this early stage of development.

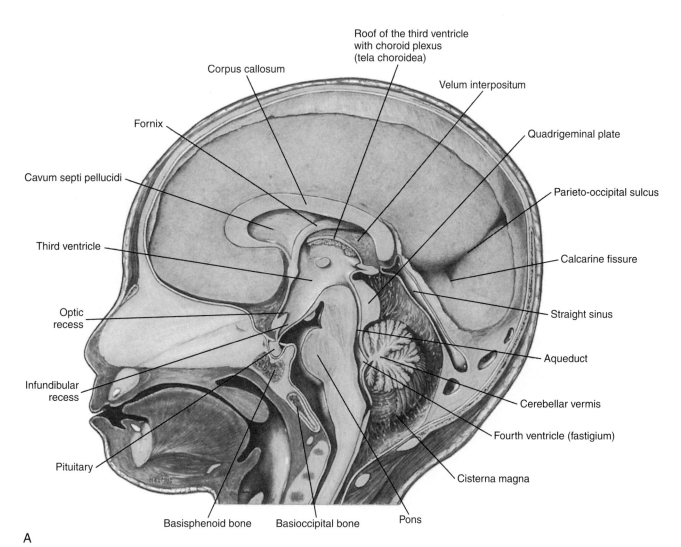

A
Figure 1–3
Normal brain of a 26-week gestation newborn. *A,* Midline section, showing the right side of the brain.

Continued

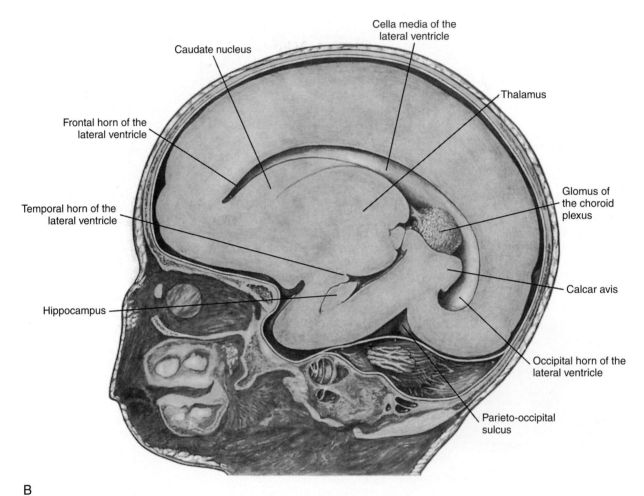

Cella media of the
lateral ventricle

Caudate nucleus

Thalamus

Frontal horn of the
lateral ventricle

Glomus of
the choroid
plexus

Temporal horn of the
lateral ventricle

Calcar avis

Hippocampus

Occipital horn of the
lateral ventricle

Parieto-occipital
sulcus

B
Figure 1–3—cont'd
B, obliquely cut parasagittal section through the long diameter of the lateral ventricle, corresponding to sonographic imaging. Right hemisphere as seen from medially.

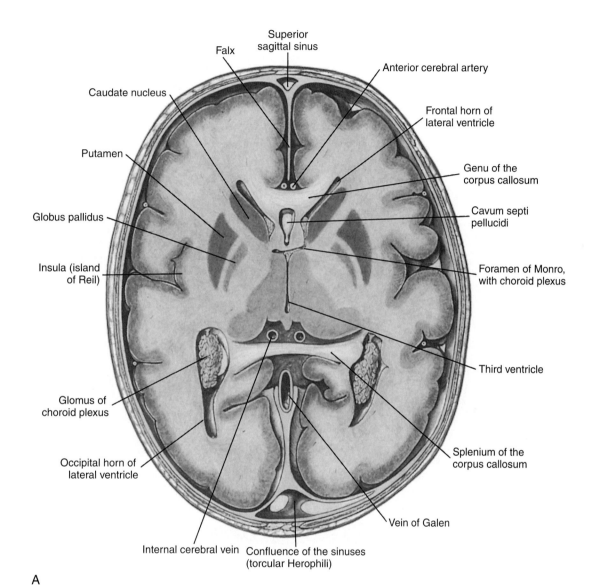

Superior
sagittal sinus

Falx

Anterior cerebral artery

Caudate nucleus

Frontal horn of
lateral ventricle

Putamen

Genu of the
corpus callosum

Globus pallidus

Cavum septi
pellucidi

Insula (island
of Reil)

Foramen of Monro,
with choroid plexus

Third ventricle

Glomus of
choroid plexus

Occipital horn of
lateral ventricle

Splenium of the
corpus callosum

Vein of Galen

Internal cerebral vein   Confluence of the sinuses
(torcular Herophili)

A

Figure 1–4
Axial sections through anatomic preparation of the brain of a 29-week gestation fetus, viewed
from above. *A,* Closest to the vertex; *D,* most basal. *A,* Axial section through the basal ganglia and the
occipital horns of the lateral ventricle, as well as the genu and the splenium of the corpus callosum.

Continued

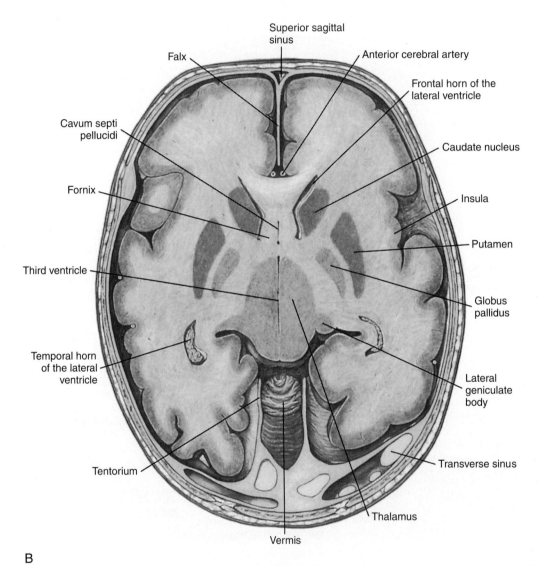

B

Figure 1–4—cont'd
B, Axial section through the inferior portion of the basal ganglia and the tentorial notch. The occipital dural sinuses are still quite wide at this stage of development.

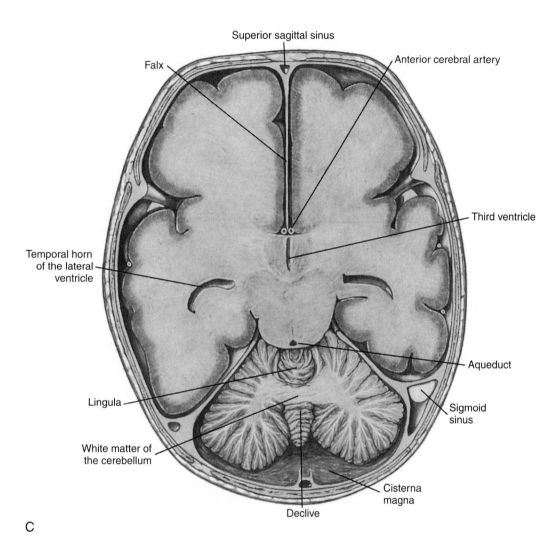

C

Figure 1–4—cont'd
C, Axial section through the hypothalamus, the midbrain, and the cerebellum.

Continued

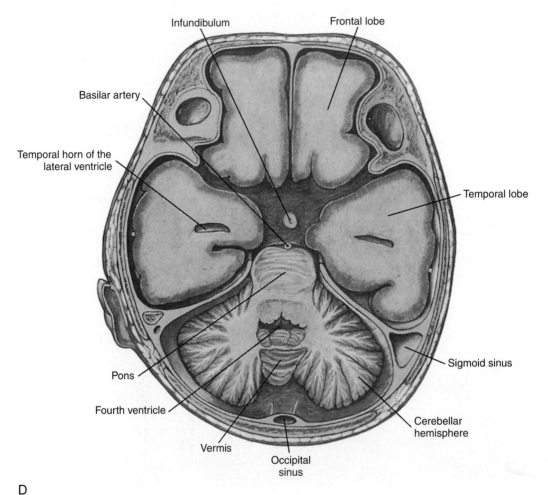

Infundibulum

Frontal lobe

Basilar artery

Temporal horn of the
lateral ventricle

Temporal lobe

Sigmoid sinus

Pons

Fourth ventricle

Cerebellar
hemisphere

Vermis

Occipital
sinus

D

Figure 1–4—cont'd
D, Axial section through the basal portions of the frontal and temporal lobes, the pons, and the
cerebellum.

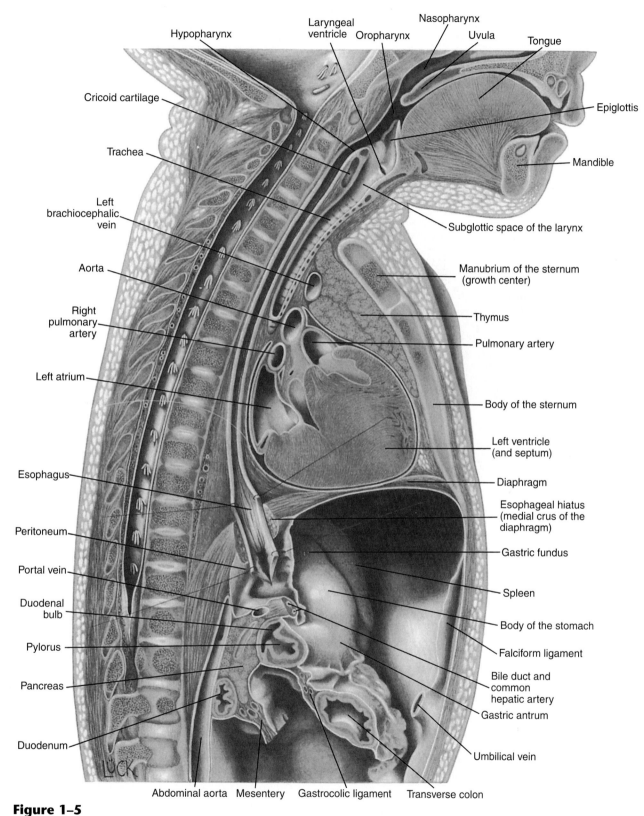

Hypopharynx

Laryngeal ventricle

Oropharynx

Nasopharynx

Uvula

Tongue

Cricoid cartilage

Trachea

Left brachiocephalic vein

Aorta

Right pulmonary artery

Left atrium

Esophagus

Peritoneum

Portal vein

Duodenal bulb

Pylorus

Pancreas

Duodenum

Epiglottis

Mandible

Subglottic space of the larynx

Manubrium of the sternum (growth center)

Thymus

Pulmonary artery

Body of the sternum

Left ventricle (and septum)

Diaphragm

Esophageal hiatus (medial crus of the diaphragm)

Gastric fundus

Spleen

Body of the stomach

Falciform ligament

Bile duct and common hepatic artery

Gastric antrum

Umbilical vein

Abdominal aorta   Mesentery   Gastrocolic ligament   Transverse colon

Figure 1–5

Midline section of a 29-week gestation premature newborn, view of the left side. The facial bones are low-lying and the neck is short. The thymus occupies the narrow upper throat, narrowing to a point. The entire length of the esophagus is shown. Both the gastroesophageal junction and antro-pyloric junction are shown.

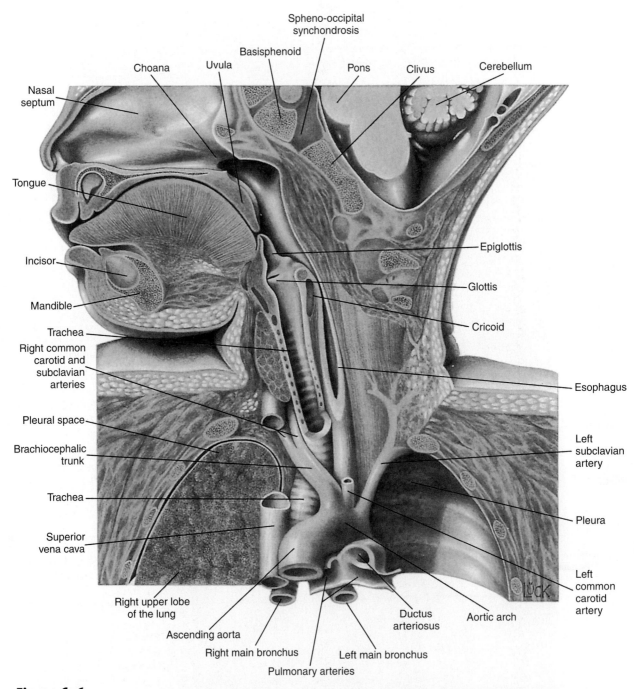

Figure 1-6

Nasal and oral cavity, pharynx, neck, and upper thorax of a 26-week gestation premature infant, with the head turned to the right. The ductus arteriosus forms part of the left upper margin of the mediastinum. The brachiocephalic trunk runs obliquely across the anterior trachea.

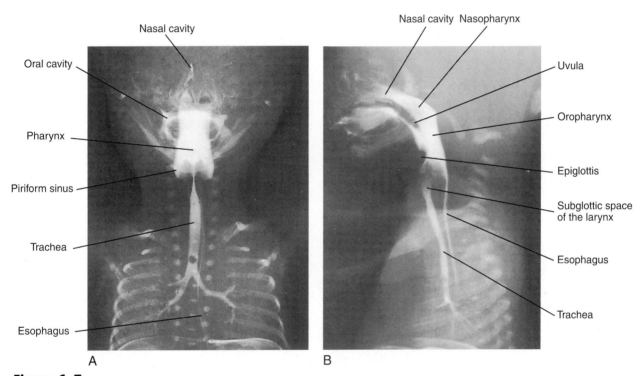

A

B

Figure 1–7
Post-mortem contrast filling of the oral cavity, pharynx, trachea, and esophagus of a 15-week gestation fetus (with peritoneum also contrast-filled).

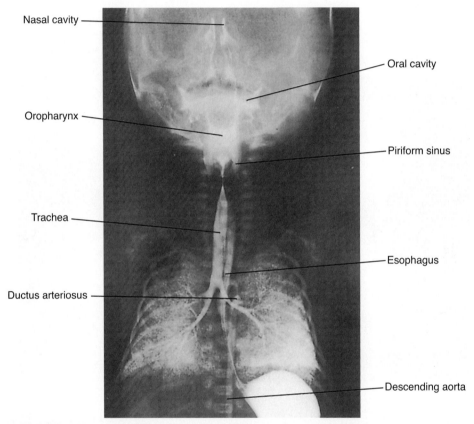

Figure 1–8
Fetus at the 20th week of gestation, with contrast filling of the respiratory tract and upper gastrointestinal tract (together with aortography).

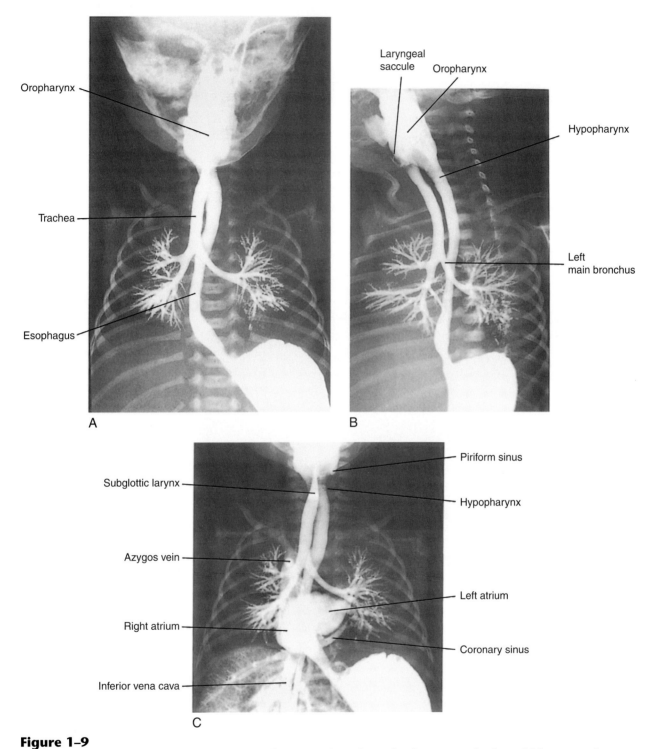

Oropharynx

Trachea

Esophagus

A

Laryngeal saccule

Oropharynx

Hypopharynx

Left main bronchus

B

Subglottic larynx

Azygos vein

Right atrium

Inferior vena cava

C

Piriform sinus

Hypopharynx

Left atrium

Coronary sinus

Figure 1–9
Premature of 32 weeks gestation, post-mortem demonstration of mouth, pharynx, tracheobronchial tree, esophagus, and stomach. *A,* Frontal; *B,* right posterior oblique; *C,* frontal with simultaneous contrast filling of the venous system as well as both atria.

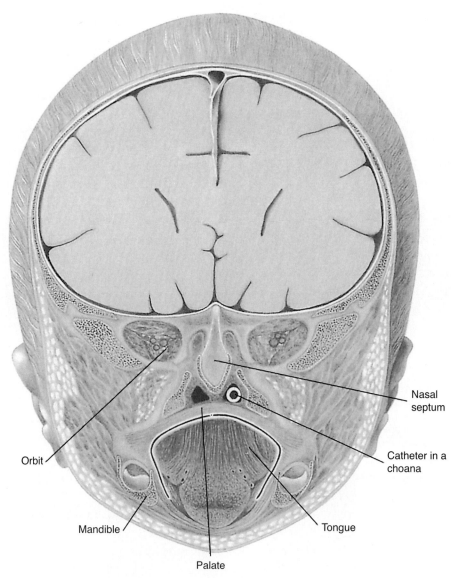

Nasal
septum

Catheter in a
choana

Orbit

Mandible

Tongue

Palate

Figure 1–10
Coronal section through the head of a premature of 28 weeks gestation. A catheter with
outer diameter of only 3 mm almost fully occludes the choana.

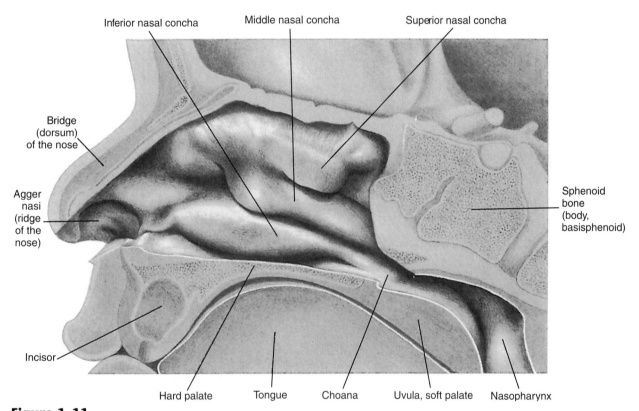

Figure 1–11
Premature of 32 weeks gestation, midline section; the same case as in Figure 1–12, following removal of the nasal septum. View of the lateral wall of the right nasal cavity, which extends far upward in front of the sphenoid. The still small choana lies basally.

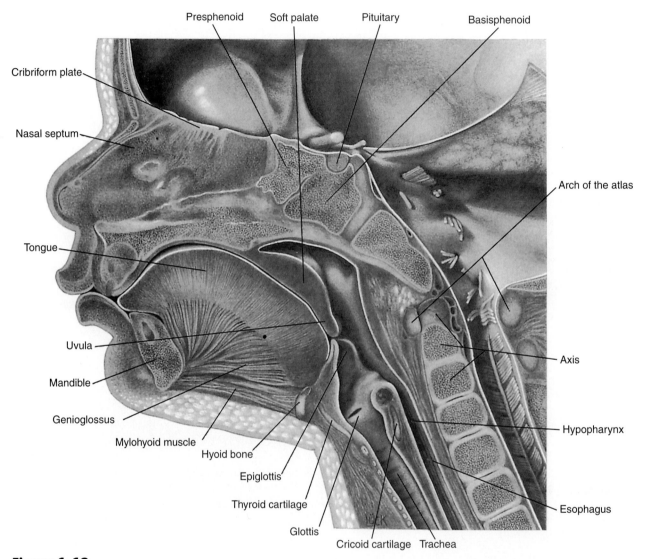

Figure 1–12

The same case as in Figure 1–11 with the nasal septum intact. The choana is obliquely positioned. The uvula and epiglottis contact each other in post-mortem condition; normally their relationship varies according to the phase of swallowing and respiration. Retropharyngeal and nasopharyngeal soft tissue do not yet lie prevertebrally, but below the clivus of the skull base (brain and spinal column have been removed).

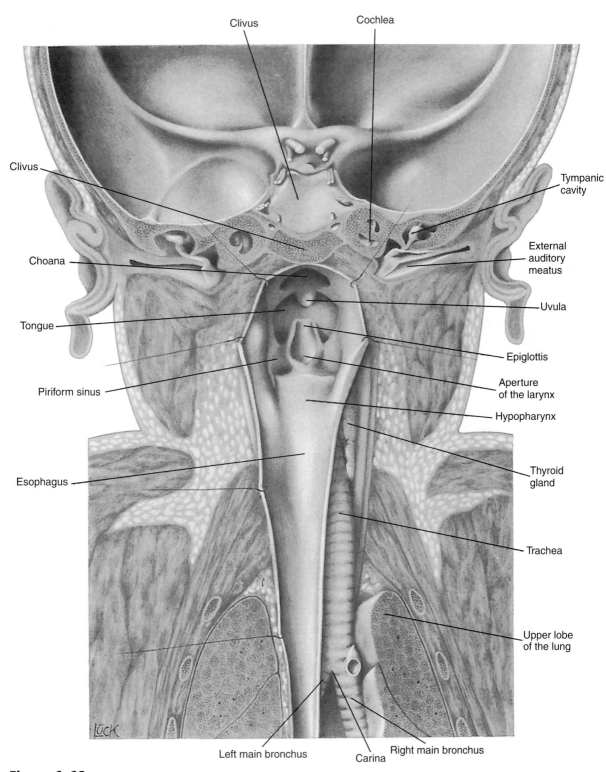

Clivus

Cochlea

Clivus

Tympanic cavity

Choana

External auditory meatus

Tongue

Uvula

Epiglottis

Piriform sinus

Aperture of the larynx

Hypopharynx

Esophagus

Thyroid gland

Trachea

Upper lobe of the lung

LÜCK

Left main bronchus

Carina

Right main bronchus

Figure 1–13

Frontal section through the head, neck, and upper thorax of a premature of 34 weeks gestation. View from behind. The pharynx and esophagus are opened, revealing nasopharynx, base of the tongue, openings of the larynx, piriform sinuses, and posterior wall of the cricoid plate.

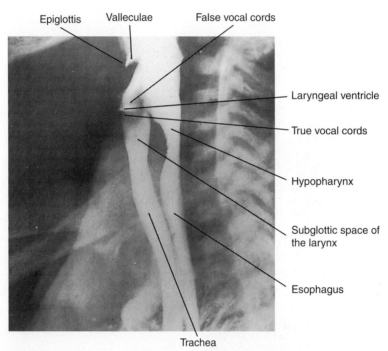

Figure 1–14
Pharynx, larynx, and upper esophagus and trachea sections on post-mortem contrast examination of a 32-week gestation premature infant. Trachea and esophagus, lateral view.

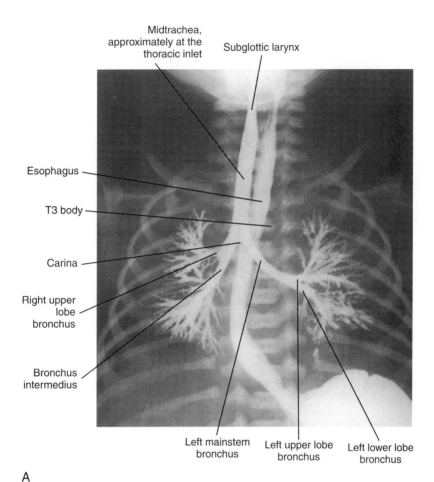

Midtrachea, approximately at the thoracic inlet

Subglottic larynx

Esophagus

T3 body

Carina

Right upper lobe bronchus

Bronchus intermedius

Left mainstem bronchus

Left upper lobe bronchus

Left lower lobe bronchus

A

Figure 1–15

Post-mortem tracheobronchogram-esophagram. Premature of 32 weeks gestation. *A*, Frontal.   *Continued*

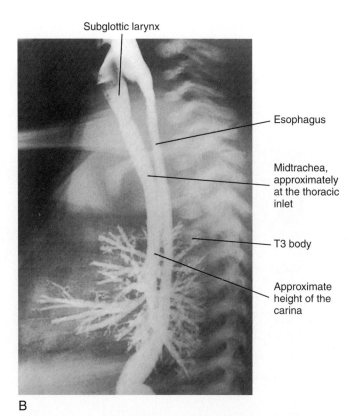

B

Figure 1–15—cont'd
B, lateral. The trachea lies to the right of the esophagus. The right mainstem bronchus passes obliquely across the middle of the esophagus. The midtrachea lies approximately at the thoracic inlet; in this case the carina lies at the T3–T4 level.

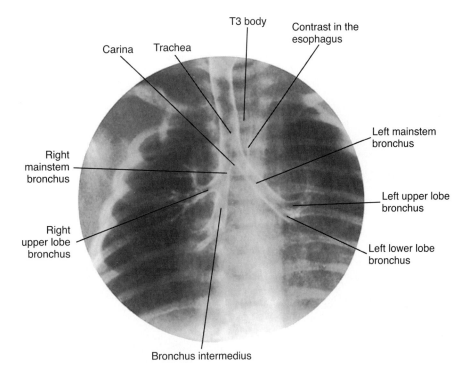

Carina   Trachea   T3 body   Contrast in the esophagus

Right mainstem bronchus

Right upper lobe bronchus

Left mainstem bronchus

Left upper lobe bronchus

Left lower lobe bronchus

Bronchus intermedius

Figure 1–16
Tracheobronchogram of a seven-week-old infant resulting from unexpected aspiration of the contact material. The right mainstem bronchus lies straighter than the left in the sense of being nearly a direct continuation of the trachea. The carina is at the T3 level. The left mainstem bronchus crosses over the esophagus, which is demonstrated by a small amount of contrast material. Right clavicle fracture.

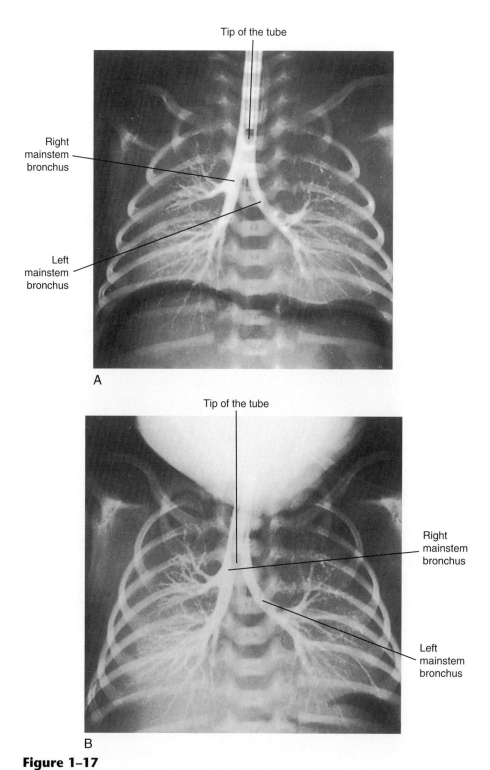

Figure 1–17

Premature, 29 weeks gestation, post-mortem demonstration of the variation of tracheal tube position with change in position of the head. *A,* Normal supine position with the neck mildly extended. The tip of the nasotracheal tube (secured outside the nostril) lies well above the carina; *B,* with flexion of the neck (head tipped forward), the tip of the tube slips into the right main bronchus.

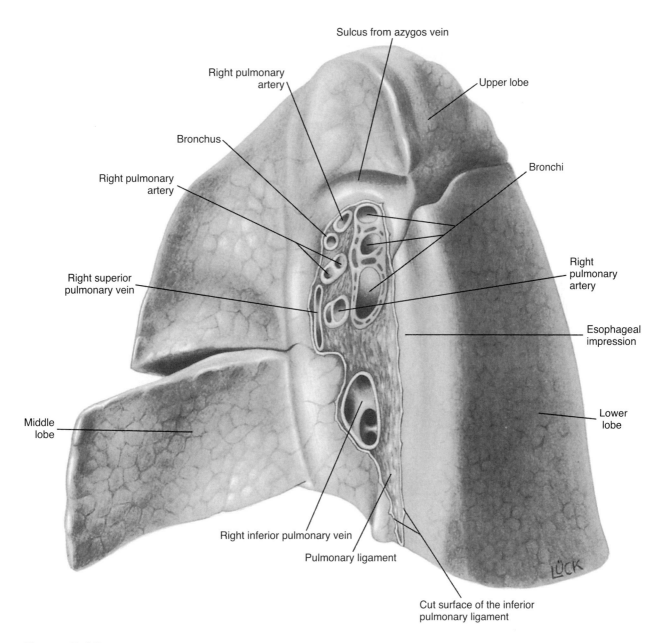

Sulcus from azygos vein

Right pulmonary artery

Upper lobe

Bronchus

Right pulmonary artery

Bronchi

Right pulmonary artery

Right superior pulmonary vein

Esophageal impression

Middle lobe

Lower lobe

Right inferior pulmonary vein

Pulmonary ligament

Cut surface of the inferior pulmonary ligament

Figure 1–18
Right lung of a term newborn, viewed medially. Relatively large sagittal diameter. The anterior step-off between the upper and middle lobes is because of the thymus. The impression of the azygos vein lies above the hilus. The surface area attributable to hilus and the pulmonary ligament is relatively large.

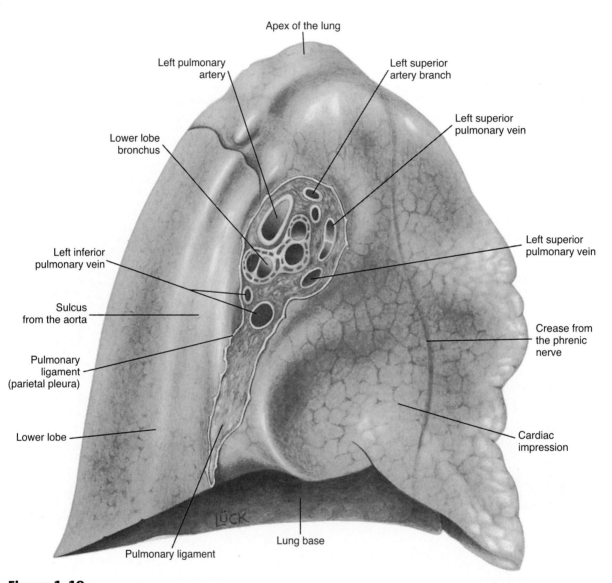

Apex of the lung

Left pulmonary artery

Left superior artery branch

Left superior pulmonary vein

Lower lobe bronchus

Left superior pulmonary vein

Left inferior pulmonary vein

Sulcus from the aorta

Crease from the phrenic nerve

Pulmonary ligament (parietal pleura)

Lower lobe

Cardiac impression

LÜCK

Pulmonary ligament

Lung base

Figure 1–19
Left lung of the same term newborn as in Figure 1–18. Impression from the aorta above and behind the hilus. Wide contact between lung and mediastinum between the two leaves of the pulmonary ligament.

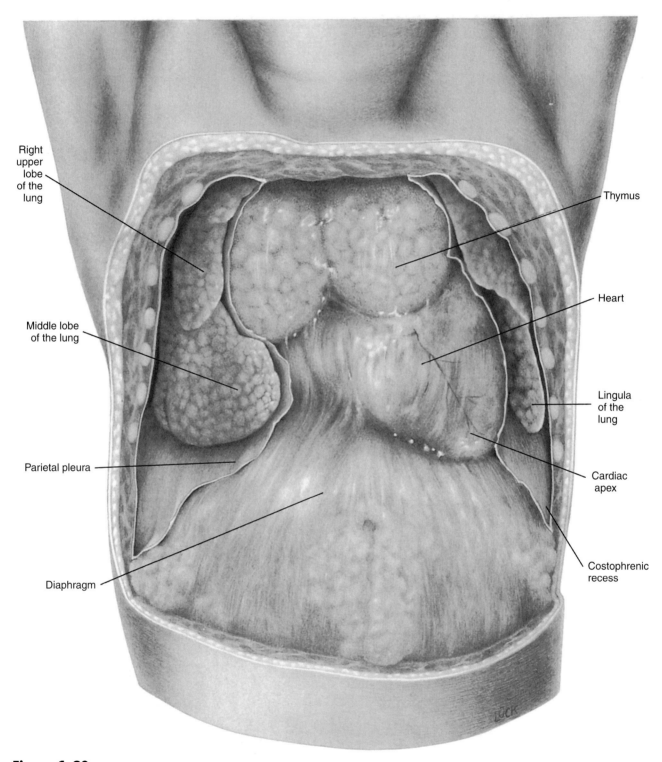

Right upper lobe of the lung

Middle lobe of the lung

Parietal pleura

Diaphragm

Thymus

Heart

Lingula of the lung

Cardiac apex

Costophrenic recess

Figure 1–20
Opened pleural space, viewed from in front, in a 35 week gestation premature. In front, a large area remains lung-free, because thymus and pericardium lie directly at the anterior thoracic wall.

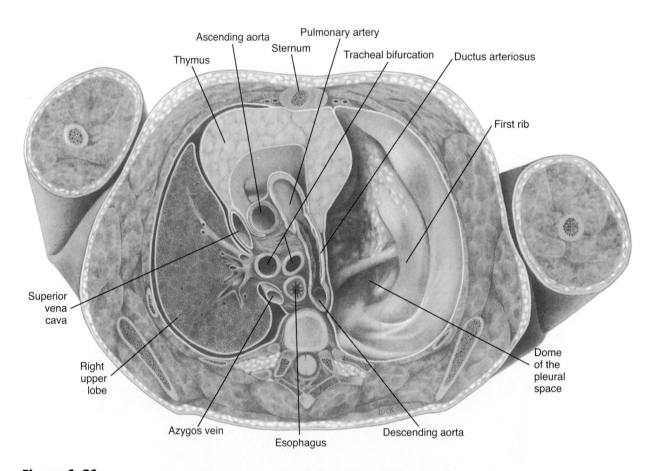

Figure 1–21

The upper thoracic region, viewed from below, in a 33 week gestation premature. Removal of the left lung permits a look at the apex of the left pleura. The right lung apex remains connected to the hilus. The upper portion of the pericardial sac, the aortic recess, is widened in the post-mortem state. The ductus arteriosus, which runs a bowed course between the pulmonary artery and the descending aorta, is long, with its intima already becoming folded.

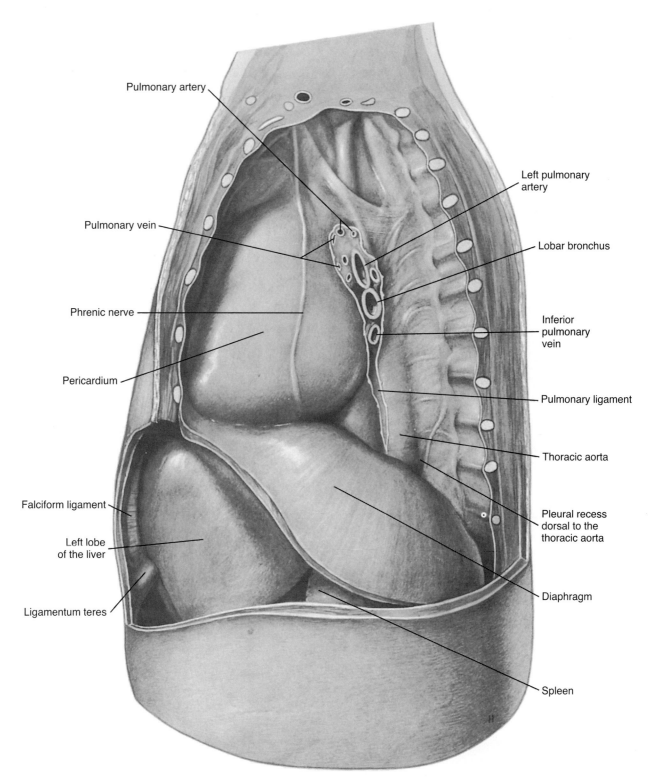

Pulmonary artery

Pulmonary vein

Phrenic nerve

Pericardium

Falciform ligament

Left lobe
of the liver

Ligamentum teres

Left pulmonary
artery

Lobar bronchus

Inferior
pulmonary
vein

Pulmonary ligament

Thoracic aorta

Pleural recess
dorsal to the
thoracic aorta

Diaphragm

Spleen

Figure 1–22
Premature of 29 weeks gestation, with opened left pleural cavity—view of the mediastinum from the left.

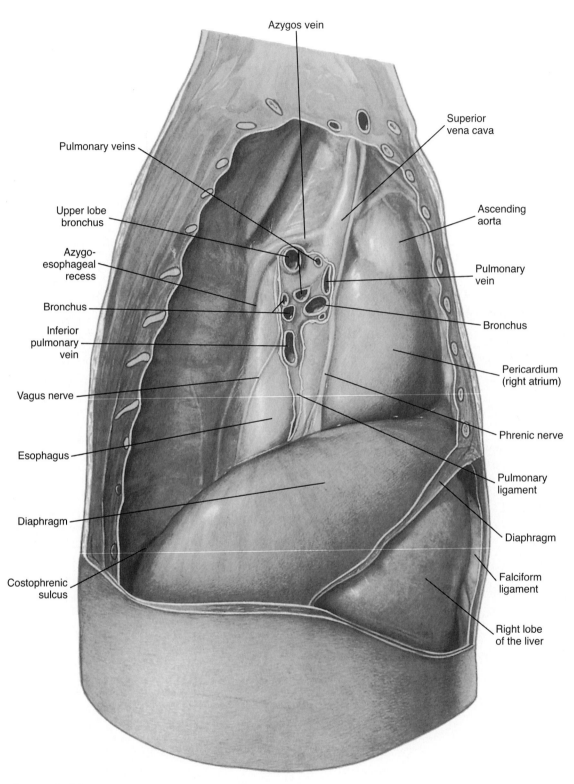

Figure 1–23
Opened right pleural space—view of the mediastinum from the right in the same case as Figure 1–22.

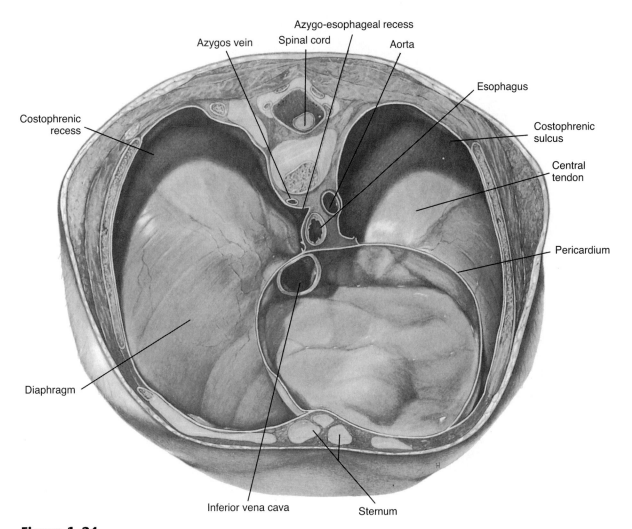

Azygo-esophageal recess

Azygos vein
Spinal cord
Aorta

Esophagus

Costophrenic
recess

Costophrenic
sulcus

Central
tendon

Pericardium

Diaphragm

Inferior vena cava
Sternum

Figure 1–24
View of the diaphragm from above: caudal portion of the pleural cavities and the pericardial sac. Posteriorly, the pleural recess extends far inferiorly. The right pleural space forms the azygo-esophageal recess between the esophagus and the azygos vein. In front, the pericardial sac has a broad interface with the anterior wall of the thorax.

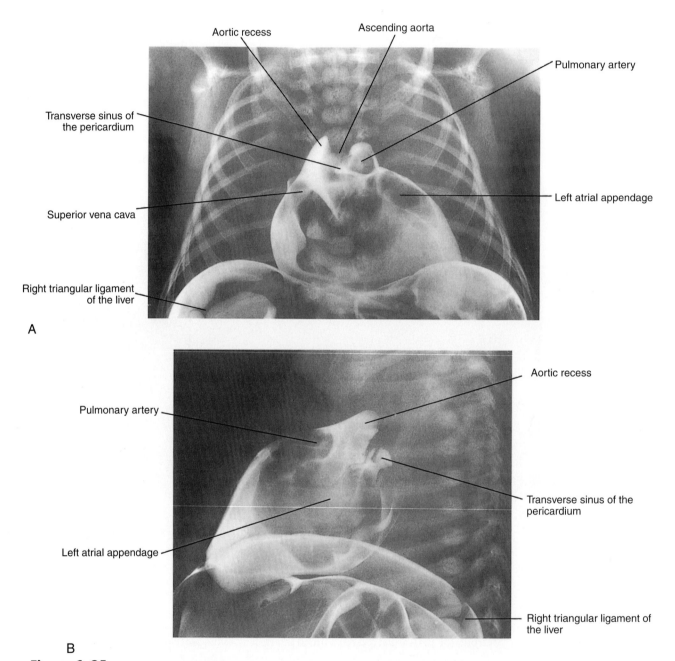

Figure 1–25
Post-mortem contrast filling of the pericardial sac (and the peritoneal cavity) in a premature of 26 weeks gestation. Intrapericardially are also found those portions of the ascending aorta, pulmonary artery, and superior vena cava nearest the heart. *A,* Frontal view; *B,* lateral view.

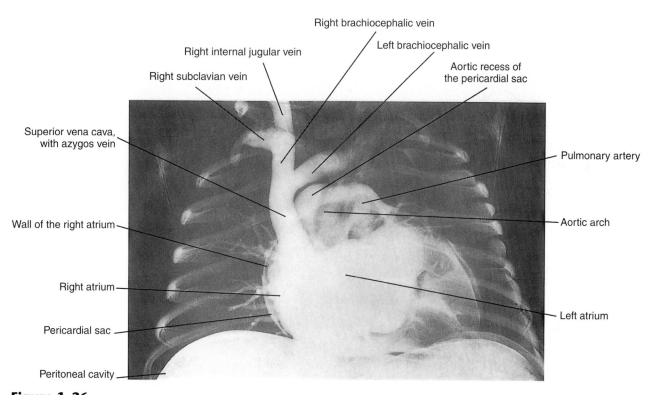

Right brachiocephalic vein

Right internal jugular vein

Left brachiocephalic vein

Right subclavian vein

Aortic recess of
the pericardial sac

Superior vena cava,
with azygos vein

Pulmonary artery

Wall of the right atrium

Aortic arch

Right atrium

Left atrium

Pericardial sac

Peritoneal cavity

Figure 1–26

The same case as in Figure 1–25. Additional contrast filling of the superior vena cava, right and left atrium, the pulmonary veins, and suggestively also the left pleural cavity. The aortic recess of the pericardial sac extends to the level of the left brachiocephalic vein. The wall of the right atrium is quite thin (compare to Figure 1–27).

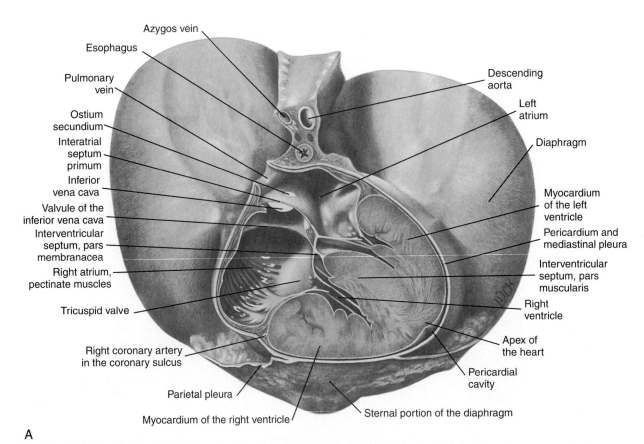

A

Figure 1–27

Heart of a 34 week gestation premature infant; section through both atria and both ventricles. *A*, Lower part of the heart, seen from above, together with pericardium, posterior mediastinum and diaphragm.

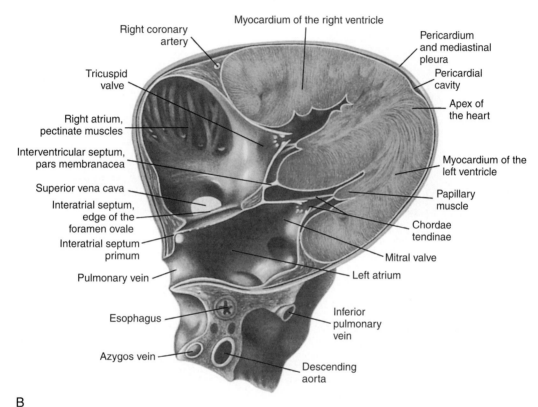

Right coronary artery

Myocardium of the right ventricle

Pericardium and mediastinal pleura

Pericardial cavity

Tricuspid valve

Apex of the heart

Right atrium, pectinate muscles

Interventricular septum, pars membranacea

Myocardium of the left ventricle

Superior vena cava

Papillary muscle

Interatrial septum, edge of the foramen ovale

Chordae tendinae

Interatrial septum primum

Mitral valve

Pulmonary vein

Left atrium

Esophagus

Inferior pulmonary vein

Azygos vein

Descending aorta

B

Figure 1–27—cont'd

B, upper part of the heart, viewed from below, with the heart valves in open position, corresponding approximately to the parasternal 4-chamber view of echocardiography. The ventricles show post-mortem contraction.

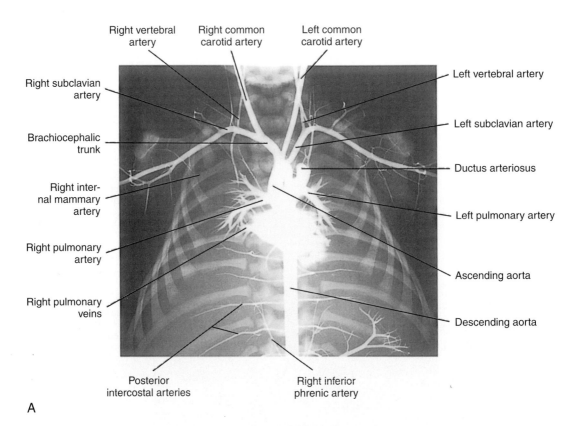

A

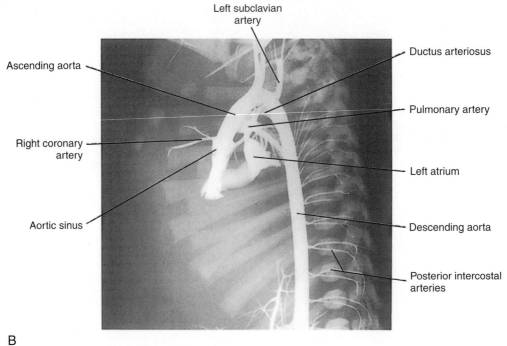

B

Figure 1–28
Post-mortem angiogram of a term newborn. *A* and *B*, frontal views.

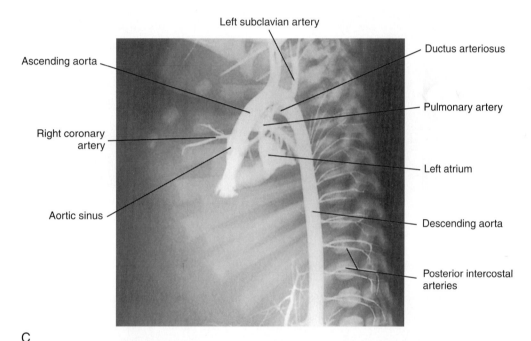

Left subclavian artery

Ductus arteriosus

Ascending aorta

Pulmonary artery

Right coronary artery

Left atrium

Aortic sinus

Descending aorta

Posterior intercostal arteries

C

Figure 1–28—cont'd

C, lateral view. The ductus arteriosus extends far superolaterally. The lung veins lie inferior to the corresponding arteries. The right brachiocephalic trunk runs obliquely upward across the trachea. The aorta and azygos vein delimit by their curved course the infraaortic and infraazygos space, respectively.

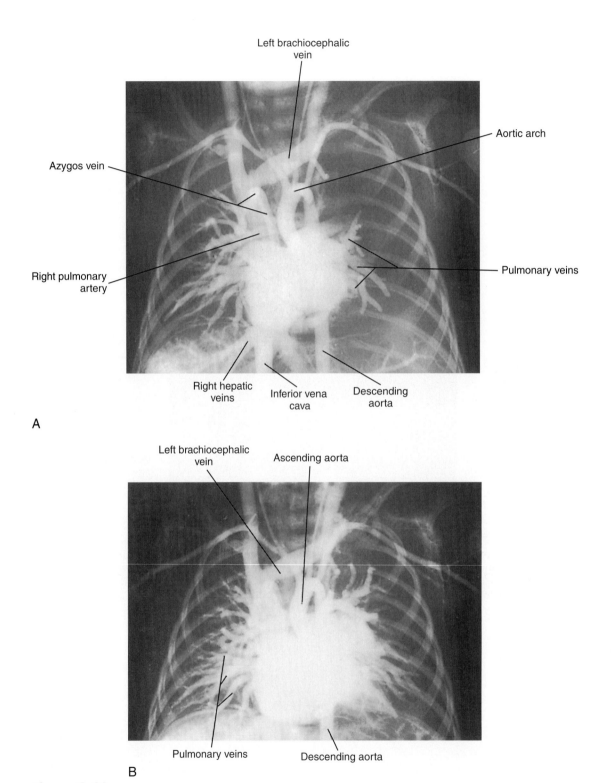

Figure 1–29

Post-mortem angiogram of a 29 weeks gestation premature. *A* and *B,* frontal views, with increasing contrast flow.

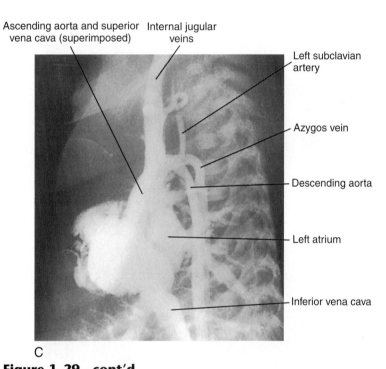

Ascending aorta and superior
vena cava (superimposed)　Internal jugular
veins

Left subclavian
artery

Azygos vein

Descending aorta

Left atrium

Inferior vena cava

C

Figure 1–29—cont'd
C, lateral. The arteries are collapsed to some extent. The aorta and
azygos vein divide the mediastinum into various sections by their curved
course.

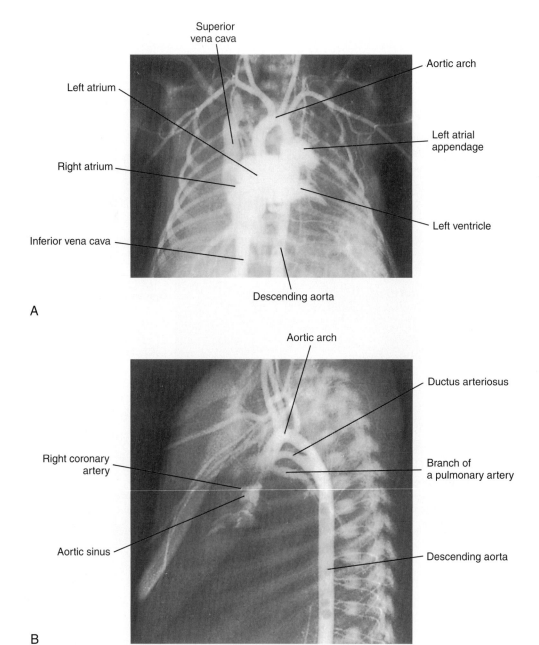

Figure 1–30
Post-mortem angiogram of a 22 week gestation fetus. *A,* frontal view; *B* and *C,* lateral views, with increasing contrast filling. Demonstration of the aortic arch. The ductus arteriosus is long, and slightly contracted in its middle portion.

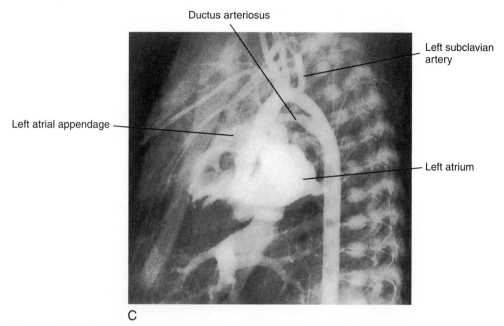

C

Figure 1–30—cont'd

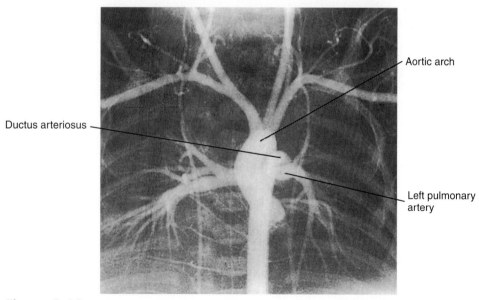

Figure 1–31
Topography of the ductus arteriosus, aorta, and pulmonary arteries, as shown on a post-mortem arteriogram of a 24 week fetus.

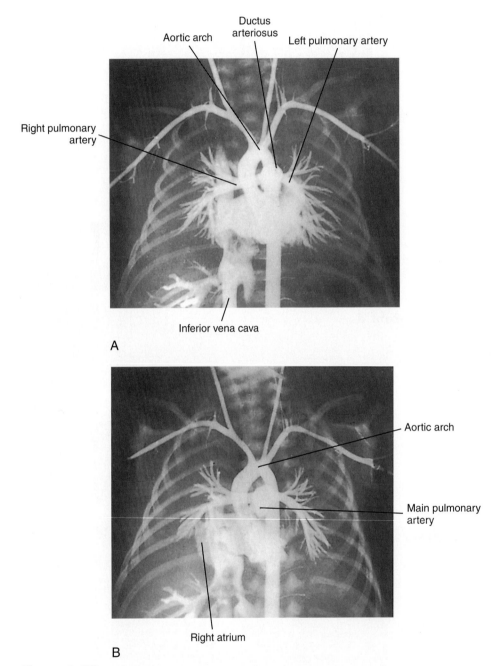

Figure 1–32
Topographic relationships between the pulmonary arteries and other vessels of the thorax, as shown on a post-mortem angiogram of a 26 week fetus. *A*, frontal view; *B*, right posterior oblique.

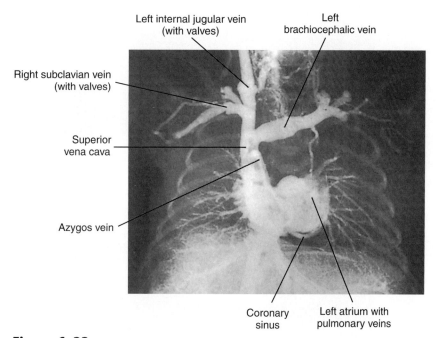

Figure 1–33
Frontal view of the veins of the thorax of a 22 week fetus on post-mortem venogram.

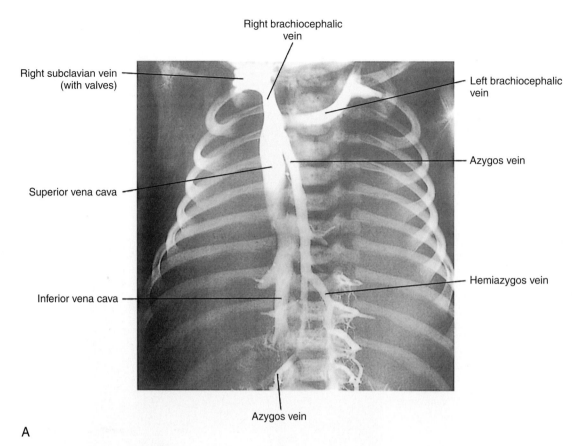

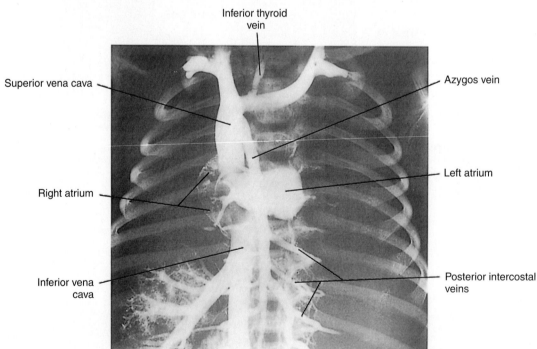

Figure 1–34
Veins of the thorax on post-mortem venogram of a term newborn. Superior vena cava and azygos vein systems. *A* and *B*, frontal.

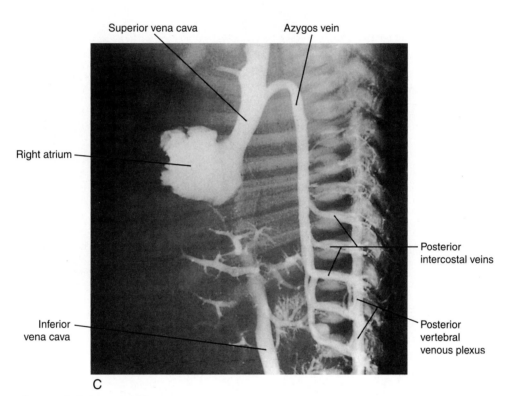

Figure 1–34—cont'd
C, lateral.

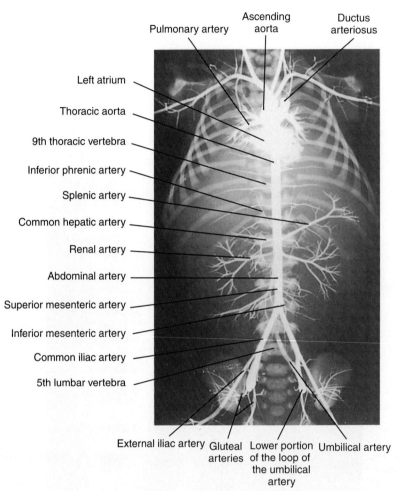

Left atrium

Thoracic aorta

9th thoracic vertebra

Inferior phrenic artery

Splenic artery

Common hepatic artery

Renal artery

Abdominal artery

Superior mesenteric artery

Inferior mesenteric artery

Common iliac artery

5th lumbar vertebra

Pulmonary artery

Ascending aorta

Ductus arteriosus

External iliac artery   Gluteal arteries   Lower portion of the loop of the umbilical artery   Umbilical artery

A

Figure 1–35

Male term newborn. Post-mortem normal angiography. *A* and *B,* frontal; *C* and *D,* lateral. Various stages of opacification: *A* and *C,* arteriogram; *B* and *D,* additional venogram. The angle between the umbilical arteries and the internal iliac arteries may make catherization via the umbilical artery more difficult. The bifurcation of the aorta lies more cranial than the confluence of the common iliac veins into the inferior vena cava. The level of the aortic bifurcation is variable; in this case it is rather more cranial than average. The inferior vena cava in its upper portion lies more anterior than the aorta; the renal veins lie anterior to the arteries. The left renal vein crosses in front of the aorta; the right renal artery lies considerably posterior to the inferior vena cava.

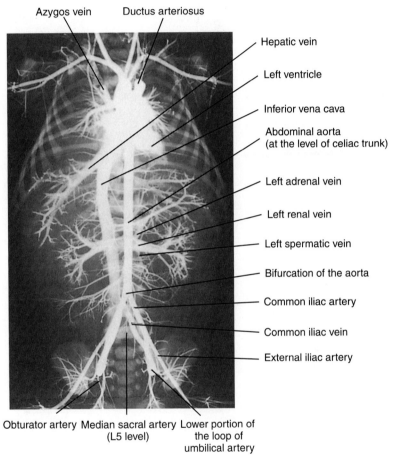

Azygos vein   Ductus arteriosus

Hepatic vein

Left ventricle

Inferior vena cava

Abdominal aorta
(at the level of celiac trunk)

Left adrenal vein

Left renal vein

Left spermatic vein

Bifurcation of the aorta

Common iliac artery

Common iliac vein

External iliac artery

Obturator artery   Median sacral artery   Lower portion of
(L5 level)   the loop of
umbilical artery

B

Figure 1–35—cont'd   *Continued*

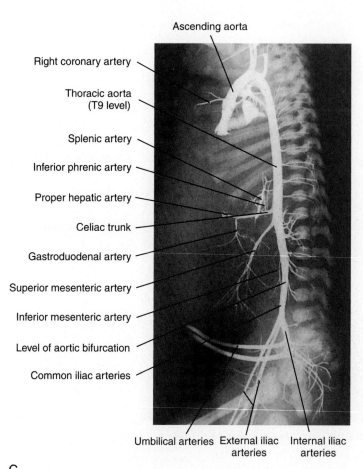

Ascending aorta

Right coronary artery

Thoracic aorta
(T9 level)

Splenic artery

Inferior phrenic artery

Proper hepatic artery

Celiac trunk

Gastroduodenal artery

Superior mesenteric artery

Inferior mesenteric artery

Level of aortic bifurcation

Common iliac arteries

Umbilical arteries   External iliac   Internal iliac
                      arteries   arteries

C

Figure 1–35—cont'd

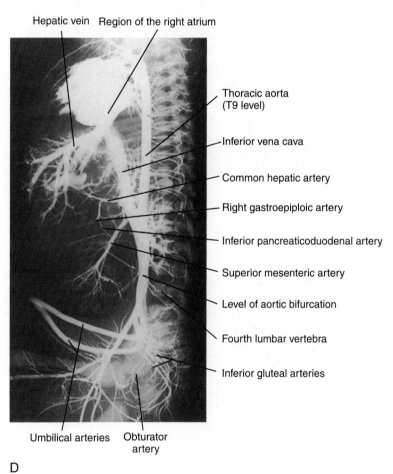

Hepatic vein   Region of the right atrium

Thoracic aorta
(T9 level)

Inferior vena cava

Common hepatic artery

Right gastroepiploic artery

Inferior pancreaticoduodenal artery

Superior mesenteric artery

Level of aortic bifurcation

Fourth lumbar vertebra

Inferior gluteal arteries

Umbilical arteries   Obturator
artery

D

Figure 1–35—cont'd

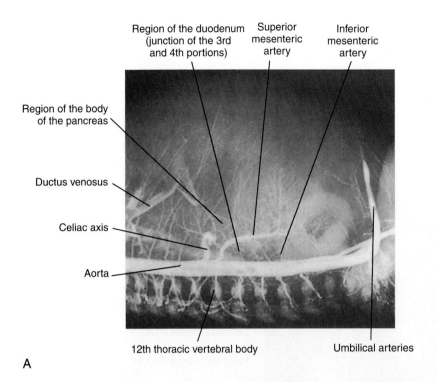

Region of the duodenum (junction of the 3rd and 4th portions)

Superior mesenteric artery

Inferior mesenteric artery

Region of the body of the pancreas

Ductus venosus

Celiac axis

Aorta

12th thoracic vertebral body

Umbilical arteries

A

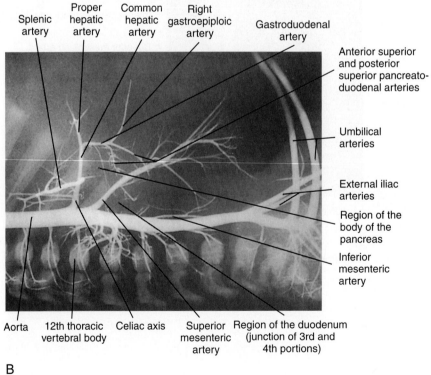

Splenic artery

Proper hepatic artery

Common hepatic artery

Right gastroepiploic artery

Gastroduodenal artery

Anterior superior and posterior superior pancreato-duodenal arteries

Umbilical arteries

External iliac arteries

Region of the body of the pancreas

Inferior mesenteric artery

Aorta

12th thoracic vertebral body

Celiac axis

Superior mesenteric artery

Region of the duodenum (junction of 3rd and 4th portions)

B

Figure 1–36

The ventral branches of the aorta on angiogram and ultrasound images—supine. Cranial is to the reader's left and caudal is to the reader's right. *A,* post-mortem aortogram of a female 31 week gestation premature infant; lateral view. *B,* postmortem aortogram of a term male newborn; lateral view.

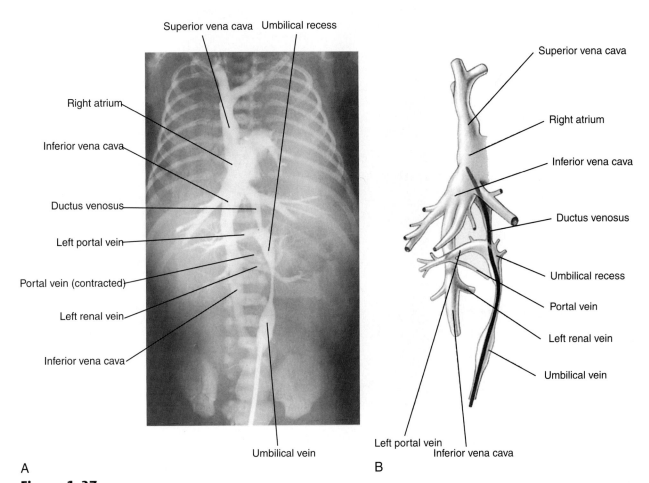

A

B

Figure 1–37
Post-mortem venogram of female premature twin of 26 weeks gestation. *A*, Frontal, relatively little contrast filling; *B*, line drawing to *A* with position of an umbilical vein catheter indicated. The tip lies at the junction of the inferior vena cava and the right atrium.

Continued

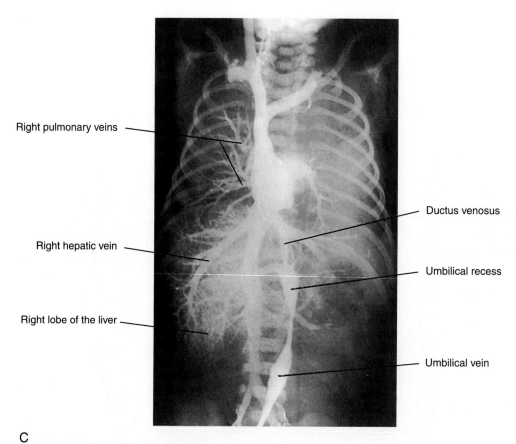

Right pulmonary veins

Right hepatic vein

Right lobe of the liver

Ductus venosus

Umbilical recess

Umbilical vein

C

Figure 1–37—cont'd
C, frontal, more complete contrast filling.

Superior vena cava   Azygos vein

Right atrium

Inferior vena cava

Hepatic vein

Ductus venosus

Umbilical recess

Portal vein

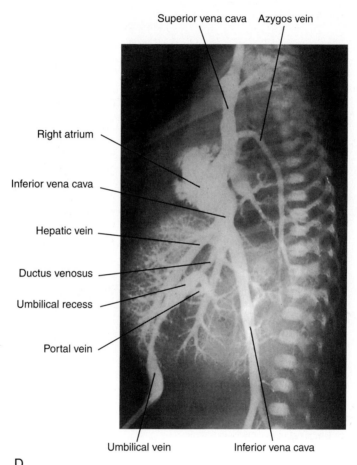

Umbilical vein   Inferior vena cava

D

Figure 1–37—cont'd
D, lateral.   *Continued*

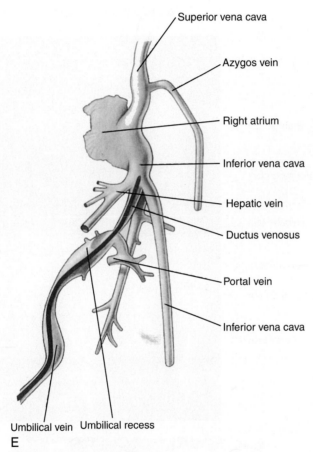

Superior vena cava

Azygos vein

Right atrium

Inferior vena cava

Hepatic vein

Ductus venosus

Portal vein

Inferior vena cava

Umbilical vein   Umbilical recess

E

Figure 1–37—cont'd
E, line drawing to *D* with umbilical vein catheter.

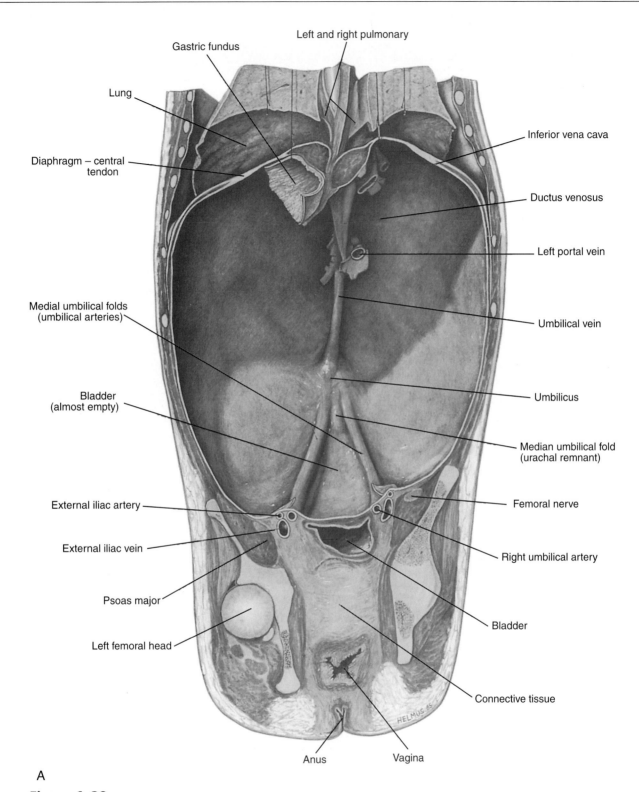

Left and right pulmonary

Gastric fundus

Lung

Diaphragm – central tendon

Inferior vena cava

Ductus venosus

Left portal vein

Medial umbilical folds (umbilical arteries)

Umbilical vein

Bladder (almost empty)

Umbilicus

Median umbilical fold (urachal remnant)

External iliac artery

Femoral nerve

External iliac vein

Right umbilical artery

Psoas major

Left femoral head

Bladder

Connective tissue

Anus

Vagina

A

Figure 1–38

Female 36 week gestation premature infant. Anatomic preparation of the anterior abdominal wall and the umbilical vessels. The liver has been removed. The falciform ligament remains intact, being detached from its hepatic attachment. The intrahepatic umbilical recess is revealed, showing many small branches in the liver parenchyma; from the right posterior, the main stem of the left portal vein flows to this site. The ductus venosus, which runs its own ligament, joins the umbilical recess to the cranial portion of the inferior vena cava. The urinary bladder is empty; it is connected to the umbilicus by the median umbilical fold. *A,* view from behind.

Continued

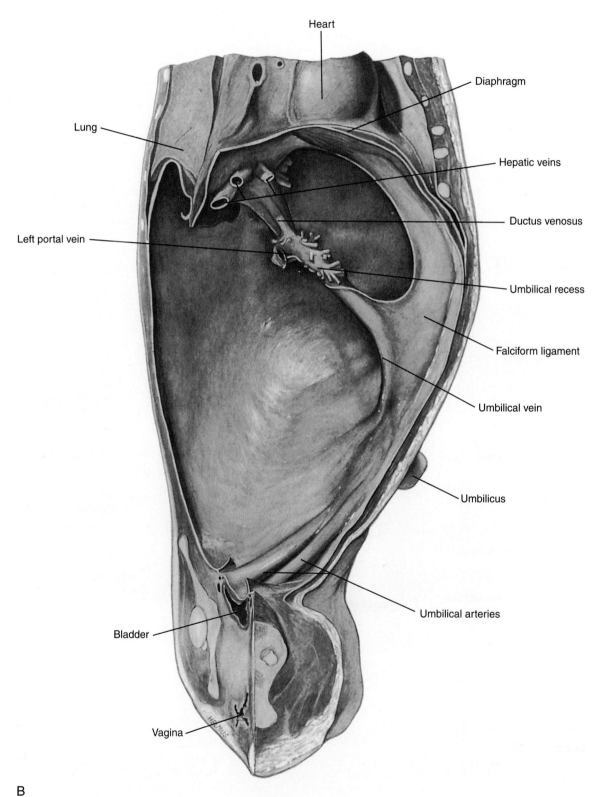

B

Figure 1–38—cont'd
B, view from the right.

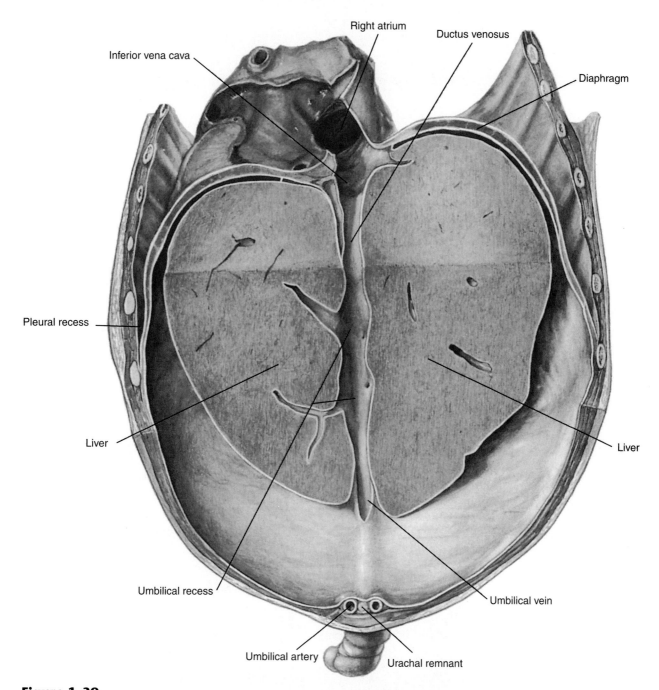

Right atrium

Ductus venosus

Inferior vena cava

Diaphragm

Pleural recess

Liver

Liver

Umbilical recess

Umbilical vein

Umbilical artery

Urachal remnant

Figure 1–39
Anatomic preparation of the umbilical vein system of a 32 week gestation newborn, seen from behind and from below. The posterior portions of the liver have been removed. The umbilical vein, umbilical recess, ductus venosus, and right atrium have been opened posteriorly. The umbilical recess comprises an extended spacious intrahepatic segment of the vein with numerous branches. The umbilical vein system describes and S-shaped curve from the umbilicus to the heart (see Figure 1–38b); the liver thus must be sectioned in two planes from full demonstration.

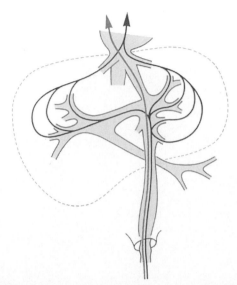

Figure 1–40
Fetal and neonatal blood flow from the umbilical vein to the heart. Approximately 50% flows through the ductus venosus (red), and 50% through the liver parenchyma (black); modified from Lind and Meyer [485].

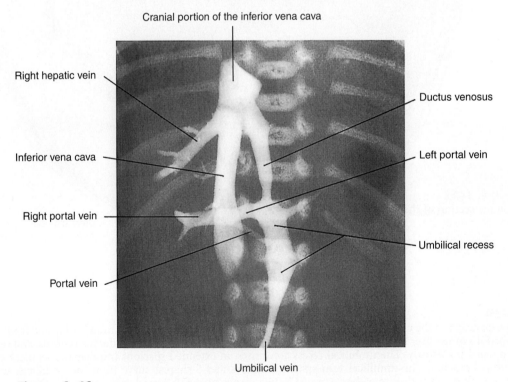

Figure 1–41
Post-mortem demonstration of the umbilical recess with its junction to the ductus venosus and the left portal vein. Twin premature, 27 weeks gestation, deceased on the first day of life.

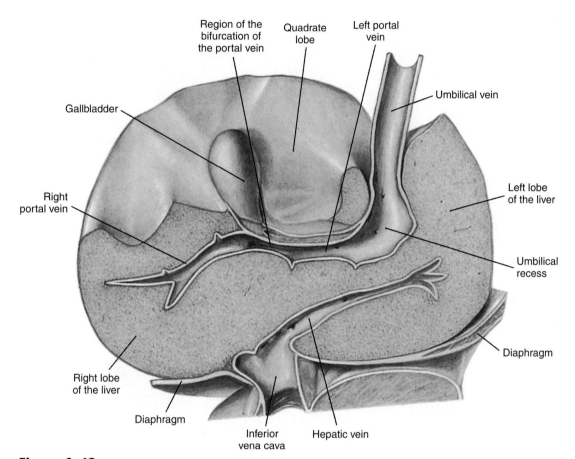

Figure 1–42

Oblique section of the liver of a 35 week gestation premature infant, viewed from below, to correspond to an ultrasound image. The wide umbilical vein enters the wide umbilical recess, which lies in contact with the main left and right portal veins. The ductus venosus and the portal vein root are not encountered in this section. A left hepatic vein is demonstrated.

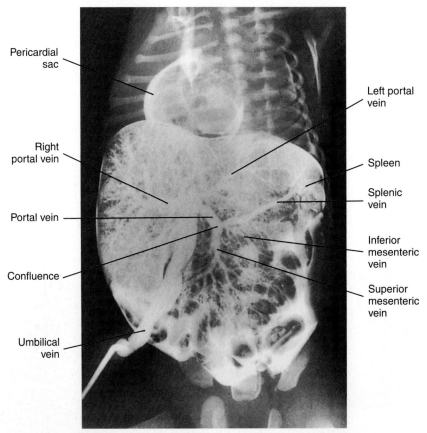

Pericardial sac

Right portal vein

Portal vein

Confluence

Umbilical vein

Left portal vein

Spleen

Splenic vein

Inferior mesenteric vein

Superior mesenteric vein

Figure 1–43
Portal venous system of a 26 week gestation premature infant. Post-mortem veno-, peritoneo-, pericardiography. Right posterior oblique position.

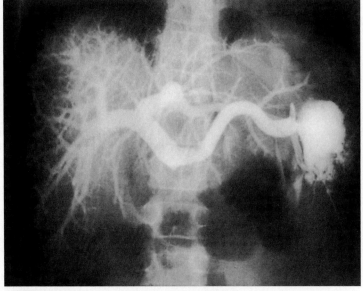

Figure 1–44
Normal direct splenoportogram of a 9 1/2-year-old boy, to compare to the fetal and neonatal relationships.

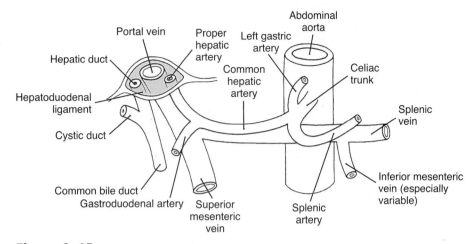

Figure 1–45
Topography of the portal system, the celiac trunk and its branches, and the bilary tract, seen from the front (modified from Lierse [479]). In the hepatoduodenal ligament the portal vein lies posteriorly, the proper hepatic artery lies anteriorly or left-anteriorly, and the common bile duct and hepatic duct lies right-anteriorly.

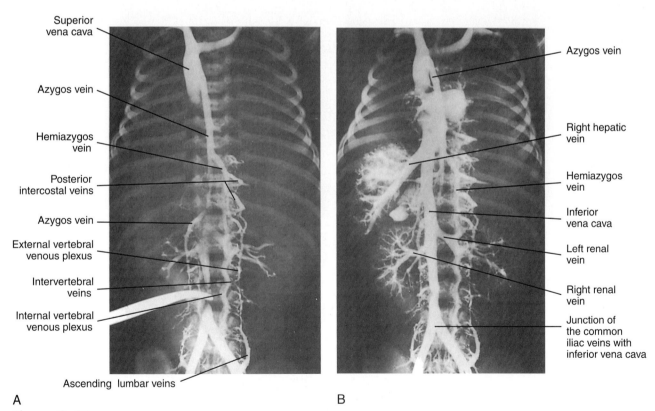

A   B

Figure 1–46
Vena cava and azygos system. Post-mortem venogram of a term female newborn. *A* and *B*, frontal; *C* and *D*, lateral, with increasing contrast filling. In *A* and *C*, with clamped inferior vena cava the hemiazygos and azygos veins are filled via the ascending lumbar veins and the vertebral venous plexus.   *Continued*

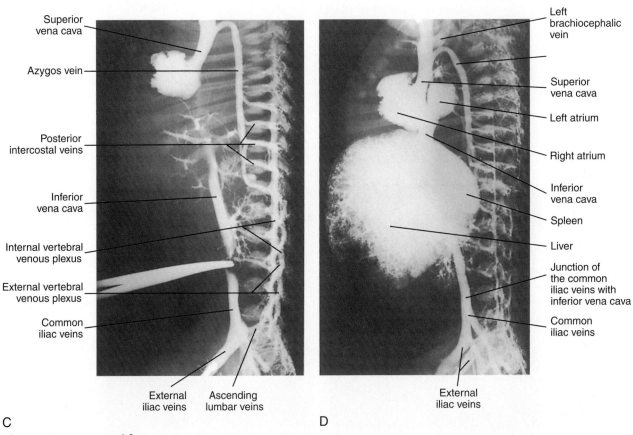

Figure 1–46—cont'd

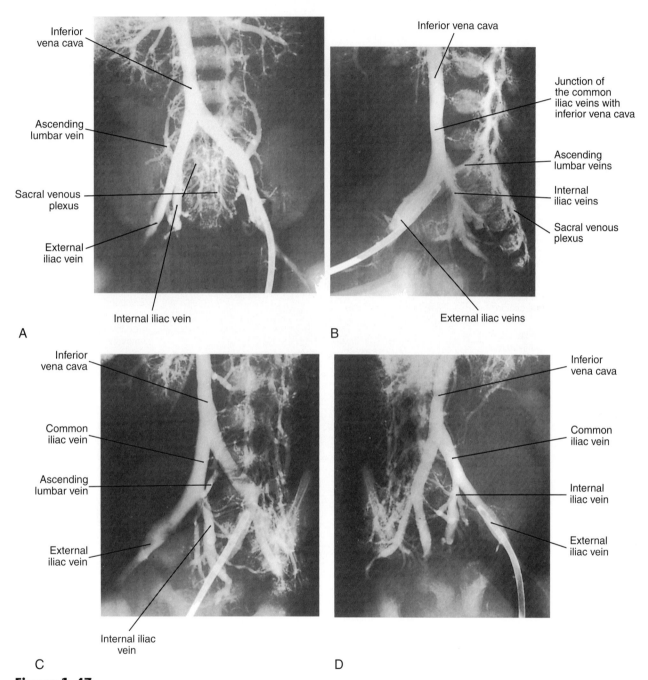

Figure 1–47
Pelvic veins on post-mortem venogram of a term female newborn. Catheter tip is in the left external iliac vein.
A, frontal; *B*, lateral; *C*, right posterior oblique; *D*, left posterior oblique.

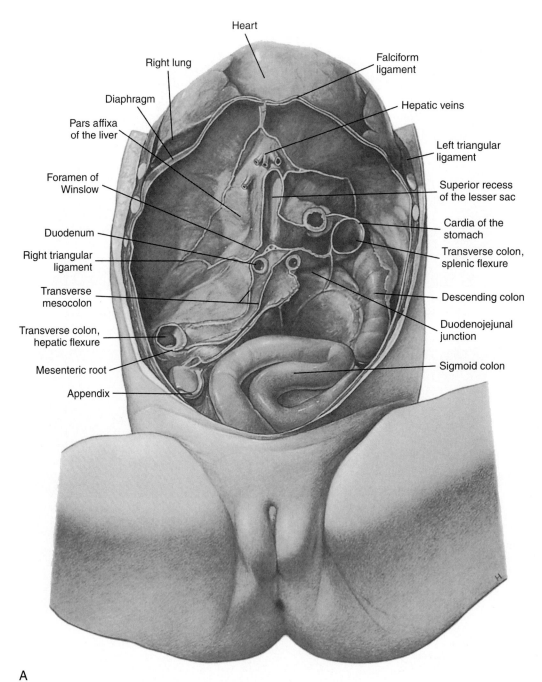

Heart

Right lung

Diaphragm

Pars affixa
of the liver

Foramen of
Winslow

Duodenum

Right triangular
ligament

Transverse
mesocolon

Transverse colon,
hepatic flexure

Mesenteric root

Appendix

Falciform
ligament

Hepatic veins

Left triangular
ligament

Superior recess
of the lesser sac

Cardia of the
stomach

Transverse colon,
splenic flexure

Descending colon

Duodenojejunal
junction

Sigmoid colon

A
Figure 1–48
Upper and posterior wall of the peritoneal cavity of the term female newborn. *A*, anatomic preparation following removal of liver, spleen, stomach, small bowel, and transverse colon.

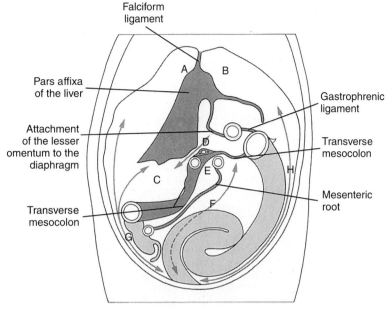

B

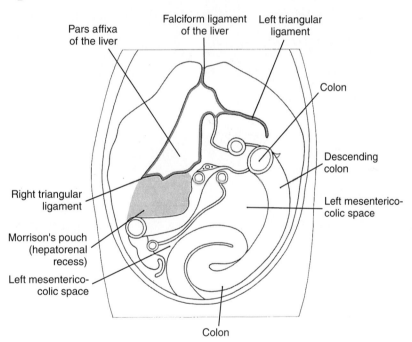

C

Figure 1–48—cont'd

B, line drawing corresponding to *A.* The arrows indicate the main junctional pathways between the regions of the peritoneal spaces (paracolic gutters, epiploic foramen of Winslow, etc.). Dark area: contact areas of the pars affixa (bare area) of the liver, as well as the ligaments of the stomach and bowel; A = right subphrenic recess; B = left subphrenic recess; C = Morison's pouch; D = lesser sac (omental bursa); E = right mesenterico-colic space; F = left mesenterico-colic space; G = right paracolic gutter (parieto-colic space); H = left paracolic gutter (parieto-colic space). *C,* shaded area: subhepatic/hepatorenal space (Morison's pouch). Free fluid in the peritoneal cavity is easily seen here in the supine subject between the right kidney and the liver; red line: coronary ligament. The lateral ends of the ligament are designated as the left and right triangular ligament. The falciform ligament is the anterior continuation of the coronary ligament.

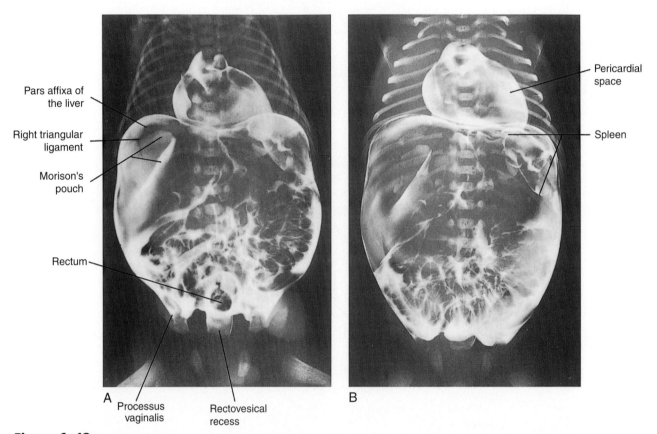

Figure 1–49
Post-mortem peritoneogram and pericardiogram of a male, 26-weeks gestation fetus. *A,* frontal, supine. Morison's pouch is contrast-filled; it borders cranially on the juncture of the bare area of the liver (pars affixa) with the diaphragm. The testes had not yet descended. *B,* with the specimen suspended (i.e., simulated upright), the abdominal viscera descend, and Morison's pouch has partially emptied.

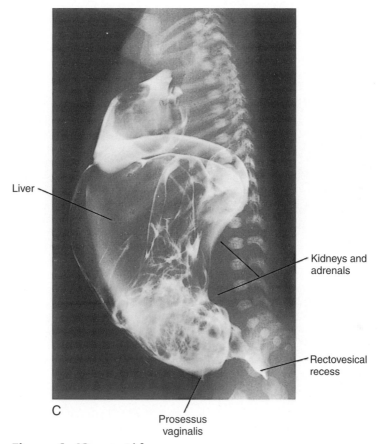

Liver

Kidneys and
adrenals

Rectovesical
recess

C

Prosessus
vaginalis

Figure 1–49—cont'd
C, lateral. The kidneys and adrenals arch forward considerably. The
testes are undescended, while the peritoneal processus vaginalis is just
beginning to point downward.

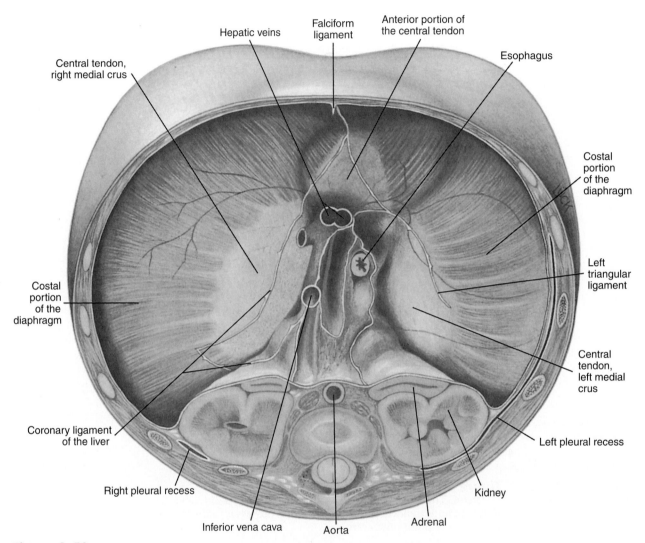

Figure 1–50
Undersurface of the diaphragm in a newborn. The central tendon forms a trifoil-shaped surface. The position of the peri-cardial sa is evident anteriorly. Between the two leaves of the hepatic coronary ligament lies the junctional surface of the diaphragm with the bare are (pars affixa) of the liver. The deep distal extent of the plural cavity recesses are seen behind both kidneys.

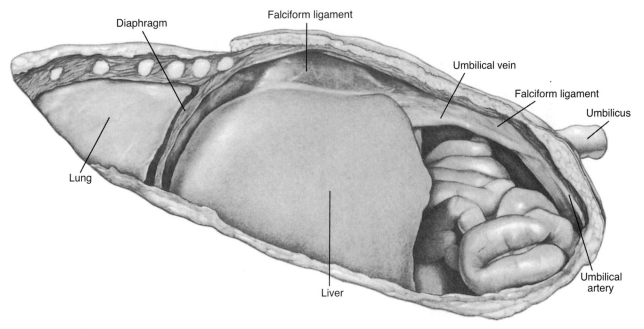

Figure 1–51
Peritoneal space of a 32-week gestation newborn, opened from the right. The falciform ligament forms an extensive transparent membrane, extending from the diaphragm to the umbilicus. The umbilical vein comprises its inferoposterior border.

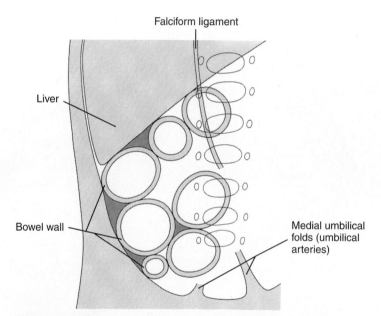

Figure 1–52
Summary of radiographic demonstration of free air in the peritoneum in the supine position: 1) the "tell-tale triangle" sign (darker shaded area); both sides of bowel wall seen; 2) visible falciform ligament; 3) visible medial umbilical folds (umbilical arteries).

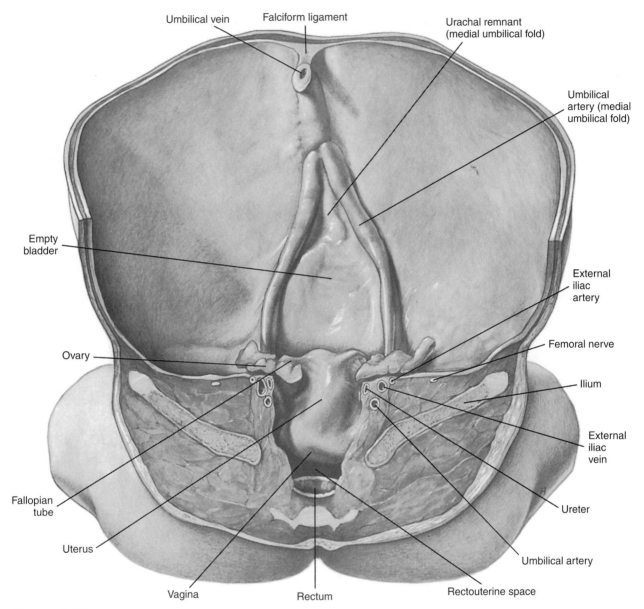

Umbilical vein   Falciform ligament   Urachal remnant (medial umbilical fold)

Umbilical artery (medial umbilical fold)

Empty bladder

External iliac artery

Ovary

Femoral nerve

Ilium

External iliac vein

Fallopian tube

Ureter

Uterus

Umbilical artery

Vagina   Rectum   Rectouterine space

Figure 1–53
Female premature infant of 28 weeks gestation. Anterior abdominal wall and pelvic organs seen from behind. The median umbilical fold (containing the urachal remnant) and especially the medial umbilical folds (containing the umbilical arteries) form quite thick cords. (The lateral umbilical folds were not prominent in this specimen.) This illustration shows that when the urinary bladder is empty there is the possibility of free air collecting between the umbilical arteries in the supine position.

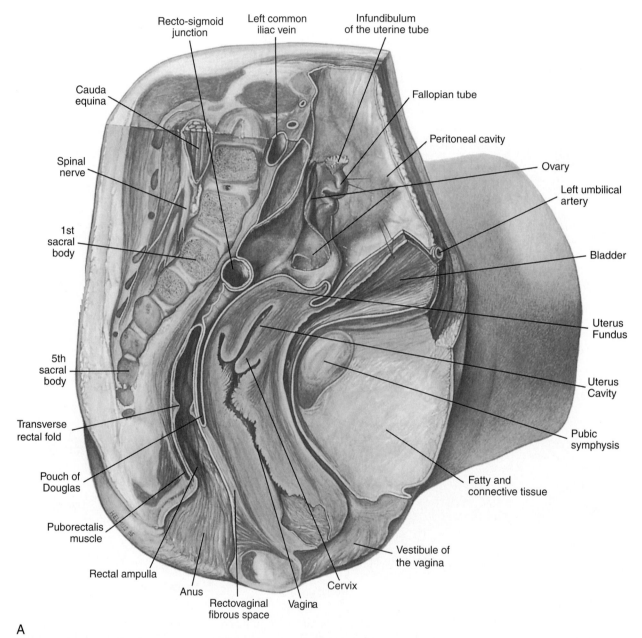

Recto-sigmoid junction

Left common iliac vein

Infundibulum of the uterine tube

Cauda equina

Fallopian tube

Peritoneal cavity

Spinal nerve

Ovary

Left umbilical artery

1st sacral body

Bladder

5th sacral body

Uterus Fundus

Transverse rectal fold

Uterus Cavity

Pouch of Douglas

Pubic symphysis

Puborectalis muscle

Fatty and connective tissue

Rectal ampulla

Vestibule of the vagina

Anus

Rectovaginal fibrous space

Cervix

Vagina

A

Figure 1–54

Female newborn. Midline section through the pelvis. The bladder is empty. The peritoneal cavity extends via its rectouterine pouch (of Douglas) considerably more caudally, behind the vagina, than in an adult. Thus, the rectovaginal fibrous space does not extend as far cranially as in the adult situation. *A,* anatomic preparation.

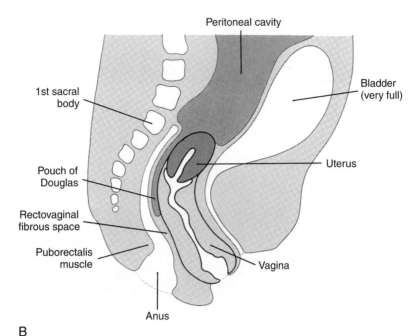

Peritoneal cavity

1st sacral
body

Bladder
(very full)

Pouch of
Douglas

Uterus

Rectovaginal
fibrous space

Puborectalis
muscle

Vagina

Anus

B

Figure 1–54—cont'd
B, the peritoneal cavity is indicated on this schematic representation.

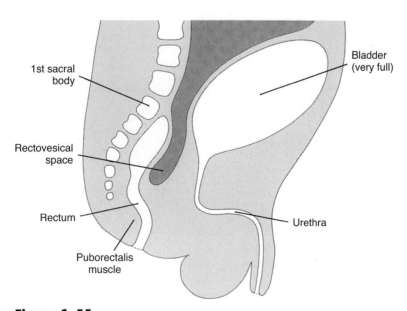

1st sacral
body

Bladder
(very full)

Rectovesical
space

Rectum

Urethra

Puborectalis
muscle

Figure 1–55
Midline section through the pelvis of a male newborn. Diagram from
anatomic preparation. Darker shaded area: peritoneal cavity. The
rectovesical space extends further caudally than in the adult.

Peritoneal cavity

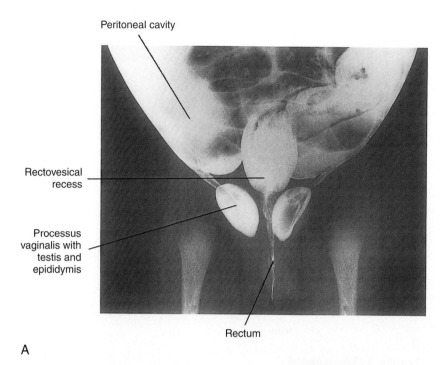

Rectovesical
recess

Processus
vaginalis with
testis and
epididymis

Rectum

A

Peritoneal cavity

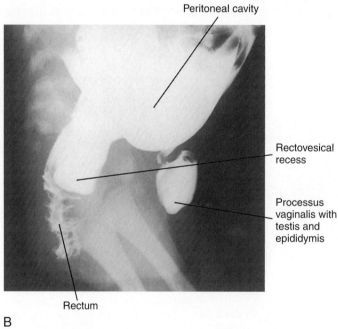

Rectovesical
recess

Processus
vaginalis with
testis and
epididymis

Rectum

B

Figure 1–56
Post-mortem peritoneography with contrast in the rectum as well, in a male
premature 30-week gestation infant. The processus vaginalis is still patent bilaterally, with testis and epididymis in the inguinal region. The rectovesical space
extends far inferiorly.

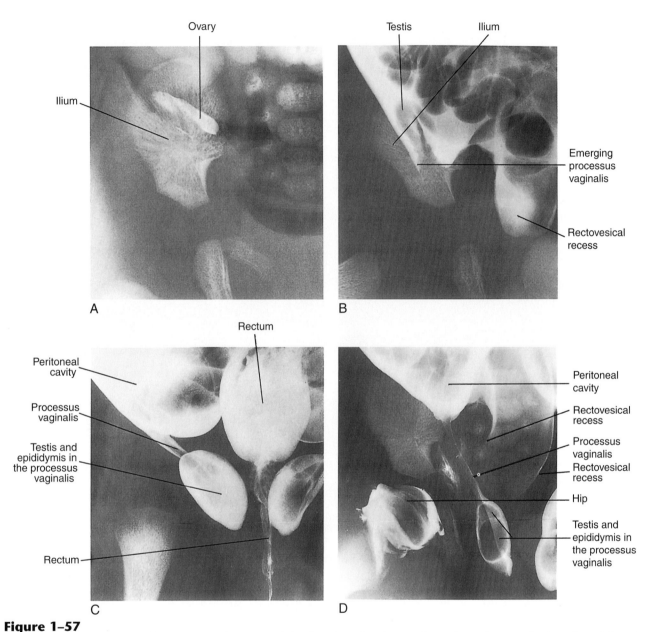

Figure 1–57
Topographic relationships of the peritoneal cavity and the female and male gonads. In the early stages both male and female gonads have the same position, projected over the iliac wing. The testes later descend with development of the processus vaginalis. *A*, ovary of a 29-week gestation fetus. In this preparation the peritoneal cavity is filled with air and the ovary coated with positive contrast; *B*, intraperitoneal position of the testis of a 26-week gestation fetus on post-mortem peritoneography; the processus vaginalis is a tiny outpouching of the peritoneum; *C*, early testicular descent in a premature 30-week gestation infant. Post mortem contrast filling of the peritoneal cavity and rectum (same case as Figure 1–56). The testis in the process vaginalis projects over the inguinal region at this stage; *D*, more advanced, but not yet complete testicular descent in a 32-week gestation premature infant on post-mortem peritoneography with hip arthrography. The still patent processus vaginalis has lengthened. Note the short distance between testis and hip.

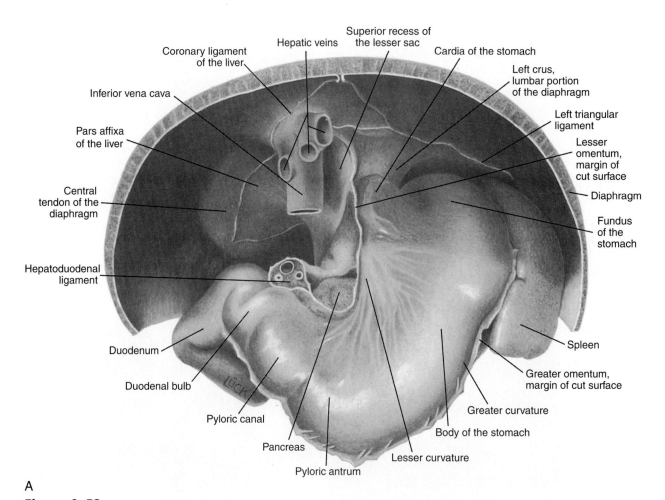

A

Figure 1–58

Stomach and duodenum of anatomic preparation of a 32-week gestation premature, showing diaphragm and spleen. *A,* Intact stomach and duodenum, lesser sac opened.

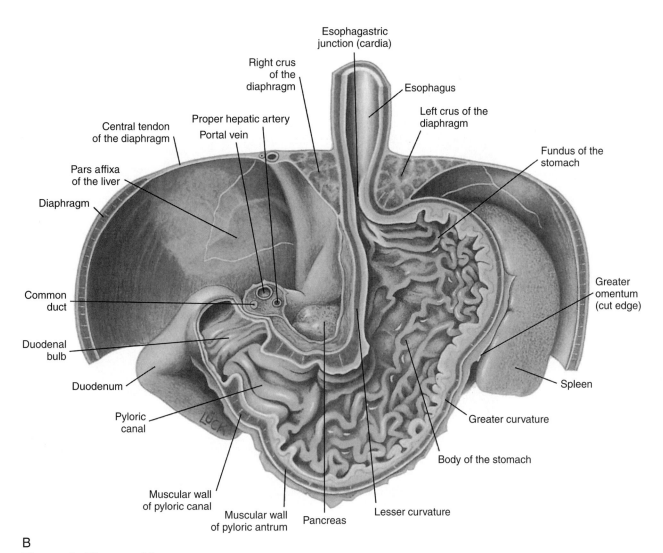

B

Figure 1–58—cont'd

B, distal esophagus, stomach, pylorus and duodenal bulb opened. The diaphragm and its crura are sectioned at the level of the esophageal hiatus. The crura are strongly developed and encompass a relatively long portion of the distal esophagus. No intraperitoneal portion of the esophagus is present in this case.

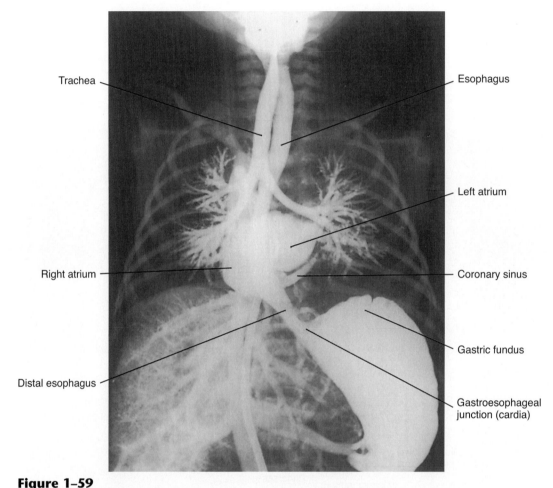

Trachea

Esophagus

Left atrium

Right atrium

Coronary sinus

Gastric fundus

Distal esophagus

Gastroesophageal
junction (cardia)

Figure 1–59
Premature infant, 32 weeks gestation; post-mortem radiologic demonstration of the normal topographic relationships of the stomach and the esophagus to other thoracic structures. The gastroesophageal junction and the gastric fundus are relatively distant from those portions of the heart which lie against the esophagus (left atrium and coronary sinus). The relatively long distal portion of the esophagus—comprising the "vestibule"—is surrounded by the powerful crura of the diaphragm. No intraperitoneal portion of the esophagus can be seen in this demonstration (see also Figure 1–58b).

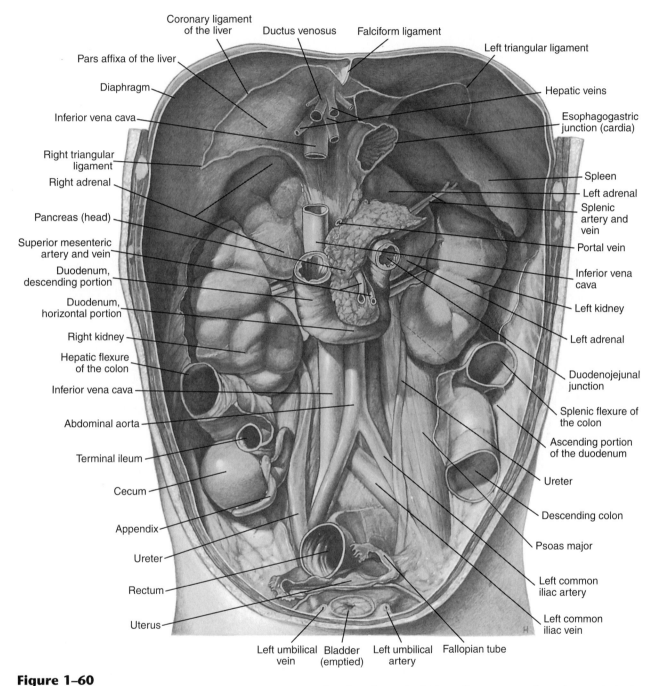

Coronary ligament of the liver
Ductus venosus
Falciform ligament
Left triangular ligament
Pars affixa of the liver
Diaphragm
Hepatic veins
Inferior vena cava
Esophagogastric junction (cardia)
Right triangular ligament
Spleen
Right adrenal
Left adrenal
Splenic artery and vein
Pancreas (head)
Superior mesenteric artery and vein
Portal vein
Duodenum, descending portion
Inferior vena cava
Duodenum, horizontal portion
Left kidney
Right kidney
Left adrenal
Hepatic flexure of the colon
Duodenojejunal junction
Inferior vena cava
Splenic flexure of the colon
Abdominal aorta
Ascending portion of the duodenum
Terminal ileum
Ureter
Cecum
Descending colon
Appendix
Psoas major
Ureter
Left common iliac artery
Rectum
Left common iliac vein
Uterus
Left umbilical vein
Bladder (emptied)
Left umbilical artery
Fallopian tube

Figure 1–60

Retroperitoneal organs of a 32 week gestation premature female infant. The kidneys have a smooth surface with fetal lobulation. The adrenals are strikingly large compared to other organs. The left adrenal lies medial to the upper half of the kidney. The relatively high position of the ileocecal region is not pathologic for either premature or term newborn.

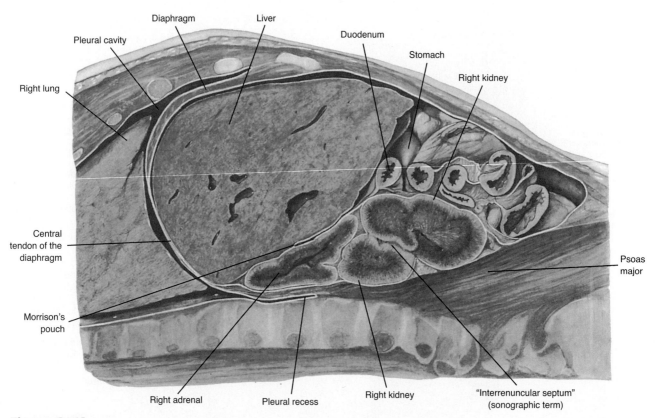

Figure 1–61

Oblique longitudinal section through the right kidney and adrenal, corresponding to a sonographic cut in a 27 week gestation fetus. Because of the lobulated surface and deep indentation in the hilar region the kidney simulates a division in this plane (sonographically the finding is termed "interrenuncular septum"). The adrenal is (as is normal) very large.

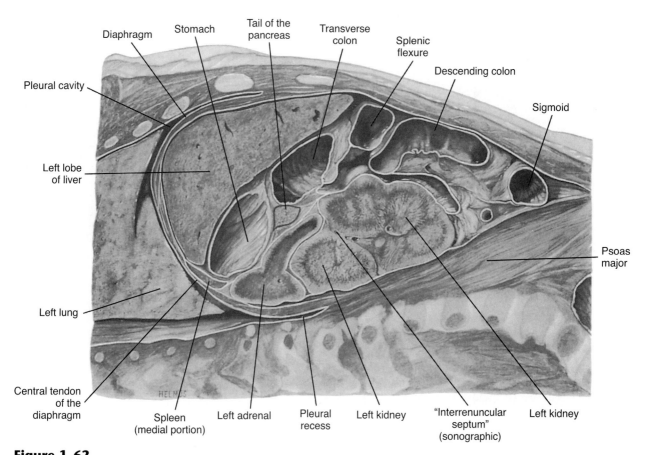

Figure 1–62
Oblique longitudinal section through the medial portion of the left kidney and adrenal corresponding to a frequent ultrasound plane. Fetus of 27 weeks gestation (same case as Figure 1–61). Because of the deep notching of the fetal (renuncular) lobulation in the hilar region, a septum formation is simulated (the sonographic "interrenuncular septum"). Normal large adrenal. The left lobe of the liver is still very large at this stage of development. In this rather medial section only a very small portion of the spleen is present. Gas in the colon can obscure the ultrasound imaging of the left kidney in this plane.

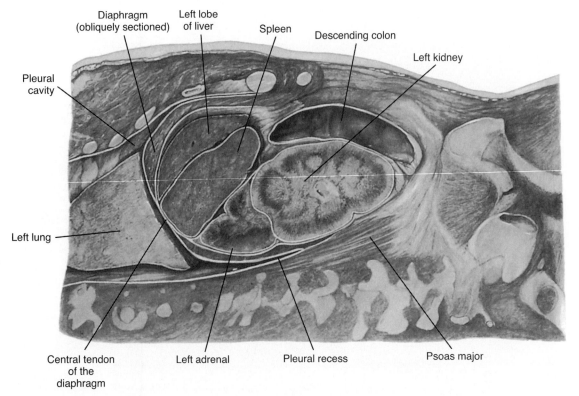

Figure 1–63

The same specimen as in Figures 1–61 and 1–62; a still more lateral oblique longitudinal section through the left kidney and adrenal. A larger portion of the spleen is now encountered, although still overlapped by the left lobe of the liver. A corresponding sonographic section could nicely show increased peritoneal fluid localized between the spleen and the left kidney and adrenal. Colon air is usually less of a disturbance than on more medial sections corresponding to Figure 1–62. Laterally, septum formation across the kidney is no longer simulated.

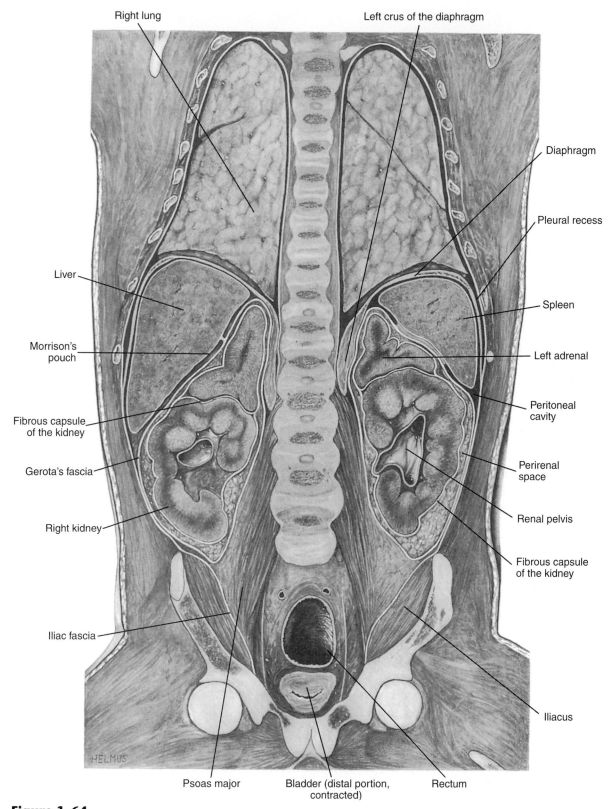

Right lung

Left crus of the diaphragm

Diaphragm

Pleural recess

Liver

Spleen

Morrison's
pouch

Left adrenal

Fibrous capsule
of the kidney

Peritoneal
cavity

Gerota's fascia

Perirenal
space

Right kidney

Renal pelvis

Fibrous capsule
of the kidney

Iliac fascia

Iliacus

Psoas major

Bladder (distal portion,
contracted)

Rectum

HELMUS

Figure 1–64

Frontal section through the trunk of a 26 week gestation male fetus. The large kidneys and adrenals are enclosed by the perirenal space, which is bounded outward by Gerota's (renal) fascia. The crus of the diaphragm is strongly developed. The caudal pleural recess extends downward medially and laterally to a remarkable extent.

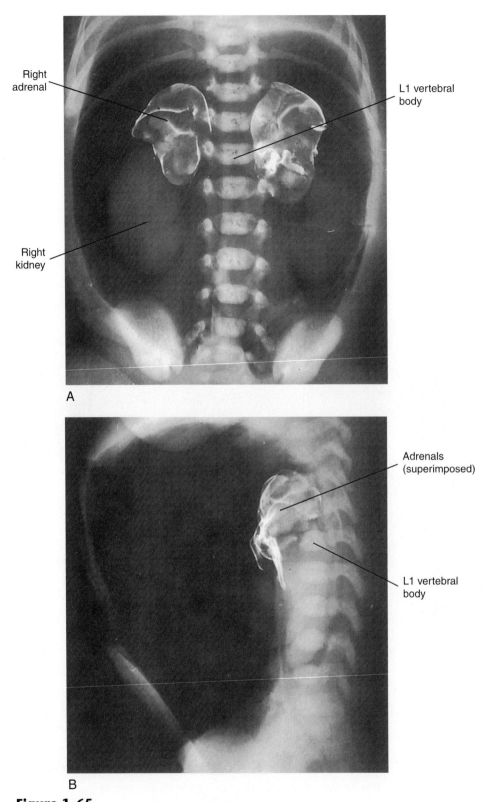

Figure 1–65
Post-mortem radiographs of a term newborn after anatomic preparation. The adrenals were dissected free and coated with contrast material. Normal findings: both adrenals are large, spanning four vertebral bodies; they lie para- and prevertebral. The left adrenal extends more medially than the right. *A,* frontal; *B,* lateral.

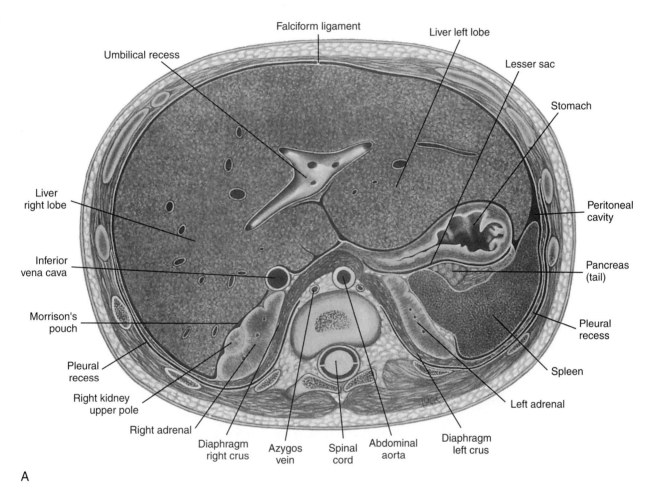

Falciform ligament

Liver left lobe

Umbilical recess

Lesser sac

Stomach

Liver right lobe

Peritoneal cavity

Inferior vena cava

Pancreas (tail)

Morrison's pouch

Pleural recess

Pleural recess

Spleen

Right kidney upper pole

Left adrenal

Right adrenal

Diaphragm right crus

Azygos vein

Spinal cord

Abdominal aorta

Diaphragm left crus

A

Figure 1–66
Axial sections through the abdomen and pelvis of a male newborn, viewed from below (corresponding to CT).
A, transverse section through the upper abdomen, including a large portion of the liver, spleen, and the adrenals.

Continued

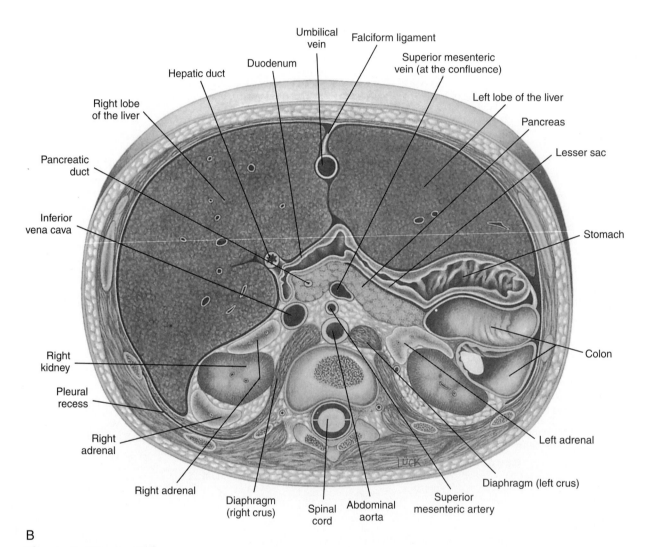

B

Figure 1–66—cont'd
B, transverse section through the liver, pancreas, and upper pole of the kidneys.

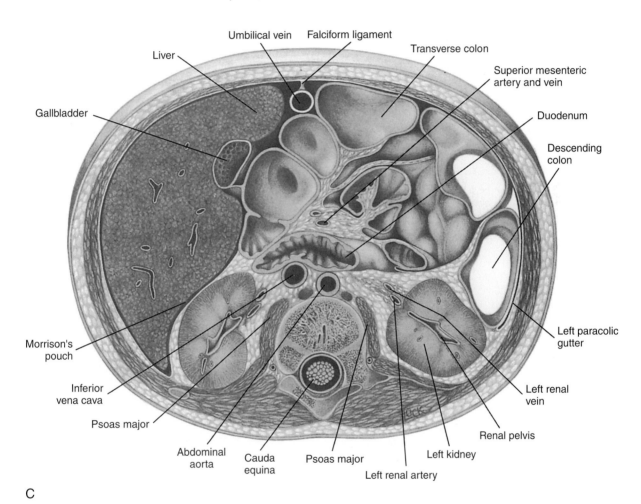

C

Figure 1–66—cont'd
C, transverse section through the right lobe of the liver, the gallbladder, and the middle portion of the kidneys.

Continued

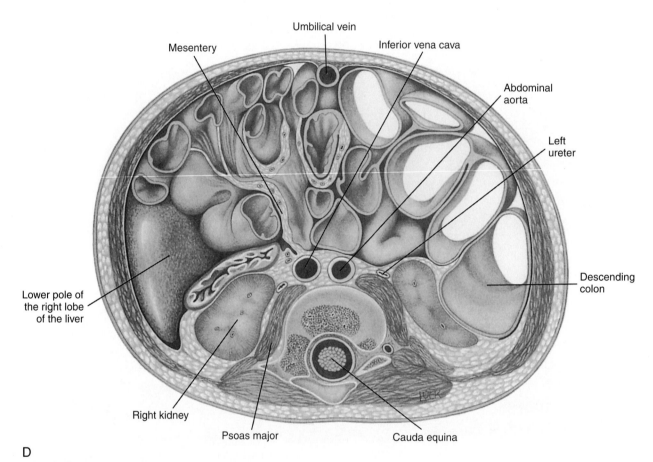

D
Figure 1–66—cont'd
D, transverse section through the intestines at the level of the lower poles of the liver and the kidneys, a short distance above the umbilicus.

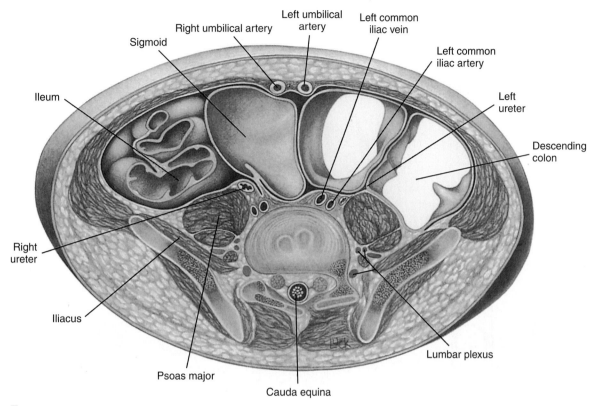

E

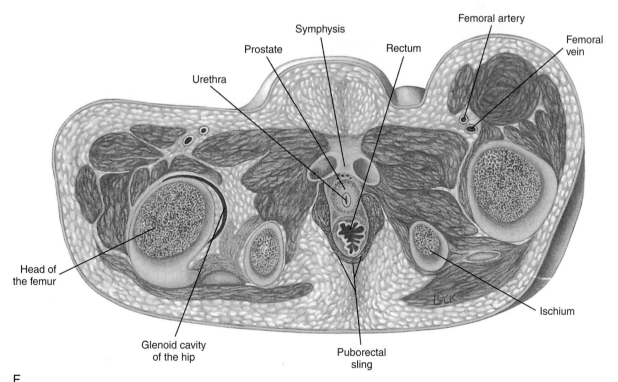

F

Figure 1–66—cont'd
E, transverse section at the level of the pelvic inlet; *F,* transverse section through the floor of the pelvis, including the puborectal sling.

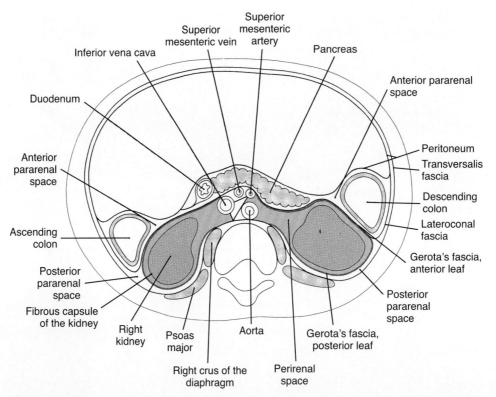

Figure 1–67

Schematic representation of the retroperitoneal space at the level of the kidneys, viewed from below (modified from Meyers [536]). Gerota's fascia (= renal fascia = perirenal fascia) surrounds the perirenal space. Anterior to it lies the anterior pararenal space, which surrounds the colon, pancreas, and duodenum. Posterior to the perirenal space lies the posterior pararenal space, a thin cleft between the posterior leaf of Gerota's fascia and the muscular fascia of the psoas major and the transversalis fascia.

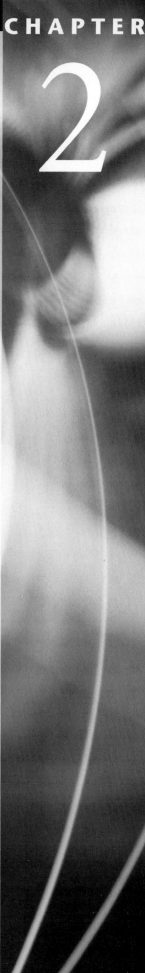

THE NEWBORN INFANT WITH RESPIRATORY DISTRESS FROM MEDICAL CAUSES

Outline

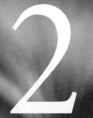

CHAPTER 2

David K. Edwards, III, MD

THE NEWBORN INFANT WITH RESPIRATORY DISTRESS FROM MEDICAL CAUSES

The newborn infant is markedly different in many important ways from older infants, children, and adults. A similar difference exists between preterm and term infants. Thus, neonatology is a unique discipline that bears only a minor resemblance to other branches of pediatrics. Similarly, the radiology of neonates is in many ways unique, different enough that many general radiologists and even some pediatric radiologists are uncomfortable when they examine films of a sick newborn infant.

There are at least three valid reasons for this discomfort. One is that sick newborn infants are fairly often in dire straits and at a distinct risk of dying if immediate, appropriate medical or surgical care is delayed. Another is that the radiographic findings in newborn infants are often difficult to interpret, nonspecific, or downright misleading. Finally, radiology is of vital importance; in probably no field of medicine other than orthopedics is there a greater immediate dependence on radiology. Thus, the findings on the films truly *matter*, often to a crucial extent. All of these factors put considerable stress on the radiologist presented with films for interpretation.

Respiratory distress in newborn infants is one of the least specific findings in pediatrics. Its causes are numerous and include central nervous system disorders, any of several metabolic disturbances, pulmonary surfactant deficiency, neonatal pneumonia, meconium aspiration syndrome, and diaphragmatic hernia, to name but a few. Despite this wide spectrum of causes, infants have relatively few ways of manifesting respiratory distress: tachypnea, grunting, flaring of the nasal alae, and substernal and intercostal retractions, with or without cyanosis, hypoxia, or hypercarbia. This stereotyped paucity of findings is frustratingly nonspecific.

Chest radiography plays an important role in narrowing the differential diagnosis of infantile respiratory distress. In fact, a chest film is the most common radiographic study requested for respiratory distress or for a diversity of other conditions such as maternal fever or prolonged rupture of the membranes (Figs. 2–1, 2–2).

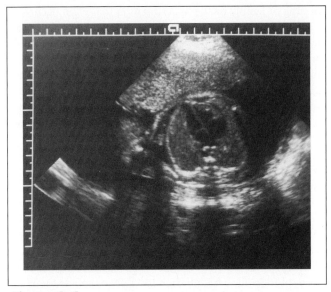

Figure 2–1
Prenatal diagnosis: normal chest. Axial image of the normal fetal chest at 26 weeks of gestation. The four cardiac chambers are normal. Note the homogeneous echogenicity of the pulmonary parenchyma.

Fortunately for the radiologist, although the number of newborn infants affected with respiratory distress is large, the number of intrathoracic causes of the distress is relatively small. Thus, knowledge of only a few important disorders permits clinically helpful and often accurate radiographic diagnosis in the great majority of neonates. This pleasant circumstance may be consolingly compared with adult chest radiology, in which the list of possible abnormalities and disorders appears nearly infinite.

This chapter describes the few important medical disorders that constitute the mainstay of neonatal chest radiography;

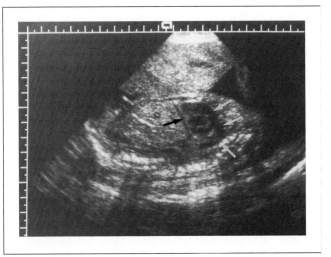

Figure 2–2
Prenatal diagnosis: normal diaphragm. Parasagittal image at 26 weeks of gestation shows the pulmonary artery and ductal arch *(white arrows)* and a normal diaphragm *(black arrow)*.

the next chapter discusses those disorders generally categorized as surgical. Although it is uncommon for a radiograph to reveal absolutely pathognomonic findings—and, admittedly, findings may overlap from disease to disease—knowledge of the major lesions described in the sections that follow will permit the radiologist to contribute substantially to diagnosis and management. Emphasis is placed on the initial chest radiographs and those taken during the first day of life, because during this initial period crucial decisions must be made (i.e., transfer to a tertiary care center, administration of exogenous surfactant therapy, insertion of a chest tube, or surgical intervention).

A close relationship between the radiologist and the referring neonatologists is vitally important.[15] The radiologist will profit by becoming a member of the "team" intimately involved in the care of sick infants; the patient will profit as well. As noted earlier, neonatology depends heavily on radiology, and a radiologist who is concerned, knowledgeable, and cooperative will improve patient care and enjoy the satisfaction of personal participation in the effort. Furthermore, moment-to-moment feedback is immensely helpful in improving diagnostic skills. A daily work conference during which the day's films are reviewed with the clinicians is an excellent way of achieving this.

However close the relationship with the neonatologists becomes though, the radiologist must remain, in Peterson's words, "first a radiologist."[70] In other words, the radiologist must discover and relate the "story" told by the films and must adhere to this story in the presence of clinical evidence to the contrary and the conflicting opinions (sometimes vigorously expressed) of the clinicians. The radiologist best serves himself, his clinical colleagues, and the patient by remaining faithful to the findings revealed on the radiographs.

MAJOR MEDICAL CONDITIONS CAUSING RESPIRATORY DISTRESS

The important disorders causing respiratory distress in newborn infants are typically divided into medical and surgical causes. Categorizing diseases according to what is done with the patient after the film is interpreted is a somewhat artificial exercise but is retained here to honor tradition.

TRANSIENT TACHYPNEA OF THE NEWBORN

In utero, the fetal lungs are filled with fluid. Replacement of the majority of this fluid with gas normally occurs immediately after delivery. Fetal lung fluid is expelled from the trachea into the hypopharynx, from which it is swallowed or leaks out of the infant's mouth. The remaining lung fluid drains through the pulmonary lymphatics in the interstitium. Transient tachypnea of the newborn (TTN) is a condition in which the clearance of lung fluid is sufficiently delayed that the infant exhibits tachypnea and often other manifestations of respiratory distress.[4] The condition is the most common cause of respiratory distress in newborn infants.[52] It is relatively frequent in infants delivered by cesarean section, and it has been speculated that it results from a lack of the thoracic compression that occurs during a normal vaginal delivery.[63] A less explicable risk factor appears to be maternal asthma.[19]

The usual course of TTN is a progressive clearing of clinical abnormalities, a process that usually occurs within the first day but may require up to 72 hours. It is curious that such tachypnea often takes a few hours to develop after delivery, although the volume of unabsorbed fluid would be expected to be greatest immediately after birth.

Some infants with TTN exhibit a phenomenon known as *persisting pulmonary hypertension of the newborn* (or *persisting fetal circulation*; see later discussion) with cyanosis and distress that may be severe.[9] Persisting pulmonary hypertension is a serious condition that may occur secondary to asphyxia, idiopathically, or, more commonly, as a result of several pulmonary disorders, most notably meconium aspiration syndrome, neonatal pneumonia, and diaphragmatic hernia. Evidently pulmonary arterial hypertension occurs in response to the pulmonary disease or other insult, resulting in right-to-left shunting at the levels of the foramen ovale and the patent ductus arteriosus.[36] The result is profound cyanosis, despite the absence of any structural cardiac anomaly. The condition may be lethal and contributes to the morbidity and mortality of affected infants; it is one of the major indications for extracorporeal membrane oxygenation.[85]

MECONIUM ASPIRATION SYNDROME

Hypoxia in utero evokes two responses in the term or post-term fetus: deep, gasping respirations of amniotic fluid and passage of meconium[20]; preterm fetuses express meconium relatively seldom. The combination of these responses results in aspiration of meconium to a varying depth in the airways. Meconium is toxic in the lungs and evokes an almost immediate inflammatory response in addition to its direct effect of obstructing smaller airways.[88] When meconium-stained amniotic fluid is encountered at delivery, it is common practice to begin suctioning the airway while the infant's head is still on the perineum. The presence of meconium below the cords worsens the prognosis.

Respiratory distress is usually immediate and of a degree reflecting the severity of the condition. Pneumothorax and pneumomediastinum are common and are possibly caused by shearing stresses between affected and nonaffected regions of lung or simply by the hyperinflation that often occurs.[102] The most ominous complication is persisting pulmonary hypertension,[33] which often results in profound cyanosis and may require extracorporeal membrane oxygenation.[85] In infants who survive meconium aspiration syndrome, clinical clearing is variable and depends on severity. Bacterial superinfection may occur but is less common; some patients require prolonged respiratory support and may develop bronchopulmonary dysplasia.

Sometimes meconium is expelled into the amniotic fluid without significant aspiration. Some distressed fetuses have gasping respirations without expelling meconium. The aspiration of "clear" amniotic fluid is not a benign process, because the fluid, even in the absence of meconium, contains irritating debris in the form of skin cells and lanugo hairs. This so-called *drowned newborn syndrome*[97] is difficult to document and has not been systematically studied, but may account for some cases of extended TTN or spontaneous air leaks. Aspiration of maternal blood also occurs, but in my experience this is usually clinically benign and short-lived.

NEONATAL PNEUMONIA

One of the most common clinical directives on requisitions for chest radiography in newborn infants is "rule out sepsis." Sepsis, or viable microorganisms in the blood or cerebrospinal fluid, is radiographically occult, and the radiograph is used to detect the neonatal pneumonia that often accompanies sepsis and may be the cause of it.

Neonatal pneumonia arises from one of three major mechanisms: ascending infection from the maternal vagina, often associated with premature or prolonged rupture of the membranes and chorioamnionitis; infection acquired during passage through the birth canal or shortly thereafter; and infection from a maternal hematogenous source.[6] In utero pneumonia with sepsis is a major cause of stillbirth and premature delivery. The infectious agents are usually bacteria, most commonly hemolytic and nonhemolytic streptococci, *Escherichia coli,* and *Staphylococcus* spp.,[3,58,69,76] although a wide variety of other bacteria have been implicated. Less commonly the infection is viral.[41,80] The organism *Ureaplasma urealyticum* has been indirectly implicated as a cause of neonatal pneumonia[58] and, following colonization of the respiratory tract, chronic lung disease and bronchopulmonary dysplasia[75].

The clinical signs of neonatal pneumonia often, but not invariably, include respiratory distress. Despite the life-threatening nature of neonatal sepsis, its clinical signs are variable and often nondescript and include lethargy, variable extremes of body temperature, a white blood cell count that ranges from leukocytosis to leukopenia, and feeding difficulties. Neonatologists have learned to suspect sepsis not only in infants with known risk factors (e.g., prolonged membrane rupture, maternal fever, and unexplained respiratory distress) but also in infants who seem even vaguely ill.

The most ominous complication of neonatal pneumonia, other than septic shock, is persisting pulmonary hypertension. Group B streptococci cause the most common type of pneumonia associated with neonatal pulmonary hypertension, but this condition has also been described with *Ureaplasma* pneumonia[90]; pneumonias from other organisms can also result in neonatal pulmonary hypertension. An uncommon but well-documented phenomenon associated with group B streptococcal pneumonia is the delayed appearance of a right diaphragmatic hernia[39,59]; the mechanism by which this occurs is uncertain.

RESPIRATORY DISTRESS SYNDROME

Respiratory distress syndrome (RDS) was formerly called *hyaline membrane disease*, a term now largely abandoned because of the pathologic nonspecificity of pulmonary hyaline membranes in infants. Sometimes RDS is called *idiopathic respiratory distress syndrome*, a term that is misleading, as the cause of RDS has been documented with great clarity. RDS results from a deficiency of pulmonary surfactant, which usually, but not invariably, is caused by prematurity. Surfactant deficiency causes instability and collapse of alveoli, producing diffuse microatelectasis, stiff lungs, impaired gas exchange, and resultant respiratory distress. Prematurity is the major predisposing factor for pulmonary surfactant deficiency, although RDS occasionally occurs in term infants, especially in those with diabetic mothers.

The most accurate diagnosis of RDS is provided by biochemical analysis of lung effluent (amniotic fluid or gastric or tracheal aspirate) to detect the presence and quantity of surfactant materials.[51] The presence of phosphatidylglycerol usually defines a mature surfactant system[10] and hence suggests the presence of some disorder other than RDS as a cause of respiratory distress. At most centers, a firm diagnosis of RDS also requires the presence of typical findings on a chest radiograph.

The maturity of the surfactant system is influenced by the endocrine glucocorticoid axis, which is activated by administering betamethasone to pregnant women during preterm labor. This treatment, when successful, may ameliorate or avoid the occurrence of RDS after preterm delivery.[35] A similar mechanism presumably accounts for the relative paucity of RDS among infants who had any of a variety of in utero stresses (see "Premature Infants with Accelerated Lung Maturity").

The complications and associations of RDS are numerous. Of particular importance are intrathoracic air leaks (related to ventilator therapy; see next chapter), left-to-right shunting through a patent ductus arteriosus (PDA), and the development (relatively late in the disease's course) of

bronchopulmonary dysplasia (BPD), which is currently the most common cause of chronic lung disease in children born in the United States.[67] Intraventricular hemorrhage remains an important nonthoracic cause of mortality and morbidity among patients with RDS.[40]

Therapy for RDS consists of supportive care, most importantly the maintenance of gas exchange using elevated inspired oxygen tension and mechanical ventilatory assistance. The endotracheal administration of exogenous surfactant also appears to improve immediate gas exchange, survival rate, and morbidity rate for BPD.[46,60] The common association of left-to-right shunting through the PDA may be controlled by fluid restriction, administration of indomethacin, or surgical ligation.

PREMATURE INFANTS WITH ACCELERATED LUNG MATURITY

Occasionally preterm infants (less than about 30 weeks' gestation) with low birth weight (less than 1500 g) "ought" to have RDS but are spared because of intrauterine stress or maternal steroid therapy. These patients have been described as having *immature lung syndrome,*[28] which is an unsatisfactory name because their lungs are actually relatively mature, at least in terms of surfactant production. We presently call such infants *PALM infants*; the acronym PALM represents *premature with accelerated lung maturity*. The most reliable way of diagnosing this condition is identifying a mature phospholipid profile in lung effluent.[10,38]

PALM infants generally fare better than infants of comparable maturity who have RDS.[28] However, they are still susceptible to intraventricular hemorrhage and symptomatic shunting through a PDA. Because they rarely require high-pressure assisted ventilation, they seldom develop intrathoracic air leaks. However, low-pressure assisted ventilation for recurrent apnea may cause mild BPD in these infants.

PERSISTING PULMONARY HYPERTENSION OF THE NEWBORN

Persisting pulmonary hypertension of the newborn (PPHN) was formerly called *persisting fetal circulation*. In affected infants, pulmonary vascular resistance, instead of rapidly falling as is usual postnatally, becomes suprasystemic. Right-to-left shunting at the levels of the PDA and the foramen ovale ensues, with subsequent cyanosis that can be profound and life threatening.[36,61] The incidence of PPHN is about 0.8 per 1000 live births with vaginal delivery and is increased substantially by cesarean delivery.[57]

Although the condition can be idiopathic, PPHN is usually secondary to lung disease, particularly meconium aspiration syndrome, neonatal pneumonia, or pulmonary hypoplasia.[32,33] An intriguing speculation is that some cases may be related to diffuse pulmonary microthrombi.[56] The occurrence of severe PPHN is a major indication for the use of extracorporeal membrane oxygenation. Less drastic therapy involves the use of pulmonary vasodilators, such as inhaled nitric oxide.[71,84]

RADIOGRAPHY OF NEWBORNS WITH RESPIRATORY DISTRESS: GENERAL

BASIC RADIOGRAPHIC TECHNIQUES

The two most important imaging modalities for newborn infants with respiratory distress are the plain chest film and the echocardiogram. The latter is beyond the scope of this chapter and will not be discussed. The plain chest film, however, forms the basis for diagnosis and for subsequent imaging and treatment.

Infants with severe respiratory distress generally require filming with a mobile ("portable") unit. Even though the radiation dose from chest films in this age group is minimal, many affected infants require a substantial number of films during their hospitalization and afterward, so it is advisable to limit the radiation dose as much as possible. The use of rare earth screens is one way of accomplishing this.[30]

In addition to avoiding unnecessary filming, careful coning of the primary beam also minimizes the radiation dose. Although "whole babygrams" are properly deplored, it must also be admitted that sometimes these convey useful information not available on a tightly coned view of the chest. Such information includes an increased view of the skeleton; the situs of the abdominal viscera; the development of dentition (making assessment of gestational age possible);[50] the location of umbilical catheters; and the detection of intra-abdominal diseases such as pneumoperitoneum, meconium peritonitis, and intestinal atresia. A compromise that others[12] and I have adopted is to use wide coning from the mouth to the umbilicus for the initial chest film only. Subsequent chest films are tightly coned to the chest (Fig. 2–3).

Because infants with respiratory distress are frequently treated with assisted ventilation and often have other tubes and catheters in place, they are best left undisturbed as much as possible during filming. For this reason, the frontal film is a supine anteroposterior (AP) view and the lateral film is a cross-Isolette supine view. Overhead lateral views markedly disturb neonates' tranquility and are confusing because the dependent lung tends to collapse and the superior lung tends to be overinflated. However, gravity-dependent views (see later discussion) are helpful in selected circumstances.

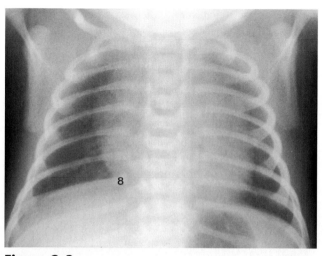

Figure 2–3
Normal frontal radiograph. The right hemidiaphragm is at the level of the eighth rib (8). A large thymus obscures much of the normal pulmonary vascularity. Note that the infant's chin is at midline, and the chest, correspondingly, is not rotated

The utility of the lateral view of the chest has been questioned.[34] I believe the lateral view is an essential part of the radiographic chest evaluation, at least for the initial film. The lateral view of the position and configuration of the diaphragm allows assessment of the degree of inflation; it permits confident recognition of cardiomegaly, which may be simulated by the thymus on the AP projection, and it provides the clearest view of the spine and the sternum. Fairly frequently, a pneumothorax may be occult on the AP view but clearly evident on the lateral projection. The retrocardiac and retrosternal regions, poorly assessed on the AP view, are well defined on the lateral view. Finally, the lateral view, when combined with the AP view, permits confident definition of the location of intrathoracic tubes, catheters, infiltrates, and masses (Figs. 2–4, 2–5).

The lateral view has its drawbacks, however. It adds to the radiation dose and disturbs the patient and accompanying staff during exposure. For this reason, the lateral view is commonly and appropriately omitted for routine follow-up studies, except in certain settings. A lateral view is necessary or at least strongly suggested in the following circumstances:

1. *The initial chest film:* Because of the information provided by this projection and the utility of knowing as much as possible about the patient at the outset, the initial chest examination should include the lateral view unless the patient is in such desperate straits that additional filming is life threatening. I advise our technologists to obtain the lateral view before the AP view, because it is then less commonly omitted.

2. *Position of tubes and catheters:* Three-dimensional assessment of the placement of tubes, especially chest tubes, requires a lateral view to see whether the tube is

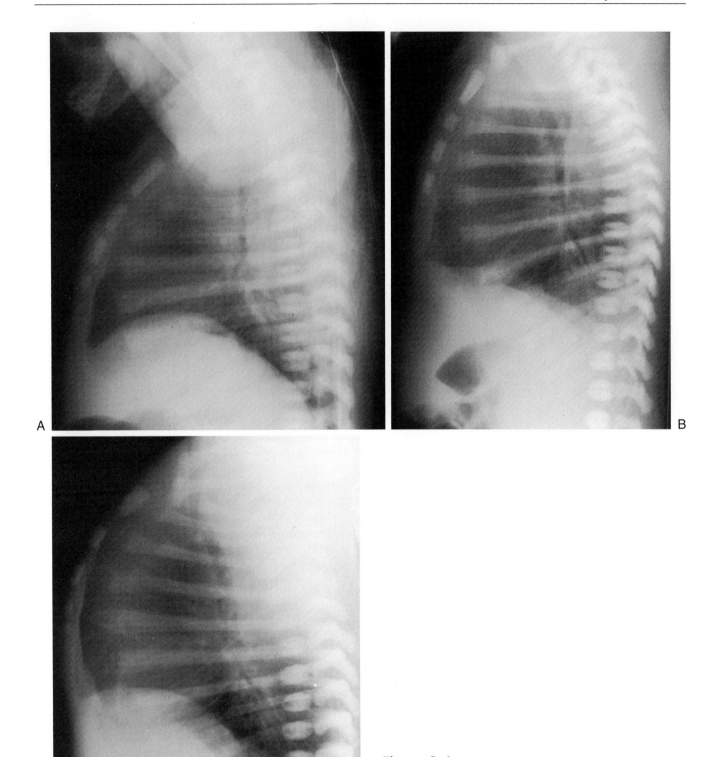

Figure 2–4
Pulmonary aeration as seen in the lateral view. *A,* Hypoaeration is present in this premature infant before surfactant administration. *B,* Mild hyperinflation. Note that the thorax is mildly expanded. *C,* Marked hyperinflation: This infant demonstrates severe, retained lung fluid. Both hemidiaphragms are everted.

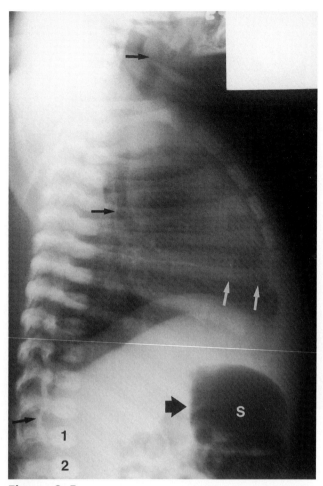

Figure 2–5

Lateral chest film showing mild hyperinflation. The *top black arrow* is at the level of the cords, and the *middle black arrow* is at the carina. An acceptable position for the endotracheal tube is in the middle third between these two points. The *white arrows* indicate the anterior ends of the fifth ribs. A perfectly positioned lateral film would have the two rib ends superimposed. Note *fat arrow* pointing to the air-fluid level in the stomach (S), indicating that the infant was supine and the beam was directed as a cross-table lateral. Free intraperitoneal air would lie anteriorly with this view. Also note the *black arrow in the lower left corner* pointing to the twelfth rib. This little rib usually is attached to the twelfth vertebral body, thereby identifying which vertebral body represents T12 and L1. Vertebral bodies L1 and L2 are identified here as *1* and *2*. The umbilical catheter position can thus be determined from the lateral view.

positioned anteriorly (to drain pneumothorax in a supine infant) or posteriorly (to drain fluid).

3. *Unexplained clinical deterioration:* If the patient's condition permits, the lateral view may add information that may explain clinical deterioration. Such settings include an unsuspected pneumothorax and malposition of an endotracheal or other tube.

4. *Localization of masses or infiltrates:* Sometimes masses, cysts, or infiltrates not seen on the initial radiograph because of lung disease or other problems may be

suspected on subsequent films; the lateral view is needed to identify and characterize these more fully.

Radiographic interpretation, especially of the AP view, is enhanced if the patient is not rotated. Rotation may be avoided by recalling that "as the head goes, so goes the chest." If the head is facing the ceiling, the chest generally is also. Lack of rotation may be achieved by having an attendant use two hands for restraint. The thumb, forefinger, and middle finger of one hand are used to clasp the infant's wrists above its head; the same digits of the other hand clasp the infant's ankles. The head and toes are positioned straight up, and the film is thus exposed (Fig. 2–6).

The endotracheal tube tip moves up and down the airway as a function of head position,[21] so placing the head in such a way as to attain a nonrotated view of the chest may change the position of this tube. If this is undesirable, the infant's head may be left in its usual position, accepting that a rotated and unsatisfactory view of the chest will result. If *only* the position of the tube tip is required, a coned view of the upper mediastinum (called a *ramogram*, in honor of Barbara Ramos, the technologist who proposed it) will provide this information with slightly less radiation and without subjecting the radiologist to a confusing and possibly misleading view of the thoracic contents.

For an infant receiving assisted ventilation with a respirator, the exposure may be made near the end of the inspiratory cycle, or the respirator may be briefly disconnected and the infant filmed during quiet respiration. Infants breathing without mechanical support should be filmed during quiet breathing. Filming should be avoided while infants are crying, because crying causes large excursions of the diaphragm, resulting in severely hypoventilatory and spuriously hyperventilatory examinations; if at all possible, a crying infant should be pacified before filming.

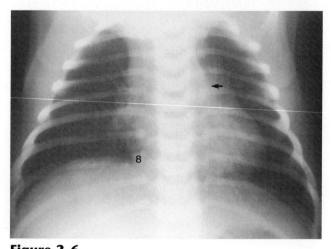

Figure 2–6

Normal anteroposterior (AP) chest radiograph; all the markings seen are normal pulmonary vessels. A large "ductus bump" is present (*arrow*). 8, Eighth rib.

SUPPLEMENTARY IMAGING TECHNIQUES

A large array of imaging modalities can be used to investigate abnormalities seen on the plain chest film. These include computed tomography (CT) and magnetic resonance imaging (MRI), which may be useful in evaluating intrathoracic masses and congenital heart disease. However, these modalities require the infant to be sufficiently stable to allow conveyance and support outside the intensive care nursery. This section describes modalities that permit the use of mobile units within the nursery.

Sonography

The major sonographic modality used in infants with respiratory distress is echocardiography. This is probably the most sensitive modality for identifying left-to-right shunting through a PDA and is also invaluable for evaluating the internal cardiac anatomy in infants with possible congenital heart disease.[79]

Sonography is also useful in characterizing masses that abut the diaphragm; in infants with suspected sequestration, for example, Doppler evaluation may reveal an aortic blood supply.[79] Large pleural effusions can also be monitored with sonography. The motion of the hemidiaphragms may also be assessed with real-time sonography; the transducer is angled up through the liver so that the motions of both hemidiaphragms are viewed simultaneously, thereby detecting paralysis or paradoxical motion, if present.

Gravity-Dependent Views

The most common gravity-dependent view is the cross-Isolette lateral view, discussed earlier. In some settings, however, a decubitus view may be useful. In infants with suspected pneumothorax, the side with the pneumothorax is placed uppermost, and a cross-Isolette decubitus film is made; in this position the lung separates from the rib cage, clearly revealing the lung edge and free gas.[94] To evaluate pleural fluid, the affected lung is placed downward. However, if the volume of pleural fluid is large, the resultant film may simply reveal an opaque dependent hemithorax. In this setting, it may be useful to place the affected side uppermost; this allows the lung to float superiorly, enabling assessment of the more medially located fluid, which layers inferiorly to the lung.

The decubitus position may enhance resorption of unilateral pulmonary interstitial emphysema[16] when the affected side is placed downward. The gravitational shift test,[103] which has been used in adults to distinguish between fixed infiltrate and excess mobilizable lung water, has not been systematically examined in infants.

Assisted Expiration View

The assisted expiration view, which is valuable to document focal air trapping in older infants and children with aspirated foreign bodies,[95] may occasionally be useful in the neonate. Manual pressure is exerted on the patient's abdomen in a posterior-superior direction to empty the lungs. A film is exposed at the end of this forced expiration. I have successfully used this maneuver to confirm air trapping in infants with congenital lobar emphysema and infants with BPD in whom airway granulomas provide a "ball valve" effect in the bronchus intermedius.[62]

ESSENTIAL DIAGNOSTIC RADIOGRAPHIC FINDINGS AND CLUES

As is implied in the later discussion of individual diseases, chest radiography of newborn infants is not entirely a simple matter. The findings in several conditions overlap, and the patient's clinical condition is not always reflected by radiographically visible abnormalities. Furthermore, the referring neonatologists are often as unsure of the patient's diagnosis as is the radiologist, so the radiologist may not be helped much by information on the requisition form, even when such information is provided. Finally, the clinical findings and history of "respiratory distress" are vastly nonspecific. Thus, it is helpful to exploit the plain chest radiograph as much as possible, because even subtle clues may prove crucial to making a diagnosis, which in turn may influence treatment and clinical outcome.

As a general rule, surgical causes of respiratory distress tend to be focal or unilateral, whereas medical causes tend to involve both lungs fairly equally. Of course, focal infiltrates, as seen in some infants with neonatal pneumonia, and conditions such as bilateral pulmonary interstitial emphysema do not follow this rule.

Severe congenital heart disease often presents in the newborn period with some combination of respiratory distress, congestive failure, and cyanosis. Usually congenital heart disease is more apparent clinically than radiographically; indeed, chest radiographs of affected infants may be deceptively normal and commonly suggest retained fetal lung fluid or diffuse pneumonia. The distinction between heart disease and parenchymal lung disease in the immediate neonatal period is notoriously difficult.[24] Chest radiographic clues indicating heart disease include an unusual morphology of the cardiac silhouette; a concave main pulmonary artery segment; tracheal displacement to the left on an AP film, suggesting a right-sided aortic arch (which also may be diagnosed by the position of an umbilical arterial catheter in the chest); abnormalities of visceral or cardiac situs; clear-cut enlarged "shunt" vessels, which often become more apparent with time as pulmonary vascular resistance decreases; and a cardiothoracic ratio exceeding about 60%.[25] Visual clues such as the "snowman" of anomalous venous return and the "egg-on-a-string" of transposition are sometimes helpful in older infants and children but are commonly masked in neonates by a large thymus. A detailed discussion of cardiac disease in newborns is beyond the scope of this chapter and the expertise of its author.

Normal Variants

The *thymus gland* is a notorious source of difficulty when interpreting chest films (particularly the AP film) of newborn infants. The two lobes of the thymus, despite being fairly thin, are often dense enough to obscure the upper and middle mediastinum and sometimes even the lower mediastinum. A thymus may be recognized by a wavy margin, where it is focally indented by the anterior ribs[66]; by a triangular or "sail" configuration[83]; and by the "notch" formed where the thymic shadow intersects the cardiac silhouette.[94] The triangular sail is sometimes best seen on the lateral projection, just behind the sternum. On the AP projection, the sail is usually on the right, ending inferiorly at the minor fissure, but it may be on the left as well, where it almost never indicates a second minor fissure. (True bilateral right-sided pulmonary anatomy suggests asplenia.[31]) The apparent "cardiomegaly" caused by large thymic lobes can be discounted by examining the lateral projection and noting a normal-sized heart.

The *trachea* is a soft, floppy structure in newborn infants and hence buckles easily when the neck is flexed and during expiration. A small anterior indentation seen on the lateral view is almost always normal. The position of the upper intrathoracic trachea on the AP view defines the situs of the aortic arch, which lies on the contralateral side from the trachea. One of the few advantages of a hypoventilatory examination is that the trachea may buckle markedly away from the aorta, thereby clearly revealing the aortic situs.

Air bronchograms are normal in the central third of the chest of newborn infants and are pathologic only if they extend peripherally. The more sharp and well defined these are, the more parenchymal abnormalities they reflect.

An *anterior lucency* in the retrosternal region on the lateral view may simply be a result of the infant's relatively short ribs not reaching the sternum. A genuine pneumothorax in this region is usually more radiolucent and is limited posteriorly by the anterior edge of the partially collapsed lung. Another retrosternal normal variant, seen inferiorly on the lateral view, is a well-defined density that may be the transverse thoracic muscles or the abutting anterior lungs.[82]

Pleural bulging at the apices and intercostal space is probably normal only in a crying infant who is vigorously exhaling or straining against a closed glottis. In an infant who is not crying, pleural bulging should raise the question of abnormal air trapping.[77]

Artifacts

Several artifacts of patient position or exposure may result in confusing or suboptimal images. Cephalic beam angulation casts the anterior ribs upward, a distortion that may suggest a bony dysplasia; furthermore, the cardiac apex may appear uptilted and the main pulmonary artery may be concealed beneath the cardiac silhouette, forming a concave pulmonary artery segment or a radiographic "pseudo-tet." These artifacts may be suspected by noting the uptilted configuration of the anterior ribs.

A rotated view of the chest often suggests asymmetric parenchymal disease when in fact the disease is symmetric. Substantial rotation may also cast the sternal ossification centers over one hemithorax, falsely suggesting masses. To evaluate rotation, the length of the lower posterior ribs is compared left to right. The infant is rotated in the direction of the longer ribs. Rotation may be suspected when the chin is included in the beam and is pointing to one shoulder; the chest follows the head.

The normal level of inspiration is the dome of the right hemidiaphragm at the posterior eighth rib, with a normal range of about seven to nine ribs.[25] A significantly hypoventilatory examination usually indicates RDS, pulmonary hypoplasia, or (most commonly) a crying infant filmed during expiration. Needless to say, adventitious hypoventilatory studies and underpenetrated studies are misleading and tend to overestimate the actual extent of parenchymal disease. The use of such films for interpretation invariably leads to overdiagnosis, overtreatment, and a rapid loss of credibility.

Skin folds often overlie the chest but usually in locations that do not parallel the pleura. A skin fold that happens to lie parallel to the pleura may simulate a pneumothorax but can usually be distinguished by perceiving lung markings beyond it or by following the line to a location incompatible with intrapleural air. If uncertainty remains, the film can simply be repeated, or a decubitus view can be exposed with the questionable side up.

The scapula is commonly cast over the lungs of infants on AP radiographs. It can thus simulate a focal upper lobe pneumonia but can usually be distinguished by deliberately locating and outlining both scapulae. Similarly, the scapular spine cast over a lung can simulate focal atelectasis.

Plastic umbilical clamps occasionally overlie the upper abdomen, but almost always their identity is apparent on inspection. Monitor leads over the chest can mask significant abnormalities; these are best placed in the axillae, where they cause problems only on the lateral view.

Although this is not an artifact, it is imperative to identify the patient correctly on the film; medical and medicolegal disasters can ensue when films are mislabeled. A common cause of this, at least in our nursery, is the situation when two or more infants of multiple gestations, with identical surnames, are ill. I encourage taping a small metal marker on the shoulder of the "B" infant of twins and using appropriate variations when there are more than two infants. The markers are 3-mm metal balls used in mammography.

Bones

The skeletal status of a neonate can be ascertained from the plain chest radiograph, and the identification of any abnormalities can be extremely helpful in making a correct diagnosis. The scope of this chapter does not permit a full description of all of the bony dysplasias and conditions that may be encountered, but examination of the skeleton in such infants will usually suggest the diagnosis of a congenital disorder. The most dramatic and clinically relevant diagnosis is thanatophoric dysplasia, in which the short ribs encase a thorax that is too small to permit normal lung development and gas exchange.

The bones may also suggest a chromosomal abnormality. The presence of wavy, hypoplastic "ribbon ribs," together with a hypoplastic sternum (seen on the lateral projection), suggests one of a few trisomies, most commonly trisomy 18.[64] A markedly bell-shaped chest, 11 rib pairs, and a bifid sternal manubrial ossification center (seen on the lateral projection) suggest trisomy 21,[23] as do relatively tall vertebral bodies[98] and flared iliac wings.[11]

A bell-shaped chest, if relatively mild, is common in infants who are generally hypotonic ("floppy") as a result of any of many causes (e.g., maternal anesthesia, asphyxia, pancuronium bromide paralysis, or central nervous system dysfunction). A markedly bell-shaped chest suggests not only trisomy 21 but also pulmonary hypoplasia, especially if accompanied by an intrathoracic air leak.[5,55] This should prompt questioning about a history of oligohydramnios and oliguria.[100]

The presence of growth lines in the bones of a newborn infant suggests intrauterine growth arrest from any of many causes,[29] one of which is maternal magnesium administration for tocolysis.[54] Such lines, as well as "celery stalk" changes at the ends of long bones, may be seen in congenital infections such as toxoplasmosis, rubella, cytomegalovirus, and herpes (collectively known as the TORCH group), as well as in congenital syphilis. Congenital syphilis, a disease presently showing a resurgence, may also cause periostitis and other distinctive changes[17,72]; I encountered an infant in whom the chest radiograph, which revealed clavicular periostitis, was the only clue to congenital syphilis.

The skeleton also provides clues about fetal maturity. The teeth may be examined if they are included in the beam[50]; the humeral head or coracoid ossification centers, when ossified, suggest a term infant.[49] The length of the thoracic spine also varies in a nearly linear way with gestational age,[48] presumably except in infants who are small for gestational age. In general, and with the help of experience, the infant's weight and gestational age can be approximated from the size of the infant's image on the radiograph. This can occasionally be useful; for example, a tiny infant with diffuse pulmonary granularity and abnormal air bronchograms probably has RDS, whereas the same parenchymal findings in a large infant more strongly suggest another process, particularly pneumonia.

Detection of an anomalous vertebral body properly raises the question of vertebral, anal, tracheal, esophageal, renal, and limb (VATERL) anomalies.[91] The major elements of this association, some of which may be absent, are vertebral anomalies, imperforate anus, tracheoesophageal fistula, and anomalies of the radius. This constellation of anomalies, which has grown over time and has thus been called the *alphabet association* (CB Graham, personal communication), presumably reflects the fact that if an embryo is injured early in development, multiple organ systems tend to be involved.

A fractured clavicle suggests a difficult delivery.[18] When a chest film is requested to "rule out clavicular fracture," it is my practice to obtain a full AP chest film (no lateral film), because associated phrenic nerve damage sometimes leads to a paralyzed hemidiaphragm. It should be noted that occasionally a clavicular fracture may not be seen because of the curved shape of the clavicle and overlap at the fracture site. If there is strong clinical suspicion of a fractured clavicle, the infant should be treated as though such a fracture were present, or a repeat film with an angled beam should be exposed. Treatment is not necessary for healing, which usually proceeds excellently in any case, but a fractured clavicle is painful, and in the early days of life the parents may label an affected infant as unduly fretful, temperamental, or a difficult feeder if they are unaware of the injury and the discomfort it can cause during normal handling.

Level of Lung Inflation

The extent of lung inflation provides an often-helpful clue about the nature of parenchymal disease. Inflation is best appreciated by the position and configuration of the hemidiaphragms on the lateral projection. Normally, the hemidiaphragms form a gentle, cephalic curve. With air trapping, the posterior portion of the hemidiaphragms flattens; with underaeration, the cephalic curve is exaggerated, and the position of the hemidiaphragms is high (Fig. 2–4).

Genuine underinflation is common in only two medical disorders: RDS and pulmonary hypoplasia. Other common medical disorders—retained fetal lung fluid, meconium aspiration syndrome, and neonatal pneumonia—typically produce hyperinflation, with hemidiaphragms that are low and flattened posteriorly. Diaphragmatic appearance is useful in distinguishing RDS from retained fetal lung fluid in its alveolar phase or diffuse pneumonia from RDS. With RDS there is diffuse atelectasis; with the other conditions there is not.

A *caveat* is necessary for infants who are already being treated with assisted ventilation when the initial film is exposed. In this setting, the position of the hemidiaphragms is as much a function of ventilator pressure as of the underlying lung disease. Thus, an infant with RDS, an atelectatic condition, can have low, flat hemidiaphragms (and thus hyperinflation) if ventilator pressure is enough to overcome the tendency of the lungs to collapse.

Pleural Fluid

Large amounts of pleural fluid are seen with chylothorax[14] and hydrops.[92] Hydrops may be related to blood incompatibility (immune hydrops) or to numerous nonimmune causes,[8] and the pleural fluid is often accompanied by ascites and anasarca. In infants without chylothorax or hydrops, smaller amounts of pleural fluid may be seen near the costophrenic angles and in the fissures; interlobar fissures are commonly visualized in newborn infants, and probably only those more than 1 mm thick should be considered abnormal.

Pleural fluid is seldom seen in infants with uncomplicated RDS but is common in infants with retained fetal lung fluid, meconium aspiration syndrome, and neonatal pneumonia. In making the sometimes-difficult distinction between RDS and other similar conditions, the presence of visible pleural fluid makes RDS less likely. Of course, RDS and pneumonia may coexist,[42] in which case the presence of pleural fluid may be the only clue to the coexistent infection.

As is discussed later, neonatal pneumonia can resemble retained fetal lung fluid radiographically. Small amounts of pleural fluid are common in infants with retained fetal lung fluid, but it is my subjective and clinical impression that the larger the amount of pleural fluid, the more likely it is that the infant has pneumonia rather than simple retained lung fluid.

The Stomach

Visceral situs inversus may be noted by a right position of the gastric gas bubble or by the direction of a nasogastric tube. This is an important observation because of the high association of visceral situs inversus with congenital heart disease.[86] The conditions of asplenia and polysplenia are also commonly associated with heart disease and may be suspected by noting a midline stomach and liver.[31,89]

RADIOGRAPHY OF MAJOR MEDICAL CONDITIONS

PATTERNS OF DISEASE

In discussing pulmonary abnormalities, it is necessary to have a firm idea of what represents "normal." In this discussion, pulmonary parenchymal normalcy is defined as the absence of any peripheral markings in the lungs except normal blood vessels. By this definition, a completely normal film of a newborn infant is relatively uncommon. At delivery, the lungs are filled with fluid that requires a finite time to drain and be absorbed. Thus, chest radiographs of infants who are perfectly normal clinically in the early hours of life often reveal this excessive fluid. Such films are not normal, however, although some radiologists conclude their comments with "normal for age." Another reason for the relative paucity

of normal chest radiographs is that clinically normal infants are not customarily radiographed.

In the chest radiographic diagnosis of newborn infants, a "pattern" approach is useful. For example, one may speak of an "RDS pattern," meaning diffuse granularity with abnormal air bronchograms, or a "wet-lung pattern," meaning diffusely increased nonvascular markings. As is emphasized in the following discussion, few, if any, absolutely pathognomonic chest radiographs are encountered among the important medical causes of respiratory distress. Instead, the various patterns exhibit considerable overlap (see Diagram), and each pattern has its own differential diagnosis (Table 2–1). However, knowledge of the relevant patterns and of the disorders that overlap with each other radiographically permits at least a fair degree of diagnostic confidence.

The five most important patterns of neonatal lung disease are as follows:

1. *Normal.* No markings except normal blood vessels are seen in the lungs.
2. *Granular pattern.* The prototype of this pattern is RDS. The lungs are diffusely and usually homogeneously involved, with a granular pattern ranging in density from slightly above normal to essentially opaque lungs. Abnormal air bronchograms (extending beyond the central third of the chest) are seen with varying degrees of clarity, ranging from barely visible to constituting virtually the only visible gas in the lungs.
3. *Streaky or wet-lung pattern.* The prototype of this pattern is retained fetal lung fluid. The lungs are diffusely and

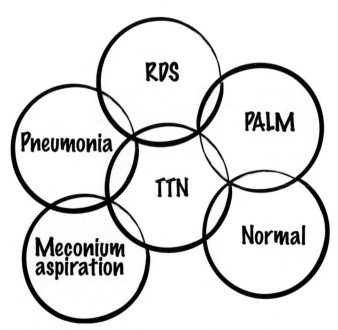

Overlap of the radiographic appearances of common neonatal lung diseases. RDS: respiratory distress syndrome; PALM: premature with accelerated lung maturity; TTN: transient tachypnea of the newborn.

> **TABLE 2-1** IMPORTANT DIFFERENT DIAGNOSTIC
> CONSIDERATIONS FOR MAJOR
> PARENCHYMAL LUNG PATTERNS
>
> **Normal lungs**
> Normal infant
> Premature with accelerated lung maturity
> Transient tachypnea of the newborn
> Sepsis (without radiographically demonstrable
>   pneumonia)
> **Respiratory distress syndrome (RDS) pattern**
> RDS
> Transient tachypnea of the newborn (when fluid is in the
>   alveolar phase)
> Premature with accelerated lung maturity
> Neonatal pneumonia (especially pneumonia caused by
>   group B *Streptococcus* and *Haemophilus influenzae,* but
>   also pneumonia caused by other organisms)
> Pulmonary hemorrhage
> Severe pulmonary venous congestion (prototype: total
>   anomalous pulmonary venous connection with
>   obstruction)
> **Wet-lung pattern**
> Transient tachypnea of the newborn
> Normal infant in early hours of life
> Diffuse pneumonia
> Meconium aspiration syndrome (mild)
> RDS (when lung fluid is in its early, alveolar phase)
> Premature with accelerated lung maturity
> Clear amniotic fluid aspiration
> Pulmonary venous congestion from variety of causes,
>   including heart lesions causing elevated left-sided
>   pressures, overhydration, and placental transfusion
> Pulmonary hemorrhage
> Hyperviscosity syndrome
> **Meconium aspiration syndrome pattern**
> Meconium aspiration syndrome
> Retained fetal lung fluid (with or without tachypnea)
> Diffuse pneumonia
> **Focal pattern (lungs inhomogeneously
> involved)**
> Neonatal pneumonia
> Focal atelectasis
> Congenital lobar emphysema (lucent upper or middle lobe)
> Intrathoracic mass, cyst, or other surgical lesion

fairly homogeneously involved with increased nonvascular, largely linear, and seemingly interstitial markings, the most prominent of which extend from the hili. This is the most commonly seen radiographic pattern among infants generally and unfortunately is the least specific.

4. *Patchy pattern.* The prototype of this pattern is meconium aspiration syndrome. The lungs show a diffuse pattern of irregular punctate or patchy abnormal densities, distributed fairly homogeneously throughout both lungs.

5. *Focal pattern.* In the previous patterns, one part of the lung looks pretty much like the other parts of the lung. With the focal pattern, the appearance is asymmetric[2]; one observes a focal region (or several regions) of abnormal density, whereas other parts of the lung are normal or substantially less abnormal. The prototype is a focal infiltrate.

As a broad generality, a condition that is radiographically severe is easier to diagnose than a milder version, because the findings tend to be more characteristic. For example, mild RDS is more easily confused with retained fetal lung fluid or PALM than is radiographically severe RDS. However, this situation is by no means invariable; for example, some infants with very severe meconium aspiration syndrome have chest radiographs that suggest RDS.

The following subsections discuss the radiographic findings in the major medical disorders that cause respiratory distress in newborn infants.

TRANSIENT TACHYPNEA OF THE NEWBORN

The typical findings on chest radiographs of infants with TTN form a pattern of diffusely increased nonvascular markings that tend to extend from the hili in a radiating fashion.[47,81,96] The excessive markings appear to be largely interstitial rather than alveolar, with an increased number and density of line shadows. Lines that may represent or be analogous to Kerley's A lines are seen; Kerley's B lines are much less common and when seen are preferentially in the retrocardiac region on the lateral view rather than at the costophrenic angles on the AP view (Fig. 2–7).

Small to moderate pleural effusions are usually noted as "companion shadows" to the inner ribs near or at the costophrenic angles and in the apices. These are thought to represent pleural fluid because they tend to disappear on subsequent films; true costal companion shadows are seldom, if ever, seen in newborn infants (Fig. 2–8).

Hyperinflation that is mild to occasionally marked usually accompanies TTN. This is best appreciated by noting the configuration of the posterior hemidiaphragms on the lateral view, which generally shows flattening instead of the normal cephalic curvature. On the AP view, hyperinflation is more difficult to evaluate but may be diagnosed when the dome of the right hemidiaphragm is below the ninth posterior intercostal space.[25] Adventitious hyperinflation (and hypoinflation) is common in infants who are filmed while crying.

These chest abnormalities are thought to represent retained fetal lung fluid, or so-called wet lung. Of course, all newborns have excessive lung fluid at birth, and it is difficult to say why some infants respond with tachypnea and respiratory distress whereas others do not. It appears that chest

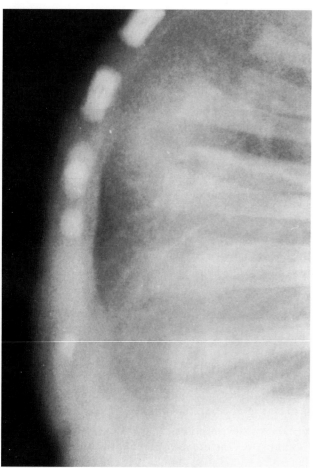

Figure 2–7
Retained lung fluid. Increased fluid in the lymphatics is best seen on the lateral view in the anterior clear space (i.e., the space between the sternum and the ribs).

radiographs are not predictive in this regard; the extent and apparent severity of the radiographic abnormalities do not correlate closely with the degree of clinical abnormality (SvW Hilton, unpublished data) or even with the clinical diagnosis.[53] Furthermore, it is a common experience to obtain an AP chest film to exclude clavicular fracture in a nontachypneic infant and to see changes that resemble "severe" retained fetal lung fluid. The radiographic diagnosis of retained fetal lung fluid or simply "wet lung" is preferable to that of TTN, because the film does not reveal the tachypnea, which may be absent (Fig. 2–9).

In the immediate and early hours after delivery, the majority of fetal lung fluid is alveolar rather than interstitial and may produce on film a reticulonodular pattern that suggests another disease, particularly RDS or pneumonia. The distinction may be made clinically by excluding sepsis and by performing surfactant analysis to exclude RDS and may be suggested radiographically by evaluating the level of inflation; RDS, a disease of diffuse atelectasis, is not

associated with hyperinflation, at least in the absence of assisted ventilation. Thus, an RDS pattern in the early hours of life, if accompanied by flat hemidiaphragms, usually reflects retained fetal lung fluid or sometimes pneumonia, but not RDS.

The radiographic hallmark of TTN is progressive clearing with sequential films,[47,81,96] reflecting removal of the excessive lung fluid out of the trachea and through absorption and thence renal excretion. Complete clearing to radiographic normalcy is common within 24 hours and nearly invariable by 72 hours. Unfortunately, this hallmark is not especially useful in the prospective sense. If there is progressive clearing, the abnormalities seen initially were probably those of excessive lung fluid. If there is not progressive clearing or if the abnormalities get worse, then the disorder is not TTN but something else, usually neonatal sepsis with pulmonary involvement or congenital heart disease.

Sometimes one cannot be certain of the diagnosis even with progressive clearing, particularly in infants in whom sepsis was clinically suspected and were treated with antibiotics. In such infants the initial abnormalities represented retained lung fluid or neonatal pneumonia that was successfully treated. Thus, the radiographic diagnostic process can be frustrating.

Occasional infants with TTN develop persisting pulmonary hypertension.[9] When this occurs, the infant may be severely ill despite having a benign underlying disease and correspondingly benign films. The chest radiographs do not identify such patients (Figs. 2–10, 2–11, and 2–12).

The radiographs of infants with TTN usually exhibit the streaky pattern of wet lung described earlier. However, this pattern may also be simulated by other disorders (see Table 2–1). Neonatal pneumonia may exactly resemble TTN, as can mild cases of meconium aspiration syndrome. The clinical setting can usually distinguish cases of meconium aspiration syndrome, but pneumonia can be both clinically and radiographically occult. The usual practice is to treat the infant empirically with antibiotics when sepsis is a possibility.

MECONIUM ASPIRATION SYNDROME

Meconium aspiration syndrome usually produces a distinct pattern of patches of abnormal density that are distributed fairly homogeneously throughout both lungs.[102] There is almost always hyperinflation, which is often marked, especially in more severe cases. Significant pleural effusions are also common. Generally speaking, the more consolidated the patches and the more opaque the lungs, the more severe the disease and the more ill the infant, although this finding is not invariable. Clearance of the parenchymal abnormalities tends to be slower with radiographically more severe disease, although for unknown reasons "severe" infiltrates may clear

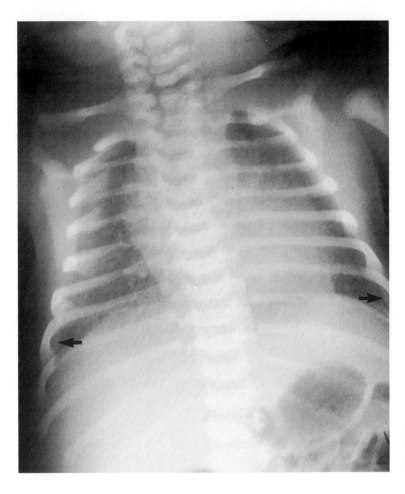

Figure 2–8
Retained lung fluid. Note the increased fluid in all compartments of the thorax: intrapleural *(arrows)*, intravascular, and intralymphatic.

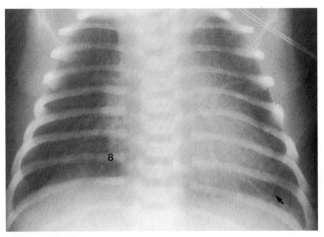

Figure 2–9
Radiographically mild retained fetal lung fluid. Only a few scattered nonvascular markings and mild hyperinflation are seen. Note the skin fold *(arrow)* and the posterior right eighth rib (8).

markedly within a day, probably owing to varying amounts of retained fetal lung fluid (Fig. 2–13).

The presence of meconium-stained amniotic fluid at delivery does not mean that there has been significant aspiration. Chest films of infants without meconium below the cords at laryngoscopy may be normal or reveal only retained fetal lung fluid. In infants with copious meconium below the cords, the radiographic and clinical abnormalities usually are both relatively severe.

In infants who require extensive "bagging" or mechanical ventilation, air leaks such as pneumothorax and pneumomediastinum are common; however, these may also occur spontaneously. Suspicious radiolucencies should be carefully scrutinized, as air leaks can substantially worsen the clinical course of an affected infant.

Probably the worst complication of meconium aspiration syndrome is PPHN, which unfortunately is not radiographically apparent. PPHN may require substantial oxygenation and assisted ventilation with high pressures; some neonates require extracorporeal membrane oxygenation in centers where this is available (Figs. 2–14, 2–15, and 2–16).

In infants with meconium aspiration syndrome and other causes of PPHN who are subjected to extremely rigorous

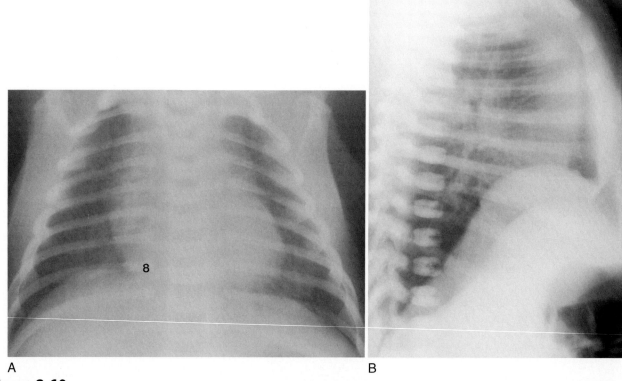

A   B

Figure 2–10
Retained fetal lung fluid. *A,* The AP projection shows a vague reticulonodular pattern but does not suggest the marked hyperinflation revealed by the inverted posterior hemidiaphragms seen on the lateral projection *(B).* The eighth posterior rib is marked (8) on *A.* Inferior beam angulation may project the dome of the right hemidiaphragm higher than when the beam is directed perpendicular to the diaphragmatic dome. The cross-table lateral view provides the most accurate depiction of pulmonary inflation.

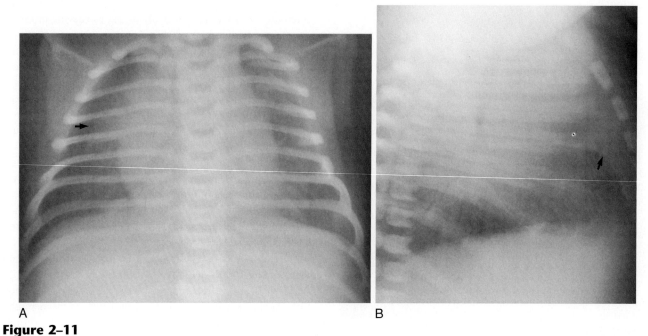

A   B

Figure 2–11
Retained fetal lung fluid simulating respiratory distress syndrome (RDS). The reticulonodular pattern on the AP projection *(A)* raises the question of RDS, but the lateral projection *(B)* shows flattened hemidiaphragms (hyperinflation) that are not suggestive of RDS, which is an atelectatic process. Note the right lobe of the thymus on both the frontal and lateral projections *(arrows).*

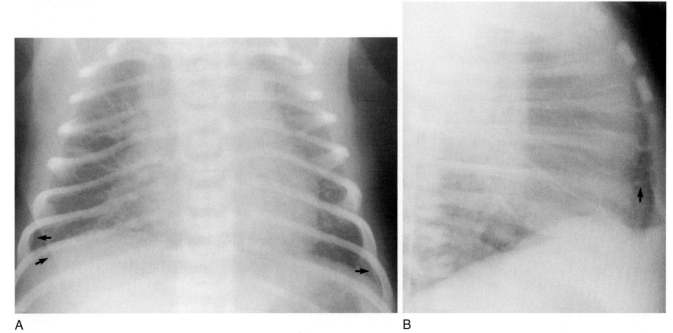

A   B

Figure 2–12
Retained fetal lung fluid showing diffuse, streaky nonvascular markings throughout both lungs *(A)*. Note the bilateral effusions *(horizontal arrows)* and a right skin fold *(slanted arrow)*. On the lateral projection *(B)*, lines just posterior to the sternum may be Kerley's B lines *(arrow)*.

assisted ventilation, a pattern of diffuse parenchymal opacity sometimes develops over several days. The radiographic findings are suggestive of RDS, with a granular, "ground-glass" appearance and air bronchograms. It is plausible that this represents adult RDS, encountered in other settings among adults and older children.[44,73] This diagnosis has been substantiated by histologic examination of the lungs in a few infants at my institution. In addition, these infants can develop chronic changes that clinically and radiographically suggest BPD.

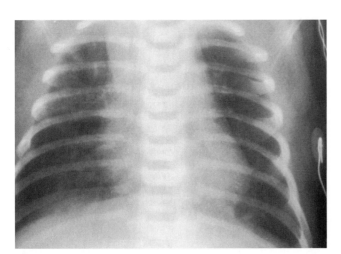

Figure 2–13
Meconium aspiration syndrome. Patchy densities are seen throughout both lungs, with some asymmetry of distribution. This radiographic picture might also be seen with neonatal pneumonia.

Aspiration of materials other than meconium is also associated with some degree of illness. The aspiration of clear amniotic fluid has not been scientifically documented, because pathologic proof is rarely available. This so-called *drowned newborn syndrome*[97] radiographically suggests severe retained fetal lung fluid; unlike infants with retained fetal lung fluid, however, spontaneous air leaks such as pneumothorax and pneumomediastinum are common. Aspiration of maternal blood may also produce a radiographic picture suggesting severe retained fetal lung fluid.

NEONATAL PNEUMONIA

One of the most common reasons chest radiography is requested in newborn infants with and without respiratory distress is to "rule out sepsis." Of course, sepsis, implying viable microorganisms in the blood or cerebrospinal fluid, is not discernible radiographically; what is meant is "rule out pneumonia," because neonatal pneumonia often causes or accompanies sepsis.

There are four important chest radiographic patterns seen in neonatal pneumonia:

1. A normal chest, which may occur in a septic infant in whom pneumonia has not become radiographically manifest.
2. The presence of focal or multiple infiltrates, which may be lobar, segmental, or nondescript in location. The presence of a focal infiltrate or infiltrates is the

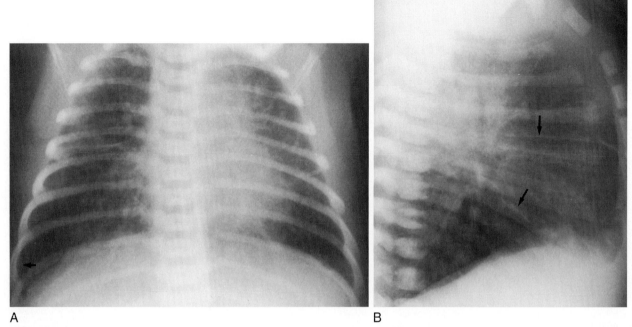

A   B

Figure 2–14
Meconium aspiration syndrome. *A,* Patchy abnormal densities are scattered throughout both lungs. An effusion is present on the right *(arrow). B,* The minor and major fissures are thickened (*upper* and *lower arrows,* respectively).

easiest neonatal pneumonia pattern to diagnose, because it looks like what it is.

3. A more common appearance of neonatal pneumonia mimics retained fetal lung fluid, with streaky, radiating densities. The only difference is that the abnormalities do not resolve; they either stay the same or, more commonly, worsen. Prospective radiographic diagnosis of this appearance of neonatal pneumonia is virtually impossible but can be

suggested if moderately severe changes of retained lung fluid are seen in a severely ill neonate. Cardiomegaly is sometimes present, and clinical as well as radiographic confusion with congenital heart disease may arise. Generally, the more pleural fluid present, the higher the likelihood that the diagnosis is pneumonia rather than simple retained lung fluid, but this clinical impression has not been studied (Figs. 2–17, 2–18).

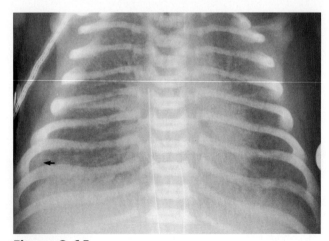

Figure 2–15
Severe meconium aspiration syndrome. The patchy densities are nearly confluent, and the radiograph almost suggests RDS. A large right pleural effusion is present in the costophrenic angle *(arrow).*

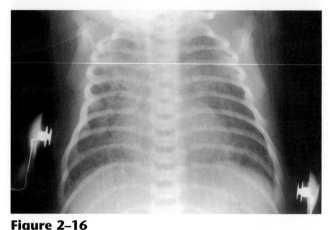

Figure 2–16
Meconium aspiration syndrome. Nine-day old infant with severe meconium aspiration syndrome demonstrates marked hyperinflation and bilaterally symmetric densities.

5

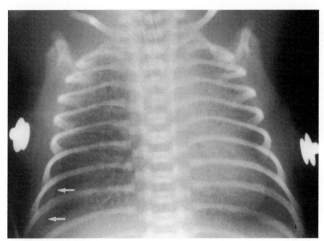

Figure 2–17
Pleural effusion. Note the large effusion *(white arrows)* in this infant with group B streptococcal sepsis. The amount of pleural fluid increases with time in pneumonia and decreases when caused by retained lung fluid or meconium aspiration.

4. A less common but radiographically treacherous manifestation of neonatal pneumonia is a diffuse, ground-glass infiltrate with air bronchograms that resembles RDS. The most common condition that presents in this manner is group B streptococcal pneumonia[1]; *Haemophilus influenzae* pneumonia is another. Clues to the correct diagnosis are (1) the unlikely presence of RDS in a term newborn; (2) pulmonary hyperinflation (underaeration is expected with RDS); and (3) the

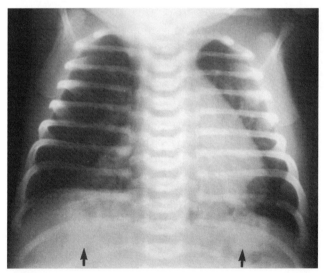

Figure 2–18
Neonatal pneumonia. The pattern is similar to that seen in older children and adults. In this neonate, the patchy densities are non-segmental. Note that foci of increased density are easily identified in the lower lobes overlying the diaphragm *(arrows)*.

presence of pleural effusions (uncommon with uncomplicated RDS). RDS and neonatal pneumonia occasionally do coexist, but the neonate is invariably premature in this setting; the presence of pleural fluid is the best radiographic clue to the coexistence of both RDS and sepsis[42] (Fig. 2–19).

Rarely, neonatal pneumonias present with a pattern of patchy infiltrates that suggests meconium aspiration syndrome. This appearance does not seem to be bacteriologically specific. A clinical history of meconium-stained amniotic fluid helps in the differential diagnosis. Regardless of the diagnosis, antibiotics are administered.

RESPIRATORY DISTRESS SYNDROME

RDS presents radiographically with a triad of findings[99]: a diffuse, homogeneous "infiltrate" with a granular, ground-glass appearance; abnormal air bronchograms; and under-aeration. Of these, underaeration is the least useful, because by the time of their first radiograph, many affected infants are already being treated briskly with assisted ventilation, and the level of the hemidiaphragms in this setting reflects the ventilator pressure as much as the intrinsic state of the lungs.

The pulmonary abnormalities are usually globally and homogeneously distributed. If there is marked asymmetry, then pneumonia, focal pulmonary hemorrhage, or ectopic air, either alone or in combination with RDS, should be suspected. Observations that RDS is worse in the lower lobes (and that differential clearing occurs from upper to lower lobes and from peripheral to central) probably reflect the physical thickness of the lungs in these regions (Fig. 2–20).

In most infants, distinctive changes of RDS are present on the initial film. In a few infants, however, the initial radiograph may be normal, and typical changes appear 1 or more hours later. It is speculated that some surfactant is present at delivery, but its production rate does not keep up with the rate of surfactant degradation.

The extent of radiographically apparent RDS on early films correlates closely with the clinical condition of the infant[45] and the pathologic severity in infants who die.[87] Indeed, radiographic scoring systems have been devised in an attempt to quantify severity; generally, the scores reflect more severe disease with increasing radiopacity and more prominent air bronchograms.[27] Such scoring systems are somewhat useful in statistical analyses and in rough prognostic estimates for individual patients (Fig. 2–21).

The usual radiographic course of uncomplicated and untreated RDS is either no change or a variable degree of worsening over the first 1 or 2 days, followed by gradual clearing over days to weeks.[93] This course is relatively seldom seen for two reasons. First, complications and associated conditions such as shunting through a PDA and air leaks are common; these complications obscure the radiographic

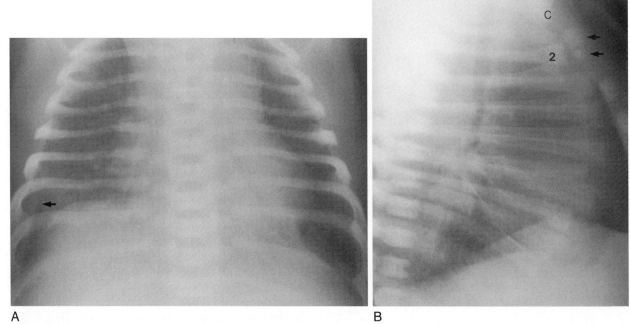

A   B

Figure 2–19
Neonatal pneumonia. Diffuse pneumonia with sepsis. The pattern of streaky nonvascular markings suggests retained fetal lung fluid; moderate pleural effusions are seen in the costophrenic angles on the AP projection *(A)*. Pleural fluid is extending into the major fissure *(arrow)*. *B,* The lateral view reveals mild hyperinflation. Note the double manubrial ossification center *(arrows)*. The manubrium is at the level of the second rib (2) and the clavicle (C).

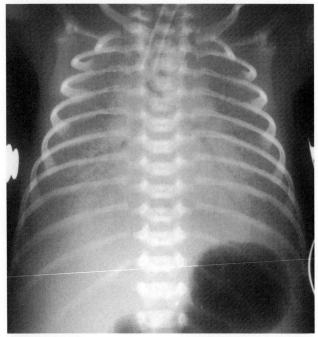

Figure 2–20
Respiratory distress syndrome (RDS). Typical findings of severe respiratory distress syndrome are seen, including hypoaeration despite mechanically assisted ventilation, air bronchograms beyond the middle third of the chest, and a reticulogranular pattern. This "classic" pattern is becoming something of a rarity, because of application of assisted ventilation and exogenous surfactant before the initial film is exposed.

visualization of the progression of RDS. Second, RDS is commonly treated with endotracheal administration of exogenous surfactant.[46,60] This treatment often produces radiographic clearing that may be marked[101]; the clearing may be transient or permanent, and multiple doses of surfactant may be administered (Figs. 2–22, 2–23). Occasionally this abrupt clearing is focal and restricted to one or more lobes of the lungs because of inadvertent focal administration of surfactant[27]; asymmetrical clearing following surfactant administration does not appear to affect clinical outcome[78] (Fig. 2–24).

Discussion of the long-term course of infants with RDS is beyond the scope of this chapter, and the pulmonary complications that occur after the first few days of life are not described. These complications include BPD, focal atelectasis from mucus plugs, superimposed infections, subglottic stenosis or cysts from endotracheal intubation, granuloma formation in the bronchus intermedius, and persisting interstitial gas. However, several pulmonary complications do occur in the first few days of life in patients with RDS, and these are discussed in the following subsection.

Complications and Associations of RDS

Probably the most important complication is left-to-right shunting through a PDA.[43] Shunting through the PDA may be present initially, but more often it becomes manifest

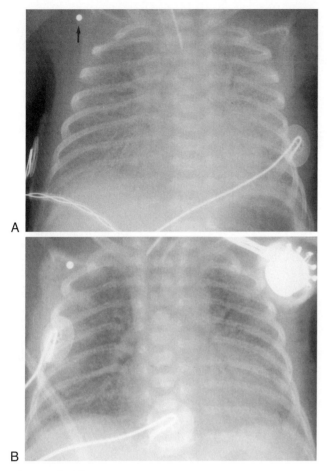

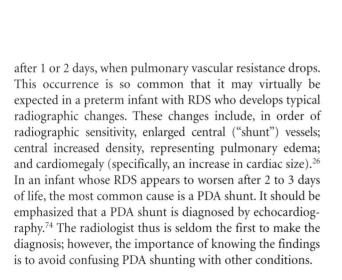

Figure 2–21

RDS. The infant is intubated, and the lungs show a dense reticulo-nodular pattern with air bronchograms *(A)*. Note the metallic ball taped to the right axilla *(arrow)*. This marker indicates that the infant is the second of twins. The markers are used in mammography to indicate masses and in adult chest radiography as nipple markers. *B,* The lung densities are only slightly clearer after surfactant therapy; retreatment was required.

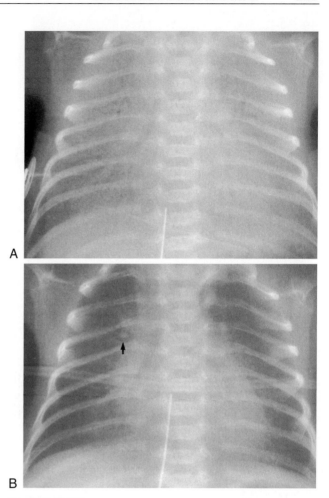

Figure 2–22

RDS with patent ductus arteriosus (PDA). *A* shows typical findings of RDS, which partially clear after surfactant therapy *(B)*. However, on *B,* large vessels are seen in the hilar regions *(arrow)*, suggesting left-to-right shunting.

after 1 or 2 days, when pulmonary vascular resistance drops. This occurrence is so common that it may virtually be expected in a preterm infant with RDS who develops typical radiographic changes. These changes include, in order of radiographic sensitivity, enlarged central ("shunt") vessels; central increased density, representing pulmonary edema; and cardiomegaly (specifically, an increase in cardiac size).[26] In an infant whose RDS appears to worsen after 2 to 3 days of life, the most common cause is a PDA shunt. It should be emphasized that a PDA shunt is diagnosed by echocardiography.[74] The radiologist thus is seldom the first to make the diagnosis; however, the importance of knowing the findings is to avoid confusing PDA shunting with other conditions.

The occurrence of a so-called "whiteout" appearance is common in patients with RDS; the lungs become much more radiopaque than on previous films. Often this is caused by the PDA shunting, but there are other causes as well; the most important of these are listed in Table 2–2.

Another common complication of RDS and its therapy is the occurrence of air leaks or collections of intrathoracic extra-alveolar gas. These can be serious and are often lethal. It is all too common to see an initial chest film that reveals severe RDS, followed by a film showing extensive bilateral pulmonary interstitial emphysema, and then to learn of the infant's death. Often in this setting, when death ensues, the emphysematous spaces are found to contain considerable

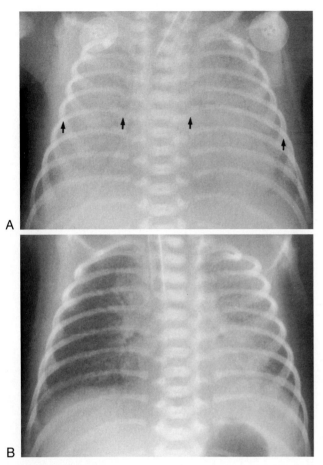

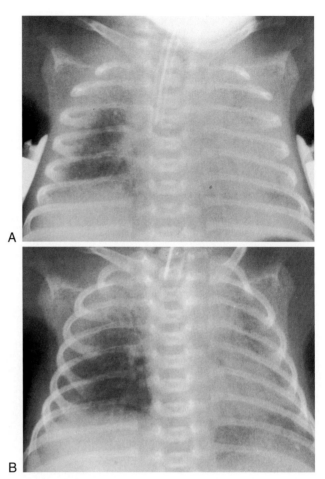

Figure 2–23
RDS. The infant is intubated, and the lungs show a dense reticulo-nodular pattern with air bronchograms *(A)*. Note how to evaluate rotation on the frontal chest: The lengths of the posterior ribs are compared from left to right *(arrows)*. Because the infant is supine, the side of the longer ribs indicates to which side the thorax is rotated. In this case, the left ribs are longer; thus this radiograph is a left posterior oblique view. Surfactant was administered, resulting in significant improvement in the density of the lung *(B)*. Note that the right lung is slightly better aerated than the left. Uneven distribution of clearing is common.

Figure 2–24
Focal deposition of exogenous surfactant. Post-treatment radiographs of an infant 5 hours *(A)* and 14 hours *(B)* after birth showing moderately severe RDS except in the right lower and middle lobes; surfactant was administered through the malpositioned endotracheal tube *(A)*. (From Edwards DK, Hilton SvW, Merritt TA, et al. Respiratory distress syndrome treated with human surfactant: radiographic findings. Radiology 157:329–334, 1985.)

blood. In survivors of air leaks, as noted earlier, the subsequent development of BPD is common.[65] Air leaks are discussed in more detail in the next chapter.

BPD is the most common chronic pulmonary sequel of prematurity and RDS. A full discussion of this complex disorder is beyond the scope of this chapter. As BPD was initially described, the chest radiograph revealed a sequence of more or less stereotyped appearances constituting four stages of disease[68]; this sequence is rarely observed with contemporary treatment techniques.[22] Changes representing BPD are histologically present in the first few days of life in some infants with RDS[7]; however, diagnosing

BPD radiographically is risky before about 2 weeks of age, at which time abnormalities that prove long-lived may appear.

PREMATURE INFANTS WITH ACCELERATED LUNG MATURITY

So-called PALM infants, who are quite small as a result of their prematurity, are seemingly spared RDS because intrauterine stress or maternal steroid administration has accelerated the development of their pulmonary

TABLE 2-2 CAUSES OF INCREASED PARENCHYMAL DENSITY IN INFANTS WITH RESPIRATORY DISTRESS SYNDROME ("WHITEOUT")

Worsening RDS (first 1 to 2 days only)
"Rebound" after surfactant administration
Left-to-right shunting through a patent ductus arteriosus
Fluid overload
"Weaning effect" from endotracheal tube removal or decreased ventilator pressure
Pulmonary hemorrhage
Superimposed pneumonia
Massive aspiration
Stage II bronchopulmonary dysplasia
Extracorporeal membrane oxygenation therapy
(Expiratory examination)*
(Underpenetrated examination)*

*Reflective of artifact rather than patient pathologic condition.

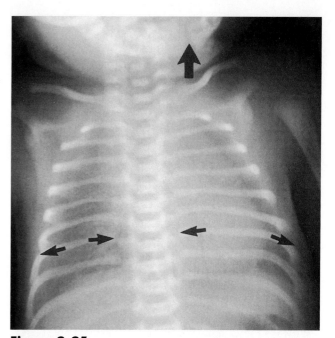

Figure 2–25
Premature infant with accelerated lung maturity (PALM). Note the hyperinflation and suggestion of retained fetal lung fluid. The infant's arms were not used to immobilize the head in the midline. The head is rotated to the left *(large arrow)*, as is the chest, as indicated by the apparent length of the posterior ribs *(arrows)*.

surfactant system.[28] The presence of sufficient surfactant prevents the widespread alveolar collapse and atelectasis characteristic of RDS. Analysis of pulmonary effluent reveals mature surfactant phospholipids.

When one interprets the chest films of small preterm infants, it is helpful to recall that "all that's premature is not RDS." Many PALM infants are erroneously diagnosed with RDS because they are quite small and their lungs are not normal. This diagnosis can be misleading, suggesting a probable course and a prognosis that are more grim than the actuality. Unfortunately, inappropriate treatment may be administered. PALM infants may require only minimal ventilation for apnea but not the aggressive ventilator therapy appropriate for infants with RDS. PALM infants are prone to other complications of prematurity, such as intracranial hemorrhage, shunting through a PDA, and the development of necrotizing enterocolitis. These complications should be carefully anticipated, because they can be life threatening (Fig. 2–25).

The distinction between a PALM infant and an infant with RDS can be crucial for several reasons. An infant with RDS often requires transfer to a tertiary care center, whereas a PALM infant may not. Treating a PALM infant with exogenous surfactant subjects the infant to an invasive, costly, and essentially needless procedure. It is possible that the statistics reported in some studies of surfactant therapy have been biased by the assumption that PALM infants have RDS. Fortunately for the radiologist, biochemical analysis of pulmonary effluent probably provides a more reliable diagnosis than does the chest film. Furthermore, neonatologists usually quickly recognize that an individual infant has few or no ventilatory requirements. However, when biochemical

analysis and highly trained neonatologists are unavailable or when the clinical situation is equivocal, the radiologist's ability to differentiate RDS from PALM may be critical to the infant's welfare.

One hallmark of a PALM infant is small size. By allowing for the fact that there is considerable variation and assuming a film-focal spot distance of 102 cm, a thoracic spine length of 70 mm represents a weight of about 1500 g. In infants smaller than this, the PALM diagnosis may be appropriate. Another hallmark is a small thymic silhouette[13,37]; infants with RDS tend to have wide (i.e., normal) thymic shadows, whereas in PALM infants these are typically small, presumably reflecting intrauterine stress or steroid therapy.

The lungs of PALM infants may be entirely normal, but more commonly they reveal a wet lung pattern of increased nonvascular markings. The lungs of some PALM infants reveal a faint pattern of fine granularity that might suggest RDS, except that the level of inflation is typically normal and there is a notable absence of abnormal air bronchograms.[28] Small pleural effusions are sometimes seen, without apparent prognostic import (Fig. 2–26).

Like infants with RDS, PALM infants often develop left-to-right shunting through a PDA. The radiographic abnormalities of PDA shunting can usually be recognized as such, although sometimes the associated pulmonary edema can be confused with late-onset RDS. As with RDS, the echocardiogram is crucial in this setting.

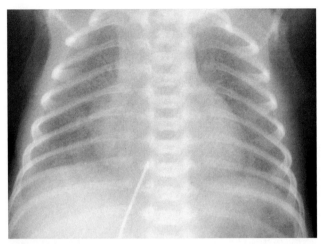

Figure 2–26
PALM. The lungs show a slightly granular pattern diffusely, without significant air bronchograms. The thymus is small, and mild cardiomegaly is present.

PERSISTING PULMONARY HYPERTENSION OF THE NEWBORN

It might be easiest (although somewhat unsatisfying) for both the author and reader to limit this section to the words, "There are no useful radiographic findings of PPHN." This statement combines the virtues of brevity and validity. In patients with right-to-left shunting at the PDA and the foramen ovale, one might expect the radiograph to reveal diminished pulmonary blood flow, but it does not. Possibly this is because diminished blood flow is more difficult to appreciate than the converse and because pulmonary vascularity is often obscured by lung disease.

The condition of PPHN occurs in two forms. The first, called *primary PPHN*, occurs in the absence of known lung disease. The more common form, known as *secondary PPHN*, occurs in the presence of and presumably in response to a variety of pulmonary diseases.[33] These include meconium aspiration syndrome, neonatal pneumonia, and, less commonly, RDS and TTN. A closely related but probably different mechanism causes right-to-left shunting in infants with pulmonary hypoplasia resulting from oligohydramnios and from diaphragmatic hernia.

The radiologist's role in infants with PPHN is limited primarily to excluding other causes of respiratory insufficiency, such as "air block" from large air leaks. In infants with secondary PPHN, the radiologist also assists in diagnosing the character of the underlying lung disease and in monitoring the state of the heart and lungs during subsequent therapy. In infants with primary PPHN, the radiologist may suggest the diagnosis after noting a benign-appearing chest radiograph in an infant who is extremely ill. Usually, however, the diagnosis is made clinically, and the most important imaging modality is the echocardiogram.

REFERENCES

1. Ablow RC, Gross I, Effmann EL, et al. The radiographic features of early onset group B streptococcal neonatal sepsis. Radiology 124:771–777, 1977.
2. Alford BA, McIlhenny J. An approach to the asymmetric neonatal chest radiograph. Radiol Clin North Am 37:1079–1092, 1999.
3. Anderson GS, Green CA, Neligan GA, et al. Congenital bacterial pneumonia. Lancet 2:585–587, 1962.
4. Avery ME, Gatewood OB, Brumley G. Transient tachypnea of the newborn. Possible delayed resorption of fluid at birth. Am J Dis Child 111:380–385, 1966.
5. Bashour BN, Balfe JW. Urinary tract anomalies in neonates with spontaneous pneumothorax and/or pneumomediastinum. Pediatrics 59:1048–1049, 1977.
6. Benirschke K. Routes and types of infection in the fetus and newborn. Am J Dis Child 99:714–721, 1960.
7. Bonikos DS, Bensch KG, Northway WH Jr, Edwards DK. Bronchopulmonary dysplasia: The pulmonary pathologic sequel of necrotizing bronchiolitis and pulmonary fibrosis. Hum Pathol 7: 643–666, 1976.
8. Boyd PA, Keeling JW. Fetal hydrops. J Med Genet 29:91–97, 1992.
9. Bucciarelli RL, Egan EA, Gessner IH, Eitzman DV. Persistence of fetal cardiopulmonary circulation: One manifestation of transient tachypnea of the newborn. Pediatrics 58:192–197, 1976.
10. Bustos R, Kulovich MV, Gluck L, et al. Significance of phosphatidylglycerol in amniotic fluid in complicated pregnancies. Am J Obstet Gynecol 133:899–903, 1979.
11. Caffey J, Ross S. Mongolism (mongoloid deficiency) during early infancy: Some newly recognized diagnostic changes in the pelvic bones. Pediatrics 17:642–651, 1956.
12. Capitanio MA, Kirkpatrick JA Jr. Roentgen examination in the evaluation of the newborn infant with respiratory distress. J Pediatr 75:896–907, 1969.
13. Chen CM, Yu KY, Lin HC, et al. Thymus size and its relationship to perinatal events. Acta Paediatr 89:975–978, 2000.
14. Chernick V, Reed MH. Pneumothorax and chylothorax in the neonatal period. J Pediatr 76:624–632, 1970.
15. Cleveland RH. A radiologic update on medical diseases of the newborn chest. Pediatr Radiol 25:631–637, 1995.
16. Cohen RS, Smith DW, Stevenson DK, et al. Lateral decubitus position as therapy for persistent focal pulmonary interstitial emphysema in neonates: A preliminary report. J Pediatr 104:441–443, 1984.
17. Cremin BJ, Fisher RM. The lesions of congenital syphilis. Br J Radiol 43:333–341, 1970.
18. Cumming WA. Neonatal skeletal fractures: Birth trauma or child abuse? J Can Assoc Radiol 30:30–33, 1979.
19. Demissie K, Marcella SW, Breckenridge MB, Rhoads GG. Maternal asthma and transient tachypnea of the newborn. Pediatrics 102:84–90, 1998.
20. Desmond MM, More J, Lindley JE, Brown CA. Meconium staining of the amniotic fluid: A marker of fetal hypoxia. Obstet Gynecol 9:91–103, 1957.
21. Donn SM, Kuhns LR. Mechanism of endotracheal tube movement with change of head position in the neonate. Pediatr Radiol 9:37–40, 1980.
22. Edwards DK. Radiographic aspects of bronchopulmonary dysplasia. J Pediatr 95:823–829, 1979.
23. Edwards DK, Berry CC, Hilton SvW. Trisomy 21 in newborn infants: Chest radiographic diagnosis. Radiology 167:317–318, 1988.
24. Edwards DK, Higgins CB. Radiology of neonatal heart disease. Radiol Clin North Am 18:369–385, 1980.
25. Edwards DK, Higgins CB, Gilpin EA. The cardiothoracic ratio in newborn infants. AJR Am J Roentgenol 136:907–913, 1981.
26. Edwards DK, Higgins CB, Merritt TA, et al. Radiographic and echocardiographic evaluation of newborns treated with indomethacin for patent ductus arteriosus. AJR Am J Roentgenol 131:1009–1013, 1978.

27. Edwards DK, Hilton SvW, Merritt TA, et al. Respiratory distress syndrome treated with human surfactant: Radiographic findings. Radiology 157:329–334, 1985.

28. Edwards DK, Jacob J, Gluck L. The immature lung: Radiographic appearance, course, and complications. AJR Am J Roentgenol 135:659–666, 1980.

29. Edwards DK III. Skeletal growth lines seen on radiographs of newborn infants: Prevalence and possible association with obstetrical abnormalities. AJR Am J Roentgenol 161:141–145, 1993.

30. Faulkner K, Barry JL, Smalley P. Radiation dose to neonates on a special care baby unit. Br J Radiol 62:230–233, 1989.

31. Forde WJ, Finby N. Roentgenographic features of asplenia, a teratologic syndrome of visceral symmetry. AJR Am J Roentgenol 86:523–533, 1961.

32. Fox WW, Duara S. Persistent pulmonary hypertension in the neonate: Diagnosis and management. J Pediatr 103:505–514, 1983.

33. Fox WF, Gewitz MH, Dinwiddie R, et al. Pulmonary hypertension in the perinatal aspiration syndromes. Pediatrics 59:205–211, 1977.

34. Franken EA Jr, Yu P, Smith WL, et al. Initial chest radiography in the neonatal intensive care unit: Value of the lateral view. AJR Am J Roentgenol 133:43–45, 1979.

35. Gamsu HR, Mullinger BM, Donnai P, Dash CH. Antenatal administration of betamethasone to prevent respiratory distress syndrome in preterm infants: Report of a UK multicentre trial. Br J Obstet Gynaecol 96:401–410, 1989.

36. Gersony WM, Duc GV, Sinclair JC. "PFC" syndrome (persistence of the fetal circulation) [Abstract]. Circulation 39:87, 1969.

37. Gewolb IH, Lebowitz RL, Taeusch HW Jr. Thymus size and its relationship to the respiratory distress syndrome. J Pediatr 95:108–111, 1979.

38. Harker LC, Merritt TA, Edwards DK III. Improving the prediction of surfactant deficiency in very low-birthweight infants with respiratory distress. J Perinatol 12:129–133, 1992.

39. Harris MC, Moskowitz WB, Engle WD, et al. Group B streptococcal septicemia and delayed-onset diaphragmatic hernia. Am J Dis Child 135:723–725, 1981.

40. Hillman K. Intrathoracic pressure fluctuations and periventricular haemorrhage in the newborn. Aust Paediatr J 23:343–346, 1987.

41. Hubbell C, Dominguez R, Kohl S. Neonatal herpes simplex pneumonitis. Rev Infect Dis 10:431–438, 1988.

42. Jacob J, Edwards D, Gluck L. Early-onset sepsis and pneumonia observed as respiratory distress syndrome. Assessment of lung maturity. Am J Dis Child 134:766–768, 1980.

43. Jacob J, Gluck L, DiSessa T, et al. The contribution of PDA in the neonate with severe RDS. J Pediatr 96:79–87, 1980.

44. Katz R. Adult respiratory distress syndrome in children. Clin Chest Med 8:635–639, 1987.

45. Kero PO, Makinen EO. Comparison between clinical and radiological classifications of infants with the respiratory distress syndrome (RDS). Eur J Pediatr 130:271–278, 1979.

46. Konishi M, Fujiwara T, Naito T, et al. Surfactant replacement therapy in neonatal respiratory distress syndrome. A multi-centre, randomized clinical trial: Comparison of high- versus low-dose of surfactant TA. Eur J Pediatr 147:20–25, 1988.

47. Kuhn JP, Fletcher BD, DeLemos RA. Roentgen findings in transient tachypnea of the newborn. Radiology 92:751–757, 1969.

48. Kuhns LR, Holt JF. Measurement of thoracic spine length on chest radiographs of newborn infants. Radiology 116:395–397, 1975.

49. Kuhns LR, Sherman MP, Poznanski AK, Holt JF. Humeral-head and coracoid ossification in the newborn. Radiology 107:145–149, 1973.

50. Kuhns LR, Sherman MP, Poznanski AK. Determination of neonatal maturation on the chest radiograph. Radiology 102:597–603, 1972.

51. Kulovich MV, Hallman MB, Gluck L. The lung profile. I. Normal pregnancy. Am J Obstet Gynecol 135:57–63, 1979.

52. Kumar A, Bhat BV. Epidemiology of respiratory distress of newborns. Indian J Pediatr 63:93–98, 1996.

53. Kurl S, Heinonen KM, Kiekara O. The first chest radiograph in neonates exhibiting respiratory distress at birth. Clin Pediatr (Phila) 36:285–289, 1997.

54. Lamm CI, Norton KI, Murphy RJC, et al. Congenital rickets associated with magnesium sulfate infusion for tocolysis. J Pediatr 113:1078–1082, 1988.

55. Leonidas JC, Fellows RA, Hall RT, et al. Value of chest radiography in the diagnosis of Potter's syndrome at birth. AJR Am J Roentgenol 123:716–723, 1975.

56. Levin DL, Weinberg AG, Perkin RM. Pulmonary microthrombi syndrome in newborn infants with unresponsive persistent pulmonary hypertension. J Pediatr 102:299–303, 1983.

57. Levine EM, Ghai V, Barton JJ, Strom CM. Mode of delivery and risk of respiratory diseases in newborns. Obstet Gynecol 97:439–442, 2001.

58. Madan E, Meyer MP, Amortegui A. Chorioamnionitis: A study of organisms isolated in perinatal autopsies. Ann Clin Lab Sci 18:39–45, 1988.

59. McCarten KM, Rosenberg HK, Borden S, Mandell GA. Delayed appearance of right diaphragmatic hernia associated with group B streptococcal infection in newborns. Radiology 139:385–389, 1981.

60. Merritt TA, Hallman M, Bloom BT, et al. Prophylactic treatment of very premature infants with human surfactant. N Engl J Med 315:785–790, 1986.

61. Merten DF, Goetzman BW, Wennberg RP. Persistent fetal circulation: An evolving clinical and radiographic concept of pulmonary hypertension of the newborn. Pediatr Radiol 6:74–80, 1977.

62. Miller KE, Edwards DK, Hilton S, et al. Acquired lobar emphysema in premature infants with bronchopulmonary dysplasia: An iatrogenic disease? Radiology 138:589–592, 1981.

63. Milner AD, Saunders RA, Hopkin IE. Effects of delivery by caesarean section on lung mechanics and lung volume in the human neonate. Arch Dis Child 53:545–548, 1978.

64. Moseley JE, Wolf VS, Gottlieb MI. The trisomy 17–18 syndrome. AJR Am J Roentgenol 89:905–913, 1963.

65. Moylan FMB, Walker AM, Kramer SS, et al. Alveolar rupture as an independent predictor of bronchopulmonary dysplasia. Crit Care Med 6:10–13, 1978.

66. Mulvey RB. The thymic "wave" sign. Radiology 81:834–838, 1963.

67. Northway WH Jr. Bronchopulmonary dysplasia: Then and now. Arch Dis Child 65:1076–1081, 1990.

68. Northway WH Jr, Rosan RC. Radiographic features of pulmonary oxygen toxicity in the newborn: Bronchopulmonary dysplasia. Radiology 91:49–58, 1968.

69. Olding L. Bacterial infection in cases of perinatal death. A morphological and bacteriological study based on 264 autopsies. Acta Paediatr Scand Suppl 171:1, 1966.

70. Peterson HO. First a radiologist. In Fischer HW, ed. The Radiologist's Second Reader. Granville, OH: Granville Medical Books, 1992, pp 155–162.

71. Roberts JD, Polaner DM, Lang P, Zapol WM. Inhaled nitric oxide in persistent pulmonary hypertension of the newborn. Lancet 340:818–819, 1992.

72. Rosen EU, Solomon A. Bone lesions in early congenital syphilis. S Afr Med J 50:135–138, 1976.

73. Royall JA, Levin DL. Adult respiratory distress syndrome in pediatric patients. 1. Clinical aspects, pathophysiology, pathology, and mechanisms of lung injury. J Pediatr 112:169–180, 1988.

74. Sahn DJ, Vaucher Y, Williams DE, et al. Echocardiographic detection of large left to right shunts and cardiomyopathies in infants and children. Am J Cardiol 38:73–79, 1976.

75. Sanchez PJ, Regan JA. Ureaplasma urealyticum colonization and chronic lung disease in low birth weight infants. Pediatr Infect Dis J 7:542–546, 1988.

76. Schaffer AJ, Markowitz M, Perlman A. Pneumonia of newborn infants. JAMA 159:663–668, 1955.

77. Schorr S, Ayalon D. Intercostal lung bulging, an early roentgen sign of emphysema in children. Radiology 75:544–551, 1960.

78. Slama M, Andre C, Huon C, Antoun H, Adamsbaum C. Radiological analysis of hyaline membrane disease after exogenous surfactant treatment. Pediatr Radiol 29:56–60, 1999.

79. Snider AR. Use and abuse of the echocardiogram. Pediatr Clin North Am 31:1345–1366, 1984.

80. Sun CC, Duara S. Fatal adenovirus pneumonia in two newborn infants, one case caused by adenovirus type 30. Pediatr Pathol 4: 247- 255, 1985.

81. Swischuk LE. Transient respiratory distress of the newborn (TRDN); a temporary disturbance of a normal phenomenon. AJR Am J Roentgenol 108:557–563, 1970.

82. Swischuk LE. Imaging of the Newborn, Infant, and Young Child. 3rd ed. Baltimore: Williams & Wilkins, 1989, pp 15, 136–139.

83. Tausend ME, Stern WZ. Thymic patterns in the newborn. AJR Am J Roentgenol 95:125–130, 1965.

84. The Neonatal Inhaled Nitric Oxide Study Group. Inhaled nitric oxide in full-term and nearly full-term infants with hypoxic respiratory failure. N Engl J Med 336:597–604, 1997.

85. Toomasian JM, Snedecor SM, Cornell RG, et al. National experience with extracorporeal membrane oxygenation for newborn respiratory failure. Data from 715 cases. ASAIO Trans 34:140–147, 1988.

86. Tucker AS, Liebman J, Bolande RP. Heterotaxy as related to congenital heart disease. Ann Radiol 9:178–184, 1966.

87. Tudor J, Young L, Wigglesworth JS, Steiner RE. The value of radiology in the idiopathic respiratory distress syndrome: A radiological and pathological correlation study. Clin Radiol 27:65–75, 1976.

88. Tyler DC, Murphy J, Cheney F. Mechanical and chemical damage to lung tissue caused by meconium aspiration. Pediatrics 62:454–459, 1978.

89. Vaughan TJ, Hawkins IF Jr, Elliott LP. Diagnosis of polysplenia syndrome. Radiology 101:511–518, 1971.

90. Waites KB, Crouse DT, Philips JB III, et al. Ureaplasmal pneumonia and sepsis associated with persistent pulmonary hypertension of the newborn. Pediatrics 83:79–85, 1989.

91. Weaver DD, Mapstone CL, Yu P. The VATER association. Am J Dis Child 140:225–229, 1986.

92. Weber AM, Philipson EH. Fetal pleural effusion: A review and meta-analysis for prognostic indicators. Obstet Gynecol 79:281–286, 1992.

93. Weller MH. The roentgenographic course and complications of hyaline membrane disease. Pediatr Clin North Am 20:381–406, 1973.

94. Wesenberg RL. The Newborn Chest. Hagerstown, MD: Harper & Row, 1973, pp 15–17, 35.

95. Wesenberg RL, Blumhagen JD. Assisted expiratory chest radiography. An effective technique for the diagnosis of foreign-body aspiration. Radiology 130:538–539, 1979.

96. Wesenberg RL, Graven SN, McCabe EB. Radiological findings in wet-lung disease. Radiology 98:69–74, 1971.

97. Wesenberg RL, Rumack CM. The drowned newborn syndrome (DNS). Presented at the 16th Annual Meeting of the Society for Pediatric Radiology, 1973.

98. Willich E, Fuhr U, Kroll W. Skeletal manifestations in Down's syndrome: Correlation between roentgenologic and cytogenetic findings. Ann Radiol 18:355–358, 1975.

99. Wohlfeld GM. Hyaline membrane disease. AJR Am J Roentgenol 93:425–427, 1965.

100. Wolf EL, Berdon WE, Baker DH, et al. Diagnosis of oligohydramnios-related pulmonary hypoplasia (Potter syndrome): Value of portable voiding cystourethrography in newborns with respiratory distress. Radiology 125:769–773, 1977.

101. Wood BP, Sinkin RA, Kendig JW, et al. Exogenous lung surfactant: Effect on radiographic appearance in premature infants. Radiology 165:11–13, 1987.

102. Yeh TF, Harris V, Srinivasan G, et al. Roentgenographic findings in infants with meconium aspiration syndrome. JAMA 242:60–63, 1979.

103. Zimmerman JE, Goodman LR, St. Andre AC, Wyman AC. Radiographic detection of mobilizable lung water: The gravitational shift test. AJR Am J Roentgenol 138:59–64, 1982.

ADDITIONAL READING

Agrawal V, David RJ, Harris VJ. Classification of acute respiratory disorders of all newborns in a tertiary care center. J Natl Med Assoc 95:585–595, 2003.

Chang EY, Menard MK, Vermillion ST, Hulsey T, Ebeling M. The association between hyaline membrane disease and preeclampsia. Am J Obstet Gynecol 191:1414–1417, 2004.

Ersch J, Fauchere JC, Bucher HU, Hebisch G, Stallmach T. The pulmonary paradox in premature infants: in-utero infected lungs do better than those with accelerated maturation. J Perinat Med. 32:84–89, 2004.

Kunduri GG. New approaches for persistent pulmonary hypertension of newborn. Clin Perinatol 31:591–611, 2004.

Ostapchuk M, Roberts DM, Haddy R. Community-acquired pneumonia in infants and children. Am Fam Physician 70:899–908, 2004.

Pierce CM: Persistent pulmonary hypertension of the newborn. Hosp Med. 65:418-421, 2004.

THE NEWBORN INFANT WITH RESPIRATORY DISTRESS FROM SURGICAL CAUSES

Outline

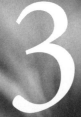

CHAPTER

3

David K. Edwards, III, MD

THE NEWBORN INFANT WITH RESPIRATORY DISTRESS FROM SURGICAL CAUSES

A
s is the case with medical conditions that cause respiratory distress in infants, surgical conditions are commonly first perceived and usually diagnosed with plain radiographs of the chest. Thus, it is useful to review the general radiographic discussion presented in the previous chapter, especially the section entitled "Radiography of Newborns with Respiratory Distress: General," pages 104–110.

MAJOR SURGICAL CONDITIONS CAUSING RESPIRATORY DISTRESS

INTRATHORACIC AIR LEAKS

Intrathoracic air leaks usually occur in the setting of mechanically assisted ventilation and thus often accompany respiratory distress syndrome (RDS), meconium aspiration syndrome, and persisting pulmonary hypertension of the newborn (PPHN). However, small air leaks are often incidentally evident on an initial chest radiograph taken for other reasons. Sometimes such spontaneous air leaks reflect pulmonary hypoplasia secondary to oligohydramnios. Very rarely, this may be the presenting symptom of an underlying genitourinary abnormality.[2] More commonly, however, genitourinary abnormalities are diagnosed by prenatal sonography.

Macklin and Macklin's[30] conventional and venerable account of the development of air leaks describes alveolar rupture with dissection of gas in the pulmonary interstitium. The air dissects along blood vessels to the hilus of the lung, with the subsequent formation of pneumomediastinum. Pneumomediastinum may then rupture into the pleural space, causing a pneumothorax. This suggests that pulmonary interstitial emphysema (PIE) is the initial lesion, with the other air leaks following in a more or less serial fashion. In practice with newborn infants, there does not seem to be any stereotyped sequence of air leaks; instead, pneumothorax, pneumomediastinum, and PIE seem to occur independently and unpredictably.

The fact remains that PIE is the most common air leak among infants treated with assisted ventilation. It has been speculated that the ectopic gas is situated in pulmonary lymphatics[26,58]; evidently the exact anatomic location of PIE is difficult to confirm pathologically. However, it is worth noting that the pulmonary lymphatics drain primarily into tracheobronchial nodes and thence into the vascular system. Central nodes distended with gas are not commonly noted in autopsies of infants with PIE, and spillage of lymphatic gas into the vascular system would be expected to produce gas embolism. Fortunately, gas embolism is a rare event, certainly much rarer than PIE, so the proposed endolymphatic location of PIE is somewhat enigmatic.

Air leaks exert their primary malignant effects simply by acting as mass lesions. They occupy space in the thorax that thus becomes unavailable for respiration, collapsing airways and alveoli and thus rendering some to many of these useless for gas exchange. The larger the air leak, the worse its clinical effects. "Tension," caused by the mass effect that shifts the diaphragm and mediastinum, is most ominous because not only does it occupy needed space, but it also compresses otherwise unaffected airways and impedes venous return to the heart, thus decreasing cardiac output. This constellation of events results in the so-called *air block*.

Air leaks are considered surgical lesions because, when focal, they can be drained with a needle or tube. This is certainly the case with pneumothorax, pneumomediastinum, and pneumopericardium. However, other loculated collections are harder to approach; these include gas in the inferior pulmonary ligament,[54] the infra-azygous pneumomediastinum,[6] and gas loculated beneath the visceral pleura.[24] PIE has been approached surgically by slicing the lung surface so that the ectopic gas reaches the relatively accessible pleural space,[27] but usually PIE is treated without surgery. Methods of treatment for unilateral PIE have included selective mainstem intubation ventilation of the normal lung[9] and use of the decubitus position, which places the affected lung inferiorly and thereby compresses the interstitial air while increasing blood flow to the affected lung.[15] With bilateral PIE, high-frequency oscillatory ventilation is sometimes useful, presumably because of its ability to reduce mean airway pressure.[4] Nonsurgical management of air leaks consists of the so-called nitrogen washout, which involves allowing the infant to breathe concentrated oxygen.[11]

The early occurrence of air leaks substantially increases the likelihood that the patient will develop bronchopulmonary dysplasia,[36] presumably because infants with air leaks tend to require more respiratory support (i.e., elevated oxygen and mechanical ventilation).

DIAPHRAGMATIC HERNIA

Large, posterior defects in the diaphragm (foramen of Bochdalek) commonly present either on prenatal sonography or, in the immediate neonatal period, with severe respiratory distress. The essential problem is pulmonary hypoplasia; during fetal life the thorax contains a variable amount of abdominal viscera, which prevents full development and expansion of the lungs. The hypoplasia is bilateral but is substantially more marked on the ipsilateral side, which is more often (in live-born infants, at least) the left side.[3] Correction requires surgery, and subsequent support may necessitate extracorporeal membrane oxygenation.[53]

The condition is visible on prenatal sonograms[12] and otherwise becomes evident at delivery if the infant has severe respiratory distress and a scaphoid abdomen. The diagnosis is confirmed by chest radiography. Immediate therapy consists of endotracheal intubation and ventilator support, and insertion of a nasogastric tube to reduce the amount of swallowed gas that might further dilate intrathoracic bowel.

INTRATHORACIC MASSES AND FOCAL PROCESSES

A wide variety of developmental and neoplastic masses may present in the neonatal period and cause respiratory distress. Most of these are rarities; the only ones that approach being common are cystic adenomatoid malformation, pulmonary sequestration, and congenital lobar emphysema. Congenital lobar emphysema may not be amenable to prenatal ultrasonic diagnosis, but the other two certainly are[37,42]; supplementing sonography with magnetic resonance (MR) imaging seems to improve diagnosis and lesion characterization.[22] The prognosis for patients with cystic adenomatoid malformation is a function of its size (with larger being worse) and its cystic components.[47] So grim is the prognosis of a large cystic adenomatoid malformation diagnosed sonographically that termination of pregnancy is a reasonable, albeit drastic, consideration.[33] Indeed, the prognosis for any fetus with a large intrathoracic tumor is so poor, because of the associated pulmonary hypoplasia, that termination of the pregnancy may be indicated.

Congenital lobar emphysema affects the upper lobes or the right middle lobe. The extent of hyperexpansion may or may not be sufficient to cause neonatal respiratory distress; thus, sometimes the condition is not diagnosed until later in life.

Pulmonary sequestrations almost always involve a lower lobe and are categorized as intralobar and extralobar; the extralobar type is invested with a separate pleura, and venous drainage is via systemic veins, whereas the intralobar type generally is invested within the pulmonary pleura and drainage is to pulmonary veins.[43] The arterial supply for both arises from the aorta, and identifying this supply is nearly diagnostic of the condition. However, in some infants cystic adenomatoid malformations also have an arterial supply,[23] and imaging maneuvers (e.g., color Doppler) to demonstrate the vascular anatomy may be useful in planning the surgical approach.

It is worth noting that lung lesions noted on prenatal sonography commonly shrink or even disappear during the course of pregnancy[29,38] and may be subtle or even invisible on plain radiographs of the infant. However, in the majority of such infants, postnatal computed tomography (CT) reveals definite persisting abnormalities.[57] A decrease in lesion size also may continue following birth.[39]

RADIOGRAPHY OF MAJOR SURGICAL CONDITIONS

GENERAL RADIOGRAPHIC CONSIDERATIONS

Episodes of air leak, defined here as intrathoracic extra-alveolar (or ectopic) gas, are common in newborn infants. The most common setting is an infant with RDS being treated with assisted ventilation; in this setting, the combination of decreased lung compliance and supra-atmospheric airway pressures makes lung rupture and air leak relatively likely. However, air leaks are also common in meconium aspiration syndrome and in other conditions in which assisted ventilation is needed. Spontaneous air leaks, which occur at or near delivery in the absence of assisted ventilation, are a common cause of tachypnea and respiratory distress; these may be related to high transpleural pressures engendered during the first few breaths of life.

Intrathoracic ectopic gas can collect in a wide variety of places, the most common of which are the pulmonary interstitium (pulmonary interstitial emphysema), the pleural spaces (pneumothorax), and the mediastinum (pneumomediastinum). Table 3–1 presents a list of the types of air leaks that may be encountered. The plain chest radiograph alone is a powerful tool for diagnosis, but occasionally other radiographic maneuvers may be needed to verify the location of the ectopic gas.

Some air leaks have supra-atmospheric pressures within the abnormal gas collection. The hallmark of this "tension" is the displacement of anatomic structures such as the mediastinum or diaphragm. An air leak under tension usually has more severe consequences than one that is not; the intrathoracic mass effect is greater, and the increased pressure may impede respiratory efforts and blood return to the heart (Figs. 3–1, 3–2, and 3–3).

TABLE 3-1 TYPES OF AIR LEAKS IN THE NEONATAL CHEST

Pulmonary interstitial emphysema
    Pseudoclearing of RDS
    "Tension" (unilateral or bilateral)
    Pseudocysts (subpleural blebs)
    Chronic interstitial emphysema or pseudocysts
Pneumomediastinum
    Ordinary (thymic lobes outlined by gas)
    Tension (heart forced backward and flattened)
    Subazygos (gas in azygoesophageal recess)
    Inferior pulmonary ligament gas (low midchest; triangular)
    Periaortic (gas dissecting to abdomen, often)
Pneumothorax
    "Ordinary" (radiographically like pneumothorax in an adult; uncommon in supine infants)
    Tension (unilateral or bilateral)
    Medial pneumothorax (lucency paralleling the mediastinum)
Gas below the visceral pleura
    At lung base (usually)
    Against a fissure, including an accessory fissure
Pneumopericardium (tension or otherwise)
Gas embolus (survivors rare; gas in chambers of heart and in blood vessels)
Unknown: "large air bubble" (usually anterior chest; rare and enigmatic)

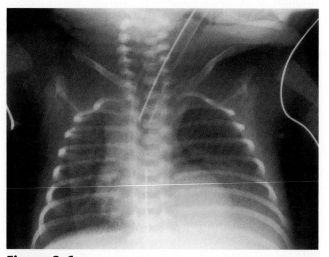

Figure 3–1
Skin fold. Premature infant with questionable interstitial pulmonary emphysema (PIE). A clear line is seen curving from the right scapula across the right lung. It extends into the abdomen, indicating that it is a skin fold. Skin folds go from one density to another to another unlike a pneumothorax, which depicts a razor-sharp line made by air surrounding both the inside and outside of the plural surface. Sliding the cassette underneath the infant before exposing the film causes skin folds on the frontal view.

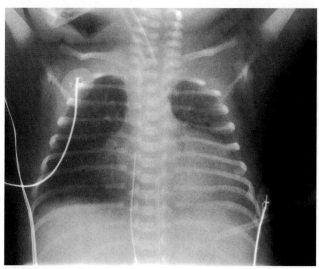

Figure 3–2
Pericardial effusion. Note the marked cardiomegaly in this premature infant with normal vascularity. The contour of the heart is typical for a pericardial effusion in newborns and adults. A malplaced line was the cause, and the diagnosis was confirmed with sonography. Surgical intervention was not needed.

SPECIFIC INTRATHORACIC AIR LEAKS

Pulmonary Interstitial Emphysema

It has been speculated that the initial lesion in all air leaks is PIE, because entry into the interstitium should follow alveolar rupture. However, air leaks commonly appear without radiographic evidence of preexisting or coexisting PIE. In these infants the interstitial air may have drained

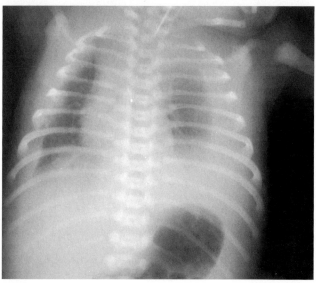

Figure 3–3
Chylothorax. Bilateral large pleural effusions are present. The etiology remained obscure and surgery was performed.

elsewhere by the time the film is exposed, or the alveolar rupture may have occurred directly into other spaces such as the pleura or mediastinum.

The most common setting for PIE is an infant with RDS being treated with assisted ventilation. The complication commonly appears full-blown, involving an entire lung or both lungs. Sometimes, however, it appears first in a lobe, usually an upper lobe. The radiographic appearance is that of abnormal lucencies that have none of the features of air bronchograms; that is, interstitial air is irregular and does not branch or taper peripherally. Instead, PIE tends to be irregular, without a discernible branching pattern, and is "too big too far out" to represent air bronchograms. PIE may have an angular appearance,[50] but sometimes it is circular, resembling bubbles. Usually interstitial air is best identified on the anteroposterior (AP) view; the lateral view, unlike that in infants with pneumothorax, usually adds little.

When the abnormal gas collections of PIE are small, the radiograph may appear deceptively benign; this has been called *pseudoclearing* of RDS,[10] because at first glance, the dense opacity caused by RDS appears to have improved and the lung seems more aerated. Close inspection of the film reveals the true situation, and the patient's prognosis is much worse than that for the patient with RDS without this complication (Fig. 3–4).

Collections of PIE may exhibit tension, depressing the diaphragm and, when unilateral or asymmetric, displacing the mediastinal contents away from the PIE. Tension PIE is clinically frustrating because there is no simple cavity into which a tube may be placed for drainage. Bilateral tension PIE is usually a serious and life-threatening condition.

The natural history of PIE varies. Probably the most common progression is resorption of the ectopic gas, which may occur spontaneously or may be facilitated by lowering the mean airway pressure. (High-frequency oscillatory ventilation has been used for this.) Resorption of unilateral PIE may be facilitated by selective intubation and ventilation of the contralateral lung[9] or by decubitus positioning with the affected side down[15] (Figs. 3–5 and 3–6).

Often, however, the interstitial gas dissects elsewhere and causes a pneumothorax or pneumomediastinum. If diagnosed promptly, this can be beneficial therapeutically, because such collections are amenable to tube drainage. The observation of PIE should alert those caring for the patient to the likelihood of another air leak, most likely a tension pneumothorax.

Less commonly, PIE forms discrete collections or bubbles of gas that have been called *pseudocysts*. These are most common next to the hili, often on the right.[13] Most likely, these collections are situated between the lung and the visceral pleura. Such pseudocysts have no prognostic implications; however, they, too, may decompress into the pleural space, causing a pneumothorax.

Rarely, PIE or associated pseudocysts may persist in a lobe or lung, causing extended respiratory compromise and

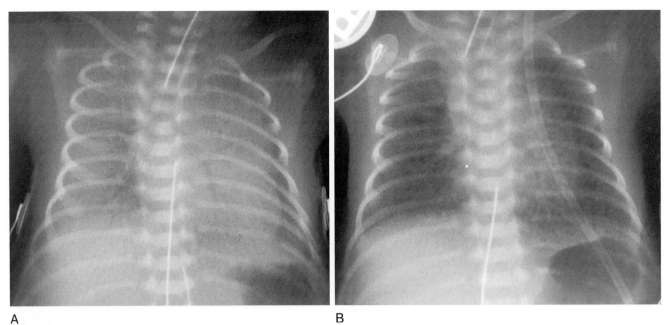

A

B

Figure 3–4

Pseudoclearing of respiratory distress syndrome (RDS). An infant had severe respiratory distress *(A)* and deteriorated clinically. On superficial inspection of a second radiograph *(B)*, the lungs appear more aerated. However, the increased lucency is caused by diffuse pulmonary interstitial emphysema.

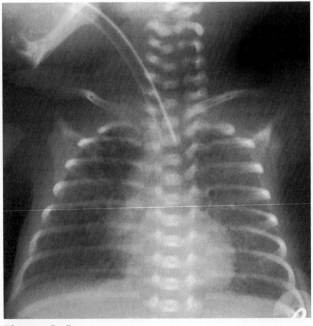

Figure 3–5

Focal pulmonary interstitial emphysema in the right upper lobe. Irregular, tubular densities extending to the pleural edge are easily identified as pulmonary interstitial gas. Notice that the head is turned to the right, as is the chest.

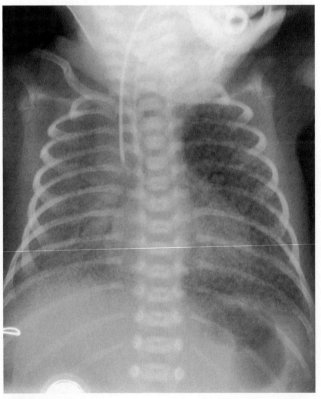

Figure 3–6

Severe PIE in the left lung. The endotracheal tube is in the right main bronchus.

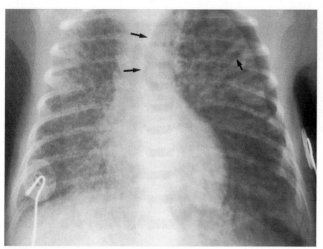

Figure 3–7

Bilateral PIE in an infant with underlying RDS. The lungs reveal multiple irregular lucencies that do not suggest air bronchograms in their configuration or distal caliber. A left pneumothorax is herniating across the midline *(arrows)*. The *arrow* in the left lung points to a lucency that is irregular, does not taper like an air bronchogram, and is too far distal to be an airway.

requiring surgical resection[46] or percutaneous catheter decompression.[1] Fortunately this behavior is rare (Figs. 3–7, 3–8, 3–9, and 3–10).

Pneumothorax

Pneumothorax is nearly as common as PIE in ventilated infants with RDS and is the most common form of air leak

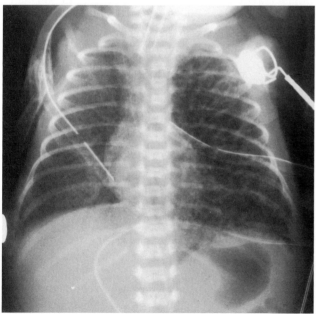

Figure 3–8

Extensive bilateral PIE. There is a greater mass effect on the left. Note displacement of the mediastinum to the right side.

to occur "spontaneously" in newborns who are not treated with assisted ventilation. Pneumothorax is simply air in the pleural space; however, as simple as this may seem, the radiographic manifestations of pneumothorax are varied and sometimes confusing.

A crucial feature to recall when diagnosing pneumothorax is the infant's position, which is generally supine. Gas in the pleural space rises and the lung falls; thus, the ectopic gas lies anteriorly in the pleural space. For this reason, gas outlining the periphery of the lung, as seen in upright adult patients, is uncommon in neonates. Even with large pneumothoraces, the AP film may reveal only a small portion of peripheral pleura or none at all. In this circumstance, the lateral view is more revealing; the ectopic gas is seen anteriorly behind the sternum, often with a discernible lung edge. The detection of small pneumothoraces may be improved by application of edge-enhancement techniques to the digital image.[19]

In addition, the neonatal lung does not collapse proportionally as much as the adult lung because of decreased compliance, especially in infants with RDS. In adults with pneumothorax, the lung may be reduced to a fist-sized hilar mass, whereas in neonates the lung volume seldom appears less than about half normal, even in the presence of a tension pneumothorax (Fig. 3–11).

The lateral view may also reveal a third line paralleling the two lines representing the hemidiaphragms; this "triple diaphragm sign" (poorly named because the adventitious line does not remotely resemble a hemidiaphragm) indicates subpulmonic gas.[17] Four lines may be seen with bilateral pneumothoraces.

Pneumothoraces may be loculated, most commonly at a lung base. Occasional gas collections in this location are large enough to suggest a cystic mass. In this setting, a decubitus view should reveal that the gas is free in the pleural space.

Gas in the minor fissure has been described as a sign of right pneumothorax in adults. This also occurs in infants, in whom the gas collection is somewhat more bulbous (leaf shaped) than in adults.[44] Gas is less commonly loculated in a major fissure.

In a supine infant with a small pneumothorax, the lung, which is tethered at the hilus, falls laterally, and the ectopic gas rises to lie adjacent to the ipsilateral mediastinum. This so-called medial pneumothorax[35] appears radiographically as a dark stripe along the mediastinum.[49] Sometimes confusion with a pneumomediastinum arises; however, pneumomediastinum is bilateral, and intrapleural gas does not outline the thymus. Usually, with awareness of these findings, the correct diagnosis is simple (Figs. 3–12, 3–13, and 3–14).

When there is doubt about the presence of a pneumothorax, the best radiographic maneuver is a horizontal beam decubitus view, with the side of the potential pneumothorax uppermost.[55] The ectopic gas rises, and the lung falls medially, so that the lung edge becomes apparent. A common

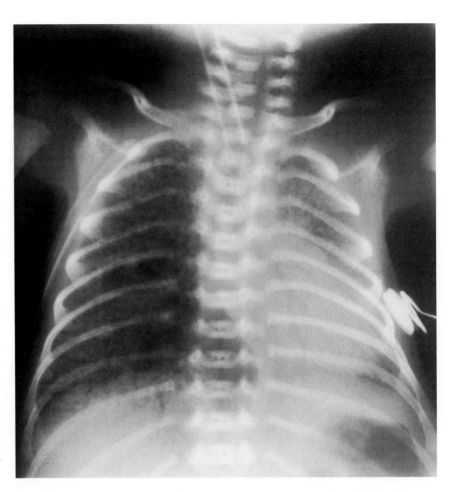

Figure 3–9
Severe PIE with mass effect on the right. Also present are loculated cysts of gas in the right lower lobe and gas in the inferior pulmonary ligament.

mimic of a pneumothorax is a skin fold running across the chest and paralleling the pleural surface. A skin fold usually has lung markings peripherally or extends to a location incompatible with the pleura (Fig. 3–1). If doubt remains, the decubitus view is diagnostic. The decubitus view is also useful when the clinicians doubt the diagnosis, which commonly occurs in the setting of a medial pneumothorax or when no convincing pleural edge is visible.

Tension pneumothorax is common in infants, especially those being treated with assisted ventilation. The usual manifestations of tension pneumothorax are depression of the ipsilateral hemidiaphragm and shift of the mediastinum away from the ectopic gas. The usual treatment of tension pneumothorax is placement of a chest tube whose tip ideally lies anterior in the midchest; adequate assessment of chest tube placement requires a lateral as well as an AP radiograph.

Several signs related to pneumothorax have been described. One of these is the "large, hyperlucent hemithorax" sign[49]; this sign is pretty much what the name implies: the affected hemithorax is large compared with the other and is hyperlucent. This is seen on an AP view in which the ectopic gas lies anterior to the lung, compressing the lung posteriorly and preventing visualization of the lateral lung edge, which

would make diagnosis simple. The "herniated tongue of pleura" sign[18] is also seen on the AP view and represents the pleura under pressure crossing the midline anteriorly and superiorly in the chest. This sign suggests a tension pneumothorax. Visualization of the anterior junctional line (normally invisible) in approximately the center or just left of the center of the chest on an AP view is a sign of bilateral pneumothoraces.[31] All of these signs may be confirmed, usually on the lateral view or by the appropriate decubitus view (Figs. 3–15, 3–16, and 3–17).

Pneumomediastinum

Pneumomediastinum is ectopic gas in the mediastinum. It is less common than PIE or pneumothorax but is nonetheless frequently seen spontaneously and in infants treated with assisted ventilation. The radiographic hallmark of pneumomediastinum is gas outlining the thymus. The two lobes of the thymus are rarely seen distinctly, as they usually blend with the overall mediastinal silhouette. With pneumomediastinum, the lobes are outlined with gas and appear in any of several configurations, depending on the size and shape of the lobes and the distribution of the ectopic gas. Often the lobes are seen as triangular densities adjacent to the upper

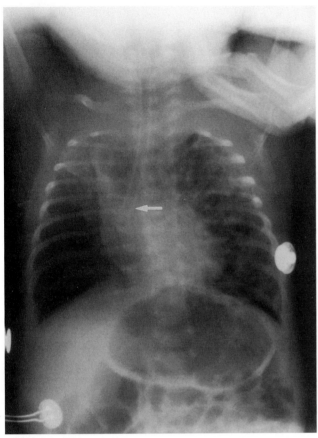

Figure 3–10
Selective intubation for severe unilateral PIE *(left)*. This patient had severe left-sided PIE that was compressing the normal left lung. A frequent complication of right-sided selective intubation is right upper lobe atelectasis. Despite these problems, this infant did well. (From Brooks JG, Bustamante SA, Koops BL, et al. Selective bronchial intubation for the treatment of severe localized pulmonary interstitial emphysema in newborn infants. J Pediatr 91:648–652, 1977.)

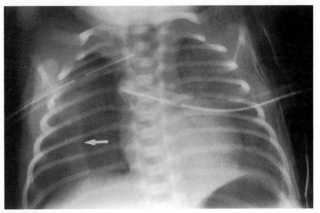

Figure 3–12
Medial pneumothorax is seen on the right *(arrow)* as the lung falls away from the mediastinum. This should not be confused with a pneumomediastinum.

mediastinum; sometimes their configuration suggests a "spinnaker sail."[34] The thymus outlined by gas is often best appreciated on the lateral view (Figs. 3–18, 3–19, and 3–20).

Rarely, a pneumomediastinum may be under tension; in this setting the thymic lobes are sometimes not seen because they are tightly pressed against other structures. The most revealing sign of a tension pneumomediastinum is seen on the lateral view, which demonstrates anterior lucency and a cardiac silhouette situated more posteriorly than is normal; on the AP view, the lungs may be compressed laterally. In my experience, a tension pneumomediastinum is typically fairly benign clinically.

Even under tension, a pneumomediastinum in an infant seldom dissects into the soft tissues of the neck, which is

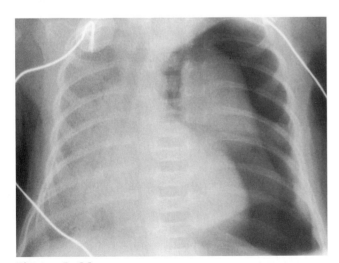

Figure 3–11
Tension left pneumothorax, with rightward displacement of the mediastinum and depression of the ipsilateral hemidiaphragm.

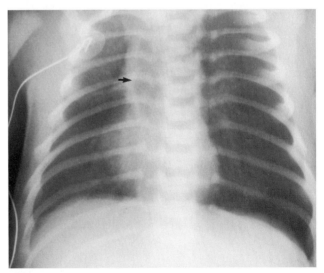

Figure 3–13
Pneumothorax. Left pneumothorax with herniation of the pleura across the midline *(arrow)*. This implies a tension pneumothorax.

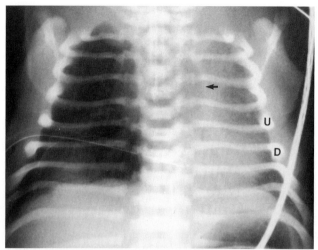

Figure 3–14

Pneumothorax. Large right pneumothorax with herniation of the pleura across the anterior upper chest (*arrow*), indicating a tension pneumothorax. As a result of beam angulation, the anterior portion of the upper ribs points upward (U), while the lower ribs point downward (D).

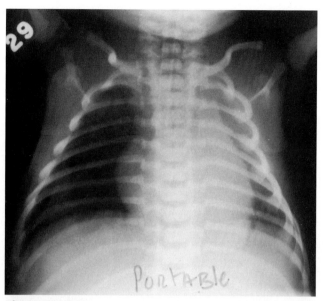

Figure 3–16

Pneumothorax. Large, hyperlucent hemithorax indicating a right pneumothorax.

notably different from a pneumomediastinum in adults and older children. The finding of free gas in the soft tissues of the neck, regardless of whether a pneumomediastinum is present, much more commonly reflects an iatrogenic hypopharyngeal tear, usually caused by attempts at endotracheal intubation.

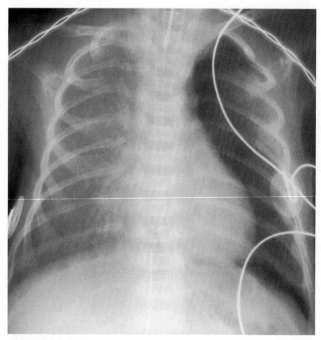

Figure 3–15

Pneumothorax. Large, hyperlucent hemithorax indicating a left pneumothorax.

A pneumomediastinum may dissect into the inferior pulmonary ligament,[54] producing a fairly distinctive ovoid or triangular lucency at the lung base. When gas is in the left pulmonary ligament, the esophagus may be seen as a linear density within the lucency. These gas collections generally occur in the setting of widespread air leaks. Tube drainage of inferior pulmonary ligament gas is virtually impossible (Figs. 3–21, 3–22, and 3–23).

A pneumomediastinum may also accumulate in the azygoesophageal recess (the so-called *infra-azygous pneumomediastinum*[6]). A gas collection here presents with a teardrop-shaped lucency in the central lower chest; its left margin is the esophagus. Unlike the usual case with pneumomediastinums, gas from the azygoesophageal recess commonly dissects into the neck and may also dissect inferiorly, causing a pneumoperitoneum.[40]

Gas from a pneumomediastinum also may lie further posteriorly, outlining the lower thoracic aorta. Gas collections in this region also commonly dissect into the peritoneal cavity.

Miscellaneous Air Leaks

Ectopic intrathoracic gas can also appear in relatively uncommon locations; these are all much rarer than PIE, pneumothorax, and pneumomediastinum. A brief discussion of several of these follows.

Gas Below the Visceral Pleura Ectopic gas may collect between the lung parenchyma and the visceral pleura.[24] Most commonly this occurs at a lung base, where the collection simulates a subpulmonic pneumothorax, except that it

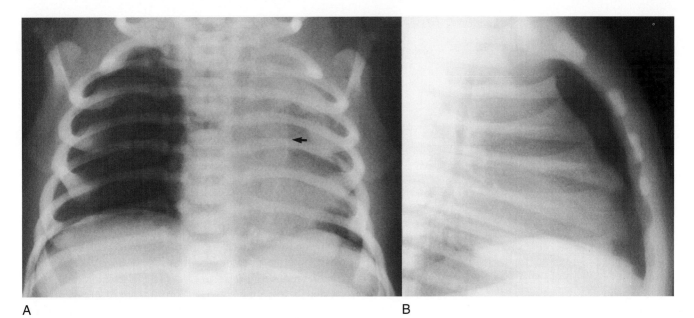

A   B

Figure 3–17
Pneumothorax. Anterior junction line seen on the anteroposterior (AP) projection *(A)*, running vertically left of midline *(arrow)*. This indicates bilateral pneumothoraces, which are more clearly demonstrated on the lateral projection *(B)* as anterior lucencies.

does not rise with decubitus positioning and is not drained with pleurocentesis. Occasionally such collections lie against a fissure, including the minor fissure; again, their radiographic hallmark is their failure to enter the lateral pleural space with decubitus positioning.

Pneumopericardium Ectopic gas in the pericardium outlines the heart, including its inferior margin, and ends superiorly as the pericardium inserts at the origin of the great vessels.[7] This appearance suggests a gas bubble with the heart at its center. The primary features distinguishing a pneumopericardium from a pneumomediastinum are (1) a pneumopericardium does not outline the thymus with gas and (2) a pneumopericardium does not extend superiorly beyond

the takeoff of the great vessels. Sometimes a pneumomediastinum dissects gas below the cardiac silhouette, and therefore gas in this location does not distinguish between the two.

A pneumopericardium may exhibit tension, best diagnosed radiographically by shrinkage of the cardiac silhouette; in a canine model, blood return to the heart began to decrease when the cardiac silhouette diminished by about one third.[21] This finding should prompt immediate pericardiocentesis.

Gas Embolus Ectopic gas from other air leaks, primarily interstitial emphysema, sometimes (fortunately rarely) enters the vascular system, producing gas embolus. The ectopic gas appears most commonly in the venous side of the circulation.[5] In this situation, the chest film, which is generally the patient's

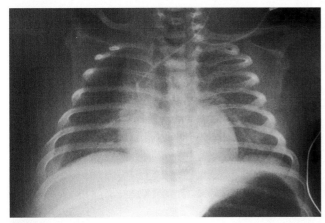

Figure 3–18
Neonatal appendicitis. A two week old infant presented with Sepsis and mild respiratory distress. Chest film revealed a large right sided pleural effusion. At autopsy the infant had appendicitis.

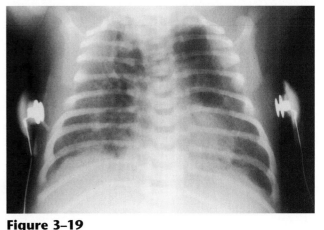

Figure 3–19
Pneumomediastinum. There are ill-defined lucencies seen bilaterally, which extend to the apex of the lungs. The air appears trapped, and neither lobe of the thymus is visible.

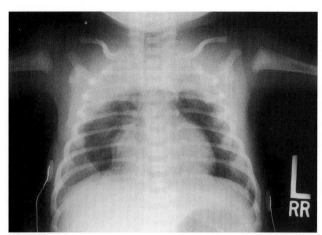

Figure 3–20
Pneumomediastinum. Air in the mediastinum is suggested by the mass of both lobes of the thymus in the apices of the lungs. The inferior aspect of both lobes of the thymus is clearly delineated.

last, often reveals gas in the chambers of the heart and in various blood vessels, nearly always including those of the liver. This complication is almost always lethal; there has been at least one reported survivor,[25] and two survivors in my experience were severely handicapped neurologically from extensive central nervous system infarction (Fig. 3–24).

DIAPHRAGMATIC HERNIA

Diaphragmatic hernias that present in the newborn period are nearly always large, posterolaterally lying hernias through the foramen of Bochdalek, more commonly (in live-born infants, at least) on the left than on the right side.[3] A variable quantity of intestinal contents, often including not only bowel but also stomach and part of the liver, enters the chest during fetal life. The chest radiograph is quite distinctive. The mediastinum appears "slumped" away from an abnormal hemithorax that is often largely opaque initially but may contain bubbles representing gas-filled bowel. When the condition is suspected clinically, as it usually is, active nasogastric suction is initiated to minimize filling of bowel loops with air. Commonly the abdomen is relatively small and narrow (Figs. 3–25, 3–26, 3–27, 3–28, and 3–29).

The radiographic appearance is so distinctive that there are rarely other diagnostic considerations, especially when the findings are combined with clinical observations. However, it is conceivable that a diaphragmatic hernia could be confused with another intrathoracic mass; for example, the gas-filled bowel loops might suggest a cystic adenomatoid malformation. In this unlikely event, introducing contrast material through a nasogastric tube demonstrates gut in the chest. A gas-filled, dilated intrathoracic stomach has in one unfortunate instance been confused with a pneumothorax.[28] A right-sided diaphragmatic hernia containing mostly liver can suggest a pulmonary mass, in which case sonography is useful (Figs. 3–30, 3–31).

Following surgical correction, there is generally a substantial and often long-lived pneumothorax on the side of the previous hernia. A small tongue of tissue may be seen extending from the hilus, representing the hypoplastic ipsilateral lung. Because of the common complication of severe pulmonary hypertension, extracorporeal membrane oxygenation (ECMO) may be required to permit gas exchange while the hypoplastic lungs develop. A largely dilated esophagus has been described in survivors of diaphragmatic hernia and ECMO therapy.[48]

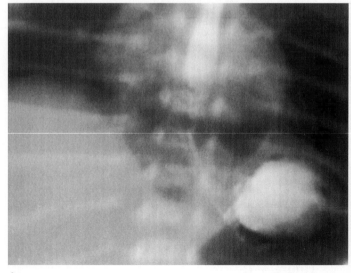

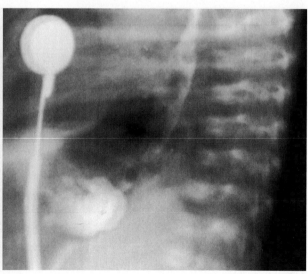

A   B

Figure 3–21
Air in the inferior pulmonary ligament. *A,* Note air at the base of both lungs. *B,* Contrast material is seen in the esophagus.

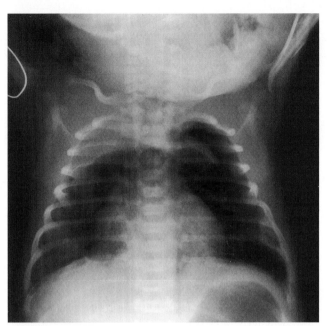

Figure 3–22
Pneumomediastinum. Note air around the left lobe of the thymus; the right lobe is in the apex of the thorax.

Other hernias are less common. Rarely, a hernia through the anteromedial foramen of Morgagni may be large enough to cause respiratory distress in an infant,[51] but usually these present later in life. Visceral hernias into the pericardium also occur; these are rare and often lethal. Eventrations of the diaphragm are relatively common and usually of no clinical significance; however, if these are large and bilateral, pulmonary hypoplasia and its associated grim consequences may result.

The late or delayed appearance of a diaphragmatic hernia following streptococcal pneumonia is a well-recognized but poorly understood phenomenon.[20,32] The radiographic

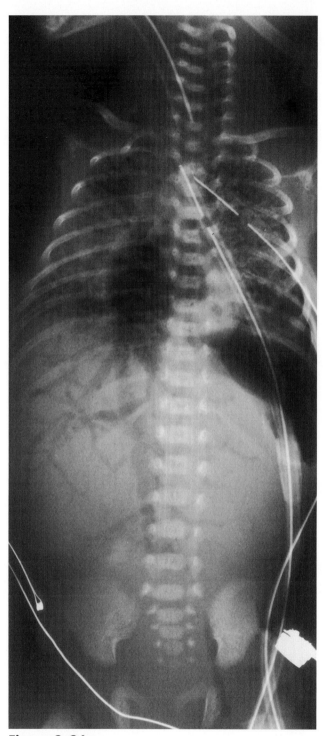

Figure 3–24
Gas embolus. Severe entry of gas into the heart and venous system is documented. Survivors have devastating neurologic deficits. Note extensive PIE.

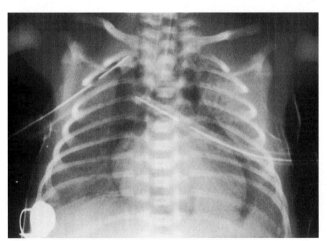

Figure 3–23
Pneumomediastinum. Pneumomediastinum, pneumothorax, and air dissecting into the tissues of the neck.

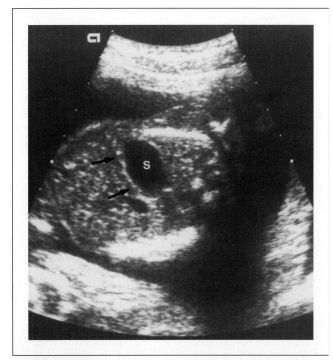

Figure 3–25

Prenatal diagnosis: congenital diaphragmatic hernia. A sagittal sonogram reveals the stomach (S) to be above the diaphragm *(arrows)*. Cardiac displacement, bowel in the chest, and a decrease in normal lung tissue are the hallmarks of prenatal diagnosis.

appearance of bowel in the chest in an infant with pneumonia may be confusing, suggesting lung blebs or a pulmonary necrotizing process.

INTRATHORACIC MASSES AND FOCAL PROCESSES

A wide variety of intrathoracic masses and cysts may cause respiratory distress in the newborn period. Only the most common of these—pulmonary sequestration, cystic adenomatoid malformation (CAM), and congenital lobar emphysema—are briefly discussed here. Pulmonary sequestrations and CAMs may be detected on prenatal sonography.[37,42] Such masses cause respiratory distress because they are space-occupying lesions, reducing the surface area available for gas exchange and because of pulmonary hypoplasia, which occurs with masses that are large enough to impede lung growth significantly (Fig. 3–32).

The severity of clinical abnormalities caused by these conditions in the newborn period ranges from none to moderate respiratory distress and seemingly is a function of the size of the mass.

Pulmonary Sequestration

A pulmonary sequestration is part of a spectrum of bronchopulmonary foregut malformations[8,51]; it is generally identified as a solid mass, nearly always at a lung base. These are classified as intrapulmonary and extrapulmonary sequestrations; those considered extrapulmonary are invested with their own pleura, and their venous drainage is systemic.

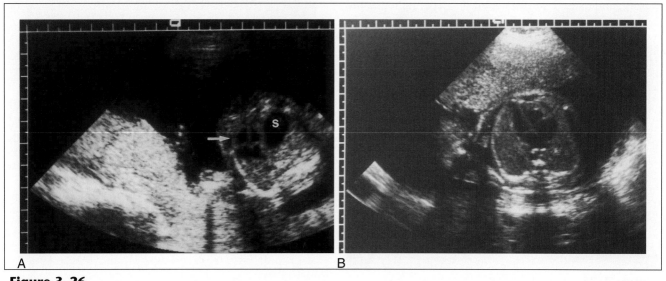

Figure 3–26

Prenatal diagnosis: congenital diaphragmatic hernia. *A,* An axial image of the fetal chest at 27 weeks shows the normal four-chamber view of the heart *(arrow)* displaced laterally by the stomach (S) in the chest. *B,* Normal heart and chest for comparison.

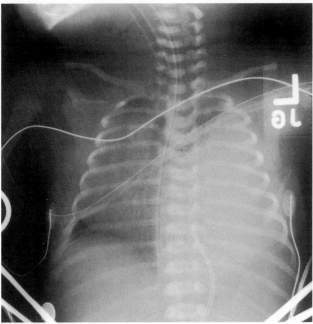

Figure 3–27
Left-sided congenital diaphragmatic hernia. Note a mass in the left hemithorax. There is a mediastinal shift to the right, and the lungs and heart are compressed in the right hemithorax. The rounded contour of the heart can be seen above the right hemidiaphragm. A paucity of gas in the intestine makes the diagnosis more challenging.

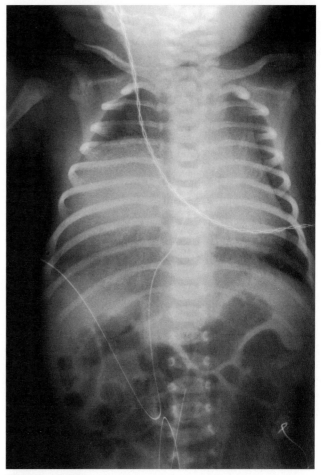

Figure 3–29
Right-sided congenital diaphragmatic hernia. Only a portion of the liver was in the right hemithorax. Note that the heart is not severely compressed.

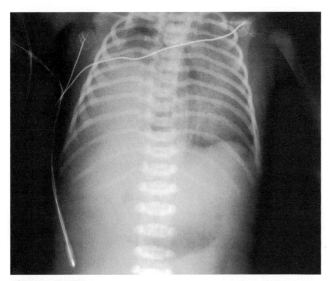

Figure 3–28
Right-sided congenital diaphragmatic hernia. Note the heart and lungs in the left hemithorax. The liver was in the right hemithorax.

Intrapulmonary sequestrations are within the lung's pleura and have pulmonary venous drainage. The clinical importance of this pathologic distinction is small. The hallmark of a sequestration is systemic blood supply, nearly always from a branch of the aorta. The distinction between sequestration and cystic adenomatoid malformation (vide infra) is not always evident, and there is considerable overlap and hybridization of the two lesions[8,39] (Fig. 3–33).

A sequestration may be investigated with ultrasound; because it abuts the diaphragm, the transducer is angled through the abdomen. The mass is generally almost entirely solid. Doppler scanning may reveal a systemic feeding artery. Systemic supply may also be detected with contrast-bolus CT or MR angiography. An old, direct, and simple technique is aortography using an existing umbilical arterial catheter; the anatomic detail provided is exquisite, and the procedure does not carry the morbidity of percutaneous angiography.

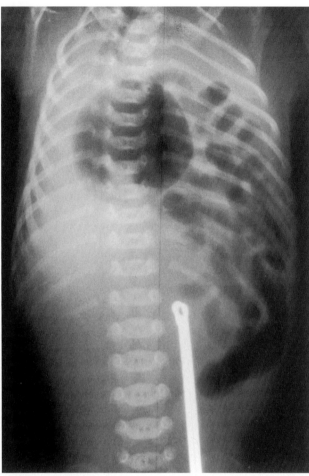

Figure 3–30
Left-sided congenital diaphragmatic hernia. Note that multiple loops of bowel are in the left hemithorax. Immediate decompression with a nasogastric tube is desirable.

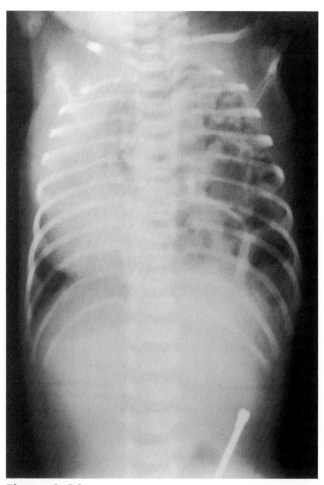

Figure 3–31
Left-sided congenital diaphragmatic hernia. Note extensive lung ompression from air in bowel. Rarely are the loops of bowel confused with cysts in an cystic adenomatoid malformation.

Cystic Adenomatoid Malformation

CAMs are hamartomatous malformations of lung tissue instead of normal bronchi and alveoli. The malformed lung can communicate with the bronchial tree, and its blood supply is the pulmonary artery. Males are afflicted more than females, and there is a right-sided preponderance for the disease. In midgestation the volume of malformed tissue peaks. From then until birth the CAM diminishes in size. The diagnosis is often made with a frontal and lateral radiograph of the chest, but CT is the examination of choice.

As with sequestrations, CAMs are most common at a lung base, making them amenable to sonographic investigation. The cystic components are fluid filled initially and may not be seen on chest radiographs; however, their extent is clearly defined with sonography or CT. After fluid has drained from the cysts, they become visible as gas-filled bubbles on chest radiographs. Of course, with CAMs that are largely solid, such bubbles will not appear (Fig. 3–34).

It is worth noting that a few CAMs have a systemic rather than pulmonary blood supply.[23] Although these are uncommon, it may be surgically useful to know of their existence preoperatively. Systemic supply may be imaged as described for a pulmonary sequestration.

Congenital Lobar Emphysema

Congenital lobar emphysema initially appears radiographically as a lobar consolidation or focal lobar "wet lung" involving an upper lobe[52] or the right middle lobe[16]; involvement of a lower lobe is almost never encountered. The cause is bronchial obstruction evoking retention of lung fluid in a defined lobar segment. The most important differential diagnostic consideration is a lobar consolidative pneumonia, which is rare in neonates and is accompanied by clinical signs of infection. The large size of the affected lobe may not be appreciated initially. Over a period usually lasting several days, the fluid is resorbed and replaced with air, at which point the diagnosis becomes more obvious; however, at least

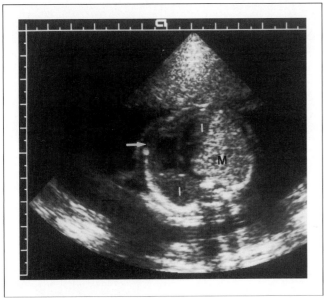

Figure 3–32
Prenatal diagnosis: pulmonary sequestration. An axial image of the fetal chest at 22 weeks of gestation. Cardiac deviation is seen *(arrow)*. Normal lung parenchyma is visible (l) as is a homogenous echogenic mass (M) occupying most of the left hemithorax. The parents elected to terminate the pregnancy, and a large pulmonary sequestration was found at autopsy.

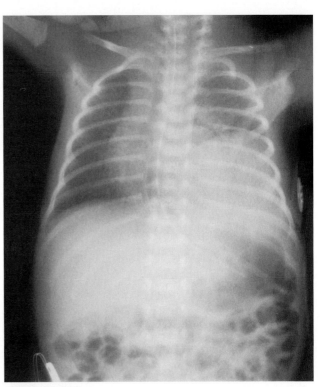

Figure 3–33
Pulmonary sequestration. Note a large mass displacing the nasogastric tube to the left and inferiorly.

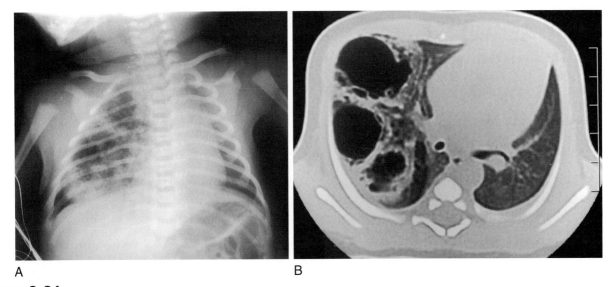

A   B

Figure 3–34
Cystic adenomatoid malformation. *A,* radiograph reveals multiple large cystic masses involving the right upper, middle, and lower lobes of the lung. *B,* Computed tomography scan confirms a normal left lung and involvement as seen on the plain film. These findings are virtually diagnostic.

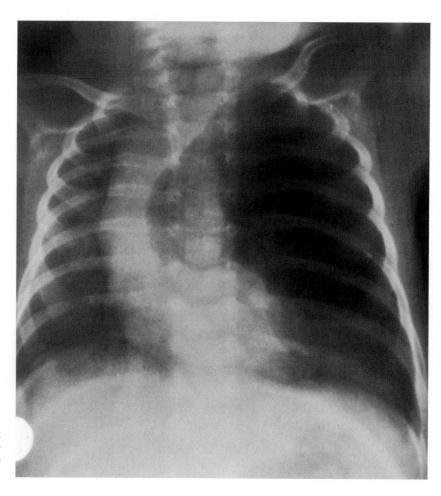

Figure 3–35
Congenital lobar emphysema. Note the marked overinflation of the left upper lobe. A severe medial shift is present, and the remainder of the left lower lobe is compressed.

one infant has been reported in whom chest CT was required for diagnosis.[41] Usually plain radiographs are sufficient to diagnose and manage patients with congenital lobar emphysema (Fig. 3–35).[45]

The only other disorder that might be confused with congenital lobar emphysema is the rarer entity of polyalveolar lobe.[14] Familiarity with the typical radiographic findings of fluid and air trapping make the radiographic diagnosis simple. An assisted expiration film is an easy method of further documenting the fact that the abnormality is caused by bronchial obstruction.[56] More sophisticated imaging modalities are usually unnecessary.

REFERENCES

1. Arias-Camison JM, Kurtis PS, Feld RS, et al. Decompression of multiple pneumatoceles in a premature infant by percutaneous catheter placement. J Perinatol 21:553–555, 2001.
2. Bashour BN, Balfe JW. Urinary tract anomalies in neonates with spontaneous pneumothorax and/or pneumomediastinum. Pediatrics 59:1048–1049, 1977.
3. Berdon WE, Baker DH, Armoury R. The role of pulmonary hypoplasia in the prognosis of newborn infants with diaphragmatic hernia and eventration. AJR Am J Roentgenol 103:413–421, 1968.
4. Blum-Hoffman E, Kopotic RJ, Mannino FL. High-frequency oscillatory ventilation combined with intermittent mandatory ventilation in critically ill neonates: 3 years of experience. Eur J Pediatr 147:392–398, 1988.
5. Booth TN, Allen BA, Royal SA. Lymphatic air embolism: A new hypothesis regarding the pathogenesis of neonatal systemic air embolism. Pediatr Radiol 25 (Suppl 1):228–229, 1995.
6. Bowen A III, Quattromani FL. Infraazygous pneumomediastinum in the newborn. AJR Am J Roentgenol 135:1017–1021, 1980.
7. Brans YW, Pitts M, Cassady G. Neonatal pneumopericardium. Am J Dis Child 130:393–396, 1976.
8. Bratu I, Flageole H, Chen MF, et al. The multiple facets of pulmonary sequestration. J Pediatr Surg 36:784–790, 2001.
9. Brooks JG, Bustamante SA, Koops BL, et al. Selective bronchial intubation for the treatment of severe localized pulmonary interstitial emphysema in newborn infants. J Pediatr 91:648–652, 1977.
10. Campbell RE, Hoffman RR Jr. Predictability of pneumothorax in hyaline membrane disease. AJR Am J Roentgenol 120:274–278, 1974.
11. Chernick V, Avery ME. Spontaneous alveolar rupture in newborn infants. Pediatrics 32:816–824, 1963.
12. Chinn DH, Filly RA, Callen PW, et al. Congenital diaphragmatic hernia diagnosed prenatally by ultrasound. Radiology 148:119–123, 1983.
13. Clarke TA, Edwards DK. Pulmonary pseudocysts in newborn infants with respiratory distress syndrome. AJR Am J Roentgenol 133:417–421, 1979.
14. Cleveland RH, Weber B. Retained fetal lung liquid in congenital lobar emphysema: A possible predictor of polyalveolar lobe. Pediatr Radiol 23:291–295, 1993.

15. Cohen RS, Smith DW, Stevenson DK, et al. Lateral decubitus position as therapy for persistent focal pulmonary interstitial emphysema in neonates: A preliminary report. J Pediatr 104:441–443, 1984.

16. Cremin BJ, Movsowitz H. Lobar emphysema in infants. Br J Radiol 44: 692–696, 1971.

17. Edwards DK. Radiology of hyaline membrane disease, transient tachypnea of the newborn, and bronchopulmonary dysplasia. In Farrell PM, ed. Lung Development: Biological and Clinical Perspectives. Vol II. New York: Academic Press, 1982, pp 47–89.

18. Fletcher BD. Medial herniation of the parietal pleura: A useful sign of pneumothorax in supine neonates. AJR Am J Roentgenol 130: 469–472, 1978.

19. Goo HW, Kim HJ, Song KS, et al. Using edge enhancement to identify subtle findings on soft-copy neonatal chest radiographs. AJR Am J Roentgenol 177:437–440, 2001.

20. Harris MC, Moskowitz WB, Engle WD, et al. Group B streptococcal septicemia and delayed-onset diaphragmatic hernia. Am J Dis Child 135: 723–725, 1981.

21. Higgins CB, Broderick TW, Edwards DK, Shumaker A. The hemodynamic significance of massive pneumopericardium in preterm infants with respiratory distress syndrome. Clinical and experimental observations. Radiology 133:363–368, 1979.

22. Hubbard AM, Adzick NS, Crombleholme TM, et al. Congenital chest lesions: Diagnosis and characterization with prenatal MR imaging. Radiology 212:43–48, 1999.

23. Hutchin P, Friedman PJ, Saltzstein SL. Congenital cystic adenomatoid malformation with anomalous blood supply. J Thorac Cardiovas Surg 62:220–225, 1971.

24. Ivey HH, Kattwinkel J, Alford BA. Subvisceral pleural air in neonates with respiratory distress. Am J Dis Child 135:544–546, 1981.

25. Kogutt M. Systemic air embolism secondary to respiratory therapy in the neonate: Six cases including one survivor. AJR Am J Roentgenol 131:425–429, 1978.

26. Leonidas JC, Bhan I, McCauley RG. Persistent localized pulmonary interstitial emphysema and lymphangiectasia: A casual relationship? Pediatrics 64:165–171, 1979.

27. Levine DH, Trump DS, Waterkotte G. Unilateral pulmonary interstitial emphysema: A surgical approach to treatment. Pediatrics 68: 510–514, 1981.

28. Liang JS, Lu FL, Tang JR, Yau KI. Congenital diaphragmatic hernia misdiagnosed as pneumothorax in a newborn. Acta Paediatr Taiwan 41:221–223, 2000.

29. MacGillivray TE, Harrison MR, Goldstein RB, Adzick NS. Disappearing fetal lung lesions. J Pediatr Surg 28:1321–1324, 1993.

30. Macklin MT, Macklin CC. Malignant interstitial emphysema of the lung and mediastinum as an important occult complication in many respiratory diseases and other conditions. Medicine (Baltimore) 23: 281–358, 1944.

31. Markowitz RI. The anterior junction line: A radiographic sign of bilateral pneumothorax in neonates. Radiology 167:717–719, 1988.

32. McCarten KM, Rosenberg HK, Borden S, Mandell GA. Delayed appearance of right diaphragmatic hernia associated with group B streptococcal infection in newborns. Radiology 139: 385–389, 1981.

33. Mendoza A, Wolf P, Edwards DK, et al. Prenatal ultrasonographic diagnosis of congenital adenomatoid malformation of the lung. Correlation with pathology and implications for pregnancy management. Arch Pathol Lab Med 110:402–404, 1986.

34. Moseley JE. Loculated pneumomediastinum in the newborn. A thymic "spinnaker sail" sign. Radiology 75:788–790, 1960.

35. Moskowitz PS, Griscom NT. The medial pneumothorax. Radiology 120:143–147, 1976.

36. Moylan FMB, Walker AM, Kramer SS, et al. Alveolar rupture as an independent predictor of bronchopulmonary dysplasia. Crit Care Med 6:10–13, 1978.

37. Nyberg DA, Mahony BS, Pretorius DH. Diagnostic Ultrasound of Fetal Anomalies: Text and Atlas. Chicago: Year Book, 1990.

38. Quinton AR, Smoleniec JS. Congenital lobar emphysema—The disappearing chest mass: Antenatal ultrasound appearance. Ultrasound Obstet Gynecol 17:169–171, 2001.

39. Roggin KK, Breuer CK, Carr SR, et al. The unpredictable character of congenital cystic lung lesions. J Pediatr Surg 35:801–805, 2000.

40. Rosenfeld DL, Cordell CE, Jadeja N. Retrocardiac pneumomediastinum: Radiographic finding and clinical implications. Pediatrics 85:92–97, 1990.

41. Rusakow LS, Khare S. Radiographically occult congenital lobar emphysema presenting as unexplained neonatal tachypnea. Pediat Pulmonol 32:246–249, 2001.

42. Sauerbrei E. Lung sequestration. Duplex Doppler diagnosis at 19 weeks gestation. J Ultrasound Med 10:101–105, 1991.

43. Savic B, Birtel FJ, Tholen W, et al. Lung sequestration: Report of seven cases and review of 540 published cases. Thorax 34:96–101, 1979.

44. Spizarny DL, Goodman LR. Air in the minor fissure: A sign of right-sided pneumothorax. Radiology 160:329–331, 1986.

45. Stigers KB, Woodring JH, Kanga JF. The clinical and imaging spectrum of findings in patients with congenital lobar emphysema. Pediatr Pulmonol 14:160–170, 1992.

46. Stocker JT, Madewell JE. Persistent interstitial pulmonary emphysema: Another complication of the respiratory distress syndrome. Pediatrics 59:847–857, 1977.

47. Stocker TJ, Madewell JE, Drake RM. Congenital cystic adenomatoid malformation of the lung: Classification and morphological spectrum. Hum Pathol 8:155–171, 1977.

48. Stolar CJ, Berdon WE, Dillon PW, et al. Esophageal dilatation and reflux in neonates supported by ECMO after diaphragmatic hernia repair. AJR Am J Roentgenol 151:135–137, 1988.

49. Swischuk LE. Two lesser known but useful signs of neonatal pneumothorax. AJR Am J Roentgenol 127:623–627, 1976.

50. Swischuk LE. Bubbles in hyaline membrane disease. Differentiation of three types. Radiology 122:417–426, 1977.

51. Swischuk LE. Imaging of the Newborn, Infant, and Young Child. 3rd ed. Baltimore: Williams & Wilkins, 1989, pp 15, 136–139.

52. Thakral CL, Maji DC, Sajwani MJ. Congenital lobar emphysema: experience with 21 cases. Pediatr Surg Int 17:88–91, 2001.

53. Toomasian JM, Snedecor SM, Cornell RG, et al. National experience with extracorporeal membrane oxygenation for newborn respiratory failure. Data from 715 cases. ASAIO Trans 34:140–147, 1988.

54. Volberg FM Jr, Everett CJ, Brill PW. Radiologic features of inferior pulmonary ligament air collections in neonates with respiratory distress. Radiology 130:357–360, 1979.

55. Wesenberg RL. The Newborn Chest. Hagerstown, MD: Harper & Row, 1973, pp 15–17, 35.

56. Wesenberg RL, Blumhagen JD. Assisted expiratory chest radiography. An effective technique for the diagnosis of foreign-body aspiration. Radiology 130:538–539, 1979.

57. Winters WD, Effmann EL, Nghiem HV, Nyberg DA. Disappearing fetal lung masses: importance of postnatal imaging studies. Pediatr Radiol 27:535–539, 1997.

58. Wood BP, Anderson WH, Mauk JE, Merritt TA. Pulmonary lymphatic air: Locating "pulmonary interstitial emphysema" of the premature infant. AJR Am J Roentgenol 138:809–814, 1982.

ADDITIONAL READING

Boloker J, Bateman DA, Wunt JT, Stoler CJ. Congenital diaphragmatic hernia in 120 infants treated consecutively with permissive hypercapnea/spontaneous respiration/elective repair. J Pediatr Surg 37:357–366, 2002.

Breysem L, Bosmans H, Dymarkowski S, et al. The value of fast MR imaging as an adjunct to ultrasound in prenatal diagnosis. Eur Radiol 13:1538–1548, 2003.

Downard CD, Jaksic T, Garza JJ, et al. Analysis of an improved survival rate for congenital diaphragmatic hernia. J Pediatr Surg 38:729–732, 2003.

Holt PD, Arkovitz MS, Berdon WE, Stolar CJ. Newborns with diaphragmatic hernia: Initial chest radiography does not have a role in predicting clinical outcomes. Pediatr Radiol 34:462–464, 2004.

Kaushik N, Cohen RA, Helton JG. 3-D CT angiographic demonstration of a neonatal ductus arteriosus aneurysm with development of ductal calcification: are the "ductus bump," ductus arteriosus aneurysm, and ductal calcification related? Pediatr Radiol 34:738–741, 2004.

Takeda S, Miyoshi S, Inoue M, et al. Clinical spectrum of congenital cystic disease of the lung in children. Eur J Cardiothorac Surg 15:11–17, 1999.

Tawil MI, Pilling DW. Congenital cystic adenomatoid malformation: Is there a difference between the antenatally and postnatally diagnosed cases? Pediatr Radiol 35:79–84, 2005.

van Leeuwen KV, Teitelbaum DH, Hirschl RB, et al. Prenatal diagnosis of congenital cystic adenomatoid malformation and its postnatal presentation, surgical indication and natural history. J Pediatr Surg 34:794–799, 1999.

THE FETUS AND NEONATE WITH URINARY TRACT ABNORMALITIES

Outline

Sandra Fernbach, MD

THE FETUS AND NEONATE WITH URINARY TRACT ABNORMALITIES

In each of the last two decades the use of prenatal sonography has been more widespread with increasing accuracy and sophistication of the diagnoses made prenatally.[16,36,64] Urinary tract anomalies diagnosed sonographically can be further explored with magnetic resonance imaging (MRI) if indicated[57]; for example, prenatal sonographic diagnosis of the rare renal tumor mesoblastic nephroma has been confirmed with MRI.[35] When urinary tract anomalies cannot be fully diagnosed initially, subsequent prenatal scans or postnatal imaging may be necessary to characterize the anomaly so that appropriate, timely treatment can begin.

Familiarity with the postnatal appearances of anomalies of the genitourinary tract assists in interpretation of the prenatal findings. Pediatric radiologists are familiar with many of the renal anomalies and the syndromes associated with renal anomalies (Table 4–1). Training in recognizing complex or unusual urinary tract anomalies greatly facilitates diagnosing such lesions in utero.

The increasing use and accuracy of prenatal sonography have important consequences. In utero treatment, both corrective and palliative, can defer or prevent additional urinary tract damage. Severe urinary tract anomalies causing oligohydramnios can be treated with replacement of amniotic fluid in an immature fetus or early delivery of a mature one. With detection of severe anomalies such as spina bifida, posterior urethral valves (PUVs), and prune belly syndrome, elective termination of the pregnancy can be an alternative.[16]

This chapter describes the sonographic findings of many anomalies that are recognizable prenatally and their prenatal treatment, if such is possible. Also discussed is the prognosis in the most important conditions. The postnatal imaging studies that may be helpful before and after corrective surgery are presented.

TABLE 4-1 SELECTED CONDITIONS ASSOCIATED WITH RENAL ANOMALIES

CONDITION	ANOMALIES
VACTERL complex (*v*ertebral, *a*norectal, *c*ardiac, *tr*acheoesophageal, *r*enal, and *l*imb anomalies; includes imperforate anus)	Renal ectopia, fusion, and agenesis
	Anomalies less severe and less frequent (4%) with low imperforate anus
	Anomalies more severe and more frequent (37%) with high imperforate anus
Vertebral anomaly (fusion, cleft, butterfly)	16% with unilateral renal agenesis, crossed ectopy, hydronephrosis, duplex
MURCS association (Müllerian duct aplasia, renal aplasia, cervical spine anomalies)	Unilateral renal agenesis
Prune belly syndrome (Eagle-Barrett syndrome)	Renal dysplasia, vesicoureteric reflux (greater than 40%) Urachal and urethral anomalies, cryptorchidism
Brachio-oto-renal syndrome	Unilateral renal agenesis or hypoplasia
Kallmann's syndrome	Unilateral renal agenesis, unilateral multicystic dysplastic kidney (in 40%)
CHARGE association (coloboma, heart anomaly, choanal, atresia, retardation, genital and ear anomalies)	Unilateral renal agenesis, hydronephrosis, renal hypoplasia Genital anomalies: micropenis, hypospadias, cryptorchidism; labial, uterine, and vaginal anomalies
Meckel-Gruber syndrome	Visible cysts, enlarged kidneys
Cerebrohepatorenal syndrome (Zellweger syndrome)	Cortical cysts
Tuberous sclerosis	Large cysts, similar to autosomal dominant polycystic kidney disease
Trisomy 21 (Down syndrome)	Renal dysplasia with or without cysts
Trisomy 13 (Patau syndrome)	Renal cortical cysts, hydronephrosis, hydroureteronephrosis
Trisomy 18 (Edward syndrome)	Ectopic, horseshoe kidney; hydronephrosis and hydroureteronephrosis
45 XO (Turner's syndrome)	Horseshoe kidney

OBSTRUCTIVE LESIONS

PRENATAL HYDRONEPHROSIS

Hydronephrosis (HN) is the most common urinary tract anomaly detected with prenatal sonography (Figs. 4–1 through 4–2).[22,29,46,63] About 1% to 2% of fetuses demonstrate some degree of HN in early pregnancy, which disappears in up to half before birth.[4,28,46,51] Additionally, longitudinal studies show that about half of kidneys with postnatal HN develop into normal nonobstructed kidneys.[48]

The diagnosis of HN in utero should be made cautiously. Normal echolucency of the medullary pyramids, regularly arrayed about the renal pelvis, can simulate HN. The "hydronephrotic" variant of multicystic dysplastic kidney (MCDK) may be difficult to distinguish from HN. Maternal hydration does not affect fetal pyelectasis and need not be considered when HN is detected.

It is important to document the degree and the progression of prenatal HN and to search for other urinary tract anomalies that might be causative. An associated hydroureter is an important finding because it shifts the probable diagnosis from ureteropelvic junction obstruction (UJPO) (almost 50%) to ureterovesical obstruction (about 20%) and a number of other lower obstructive and nonobstructive processes (Tables 4–2 and 4–3).[48] HN in the fetus may be caused by vesicoureteric reflux (VUR) and in utero resolution of reflux may be one reason why the prevalence of HN decreases in late pregnancy (Fig. 4–3). Observation of increasing HN during voiding suggests VUR, but its absence does not exclude VUR.

A commonly used grading system for prenatal HN is that developed by Grignon et al.[28] In this system, the five grades of dilatation are related to the size of the anteroposterior diameter of the renal pelvis, the amount of dilatation of the pelvicaliceal system, and the presence of cortical atrophy on studies performed at 20 weeks of gestational age. Grades III through V HN all have a renal pelvis of greater than 15 mm

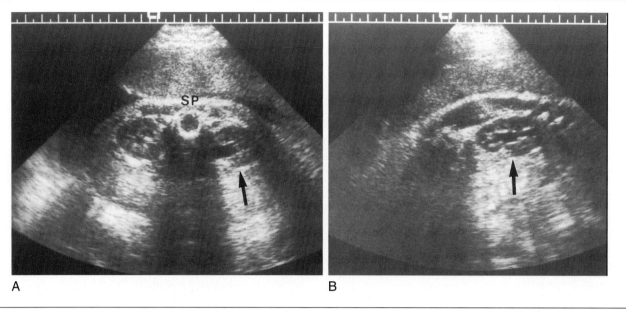

Figure 4–1
Prenatal diagnosis: mild hydronephrosis. *A,* A prone axial image of fetal kidneys at 34 weeks of gestation shows a normal left kidney and mild upper tract dilatation on the right *(arrow). B,* Longitudinal image of the right kidney with mild dilation of the pelvicaliceal system *(arrow).* Unilateral vesicoureteral reflux was proven to be the cause of the collecting system dilatation. SP, spine.

and increasing degrees of caliceal dilatation, with a corresponding 80% likelihood of necessary surgical correction.[28] Other sonographers have used measurements of greater than or equal to 4 mm in the second trimester and greater than or equal to 7 mm in the third trimester as signs of pathologic dilatation.[2,4,13,48,51] Before 23 weeks of gestation, there may be no renal pelvis dilatation in kidneys that later dilate and demonstrate obstruction postnatally.[2] Increasing size of the renal pelvis throughout pregnancy also implies the likelihood of postnatal obstruction.[4] Renal pelvis size may increase in utero with bladder distention; thus, abnormal measurements should be verified with repeat studies.[54]

The gender of the fetus is important because many urologic diagnoses have a male predominance, and some (PUVs and prune belly syndrome) occur exclusively in male fetuses. The echogenicity of the kidneys is helpful diagnostically. Increased renal echogenicity favors an obstructive process, particularly in association with oligohydramnios, although not all echogenic kidneys exhibit diminished renal function postnatally.[38] The development of cortical cysts within echogenic hydronephrotic kidneys indicates relatively

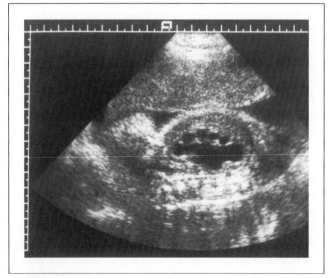

Figure 4–2
Prenatal diagnosis: moderate hydronephrosis. This coronal image of a 27-week fetus suggests ureteropelvic junction (UPJ) obstruction. Ureteral dilatation was not seen. The diagnosis of UPJ was confirmed at birth.

TABLE 4-2 PRENATAL AND POSTNATAL HYDRONEPHROSIS
Extrarenal pelvis
Megacalycosis
Retrocaval ureter
Ureteropelvic junction obstruction (10% to 15% bilateral)
Ureteral valve or polyp
Vesicoureteric reflux

TABLE 4-3 PRENATAL AND POSTNATAL
HYDROURETERONEPHROSIS

Bladder outlet obstruction
    Anterior urethral valve
    Urethral polyp
    Posterior urethral valves
    Urethral atresia
Duplicated ureters
    Upper pole obstructed (ectopic ureterocele, ectopic
      distal insertion)
    Lower pole (vesicoureteric reflux, ureteropelvic
      junction obstruction)
Megaureter-megacystis syndrome
Neurogenic bladder
Primary megaureter
Prune belly syndrome
Simple ureterocele
Vesicoureteric reflux

---

severe obstruction. It is crucial to estimate the amount of amniotic fluid, because this value is diagnostically useful, pragmatically valuable, and possibly suggestive of a need for prenatal intervention. Bilaterally large and echogenic kidneys, in the absence of HN or enlarged ureters, suggest autosomal recessive kidney disease. Amniotic fluid volume may be normal or decreased, because some of these kidneys retain function even into the neonatal period. Prenatally, echogenic pyramids may be an unusual manifestation of autosomal recessive polycystic renal disease; postnatally, echogenic pyramids may reflect renal tubular acidosis, Bartter's syndrome, and transient neonatal nephropathy.

The retrovesical region is evaluated for dilatation of the distal ureter, an inconsistent finding in fetuses and infants with VUR and more suggestive of primary megaureter or ureterocele. Sonography of the bladder should include a search for an intravesical structure (ureterocele) and measurement of bladder wall thickness, which increases with outlet obstruction.

The use of prenatal sonography has brought to the pediatric radiologist and urologist a patient distinct from those studied for HN in the past: the fetus or infant who is as yet asymptomatic. This situation has necessitated diagnostic tests directed to answer previously unasked questions: Is the HN significant? Might it resolve without treatment? When should the child be treated?

The differential diagnosis of prenatally detected HN is broad (see Table 4–2). The initial postnatal imaging study to confirm the prenatally detected abnormality is usually sonography. Early researchers cautioned against performing a sonography in the first 24 hours of life, a period of relative oliguria in many infants.[28] However, delaying the first postnatal renal sonogram for a few days to weeks has been challenged on both scientific and practical grounds.[13,20]

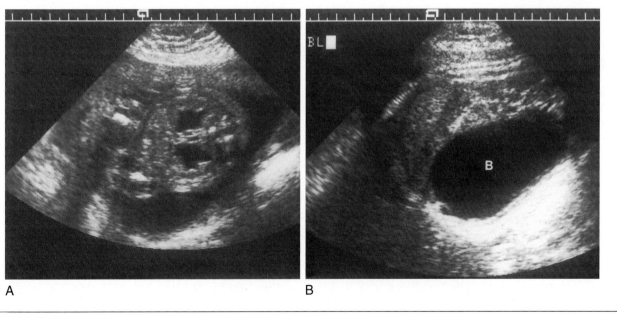

A   B

Figure 4–3
Prenatal diagnosis: primary grade V reflux. *A,* This prone axial image of a 38-week fetus shows bilaterally symmetric upper tract dilatation. During the study the degree of dilatation varied from mild to severe. *B,* The bladder (B) of this female infant also changed in size during the study. The diagnosis of severe reflux was made prenatally and confirmed at birth.

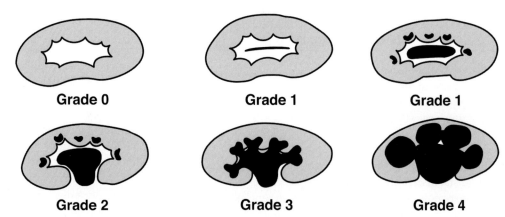

Figure 4–4
Society of Fetal Urology grading system for hydronephrosis.

Examining the neonate before discharge prevents loss of a patient with treatable HN to follow-up. In pilot studies the quality of the sonographic information obtained in this early period appears to be as reliable for "significant" HN as the information obtained at later studies. The definition of "significant" HD is likely to cause clinical problems.[13,20]

Postnatal sonography, like prenatal sonography, includes careful evaluation of the bladder. Bladder wall thickening may be a sign of PUVs or less common causes of urethral obstruction. Dilation of the distal ureter should prompt a search for a ureterocele, the absence of which suggests vesicoureteral reflux or primary (aperistaltic) megaureter.

Sonography-detected HN is commonly graded using a system developed by the Society for Fetal Urology (Fig. 4–4).[26,45] There are five grades: 1–4. Grade 4 has been divided into A and B, with A referring to those fetuses with focal cortical thinning and B to those with diffuse cortical loss.[67] The standardized grading of HN has improved communication among pediatricians, radiologists, and urologists and has facilitated comparative studies of treatment outcomes.

Reflux is noted in about 20% of infants with prenatally diagnosed HN, even when the HN has resolved by birth.[3,22] Voiding cystourethrography (VCUG) is routine in male neonates with persistent prenatal HN. Its value in those whose HN has resolved could be questioned, although a normal renal sonogram does not exclude high-grade reflux.[8] The entire urethra must be visualized to exclude obstructing lesions: ectopic ureterocele, PUV, fibrovascular polyp, and anterior urethral valve. In infants, cyclic VCUG is generally preferable; the urethra is visualized only on one cycle of voiding, with the renal fossa imaged at the end of each. Because bladder anomalies are rare and urethral anomalies are virtually nonexistent in girls, nuclear cystography may instead be used to screen them for reflux. Cystosonography using commercially available contrast agents is being developed as a sensitive technique to detect reflux and is showing promise as a technique to evaluate the male urethra.[7,11,18] Its main advantage is the absence of ionizing radiation; bladder catheterization remains necessary to instill the sonographic contrast agent.

Reflux is graded using the classification of the International Reflux Study, which has predictive value except with neurogenic bladder or a diverticulum underlying the affected ureter ("secondary reflux," Fig. 4–5). In neonates, low grades of VUR often resolve within a few years. Higher grades of VUR resolve less frequently and more slowly. A notable exception to this rule is seen in male neonates who, for unknown reasons, may rapidly outgrow grade V VUR.[3,23,29] Many patients in whom neonatal HN resolves are boys whose HN is caused by severe VUR.

Even when reflux is present, additional imaging may be needed to distinguish nonobstructive from obstructive HN, because VUR can coexist with either ureteropelvic junction or ureterovesical junction obstruction. UPJO is about seven times more common than ureterovesical junction obstruction, but the exact incidence of either is uncertain because of sampling bias.

Imaging is also helpful in assessing the degree of obstruction and kidney function as the child grows. This information, usually obtained with renal scintigraphy, can help the urologist decide whether and when a hydronephrotic kidney requires surgery. Diuretic renal scintigraphy can be performed using technetium-99m mercaptoacetyltriglycine (MAG3) or, less commonly, technetium-99m diethyltriaminepentaacetic acid (DTPA). Reproducible, high-quality information is obtained when specific study protocols are followed.[15] For example, supravesical obstruction is more apparent when urine production is maximized by hydrating the infant and then administering a diuretic at a predetermined stage of the study. Keeping the bladder drained by catheter eliminates the confounding problem of secondary HN produced by a full bladder or VUR. Two main parameters, each with prognostic significance, are used to evaluate the degree of obstruction: the appearance of the washout curves and the $T_{1/2}$.[71] Both reflect the ability of the kidney to excrete isotope after a diuretic. Washout curves are described as nonobstructive, indeterminate, or obstructive. $T_{1/2}$ is the time when

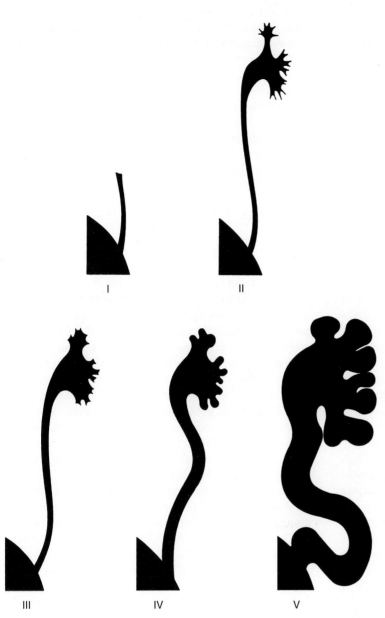

Figure 4–5

Grading of vesicoureteral reflux. Grade I reflux: reflux into the distal portion of the ureter only. Grade II reflux: reflux into the renal collecting system, without distention of the collecting system (as compared with excretory urography). Grade III reflux: reflux into the distal renal collecting system, causing mild distention of the renal collecting system and mild evidence of ureteral tortuosity. Grade IV reflux: moderate reflux into the renal collecting system, causing moderate distention of the intrarenal collecting system as well as tortuosity of the ureter. Grade V reflux: severe reflux into the renal collecting system, causing severe distention of the intrarenal collecting system and pronounced tortuosity of the ureter.

half of the isotope has been eliminated from the kidney. Scintigraphy is also used to evaluate renal function after surgery.

Those with prenatally detected HN have at least three possible outcomes. In about 50% the HN resolves before birth, and results of other studies are normal.[28] Some have stable postnatal HN with no loss of renal function, and others will have progression of HN and diminished renal function on scintigraphy, prompting surgery.

URETEROPELVIC JUNCTION OBSTRUCTION

UPJO is the most common etiology of prenatally diagnosed obstructive HN, occurring in about 3 per 1000 births.[46]

Approximately 60% to 65% of the patients are male, and 60% to 65% of cases involve the left kidney. UPJO occurs in single systems and in the lower pole of kidneys with incompletely or completely duplicated ureters and has an increased incidence in horseshoe kidneys. In 10% to 20% of patients, UPJO is bilateral. Of children with a MCDK, 15% have a contralateral UPJO.

The obstruction may result from intrinsic narrowing of the ureteropelvic junction or extrinsic compression of the proximal ureter, usually from vessels about the renal hilum.[58,59] Extrinsic compression by vessels is an uncommon cause of prenatal and neonatal HN and more often presents in later childhood.[59] Much less often, the UPJO is caused by intraluminal processes such as ureteral valves or polyps. Insertion of the ureter above the most dependent portion of the renal pelvis may be a primary or secondary lesion that impedes urine flow from the kidney. A retrocaval ureter, an anomaly of development of the inferior vena cava, is often associated with right-sided hydroureteronephrosis but is not considered a true UPJO. Sonography may demonstrate only the dilated renal pelvis with a retrocaval ureter, which may simulate a UPJO.

UPJO is a possible diagnosis when HN is detected prenatally but may not become manifest until later when the child presents with a urinary tract infection or flank mass. The dilated renal pelvis is sensitive to trauma, and the child may develop hematuria after a minor injury. Less commonly, a child may present with intermittent nausea, vomiting, and upper abdominal pain. This situation occurs when copious diuresis is induced by ingestion of a large volume of a preferred and tasty beverage. These symptoms suggest a UPJO due to extrinsic vascular compression.[58]

Imaging studies include sonography, diuretic-enhanced renal scintigraphy, and VCUG (Fig. 4–6). Excretory urography, which is rarely performed, typically reveals ipsilateral delayed function, caliceal crescents, delayed contrast material excretion, a dilated pelvicaliceal system, and a variable amount of parenchymal loss. Corresponding changes are noted on contrast-enhanced computed tomography (CT) scans. When a small segment of dilated proximal ureter is identified on contrast studies, extrinsic vascular compression is the likely etiology.[58] CT or magnetic resonance angiography may be useful preoperatively when the child's findings suggest a crossing vessel as a cause of the UPJO. Retrograde ureterography and the Whitaker test have been largely supplanted by high-quality imaging studies.

Reflux accompanies UPJO in about 10% of children and may hasten corrective surgery. Diagnosis of reflux is usually made with a VCUG or nuclear cystogram. In the presence of reflux, UPJO is suggested by a number of findings: dilution of contrast material entering the renal pelvis, dissimilarity of the reflux grade in the ureter and the renal pelvis, and failure of the renal pelvis to drain on a delayed image.

Pyeloplasty to correct UPJO can be performed endoscopically or with open surgery. Postoperatively, drainage from the renal pelvis is improved, but renal function is usually stabilized rather than improved.[47] A small percentage of children continue to have decreased function despite technically successful pyeloplasty.[71]

PRIMARY (APERISTALTIC) MEGAURETER

Primary megaureter is a term that describes a dilated ureter that drains poorly in the absence of a discernible mechanical obstruction such as a stricture or ureterocele. Other causes of ureteral dilatation (polyuria or infection) are relevant after, but not before, birth. A number of pathologic processes have been implicated in the development of primary megaureter, but none has been established with certainty. Primary megaureter is the second most common obstructive process producing fetal HN. Boys account for 60% to 80% of occurrences. Bilateral involvement occurs in 25% and more often in those diagnosed prenatally or in infancy. Reflux can occur in up to 10% of affected ureters and may confound the diagnosis. Ipsilateral UPJO complicates the lower obstruction in about 10%. Such tandem obstruction is easier to diagnose with renal scintigraphy than sonographically.[50,66]

The resultant hydroureteronephrosis may be detected pre- or postnatally. The postnatal imaging sequence is sonography, which, if results are still positive, is followed by a VCUG and diuretic renal scintigraphy (Fig. 4–7). Both the postnatal sonogram and scintigram demonstrate the dilated ureter. When VUR is present, a delayed VCUG image depicts the lack of drainage from the ureter.

Surgical correction requires excision of the nondilated, aperistaltic distal segment and reimplantation of the remaining ureter. This procedure also corrects concomitant reflux.

POSTERIOR URETHRAL VALVES (PUV)

PUVs occur in about 1 in 10,000 live male births. In about half, the diagnosis is made or suspected on prenatal sonography (Fig. 4–8 and 4–9). Otherwise, diagnosis follows a presentation of urinary tract infection, abdominal distention, failure to thrive, or difficulty voiding. In approximately 70%, the obstruction is diagnosed before 1 year of age.

The usual prenatal sonographic description of PUV includes visualization of a dilated bladder with a thickened wall and the less commonly seen "keyhole" deformity of the

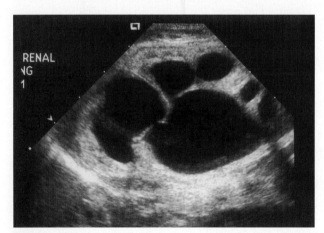

Figure 4–6
Severe hydronephrosis (Grade 4) in a 2-month-old girl with a urinary tract infection (UTI). Note marked caliectasis. Grade 3 reflux was present in addition to the UPJO.

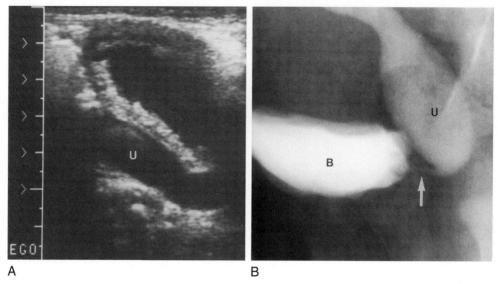

Figure 4–7
Primary megaureter: incidental finding during a workup for UTI. *A,* This sonogram reveals marked distal ureteral dilatation. *B,* Note severe narrowing of the distal left ureter as defined with a VCUG *(arrow).* This congenital disorder is the most common cause of obstruction at the lower end of the ureter. The left side is more commonly affected, and 20% of cases are bilateral. There is a marked male predominance.

dilated prostatic urethra beneath the bladder base. Two additional findings are thickening of the posterior urethra and visualization of the valves themselves as bright echogenic lines in the posterior urethra.[14] HN or hydroureteronephrosis is common, may be uni- or bilateral, and develops secondary to reflux or to obstruction produced by the thickened bladder wall. Bilateral moderate or severe hydroureteronephrosis is associated with a poor outcome, defined as perinatal death

or end-stage renal disease.[34] The diagnosis of PUV must be approached with caution because about half of those thought to have PUV in utero may prove to have other urinary tract anomalies: prune belly syndrome, urethral atresia/duplication, megacystis-megaureter, MCDK, or reflux.[1]

The amount of amniotic fluid is important. Oligohydramnios presages development of Potter's sequence with pulmonary hypoplasia if prenatal intervention is not accomplished.

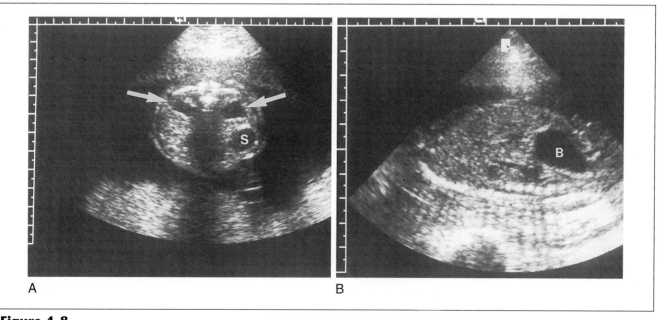

Figure 4–8
Prenatal diagnosis: posterior urethral valves (PUV). *A,* Axial view of a prone 22-week fetus. Note upper tract dilatation *(arrows).* S, stomach. *B,* The sagittal view reveals moderately severe dilatation of the bladder. The diagnosis of PUV was confirmed at birth.

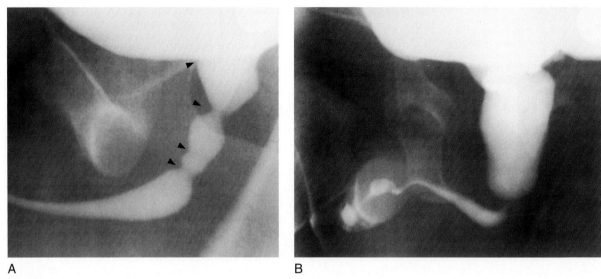

A   B

Figure 4–9

Normal male urethra. *A,* Note the very prominent intermuscular incisura (junction of striated and smooth muscle) across the midportion of the verumontanum *(top arrowhead).* A circumferential indentation is produced by the urogenital diaphragm *(bottom arrowhead).* The levator sling *(middle arrowhead)* is seen as a distinct indentation between the intermuscular incisura and the urogenital diaphragm. *B,* PUVs. There is marked elongation and dilatation of the posterior urethra secondary to PUVs.

Perirenal urinoma may develop and appear as a focal fluid collection, simulating an obstructed upper pole, or urine may dissect beneath the renal capsule producing a lucent rim around the kidney. The urinoma may contain septations and thus simulate other cystic masses (Fig. 4–10). Because the kidney has decompressed into the urinoma, it may not demonstrate HN. Secondary urinary ascites may ensue as the retroperitoneal fluid enters the peritoneal space; its

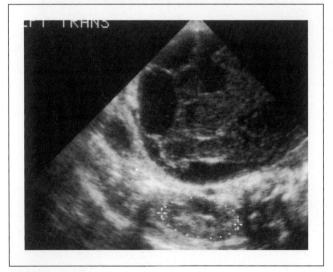

Figure 4–10

Postnatal transverse renal sonogram: PUV with urinoma: The septated urinoma is ventral to the nonhydronephrotic underlying kidney.

appearance is the same as prenatal ascites from other causes. Associated renal dysplasia should be suspected when the renal parenchyma is unusually echogenic or contains small cysts.[38]

Two types of PUV are commonly seen: types I and III. Type I is the most common, accounting for more than 90% of PUV. Type I valves originate on the verumontanum and extend distally for one or two leaflets. Type III is a fenestrated membrane across the urethra at the level of the urogenital diaphragm; the extent of symptoms is related to the size of the central opening.

The urethra proximal to both type I and III PUVs dilates and elongates. The obstruction also evokes hypertrophy of the bladder wall, which can progress to marked cellule or diverticulum formation. The changes in the urethra and the bladder interact at the level of the bladder neck producing a focal indentation or kinking. Reflux is identified in about one third of patients with PUV. Massive unilateral reflux associated with a nonfunctional kidney is a well-recognized entity. However, the refluxing kidney may function well and should be carefully assessed when nephrectomy is being considered.[17,21] The results of bilateral VUR are quite variable.[25] A kidney with VUR *and* urinoma tends to have better renal function than a contralateral refluxing kidney, but poorer function than a kidney with no VUR.[25]

Prenatal intervention involves placing a catheter in the bladder via fetoscopy. This vesicoamniotic shunt allows the kidneys to drain at a level above the obstruction and reverses the oligohydramnios but, unfortunately, does not necessarily preserve pulmonary or renal function.[32,49] Also, vesicoamniotic shunts may dislodge and require replacement. Prenatal correction of PUV is presently experimental. Other infrequently performed in utero procedures include cutaneous ureterostomy and bladder marsupialization. The rationale for prenatal intervention was questioned by a review of 36 fetuses: the fetal mortality rate was 43% and the long-term outcome differed little from that for those treated postnatally.[32] Postnatally, valve ablation is the most common treatment; vesicostomy is used in very small infants. Markedly dilated ureters above an extremely thickened bladder may necessitate high ureterostomy or a loop cutaneous ureterostomy.

The prognosis for affected fetuses is variable, and the diagnosis must be viewed with uncertainty in the prenatal period.[40] With confident diagnosis in the presence of oligohydramnios, the prognosis is grim, with a mortality of more than 60%. Most of these deaths result from the pulmonary hypoplasia evoked by severe oligohydramnios. Some infants with oligohydramnios survive the neonatal period but have profound renal failure in later infancy. Only one third of neonates with PUV have normal renal function in the neonatal period.[6] Half of the remainder recover normal renal function after treatment of the PUV.[6] Infants with a large, loculated urinoma or copious ascites may also have severe respiratory distress at birth that resolves when the excess fluid is removed or is resorbed following relief of the obstruction. Many infants with PUV have little or no respiratory distress at birth and no immediate urinary tract sequelae once the valves are treated. Long-term renal function is more problematic. Renal function may be adversely affected by the high bladder pressures that precede treatment of the PUV, by the associated VUR, or by secondary bladder problems. Renal failure ultimately develops in 30% to 60%, possibly reflecting prenatal dysplasia instead of the timing and type of surgery.[23,32] About 6% of those who survive the neonatal period have significant problems of both the upper and lower urinary tract and may die of chronic renal failure and its complications. Those with moderate to severe hydroureteronephrosis have a particularly grim outcome, with close to 90% (in a small series) either dying or having chronic renal failure.[34] Patients who are seen in infancy do better but still face the complications of renal dysplasia, VUR, and "valve bladder." Children whose PUVs are diagnosed later are not spared compromised renal function.[6] About 10% have renal insufficiency and require transplantation by age 11; in another 20% to 30% end-stage renal disease does not develop until the end of the second decade or slightly thereafter. Boys whose PUVs present after infancy have less severe symptoms and less sequelae.

Immediate postnatal evaluation of the urinary tract is focused on answering two questions. What is the status of the kidneys? Is the bladder obstructed by PUV or is a different process present? A plain film may show the mass effect of a dilated pelvicaliceal system or urinoma. Sonography determines the presence or absence of HN or cystic renal disease and demonstrates bladder wall thickness. VCUG permits visualization of the urethra and detection of VUR. Other obstructive processes, such as a prolapsing ectopic

ureterocele (unusual in a male) or an anterior urethral valve, are excluded.

Despite the valves, bladder catheterization is usually accomplished readily using a small feeding tube. In neonates with PUV, the first bladder filling may result in voiding at unexpectedly low volume. The second (and third) voids of the cyclic VCUG may follow instillation of normal or greater than normal neonatal bladder volumes. The bladder wall may be thickened and irregular with multiple cellules and diverticula. The bladder neck is also thickened and impinges on the superior aspect of the dilated and elongated prostatic urethra. The high pressure of voiding may also force contrast material into the prostate gland, even in neonates (Fig. 4–11). The abrupt change in urethral caliber in the posterior urethra is diagnostic of PUV, even when their direct visualization is obscured by the catheter. The findings of PUV do not overlap with those of normal urethrograms, even those that demonstrate prominence of the incisura or plicae colliculi (see Figs. 4–11 and 4–12).

To evaluate differential renal function, imaging usually involves ^{99m}Tc-MAG3 or other renal system–specific technetium chelates. Scintigraphy may be most helpful in evaluating the potentially dysplastic kidney with VUR.

After valve ablation, most boys are free of obstruction and require little imaging after the first postoperative studies. The posterior urethra may remain dilated initially and return to a normal size over months or years. Those with persistent VUR or a voiding problem may need to undergo cystometrography, which measures bladder pressures, the rate of bladder emptying, and other physiologic parameters.[19] Hypocontractility of the bladder can manifest as high bladder volumes that may inhibit ureteral drainage, transmit elevated pressure to the kidneys, and result in progressive renal disease severe enough to require renal transplantation.[19] Incomplete emptying produces abdominal distention, urinary tract infection, and overflow incontinence. Pharmacologic manipulation of bladder pressures and clean intermittent catheterization are used in this setting. Children with high-pressure bladders may also present with incontinence. When diagnosed early, the bladder abnormalities can be managed with bladder augmentation or a pharmacologic decrease of bladder pressure. Incontinence may also diminish or disappear at adolescence, a change that may result from development of the prostate gland.

MULTICYSTIC DYSPLASTIC KIDNEY (MCDK)

MCDK is noted in about 1 per 3000 to 4000 live births. It is the most common "incidental" finding on prenatal sonography.[43] The cystic component is derived from dilatation of obstructed distal tubules and glomeruli. The parenchymal dysplasia, associated with a drastic reduction

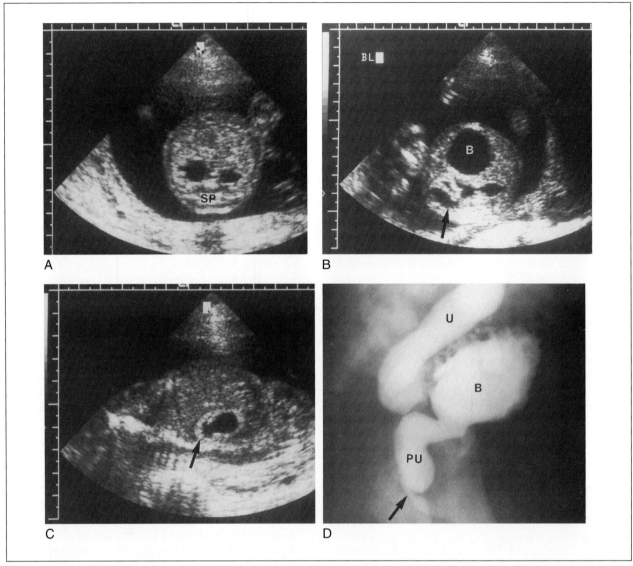

Figure 4–11
Prenatal diagnosis: PUV causing obstruction. *A,* This axial image of fetal kidneys reveals bilateral hydronephrosis. SP, spine. *B,* A more caudal axial image reveals an enlarged bladder (B) and a urinoma surrounding the right kidney *(arrow). C,* A longitudinal image of the left kidney shows severe dilatation of the collecting system and marked echogenicity of the renal parenchyma *(arrow),* suggesting early dysplastic changes. Repair of the PUV was uneventful. When last seen at 3 years of age, the boy's serum creatinine level remained elevated. *D,* Postnatal VCUG reveals PUV *(arrow),* a dilated posterior urethra (PU), a trabeculated bladder (B), and reflux into a dilated ureter (U).

in the number of functioning nephrons, usually develops secondary to focal atresia of the ipsilateral renal pelvis or ureter. MCDK may develop above a dilated patent ureter obstructed distally by a ureterocele in nonduplicated or duplicated systems.[9,39,74] Segmental MCDK has been reported in duplex, horseshoe, and crossed ectopic kidneys. MCDK may occur as part of some syndromes and in some families is an inherited trait, variously manifested as uni- or bilateral renal agenesis or MCDK (see Table 4–1).

Although the varied prenatal appearance of MCDK may make prenatal diagnosis difficult, it is diagnosed prenatally (75% of cases) more often than postnatally.[30] After birth, MCDK may be detected as a flank mass or, much less often, incidentally when the kidneys are imaged because of infection or trauma. When the typical appearance (cysts of varying size distributed randomly throughout abnormally echogenic parenchyma) is present, the diagnosis can be made with confidence (Fig. 4–13). Occasionally, the MCDK consists entirely of

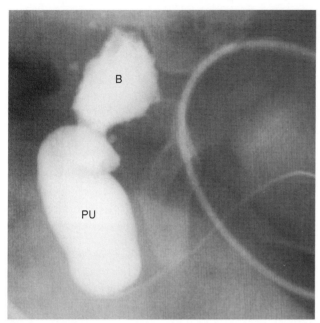

Figure 4–12
PUV in an 8-month-old boy who presented with a UTI. The bladder (B) is relatively empty and trabeculated. The fusiform, dilated chamber inferior to the bladder is the enlarged posterior urethra (PU). The urinary stream distal to the valves is markedly attenuated.

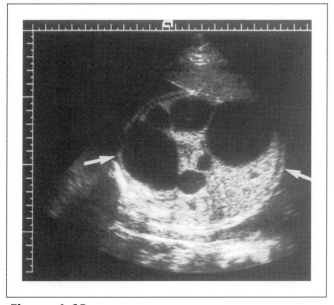

Figure 4–13
Prenatal diagnosis: multicystic dysplastic kidney (MCDK). This axial view of a fetus at 32 weeks of gestation reveals noncommunicating cysts of varying size (arrows). The contralateral kidney was normal.

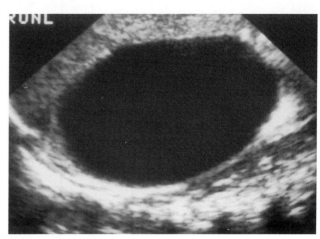

Figure 4–14
Postnatal coronal renal sonogram: atypical MCDK. The entire kidney is a single large cyst without any internal architecture.

a large solitary cyst (Fig. 4–14). When there are multiple cysts of similar size arrayed symmetrically, (the "hydronephrotic" variant), true HN may be difficult to exclude. Careful evaluation of the bladder may help detect causes of HN or hydroureteronephrosis. In utero the MCDK usually measures larger than gestational norms and, because of compensatory hypertrophy, the contralateral kidney may also be large.[31,37,60] The fetus with unilateral MCDK and a well-functioning contralateral kidney usually has a normal amount of amniotic fluid. Rarely, a large MCDK can impinge on the stomach and cause polyhydramnios suggesting gastrointestinal tract atresia.

Sequential prenatal studies reveal changes in the appearance of the affected kidney.[30,37,41,61,62,70] The cysts may enlarge, decrease, or remain stable; similarly, the kidney size may remain stable, increase, or decrease (Fig. 4–15). The kidney,

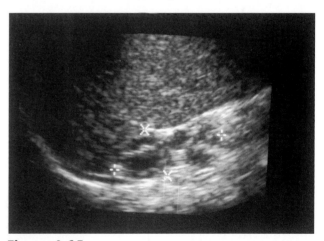

Figure 4–15
Postnatal sagittal renal sonogram. An involuting MCDK (between calipers) still contains a few small cysts.

along with its vascular pedicle, may completely involute, simulating unilateral renal agenesis.

Bilateral involvement, uniformly fatal, occurs in about 25% of infants and is associated with profound oligohydramnios.[42,43] About two thirds of affected children have anomalies of other organ systems, and stillbirths are more common than live births with subsequent death.[42,43] Although males have unilateral MCDK twice as often as females, bilateral disease is twice as common in females.[43] Another lethal variant is seen in the 10% of fetuses in whom the MCDK is the only kidney. These fetuses demonstrate Potter's (oligohydramnios) sequence: abnormal facies (micrognathia, flattened nose, creases beneath the eyes, and low and crumpled ears) and pressure effects on the limbs (closed apposed fingers, dislocated hips, and club or rocker bottom feet).

Contralateral renal anomalies are present in about 30% of infants with MCDK.[37,43] These include UPJO (in 15%), ureterovesical junction obstruction (in 6%), and ipsi- and contralateral VUR (in 10% to 25%).[37,42,70,75] Severe contralateral UPJO can result in oligohydramnios with its deformational consequences (Fig. 4–16).

Postnatal studies to confirm the prenatal diagnosis and to assess the contralateral kidney are usually limited to sonography and cystography. When there is a question about the diagnosis, as may occur in children with the hydronephrotic appearance of MCDK, renal scintigraphy can provide key information. In general, the MCDK does not function and appears as an isotope-free region. An occasional MCDK may have faint uptake of isotope, indicating that a few viable nephrons remain, but the appearance does not suggest a poorly functioning obstructed kidney.

Voiding cystourethrography is necessary because of the increased incidence of contralateral reflux and lower urinary tract anomalies[39,75] (Fig. 4–17). Lower urinary tract anomalies are reported in 32% and include ipsilateral reflux, ipsilateral ureterocele, and bladder diverticula. Cystic dysplasia of the rete testis occurs in boys with MCDK and has also been reported in association with only one other anomaly of the kidney: unilateral renal agenesis.[56,68,73] It is tempting to speculate that those children with cystic dysplasia of the rete testis and unilateral renal agenesis may have had a MCDK that involuted.

Before 1980, the MCDK was always removed surgically because diagnosis was limited by the imaging techniques available and because of concern about malignancy. Later, when sonography and, in unusual cases, CT imaging allowed confident exclusion of other mass lesions, the MCDK was usually left in place. Longitudinal studies document that within the first 5 to 10 years 48% involute completely and another 33% become smaller.[37] Physicians in many institutions still prefer to remove the abnormal kidney, citing the cost effectiveness of surgery compared with multiple sequential imaging procedures.[55] Two associations or complications, one infrequent (hypertension) and the other rare (possible malignant change), are also cited as reasons for nephrectomy. The hypertension may disappear following nephrectomy but does not always do so.[62] The paucity of case reports of malignancy in MCDK suggests that this is a real but

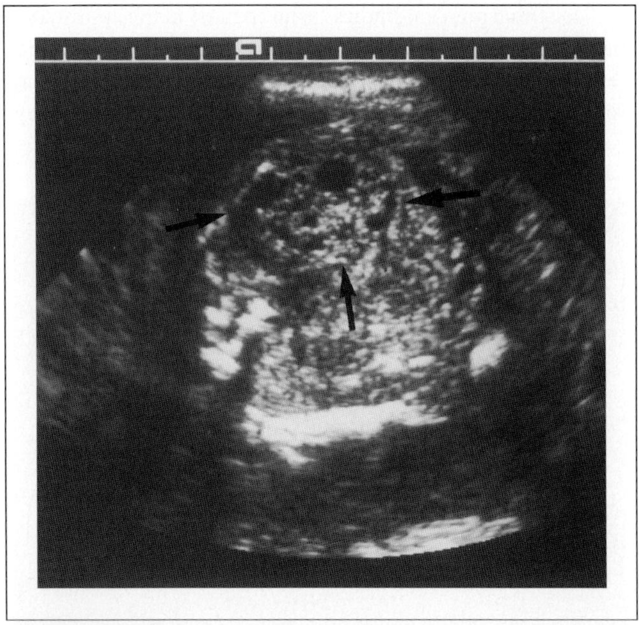

Figure 4–16
Prenatal diagnosis: single MCDK. Endovaginal scan of an 18-week fetus with a single MCDK *(arrows).* Severe oligohydramnios makes visualization difficult. The pregnancy was terminated, and the diagnosis was verified.

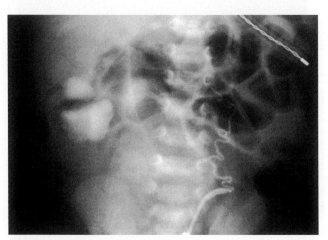

Figure 4–17
Bilateral retrograde ureterography: unilateral (L) MCDK with contralateral ureteropelvic junction obstruction. The tortuous right ureter is distended by the retrograde injection of contrast material. The small, poorly defined collection of contrast material above and medial to the ureter is a portion of the dilated renal pelvis.

very rare phenomenon. One longitudinal collaborative study of 600 patients with MCDK has yet to yield a malignancy.[70]

OTHER KIDNEY CYSTS

Prenatal diagnosis of a single renal cyst suggests several diagnoses: simple cyst, obstructed upper pole, unusual MCDK, and, very rarely, autosomal dominant polycystic renal disease or tuberous sclerosis. A search for associated or secondary findings or sequential studies usually facilitates distinction of these.

Simple cysts are commonly recognized at all ages as well as in utero, particularly on sonograms performed between 14 and 16 weeks of gestation and usually disappearing in late pregnancy or by birth.[10] Autosomal dominant polycystic disease should be diagnosed with extreme caution in utero and should be considered only when there is an affected parent. Asymmetric involvement of the kidneys may make the diagnosis more difficult, so cytogenetic analysis may be useful.

COMPLICATED RENAL DUPLICATION

Duplication of the ureters, commonly referred to as renal duplication, is a common renal anomaly. Autopsy series indicate that about 1% of the population has some form of duplication. In most cases, the duplication is incomplete with the two ipsilateral ureters joining above the bladder. However, about 0.2% of the population has two separate ureters extending from the kidney to the bladder or to ectopic sites (wolffian derivatives) in the pelvis and on the perineum. Bilaterality of duplication, without parallelism of complications, occurs in 12%. Although boys and girls have a similar incidence of duplication, complications of duplication are 6 to 8 times more frequent in girls than boys.

When both ureters enter the bladder in a normal location on the trigone, complications are rare. Otherwise, there are four main complications of ureteral duplication:

1. Obstruction of the upper pole associated with an ectopic insertion of the ureter with an associated ureterocele
2. Obstruction of the upper pole associated with an ectopic ureteral insertion
3. VUR into the lower pole and, least commonly
4. UPJO of the lower pole[24,27]

Of these, VUR is the most common.

The prenatal appearance of the renal duplication depends upon the associated complications, if any.[5,33] More than one complication may exist in a single kidney. A duplicated kidney without complications can be suspected when an otherwise normal appearing kidney has a length greater than the 95th percentile for gestational age.

In the setting of possible duplication, sonography of the bladder and pelvis should exclude a ureterocele or retrovesical extension of an ectopic ureter. Because the obstructed upper pole usually has little parenchyma, its fluid-filled infundibulum and calices can simulate an upper pole cyst, especially when the ureter extending inferiorly from it is not recognized. The fluid-filled upper pole can also suggest an adrenal cyst.

Lower pole dilatation should raise the possibility of reflux or lower pole UPJO or both.[27] The lower pole pelvis can also dilate when its ureter is extrinsically compressed by a dilated upper pole ureter or when the lower pole ureteral orifice is obstructed by an ispi- or contralateral upper pole ureterocele. Uncommonly, the appearance of a dilated upper above a dilated lower pole can simulate the appearance of a MCDK (Fig. 4–17). Results of prenatal detection are varied, with some authors claiming decreased postnatal morbidity and others disputing this.[5,65,72]

When not detected prenatally, complicated duplications usually present with urinary tract infection due to the stasis produced by obstruction and reflux. Sonographic evaluation of the bladder is key. An intravesical fluid-filled ureterocele may have a thick or thin wall. If large, it additionally may obstruct (1) the adjacent lower pole ureteric orifice and the contralateral ureteric orifice(s), producing dilation of the ureters above, or (2) the bladder outlet, resulting in bladder wall thickening. Infected fluid within the ureter appears echogenic, and a debris-urine level can develop in both the ureter and ureterocele.

The postnatal sonographic findings of duplication may be subtle: increased renal length and a split of the central renal echo complex into an upper and lower component. Despite the relatively normal appearance of the kidney, reflux may be present. Reflux, when present, is in the lower system in 95% of cases and produces the well known "drooping lily" appearance. Lower pole reflux is graded using the International Reflux Study system. Reflux into a dilated upper pole may develop after transurethral incision of a ureterocele, a procedure done to improve upper pole drainage.

Children (90% female) with ectopic ureteral insertion often present with wetness because most of the insertions are extra- or infrasphincteric (Table 4–4; Fig. 4–18). The ectopic ureter may drip urine continuously or maintain some reservoir function when the patient is supine. Renal sonography usually demonstrates an upper pole that is almost entirely composed of fluid. The dilated upper pole ureter cannot be followed into the bladder. Transperineal sonography may permit visualization of the distal segment. In boys, the ectopic ureteral orifice enters above the external sphincter (Table 4–4), and presentation involves urinary tract infection, orchitis, or epididymitis rather than enuresis or wetness (Fig. 4–19).

TABLE 4-4 Sites of Ectopic Ureteral Insertion
Female Urethrovaginal septum Vagina Urethra (distal to sphincter) **Male** Epididymis Vas deferens Seminal vesicle Prostatic urethra

Treatment and prognosis depend on the associated complication(s).

RENAL AGENESIS

BILATERAL RENAL AGENESIS

This lethal anomaly occurs in about 1 to 3 per 10,000 births. Prenatally, it is diagnosed when no renal tissue is present in a normal or ectopic location after about 12 weeks of gestation, the time when the kidneys are usually first identified.[44] A most telling prenatal sonographic finding is the failure of the bladder to fill and empty in the usual 30- to 60-minute cycle. Prolonged observation (up to 90 minutes) is recommended when neither bladder nor kidneys are seen. Color Doppler sonography can be used to look for renal arteries or

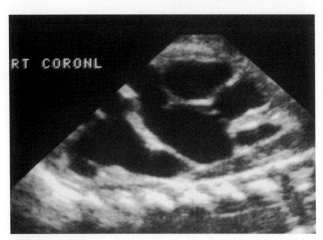

RT CORONL

Figure 4–18
Postnatal sagittal renal sonogram: duplex kidney simulating the "hydronephrotic" variant of MCDK. The dilated upper and lower poles do not communicate with each other. The slight asymmetry in the size of the calices also suggests cysts rather than typical dilated calices.

an ectopic kidney. When no renal parenchyma is visualized, other diagnoses to consider include renal hypoplasia and dysplasia.[44]

The adrenal glands have a characteristic abnormal appearance when the kidney is absent or ectopic: they are elongated rather than folded into their normal triangular or V-shape. Occasionally the adrenal glands may "roll up," fill the renal fossa, and simulate renal parenchyma. Bowel loops may also enter the empty renal fossa and suggest a hydronephrotic kidney, which is excluded by noting bowel peristalsis.

Despite renal agenesis, amniotic fluid volume may be normal in the first trimester because in this period the fluid is maternal in origin. As pregnancy progresses, the amniotic fluid volume diminishes and the absence of renal parenchyma becomes more obvious. In utero death (or elective termination of pregnancy) is common; fetuses manifesting Potter's sequence are stillborn or die in the immediate perinatal period.

In most families, the birth of an anephric infant is an isolated occurrence, but familial instances have been reported in which affected pregnancies demonstrate bilateral renal agenesis, unilateral renal agenesis, or renal dyplasia.

UNILATERAL RENAL AGENESIS

Unilateral renal agenesis is noted in about 1 per 450 to 1000 autopsies and occurs slightly less often in clinical studies. It appears to develop in one of two pathways. The first is a severe in utero insult to the ureteral bud or wolffian duct, which then fails to induce the adjacent metanephros. This may occur in conjunction with disrupted embryogenesis of other organs. The second pathway involves complete in utero involution of a MCDK. The variation in the incidence and pattern of associated anomalies and the presence/absence of the ipsilateral ureter and trigone may reflect these two differing pathways. Those children with the more pronounced associated anomalies are more likely to have primary renal agenesis. Occasionally, the solitary kidney itself is ectopic or malrotated, reflecting the prenatal insult to the developing metanephros. The association of cystic dysplasia of the rete testis with unilateral renal agenesis and a MCDK is another suggestion that, in some, the pathway to unilateral renal absence may be a MCDK.[56,68,73]

Amniotic fluid volume is normal unless the contralateral kidney is absent or abnormal. Absence of the kidney may not be sonographically apparent when the bowel or adrenal gland simulates a kidney. When a single kidney is present in a normal location, the other kidney should be sought in an ectopic location, from the pelvis to the thorax.

Anomalies of other organs systems are frequently seen (see Table 4–1). Some children with agenesis manifest the ever-expanding VACTERL (*v*ertebral, *a*norectal, *c*ardiac,

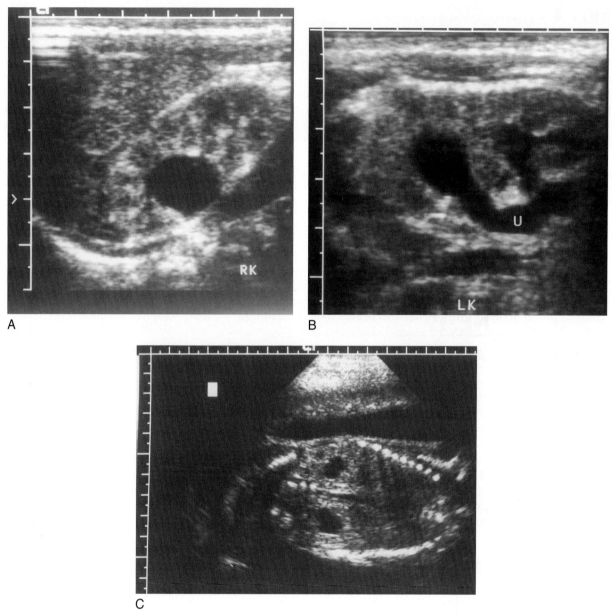

Figure 4–19

Prenatal diagnosis: renal duplication with bilateral upper moiety obstruction and ectopic ureteric insertion into the urethra. *A,* This coronal view of the left kidney shows upper moiety obstruction. *B,* A second coronal view of the left kidney (LK) shows upper moiety and proximal ureteral dilatation (U). Both upper pole ureters inserted ectopically into the urethra. *C,* Bilateral hydronephrosis had been detected prenatally at 24 weeks of gestation.

*t*racheo*e*sophageal, *r*enal, and *l*imb anomalies) association. Others have unilateral renal agenesis associated with only a single additional anomaly, commonly of the heart or skeleton. Renal ectopia may be present; indeed, 10% of children with a pelvic kidney have no other kidney.

In many children the solitary kidney is detected prenatally or postnatally when associated anomalies prompt evaluation of the genitourinary system.[69] A single kidney may also be detected only when urinary tract infection or trauma requires renal imaging. In some girls, the renal anomaly is identified at puberty when associated anomalies of the ipsilateral genital tract (the Mayer-Rokitansky syndrome) are noted, and the kidneys are imaged (Table 4–5). Searching for uterine anomalies in prepubertal girls with known unilateral renal agenesis is sonographically difficult and prone to error; MRI has been advocated in this setting and may provide clearer definition of the abnormal internal anatomy.[52] Ipsilateral genital anomalies are also present in boys, but

TABLE 4-5 GENITAL ANOMALIES ASSOCIATED
WITH UNILATERAL RENAL AGENESIS
IN GIRLS

Ovary
Absence
Fallopian tube-Absent, obstructed
Uterus
Bicornuate/duplicated
Unicornuate
Vagina
Atresia
Blind ending hemivagina
Hypoplasia

many are clinically subtle or without imaging findings
(Table 4–6). The one anomaly frequently imaged in association with unilateral renal agenesis is a seminal vesicle cyst,
but this is rarely seen until the second decade or much later.
Absence of the ipsilateral testis occurs in 1% to 5% of
children.

Treatment is focused on maintaining the function of
the solitary kidney.[53] A cystogram should be performed to
diagnose VUR, present in about 30% to 40% of children.[53,69]
Such VUR is managed as it would be in children with two
kidneys: by the grade of reflux, the age of the patient, and the
presence of complicating factors. When any degree of HN is
present, renal drainage should be assessed via diuretic renography, because obstruction of the ureteropelvic junction, the
ureterovesical junction, or both is noted in about 20% of
patients.[12]

TABLE 4-6 GENITAL ANOMALIES ASSOCIATED
WITH UNILATERAL RENAL AGENESIS
IN BOYS (IPSILATERAL ANOMALIES)

Ejaculatory duct
Absence
Seminal vesicle
Absence
Cyst
Testes
Absence
Hypoplasia
Cystic dysplasia of the rete testis
Vas deferens
Absence

SUMMARY

Prenatal detection of renal anomalies is common. When an
anomaly is suggested, several imaging maneuvers are necessary:
1. The contralateral kidney is assessed.
2. The condition of other portions of the urinary tract
   (ureter and bladder) is noted.
3. The fetal gender is determined.
4. The amount of amniotic fluid is estimated.
5. The presence or absence of anomalies of other organ
   systems is assessed.

This information is correlated with specific clinical information including chromosomal studies and family history.
Occasionally MRI may be warranted, especially if anomalies
may be severe enough to warrant elective termination of the
pregnancy. Sequential prenatal studies may also clarify the
urinary tract anomaly. Postnatal imaging often confirms
the prenatal diagnosis and can be used to plan appropriate
treatment.

REFERENCES

1. Abbott JF, Levine D, Wapner R. Posterior urethral valves: Inaccuracy
   of prenatal diagnosis. Fetal Diagn Ther 13:179–183, 1998.
2. Anderson N, Clautice-Engle T, Allan R, Abbott GD. Detection of
   obstructive uropathy in the fetus: Predictive value of sonographic
   measurements of renal pelvic diameter at various gestational ages.
   AJR Am J Roentgenol 164:719–723, 1995.
3. Arena F, Romeo C, Crucetti A, et al. Fetal vesicoureteral reflux: Neonatal
   findings and follow-up study. Pediatr Med Chir 23:31–34, 2001.
4. Aviram R, Pomeran A, Sharony R, Beyth Y, Rathaus V, Tepper R. The
   increase of renal pelvis dilatation in the fetus and its significance.
   Ultrasound Obstet Gynecol 16:60–62, 2000.
5. Avni EF, Dacher JN, Stallenberg B, Collier F, Hall M, Schulman CC.
   Renal duplications: The impact of perinatal ultrasound on diagnosis
   and management. Eur Urol 20:43–48, 1991.
6. Bajpai M, Dave S, Gupta DK. Factors affecting outcome in the
   management of posterior urethral valves. Pediatr Surg Int 17:11–15,
   2001.
7. Berrocal T, Gaya F, Arjonilla A, Lonergan GJ. Vesicoureteral reflux:
   Diagnosis and grading with echo-enhanced cystosonography versus
   voiding cystourethrography. Radiology 221:359–365, 2001.
8. Blane CE, DiPietro MA, Zerin JM, Sedman AB, Bloom DA. Renal
   sonography is not a reliable screening examination for vesicoureteral
   reflux. J Urol 150:752–755, 1993.
9. Blane CE, Ritchey ML, DiPietro MA, Sumida R, Bloom DA. Single
   system ectopic ureters and ureteroceles associated with dysplastic
   kidneys. Pediatr Radiol 22:212–220, 1991.
10. Blazer S, Zimmer EZ, Blumenfeld Z, Zelikovic I, Bronshtein M.
    Natural history of fetal simple cysts detected in early pregnancy. J Urol
    162:812–814, 1999.
11. Bosio M. Cystosonography with echocontrast: A new imaging
    modality to detect vesicoureteric reflux in children. Pediatr Radiol
    28:250–255, 1998.
12. Cascio S, Paran S, Puri P. Associated urological anomalies in children
    with unilateral renal agenesis. J Urol 162:1081–1083, 1999.
13. Clautice-Engle T, Anderson NG, Allan RB, Abbott GD. Diagnosis of
    obstructive hydronephrosis in infants: Comparison sonograms

performed at 6 days and 6 weeks after birth. AJR Am J Roentgenol 164:963–967, 1994.

14. Cohen HL, Zinn HL, Patel A, Zinn DL, Haller JC. Prenatal sonographic diagnosis of posterior urethral valves: Identification of valves and thickening of the posterior urethral wall. J Clin Ultrasound 26:366–370, 1998.

15. Conway JJ, Maizels M. The "well tempered" diuretic renogram: a standard method to examine the asymptomatic neonate with hydronephrosis or hydroureteronephrosis. A report from the combined meetings of The Society for Fetal Urology and members of The Pediatric Nuclear Medicine Council-The Society of Nuclear Medicine J Nucl Med 33:2047–2051, 1992.

16. Cromie WJ, Lee K, Houde K, Holmes L. Implications of prenatal ultrasound screening in the incidence of major genitourinary malformations. J Urol 165:1677–1680, 2001.

17. Cuckow PM, Dinneen MD, Risdon RA, Ransley PG, Duffy PG. Long-term renal function in the posterior urethral valves, unilateral reflux and renal dysplasia syndrome. J Urol 158:1004–1007, 1997.

18. Darge K, Troeger J, Duetting T, et al. Reflux in young patients: Comparison of voiding US of the bladder and retrovesical space with echo enhancement versus voiding cystourethrography for diagnosis. Radiology 210:201–207, 1999.

19. De Gennaro M, Capitanucci ML, Silveri M, Morini FA, Mosiello G. Detrusor hypocontractility evolution in boys with posterior urethral valves detected by pressure flow analysis. J Urol 165:2248–2252, 2001.

20. Docimo SG, Silver RI. Renal ultrasonography in newborns with prenatally detected hydronephrosis: Why wait? J Urol 157:1387–1389, 1997.

21. Donnelly LF, Gylys-Morin VM, Wacksman J, Gelfand MJ. Unilateral vesicoureteral reflux: Association with protected renal function in patients with posterior urethral valves. AJR Am J Roentgenol 168:823–826, 1997.

22. Ebel KD. Uroradiology in the fetus and newborn: diagnosis and follow-up of congenital obstruction of the urinary tract. Pediatr Radiol 28:630–635, 1998.

23. Farhat W, McLorie G, Geary D, et al. The natural history of vesicoureteral reflux associated with antenatal hydronephrosis. J Urol 164:1057–1060, 2000.

24. Fernbach SK, Feinstein KA, Spencer K, Lindstrom CA. Ureteral duplication and its complications. Radiographics 17:109–127, 1997.

25. Fernbach SK, Feinstein KA, Zaontz MR. Urinoma formation in posterior urethral valves: Relationship to later renal function. Pediatr Radiol 20:543–545, 1990.

26. Fernbach SK, Maizels M, Conway JJ. Ultrasound grading of hydronephrosis: Introduction to the system used by the Society for Fetal Urology. Pediatr Radiol 23:478–480, 1993.

27. Fernbach SK, Zawin JK, Lebowitz RL. Complete duplication of the ureter with ureteropelvic junction obstruction of the lower pole of the kidney: Imaging findings. AJR Am J Roentgenol 164:701–704, 1995.

28. Grignon A, Filion R, Filiatrault D, et al. Urinary tract dilatation in utero: Classification and clinical applications. Radiology 160:645–647, 1986.

29. Herndon CD, McKenna PH, Kolon TF, Gonzales ET, Baker LA, Docimo SG. A multicenter outcomes analysis of patients with neonatal reflux presenting with prenatal hydronephrosis. J Urol 162:1203–1208, 1999.

30. Heymans C, Breysem L, Proesmans W. Multicystic kidney dysplasia: A prospective study on the natural history of the affected and the contralateral kidney. Eur J Pediatr 156:673–675, 1998.

31. Hill LM, Nowak A, Hartle R, Tush B. Fetal compensatory hypertrophy with a unilateral functioning kidney. Ultrasound Obstet Gynecol 15:191–193, 2000.

32. Holmes N, Harrison MR, Baskin LS. Fetal surgery for posterior urethral valves: Long-term postnatal outcomes. Pediatrics 108:E7, 2001.

33. Hulbert WC, Rabinowitz R. Prenatal diagnosis of duplex system hydronephrosis: Effect on renal salvage. Urology 51(5A Suppl):23–26, 1998.

34. Hutton KAR, Thomas DFM, Davies BW. Prenatally detected posterior urethral valves: Qualitative assessment of second trimester scans and prediction of outcome. J Urol 158:1022–1025, 1997.

35. Irsutti M, Puget C, Baunin C, Duga I, Sarramon MF, Guitard J. Mesoblastic nephroma: Prenatal ultrasonographic and MRI features. Pediatr Radiol 30:147–150, 2000.

36. Isaksen CV, Eik-Nes DH, Blaas HG, Torp SH. Fetuses and infants with congenital urinary system anomalies: Correlation between prenatal ultrasound and postmortem findings. Ultrasound Obstet Gynecol 15:177–185, 2000.

37. John U, Rudnik-Schoneborn S, Zerres K, Misselwitz J. Kidney growth and renal function in unilateral multicystic dysplastic kidney disease. Pediatr Nephrol 12:567–571, 1998.

38. Kaefer M, Peters CA, Retik AB, Benacerref BB. Increased echogenicity: A sonographic sign for differentiating between obstructive and nonobstructive etiologies of in utero bladder distension. J Urol 158:1026–1029, 1997.

39. Karmazyn B, Zerin JM. Lower urinary tract abnormalities in children with multicystic dysplastic kidney. Radiology 203:223–226, 1997.

40. Karmarkar SJ. Long-term results of surgery for posterior urethral valves: A review. Pediatr Surg Int 17:8–10, 2001.

41. Kessler OJ, Ziv N, Livne PM, Merlob P. Involution rate of multicystic renal dysplasia. Pediatrics 102:E73, 1998.

42. Kleiner B, Filly RA, Mack L, Callen PW. Multicystic dysplastic kidney: Observation of contralateral disease in the fetal population. Radiology 161:27–29, 1986.

43. Lazebnik N, Bellinger MF, Ferguson JE 2nd, Hogge JS, Hogge WA. Insights into the pathogenesis and natural history of fetuses with multicystic dysplastic kidney disease. Prenat Diagn 19:418–423, 1999.

44. Latini JM, Curtis MR, Cendron M, Crow HC, Baker E, Marin-Padilla M. Prenatal failure to visualize the kidneys: A spectrum of disease. Urology 52:306–311, 1998.

45. Maizels M, Mitchell B, Kass E, Fernbach SK, Conway JJ. Outcome of nonspecific hydronephrosis in the infant: A report from the Registry for Fetal Urology. J Urol 152:2324–2327, 1994.

46. Mandell J, Blyth BR, Peters CA, Retik AB, Estroff JA, Benacerraf BR. Structural genitourinary defects detected in utero. Radiology 178:193–196, 1991.

47. McAleer IM, Kaplan GW. Renal function before and after pyeloplasty: Does it improve? J Urol 162:1041–1044, 1999.

48. McIlroy PJ, Abbott GD, Anderson NG, Turner JG, Mogridge N, Wells JE. Outcome of primary vesicoureteric reflux detected following fetal renal pelvic dilatation. J Paediatr Child Health 26:569–573, 2000.

49. McLorie G, Farhat W, Khoury A, Geary D, Ryan G. Outcome analysis of vesicoamniotic shunting in a comprehensive population. J Urol 166:1036–1040, 2001.

50. Meyer JS, Lebowitz RL. Primary megaureter in infants and children: A review. Urol Radiol 14:296–305, 1992.

51. Morin L, Cendron M, Crombleholme TM, Garmel SH, Klauber GT, D'Alton ME. Minimal hydronephrosis in the fetus: Clinical significance and implications for management. J Urol 155:2047–2049, 1996.

52. O'Neill MJ, Yoder IC, Connolly SA, Mueller PR. Imaging evaluation and classification of developmental anomalies of the female reproductive system with an emphasis on MR imaging. AJR Am J Roentgenol 273:407–416, 1999.

53. Palmer LS, Andros GJ, Maizels M, Kaplan WE, Firlit CF. Management considerations for treating vesicoureteral reflux in children with solitary kidneys. Urology 49:604–608, 1997.

54. Persutte WH, Hussey M, Chyu J, Hobbins JC. Striking findings concerning the variability in the measurement of the fetal renal collecting system. Ultrasound Obstet Gynecol 15:186–190, 2000.

55. Perez LM, Naidu SI, Joseph DB. Outcome and cost analysis of operative versus nonoperative management of neonatal multicystic dysplastic kidneys. J Urol 160:1207–1211, 1998.

56. Piotto L, Lequesne GW, Gent R, Bourne AJ, Freeman J, Ford WD. Congenital dysplasia of the rete testis. Pediatr Radiol 31:724–726, 2001.

57. Poutamo J, Vanninen R, Partanen K, Kirkinen P. Diagnosing fetal urinary tract abnormalities: Benefits of MRI compared to ultrasonography. Acta Obstet Gynecol Scand 79:65–71, 2000.

58. Rooks VJ, Lebowitz RL. Extrinsic ureteropelvic junction obstruction from a crossing renal vessel: Demography and imaging. Pediatr Radiol 31:120–124, 2001.

59. Ross JH, Kay R, Knipper NS. The absence of crossing vessels in association with ureteropelvic junction obstruction detected by prenatal ultrasonography. J Urol 160:973–975, 1998.

60. Rottenberg GT, DeBruyn R, Gordon I. Sonographic standards for a single functioning kidney in children. AJR Am J Roentgenol 167:1255–1259, 1996.

61. Rottenberg GT, Gordon I, De Bruyn R. The natural history of the multicystic dysplastic kidney in children. Br J Radiol 70:347–350, 1997.

62. Rudnik-Schoneborn S, John U, Deget F, Ehrich JH, Misselwitz J, Zerres K. Clinical features of unilateral multicystic renal dysplasia in children. Eur J Pediatr 157:666–672, 1998.

63. Sairam S, Al-Habib A, Sasson S, Thilaganathan B. Natural history of fetal hydronephrosis diagnosed on mid-trimester ultrasound. Ultrasound Obstet Gynecol 17:191–196, 2001.

64. Schild RL, Plath H, Hofstaetter C, Hansmann M. Diagnosis of a fetal mesoblastic nephroma by 3-D ultrasound. Ultrasound Obstet Gynecol 15:553–556, 2000.

65. Shankar KR, Vishwanath N, Rickwood AM. Outcome of patients with prenatally detected duplex system ureterocele; natural history of those managed expectantly. J Urol 165:1226–1228, 2001.

66. Shokeir AA, Nijman RJ. Primary megaureter: Current trends in diagnosis and treatment. BJU Int 86:861–868, 2000.

67. Sibai H, Salle JL, Houle AM, Lambert R. Hydronephrosis with diffuse or segmental cortical thinning: Impact on renal function. J Urol 165:2293–2295, 2001.

68. Simoneaux SF, Atkinson GO, Ball TI. Cystic dysplasia of the testis associated with multicystic dysplastic kidney. Pediatr Radiol 25:379–380, 1995.

69. Song JT, Ritchey ML, Zerin JM, Bloom DA. Incidence of vesicoureteral reflux in children with unilateral renal agenesis. J Urol 153:1249–1251, 1995.

70. Sukthankar S, Watson AR. Unilateral multicystic dysplastic kidney: Defining natural history. Anglia Paediatric Nephrology Group. Acta Paediatr 89:811–813, 2000.

71. Takla NV, Hamilton BD, Cartwright PC, Snow BW. Apparent unilateral ureteropelvic junction obstruction in the newborn: Expectations for resolution. J Urol 160:2175–2178, 1998.

72. Van Savage JG, Mesrobian HG. The impact of prenatal sonography on the morbidity and outcome of patients with renal duplication anomalies. J Urol 153:768–770, 1995.

73. Wojcik LJ, Hansen KM, Diamond DA, et al. Cystic dysplasia of the rete testis: A benign congenital lesion associated with ipsilateral urological anomalies. J Urol 158:600–604, 1997.

74. Zerin JM, Baker DR, Casale JA. Single-system ureteroceles in infants and children. Pediatr Radiol 30:139–146, 2000.

75. Zerin JM, Leiser J. The impact of vesicoureteral reflux on contralateral renal length in infants with multicystic kidney. Pediatr Radiol 28:683–686, 1998.

ADDITIONAL READING

Fagerquist M, Fagerquist U, Oden A, Blomberg SG. Fetal urine production and accuracy when estimating fetal urinary bladder volume. Ultrasound Obstet Gynecol 17:132–139, 2001.

Toiviainen-Salo S, Garel L, Grignon A, et al. Fetal hydronephrosis: Is there hope for consensus? Pediatr Radiol 34:519–529, 2004.

Berrocal T, Gaya F, Arjonilla A. Vesicoureteral reflux: can the urethra be adequately assessed by using contrast-enhanced voiding US of the bladder? Radiology 234:235–241, 2005.

Berrocal T, Lopez-Pereira P, Arjonilla A, Gutierrez J. Anomalies of the distal ureter, bladder, and urethra in children: embryologic, radiologic, and pathologic features. Radiographics 22:1139–1164, 2002.

Coplen DE, Austin PF. Outcome analysis of prenatally detected ureteroceles associated with multicystic dysplasia. J Urol 172:1637–1639, 2004.

Giorgi LJ Jr, Bratslavsky G, Kogan BA. Febrile urinary tract infections in infants: renal ultrasound remains necessary. J Urol 173:568–570, 2005.

Gordon I, Riccabona M. Investigating the newborn kidney: update on imaging techniques. Semin Neonatol 8:269–278, 2003.

Ismaeli K, Avni FE, Martin Wissing K, Hall M. Long-term clinical outcome of infants with mild and moderate fetal pyelectasis: validation of neonatal ultrasound as a screening tool to detect significant nephrouropathies. J Pediatr 144:759–765, 2004.

Miller DC, Rumohr JA, Dunn RL, Bloom DA, Park JM. What is the fate of the refluxing contralateral kidney in children with multicystic dysplastic kidney? J Urol 172:1630–1634, 2004.

Moorthy I, Joshi N, Cook JV, Warrant M. Antenatal hydronephrosis: negative predictive value of normal postnatal ultrasound—a 5 year study. Clin Radiol 58:964–970, 2003.

Nijs E, Callahan MJ, Taylor GA. Disorders of the pediatric pancreas: imaging features. Pediatr Radiol 35:358–373, 2005.

Odibo AO, Raab E, Elovitz M, Merrill JD, Macones GA. Prenatal mild pyelectasis. Evaluating the thresholds of renal pelvic diameter associated with normal postnatal renal function. J Ultrasound Med 23:513–517, 2004.

Ozcan Z, Anderson PJ, Gordon I. Prenatally diagnosed unilateral renal pelvic dilatation: a dynamic condition on ultrasound and diuretic renography. J Urol 172:1456–1459, 2004.

Perez-Brayfield MR, Kirsch AJ, Jones RA, Grattan-Smith JD. A prospective study comparing ultrasound, nuclear scintigraphy and dynamic contrast enhanced magnetic resonance imaging in the evaluation of hydronephrosis. J Urol 170:1330–1334, 2003.

Phan V, Traubici J, Hershenfield B, Stephens D, Rosenbloom ND, Geary DF. Vesicouretal reflux in infants with isolated antenatal hydronephrosis. Pediatr Nephrol 18:1224–1228, 2003.

Rabelo EA, Oliveira EA, Silva GS, Pezzuti IL, Tasuo ES. Predictive factors of ultrasonographic involution of prenatally detected multicystic dysplastic kidney. BJU Int 95:868–871, 2005.

Riccabona M, Koen M, Beckers G, Schindler M, Heinisch M, Maier C, Langsteger W, Lusuardi L. Magnetic resonance urography: a new gold standard for the evaluation of solitary kidneys and renal buds? J Urol 171:1642–1646, 2004.

Riccabona M. Assessment and management of newborn hydronephrosis. World J Urol 22:73–78, 2004.

Shukla AR, Kiddoo D, Kolon TF, Canning DA. The neonatal vanishing kidney: congenital and vascular etiologies. J Urol 172:317–318, 2004.

Toivianinen-Salo S, Garel L, Grignon A, Dubois J, Rypens F, et al (12 authors) Fetal hydronephrosis: is there hope for consensus? Pediatric Radiol 34:519–529, 2004.

Ylinen E, Ala-Houhala M, Wikstrom S. Prognostic factors of posterior urethral valves and the role of antenatal detection. Pediatr Nephrol 19:874–879, 2004.

Zurawin RK, Dietrich JE, Heard MJ, Edwards CL. Didelphic uterus and obstructed hemivagina with renal agenesis: case report and review of the literature. J Pediatr Adolesc Gynecol 17:137–141, 2004.

SPINAL ULTRASONOGRAPHY

Outline

CHAPTER

5

Rita Littlewood Teele, MD

SPINAL ULTRASONOG- RAPHY

EMBRYOLOGIC DEVELOPMENT OF THE SPINE

Much of our knowledge about anomalies of the spinal cord and vertebrae is theoretic and based in classical embryology. The timing of insults that result in maldevelopment is discussed here as an introduction to the ultrasonography of the spinal canal and its contents.

At 7 to 17 days postovulation, development of the notochord occurs with *gastrulation:* the "stomach-like" appearance of the three-layered embryo gives rise to this term. It is possible that anomalies of vertebral segmentation and malformations associated with split cord (diastematomyelia/diplomyelia) are caused by flawed signals between the notochord and neural tube and result in a duplicated neural tube.[8]

Abnormalities in primary neurulation (18 to 27 days postovulation) result in the spectrum of neural tube defects that includes rachischisis (failure of closure of much or all of the neural tube), anencephaly, cephalocele, open spina bifida, or meningomyelocele.[11,20]

Ectodermal dysjunction from neural tissue (27 to 28 days postovulation) may result in a dermal sinus between the skin surface and posterior spinal cord.

The distal cord and sacral vertebral segments, S2 through S5, are formed from totipotential germ cells and not from the primary neurulation. Proliferation of cells and tissues occurs with development; so, too, does apoptosis that results in regression of structures such as the rudimentary tail.[14] Defects in the process of secondary neurulation and failures in retrogressive differentiation occur at 28 to 56 days postovulation, which is equivalent to 6 to 10 weeks' gestational age[20] (Table 5–1). At the same time that secondary neurulation is occurring, other nearby systems are evolving; in particular, renal and cloacal differentiation is in process. Therefore, the association between anorectal anomalies, renal anomalies, and anomalies of the distal cord can be

TABLE 5-1 DEFECTS IN SECONDARY NEURULATION AND RETROGRESSIVE DIFFERENTIATION (28 TO 56 DAYS POSTOVULATION)

Lipomyelomeningocele
Tethered cord
Rudimentary tail
Caudal agenesis
Myelocystocele (often associated with cloacal malformations)
Sacrococcygeal teratoma

TABLE 5-2 INDICATIONS FOR SPINAL ULTRASONOGRAPHY OF THE NEONATE

Sacral agenesis (shallow intergluteal cleft and flat glutei)
Vertebral segmentation anomalies, especially sacral
Abnormal rectum or anus
Sacrococcygeal cleft or dimple that is deep, atypical, or both
Mass, dermal abnormality, or hairy patch over spine
Abnormal neurologic examination of legs or talipes
Sacrococcygeal teratoma
Paraspinal mass in chest or abdomen
Difficulty in accessing cerebrospinal fluid with lumbar puncture
Distraction injury when magnetic resonance imaging is unavailable

explained by an insult that affects these neighboring structures. Sacrococcygeal teratoma probably results from some of the totipotential cells developing in runaway fashion to become an exophytic (and variably intrapelvic) mass associated with the coccyx.

ULTRASONOGRAPHY OF THE NORMAL NEONATAL SPINE

When clinically indicated, scans of the infant's spinal canal and contents should be performed as soon as possible after birth. The sagittal window to the spine is through the cartilaginous synchondroses of the posterior spinous processes and the longitudinal ligament. Ossification of the laminae and posterior spinous processes prevents good visualization of the cord after 4 to 6 weeks of age. Scans can be used in older infants and children to localize the conus medullaris and to display other anatomic features but are difficult to perform and, importantly, are rarely convincing to clinicians who are accustomed to the elegant imaging available with magnetic resonance imaging (MRI) in older age groups. In the neonate, especially the premature infant, the sonographic images available with a 10 to 12 MHz linear transducer are equal to or better than some magnetic resonance images.[23] Clinical indications for spinal ultrasonography are listed in Table 5–2.

The infant should be fed or pacified; a moving target is not ideal. For views of the mid and lower spine, the baby is placed prone, across a small pillow or rolled blanket, with the back flexed and the head elevated relative to the lower spine. The cervical cord is best imaged by placing the infant in the decubitus position with the neck flexed. Sagittal views must be accompanied by transverse views. The craniospinal axis is considered as a unit. Scans of the brain are appropriate when an abnormality of the cord is documented.

The ultrasonographic examination should answer the following questions (Fig. 5–1):
1. Are vertebrae uniform in appearance and normal in number?
2. Is the cord of normal caliber and centrally placed in the canal?
3. Does the cord terminate in a normal conus medullaris above L2–L3?
4. Is the central echo complex a thin line within the cord?
5. Is the filum a thin thread extending from the conus to meld with the dorsal dura?
6. Does the thecal sac end at S2?

In some centers, radiographs of the spine are acquired before ultrasonographic scanning. If the clinical indication is such that scans are likely to be normal, for example, a dimple low in position that is unaccompanied by any other finding, it is best to obtain radiographs only if the ultrasonographic study is abnormal. Then, a BB or other metallic marker is placed directly over the termination of the conus medullaris so that the vertebral level can be confirmed radiographically. This ultrasonographic-radiologic correlation is also helpful in infants with segmentation anomalies (Fig. 5–2). Accurate numbering of vertebral bodies requires radiographs that include the entire thoracic and lumbar spine.

The cord changes subtly in size and shape throughout its course. The cervical cord is wider and slightly more oval than the thoracic cord, which is quite round. The lumbar cord swells out into a wider, oval shape before tapering at the conus medullaris. In normal neonates, termination of the distal cord is above the L2–L3 interspace.[2,3,13,16] The central echo complex is a dot or short dash on the transverse scans. It is a fine line on sagittal scans. This echogenic interface is generally considered to represent the myelinated ventral commissure abutting the anterior median fissure.[21] The filum terminale is a fibrous-glial thread that extends from the tip of the spinal cord. Its normal thickness is 1 to 2 mm.

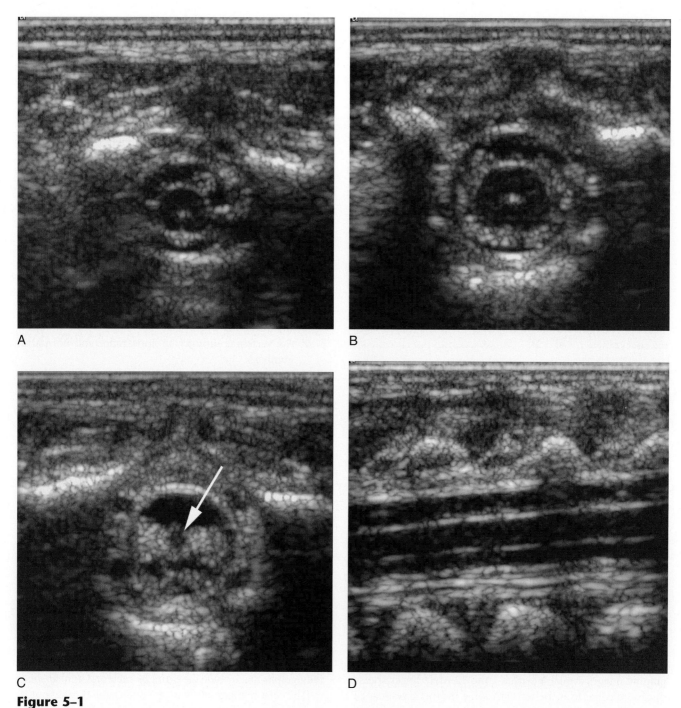

A

B

C

D

Figure 5–1

Normal scans of the neonatal spine. The transverse scan of the normal thoracic cord *(A)* shows the cord to be an echolucent structure with a central echo complex. The diameter of the thoracic cord is less than that of the lumbar cord, which is seen in transverse view *(B)*. A transverse view of the conus *(C)* shows a small, centrally positioned echolucent structure *(arrow)*.

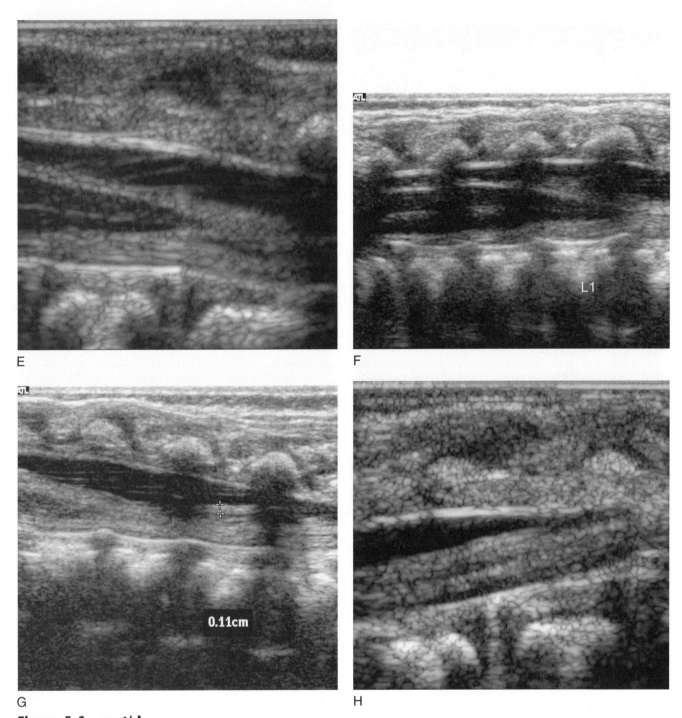

E

F

L1

G

0.11cm

H

Figure 5–1—cont'd

A sagittal view of the thoracic cord *(D)* shows a relatively echolucent structure with a central linear echo. The sagittal view of the lumbar cord *(E)* shows the tapering conus medullaris. The normal conus terminates above the level of the L2–L3 interspace *(F)*. On a sagittal view of the thecal sac *(G)*, the filum terminale is separable from nerve roots and mea-sured as being 1.1 mm in diameter. The normal diameter is less than 2 mm. The thecal sac terminates at the S2 level *(H)*.

Continued

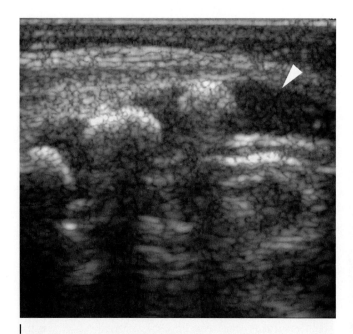

Figure 5-1—cont'd
A sagittal view of the lower sacral spine and coccyx *(I)* shows the coccyx as an unossified and therefore relatively echo-poor ovoid mass *(arrowhead)* at the inferior aspect of the spine.

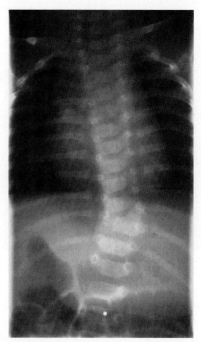

Figure 5-2
The vertebral level at which the cord terminated in this infant was difficult to assess on ultrasonography because of the vertebral anomalies. Therefore, following the scans, a BB was placed on the back at the termination of the cord, and this radiograph was obtained.

The filum intermingles with nerve roots but may be identified as a separate structure because it gradually melds with the dorsal dura in the distal thecal sac (see Fig. 5–1*G*). The sac itself ends in a tapering manner at the level of S2 (see Fig. 5–1*H*). In some infants, there may be a double interface in the distal cord or fusiform cystic inclusion in the conus medullaris. This is considered to be the ventriculus terminalis, occasionally termed the fifth ventricle and, if an isolated finding, is an embryologic remnant of no clinical significance[18,19,31,32] (Fig. 5–3*A*). Cerebrospinal fluid (CSF) may be trapped in shreds of arachnoid within the distal thecal sac (Fig. 5–3*B*). This, too, appears to have no clinical significance.[26]

ABNORMALITIES OF PRIMARY NEURULATION

Abnormalities of primary neurulation are clinically obvious in the newborn. The anatomy of the neural placode is predictable. Therefore, open spina bifida (aperta) should not be scanned because scanning adds nothing to the diagnosis and causes a risk of contamination of the site. Likewise, classic myelomeningocele, which has a covering of epithelial cells and thus can accumulate fluid, has the same underlying neural placode, which represents the unfurled neural tube. There are, however, abnormalities that affect the more proximal spinal cord and brain in infants who have open or closed primary neurulation defects.[4] The proximal spinal cord may be abnormal in 15% of affected infants. Hypoplasia of the cord, syrinx, and diastematomyelia may be present proximal to the primary anomaly (Fig. 5–4). One explanation for the concurrence of diastematomyelia with myelomeningocele is the occurrence of partial duplication of the neural tube and widening of the canal—an early embryologic event—that prevents normal closure of the neural tube and canal at another level.[8] Chiari II malformation, which accompanies abnormalities of primary neurulation, is discussed in Chapter 6.

One particular condition mimicking classic myelomeningocele may be confusing in its presentation. Rupture of the amnion early in pregnancy is thought to be responsible for amniotic bands that may constrict limbs and cause defects in the trunk and head. Interference with the developing posterior ectoderm can produce meningocele or myelomeningocele.

The ultrasonographic features of the amniotic band syndrome include (1) normal cord, *not* a neural placode at site of meningocele or myelomeningocele; (2) normal brain; and (3) other evidence of bands, for example, amputation of fingers or toes, or band-like constrictions around the limbs.

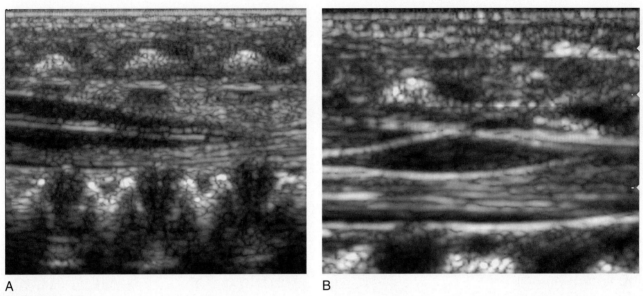

A   B

Figure 5–3
The ventriculus terminalis, an embryologic remnant of secondary neurulation, presents as a channel in the distal cord as shown on a sagittal *(A)* scan. As a solitary finding, it has no clinical significance. It may coexist with more extensive anomalies of the spinal cord (see also Fig. 5–7). Cerebrospinal fluid (CSF), trapped in shreds of arachnoid *(B)*, is another innocuous finding on ultrasonography.

CERVICAL MENINGOCELE OR MYELOCYSTOCELE

Cervical meningocele or myelocystocele is a singular malformation that affects the upper spine and may be confused with cephalocele on prenatal scans. Failure of the posterior cord to fuse in the cervical area and a gap in the adjacent mesoderm allow the central canal to balloon outwards into a cyst, contained by a second cyst, bounded by skin, of CSF from around the cord. If the walls of the central canal collapse together, a cord persists between the spinal cord and the wall of the outer cyst. This ependymal-neuroglial cord may be central, eccentric, or applied along the lateral wall of the outer cyst. The resulting images may be of a cyst within a cyst, a septated cyst, or a unilocular cyst[28] (Fig. 5–5). A Chiari II malformation may be present in some infants, presumably because enough decompression of posterior fossa occurs at a crucial time in its development. Many infants with cervical meningoceles have no intracranial abnormality, however, suggesting that the insult occurs later than is typically the case in an abnormality of primary neurulation (such as classic meningomyelocele). The cervical spinal cord may be deficient or dysplastic at the site of the defect, and local hydromyelia may develop after surgical repair of the meningocele. Close neurologic follow-up is warranted.

ABNORMALITIES OF SECONDARY NEURULATION

Lesions of the distal cord associated with mishaps in secondary neurulation are often accompanied by dermal abnormalities such as capillary vascular malformation in the midline of the back, a hairy patch, a skin tag, a deep dimple, or a cleft.[10,17] Central dimples or shallow pits below the gluteal cleft, typically at the level of the coccyx, are not associated with intraspinal anomalies and do not require investigation. A mass in the midline usually represents a lipoma and may be associated with dermal changes.[29] The appearance of some lipomas on physical examination is actually quite subtle. They tend to be rather diffuse, merging with normal subcutaneous fat. The term *lumbosacral lipomyelomeningocele* is an unfortunate choice because it includes some of the same terminology (i.e., myelomeningocele) that associated with defects of primary neurulation. In general, defects of primary neurulation have a worse neurologic prognosis than those of secondary neurulation. Importantly, abnormalities of secondary neurulation are *not* associated with Chiari II malformations of the brain.

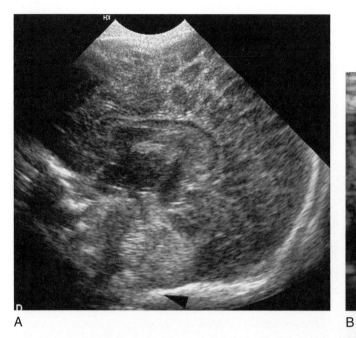

A

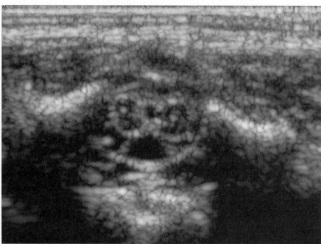

B

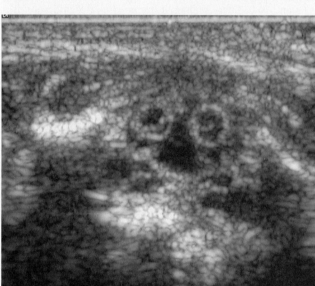

C

Figure 5–4
This neonate had had closure of a lumbosacral meningomyelocele. A Chiari II malformation of the posterior fossa accompanied the neural tube defect. The cerebellum extends below the level of the posterior fossa as marked by edge of occiput (*A, arrowhead*). Diastematomyelia, as shown on transverse views (*B and C*), was present proximal to the neural placode.

LUMBOSACRAL CORD LESIONS

Lesions of the lumbosacral cord include low termination of the cord (tethering), fatty filum (filum that is thicker than 2 mm or between 1 and 2 mm and very echogenic),

blunt or chiseled conus medullaris, syrinx, fatty tissue extending along the dorsal cord from a subcutaneous lipoma, meningocele, dermal sinus, dermoid cyst,[15] duplication of the cord, myelocystocele,[5] or combinations of these problems (Fig. 5–6). It is absolutely necessary, therefore, to be careful and thorough in scanning the spinal contents, correlating the findings from transverse scans with those from

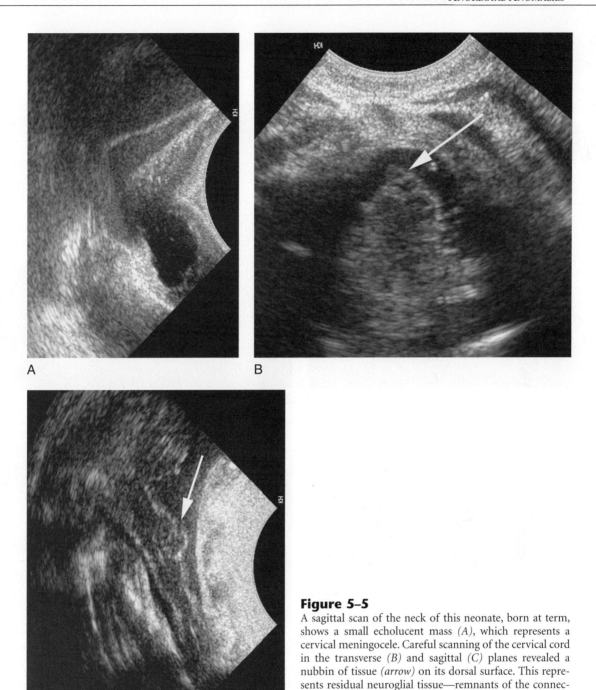

Figure 5–5
A sagittal scan of the neck of this neonate, born at term, shows a small echolucent mass *(A)*, which represents a cervical meningocele. Careful scanning of the cervical cord in the transverse *(B)* and sagittal *(C)* planes revealed a nubbin of tissue *(arrow)* on its dorsal surface. This represents residual neuroglial tissue—remnants of the connection between the meningocele sac and central canal (see text for full explanation).

sagittal scans, and documenting the correct level of termination of the cord or hemicords. Caudal agenesis refers to the failure of development of secondary neurulation or of exaggerated caudal regression. Sacral agenesis, typically below the level of S1, is part of this spectrum and is associated with agenesis of the distal cord, conal truncation, or tethering.[9,12]

ANORECTAL ANOMALIES

Screening of the infant who has an anorectal anomaly includes scans of the spine and of the kidneys because the timing of the insult often affects each of these locally developing organ systems.[7,27,30] Infants with low imperforate anus have a 17% chance of having a tethered cord or other anomaly

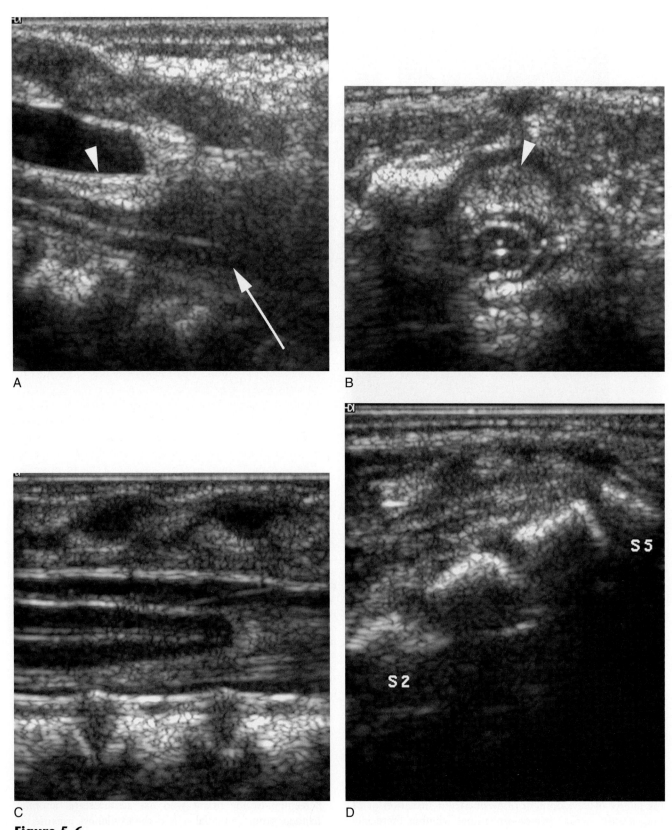

Figure 5–6
Lipomyelomeningocele with a tethered cord *(arrow)* and intracanalicular lipoma *(arrowhead)* is demonstrated on the sagittal *(A)* and axial *(B)* scans. A blunt conus in association with the ventriculus terminalis *(C)* and sacral anomaly at S5 *(D)* occurred in a patient with low imperforate anus.

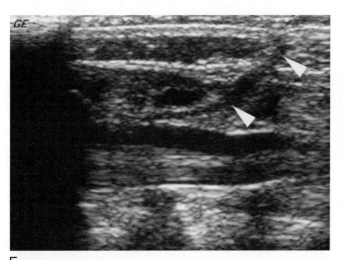
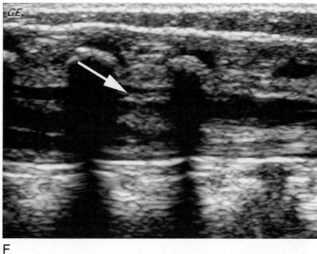

E

F

Figure 5–6—cont'd
In a third patient, a sinus tract through soft tissues *(E, arrowheads)* was continuous with a thread of tissue—dermal sinus *(arrow)*—that melded with the posterior cord *(F)*.

of the lower cord. The risk for those with high imperforate anus is double—34% (Fig. 5–7). In infants who have a cloacal anomaly, there is at least a 50% chance of an anomalous spinal cord.[2] All infants with cloacal extrophy typically have major accompanying vertebral anomalies and significant anomaly of the cord and may have myelocystocele as part of that anomaly.[1] Lumbosacral myelocystocele is defined as cystic expansion of the terminal spinal canal, low termination of the cord, and often a meningocele in association with the malformation (Fig. 5–8). In infants who have a major anomaly of the distal cord, scanning of hips in addition to the renal and reproductive tracts is worth considering.

SPLIT CORD ANOMALIES (DIASTEMATOMYELIA)

Diastematomyelia, or split cord, as an isolated abnormality has a predilection for the lower thoracic spine and lumbar spine. It may be diagnosed prenatally because an echogenic focus, representing the bony, cartilaginous, or fibrous bar, is present in the center of the spinal canal.[22] In addition, the canal is widened at the site of anomaly, disc spaces tend to be thinner, and there may be segmented or butterfly vertebrae in the same location. As noted in the Introduction, diastematomyelia may arise from an early embryologic insult to the notochord. If isolated, it is unassociated with intracranial anomalies. The amount of mesenchymal tissue trapped between the neural tissues determines whether there is a discrete bar and two cords ("diplomyelia") or a fibrous band and two hemicords (see Figs. 5–4 and 5–9). The cords may continue distally or fuse back into a single cord. A syrinx

may be present above the anomaly or within one of the hemicords. The fibrous band separating the two hemicords typically has a large arterial vessel that is obvious on color Doppler scans. In infants, in particular, plain radiographs may be subtly abnormal. Unless a bony bar is present, nothing can be seen in the central canal, and only slight widening at the site of the diastematomyelia may be recognized. Dermal changes may be present as a clue to an underlying anomaly.

SACROCOCCYGEAL TERATOMA

A sacrococcygeal teratoma is usually quite obvious on examination of the newborn, although some teratomas are occult and present later in infancy. A Currarino triad is the combination of a sacral vertebral anomaly—often a scimitar sacrum—anal stenosis, and a presacral mass that may be a meningocele, a teratoma, or other tissue type. This combination may be overlooked early in the infant's life, but, generally, the usual sacrococcygeal teratoma is quite obvious at birth as an exophytic mass anchored to the coccyx. Diagnosis may be made on prenatal scans, but the lesion may be occult in early gestation. We evaluated one baby who had had a normal scan at 18 weeks of gestational age, with good views of the distal spine and pelvis, whose large tumor was diagnosed as an incidental finding on a scan in the third trimester. In theory, pluripotential cells in the caudal cell mass fail to complete their retrogressive differentiation and develop into a teratoma related to the coccyx. The ultrasonographic features in the fetus, neonate, or both include (Fig. 5–10) (1) a generally

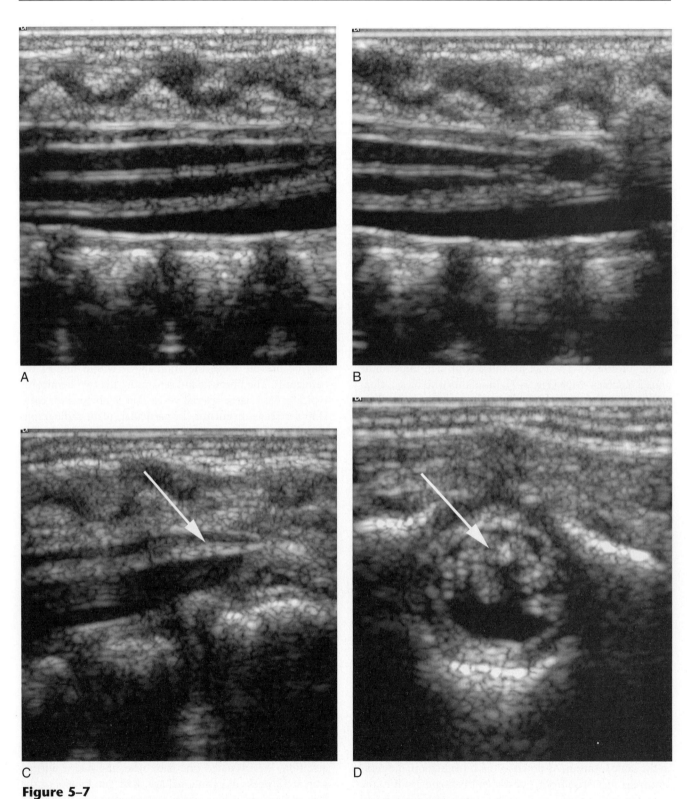

A

B

C

D

Figure 5–7
This neonate had high imperforate anus. Note the dorsal position of the distal cord in the spinal canal on this sagittal scan *(A)*. There is a pronounced ventriculus terminalis, a cyst at the termination of the conus *(B)*, and a fatty filum *(arrow)* on the sagittal *(C)* and transverse *(D)* views. Discovery of a tethered cord with low termination and a fatty filum requires a neurosurgical opinion and operative intervention for release.

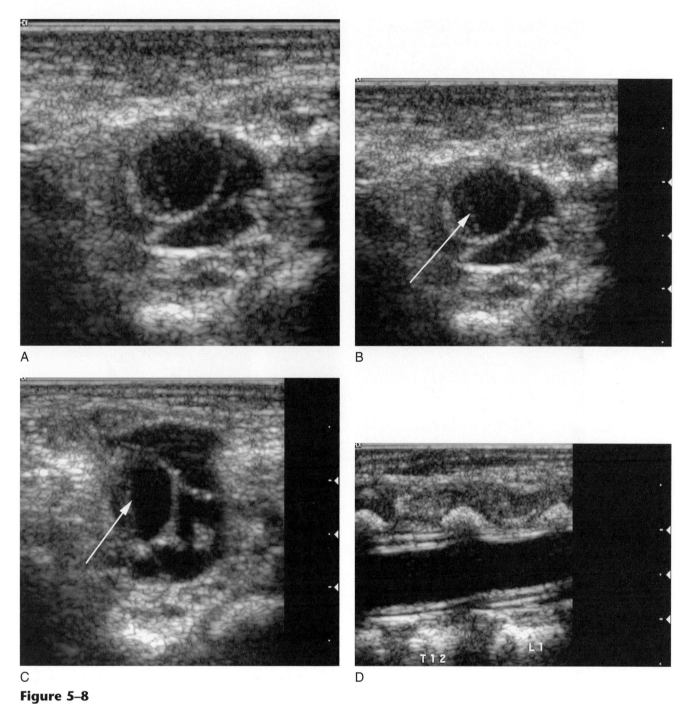

A

B

C

D

Figure 5–8

Myelocystocele refers to a dilated central canal that extends into a meningocele. Transverse scans *(A–C)* of the distal cord of this neonate show dilatation of the central canal *(arrow)*, which develops into a large sac that is contiguous with the meningocele sac. Sagittal view of the lumbar cord *(D)* demonstrate the dilated central canal.

Continued

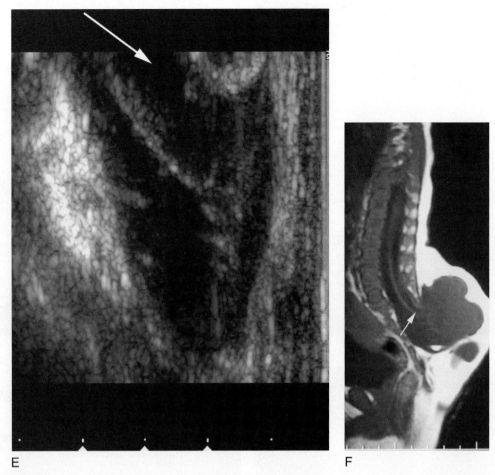

Figure 5–8—cont'd
Compare the sagittal scan of the myelocystocele *(E)* to the magnetic resonance imaging scan *(F)*. The *arrow* indicates the central canal.

large exophytic mass, contiguous with the distal spine; (2) a mass that may be cystic, solid, or both; (3) a mass that may be extremely vascular and associated with fetal hydrops; (4) an intrapelvic mass of variable size; and (5) a large intrapelvic component that can obstruct bladder outlet and ureters.

It is of interest that anomalies of the spinal cord rarely are associated with sacrococcygeal teratoma, but it is best to screen affected infants before surgery with ultrasonography or MRI. The major focus of preoperative imaging is to discover the extent of the intra-abdominal component of the tumor, and its effects on the urinary tract.

PARASPINAL MASS IN THE CHEST OR ABDOMEN

Discovery of a paraspinal mass in a neonate's chest or abdomen warrants careful evaluation of the adjacent spine and its contents. Neuroblastoma can be associated with an intraspinal abnormality. A duplication cyst of the foregut, of neurenteric origin, may present as a paraspinal mass and cervicothoracic vertebral anomalies. MRI is the imaging method of choice in such situations, with computed tomography scanning being a secondary option. Ultrasonography can be used to determine whether a mass is cystic or solid or vascular or avascular and associated with an intracanalicular mass or other finding relative to the spinal axis.

DIFFICULTY IN ACCESSING CEREBROSPINAL FLUID

Bleeding into the subarachnoid space around the cord occurs when there is an intracranial hemorrhage that pours through the foramina of Magendie and Luschka at the base of the skull. Blood in the upper cervical canal and even in the inferior thecal sac can be identified with ultrasonography in

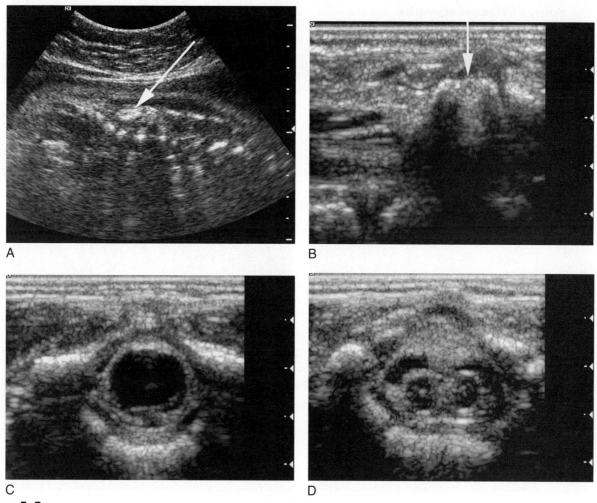

A   B

C   D

Figure 5–9
Diastematomyelia was diagnosed prenatally in this neonate because of a central echogenic focus in the lower spinal canal *(A, arrow)*. A sagittal postnatal scan *(B)* confirmed the bony spur *(arrow)* that shadowed the contents of the spinal canal. Transverse views above the bony spur show a syrinx in the cord *(C)* just proximal to duplication of the cord *(D)*.

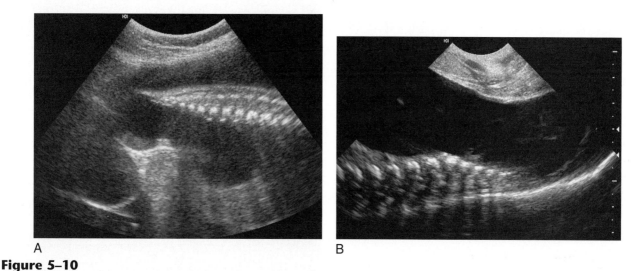

A   B

Figure 5–10
A sacrococcygeal teratoma was diagnosed prenatally in this girl. A prone sagittal scan of the fetus *(A)* shows the echogenic distal vertebral ossification centers with a large cystic mass anterior to the spine, extending inferiorly below the level of the expected pelvis. After delivery, a sagittal scan through the abdomen and pelvis *(B)* shows the large internal cystic component of this sacrococcygeal teratoma. The bladder, decompressed by urinary catheter, is not visible. No abnormality of the spinal cord was demonstrated with ultrasonography. Abdominal perineal resection of the mass was successful.

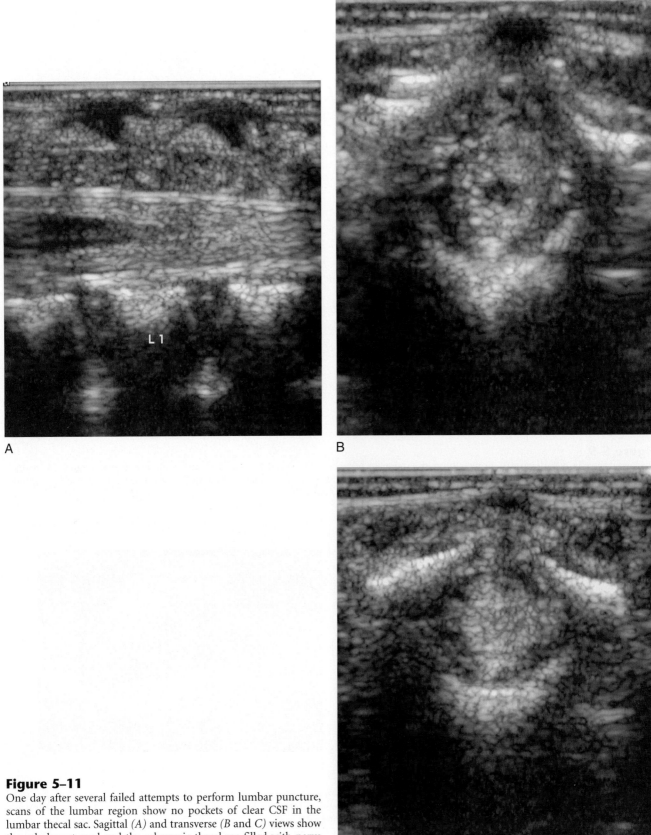

Figure 5–11
One day after several failed attempts to perform lumbar puncture, scans of the lumbar region show no pockets of clear CSF in the lumbar thecal sac. Sagittal *(A)* and transverse *(B and C)* views show the echolucent cord and the echogenic thecal sac filled with nerve roots and clotted blood.

such situations.[24,25] That lumbar puncture can fill the canal with blood has also been recognized. A common reason for repeated failure in accessing CSF from lumbar puncture in a neonate is clot from the original attempt. Subarachnoid or subdural blood in the distal thecal sac may take days to resolve (Fig. 5–11). Ultrasonography can localize pockets of CSF for aspiration.[6]

▌DISTRACTION INJURY

Distraction of the cervical cord can occur in difficult breech delivery of the neonate. Contusion of the cord may be evident on ultrasonography as a change in echogenicity of the cord. MRI is more revealing in this circumstance, but ultrasonography can establish the diagnosis if MRI is unavailable.

REFERENCES

1. Appignani BA, Jaramillo D, Barnes PD, Poussaint TY. Dysraphic myelodysplasias associated with urogenital and anorectal anomalies: Prevalence and types seen with MR imaging. AJR Am J Roentgenol 163:1199–1203, 1994.
2. Beek FJ, deVries LS, Gerards LJ, Mali WP. Sonographic determination of the position of the conus medullaris in premature and term infants. Neuroradiology 38 (Suppl 1):S174–S177, 1996.
3. Beek FJ, van Leeuwen MS, Bax NM, Dillon EH, Witkamp TD, van Gils AP. A method for sonographic counting of the lower vertebral bodies in newborns and infants. AJNR Am J Neuroradiol 15:445–449, 1994.
4. Brezner A, Kay B. Spinal cord ultrasonography in children with myelomeningocele. Dev Med Child Neurol 41:450–455, 1999.
5. Byrd SE, Harvey C, McLone DG, Darling CF. Imaging of terminal myelocystoceles. J Natl Med Assoc 88:510–516, 1996.
6. Coley BD, Shiels WE 2nd, Hogan MJ. Diagnostic and interventional ultrasonography in neonatal and infant lumbar puncture. Pediatr Radiol 31:399–402, 2001.
7. De Filippo RE, Shaul DB, Harrison EA, et al. Neurogenic bladder in infants born with anorectal malformations: Comparison with spinal and urologic status. J Pediatr Surg 34:825–827, 1999.
8. Dias MS, Pang D. Split cord malformations. Neurosurg Clin North Am 6:339–358, 1995.
9. Estin D, Cohen AR. Caudal agenesis and associated caudal spinal cord malformations. Neurosurg Clin North Am 6:377–391, 1995.
10. Gibson PJ, Britton J, Hall DM, Hill CR. Lumbosacral skin markers and identification of occult spinal dysraphism in neonates. Acta Paediatr 84:208–209, 1995.
11. Hahn YS. Open myelomeningocele. Neurosurg Clin North Am 6: 231–241, 1995.
12. Harlow CL, Partington MD, Thieme GA. Lumbosacral agenesis: Clinical characteristics, imaging and embryogenesis. Pediatr Neurosurg 23:140–147, 1995.
13. Hill CA, Gibson PJ. Ultrasound determination of the normal location of the conus medullaris in neonates. AJNR Am J Neuroradiol 16: 469–472, 1995.
14. James HE, Canty TG. Human tails and associated spinal anomalies. Clin Pediatr 34:286–288, 1995.
15. Kanev PM, Park TS. Dermoids and dermal sinus tracts of the spine. Neurosurg Clin North Am 6:359–366, 1995.
16. Kawahara H, Andou Y, Takashima S, Takeshita K, Maeda K. Normal development of the spinal cord in neonates and infants seen on ultrasonography. Neuroradiology 29:50–52, 1987.
17. Kriss VM, Desai NS. Occult spinal dysraphism in neonates: Assessment of high-risk cutaneous stigmata on sonography. AJR Am J Roentgenol 171:1687–1692, 1998.
18. Kriss VM, Kriss TC, Babcock DS. The ventriculus terminalis of the spinal cord in the neonate: A normal variant on sonography. AJR Am J Roentgenol 165:1491–1493, 1995.
19. Kriss VM, Kriss TC, Coleman RC. Sonographic appearance of the ventriculus terminalis cyst in the neonatal spinal cord. J Ultrasound Med 19:207–209, 2000.
20. Moore KL, Persaud TVN. Before We Are Born: Essentials of Embryology and Birth Defects. 5th ed. Philadelphia: WB Saunders, 1998, pp 424–452.
21. Nelson MD Jr, Sedler JA, Gilles FH. Spinal cord central echo complex: Histoanatomic correlation. Radiology. 170:479–481, 1989.
22. Raghavendra BN, Epstein FJ, Pinto RS, Genieser NB, Horii SC. Sonographic diagnosis of diastematomyelia. J Ultrasound Med 7:111–113, 1988.
23. Rohrschneider WK, Forsting M, Darge K, Troger J. Diagnostic value of spinal US: Comparative study with MR imaging in pediatric patients. Radiology 200:383–388, 1996.
24. Rudas G, Almassy Z, Papp B, Varga E, Meder U, Taylor GA. Echodense spinal subarachnoid space in neonates with progressive ventricular dilatation: a marker of noncommunicating hydrocephalus. AJR Am J Roentgenol 171:1119–1121, 1998.
25. Rudas G, Varga E, Meder U, Pataki M, Taylor GA. Changes in echogenicity of spinal subarachnoid space associated with intracranial hemorrhage: New observations. Pediatr Radiol 30:739–742, 2000.
26. Rypens F, Avni EF, Matos C, Pardou A, Struyven J. Atypical and equivocal sonographic features of the spinal cord in neonates. Pediatr Radiol 25:429–432, 1995.
27. Shaul DB, Harrison EA. Classification of anorectal malformations— Initial approach, diagnostic tests, and colostomy. Semin Pediatr Surg 6:187–195, 1997.
28. Steinbok P. Dysraphic lesions of the cervical spinal cord. Neurosurg Clin North Am 6:367–376, 1995.
29. Sutton LN. Lipomyelomeningocele. Neurosurg Clin North Am 6:325–338, 1995.
30. Tsakayannis DE, Shamberger RC. Association of imperforate anus with occult spinal dysraphism. J Pediatr Surg 30:1010–1012, 1995.
31. Unsinn KM, Mader R, Gassner I, Kreczy A. Ventriculus terminalis of the spinal cord in the neonate: A normal variant on sonography. AJR Am J Roentgenol 167:1341, 1996.

ADDITIONAL READING

Johnson MP, Sutton LN, Rintoul NE, et al. Fetal myelomeningocele repair: Short-term clinical outcomes. Am J Obstet Gynecol 189:482–487, 2003.
Mangels KJ, Tulipan N, Tsao LY, Alarcon J, Bruner JP. Fetal MRI in the evaluation of intrauterine myelomenigocele. Pediatr Neurosurg 32:124–131, 2000.
Midrio P, Silberstein HJ, Bilaniuk LT, Adzick NS, Sutton LN. Prenatal diagnosis of terminal myelocystocele in the fetal surgery era: Case report. Neurosurgery 50:1152–1154; discussion 4–5, 2002.
Naidich T, Zimmerman RA, McLone DG, et al. Congenital anomalies of the spine and spinal cord—Embryology and malformations. In Atlas S, ed. Magnetic Resonance Imaging of the Brain and Spine. Philadelphia, Lippincott, 2002, pp 1527–1631.

Simon EM. MRI of the fetal spine. Pediatr Radiol 34:712–719, 2004.

Simon EM, Goldstein RB, Coakley FV, et al (2000) Fast MR Imaging of fetal CNS anomalies in utero. AJNR 21:1688-1698.

Tulipan N, Sutton LN, Bruner JP, Cohen BM, Johnson M, Adzick NS. The effect of intrauterine myelomeningocele repair on the incidents of shunt-dependent hydrocephalus. Pediatr Neurosurg 38:27–33, 2003.

CRANIAL ULTRASONOGRAPHY

Outline

Rita Littlewood Teele, MD

CRANIAL ULTRASONOG-RAPHY

NORMAL ULTRASONOGRAPHIC ANATOMY

Standard views of the neonatal brain include coronal and sagittal scans through the anterior fontanelle at appropriate anatomic landmarks (Figs. 6–1 to 6–9). A cavum septum pellucidum or cavum vergae is present in all infants to 34 weeks' gestational age and in 36% of infants at term.[78] A small cyst of the choroid plexus is common and clinically insignificant.

The posterior fontanelle is a window[6,41] to the posterior occipital cortex, posterior horns of the lateral ventricles, and posterior fossa (Fig. 6–10). The suboccipital or foramen magnum view allows inspection of the lower portion of the posterior fossa (Fig. 6–11). It is especially helpful in infants with Chiari malformation and Dandy-Walker variants.[34,102] The asterion, or posterolateral fontanelle, is the window used during obstetric scanning for axial views of the fetal brain and measurements of biparietal diameter and head circumference. It is also valuable for neonatal scans. Axial and coronal views through the asterion allow better inspection of the posterior fossa than do views through the anterior fontanelle. This is an excellent window through which to view the third ventricle, aqueduct of Sylvius, fourth ventricle and adjacent structures, and the contralateral extra-axial space[24,41,68] (Fig. 6–12).

Small linear array transducers, 10 to 15 MHz, allow excellent resolution of structures in the near field. Through the anterior fontanelle, such structures include the sagittal sinus, meningeal spaces, cortical surface of the brain, bridging vessels, and frontal and parietal cortex[107] (Fig. 6–13). Using this technique, we have shown that premature infants of low gestational age have wider subarachnoid spaces than later-born premature infants when both groups are scanned at the same corrected age.[7]

Text continued on page 192

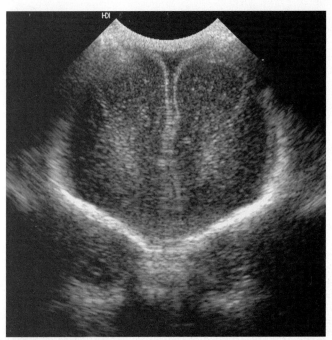

Figure 6–1
Coronal scan of the most anterior portion of the brain. Note the midline interhemispheric subarachnoid space, orbital roofs, and speckled echoes from the most anterior portion of the centrum semiovale, the frontal white matter.

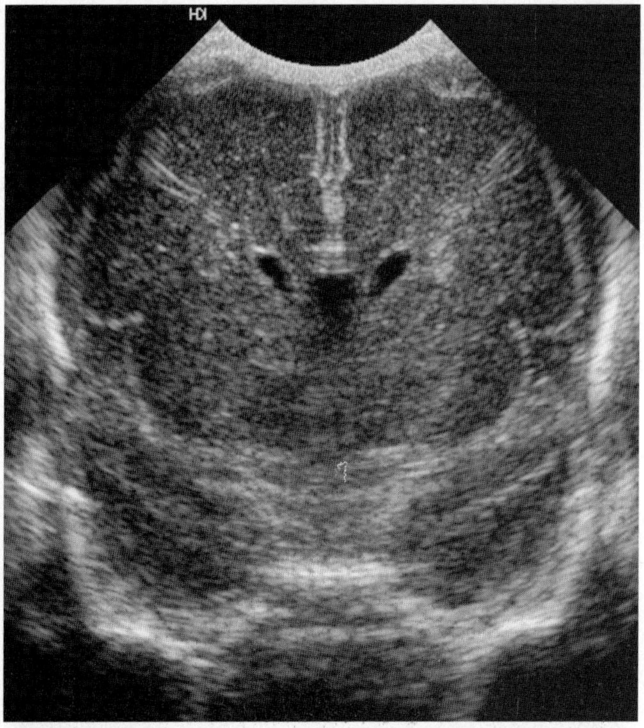

Figure 6–2
Coronal scan at the level of takeoff of the middle cerebral arteries from the internal carotid arteries is also in the same plane as the caudate nuclei. The anterior horns of the lateral ventricles, cavum septum pellucidum, and corpus callosum and anterior portions of the temporal lobes are all viewed in this plane.

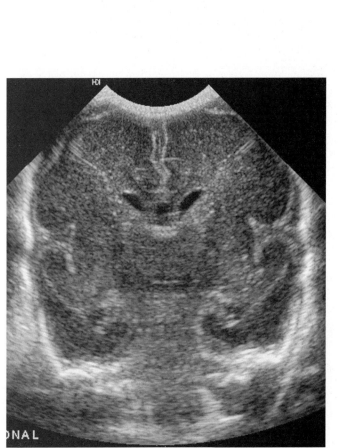

Figure 6–3
Coronal view of the brain through the foramen of Munro and anterior third ventricle. Note the T-shaped structure on each side that represents the Sylvian fissure, lateral ventricles, third ventricle with choroid plexus in its roof, temporal lobes with hippocampal gyri, and thalami at each side of the third ventricle. The normal third ventricle is slit-like.

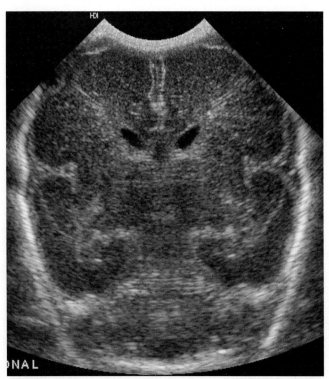

Figure 6–4

Coronal view through the cerebrum and posterior fossa at the level of the fourth ventricle. In this section, the lateral ventricles, posterior choroidal fissure, tentorium, and cerebellar hemispheres are visible. The normal fourth ventricle is difficult to identify. It may be visualized as a linear interface in the midline of the posterior fossa structures.

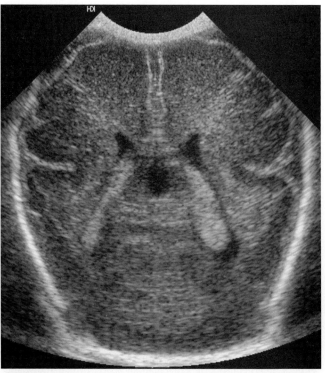

Figure 6–5

This coronal scan is angled posteriorly along the choroid plexus in both lateral ventricles. Continuation of the cavum septum pellucidum into the cavum vergae is evident. The cavum vergae presents as a central midline echolucent structure. This view is the best for evaluating the peritrigonal white matter.

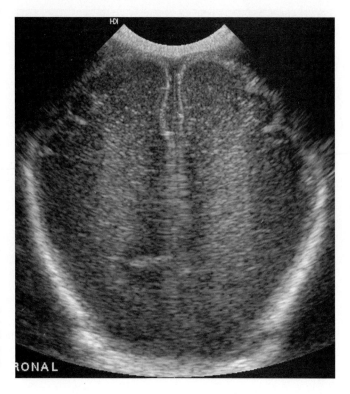

Figure 6–6

The final coronal scan is angled posteriorly and thus is close to an axial view of the brain superior to the lateral ventricles. The parieto-occipital sulcus is evident as an interface ending from the central midline interhemispheric fissure. The centrum semiovale, which represents the white matter, should be symmetric and uniform, and it appears as a speckled pattern on each side of the midline.

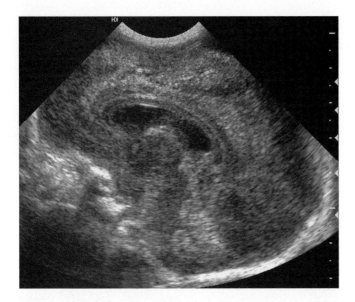

Figure 6–7

This midline sagittal scan shows the normal "Frisbee" shape of the corpus callosum. The corpus callosum is bounded on its inferior aspect by the cavum septum pellucidum anteriorly and the cavum vergae posteriorly. The normal third ventricle is essentially seen in outline. Only when dilated does it become evident on sagittal scans as an echolucent structure. The midbrain merges with the brainstem, both of which are relatively echolucent on scans through the anterior fontanelle. The pons, anterior to the medulla oblongata, is a more echogenic structure because of crossing fibers that are at 90 degrees to the interrogating beam of ultrasound. The vermis of the cerebellum is echogenic. The fourth ventricle is a subtle V-shaped defect in the anterior aspect of the cerebellum.

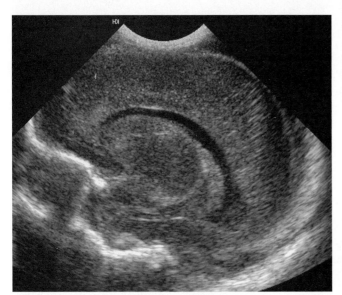

A

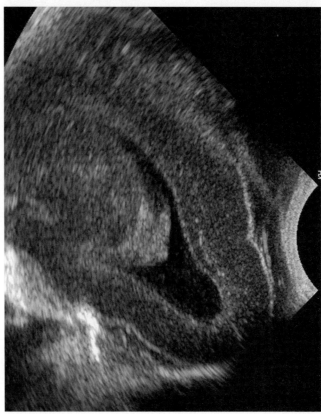

B

Figure 6–8

Parasagittal view of the lateral ventricle through the anterior fontanelle *(A)* and the posterior fontanelle *(B)*. The view through the posterior fontanelle is oriented to be similar to that through the anterior fontanelle. Note that the definition of the occipital horn is better on the view through the posterior fontanelle. The lateral ventricle has the appearance of a hand grasping the caudate nucleus and thalamus. The choroid plexus hugs the floor of the lateral ventricle.

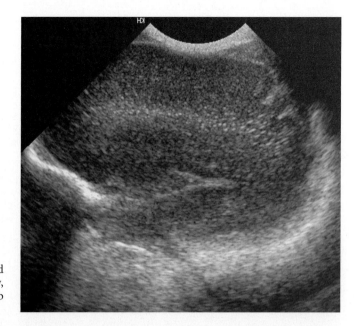

Figure 6–9
A parasagittal view angled laterally shows the frontal, parietal, and temporal lobes well. The appearance of the brain in this view, especially when it is immature, resembles a mitten, with the thumb at the position of the temporal lobe.

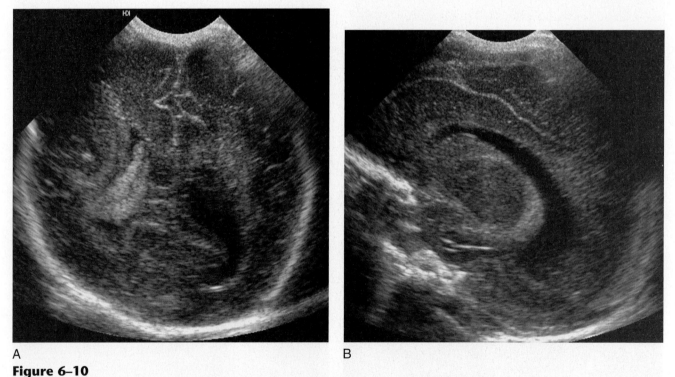

A

B

Figure 6–10
These views of the left lateral ventricle through the anterior fontanelle (*A* and *B*) show an ill-defined posteriomedial border. When viewed from the posterior fontanelle (*C* and *D*), the ill-defined border is identified as the occipital calcar avis.

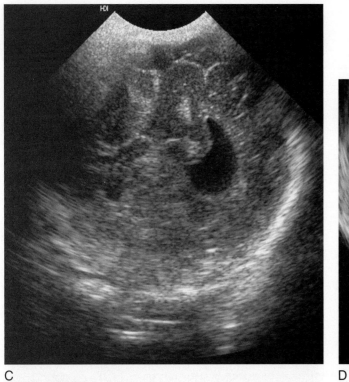

C

Figure 6–10—cont'd

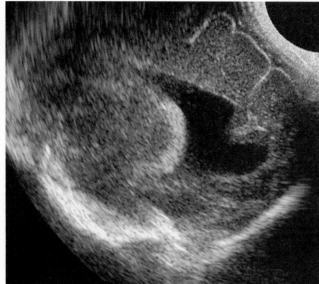

D

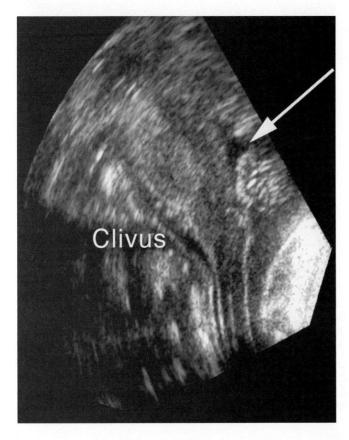

Clivus

Figure 6–11

This sagittal scan via the foramen magnum is oriented in anatomic position to coincide with other midline sagittal views of the neonatal brain. This view demonstrates the fourth ventricle *(arrow),* inferior cerebellar vermis, cisterna magna, and upper cervical cord.

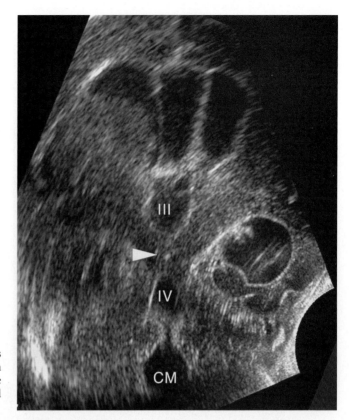

Figure 6–12
A coronal view through the posterolateral fontanelle in this premature neonate who had a dilated ventricular system following an intraventricular hemorrhage shows the anatomy of the third ventricle (III), aqueduct of Sylvius *(arrowhead),* fourth ventricle (IV), and cisterna magna (CM).

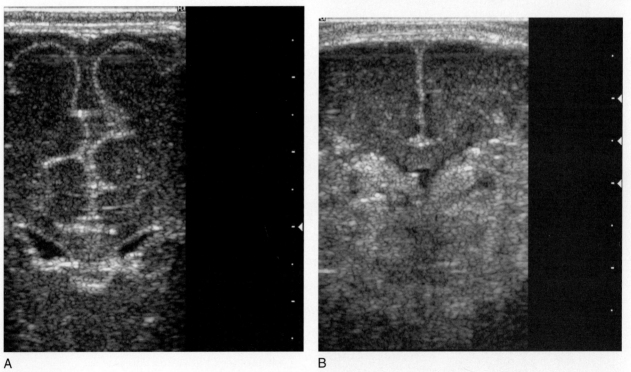

A   B

Figure 6–13
A detailed coronal view of the extra-axial spaces and cerebral parenchyma is achieved by using a linear array transducer of high frequency. The superior sagittal sinus is triangular on the coronal cross-section. It can be effaced with only minimal compression. Compare the normal scan *(A)* with that of a neonate born prematurely who had a marked abnormality of the cerebral parenchyma associated with hypoxic ischemic insult *(B).* The subarachnoid spaces have been effaced.

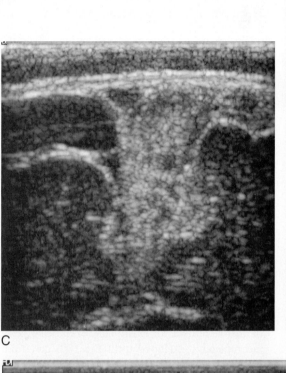

C

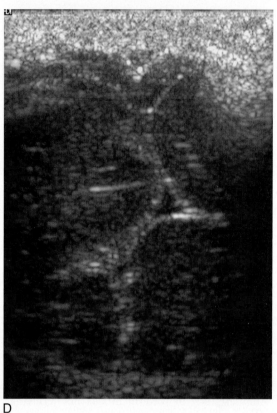

D

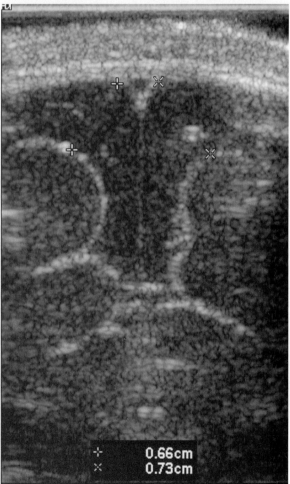

E

÷ 0.66cm
✕ 0.73cm

Figure 6–13—cont'd
A third neonate had a subdural hemorrhage on the left, resulting in increased echogenicity in the left extra-axial space *(C)*. Absence of the falx associated with indigitation of gyri *(D)* is a manifestation of trisomy 13. A detailed coronal view of the extra-axial spaces and cerebral parenchyma is achieved by using a linear array transducer of high frequency. The superior sagittal sinus is triangular on the coronal cross-section. It can be effaced with only minimal compression. Compare the normal scan *(A)* with that of a neonate born prematurely who had a marked abnormality of the cerebral parenchyma associated with hypoxic ischemic insult *(B)*. The subarachnoid spaces have been effaced. A third neonate had a subdural hemorrhage on the left, resulting in increased echogenicity in the left extra-axial space *(C)*. Absence of the falx associated with indigitation of gyri *(D)* is a manifestation of trisomy 13. Large subarachnoid spaces (greater than 5 mm in width) are common in infants who are born very prematurely and undergo scanning near their expected date of birth *(E)*.

Doppler ultrasonography of the neonatal brain is an adjunctive technique.[33] A description of cerebral blood flow is usually achieved by acquiring the resistive index (RI) of an insonated artery:

$$RI = (S - D)/S,$$

where S is peak systole and D is end diastole in centimeters per second or kilohertz.

Because the RI is a relationship, the angle of insonation is unnecessary for calculations. The anterior cerebral artery and basilar artery are each parallel to the interrogating beam via the anterior fontanelle, and, therefore, a Doppler waveform can be registered quite easily (Fig. 6–14). It is important to note that changes in the RI in a cerebral artery reflect not only intracerebral resistance but also the central pumping mechanism. A study of normal neonates born at term revealed a mean RI of 0.726 (0.057).[4] In a group of preterm infants receiving mechanical ventilation, continuous wave Doppler ultrasonography showed that central blood flow velocity increased during the first 6 hours of life to plateau at 16 hours of age.[27] Another study of preterm infants not receiving mechanical ventilation showed a mean decrease of 29% in mean flow velocity.[117] Because there are many confounding factors in considering the physiologic state of the preterm infant, "normal premature" is difficult to define. When a ductus arteriosus is widely patent—a common situation in the premature infant—the RI increases to 1.0 or higher because runoff through the ductus allows decreased antegrade flow or even reversal of flow in diastole. Where possible, documentation of scans should be on radiographic film or secure digital storage. Videotaping certain examinations, e.g. demonstration of vascular flow through an arteriovenous malformation/Vein of Galen aneurysm or documenting lack of vascular flow in an area affected by stroke, can be very helpful for demonstration to clinicians. The written report that is issued should be descriptive but concise.

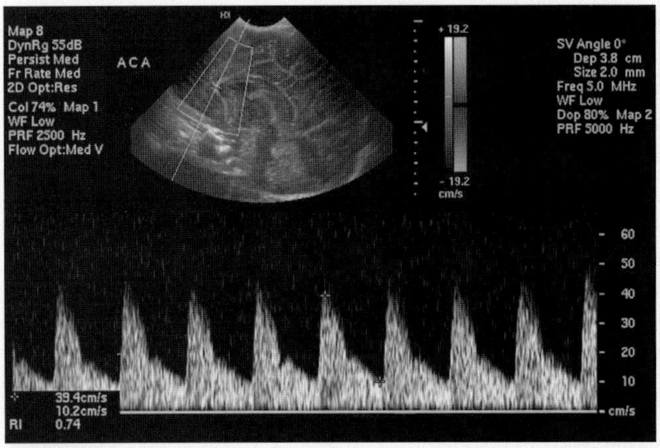

PRENATAL EVALUATION OF THE BRAIN

Prenatal obstetric sonograms, if performed as a screening procedure for estimation of gestational age and detection of anomalies, tend to be scheduled for the 18th week of gestation. These scans provide a reasonable estimation of fetal size and, by extrapolation, confirmation of gestational age (Table 6–1). They are taken late enough in gestation to allow adequate assessment of fetal anatomy. Some experts advocate screening for anomalies in the first trimester. The development of organs and, in particular, the brain is so rudimentary in the first 13 gestational weeks that a firm diagnosis of normalcy or anomaly is impossible from such a scan. In normal fetuses, for example, the cerebellar vermis may be incompletely developed until the 18th gestational week.[22] Prenatal sonographic screening of a fetus, at 18 or more weeks of gestational age, includes the following images and measurements of the craniospinal axis (Fig. 6–15): (1) documentation of size and shape of the head by use of measurements of biparietal diameter and head circumference; (2) width of the lateral ventricles; (3) appearance of the choroid plexuses; (4) cerebellar vermis and hemispheres; (5) width of the cisterna magna; (6) documentation of cavum septum pellucidum; (7) spinal ossification centers, and (8) skin line from occiput to sacrum.

Figure 6–14
The resistive index (RI) in the anterior cerebral artery is calculated by locating one of the paired arteries with color Doppler imaging, interrogating the artery with pulsed-wave Doppler, and identifying with electronic calipers the peak systolic and end-diastolic flow on the waveform. Normal is usually 0.7 to 0.75, as in this infant.

TABLE 6-1 MAJOR INDICATIONS FOR ULTRASONOGRAPHIC SCANNING OF NEONATES

Screening for germinal matrix intraventricular hemorrhage in preterm infants
Hypoxic-ischemic injury suspected, computed tomography and magnetic resonance imaging unavailable
Meningitis
Abnormal prenatal scan
Intracranial anomaly suspected
Unexplained blood loss
Preoperative screening, e.g., cardiac surgery, extracorporeal membrane oxygenation (ECMO)
Follow-up of documented abnormality
Research studies in designated units

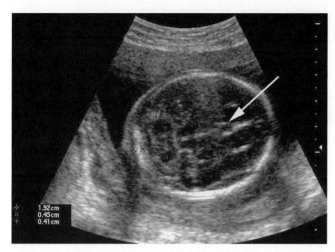

Figure 6–15
A normal axial scan of the fetal brain at 19 weeks shows the cerebellum, cisterna magna, and nuchal thickness, each measured by electronic calipers. In this view, the cavum septum pellucidum *(arrow)* is apparent in the midline.

During the first and second trimesters, the normal cerebral parenchyma is featureless, and the surface of the brain is smooth. At 18 weeks' gestational age, an invisible migration of cells from the germinal matrix is in progress; the neurons that will comprise the cerebral gray matter have not yet completed their climb along the radial glial fibers.[47]

Good views of the fetal intracranial contents are best obtained when there is a mother of normal weight, a fetus whose intrauterine position is conducive to viewing, the availability of good ultrasound equipment, and, importantly, an experienced sonographer. All prenatal scans are not created equal.

CONGENITAL ANOMALIES

Follow-up of an abnormal prenatal scan should include a review of those images before a neonatal scan is initiated. The brain is a complex, evolving organ throughout the pre- and postnatal periods.[11,12,58] Anomalies usually become more obvious with time; however, occasionally, they may be less obvious postnatally. In an example from experience, a subtle Dandy-Walker variant in association with a mid-cerebellar dermoid was occult on postnatal scans. The baby presented later with neurologic signs and symptoms that confirmed the obstetric sonologist's observation of a cerebellar abnormality.

Parents who have been told of a fetal intracranial abnormality are understandably concerned and sometimes frantic when scans are performed on their neonate. It is usually easier for all concerned if the family is not present during the procedure. A discussion with the parents, alongside the clinical staff involved with the family's care, can follow.

Ultrasonography is a method of evaluating anatomy. It is not a method with which to assess physiology. Other modalities such as computed tomography (CT) or magnetic resonance imaging (MRI) may also be needed for diagnostic certainty. The questions that families ask are rarely concerned with the anatomy of an abnormality; they are concerned with functional implications and prognosis. Such questions require considered, thoughtful replies from the imager and clinician.

It should be emphasized that an anomaly or abnormality of brain development may go undiagnosed prenatally and be suspected in the neonatal nursery because the affected infant has features of dysmorphism, a suspected syndrome, seizure activity, microcephaly, or evidence of congenital infection. Some anomalies, for example, isolated agenesis of the corpus callosum, may be clinically undetectable at birth.

ANENCEPHALY

Malformations of the brain that can be diagnosed with ultrasonography are best discussed in parallel with an outline of the normal development of brain. The formation of the neural tube in the first weeks of gestation involves its closure centrally, then rostrally, and then caudally. Failure of closure of the rostral end results in anencephaly (Fig. 6–16).

CEPHALOCELE

Partial or incomplete closure of the rostral neuropore may be indicted in the formation of cephaloceles (also called encephaloceles), defined as hernias of part of the brain through a skull defect and characterized by their position, contents, and associated malformations.[31] In most Caucasian populations, the occipital location is most common; other racial groups do not have this occipital predilection. For example, frontoethmoidal cephalocele is more common in groups such as Australian Aborigines and Igbos Nigerians.[81] Cephaloceles usually are covered by skin; neural tissue within the sac connects with the underlying brain (Fig. 6–17). The tissue may be relatively normal, recognizable brain, or it may appear as disorganized clumps of glioneuronal tissue. Intracranial malformations are common. In one series, absence of the anterior commissure, septum pellucidum, and fornices was documented in 80% of cases of occipital cephalocele examined pathologically.[81] Hydrocephalus is common, particularly with cephaloceles of the posterior fossa. Hydrocephalus may become evident only after birth, when the sac no longer functions as a storage chamber for cerebrospinal fluid (CSF).

The role of ultrasonography is to determine whether the sac contains only fluid (meningocele) or tissue plus fluid (meningoencephalocele). The prognosis is better for

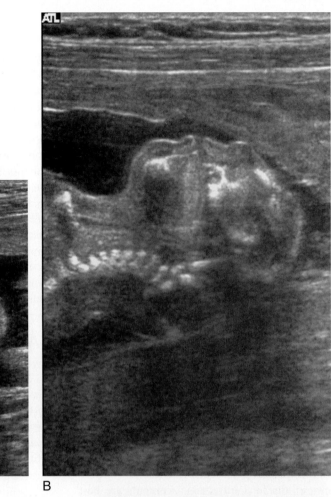

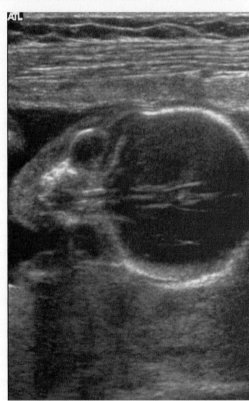

Figure 6–16
Sagittal *(A)* and coronal *(B)* images of an anencephalic fetus were obtained at 18 weeks' gestational age. A normal coronal scan of an 18-week fetus *(C)* is shown for comparison.

A

B

C

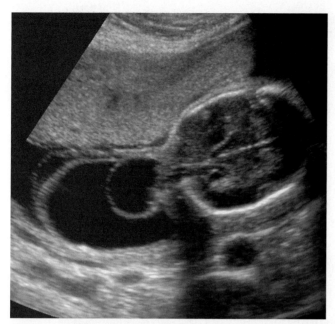

Figure 6–17
Scans of this fetus in utero at 18 weeks' gestational age show a large encephalocele of the posterior fossa. The skin-covered sac contains cerebrospinal fluid (CSF) and neural tissue of indeterminate origin. The family elected to terminate the pregnancy based on the ultrasonographic findings.

the child with an isolated meningocele. If tissue is present, ultrasound examination may be used to attempt to identify the neural structure(s) if possible. Blood supply or drainage of the tissue, as outlined with color or power Doppler ultrasonography may be helpful. Draining veins are often aberrant. Ultrasonography will also make it possible to check carefully for other malformations of the brain and to quantify hydrocephalus, if present, as a baseline for future scans. Results of ultrasonography may also help the clinician to consider syndromic associations, for example, Meckel syndrome, which is associated with occipital cephalocele, polydactyly, and renal cystic disease, or Knobloch syndrome, which is associated with occipital cephalocele and retinal abnormalities.

Definitive imaging is best achieved with MRI, but ultrasonography, used as suggested here, can delineate the major features of the anomaly and provide a working diagnosis if other imaging is delayed or unavailable.

CHIARI II MALFORMATION

Failure of fusion of the caudal end of the neural tube results in spina bifida—myelomeningocele—of the primary neurulation type. According to McClone and Knepper,[70] the leakage of CSF through the open caudal defect occurs at the same time as the rhombencephalic vesicle, the primitive

fourth ventricle, is developing. Leakage leads to collapse of this primitive ventricle and inadequate stimulation of the adjacent mesenchyme that will become the meninges and bone of the posterior fossa. Therefore, the volume of the resultant posterior fossa is smaller than normal.[71] When the cerebellum begins to enlarge, at 11 to 13 weeks, there is suboptimal room for its normal development, and it assumes the banana shape we associate with Chiari II malformation on transaxial scans of the fetus[9] (Fig. 6–18). The cisterna magna is small or obliterated, the quadrigeminal plate becomes distorted (beaked tectum) and lateral, and the third ventricles increase in volume because flow of CSF is impeded through the aqueduct, fourth ventricle, and small posterior fossa. Credence is given to this theory by results from intrauterine surgery. Patching the myelomeningocele in utero results in increasing subarachnoid spaces around the cerebellum and decreases the need for shunting of hydrocephalus in the neonatal period.[109]

Cranial ultrasonography of the neonate who has myelomeningocele includes (1) quantification of the degree of ventricular dilatation, (2) a search for other intracranial anomalies (mechanical support by the primitive ventricular system appears to be essential to normal organization of the cerebral cortex; decompression of this system predisposes to dysgenesis of corpus callosum, abnormal gyri, and gray matter heterotopia), and (3) views of the posterior fossa via suboccipital window or asterion to show the fourth ventricle, cerebellum, tonsillar position, and upper cervical cord.

The glomus of the choroid plexus in the lateral ventricles often looks particularly lumpy or prominent in neonates who have a myelomeningocele. In addition, the interthalamic adhesion (massa intermedia) is prominent in size, assumed to be due to close approximation of the thalami during the period of failure of distention of the primitive ventricular system. It is important to note that there is a spectrum of Chiari II malformations associated with meningomyelocele. Some infants have severely dysmorphic contents of the posterior fossa; others have quite subtle abnormalities (Fig. 6–19). Ventricular dilatation may be mild at birth and increase after closure of the spinal defect (Fig. 6–20).

HOLOPROSENCEPHALY

After the primary neural tube has closed, the face and the forebrain (prosencephalon) develop. The prosencephalon then cleaves to produce two cerebral hemispheres (telencephalon). Failure of cleavage results in the anomaly termed *holoprosencephaly*. Depending on the degree of failed cleavage, the adjectives *alobar, semilobar,* and *lobar* are applied as descriptors. The cross-sectional coronal view of alobar holoprosencephaly is that of a mushroom with a thick stem, representing fused thalami. A common ventricle arches over

Text continued on page 198

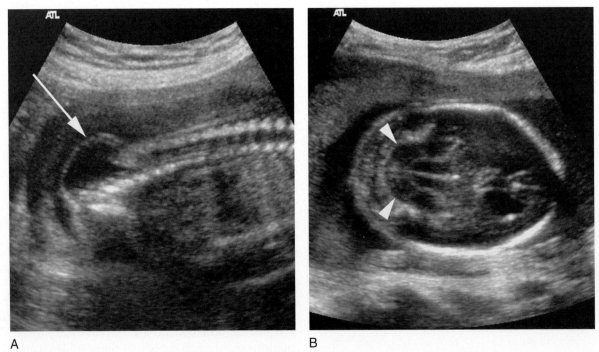

A   B

Figure 6–18
Prenatal scans of this fetus who has a myelomeningocele *(A, arrow)* also demonstrate the "banana sign" *(B, arrowheads)* of a Chiari II malformation. The abnormal cerebellar shape results from crowding of structures in the posterior fossa. The cerebellum is wrapped around the brainstem; the cisterna magna is effaced. Compare with a normal cerebellum as shown in Figure 6–15.

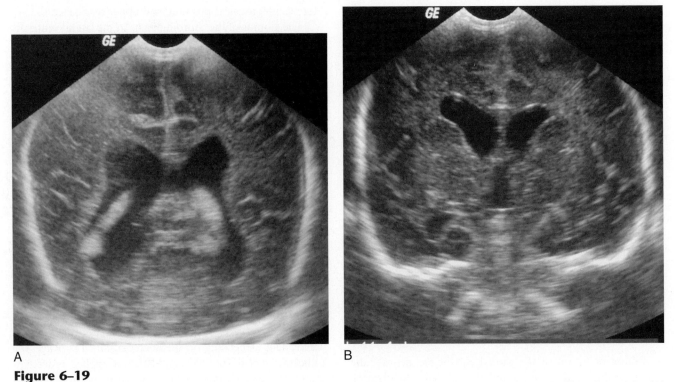

A   B

Figure 6–19
Coronal views at the level of the foramen of Munro *(A)*, massa intermedia in the third ventricle *(B)*, and the trigones of lateral ventricles *(C)* show the ventricular dilatation associated with a Chiari II malformation in this child who also had a myelomeningocele. A midline sagittal scan *(D)* shows the prominent massa intermedia in the dilated third ventricle, the beaked tectum, the low lying cerebellum, and effaced cisterna magna.

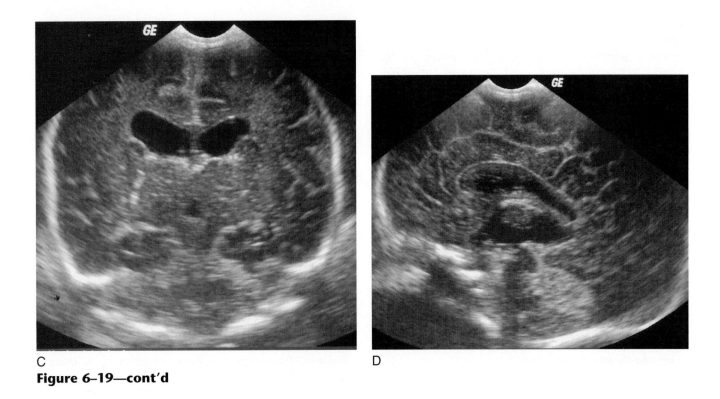

C

D

Figure 6–19—cont'd

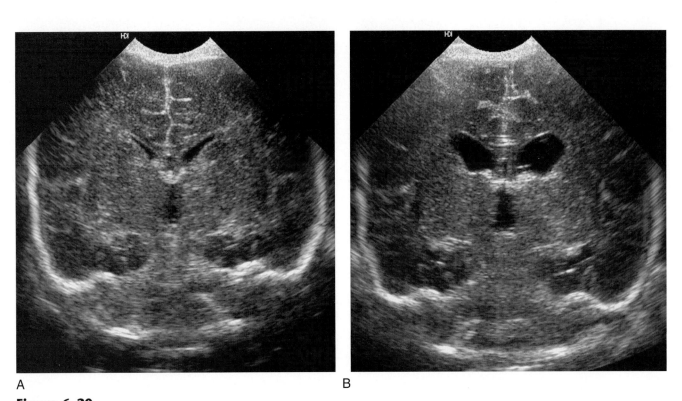

A

B

Figure 6–20

In this patient, who had a myelomeningocele and Chiari II malformation of the brain, a coronal view of the ventricles at birth shows mild dilatation of the anterior horns and third ventricle (*A*). One week later, after closure of the spinal defect, the ventricular system has increased in volume (*B*). A ventriculoperitoneal shunt was placed after these scans.

the mass of basal ganglia; typically the head is small, and the anterior fontanelle is small, making scanning difficult. Semilobar holoprosencephaly is true to its descriptor—the posterior portion of the brain is partially cleaved. Lobar holoprosencephaly has a more well-defined cleavage plane between hemispheres, but the thalami are fused as in the more severe forms.[14] Holoprosencephaly is often associated with chromosomal abnormality, particularly trisomy 13 (Fig. 6–21).

DYSGENESIS OF THE CORPUS CALLOSUM

Abnormalities of midline development include dysgenesis of the corpus callosum and absence of the septum pellucidum.[12] Dysgenesis of the corpus callosum results in a spectrum of ultrasonographic findings, depending on the severity of the lesion and whether a dorsal cyst or lipoma is also present. Callosal agenesis and hypogenesis appear to result from the absence of normal glial slings, which unite the hemispheres and guide the pioneer callosal axons transversely. Instead, fibers course parallel to the interhemispheric fissure to become the bundles of Probst.[12]

When the callosal fibers do not cross the midline, the splenium is absent as a pad compressing the trigone and posterior horns. The classic ultrasonographic features of callosal agenesis include (1) steerhead configuration of the lateral ventricles on coronal scans because of laterally displaced lateral ventricles and the medial bundles of Probst, (2) dilatation of the occipital horns of the lateral ventricles (termed *colpocephaly*) caused by absent splenium, (3) a high-riding capacious third ventricle that may have dorsal extension into a cyst, (4) sulci and gyri that radiate into the roof of the third ventricle on a midline sagittal scan, and (5) absence of the "Frisbee" (representing the rostrum, genu, body, and splenium in cross-section) that is the normal appearance of the corpus callosum on a midline sagittal scan (Fig. 6–22).

When a lipoma is present, the ultrasound beam is reflected, and there is a dense shadow beyond the echogenic mass in the midline. The lipoma may involve choroid plexus in the lateral ventricles[40] (Fig. 6–23). Heterotopia of gray matter or other subtle migrational abnormalities may be present and unrecognized on ultrasonography. MRI adds information to the ultrasonographic diagnosis; the prognosis is associated more with the ancillary findings than with the agenesis itself. Agenesis of the corpus callosum in a girl who has infantile spasms and chorioretinal lacunae is termed *Aicardi syndrome*. The neurologic outcome is particularly poor in this group.

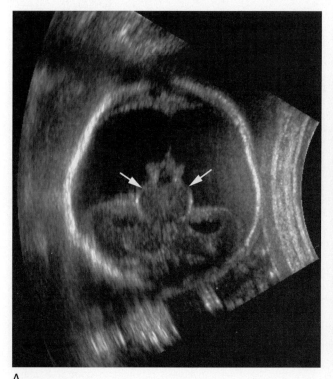

A

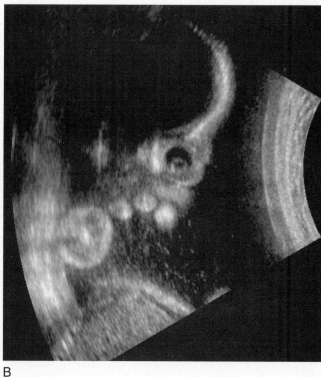

B

Figure 6–21
Prenatal scans of this fetus, later confirmed as having trisomy 13, show the fused thalami *(A, arrows)* typical of holoprosencephaly. This fetus also had bilateral cleft lip *(B)* and polydactyly (not shown). The views are oriented to provide an anatomic coronal view of the brain and en face view of the clefts.

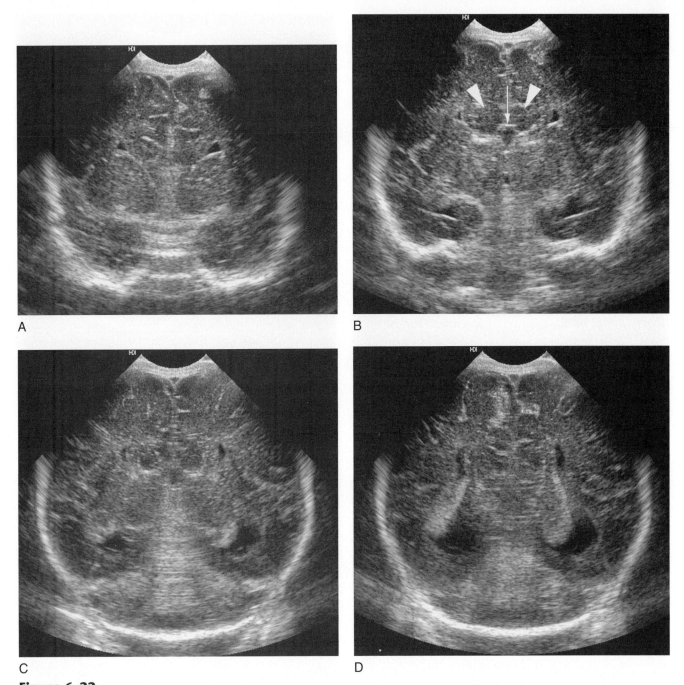

Figure 6–22

This series of coronal scans (A–E) shows the typical features of agenesis of the corpus callosum. The lateral ventricles are parallel in orientation and the occipital horns are dilated (colpocephaly). The *arrowheads (B)* point to the bundles of Probst, which represent the aberrantly oriented callosal tissue. The *arrow (B)* points to the roof of the high-riding third ventricle. A midline sagittal view *(E)* shows sulci and gyri converging onto the roof of the third ventricle with no normal pericallosal or cingulate sulcus present (see also Fig. 6–27F).   *Continued*

ABSENCE OF THE SEPTI PELLUCIDI

Absence of the septi pellucidi, when associated with optic nerve hypoplasia, and variable defects of hypothalamic dysfunction is also known as *de Morsier syndrome.*[63,90]

Absence of the septi pellucidi results in a common lateral ventricle in whole or in part. The frontal horns of the lateral ventricles tend to be inferiorly pointed (Fig. 6–24). Ultrasonography cannot identify the normal anterior commissure or hippocampal commissure, and both may be

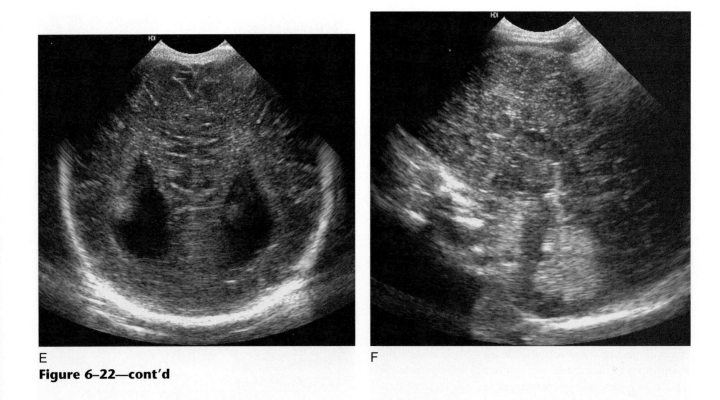

E

F

Figure 6–22—cont'd

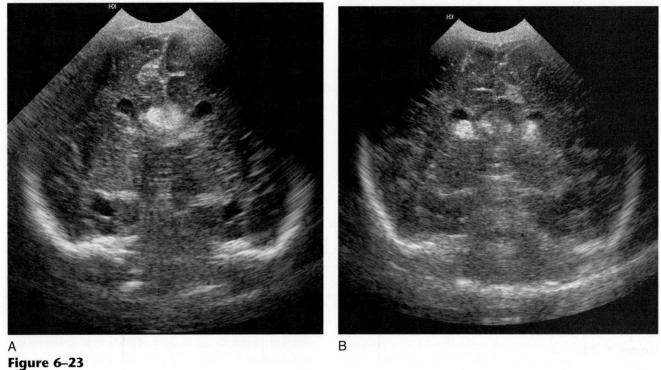

A

B

Figure 6–23
Lipoma of the corpus callosum produces a shadowing echogenic focus in the midline on the coronal scans *(A and B)* and sagittal scan *(C)*. Note involvement of the choroid plexus in each lateral ventricle *(B)*.

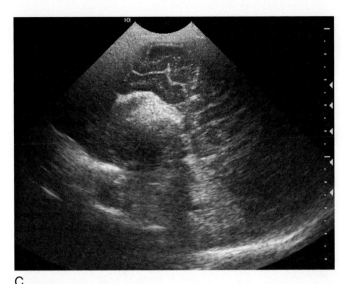

C
Figure 6–23—cont'd

absent as part of the spectrum. Closed-lip schizencephaly, which may be associated with absence of the septum pellucidum, may also go unrecognized. It is reasonable, therefore, to consider further examination with MRI when the ultrasonographic diagnosis of absent septum pellucidum is made in the neonate.[94]

SCHIZENCEPHALY

As emphasized throughout this section, the timing of neuronal migration is synchronous with the developing midline structures. For this reason, schizencephaly may coexist with the absence of the septum pellucidum. Agenesis of a section of the germinative zone is thought to be responsible for the schizencephalic defect. If CSF is present in the cleft, it is considered to be open lipped.[11] If only a pial-ependymal seam separates the cleft brain, it is considered to be closed lipped. On ultrasonography, a subtle notch in the lateral ventricular contour may be all that is recognized with the closed-lip type of schizencephaly. Open-lipped lesions are much easier to diagnose (Fig. 6–25). Communication of the lateral ventricle with a capacious subarachnoid space and gradual development of hydrocephalus is common. One third of patients have bilateral clefts. MRI is diagnostic because of the ability to discriminate between gray and white matter. The seam, whether open or closed, is lined with gray matter.

LISSENCEPHALY

Lissencephaly (smooth brain) is another neuromigrational disorder. Type I lissencephaly is associated with a

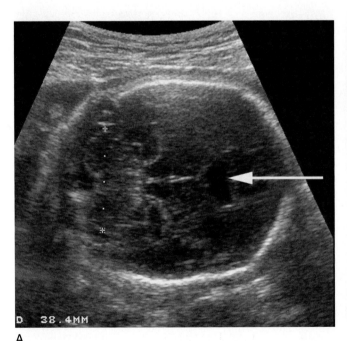

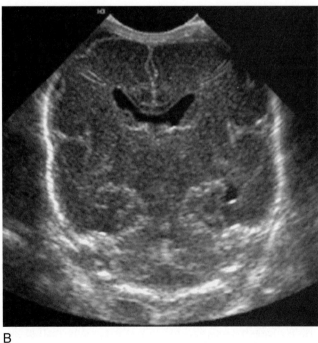

A   B
Figure 6–24
In utero, a common ventricle signifying the absence of cavum septum pellucidum *(A, arrow)* is a clue to the presence of a midline anomaly. Measurement refers to the cerebellar width, which is normal for this gestation. The coronal scan in the neonate *(B)* confirms the absence of septal tissue.

Continued

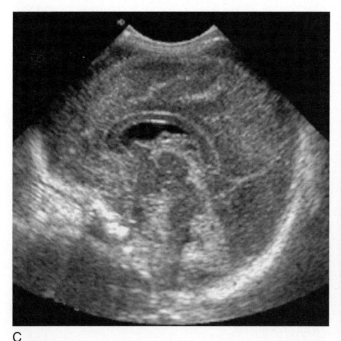

C

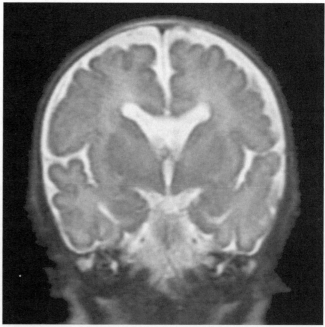

D

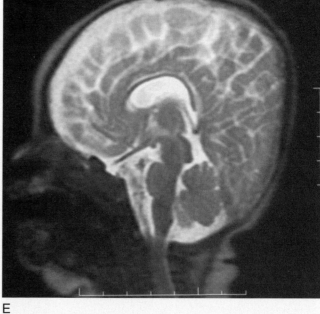

E

Figure 6–24—cont'd
The midline sagittal scan (C) may be relatively normal. Magnetic resonance imaging should be considered in all such infants, as other anomalies are often present. In this neonate, the coronal, T2-weighted scan confirms the absence of the septi pellucidi (D). The sagittal view (E) also demonstrates the absence of the anterior commissure.

deletion in chromosome 17 and the Miller-Dieker syndrome. Type II lissencephaly has a different neuropathology than type I, and the surface of the brain is more pebbled. An associated anomaly of the posterior fossa (e.g., vermian dysgenesis, cerebellar hypoplasia, or Dandy-Walker malformation) is characteristic of type II lissencephaly. The genetic abnormality has not yet been discovered; Walker-Warburg syndrome includes type II lissencephaly, retinal dysplasia, and severe hypotonia.[11] A lissencephalic neonate, born at term, has a brain similar in topography to that of a fetal brain of

18 to 20 weeks' gestational age. Midline structures may be hypoplastic. As in other neuromigrational disorders, far more diagnostic detail is available with MRI.[57]

MICROLISSENCEPHALY

Microlissencephaly has been proposed as the term to describe malformations in which children are born with head circumferences of 3 standard deviations or more below

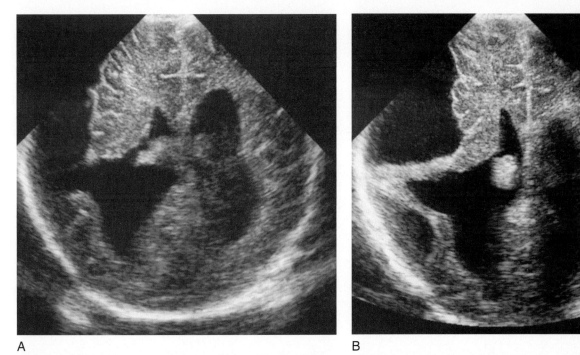

A   B

Figure 6–25
Coronal views *(A and B)* of a neonate who had open-lipped schizencephaly show the abnormal configuration of the lateral ventricle and the communication with the subarachnoid space *(A)*. This child later needed shunting of CSF because of increasing head circumference and ventricular dilatation.

the norm and their imaging studies show too few gyri and shallow sulci (Fig. 6–26). Five groups of such patients are listed by Barkovich.[10] Categorization depends on the neonatal course and imaging findings, specifically the MRI appearance. Ultrasonography has little to offer in such infants. Calcification in the parenchyma of a profoundly microcephalic infant suggests infection as a cause of the disturbance of brain growth.

DANDY-WALKER MALFORMATIONS AND VARIANTS

Walter Dandy was the neurosurgeon who followed Harvey Cushing in chairing the department of neurosurgery at Johns Hopkins University. Earl Walker was Dandy's successor in 1947. Together, they left their names on a malformation that is much more of a spectrum than the severe conditions they described in 1914 and 1942, respectively. The Dandy-Walker complex of anomalies is thought to result from abnormal incorporation of developing plates of tissues over the fourth ventricle, ballooning of the fourth ventricle into a cyst, failure of development of the foramen of Magendie, and vermian hypoplasia or aplasia.[5]

Ultrasonographic features of Dandy-Walker malformation are (1) a cyst in the posterior fossa that is the distended fourth ventricle ballooning behind the cerebellum, (2) hypoplasia

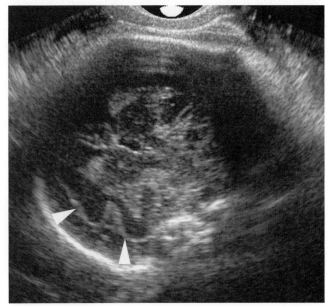

Figure 6–26
An axial scan of this fetus in utero, at 36 weeks' gestational age, shows the smooth cerebral surface *(arrowheads)* of lissencephaly. This fetus also had microcephaly; the head circumference measurement lagged 3 months behind the normal value for gestational age.

or aplasia of the vermis, (3) thin brainstem from compression or hypoplasia, (4) hypoplasia of the cerebellar hemispheres, (5) elevation of the straight sinus and torcula, and (6) hydrocephalus (Fig. 6–27A–D). Other intracranial anomalies may be present; occipital cephalocele may be associated.

Dandy-Walker variant is the name assigned to lesser degrees of vermian hypoplasia and fourth ventricular distention (Fig. 6–27 E–G). The posterior fossa is usually normal in volume and hydrocephalus is variable in degree. Dermal sinus and dermoid may be associated in rare infants. Supratentorial anomalies usually dictate the degree of neurologic impairment. Prenatal diagnosis of Dandy-Walker variant cannot be made in early gestation because the normal vermis is incomplete until 18 weeks' gestational age. Of note, chromosomal anomalies are associated with both classic Dandy-Walker malformation and Dandy-Walker variant.[28]

Mega-cisterna magna probably represents the far end of the spectrum from classic Dandy-Walker malformation.[101] It is differentiated from arachnoid cyst of the posterior fossa in that it has no mass effect on the cerebellum, and it communicates with the fourth ventricle. Mega-cisterna magna is often found in association with trisomy 18. If steeply axial views of the fetal head are obtained, one may mistake the normal foramen of Magendie and apparent widened cisterna magna as part of the spectrum of Dandy-Walker variant and mega-cisterna magna.[64] Any prenatal diagnosis should be confirmed with careful postnatal scans. Views of the posterior fossa via the asterion, posterior fontanelle, and suboccipital window are helpful.

ARACHNOID CYST

Arachnoid cysts are collections of CSF that are generally isolated anomalies (Fig. 6–28). Up to one third involve the posterior fossa. They can be associated with hydrocephalus if strategically positioned in the pathway of CSF flow.[72,113,114] There is no way to predict which cysts will increase in size. Close follow-up with imaging is needed.

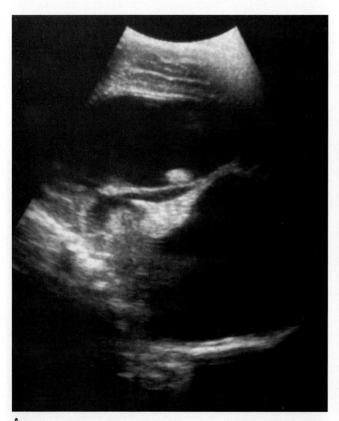

A

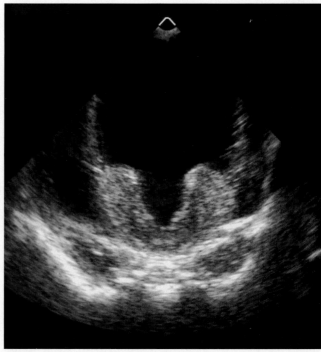

B

Figure 6–27
Dandy-Walker malformation and Dandy-Walker variant include a spectrum of anomalies involving the posterior fossa. The Dandy-Walker malformation (A–D) consists of cerebellar hypoplasia, a large posterior fossa cyst communicating with the fourth ventricle, and hydrocephalus. A sagittal scan through the anterior fontanelle shows continuity of the fourth ventricle with a large cyst in the posterior fossa (A). The coronal view through the posterior fossa (B) shows the laterally displaced, small cerebellar hemispheres, enlargement of the fourth ventricle, and its communication with the cyst in the posterior fossa.

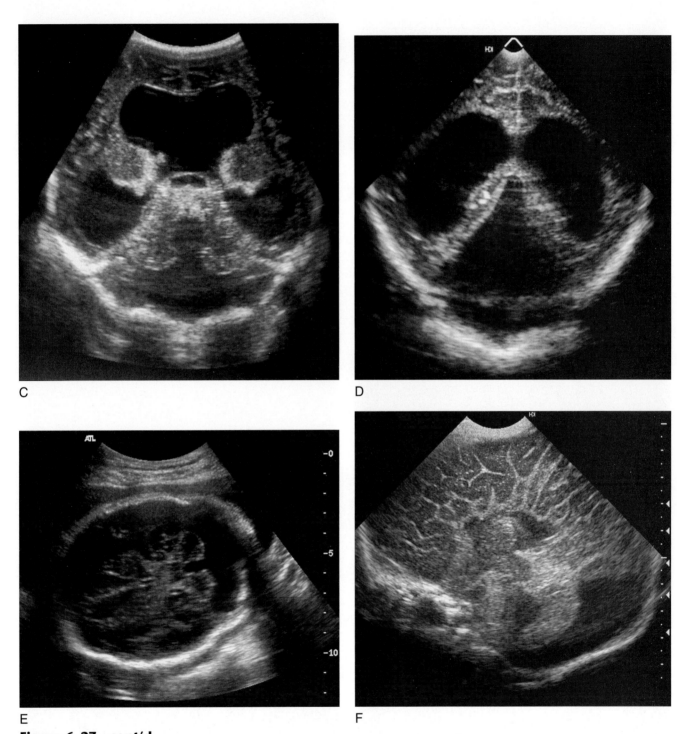

C

D

E

F

Figure 6–27—cont'd

Coronal scans *(C and D)* demonstrate the associated hydrocephalus and, in this case, absence of the posterior portion of the septi pellucidi. The less severe malformation, Dandy-Walker variant, is shown *(E to G)* on prenatal scans of a fetus who had both agenesis of the corpus callosum and a posterior fossa anomaly consisting of cerebellar hypoplasia and absence of the inferior vermis. Note the communication between the fourth ventricle and cisterna magna on the prenatal axial scan *(E)*. A midsagittal scan after the infant was delivered *(F)* shows the radiating gyri from the roof of the third ventricle, typical of agenesis of the corpus callosum, large fourth ventricle, and capacious cisterna magna.

Continued

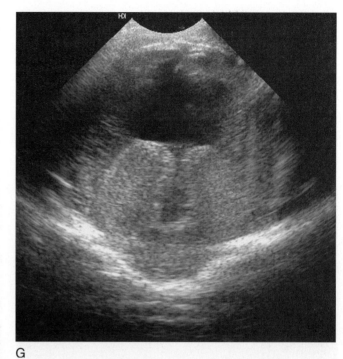

G

Figure 6–27—cont'd

A view through the posterior fontanelle *(G)* demonstrates the communication of the fourth ventricle with the cisterna magna through a defect in the inferior cerebellar vermis.

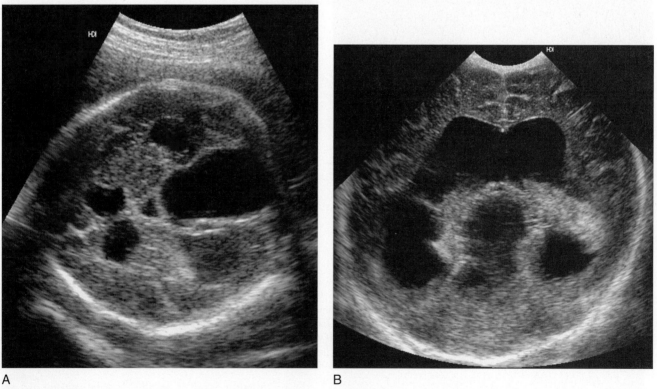

A

B

Figure 6–28

Two examples of arachnoid cysts are shown. In the first infant *(A–C)*, a prenatal scan *(A)* shows a cyst in the posterior fossa. After birth, neonatal scans confirmed that the cyst was unassociated with the fourth ventricle and therefore was not a Dandy-Walker malformation. The coronal view *(B)* shows the dilated lateral ventricles caused by obstruction to normal flow of CSF. The cyst is below the tentorium.

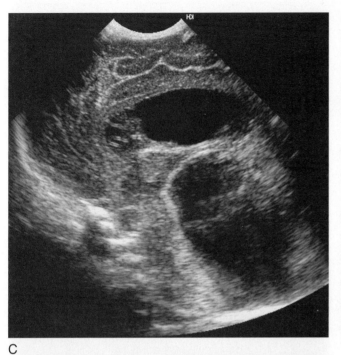

C

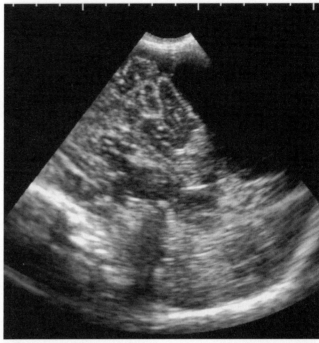

D

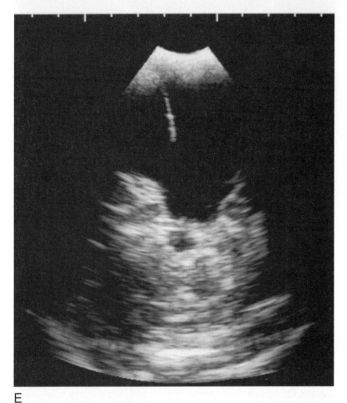

E

Figure 6–28—cont'd
The midline sagittal view *(C)* shows the cerebellum deviated anteriorly by the arachnoid cyst. This child required shunting of the ventricular system and of the cyst. In the second infant *(D and E)*, images show the arachnoid cyst to be supratentorial in location. A view through the anterior fontanelle *(D)* shows it to be posterior in location. The relationship of the cyst to the parietal occipital cortex is shown to better advantage in the view through the posterior fontanelle *(E)*. This infant developed progressive hydrocephalus, requiring shunting.

HYDRANENCEPHALY

Hydranencephaly (water brain) is an acquired anomaly that results from severe intrauterine ischemic insult. There is subsequent dissolution of the cerebral parenchyma of both hemispheres and replacement by large sacs containing CSF (Fig. 6–29). In most occurrences of hydranencephaly, the precipitating insult is occult. Maternal cocaine use has been indicted as a causative factor in one reported patient.[113] Hydranencephaly represents the most severe outcome of infarction. Thrombotic predispositions, such as protein C or S deficiency, may play a causative role in some fetuses.

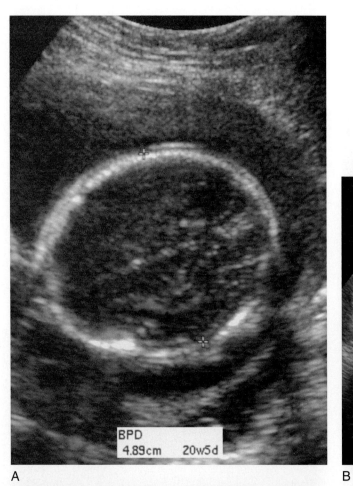

A

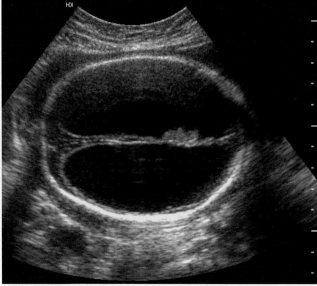

B

C

Figure 6–29

This sequence of scans shows the development of hydranencephaly in utero. At 20 weeks' gestational age, the fetal scan was completely normal with normal views of the brain (A). At 21 to 22 weeks' gestational age, the mother required emergency cardiac surgery and valve replacement for acute decompensation of her rheumatic heart disease. This resulted in a severe hypoxic insult to the fetal brain, with development of hydranencephaly in the third trimester (B and C). Note preservation of structures in the posterior fossa.

FETAL INTRACRANIAL HEMORRHAGE

Intracranial hemorrhage in the fetus has been documented on obstetric ultrasonography, usually as an unexpected finding, and with no known antecedent insult to mother or fetus. MRI has been used for confirmatory imaging. Some intracranial hemorrhages have resolved, others have resulted in hydrocephalus from obstruction at the aqueduct of Sylvius or cisternal-subarachnoidal obstruction to the flow of CSF. Alloimmune thrombocytopenia occurs in 1 per 2000 to 5000 pregnancies with intracranial hemorrhage being the result in 15% to 20% of these.[43] Maternal seizure, preeclampsia, placental abruption, infection, and trauma have been causally implicated in individual infants (Table 6–2). Trauma related to traditional "massage" of the pregnant mother has been considered in Pacific Island neonates who have been shown to have subdural and intracerebral hemorrhages[17] (Fig. 6–30). Twin-twin transfusion or death, or both, of a monochorionic twin is associated with intracerebral pathologic changes.[52] The etiology of ventriculomegaly or porencephaly in late pregnancy or in the neonate should include the possibility of prior hemorrhage and its sequelae (Fig. 6–31). Ventriculomegaly may be ex vacuo if there is significant destruction of brain at the time of the hemorrhagic insult. It seems likely that hydranencephaly is at the far end of the spectrum of ischemic-hemorrhagic intrauterine insult.

CONGENITAL INFECTION

Ventriculomegaly can occur in association with congenital infections. The acronym TORCH has evolved into to STARCH: syphilis, toxoplasmosis, acquired immunodeficiency syndrome (AIDS), rubella, cytomegalovirus, and herpes simplex (Figs. 6–32 to 6–34). To include the enteroviruses, the acronym can be stretched to STARCHES. Effects of infection on the developing brain are variable because they depend on the gestational age of the fetus at the time of infection and the target cells for the virus. Ventriculomegaly, in association with microcephaly and

TABLE 6-2 RISK FACTORS FOR INTRACRANIAL HEMORRHAGE

Very low birth weight
Hypoplastic left heart
Large patent ductus arteriosus
ECMO
Perinatal infection
Large pneumothorax
Apnea

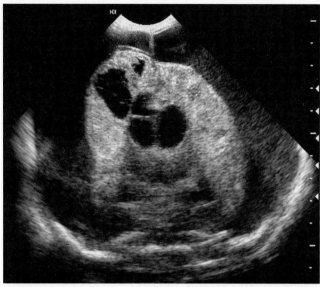

A

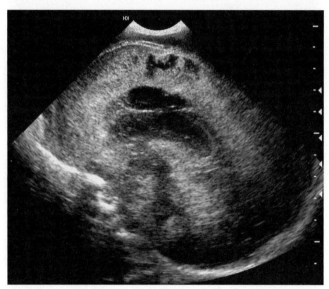

B

Figure 6–30
Trauma to the fetus via traditional abdominal "massage" of the mother's abdomen was thought to be a possible cause of the subdural collections and severe cerebral damage documented on immediate postnatal scans done in coronal *(A)*, midsagittal *(B)*, and axial *(C)* planes.   *Continued*

parenchymal calcification, is diagnostic of congenital infection that has occurred early in pregnancy. It must be noted that diagnosis of intrauterine infection early in gestation may escape notice and appropriate diagnostic studies. Therefore, in some infants, "idiopathic" microcephaly, malformations, and aqueductal stenosis recognized after birth may have been caused by occult intrauterine infections that affected the developing brain.

Text continued on page 214

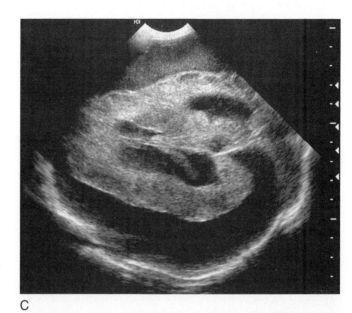

C

Figure 6–30—cont'd

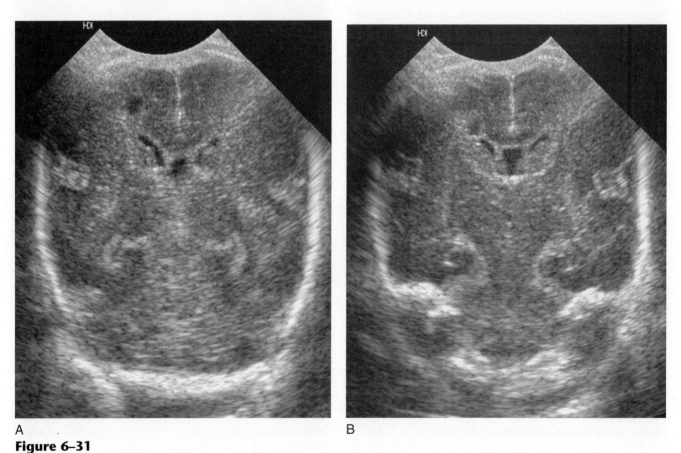

A

B

Figure 6–31

Coronal scans (*A* and *B*) of a neonate shortly after birth at 25 weeks' gestational age show an echo-poor region immediately adjacent to the lateral ventricle on the right. An oblique sagittal scan (*C*) shows a cystic lesion extending from the right lateral ventricle, or porencephaly. In reviewing the mother's history, she had sustained major trauma 2 weeks before delivery, which probably resulted in an intracranial insult to the fetus and subsequent development of porencephalic cyst.

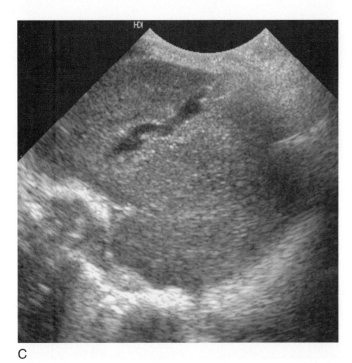

C

Figure 6–31—cont'd

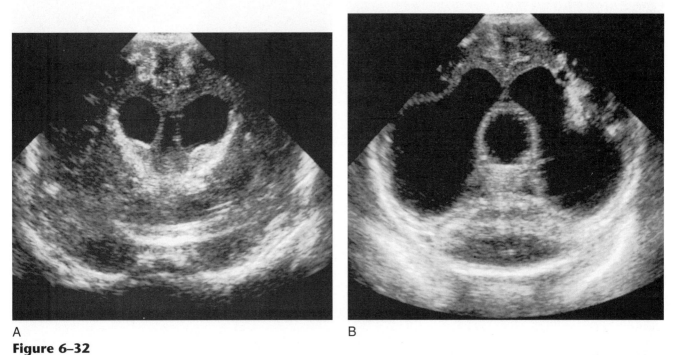

A

B

Figure 6–32

The typical features of congenitally acquired toxoplasmosis are demonstrated in these coronal *(A and B)* and midline sagittal *(C)* scans. Calcifications in the cerebral parenchyma are associated with ventriculomegaly. There is probably obstruction at the level of the aqueduct.

Continued

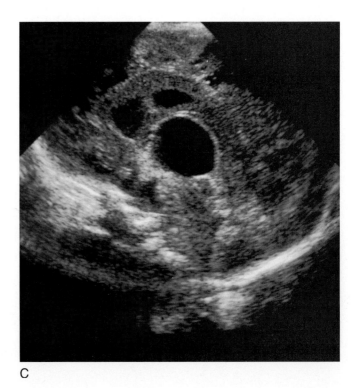

Figure 6–32—cont'd   C

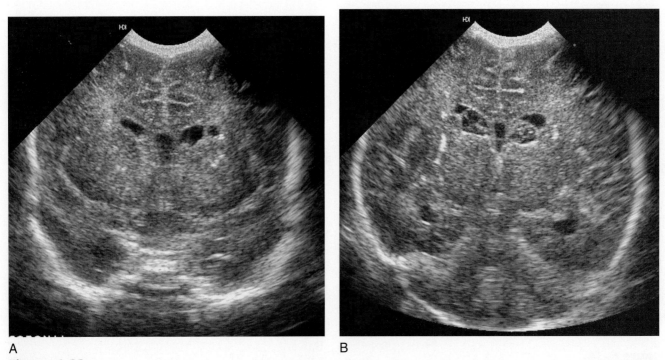

A

B

Figure 6–33
In this neonate, who had a congenital infection with cytomegalovirus, coronal views of the brain *(A and B)* show abnormal germinal matrix and echogenic foci in the basal ganglia that represent mineralizing vasculopathy.

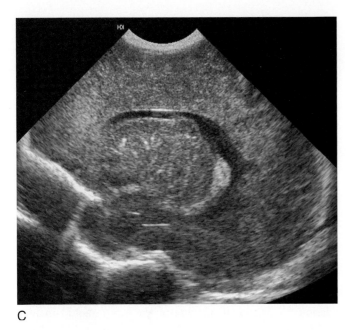

C

Figure 6–33—cont'd
The parasagittal view *(C)* further demonstrates this vasculopathy as linear branching densities extending from the Sylvian fissure.

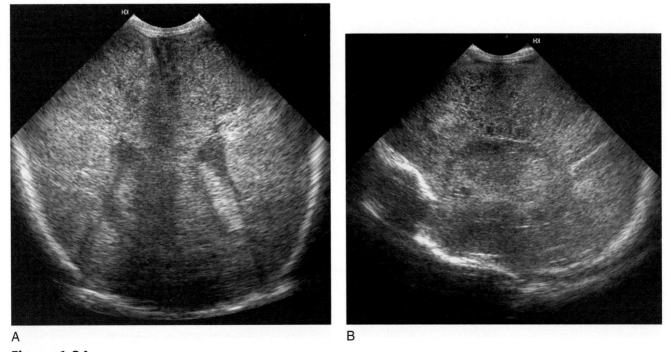

A   B

Figure 6–34
The coronal view *(A)* through the trigones of the lateral ventricles and parasagittal view of the left lateral ventricle *(B)* show loss of normal sulcal and gyral patterns and a ghostly outline of the lateral ventricles. This full-term neonate was infected with herpes simplex virus at the time of delivery and later developed severe meningoencephalitis.

AQUEDUCTAL STENOSIS

Aqueductal stenosis with consequent ventriculomegaly is often a diagnosis without a known cause (Fig. 6–35). X-linked aqueductal stenosis is a recognized genetic disorder, but the majority of occurrences are idiopathic, and the possibility of intrauterine infection, intrauterine hemorrhage, or other process obstructing the narrow channel through the mesencephalon is always a consideration. If diagnosed prenatally, death or developmental delay is the usual outcome.[67]

LENTICULOSTRIATE VASCULOPATHY

Echogenic lenticulostriate vessels are associated with congenital infections—notably cytomegalovirus[106] and rubella[29]—but may also accompany hypoxic-ischemic conditions,[32] maternal systemic lupus erythematosus, twin-twin transfusion in utero, fetal alcohol syndrome, and trisomy 13.[60,97] On parasagittal scans, the branching vessels with their echogenic walls have the appearance of candelabra (see Fig. 6–33). Probably intragestational insults of many types follow a common pathway to produce this vascular abnormality. Mineralizing vasculopathy was present in a few infants in whom neuropathologic examination was possible.

INTRACRANIAL MASS

CONGENITAL TUMORS

Congenital or neonatal tumors of the brain are extremely rare and, in general, have a dismal prognosis (Table 6–3). Of all the tumors, choroid plexus papilloma has the best rate of cure following surgical excision (Fig. 6–36). Hemorrhage into a parenchymal tumor may obscure the underlying pathologic condition. A midline germ cell tumor may coexist with a rhabdoid tumor of the kidney.

Although not neoplasms, the hamartomas of tuberous sclerosis are intracerebral masses.[66,76] They may be subependymally or cortically. When they can be identified on ultrasonography, hamartomas are echogenic (Fig. 6–37). Prenatal diagnosis of tuberous sclerosis is based on the presence of a cardiac mass or masses and an intracranial lesion.[36,95] Postnatal imaging of the brain should include MRI, which is more sensitive to small tubers in all locations throughout the brain.

VEIN OF GALEN ANEURYSM

Most texts specifically explain that "aneurysm of the vein of Galen" is a misnomer. An aneurysm refers to an artery, not a vein; the median prosencephalic vein of Markowski

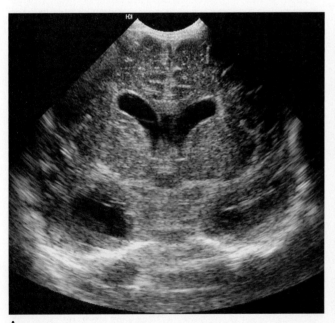
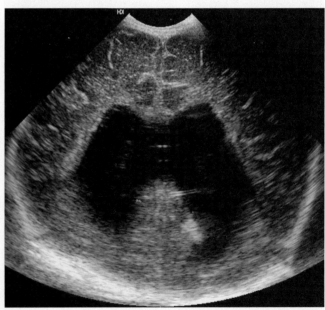

A   B

Figure 6–35
Ventriculomegaly involving the lateral and third ventricles, as shown on coronal (*A and B*) and midline (*C*) and right (*D*) sagittal scans, was unassociated with other findings in this neonate. Computed tomography (CT) scanning confirmed the ultrasonographic findings and the diagnosis of aqueductal stenosis.

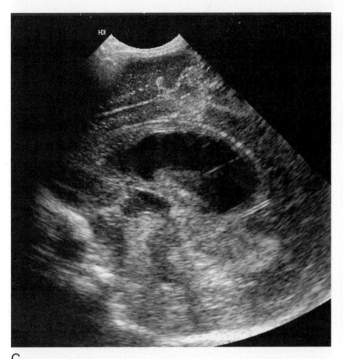

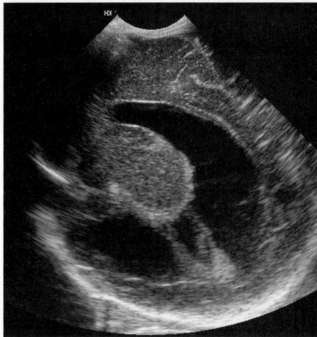

C

D

Figure 6–35—cont'd

rather than the vein of Galen may be dilated, and the actual pathologic lesion is an arteriovenous malformation: dilatation of the draining vein is a secondary feature.[23,88] The label *aneurysm of the vein of Galen* is unlikely to change, perhaps because Galen's name links it to medical history. Ultrasonography contributes to the confusion with the label because scans with color Doppler images are dramatic in demonstrating swirling flow in the dilated spherical venous chamber located posterior to the third ventricle.

<table>
<tr><td colspan="2">**TABLE 6-3** SONOGRAPHY FOR NEONATAL INTRACRANIAL MASSES AND CONGENITAL TUMORS</td></tr>
<tr><td>**CONGENITAL TUMOR**</td><td>**SITE OF INVOLVEMENT**</td></tr>
<tr><td>Teratoma/germ cell tumor</td><td>Usually supratentorial</td></tr>
<tr><td>Primitive neuroectodermal tumor/medulloblastoma</td><td>Infratentorial</td></tr>
<tr><td>Astrocytoma</td><td>Supratentorial and infratentorial</td></tr>
<tr><td>Choroid plexus papilloma</td><td>Supratentorial</td></tr>
<tr><td>Ependymoma/ ependymoblastoma</td><td>Supratentorial and infratentorial</td></tr>
<tr><td>Craniopharyngioma</td><td>Supratentorial</td></tr>
<tr><td>Miscellaneous</td><td>Supratentorial and infratentorial</td></tr>
</table>

Posterior choroidal arteries are most commonly the feeding arterial supply, but any of the major cerebral arteries can be feeding vessels.[39] The neuropathologic effects result from ischemia due to arterial steal or cardiac failure and in some infants to hydrocephalus from obstruction of CSF distal to the third ventricle by the mass of the dilated vein. Less commonly, thrombosis of the vein results in infarction. The typical clinical presentation in the neonatal period is cardiac failure in the presence of a structurally normal heart. The echocardiographer may notice a dilated superior vena cava. Prenatal diagnosis has been reported.[54] Features apparent on ultrasonography include (1) a cystic mass of variable size in the quadrigeminal plate cistern, (2) color flow, usually circular or swirling, in the "cyst" that is the dilated draining vein, (3) a pulsed Doppler waveform that shows pulsatile flow in the vein, (4) a low RI (i.e., high antegrade diastolic flow) in the arterial component of the malformation, (5) a variable degree of ventriculomegaly above the aqueduct, (6) an abnormal ultrasonic pattern of cerebral parenchyma (from ischemia), and (7) occasionally, parenchymal calcification from severe ischemia in utero (Fig. 6–38).

MRI angiography is a noninvasive means of outlining the vascular malformation in more detail than is available with ultrasonography. Treatment is focused on stopping the shunting, either by obstructing the arterial supply or the venous runoff. Ultrasonography has been used in the latter approach, by guiding transtorcular embolization of the dilated vein.[1]

Text continued on page 218

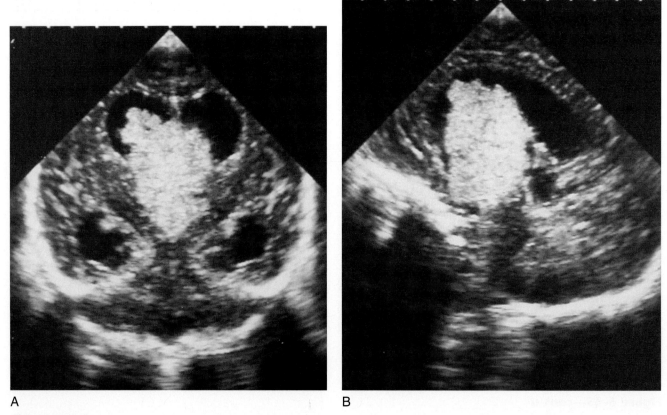

A   B

Figure 6–36
This neonate, who presented with increasing head circumference, had a choroid plexus papilloma arising from the choroid plexus in the third ventricle as seen on coronal *(A)* and sagittal *(B)* scans of the brain.

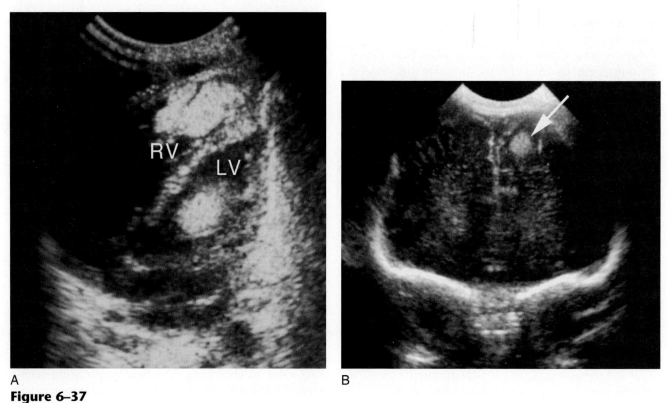

A   B

Figure 6–37
Tuberous sclerosis was suspected in this neonate, who had intracardiac tumors (probably rhabdomyomas). A short-axis view of the heart demonstrates a mass in each ventricle *(A)*. RV, right ventricle; LV, left ventricle. Coronal *(B)* and sagittal *(C)* views of the frontal lobe demonstrate an echogenic focus *(arrow)*, which represents a tuber in the cerebral gray matter. This finding confirmed the diagnosis of tuberous sclerosis.

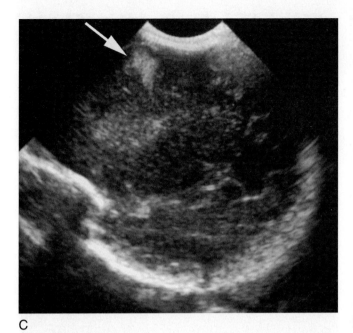

C

Figure 6–37—cont'd

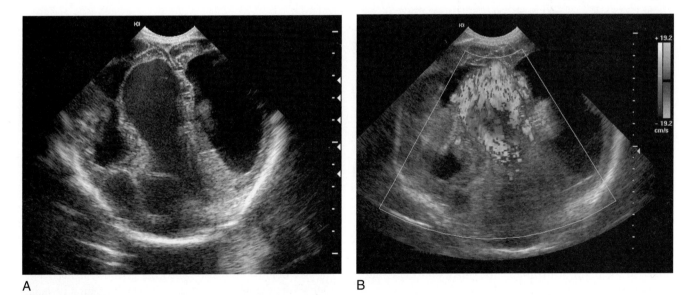

A

B

Figure 6–38

Aneurysm of the vein of Galen had been diagnosed prenatally in this neonate. These postnatal scans show a hugely dilated vein on the coronal scans (*A* and *B*) and on the midsagittal view (*C* and *D*). A pulsed-wave Doppler scan (*E*) demonstrates the turbulent flow through the vein. The arteriovenous steal was associated with severe ischemic damage to the brain in this infant whose survival was short following delivery.

Continued

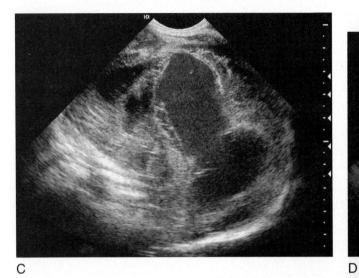

C

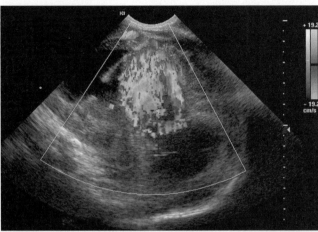

D

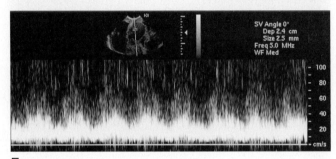

Figure 6–38—cont'd   E

THE PREMATURE INFANT WITH HYPOXIC-ISCHEMIC INJURY

Hypoxia refers to decreased oxygenation of tissue. Ischemia is decreased perfusion of tissue. The brain is exquisitely sensitive to both hypoxia and ischemia. In the clinical setting, it is often difficult to establish which process is responsible for injury and so the two are linked together—to the despair of purists—as hypoxic-ischemic injury. We consider here the sonographic features of hypoxic-ischemic injury to the brain of the premature infant and the infant born at term.

Prematurity is defined as being born at a gestational age less than 37 weeks. Generally, a good outcome can be assumed if birth weight is 1500 g or more. This usually correlates with a mean gestational age of 31 weeks. Infants weighing 1500 g or less are referred to as very low birth weight. Extremely low birth weight refers to neonates weighing less than 1000 g, which is generally 28 gestational weeks.[8] In the infant born early, the two major organs most at risk are the lungs and

the brain. A decrease in respiratory morbidity and mortality for premature infants occurred with the development and administration of exogenous surfactant and the institution of continuous positive airway pressure via nasal prongs and therefore without endotracheal intubation. Improvements in treatment of persistent patent ductus arteriosus with medication rather than surgical ligation have also played a part. Postnatally, one cannot accelerate the maturation of the premature brain to protect it from injury.[49] However, improvements in respiratory and circulatory care of premature infants have decreased the risk of injury in larger infants.

The premature infant's brain contains the remnants of the neuroepithelium, also called the germinal matrix. This highly vascular gelatinous tissue, filled with neural and glial precursors, lies in the subependymal region adjacent to the lateral ventricles and also adjacent to the fourth ventricle. From approximately 10 to 20 gestational weeks, supratentorial neuronal migration occurs from the germinal matrix. The neurons follow a path established by radial glial cells, which later differentiate into astrocytes. A second population of astrocytes arises from the germinal matrix after neural migration has occurred. Astrocytes not only provide a supportive framework, but they also appear to have important nutritive and organizational roles in relationship to neurons. The last cells to develop from neuroepithelium are the oligodendrocytes, the cells that produce myelination. Therefore, the germinal matrix that is present in the brains of premature infants has already spun out its neural cells to the layered cerebral gray matter but is in the process of supporting that neural network with astrocytes and oligodendrocytes. It is also important to note that during this same period, from 20 weeks' gestational age to term, the cortical gray matter is evolving from a layered mat to a textured carpet via the process of dendritic proliferation between neurons. The cortical gray matter, anchored by its axons in the corona radiata, increases its volume fourfold, as measured by quantitative MRI, to the extent that the smooth brain of the 20-week fetus becomes the convoluted surface, with gyri and sulci, that characterizes the normal brain of the term infant[61] (Fig. 6–39). Thus, an insult to the developing brain can affect the germinal matrix, the rapidly evolving neurons, and their potential in terms of organization via synaptic connections.

Because ultrasonography and CT have been the major diagnostic modes of imaging and because both modalities can identify hemorrhage within the brain, hemorrhagic lesions have been the focus of interest since the early 1970s.[45] However, hypoxic-ischemic injury to the developing brain is not always associated with hemorrhage.

Some nonhemorrhagic insults are identified with ultrasonography, but significant abnormalities of the parenchyma are missed that can be identified on MRI or neuropathologic examination.[2,13,98] It is apparent, however, that the plasticity of the brain is such that recruitment of idle neuronal units when others have been damaged or destroyed often permits the brain to maintain function. It has been suggested that ultrasonography produces false-negative results, whereas MRI produces false-positive results in terms of neurodevelopmental prognosis.[73]

INJURY TO THE PREMATURE INFANT'S BRAIN

GERMINAL MATRIX HEMORRHAGE

The premature infant who has respiratory failure from pulmonary immaturity and deficiency of surfactant is a prime candidate for hypoxic-ischemic insult to the brain. Bleeding into the germinal matrix occurs as a result. Insults that are associated with bleeding from the thin-walled vessels in the germinal matrix include fluctuating blood pressure and flow, hypoxia, hypercarbia, abnormalities of platelets and

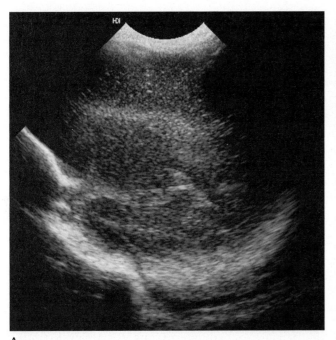

A

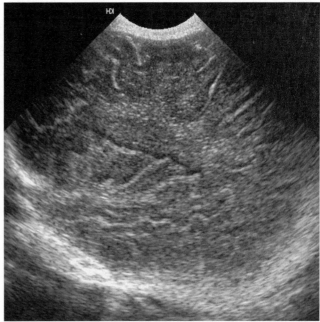

B

Figure 6–39
The parasagittal view *(A)* of the temporal lobe in a neonate of 24 weeks' gestational age shows a smooth surface of the brain with only the Sylvian fissure and early demarcation of the superior temporal sulcus visible. The presence of this sulcus indicates that the infant is greater than 24 weeks' gestational age. Compare with a parasagittal view of a full-term infant *(B)*.

coagulation, maternal infection, and placental failure.[110–112,115] Heavy maternal usage of cocaine has been associated with a higher frequency of intracranial hemorrhage.[44] The residual germinal matrix occupies the region that is later the head of the caudate nucleus. Therefore, bleeding into the germinal matrix typically presents as an echogenic focus inferolateral to the lateral ventricle on a coronal scan. Choroid plexus lying on the floor of the lateral ventricle is also an echogenic structure. The caudothalamic groove, an ultrasonographic landmark evident on a sagittal scan, is useful in distinguishing between hemorrhage in the germinal matrix and the normal choroid plexus. The choroid plexus does not extend anterior to the caudothalamic groove whereas hemorrhage into germinal matrix usually does (Fig. 6–40). If the hemorrhage is not contained within the germinal matrix, it breaks through the fragile ependymal roof into the ipsilateral lateral ventricle (Fig. 6–41). Blood in the ventricular system is often classified as grade II germinal matrix or intraventricular hemorrhage (Table 6–4). Blood may flow across into the other lateral ventricle, into the third ventricle and via the aqueduct and fourth ventricle into the cisterna magna. Distention of the ventricles with blood is considered grade III intraventricular hemorrhage (Fig. 6–42). If the amount of blood is such that clot can be imaged in the cisterna magna, there is a high correlation with subsequent hydrocephalus (see earlier discussion). If a parenchymal abnormality is recognized, it is associated with the instigating hypoxic-ischemic insult. It is not caused by extravasation of blood from the ventricle into the adjacent cerebral parenchyma, as suggested in the older literature and in the original grading systems of intracerebral hemorrhage.[26,83,96]

PERIVENTRICULAR VENOUS INFARCTION

Two vascular mechanisms probably result in parenchymal damage: arterial infarction via perfusion failure and venous infarction via obstructed drainage. Volpe[113] advocated a theory of peritrigonal venous infarction caused by ipsilateral hemorrhage, which suggests the following pathogenesis: (1) hemorrhage in the germinal matrix and leakage of blood into the lateral ventricle; (2) distention of the ipsilateral lateral ventricle with blood; (3) displacement and obstruction of the terminal vein, which drains medullary veins; and (4) venous infarction in the region (peritrigonal white matter) that is drained by the medullary veins.

The unusual anatomy of the venous system may also predispose to obstruction of venous drainage: the terminal vein, which drains medullary, choroidal, and thalamostriate veins, makes an abrupt U-turn to join the internal cerebral vein.[103] As the intraparenchymal hemorrhage resolves, it typically cavitates and becomes contiguous with the ipsilateral ventricle. Localized ectasia of the ventricle or a discrete porencephalic cyst is the end result (Fig. 6–43). Hemiplegia is the typical neurologic outcome.[30]

Text continued on page 223

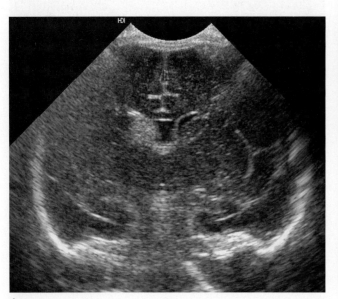
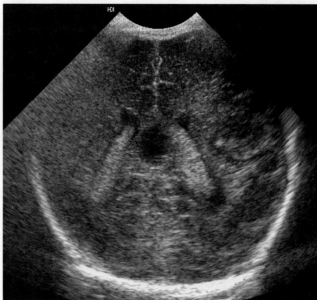

A   B

Figure 6–40

Coronal *(A and B)*, right parasagittal *(C)*, and left parasagittal *(D)* scans of this premature neonate show an echogenic focus in the right-sided germinal matrix. No intraventricular hemorrhage was documented. Note the normal ventricles and prominent central cavum vergae on the coronal view *(B)*. This infant had a grade I hemorrhage.

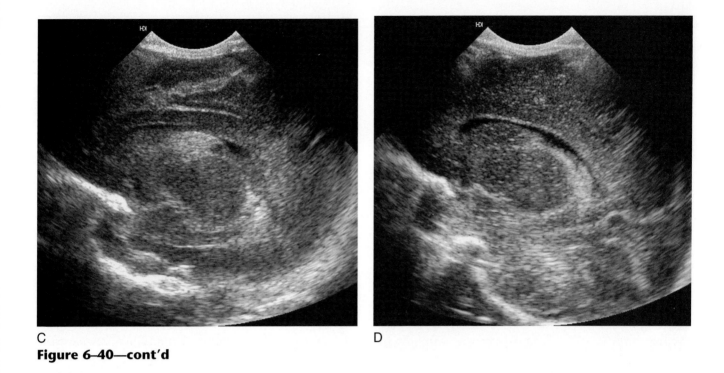

C

Figure 6–40—cont'd

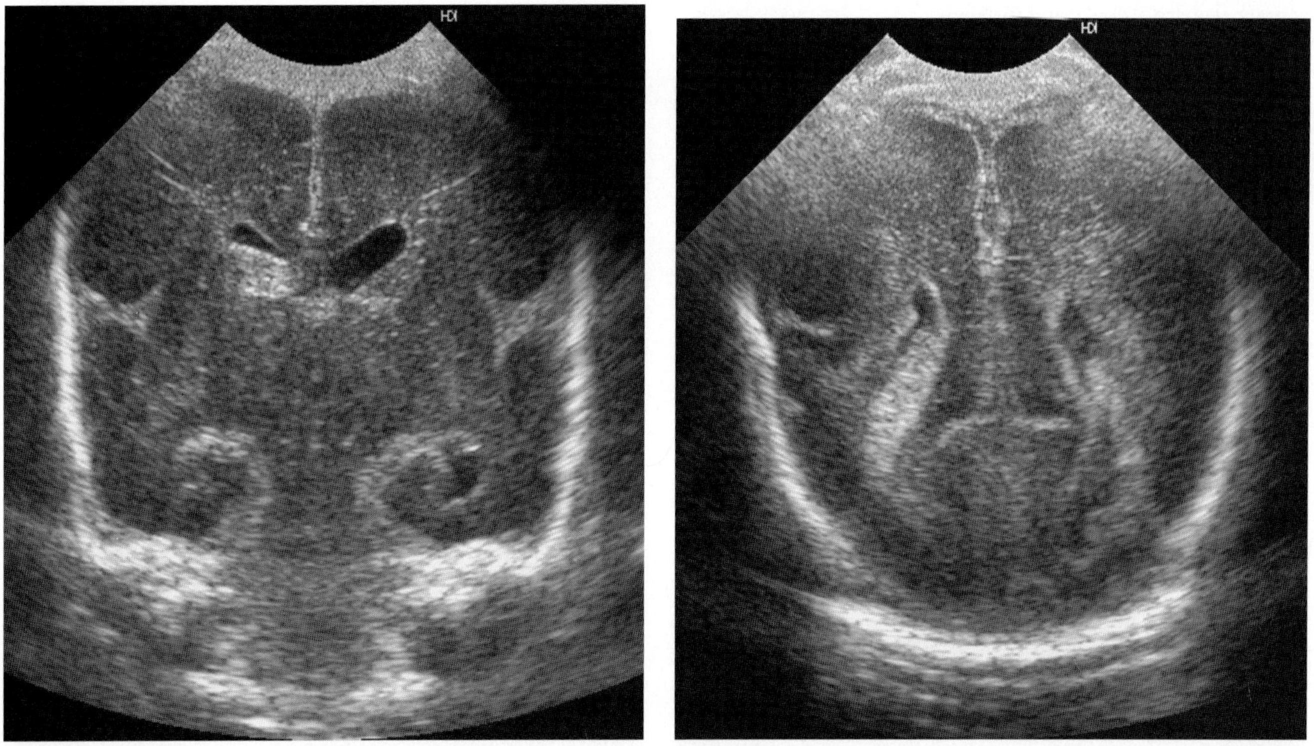

A

B

Figure 6–41

Coronal views *(A and B)* show a germinal matrix hemorrhage on the right and a clot in the posterior horn, left lateral ventricle, that is confirmed on a sagittal view of the left ventricle via the posterior fontanelle *(C)*. The ventricles are not dilated. This is classified as a grade II hemorrhage.

Continued

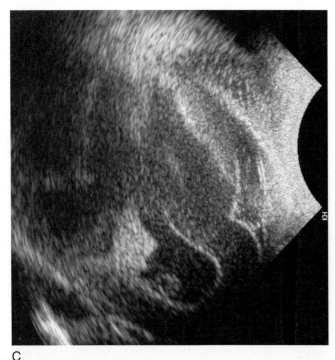

C

Figure 6–41—cont'd

TABLE 6-4 GRADING SYSTEM IN USE FOR GERMINAL MATRIX–INTRAVENTRICULAR HEMORRHAGE	
Grade I	Subependymal (germinal matrix) hemorrhage
Grade II	Intraventricular extension without ventricular dilatation
Grade III	Intraventricular extension with ventricular dilatation
Grade IV	Intraparenchymal hemorrhage with or without intraventricular dilatation

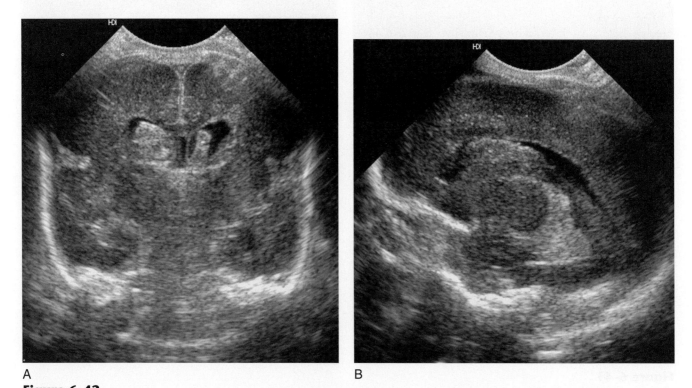

A   B

Figure 6–42

Coronal (A), left parasagittal (B), and right parasagittal (C) scans of this neonate show blood within the ventricular system that is dilated. This is classified as a grade III intraventricular hemorrhage. The source of bleeding was probably a right-sided germinal matrix.

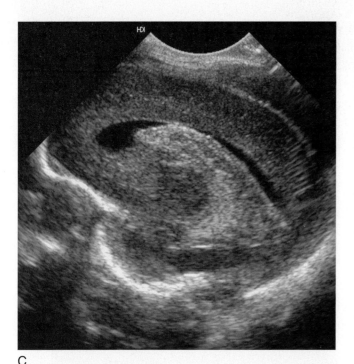

C

Figure 6–42—cont'd

CEREBELLAR HEMORRHAGE

The occurrence of cerebellar hemorrhage in the preterm infant has been underestimated to date, because the cerebellar hemispheres are naturally echogenic on ultrasonography and because ancillary views of the posterior fossa have not accompanied the standard views obtained via the anterior fontanelle.[16,75] The views of the cerebellum via the asterion seem to be the most valuable in diagnosis of cerebellar hemorrhage. These views also show the third ventricle, aqueduct, and fourth ventricle well (Fig. 6–44).

PERIVENTRICULAR LEUKOMALACIA

Arterial or ischemic-reperfusion damage results in periventricular leukomalacia (PVL). The term results from the neuropathologic findings of white (*leuko*), soft (*malacia*) brain. It is apparent, that there is a spectrum of damage to the developing brain that can be recognized on neuropathologic examination. The damage must be moderate or severe, however, for recognition with ultrasonography. In addition, confusion in the ultrasonographic literature abounds, depending on the author's ultrasonographic definition of PVL. In many cases, the definition of PVL is limited to the identification of small cysts in the periventricular white matter. A review of the theories for pathogenesis of PVL may help in interpretation of ultrasonographic findings. The vascular supply to the white matter is the short and long penetrating arteries from the cerebral cortex. The blood flow to the white matter is low compared with that to the gray matter. The cells at the receiving end of a long artery (i.e., those cells close to the lateral ventricle) will die if the flow is diminished below a critical level. Ischemia is followed by necrosis, which may be followed by hemorrhage.[77,98] With or without hemorrhage, the tissue dissolves and cavitates, which results in small cysts. On ultrasonography, one may be able to recognize an increase in periventricular blush—especially if it is asymmetric—that is the acute ischemic phase.

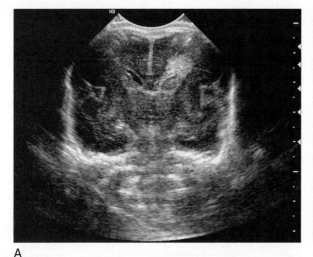

A

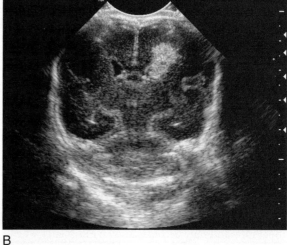

B

Figure 6–43

This sequence of images shows the evolution of hemorrhage in the germinal matrix, ventricles, and parenchyma in a premature infant, classified as a grade IV hemorrhage. At 2 days of life, coronal views (*A and B*) show intraventricular hemorrhage on the left and a left-sided intraparenchymal hemorrhage.

Continued

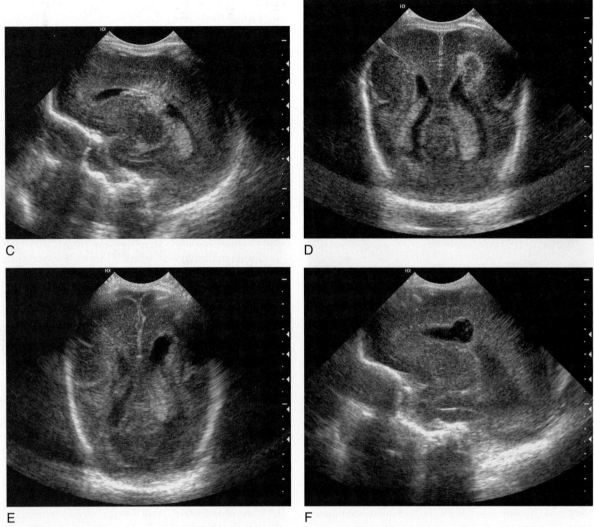

Figure 6–43—cont'd
A sagittal view of the left ventricle *(C)* shows the germinal matrix hemorrhage, some intraventricular clot, and fanlike density typical of a venous infarct, extending into the parietal parenchyma. By 6 days of age, a coronal scan *(D)* shows evolution of the intraparenchymal hemorrhage. At 38 days, the infant has developed a porencephalic cyst on the left, as shown on the coronal *(E)* and sagittal *(F)* scans.

Hemorrhagic involvement typically causes very echogenic, flame-like foci. The cysts are easiest of all to recognize (usually 7 to 14 days after the insult) and may occur without a prior, appreciable ultrasonographic abnormality (Fig. 6–45). Over time, the cysts tend to collapse and disappear from ultrasonic view.

If there is low arterial flow throughout the white matter, but without focal infarction as described earlier, it appears that the oligodendrocyte or its precursor is the cell most at risk for destruction. This cellular death is not apparent on ultrasonography and only becomes known much later when myelination is impaired because the population of remaining oligodendrocytes is so diminished. Then, the sulci are closely juxtaposed to the ventricles, and the ventricles themselves are large because the white matter is deficient of myelin. An infant, therefore, can have significant parenchymal injury in the neonatal period that is unrecognized on ultrasonography. It should be noted that the development of cortical gray matter may depend on normal function of the cells and the axons that support it. Although peripheral neurons may be protected from ischemia, they may suffer as a result of the insult to white matter. An analogy is the case of the upper floor of a building losing both its telephone links and its elevators to the floors below: it cannot function well in isolation. PVL, as a rule, is much more damaging in terms of neurologic sequelae than the pure, unilateral venous infarction that accompanies germinal matrix hemorrhage.[15,89] Usually, the intraparenchymal insult can be characterized on ultrasonography, but PVL can coexist with germinal matrix–related hemorrhage. When there is extensive parenchymal

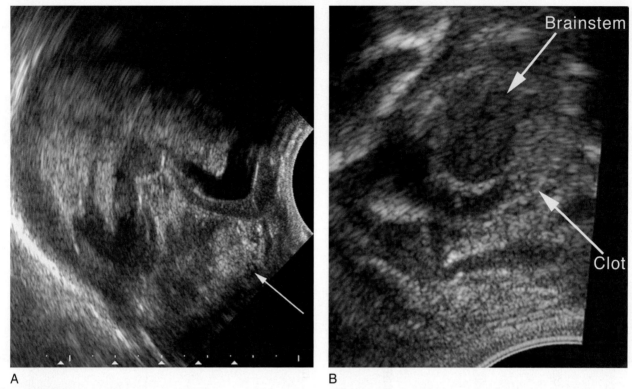

A   B

Figure 6–44

Cerebellar hemorrhage is probably underestimated in the population of premature infants who experience a severe hypoxic ischemic insult. The view through the posterolateral fontanelle *(A)*, oriented to show the cerebellum in the anatomic coronal plane, shows an echogenic focus *(arrow)* representing hemorrhage in the left cerebellar hemisphere in this infant of 25 weeks' gestational age. This infant had a coexistent severe intraventricular and cerebral intraparenchymal hemorrhage. Note the clot in the cisterna magna *(B)* on an axial view through the foramen magnum.

hemorrhage, it is difficult to be sure which etiologic mechanism—venous, or arterial, or a combination of the two—is responsible for the resulting damage[62] (Fig. 6–47). It should be noted that inflammation from either prenatal or postnatal infection is a synergistic factor in promoting intracerebral insults of all types.[38,56]

PARAVENTRICULAR CYSTS

It is not unusual to see tiny cysts paralleling the anterior frontal horns of lateral ventricles in neonates being screened for possible intracerebral hemorrhage (Fig. 6–47). The prevalence of this abnormality has been estimated to be 0.5% to 5.2%.[69] True incidence figures are unknown because the scanning is not performed for normal neonates. These cysts probably signal the occurrence of an intrauterine insult. The neurodevelopmental outcome of affected infants is associated more with other factors such as the degree of intrauterine growth retardation, infection, and other findings.[69] Over time, most cysts disappear with a mildly ectatic frontal horn being the result. These "benign" cysts occur inferior to

the angle of the lateral ventricle. PVL occurs superior to the angle of the lateral ventricle.

SCREENING PROTOCOL

The lack of clinical findings in many neonates who have intracranial pathologic lesions has led to the advocacy of performing screening ultrasonography in all premature infants at risk: those younger than 32 gestational weeks or weighing less than 1500 g.[84] In one series, severe intraventricular hemorrhages were clinically unsuspected in 65% of affected premature infants.[85] There has been a decrease in intracerebral hemorrhage in the premature population coincident with improvements in neonatal care. The prevalence of intracerebral abnormality in the 1970s was 30% to 40%.[3] Scans from National Women's Hospital, Auckland, New Zealand, the largest neonatal nursery in the South Pacific region, showed germinal matrix–related hemorrhage in 25 of 172 (15%) of infants weighing less than 1500 g. Eleven of 172 (6.4%) had severe (grades 3 and 4) hemorrhage, and 8 of 11 of those infants weighed less than 1000 g at birth.

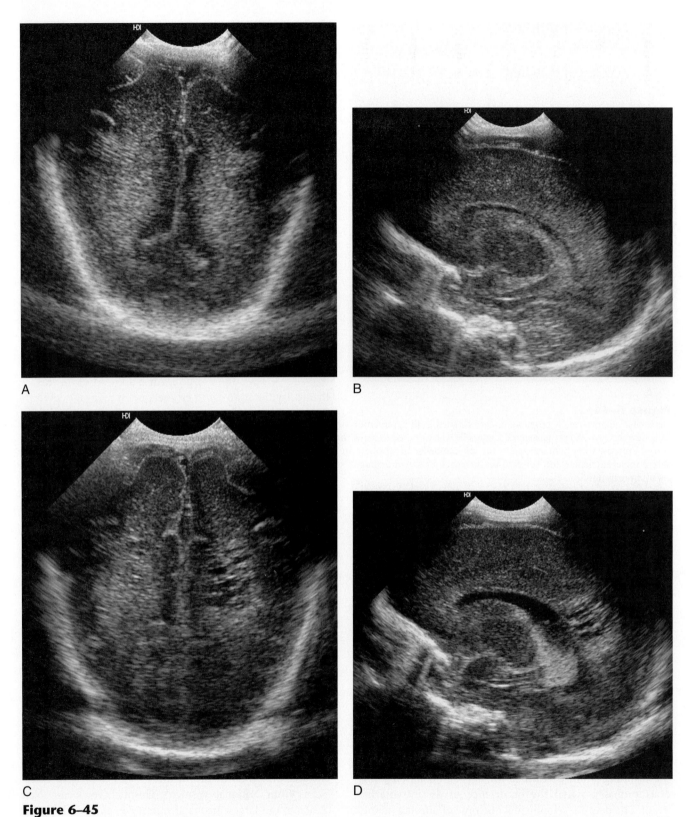

A

B

C

D

Figure 6–45

Routine ultrasonographic screening of this baby at 5 days of age shows normal brain on both a coronal scan (A) and left parasagittal view (B). At 5 weeks of age, periventricular leukomalacia, as manifest by multiple small cystic spaces, was present bilaterally. It is particularly evident on the left on this coronal scan (C) and left parasagittal view (D).

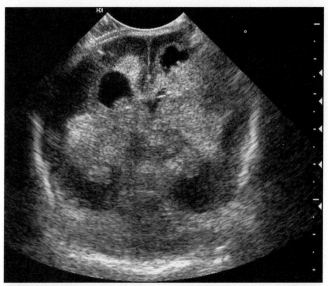

Figure 6–46
Coronal view of this neonate 6 days after birth shows extensive hemorrhage within and around the ventricles related to severe hypoxic ischemic insult.

Our suggested current protocol includes (1) screening ultrasonographic scans at 5 days of age for infants weighing less than 1500 g, (2) repeat ultrasonographic scans at 28 days, (3) a follow-up scan at discharge or at "term," whichever is earlier, (4) an immediate scan for a premature neonate who has unexplained blood loss or neurologic signs indicating an intracerebral event or who has had a significant perinatal event (such as prolonged rupture of membranes, a low Apgar score, or a need for resuscitation), and (5) if scans are abnormal, follow-up ultrasonography or other imaging, depending on the severity of findings or clinical course.

Screening protocols tend to be institutionally generated with good reasons. Some neonatal nurseries care only for infants born on site. Others have a large or exclusively referral population of neonates. Tertiary centers may receive infants with complex cardiac, surgical, or genetic abnormalities. Infants born at another site have a greater risk for intracranial insult because, with transport, they are subjected to environmental stress to which inborn infants are not. One group, in an attempt to lessen the economic burden of screening, advocated that initial scans be scheduled between days 10 and 14 of life, instead of on day 4 or 5 and again on day 14.[19] We continue to perform a scan on day 5, rather than delay the study another week, because in our environment, it gives clinicians additional information that directly affects treatment and transfer of infants. We also screen

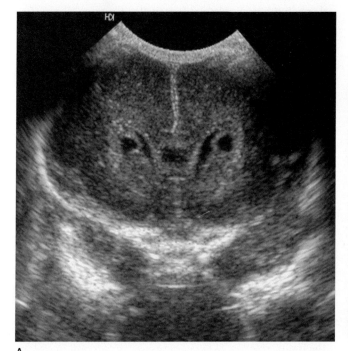

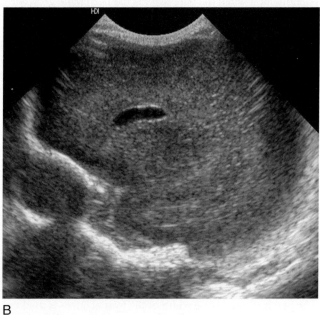

A   B

Figure 6–47
"Congenital" paraventricular cysts, when present, usually are adjacent to the frontal horns of the lateral ventricles. In this premature infant, the paraventricular cysts, an incidental finding, are bilateral and are clearly defined on a coronal view of the anterior brain *(A)*. On the left *(B)* and right *(C)* sagittal views, the cysts appear as small lucent beads paralleling the lateral ventricles.
Continued

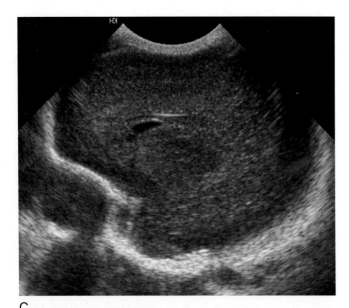

C

Figure 6–47—cont'd

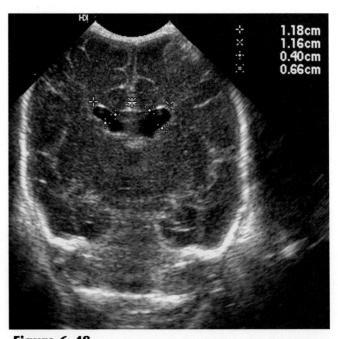

Figure 6–48
This coronal view at the level of the third ventricle, shows methods of measuring lateral ventricular size. It is apparent from this scan that transverse measurements of the maximal width of the lateral ventricle are more representative of ventricular size than is measurement from the midline.

neonates at 1 month of age. Others have emphasized that scans at or beyond 28 days of age may show ventricular enlargement or PVL despite earlier normal results.[108] Ventriculomegaly following hemorrhage in the ventricular system results from three possible mechanisms, singly or in combination: (1) overproduction of CSF (unproven as a mechanism to date), (2) obstruction of normal CSF flow and resorption,[35,92,93,116] and (3) dilatation as an ex vacuo phenomenon when the parenchyma has been damaged. The more severe the hemorrhage is, the greater the risk of posthemorrhagic ventriculomegaly.

Taylor[104] listed six goals of sonographic assessment in affected patients: (1) determining the presence of ventricular dilatation; (2) establishing the severity of ventricular dilatation; (3) localizing the obstruction; (4) demonstrating the cause of obstruction; (5) monitoring the adequacy of treatment, and (6) identifying the complications of treatment.

Measurements of ventricular size can be used as quantitative tools, but the comparison of standard coronal views from several examinations is most revealing for assessing changes in size over time. Measurements tend to be unidimensional; software for routine assessment of ventricular volume is unavailable to date. The distance between the falx and lateral extent of the frontal horns is one measurement. It includes the cavum septum pellucidum and thus is not a measure of absolute lateral dimension. In addition, it does not take into account the shape of the ventricle. The maximal transverse width of the frontal horns is used in some series and research studies (Fig. 6–48). The normal width is no more than 3 mm.[37] The width of the third ventricle cannot be adequately assessed on coronal scans because the walls are parallel to the ultrasonic beam. Accurate axial

measurement is achieved with a transverse or coronal view through the posterolateral fontanelle (asterion) (Fig. 6–49). The normal width is 0 to 2.6 mm.[37] The aqueduct is usually not evident as a discrete channel unless it is dilated from distal obstruction. Color or power Doppler ultrasonography may show the actual flow of CSF within the aqueduct if there are enough reflectors, or blood cells, within the CSF[118] (Fig. 6–50). The fourth ventricle is irregular in shape and best viewed through the asterion or posterior fontanelle. Enlargement of the fourth ventricle can occur as part of generalized blockage of the ventricular system from a subarachnoid clot but, on rare occasions, may also result from obstruction at both its inlet through the aqueduct and at its outlet foramina.[50] The choroid plexus within the fourth ventricle persists in producing CSF that cannot escape the confines of the fourth ventricle. A trapped fourth ventricle results in symptoms and signs of brainstem compression (Fig. 6–51). Several observers have recognized that ultrasonographic documentation of a clot in the cisterna magna and upper cervical canal is associated with obstructive ventriculomegaly.[35,51] An echogenic subarachnoid space around the temporal lobes is also a sign of blood around the brain.

In infants with obstructive ventriculomegaly, that is, hydrocephalus with ventricles at increased pressure, it appears that a compression stress test is valuable for diagnosis.[104,105] The RI from the anterior cerebral artery is measured before

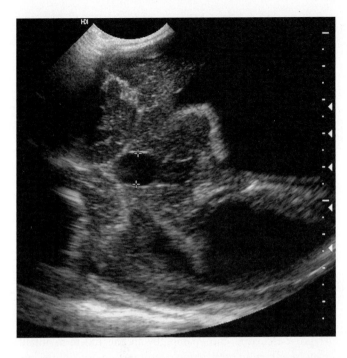

Figure 6–49
This axial scan through the posterolateral fontanelle *(asterion)* shows a widened third ventricle measured by electronic calipers. This approach is far more accurate for measurement of third ventricular width than scans through the anterior fontanelle.

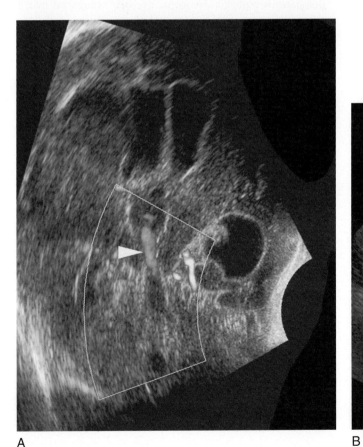

A

B

Figure 6–50
On the coronal scan via the posterolateral fontanelle, power Doppler scanning *(A)* can show flow of CSF if there are sufficient reflectors in the fluid. In this premature infant who had a preceding intraventricular hemorrhage, there was obstruction at the level of the fourth ventricle. Flow of CSF to and fro in the aqueduct, is demonstrated with blue *(B)* red.

Continued

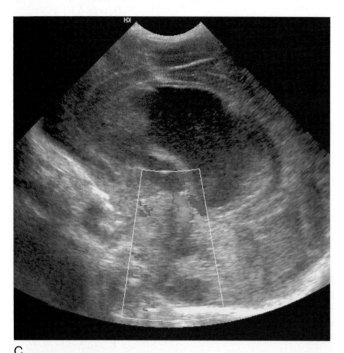

C

Figure 6–50—cont'd
(C) color signals.

and after 5 seconds of compression (with the examining transducer) over the anterior fontanelle of the neonate (Fig. 6–52). The percentage change in the RI—(compression RI − baseline RI)/baseline RI—correlated with intracranial pressure, as determined by manometry in a combined ultrasonographic and neurosurgical effort. A percentage change of 45% or greater was associated with the need for a ventriculoperitoneal shunt.

Although serial lumbar puncture is a controversial therapeutic procedure, it is used in some nurseries to treat progressive ventriculomegaly.[59,79,116] Ultrasonography can be used to monitor changes in the ventricular system following intervention. If ventriculoperitoneal shunting is deemed appropriate for an infant with posthemorrhagic or postmeningitic hydrocephalus, ultrasonography can be used during the actual surgical procedure or on follow-up scans to document the position of the shunt and to monitor complications if present. The ultrasonographic finding of persistent ventriculomegaly is an important predictor of poor neurodevelopmental outcome.[74]

INJURY TO THE TERM INFANT'S BRAIN

HYPOXIC-ISCHEMIC ENCEPHALOPATHY

Hypoxic-ischemic encephalopathy in the full-term infant may result from prepartum, intrapartum, or immediate postpartum asphyxia. Neuronal necrosis, watershed infarction in the parasagittal cortex, periventricular leukomalacia, focal ischemic injury, and venous sinus thrombosis are the neuropathologic sequelae. Ultrasonography is not as revealing as CT scanning, and neither technique is as useful as MRI in the delineation of injury. A linear array transducer of high resolution can be used to view the superficial cortex of the hemispheres. Edema or hemorrhage that may accompany parasagittal infarction is more obvious on such scans.[107] Additionally, slow or absent flow in the sagittal sinus can be diagnosed with the addition of color and pulsed-wave Doppler ultrasonography[18,65,107] (Fig. 6–53). Diffuse edema

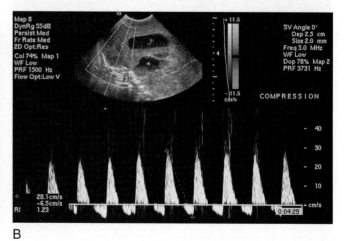

A   B

Figure 6–51
Doppler ultrasonography of the anterior cerebral artery without *(A)* and with *(B)* compression over the anterior fontanelle shows a change in the RI in this neonate who had a preceding severe intracranial hemorrhage. Views of the posterior fossa from the anterior fontanelle were poor.

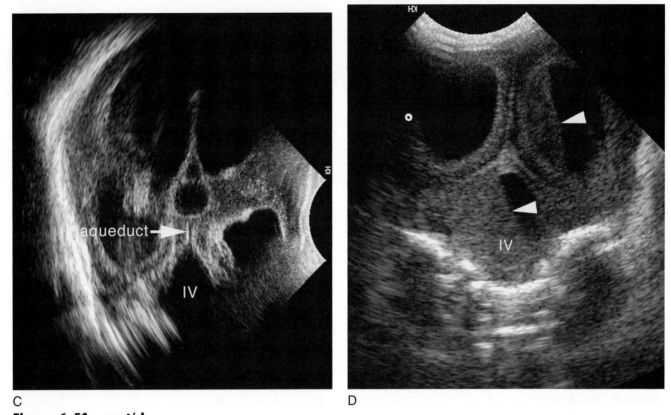

C

D

Figure 6–51—cont'd

The coronal view from the posterolateral fontanelle *(C)* shows marked enlargement of the fourth ventricle. The scan is oriented to show the third ventricle, aqueduct, and fourth ventricle (IV). The view through the posterior fontanelle *(D)* shows a fluid debris level in the occipital horn of the left lateral ventricle *(arrowhead)* and in the obstructed fourth ventricle (IV, *arrowhead*). This infant later required ventriculoperitoneal shunting.

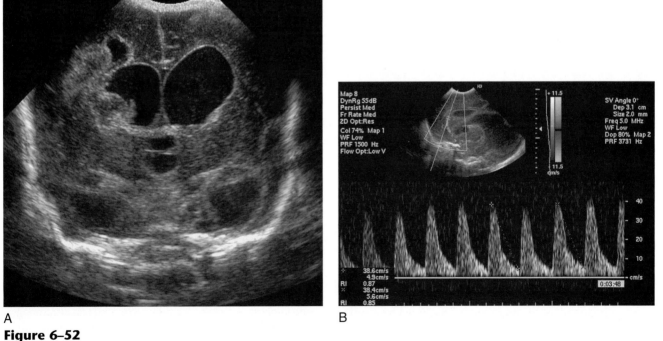

A

B

Figure 6–52

A coronal image of the brain *(A)* shows dilated ventricles several weeks after an intraventricular hemorrhage. The RI of the anterior cerebral artery without compression is 0.85 *(B).*

Continued

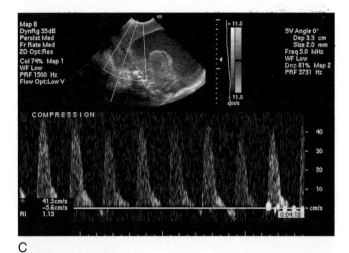

C

Figure 6–52—cont'd
After 5 seconds of compression over the anterior fontanelle, the RI increases to 1.13 *(C)*, indicating that the ventricular system is under pressure. This neonate later required ventriculoperitoneal shunting.

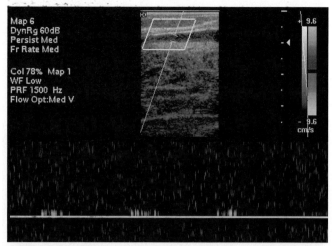

Figure 6–53
Power and pulsed-wave Doppler interrogation of the superior sagittal sinus shows minimal venous flow in this neonate who had severe hypoxic ischemic encephalopathy after birth.

tends to result in a snowy pattern of cerebral parenchyma and poor delineation of sulci and gyri. Ventricles are often slit-like (Fig. 6–54). This is a very subjective impression, however, and the lack of any appreciable abnormality on conventional ultrasonography does not rule out a significant intracranial insult.[20] Ischemic damage to periventricular white matter usually presents as an asymmetric peritrigonal blush that, with time, may cavitate. Typically, the injured area gradually contracts with the resultant ventriculomegaly being ex vacuo.

It has been generally accepted that a low RI (less than 0.6) measured from the anterior cerebral artery is a sign of loss of cerebrovascular tone, signaling a poor prognosis (Fig. 6–55). Reported series have been quite selective, however, and it is likely that multiple factors must be considered when one assesses prognosis for an asphyxiated infant and not just the waveform from a single artery.[100] Hypoxia has a major effect on cardiac function as well as on the brain. Likewise, the high RI that may be identified in some infants does not necessarily reflect only the state of the intracranial vasculature. The infant with a large patent ductus arteriosus will have significant diastolic runoff through the duct and thus a high RI.

NEONATAL STROKE

Neonatal stroke was identified in 12% of infants presenting with neonatal seizures in a large series collected from 1987 to 1993 in Oxford, England.[42] Thromboembolic disease resulting in acute infarction of the brain can be diagnosed by identifying a change in parenchymal echogenicity in a focal area of the brain in association with decreased vasculature or changes in the velocity of cerebral blood flow[55,82] (Fig. 6–56).

A thrombotic tendency was identified in 30% of infants who presented with stroke in one study.[21] Approximately one third of survivors make a complete recovery.[99]

SINOVENOUS THROMBOSIS

Thrombosis of the superior sagittal sinus or other venous sinuses has been associated with a thrombogenic tendency in 50% of infants from a reported study.[21] Venous thrombosis is also associated with hypoxia-ischemia. The true prevalence is unknown because a concerted effort to diagnose the condition must be made. Linear array transducers are best for the evaluation of the superior sagittal sinus. Bulging of the sinus beyond its normal triangular shape on coronal scans, echogenic material within the sinus, failure of the sinus to change with compression, and lack of identifiable flow within the superior sagittal sinus are all signs of thrombosis or incipient thrombosis[18,65] (Fig. 6–57).

EXTRA-AXIAL HEMORRHAGE

It is surprising that more neonates do not have clinically discernible subarachnoid and subdural hemorrhage simply from being born. Molding and pressure on the fetal skull can cause spontaneous hemorrhage in the extra-axial spaces. Subdural hematoma is associated with vigorous extraction such as vacuum and forceps deliveries but also can follow uncomplicated delivery. It can be quite subtle on ultrasonography. Careful attention to the symmetry of the brain is important in recognizing a frontoparietal subdural hemorrhage because the extra-axial collection is at the edge of the scanning

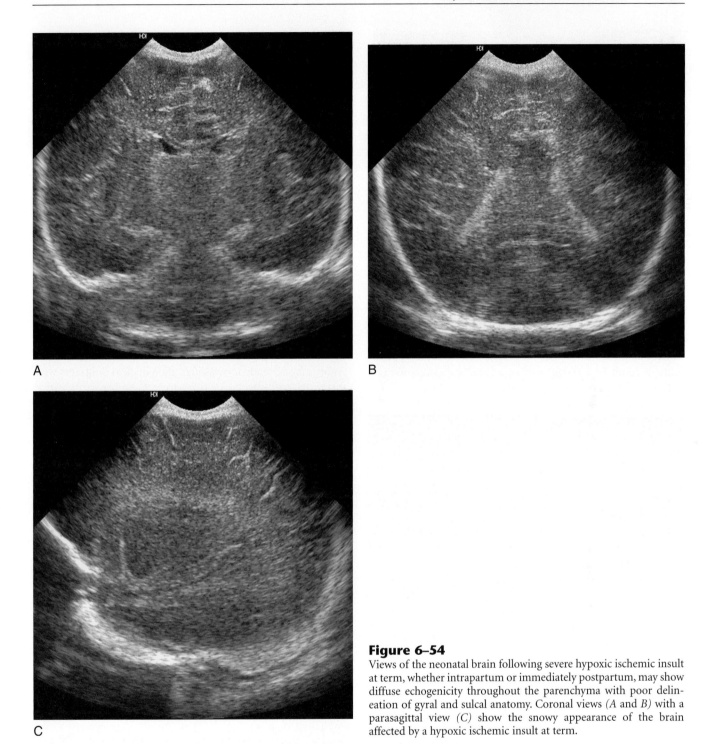

A

B

C

Figure 6–54
Views of the neonatal brain following severe hypoxic ischemic insult at term, whether intrapartum or immediately postpartum, may show diffuse echogenicity throughout the parenchyma with poor delineation of gyral and sulcal anatomy. Coronal views *(A and B)* with a parasagittal view *(C)* show the snowy appearance of the brain affected by a hypoxic ischemic insult at term.

plane. Sector scans through the anterior fontanelle must be angled out to the surface of the brain to recognize a collection of blood over the convexity. The midline of the brain may be shifted (Fig. 6–58). The ipsilateral lateral ventricle may be smaller. Transaxial scans via the asterion show a lateral supratentorial collection clearly. The involved side must be contralateral to the position of the transducer and not in

the near field. A subtemporal subdural collection can be quite difficult to recognize. Asymmetry in the appearance of the temporal lobes is the key finding. Often, there is no midline shift. A subdural collection in the posterior fossa is the most difficult diagnosis of all and can be completely overlooked on ultrasonography. It tends to silhouette the cerebellum so
Text continued on page 236

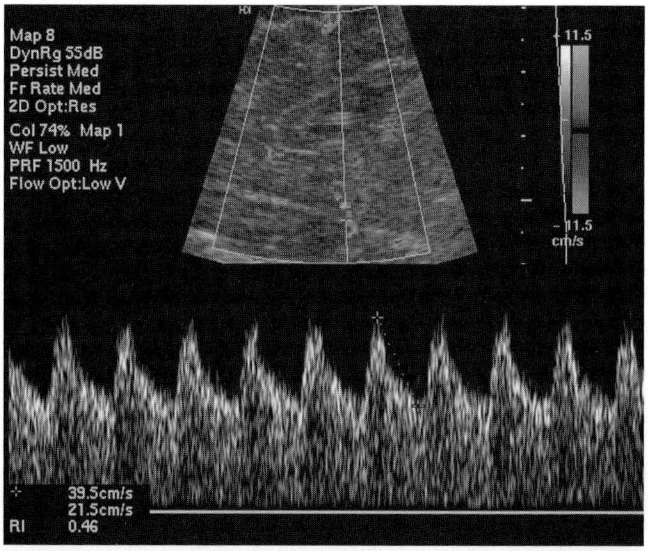

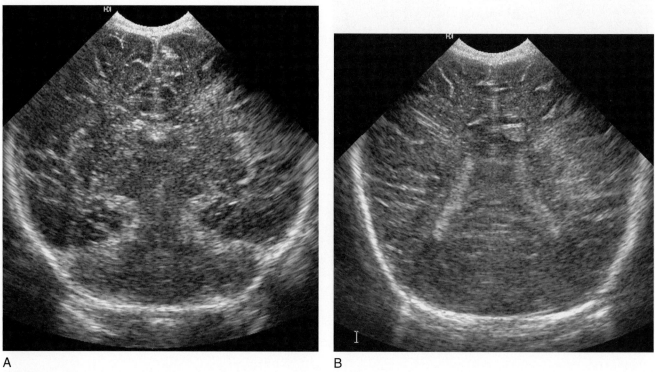

Figure 6–55
A midline sagittal scan shows the anterior cerebral artery being sampled with pulsed-wave Doppler imaging and the resulting waveform. A RI of 0.46 supports a diagnosis of severe hypoxic ischemic insult.

A   B

Figure 6–56
A neonate born at term presented with seizures during the first day of life. These were focal and right-sided. Ultrasonography shows an ill-defined area of echogenicity on the left on the coronal scans (A and B).

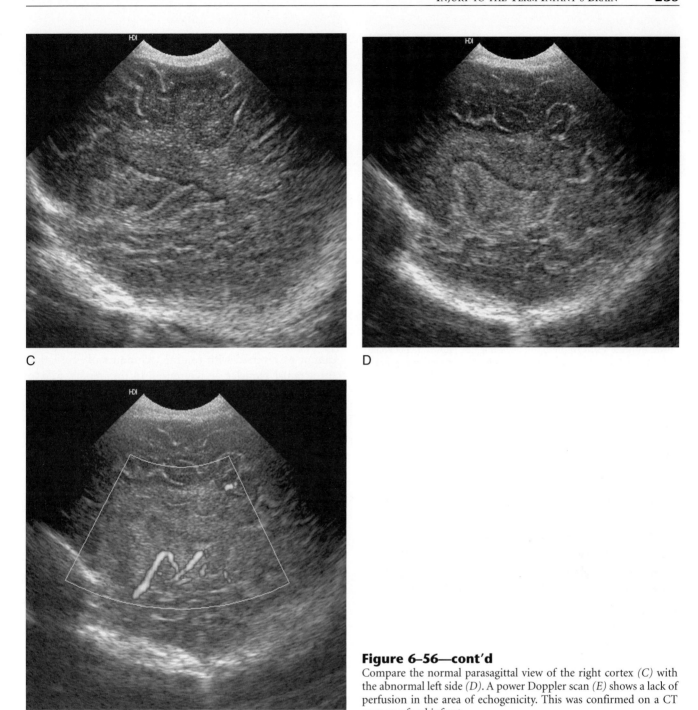

Figure 6–56—cont'd
Compare the normal parasagittal view of the right cortex *(C)* with the abnormal left side *(D)*. A power Doppler scan *(E)* shows a lack of perfusion in the area of echogenicity. This was confirmed on a CT scan as a focal infarct.

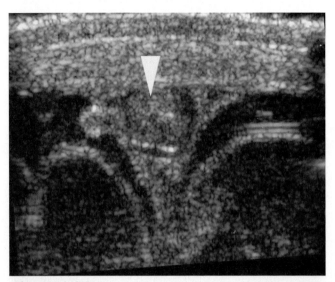

Figure 6–57
A clot in the superior sagittal sinus was unexpected in this prematurely delivered infant. She presented with seizures 7 days after birth. Routine scans of the brain were normal. However, a coronal scan through the anterior fontanelle with a linear array transducer, 10 MHz in frequency, shows a clot *(arrowhead)* distending the superior sagittal sinus. The infant was treated with anticoagulation and had an uneventful recovery.

that the edges are indistinct. Views through the posterior fontanelle or suboccipital window are very helpful. The clinical situation is usually quite alarming in affected infants because of compression of the brainstem. Decompression of the collection must be performed as soon as possible.[86] CT scanning is

diagnostic and, if available, is the study of choice in suspected subdural hematoma in all locations.

CHOROID PLEXUS HEMORRHAGE

Hemorrhage originating in the choroid plexus can occur as an isolated event or concurrent with other intracerebral bleeding in premature and full-term neonates.[48] Asymmetry of the choroid plexus is a clue to its presence (Fig. 6–59). The functional implications are unclear.

EXTRACORPOREAL MEMBRANE OXYGENATION

Extracorporeal membrane oxygenation (ECMO) is a technique of cardiopulmonary bypass. It is available in some tertiary centers for infants who have severe hypoxemia that cannot be reversed with routine techniques of ventilation. Intracranial sequelae are common. In one report, 52% of survivors of a cohort of 386 treated infants had an intracranial abnormality on ultrasonography or a CT scan. Hemorrhage, isolated or in combination with other findings, was present in 30%.[25] Almost all major hemorrhagic insults were identified on ultrasonography. Outcomes from centers that use ECMO must be carefully analyzed in terms of the type of ECMO used and the characteristics of the cohort. The infant's primary disease is highly associated with morbidity and

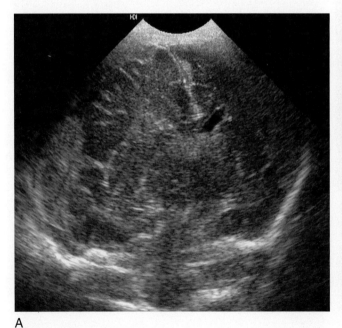
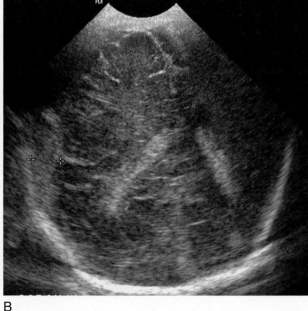

A   B

Figure 6–58
This subdural hematoma over the right frontoparietal lobe is large enough to produce a midline shift and is obvious on coronal views *(A and B)* through the anterior fontanelle.

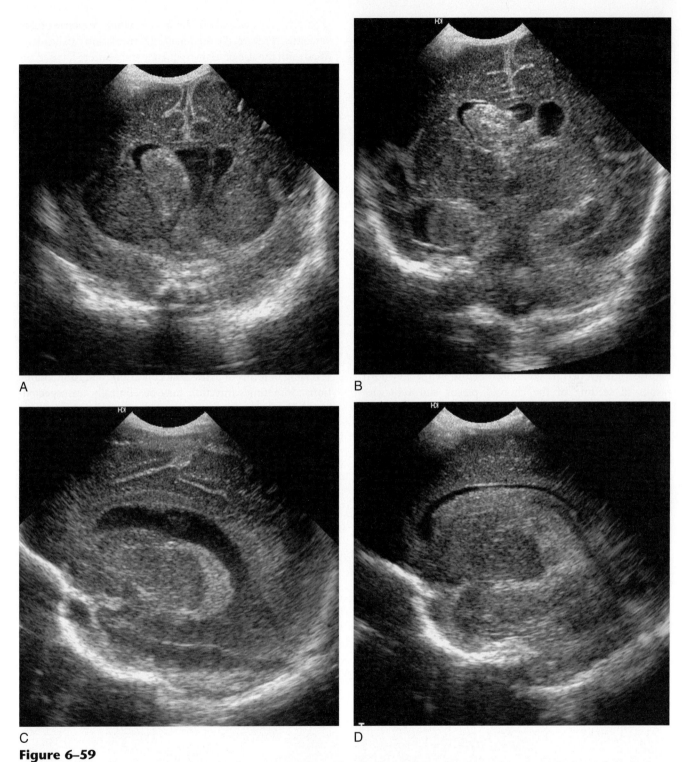

A

B

C

D

Figure 6–59
A choroid plexus hematoma may be isolated or may coexist with other hemorrhages. In this patient, coronal views of the brain at the level of the middle cerebral arteries *(A)* and third ventricle *(B)* showed a large echogenic mass representing a hemorrhage within the choroid plexus in the right lateral ventricle. No other site of hemorrhage was documented. Note the midline shift to the left. The normal left lateral ventricle *(C)* is shown for comparison with the abnormal right lateral ventricle *(D)*.

TABLE 6-5 Ultrasonographic Findings in Meningitis-Encephalitis

No anatomic abnormality (common in early stages and if prompt treatment given)
Diffuse edema
Echogenic subdural and subarachnoid space
Pial thickening/echogenicity
Stranding within ventricular system
Concomitant intracranial hemorrhage in premature
Periventricular leukomalacia
Focal infarcts
Intracranial abscess/liquefaction in certain infections

mortality with diaphragmatic hernia yielding the most pessimistic outcome figures.[46]

MENINGITIS-ENCEPHALITIS

Ultrasonographic findings in meningitis reflect the neuropathology of this condition. Sepsis in the newborn results in seeding of the choroid plexus and ventricles with bacteria. The CSF then carries the bacteria to the subarachnoid space where the inflammatory response causes vasculitis. If severe, the meningeal inflammation can be identified with the use of high-frequency transducers focused on the near field. Echogenic subarachnoid space and pial accentuation result. Cortical venous thromboses and arteritis are the result of inflammation of the ependymal and meningeal surfaces; therefore, in this phase, the findings of meningitis overlap with those of aseptic hypoxic-ischemic insult. Edema is a prominent feature of acute meningitis. Late complications include extra-axial collections of fluid and obstructive ventriculomegaly due to the scarring and destruction of normal pathways of CSF resorption (Table 6–5).

The most common organism isolated in infants with neonatal meningitis is group B streptococcus. Organisms that have a particularly devastating effect, with destruction and cavitation of brain resulting, are *Bacillus cereus, Serratia marcescens,* and *Citrobacter, Proteus, Pseudomonas,* and *Enterobacter* species[53,113(p29)] (Fig. 6–60). Typically, meningitis is diagnosed clinically, and ultrasonography plays a minor role. It should be emphasized that results of ultrasonography are often normal in neonates who have encephalitis-meningitis and is not a means of diagnosis. CT scans are usually more revealing in terms of extra-axial collections and focal infarctions. Sometimes infection may be clinically unsuspected, but clues to its presence may be evident on ultrasonography.

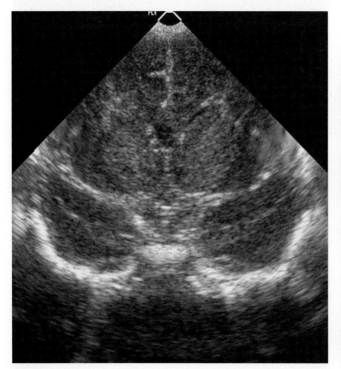

A

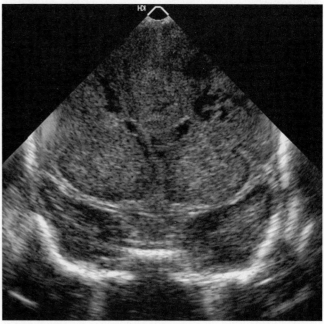

B

Figure 6–60
Coronal scan of this neonate performed 5 days after birth shows normal intracerebral anatomy *(A)*. At 1 month of age and several days after onset of encephalitis caused by *Bacillus cereus,* there was early liquefaction of the brain *(B)*.

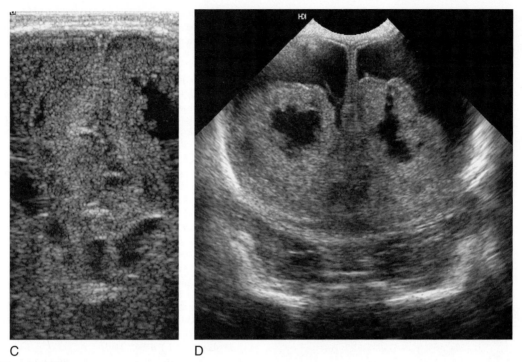

C   D

Figure 6–60—cont'd

The parenchymal involvement is shown well in a scan performed with a 10 MHz linear array transducer *(C)*. Ten days later, a coronal scan *(D)* shows severe cystic encephalomalacia associated with this infection. Collapse of the brain has resulted in marked widening of the extra-axial spaces.

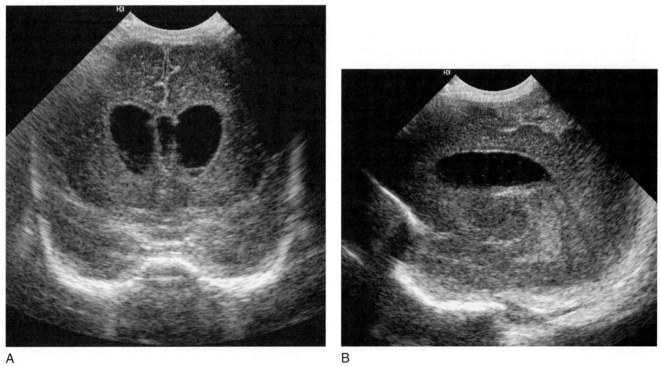

A   B

Figure 6–61

Sepsis from *Escherichia coli* was associated with meningitis, ventricular dilatation, and ventricular debris *(A and B)* in this premature infant. Two weeks after the acute event, scans revealed fine fibrinous strands, like cobwebs, throughout the ventricular system *(C)*. This appearance is typical of infection and atypical of intraventricular hemorrhage.

Continued

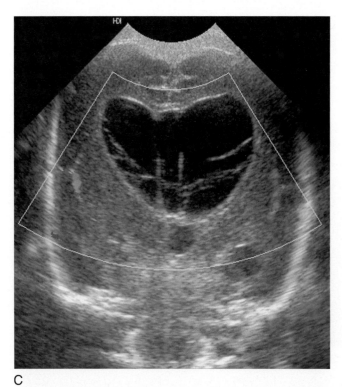

C

Figure 6–61—cont'd

In particular, the finding of stranding in the ventricular system is a sign of infection. Often this occurs with prematurity and known intraventricular hemorrhage. However, lysis of aseptic blood clots in ventricles does not produce the same pattern of sheets of tissue that may, in fact, represent glial bridges after ependymal disruption[113(p29)] (Fig. 6–61).

REFERENCES

1. Abbitt PL, Hurst RW, Ferguson RD, McIlhenny J, Alford BA.The role of ultrasound in the management of vein of Galen aneurysms in infancy. Neuroradiology 32:86–9, 1990.
2. Adcock LM, Moore PJ, Schlesinger AE, Armstrong DL. Correlation of ultrasound with postmortem neuropathologic studies in neonates. Pediatr Neurol 19:263–71, 1998.
3. Ahmann PA, Lazzara A, Dykes FD, Brann AW Jr, Schwartz JF. Intraventricular hemorrhage in the high-risk preterm infant: incidence and outcome. Ann Neurol 7:118–24, 1980.
4. Allison JW, Faddis LA, Kinder DL, Roberson PK, Glasier CM, Seibert JJ. Intracranial resistive index (RI) values in normal term infants during the first day of life. Pediatr Radiol 30:618–20, 2000.
5. Altman NR, Naidich TP, Braffman BH. Posterior fossa malformations. AJNR 13:691–724, 1992.
6. Anderson NG, Hay R, Hutchings M, Whitehead M, Darlow B. Posterior fontanelle cranial ultrasound: anatomic and sonographic correlation. Early Hum Dev 42:141–152, 1995.
7. Armstrong DL, Bagnall C, Harding JE, Teele RL. Measurement of the subarachnoid space by ultrasound in preterm infants. Arch Dis Child Fetal Neonatal Ed 86:F124–F126, 2002.
8. Avery ME, First LR, eds. Pediatric Medicine. Williams & Wilkins, Baltimore, MD. pp 130–134, 1989.
9. Babcook CJ. Ultrasound evaluation of prenatal and neonatal spina bifida. Neurosurg Clin N Am 6:203–18, 1995.
10. Barkovich AJ. Pediatric Neuroimaging, 3rd Edition. Lippincott Williams & Wilkins. Philadelphia, PA. pp 285–6, 2000.
11. Barkovich AJ, Gressens P, Evrard P. Formation, maturation and disorders of brain neocortex. AJNR 13:423–446, 1992.
12. Barkovich AJ, Lyon G, Evrard P. Formation, maturation and disorders of white matter. AJNR 13:447–461, 1992.
13. Barnes PD. Neuroimaging and the timing of fetal and neonatal brain injury. J Perinatol 21:44–60, 2001.
14. Barr LL. Neonatal cranial ultrasound. Radiol Clin North Am 37: 1127–1146, 1999.
15. Bass WT, Jones MA, White LE, Montgomery TR, Aiello F 3rd, Karlowicz MG. Ultrasonographic differential diagnosis and neurodevelopmental outcome of cerebral white matter lesions in premature infants. J Perinatol 19:330–6, 1999.
16. Baumeister FA, Hofer M. Cerebellar hemorrhage in preterm infants with intraventricular hemorrhage: a missed diagnosis? A patient report. Clin Pediatr 39:611–3, 2000.
17. Becroft DM, Gunn TR. Prenatal cranial haemorrhages in 47 Pacific Islander infants: is traditional massage the cause? NZ Med J 102: 207–10, 1989.
18. Bezinque SL, Slovis TL, Touchette AS, Schave DM, Jarski RW, Bedard MP, Martino AM. Characterization of superior sagittal sinus blood flow velocity using color flow Doppler in neonates and infants. Pediatr Radiol 25:175–9, 1995.
19. Boal DK, Watterberg KL, Miles S, Gifford KL. Optimal cost-effective timing of cranial ultrasound screening in low-birth-weight infants. Pediatr Radiol 25:425–8, 1995.
20. Boo NY, Chandran V, Zulfiqar MA, Zamratol SM, Nyein MK, Haliza MS, Lye MS. Early cranial ultrasound changes as predictors of outcome during first year of life in term infants with perinatal asphyxia. J Paediatr Child Health 36:363–369, 2000.
21. Bonduel M, Sciuccati G, Hepner M, Torres AF, Pieroni G, Frontroth JP. Prethrombotic disorders in children with arterial ischemic stroke and sinovenous thrombosis. Arch Neurol 56: 967–71, 1999.
22. Bromley B, Nadel AS, Pauker S, Estroff JA, Benacerraf BR. Closure of the cerebellar vermis: evaluation with second trimester US. Radiology 193:761–3, 1994.
23. Brunelle F. Arteriovenous malformation of the vein of Galen in children. Pediatr Radiol 27:501–13, 1997.
24. Buckley KM, Taylor GA, Estroff JA, Barnewolt CE, Share JC, Paltiel HJ. Use of the mastoid fontanelle for improved sonographic visualization of the neonatal midbrain and posterior fossa. AJR 168:1021–25, 1997.
25. Bulas DI, Taylor GA, O'Donnell RM, Short BL, Fitz CR, Vezina G. Intracranial abnormalities in infants treated with extracorporeal membrane oxygenation: update on sonographic and CT findings. AJNR 17:287–94, 1996.
26. Burstein J, Papile LA, Burstein R. Intraventricular hemorrhage and hydrocephalus in premature newborns: a prospective study with CT. AJR 132:631–35, 1979.
27. Calvert SA, Ohlsson A, Hosking MC, Erskine L, Fong K, Shennan AT. Serial measurements of cerebral blood flow velocity in preterm infants during the first 72 hours of life. Acta Paediatr Scand 77:625–31, 1988.
28. Chang MC, Russell SA, Callen PW, Filly RA, Goldstein RB. Sonographic detection of inferior vermian agenesis in Dandy-Walker malformations: prognostic implications. Radiology 193:765–70, 1994.
29. Chang YC, Huang CC, Liu CC. Frequency of linear hyperechogenicity over the basal ganglia in young infants with congenital rubella syndrome. Clin Infect Dis 22:569–71, 1996.
30. Cioni G, Bos AF, Einspieler C, Ferrari F, Martijn A, Paolicelli PB, Rapisardi G, Roversi MF, Prechtl HF. Early neurological signs in preterm infants with unilateral intraparenchymal echodensity. Neuropediatrics 31:240–51, 2000.

31. Cohen MM Jr, Lemire RJ. Syndromes with cephaloceles. Teratology 25:161–72, 1982.

32. Coley BD, Rusin JA, Boue DR. Importance of hypoxic/ischemic conditions in the development of cerebral lenticulostriate vasculopathy. Pediatr Radiol 30:846–55, 2000.

33. Couture A, Veyrac C, Baud C, Saguintaah M, Ferran JL. Advanced cranial ultrasound: transfontanellar Doppler imaging in neonates. Eur Radiol 11:2399–410, 2001.

34. Cramer BC, Jequier S, O'Gorman AM. Sonography of the neonatal craniocervical junction. AJR 147:133–9, 1986.

35. Cramer BC, Walsh EA. Cisterna magna clot and subsequent post-hemorrhagic hydrocephalus. Pediatr Radiol 31:153–9, 2001.

36. Czechowski J, Langille EL, Varady E. Intracardiac tumour and brain lesions in tuberous sclerosis. A case report of antenatal diagnosis by ultrasonography. Acta Radiol 41:371–4, 2000.

37. Davies MW, Swaminathan M, Chuang SL, Betheras FR. Reference ranges for the linear dimensions of the intracranial ventricles in preterm neonates. Arch Dis Child Fetal Neonatal Ed 82:F218–23, 2000.

38. De Felice C, Toti P, Laurini RN, Stumpo M, Picciolini E, Todros T, Tanganelli P, Buonocore G, Bracci R. Early neonatal brain injury in histologic chorioamnionitis. J Pediatr 138:101–104, 2001.

39. de Koning TJ, Gooskens R, Veenhoven R, Meijboom EJ, Jansen GH, Lasjaunias P, de Vries LS. Arteriovenous malformation of the vein of Galen in three neonates: emphasis on associated early ischemic brain damage. Eur J Pediatr 156:228–9,1997.

40. Demaerel P, Van de Gaer P, Wilms G, Baert AL. Interhemispheric lipoma with variable callosal dysgenesis: relationship between embryology, morphology and symptomatology. Eur Radiol 6:904–909, 1996.

41. Di Salvo DN. A new view of the neonatal brain: clinical utility of supplemental neurologic US imaging windows. Radiographics 21:943–55, 2001.

42. Estan J, Hope P. Unilateral neonatal cerebral infarction in full term infants. Arch Dis Child Fetal Neonatal Ed 76:F88–93, 1997.

43. Fogarty K, Cohen HL, Haller JO. Sonography of fetal intracranial hemorrhage: unusual causes and a review of the literature. J Clin Ultrasound 17:366–70, 1989.

44. Frank DA, McCarten KM, Robson CD, Mirochnick M, Cabral H, Zuckerman B. Level of in utero cocaine exposure and neonatal ultrasound findings. Pediatrics 104:1101–5, 1999.

45. Gherpelli JL, Santos Filho AS, Silveira JD, Tani ME, Costa HP. Incidence of peri-intraventricular hemorrhage in preterm newborn infants with birth weight less than 1500gm: evaluation of brain ultrasonographic studies and necropsy. Arq Neuropsiquiatr 50:284–88, 1992.

46. Graziani LJ, Gringlas M, Baumgart S. Cerebrovascular complications and neurodevelopmental sequelae of neonatal ECMO. Clin Perinatol 24:655–75, 1997.

47. Gressens P. Mechanisms and Disturbances of Neuronal Migration. Pediatr Res 8:725–30, 2000.

48. Haataja L, Mercuri E, Cowan F, Dubowitz L. Cranial ultrasound abnormalities in full term infants in a postnatal ward: outcome at 12 and 18 months. Arch Dis Child Fetal Neonatal Ed 82:F128–33, 2000.

49. Hack M, Fanaroff AA. Outcomes of children of extremely low birth-weight and gestational age in the 1990s. Semin Neonatol 5:89–106, 2000.

50. Hall TR, Choi A, Schellinger D, Grant EG. Isolation of the fourth ventricle causing transtentorial herniation: Neurosonographic findings in premature infants. AJR 159:811–15, 1992.

51. Hansen AR, DiSalvo D, Kazam E, Allred EN, Leviton A. Sonographically detected subarachnoid hemorrhage: an independent predictor of neonatal posthemorrhagic hydrocephalus? Clin Imaging 24:121–9, 2000.

52. Haverkamp F, Lex C, Hanisch C, Fahnenstich H, Zerres K. Neurodevelopmental risks in twin-to-twin transfusion syndrome, preliminary findings. Europ J Paediatr Neurol 5:21–27, 2001.

53. Hedlund GL, Boyer RS. Neuroimaging of postnatal pediatric central nervous system infections. Semin Pediatr Neurol 6:299–317, 1999.

54. Heling KS, Chaoui R, Bollmann R. Prenatal diagnosis of an aneurysm of the vein of Galen with three-dimensional color power angiography. Ultrasound Obstet Gynecol 15:333–6, 2000.

55. Hernanz-Schulman M, Cohen W, Genieser NB. Sonography of cerebral infarction in infancy. AJR 150:897–902, 1988.

56. Hollier LM. Can neurological injury be timed? Semin Perinatol 24:204–14, 2000.

57. Hoon AH Jr, Melhem ER. Neuroimaging: applications in disorders of early brain development. J Dev Behav Pediatr 21:291–302, 2000.

58. Huang CC. Sonographic cerebral sulcal development in premature newborns. Brain Dev 13:27–31, 1991.

59. Hudgins RJ. Posthemorrhagic hydrocephalus of infancy. Neurosurg Clin N Am 12:743–51, 2001.

60. Hughes P, Weinberger E, Shaw DW. Linear areas of echogenicity in the thalami and basal ganglia of neonates: an expanded association. Work in progress. Radiology 179:103–5, 1991.

61. Huppi PS, Warfield S, Kikinis R, Barnes PD, Zientara GP, Jolesz FA, Tsuji MK, Volpe JJ. Quantitative magnetic resonance imaging of brain development in premature and mature newborns. Ann Neurol 43:224–35, 1998.

62. Kuban KC, Allred EN, Dammann O, Pagano M, Leviton A, Share J, Abiri M, DiSalvo D, Doubilet P, Kairam R, Kazam E, Kirpekar M, Rosenfeld DL, Sanocka UM, Schonfeld SM. Topography of cerebral white-matter disease of prematurity studied prospectively in 1607 very-low-birthweight infants. J Child Neurol 16:401–8, 2001.

63. Kuban KC, Teele RL, Wallman J. Septo-optic-dysplasia-schizencephaly. Radiographic and clinical features. Pediatr Radiol 19:145–50, 1989.

64. Laing FC, Frates MC, Brown DL, Benson CB, Di Salvo DN, Doubilet PM. Sonography of the fetal posterior fossa: false appearance of mega-cisterna magna and Dandy-Walker variant. Radiology 192:247–51, 1994.

65. Lam AH. Doppler imaging of superior sagittal sinus thrombosis. J Ultrasound Med 14:41–6, 1995.

66. Levine D, Barnes P, Korf B, Edelman R. Tuberous sclerosis in the fetus: second-trimester diagnosis of subependymal tubers with ultrafast MR imaging. AJR 175:1067–9, 2000.

67. Levitsky DB, Mack LA, Nyberg DA, Shurtleff DB, Shields LA, Nghiem HV, Cyr DR. Fetal aqueductal stenosis diagnosed sonographically: how grave is the prognosis? AJR 164:725–30, 1995.

68. Luna JA, Goldstein RB. Sonographic visualization of neonatal posterior fossa abnormalities through the posterolateral fontanelle. AJR 174:561–7, 2000.

69. Makhoul IR, Zmora O, Tamir A, Shahar E, Sujov P. Congenital subependymal pseudocysts: own data and meta-analysis of the literature. Isr Med Assoc J 3:178–83, 2001.

70. McClone DG, Knepper PA. The cause of Chiari II malformation: a unified theory. Pediatr Neurosci 13:1–12, 1989.

71. McClone DG, Naidich TP. Developmental morphology of the subarachnoid space, brain vasculature, and contiguous structures, and the cause of the Chiari II malformation. AJNR 13:463–482, 1992.

72. Menezes AH, Bell WE, Perret GE. Arachnoid cysts in children. Arch Neurol 37:168–72, 1980.

73. Ment LR, Schneider KC, Ainley MA, Allan WC. Adaptive mechanisms of developing brain. The neuroradiologic assessment of the preterm infant. Clin Perinatol 27:303–23, 2000.

74. Ment LR, Vohr B, Allan W, Westerveld M, Katz KH, Schneider KC, Makuch RW. The etiology and outcome of cerebral ventriculomegaly at term in very low birth weight preterm infants. Pediatrics 104:243–8, 1999.

75. Merrill JD, Piecuch RF, Fell SC, Barkovich AJ, Goldstein RB. A new pattern of cerebellar hemorrhages in preterm infants. Pediatrics 102:E62, 1998.

76. Mitra AG, Dickerson C. Central nervous system tumor with associated unilateral ventriculomegaly: unusual prenatal presentation of subsequently diagnosed tuberous sclerosis. J Ultrasound Med 19:651–4, 2000.

77. Miyawaki T, Matsui K, Takashima S. Developmental characteristics of vessel density in the human fetal and infant brains. Early Hum Dev 53:65–72, 1998.

78. Mott SH, Bodensteiner JB, Allan WC. The cavum septum pellucidi in term and preterm infants. J Child Neurol 7:35–8, 1992.

79. Muller W, Urlesberger B, Maurer U, Kuttnig-Haim M, Reiterer F, Moradi G, Pichler G. Serial lumbar tapping to prevent posthaemorrhagic hydrocephalus after intracranial haemorrhage in preterm infants. Wien Klin Wochenschr 2:631–64, 1998.

80. Muller-Scholden J, Lehrnbecher T, Muller HL, Bensch J, Hengen Sorensen N, Stockhausen HB. Radical surgery in a neonate with craniopharyngioma. Report of a case. Pediatr Neurosurg 33:265–69, 2000.

81. Naidich TP, Altman NR, Braffman BH, McLone DG, Zimmerman RA. Cephaloceles and related malformations. AJNR 13:655-690, 1992.

82. Nishimaki S, Seki K, Yokota S. Cerebral blood flow velocity in two patients with neonatal cerebral infarction. Pediatr Neurol 24: 320–323, 2001.

83. Papile LA, Burstein J, Burstein R, Koffler H. Incidence and evolution of subependymal and intraventricular hemorrhage: a study of infants with birth weights less than 1500gm. J Pediatr 92:529–34, 1978.

84. Paul DA, Pearlman SA, Finkelstein MS, Stefano JL. Cranial sonography in very-low-birth-weight infants: do all infants need to be screened? Clin Pediatr (Phila) 38:503–9, 1999.

85. Perlman JM, Rollins N. Surveillance protocol for the detection of intracranial abnormalities in premature neonates. Arch Pediatr Adolesc Med 154:822–6, 2000.

86. Perrin RG, Rutka JT, Drake JM, Meltzer H, Hellman J, Jay V, Hoffman HJ, Humphreys RP. Management and outcomes of posterior fossa subdural hematomas in neonates. Neurosurgery 40:1190–99, 1997.

87. Pierrat V, Duquennoy C, van Haastert IC, Ernst M, Guilley N, de Vries LS. Ultrasound diagnosis and neurodevelopmental outcome of localised and extensive cystic periventricular leucomalacia. Arch Dis Child Fetal Neonatal Ed 84:F151–6, 2001.

88. Raybaud CA, Strother CM, Hald JK. Aneurysms of the vein of Galen: embryonic considerations and anatomical features relating to the pathogenesis of the malformation. Neuroradiology 31:109–28, 1989.

89. Resch B, Vollaard E, Maurer U, Haas J, Rosegger H, Muller W. Risk factors and determinants of neurodevelopmental outcome in cystic periventricular leucomalacia. Eur J Pediatr 159:663–70, 2000.

90. Roessmann U. Septo-optic dysplasia (SOD) or DeMorsier syndrome. J Clin Neuroophthalmol 9:156–9, 1989.

91. Rorke LB. Anatomical features of the developing brain implicated in pathogenesis of hypoxic-ischemic injury. Brain Pathol 2:211–21, 1992.

92. Rudas G, Almassy Z, Papp B, Varga E, Meder U, Taylor GA. Echodense spinal subarachnoid space in neonates with progressive ventricular dilatation: a marker of noncommunicating hydrocephalus. AJR 171:1119–21, 1998.

93. Rudas G, Varga E, Meder U, Pataki M, Taylor GA. Changes in echogenicity of spinal subarachnoid space associated with intracranial hemorrhage: new observations. Pediatr Radiol 30:739–42, 2000.

94. Sener RN. Septo-optic-dysplasia associated with cerebral cortical dysplasia (cortico-septo-optic-dysplasia). J Neuroradiol 23:245–7, 1996.

95. Sgro M, Barozzino T, Toi A, Johnson J, Sermer M, Chitayat D. Prenatal detection of cerebral lesions in a fetus with tuberous sclerosis. Ultrasound Obstet Gynecol 14:356–9, 1999.

96. Shankaran S, Slovis TL, Bedard MP, Poland RL. Sonographic classification of intracranial hemorrhage. A prognostic indicator of mortality, morbidity, and short-term neurologic outcome. J Pediatr 100:469–75,1982.

97. Shefer-Kaufman N, Mimouni FB, Stavorovsky Z, Meyer JJ, Dollberg S. Incidence and clinical significance of echogenic vasculature in the basal ganglia of newborns. Am J Perinatol 16:315–9, 1999.

98. Sie LT, van der Knapp MS, van Wezel-Meijler G, Taets van Amerongen AH, Lafeber HN, Valk J. Early MR features of hypoxic-ischemic brain injury in neonates with periventricular densities on sonograms. AJNR 21:852–61, 2000.

99. Sreenan C, Bhargava R, Robertson CM. Cerebral infarction in the term newborn: clinical presentation and long-term outcome. J Pediatr 137:351–55, 2000.

100. Stark JE, Seibert JJ. Cerebral artery Doppler ultrasonography for prediction of outcome after perinatal asphyxia. J Ultrasound Med 13:595–600, 1994.

101. Strand RD, Barnes PD, Poussaint TY, Estroff JA, Burrows PE. Cystic retrocerebellar malformations: unification of the Dandy-Walker complex and the Blake's pouch cyst. Pediatr Radiol 23:258–60, 1993.

102. Sudakoff G, Montazemi M, Rifkin M. The foramen magnum: the underutilized acoustic window to the posterior fossa. J Ultrasound Med 4:205–215, 1993.

103. Taylor GA. Effect of germinal matrix hemorrhage on terminal vein position and patency. Pediatr Radiol 25:S37–40, 1995.

104. Taylor GA. Sonographic assessment of posthemorrhagic ventricular dilatation. Radiol Clin North Am 39:541–51, 2001.

105. Taylor GA, Madsen JR. Hemodynamic response to fontanelle compression in neonatal hydrocephalus. Correlation with intracranial pressure and need for shunt placement. Radiology 201:685–9, 1996.

106. Teele RL, Hernanz-Schulman M, Sotrel A. Echogenic vasculature in the basal ganglia of neonates: a sonographic sign of vasculopathy. Radiology 169:423–7, 1988.

107. Thomson GD, Teele RL. High-frequency linear array transducers for neonatal cerebral sonography. AJR 176:995–1001, 2001.

108. Townsend SF, Rumack CM, Thilo EH, Merenstein GB, Rosenberg AA. Late neurosonographic screening is important to the diagnosis of periventricvular leukomalacia and ventricular enlargement in preterm infants. Pediatr Radiol 29:347–52, 1999.

109. Tulipan N, Hernanz-Schulman M, Lowe LH, Bruner JP. Intrauterine myelomeningocele repair reverses preexisting hindbrain herniation. Pediatr Neurosurg 31:137–142, 1999.

110. Vergani P, Patane L, Doria P, Borroni C, Cappellini A, Pezzullo JC, Ghidini A. Risk factors for neonatal intraventricular haemorrhage in spontaneous prematurity at 32 weeks gestation or less. Placenta 21:402–7, 2000.

111. Vermeulen GM, Bruinse HW, Gerards LJ, de Vries LS. Perinatal risk factors for cranial ultrasound abnormalities in neonates born after spontaneous labour before 34 weeks. Eur J Obstet Gynecol Reprod Biol 94:290–95, 2001.

112. Viscardi RM, Sun CC. Placental lesion multiplicity: risk factor for IUGR and neonatal cranial ultrasound abnormalities. Early Hum Dev 62:1–10, 2001.

113. Volpe JJ. Neurology of the Newborn, 4th Edition. WB Saunders Co., Philadelphia, PA, 2001.

114. Wang PJ, Lin HC, Liu HM, Tseng CL, Shen YZ. Intracranial arachnoid cysts in children: related signs and associated anomalies. Pediatr Neurol 19:100–4, 1998.

115. Wheater M, Rennie JM. Perinatal infection is an important risk factor for cerebral palsy in very-low-birthweight infants. Dev Med Child Neurol 42:364–7, 2000.

116. Whitelaw A. Intraventricular haemorrhage and posthaemorrhagic hydrocephalus: pathogenesis, prevention and future interventions. Semin Neonatol 6:135–46, 2001.

117. Winberg P, Sonesson SE, Lundell BP. Postnatal changes in intracranial blood flow velocity in preterm infants. Acta Paediatr Scand 79:1150–55, 1990.

118. Winkler P: Colour-coded echographic flow imaging and spectral analysis of cerebrospinal fluid (CSF) in infants. Part II. CSF-dynamics. Pediatr Radiol 22:31–42, 1992.

ADDITIONAL READING

Adamsbaum C, Merzoug V, Andre C, et al. Prenatal diagnosis of isolated posterior fossa anomalies: Attempt at a simplified approach. J Radiol 83:321–328, 2002.

Adamsbaum C, Moutard ML, Andre C, et al. MRI of the fetal posterior fossa. Pediatr Radiol 35:124–140, 2005.

Baldoli C, Righini A, Parazzini C, Scotti G, Triulzi F. Demonstration of acute ischemic lesions in the fetal brain by diffusion magnetic resonance imaging. Ann Neurol 52:243–246, 2002.

Bui T, Daire JL, Alberti C, et al. (2003) Microstructural development of fetal brain assessed in utero by diffusion tenor imaging [Abstract]. Pediatr Radiol 33(2), 2003.

Ecker JL, Shipp TD, Bromley B, Benacerraf B. The sonographic diagnosis of Dandy-Walker and Dandy-Walker variant: Associated findings and outcomes. Prenat Diagn 20:328–332, 2000.

Garel C. Abnormalities of proliferation, neuronal migration and cortical organization. In Garel C, ed. MRI of the Fetal Brain. Normal Development and Cerebral Pathologies. New York: Springer, 2004, pp 151–174.

Garel C. The role of MRI in the evaluation of the fetal brain with an emphasis on biometry, gyration and parenchyma. Pediatr Radiol 34:694–699, 2004.

Garel C. Methodology and results. In Garel C, ed. MRI of the Fetal Brain. Normal Development and Cerebral Pathologies. New York: Springer, 2004, pp 13-114.

Garel C. MRI of the Fetal Brain. Normal Development and Cerebral Pathologies. New York: Springer, 2004.

Garel C, Chantrel E, Brisse H, et al. Fetal cerebral cortex: normal gestational landmarks identified using prenatal MR imaging. AJNR Am J Neuroradiol 22:184–189, 2001.

Girard N, Gire C, Sigaudy S, et al. MR imaging of acquired fetal brain disorders. Childs Nerv Syst 19:490–500, 2003.

Girard N, Raybaud C, Gambarelli D, Figarella-Branger D. Fetal brain MR imaging. Magn Reson Imaging Clin North Am 9:19–56, 2001.

Gressens P, Luton D. Fetal MRI: Obstetrical and neurological perspectives. Pediatr Radiol 34:682–684, 2004.

Gressens P, Rogido M, Paindaveine B, Sola A. The impact of frequent neonatal intensive care practices on the developing brain. J Pediatr 140:646–653, 2002.

Guibaud L. Practical approach to prenatal posterior fossa abnormalities using MRI. Pediatr Radiol 34:700–711, 2004.

Guibaud L. Anomalies de la fosse cerebrale posterieure. In Garel C, Delezoide AL, Guibaud L, eds. Imagerie du cerveau foetal pathologique. Montpellier, Sauramps Medical, 2002, pp 99–118.

Heerschap A, Kok RD, Van den Berg PP. Antenatal proton MR spectroscopy of the human brain in vivo. Childs Nerv Syst 19:418–421, 2003.

Ismail KM, Ashworth JR, Martin WL, et al. Fetal magnetic resonance imaging in prenatal diagnosis of central nervous system abnormalities: 3-year experience. J Matern Fetal Neonatal Med 12:185–190, 2002.

Kostovic I, Judas M, Rados M, Hrabac P. Laminar organization of the human fetal cerebrum revealed by histochemical markers and magnetic resonance imaging. Cereb Cortex 12:536–544, 2002.

Levine D, Barnes P, Korf B, Edelman R. Tuberous sclerosis in the fetus: Second-trimester diagnosis of subependymal tubers with ultrafast MR imaging. AJR Am J Roentgenol 175:1067–1069, 2000.

Levine D, Barnes P, Robertson RR, Wong G, Mehta TS. Fast MR imaging of fetal central nervous system abnormalities. Radiology 229:51–61, 2003.

Murphy BP, Inder TE, Huppi PS, et al. Impaired cerebral cortical gray matter growth after treatment with dexamethasone for neonatal chronic lung disease. Pediatrics 107:217–221, 2001.

Nelson MD, Maher K, Gilles FH. A different approach to cysts of the posterior fossa. Pediatr Radiol 34:720–732, 2004.

Raybaud C, Levrier O, Brunel H, Girard N, Farnarier P. MR imaging of fetal brain malformations. Childs Nerv Syst 19:455–470, 2003.

Righini A, Bianchini E, Parazzini C, et al. Apparent diffusion coefficient determination in normal fetal brain: A prenatal MR imaging study. AJNR Am J Neuroradiol 24:799–804, 2003.

ten Donkelaar HJ, Lammens M, Wesseling P, Hori A, Keyser A, Rotteveel J. Development and development disorders of the human cerebellum. J Neurol 250:1025–1036, 2003.

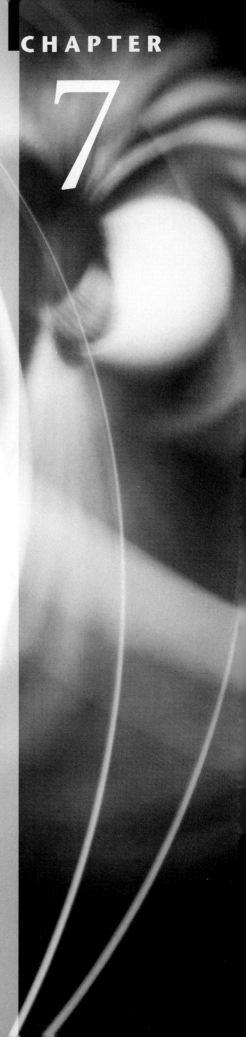

THE CHILD WITH STRIDOR

Outline

David K. Edwards, III, MD

THE CHILD WITH *STRIDOR*

The Latin word *stridor,* as used by authors such as Ovid and Cicero, meant a creaking, grating, hissing, or whistling noise, such as might be made by the wind, a door hinge, or a saw or by various animals. The medical word *stridor* has a quite similar meaning but is limited to abnormal sounds made by a human being during the process of breathing. Thus, stridor is noisy breathing, which is abnormal, because normal breathing is silent to the unaided ear. Stridor is distinguished from lung sounds such as rales or wheezes, which usually require stethoscopic examination for detection, and from vocal sounds such as grunting and crying. Like these other sounds, stridor is a symptom or finding, not a disease.

Stridor is produced by a focus or foci of turbulent gas flow in the upper airways, between the nose and trachea. The turbulent flow is created by a partial obstruction of the airway that disrupts the smooth passage of gas and produces audible eddies and vibrations. Stridor may be low- or high-pitched, loud or quiet, musical or harsh, and inspiratory or expiratory, depending on the nature and extent of the obstructing lesion and the ensuing dynamics of gas flow. Although the auditory characteristics of stridor may be of some diagnostic utility (see later), the most important feature of stridor is its implication of partial airway obstruction. The existence of such an obstruction is potentially life threatening and demands immediate diagnosis and often immediate therapy. In children, the airway is small, soft, and easily occluded; thus, the finding of stridor must be regarded with considerable gravity. Stridor is not an especially common finding, accounting for only 1% to 2% of pediatric medical hospital admissions,[1] but its seriousness in reflecting a possibly lethal disease outweighs its relative rarity.

DIFFERENTIAL DIAGNOSIS OF STRIDOR

GENERAL CONSIDERATIONS

Stridor may be caused by a variety of conditions and lesions. For differential diagnostic purposes, lesions may be categorized in several different ways, such as by pathologic category, patient age, congenital versus acquired lesions, or anatomic site of obstruction; categorization by anatomic site is perhaps easiest. The important anatomic regions involved in obstructive lesions that produce stridor are diagrammed in Figure 7–1; these include the jaw, tongue and tongue base, nasopharynx and oropharynx, retropharyngeal soft tissues, cervical soft tissues, epiglottis, glottis, larynx, subglottic airway and trachea, and esophagus. These divisions are admittedly somewhat arbitrary, and there is considerable overlap; for example, the epiglottis is part of the larynx, and the glottis (the vocal cords and the space between them) is contained within the laryngeal structures. In addition, specific lesions may occur in more than one region, and individual lesions frequently involve more than one anatomic region. Despite these difficulties, the anatomic regions may readily be recalled in stepwise fashion, and knowledge of the most important lesions occurring in each region facilitates sensible differential diagnosis in the clinical setting.

It is also reasonable to divide lesions into those that are congenital and those that are acquired[24]; however, there are many lesions (e.g., tumors) in which this distinction is unclear and possibly irrelevant. It is of greater clinical utility to combine congenital lesions with lesions producing chronic stridor and to contrast these with lesions producing acute or subacute stridor. This is because in the majority of patients, chronic or long-term stridor permits a relatively leisurely diagnostic evaluation, whereas acute stridor, which is usually of infectious or traumatic origin, often demands emergency action. Of course this distinction, although useful in differential diagnosis, may not be relevant for individual patients. Congenital abnormalities, for example, may not be manifest at birth; often these are unmasked by an intercurrent infection, at which time the patient may present with acute stridor. Relatively slow-growing tumors, particularly of the mediastinum, notoriously produce no symptoms until the airway is dangerously narrow, at which time the patient may present with acute stridor and a precarious condition (Fig. 7–2). Thus, lesions that are considered to be congenital or chronic may first appear with acute respiratory distress, and this possibility must always be kept in mind when considering diagnostic possibilities.

Tables 7–1 and 7–2 present a differential diagnosis of most conditions causing stridor in the pediatric age group. The conditions are categorized primarily according to congenital or chronic causes (Table 7–1) and acute or subacute causes (Table 7–2). Within these groups lesions are categorized according to the most important anatomic sites of occurrence. A small list of lesions that frequently produce recurring stridor is also included in Table 7–2. The most important conditions are indicated by italics; many of the remaining lesions are rare and are included for the sake of completeness. In examining these lists, it should be recalled that certain types of lesions, such as sarcomas and lymphomas, can occur virtually anywhere; the same is true of gunshot wounds and other penetrating injuries.

Table 7–3 presents a shorter differential diagnosis of stridor arranged according to patient age and including only the more common lesions. These lesions usually present at specific ages, but there is considerable overlap. Laryngomalacia,

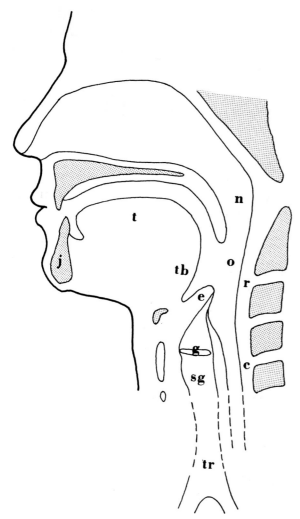

Figure 7–1
Diagram of the upper airway showing the regions at which obstructions producing stridor can occur. c, Cervical soft tissues; e, epiglottis; g, glottis; j, jaw, n, nasopharynx; o, oropharynx; r, retropharyngeal soft tissues; sg, subglottic area; t, tongue; tb, tongue base; tr, trachea.

Text continued on page 250

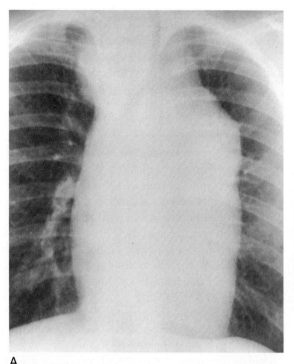
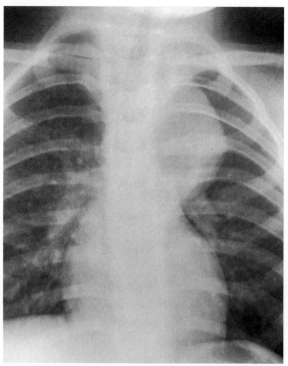

A   B

Figure 7–2
Large mediastinal tumors, both of which caused presenting symptoms of acute stridor and respiratory distress. *A,* Radiograph of a 16-year-old boy with a thymoma severely compressing and deviating the intrathoracic trachea. *B,* Frontal chest radiograph of a 3-year-old girl with a ganglioneuroma.

TABLE 7-1 CAUSES OF CONGENITAL OR CHRONIC STRIDOR IN PEDIATRIC PATIENTS*

Jaw
1. Micrognathia
   Pierre Robin syndrome N
   Treacher Collins syndrome
   (mandibulofacial dysostosis)
   Cerebrocostomandibular syndrome
   Cri du chat syndrome
   Freeman-Sheldon syndrome
   (whistling face syndrome)
   Goldenhar's syndrome
   Hallermann-Streiff syndrome
   Hanhart's syndrome
   Trisomy 13–15
   Trisomy 18
2. Temporomandibular joint ankylosis
   Juvenile rheumatoid arthritis
   Secondary to trauma

Tongue and Base of Tongue
1. Macroglossia
   Beckwith-Wiedemann syndrome
   Congenital hypothyroidism
   Trisomy 21
   Mucopolysaccharidosis I, II
   Diffuse muscular hypertrophy
   of tongue

Lingular tumors, especially hemangioma,
   lymphangioma, endothelioma
2. Lesions at base of tongue
   Thyroglossal duct cyst
   Lingual thyroid
   Congenital lingual cyst
   Dermoid, other tumors

Nasopharynx and Oropharynx
1. *Enlarged tonsils and/or adenoids*
2. *Nasal congestion*
3. Deviated nasal septum
4. Turbinate hypertrophy
5. Cleft palate
6. Congenital narrowing of pharynx in Crouzon's
   disease
7. Enlarged masses of lymphoid tissue in metabolic
   storage diseases
8. Obstetric trauma to nose
9. Tumors (newborns and infants)
   Teratoma, hamartoma, dermoid
   Neurofibroma, neuroblastoma
   Hemangioma
   Benign polyps
   Basal encephalocele
   Heterotopic gastric tissue

*The most important conditions are indicated by italics.

10. Tumors (older children)
    Juvenile angiofibroma
    Sarcomas, especially rhabdomyosarcoma
    Lymphendothelioma

Retropharyngeal Soft Tissues
1. *Lymphadenopathy*
2. *Trisomy 21* (thick prevertebral tissues)
3. Myxedema in congenital hypothyroidism
4. Tumors
    Cystic hygroma (usually originating elsewhere in neck)
    Retropharyngeal goiter
    Neurofibroma, neuroblastoma
    Hemangioma
    Lymphoma

Cervical Soft Tissues
1. *Tuberculous adenitis* (*scrofula*)
2. Cystic hygroma
3. Goiter
4. Thyroiditis
5. Thyroid tumor
6. Lymphoma
7. Klippel-Feil syndrome (brevicollis, causing crowding of structures)
8. Fibromatosis of the neck ("aggressive fibromatosis")
9. Redundant aryepiglottic folds

Epiglottis
1. Congenital floppy epiglottis
2. Bifid epiglottis
3. Chronic epiglottitis, including tuberculous

Glottis
1. *Congenital vocal cord paralysis, unilateral or bilateral*
2. Vocal cord paralysis related to hydrocephalus, Arnold-Chiari malformation, brain tumor
3. Glottic web
4. Partial glottic atresia
5. Pelizaeus-Merzbacher syndrome
6. Leigh's syndrome
7. Mobius syndrome

Larynx
1. *Laryngomalacia* (*congenital flaccid larynx*)
2. *Laryngeal papillomatosis*
3. Aryepiglottic cyst
4. Laryngotracheoesophageal cleft
5. Laryngeal stenosis, atresia
6. Laryngeal webs
7. Laryngocele
8. Hypertrophic cricoid cartilage
9. Congenital cleft arytenoids
10. Branchiogenic cyst
11. Lymphangioma
12. Other tumors

Hemangioma
Fibroma
Dermoid polyps
Granular cell myoblastoma

13. Fourth branchial pouch sinus
14. Cricoarytenoid arthritis in juvenile rheumatoid arthritis

Subglottic Region and Trachea
1. *Acquired subglottic stenosis, granuloma, or subglottic cyst secondary to intubation*
2. *Tracheomalacia (congenital flaccid trachea)*
3. *Vascular rings and slings*
4. *Subglottic hemangioma*
5. *Mediastinal and cervical tumors*
    Leukemia, lymphoma
    Thymoma
    Teratoma
    Neural tumors, especially neurofibroma, neuroblastoma, ganglioneuroma
    Neurenteric cyst; duplication cyst
    Bronchogenic cyst
6. Enlarged thyroid and other neck masses (see "Cervical Soft Tissues")
7. *Compression from aberrant innominate artery*
8. *Tracheoesophageal fistula; narrowing at site of fistula repair*
9. *Congenital subglottic stenosis*
10. *Granuloma, stricture, or subglottic cysts at site of previous tracheostomy*
11. *Papillomata seeded from above*
12. Subglottic coccidioidomycosis
13. Miscellaneous tracheal anomalies
    Tracheal diverticulum
    Tracheal duplication
    Tracheal web
    Tracheal cyst
    Cartilage ring anomalies ("segmental malacia")
    Calcification of the tracheal cartilages
    Mounier-Kuhn syndrome
14. Lobar emphysema
15. Mediastinal abscess
16. Bronchomalacia
17. Relapsing polychondritis
18. Cervical lung herniation

Esophagus
1. *Occult impacted foreign body*
2. *Proximal pouch of esophageal atresia*
3. Retroesophageal abscess or mass
4. Esophageal duplication
5. Esophageal diverticulum
6. Esophageal inflammatory disease; gastroesophageal reflux

*The most important conditions are indicated by italics.

TABLE 7-2 Causes of Acute, Subacute, and Recurring Stridor*

Acute or Subacute Stridor
Nasopharynx and Oropharynx
1. Severe facial trauma, fractures
2. Pharyngeal foreign bodies
3. Peritonsillar abscess
4. Parapharyngeal abscess
5. Swelling of uvula with angioneurotic edema
6. Mucous membrane pemphigus
Retropharyngeal Soft Tissues
1. *Retropharyngeal or parapharyngeal abscess*
2. Retropharyngeal bleeding
3. Edema following cervical spine trauma
4. Thermal and chemical trauma
Cervical Soft Tissues
1. Hematoma from trauma, iatrogenic
2. Ludwig's angina (submandibular cellulitis)
Epiglottis
1. *Acute epiglottitis*
2. Traumatic epiglottic swelling
3. Acute swelling from food (especially nuts, fish) or other allergy (*Hymenoptera* venom, vaccines, penicillin)
Glottis
1. Traumatic injury, usually iatrogenic
2. Cord paralysis secondary to surgery (often recurrent laryngeal nerve injury)
Larynx
1. *Acute laryngitis*
2. *Angioneurotic edema; laryngospasm*
3. *Foreign body*

4. Tetany (laryngismus stridulus) from hypocalcemia (rickets, celiac disease, renal failure, hypoparathyroidism)
5. External trauma, fracture, edema, local hematoma
6. Obstetric trauma; edema, or dislocation of cricothyroid or cricoarytenoid cartilages
7. Chemical or thermal injury
8. Membranous exudate of diphtheria
9. Membranous exudate of infectious mononucleosis
10. Laryngeal abscess
11. Chondritis
Subglottic Region and Trachea
1. *Croup*
2. *Foreign body*
3. Iatrogenic edema following intubation, instrumentation, operation
4. Membranous croup (bacterial tracheitis)
5. Pertussis
Esophagus
1. Esophageal foreign body
2. Acute aspiration of vomited material
Recurring Stridor
1. Allergic rhinitis
2. Laryngomalacia
3. Subglottic hemangioma
4. Allergic croup; food allergy
5. Respiratory infections in child with otherwise asymptomatic airway narrowing
6. Hereditary angioneurotic edema
7. Functional (psychogenic) stridor

*The most important conditions are indicated by italics.

subglottic stenosis, and vocal cord paralysis tend to present in the newborn period, and most congenital anomalies appear during the first year of life. Choanal atresia, an important cause of airway obstruction in neonates, is not listed because it rarely produces stridor. Retropharyngeal abscess also tends to occur in the first year of life, except for those abscesses that are secondary to foreign bodies. Foreign bodies and croup are usually first seen near the end of the first year and become more frequent in the second year. Epiglottitis is usually first encountered during the end of the second year of life, although there is a large age range.[39] By 3 to 6 years of age, enlarged tonsils and adenoids and nasal congestion become increasingly common causes of noisy breathing; epiglottitis and foreign bodies constitute the most common serious causes of stridor in this age group.

DIFFERENTIAL DIAGNOSTIC CLUES

The Timing and Characteristics of Stridor

For much of its anatomic course, the airway in pediatric patients is not a fixed tube but instead is a fairly flexible conduit whose luminal cross-sectional area changes as a result of pressure differentials. Such luminal changes are minor during normal respiration but can assume considerable importance when obstructing lesions are present. In normal respiration, the pressure differences acting on the airway are directly opposite inside and outside the thoracic cage. During inspiration, within the thorax, the airway walls are acted on by surrounding decreased pressure, and the intrathoracic airways tend to widen. During expiration, the surrounding increased pressure tends to narrow these

TABLE 7-3 MAJOR CAUSES OF STRIDOR IN DIFFERENT AGE GROUPS

Newborn and Young Infant
Laryngomalacia
Subglottic stenosis
Vocal cord paralysis
Tracheomalacia
Vascular anomalies
Hemangioma
Infant to 1 Year
Congenital anomalies (as above)
Croup
Retropharyngeal abscess
Anatomic defects revealed by intercurrent infection
Foreign bodies
1 to 2 Years
Croup
Foreign bodies
Epiglottitis
3 to 6 Years
Enlarged tonsils and adenoids
Nasal congestion
Epiglottitis
Foreign bodies

If a partial obstruction occurs in a region where the airway can change caliber, the obstruction will be greatest when the caliber is the least. Decreased airway caliber slows and disrupts gas flow, producing stridor. Thus, all things being equal, obstructions in the extrathoracic airway will tend to produce inspiratory stridor, whereas obstructions within the thorax will tend to produce expiratory stridor. A lesion that produces a fixed, unchanging obstruction (e.g., in an area surrounded by bone, such as the nasopharynx, or by an encircling vascular ring or tumor) will tend not to produce this inspiratory-expiratory distinction. A lesion that is large in relation to the cross-sectional area of the airway in any location will tend to produce significant obstruction to both inspiratory and expiratory gas flow, resulting in biphasic (to-and-fro) stridor. Biphasic stridor is generally of more immediate clinical seriousness than stridor that is purely inspiratory or expiratory.

The larynx is a fixed structure whose caliber does not vary appreciably with respiration. The narrowest part of the larynx in infants is at the vocal cords, where the cross-sectional area is 14 to 15 mm^2. It has been pointed out[30] that mucosal edema only 1 mm thick in this region, which would produce only mild hoarseness in an adult, reduces the infant airway area by 65%. Thus, this region is a critical area in infants, as relatively small lesions can produce significant obstructions; a clinical correlate of this is that lesions in this region relatively commonly produce biphasic stridor.

None of these rules is without exception, of course, and the dynamics of gas flow past particular obstructions may have auditory characteristics that are paradoxical. Nevertheless, the timing of stridor relative to the respiratory cycle may offer useful hints as to the location and severity of the obstruction. Table 7–4 lists several conditions that tend to present with inspiratory, biphasic, or expiratory stridor. It must be emphasized that stridor is usually accentuated by rapid gas flow; a

airways; this mechanism accounts for the ball valve or flapper valve air trapping observed with many endobronchial lesions. In the extrathoracic airway, during inspiration, the surrounding soft tissues remain at the same approximate pressure, while the pressure in the lumen is reduced, which tends to narrow the airway. In expiration, the increased intraluminal pressure tends to widen the extrathoracic airway (Fig. 7–3).

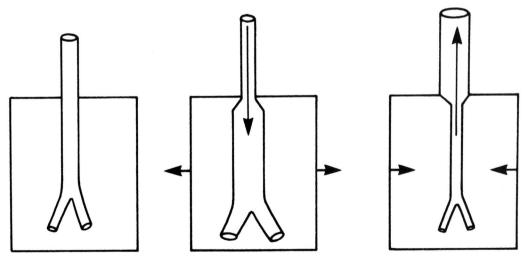

Figure 7–3
Extrathoracic and intrathoracic caliber change with respiration: diagrammatic representation.

TABLE 7-4 Respiratory Phase of Stridor Produced by Various Lesions

Lesions Tending to Produce Inspiratory Stridor
Congenital vocal cord paralysis
Laryngomalacia
Postintubation stridor
Acute laryngitis
Micrognathia, macroglossia
Thyroglossal duct cysts
Supraglottic and glottic webs
Subglottic hemangiomas (some)
Croup
Epiglottitis
Retropharyngeal abscess
Diphtheria

Lesions Frequently Producing Biphasic Stridor
Congenital subglottic stenosis
Tracheal stenosis
Vascular rings, slings
Subglottic hemangioma
Subglottic web

Lesions Tending to Produce Expiratory Stridor
Tracheomalacia
Tracheal foreign body
Mediastinal masses

---

sleeping infant breathing quietly may show a deceptive absence of stridor, even in the presence of a significant lesion. For this reason, the physical examination should include stressing the infant to provoke vigorous respiration. However, the stridor produced by many nasopharyngeal and oropharyngeal obstructions is more marked during sleep, so it is preferable to observe infants both during sleep and while breathing vigorously.

The auditory characteristics of stridor may also be diagnostically helpful. For example, the stridor of laryngomalacia is usually a high-pitched, "crowing" inspiratory sound. Glottic obstructions generally tend to produce high-pitched stridor (often crowing), whereas supraglottic lesions usually produce stridor that is low pitched and sonorous. Coarse snoring often accompanies pharyngeal obstruction. Acoustic analyses of the frequency spectra of stridor provide an objective analysis of the abnormal sounds.[41]

Vocal Characteristics

Characteristics of the voice, as manifested by speaking or crying, also offer diagnostic clues to the etiology of stridor. Obviously, lesions affecting the glottis and vocal cords tend to produce vocal abnormalities, including hoarseness, weakness of the voice, abnormalities of pitch, and aphonia. Lesions involving the adjacent larynx often produce similar vocal abnormalities (Fig. 7–4). With nasopharyngeal obstructions, the cry is unaffected in infants, but nasal (adenoidal) speech is evident in older children. Oropharyngeal obstructions either do not affect the voice or produce throaty or muffled phonation. Supraglottic laryngeal obstructions also produce a muffled, subdued, or throaty voice, whereas subglottic laryngeal obstructions produce hoarse, harsh, or husky phonation. With tracheal obstruction, tracheomalacia, and laryngomalacia, the voice is usually unaffected, but the cry may be weakened if the airway caliber is very diminished. Unilateral vocal cord paralysis tends to produce a weak cry, with little respiratory distress, whereas bilateral cord paralysis is usually associated with a nearly normal cry and severe respiratory distress. Table 7–5 presents a list of lesions that frequently produce vocal abnormalities.

Cough

Cough frequently accompanies stridor, and the character of the cough may be of diagnostic significance. Because of this, some authorities recommend eliciting coughing in infants by manual stimulation of the posterior pharynx; however, coughing that is significant is generally elicited spontaneously. Obstructions in the nasopharynx are not usually associated with cough except in infants in whom an associated feeding difficulty may produce aspiration with choking, coughing, and, often, aspiration pneumonitis. With oropharyngeal lesions and lesions at the base of the tongue, similar feeding difficulties, as well as aspiration of pooled saliva with associated coughing, may exist; the cough, when it occurs, usually sounds "wet."

A barking, seal-like cough is very suggestive of subglottic disease. The prototype of this type of cough is that associated with croup. A "croupy" or barking cough also frequently accompanies childhood laryngitis, membranous croup (tracheitis), and postintubation croup (edema secondary to intubation). Epiglottitis may also have an associated cough that is sometimes croupy, but usually with a more rasping character.

A "brassy" cough is very frequently associated with tracheal lesions. Such a cough commonly accompanies vascular rings, as may a more barking cough. An endotracheal foreign body may also produce a brassy or barking cough. With such foreign bodies, paroxysms of coughing frequently occur as the object is blown about in the airway impinging on the larynx. The cough may subside when the foreign body becomes fixed in place, or a continuing, grunting cough associated with expiration may persist. Recurring respiratory symptoms, including cough, are frequently seen with foreign bodies impacted in the esophagus, with associated esophageal obstruction, and with aspiration of swallowed materials.

Feeding Difficulties

Because of the proximity (and proximal identity) of the upper airway and upper gastrointestinal tracts, it is not surprising that lesions producing stridor may also produce

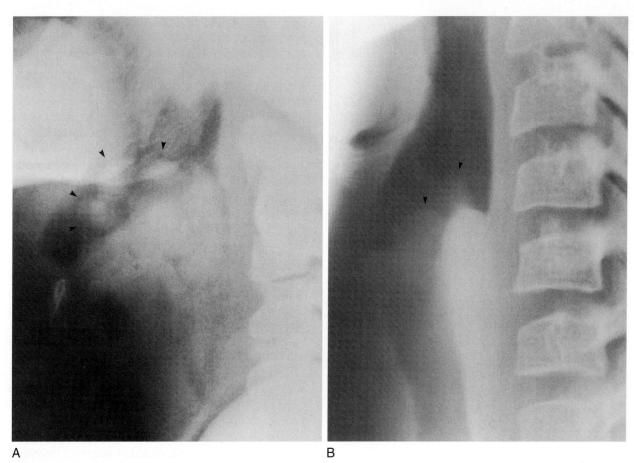

A   B

Figure 7–4
Papillomata in two patients who presented with stridor accompanied by vocal changes; laryngeal papillomata are indicated by *arrowheads*. *A,* Extensive papillomata in a 7-year-old boy. *B,* Papillomata in a 10-year-old girl.

TABLE 7-5 LESIONS COMMONLY AFFECTING PHONATION

Unilateral vocal cord paralysis (weak aspirate or breathy cry)
Obstetric injury to larynx (hoarse cry)
Laryngeal edema from instrumentation (hoarseness)
Laryngeal web (weak or absent cry)
Acute laryngitis (hoarseness)
Croup (hoarseness)
Epiglottitis (voice muffled or unaltered)
Diphtheria (hoarseness)
Laryngeal foreign body (voice hoarse or absent)
Laryngeal papillomatosis (hoarseness)
Esophageal foreign body compressing larynx
Cyst of aryepiglottic fold and other laryngeal cysts
Laryngotracheoesophageal cleft

difficulties with feeding. A list of the most important such lesions is presented in Table 7–6. Feeding difficulties are often associated with aspiration of secretions or food, which results in airway irritation, pneumonitis, and increased respiratory difficulty. In infants, nasopharyngeal obstructions cause difficulty in feeding, often with choking and aspiration, because nose breathing is impaired. Oropharyngeal obstructions, especially lesions at the base of the tongue, interfere with swallowing, as do supraglottic laryngeal lesions. Laryngomalacia and bilateral cord paralysis are often associated with choking on food. Feeding is usually normal with tracheal lesions except when the obstruction is very severe or when extrinsic pressure also involves the esophagus. With vascular rings, there is frequently little evidence of dysphagia, but frequent regurgitation and episodes of increased stridor and, occasionally, cyanosis are noted with feeding. Severe dysphagia generally accompanies retropharyngeal abscess and supraglottic inflammations, such as epiglottitis, in which a strong avoidance of swallowing results in drooling. A foreign body in the esophagus would be expected to produce feeding difficulties, but surprisingly

TABLE 7-6 LESIONS COMMONLY ASSOCIATED
WITH FEEDING DIFFICULTIES

Micrognathia, macroglossia
Nasopharyngeal obstruction in infants
Masses at base of tongue
Cyst of aryepiglottic fold and other laryngeal masses
Cystic hygroma
Laryngomalacia
Bilateral vocal cord paralysis
Tracheoesophageal fistula; esophageal atresia
Laryngotracheoesophageal cleft
Vascular ring
Masses compressing trachea and esophagus
  (bronchogenic cyst)
Esophageal foreign body
Epiglottitis
Retropharyngeal abscess

often, the gastrointestinal symptoms are masked by respiratory difficulties (Fig. 7–5). One reason for this may be the tendency for "overflow" aspiration to occur; another reason may be that the soft or pureed foods usually given to children in this age group may pass partially obstructing foreign bodies without becoming impacted or regurgitated.

Respiratory Distress

Signs of respiratory distress are usually fairly nonspecific and tend to reflect the severity of the obstruction more than

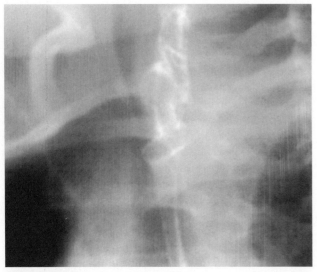

Figure 7–5
Esophageal foreign body: esophagram. A radiolucent esophageal foreign body is outlined by barium in a 2-year-old boy with the sole symptom of stridor of 6 months' duration. Dysphagia is often conspicuously absent in these children, and barium examination of the esophagus is frequently inappropriately delayed. Tracheal narrowing is evident at the level of the esophageal foreign body.

its location. Inspiratory retractions of the sternum, intercostal spaces, and suprasternal and supraclavicular regions are fairly reliable indices of respiratory distress in infants and young children, as is flaring of the nasal alae in infants. Retractions are commonly seen in obstructions above the tracheal level; only very severe tracheal obstructions cause xiphoid retractions. Retractions vanish in infants with nasopharyngeal obstructions when their mouths are open. Retractions are commonly described with laryngomalacia, vocal cord paralysis, laryngeal webs and cysts, croup, and epiglottitis. Retractions suggest a relatively severe obstruction, as do cyanosis and blood gas evidence of impaired respiratory function. Thoracoabdominal asynchrony ("rocker breathing") during respiration, which also occurs in upper airway obstruction, is a feature that appears amenable to objective measurement.[40]

Miscellaneous Diagnostic Clues

Whenever a child with congenital stridor is encountered, the physician must keep in mind that as many as 45% of such children have other congenital abnormalities and that many of these other abnormalities may contribute to the stridor.[19] A slight, but definite, male preponderance in the incidence of stridor exists; this preponderance is more marked with congenital lesions but is also observed with acquired lesions.

The stridor that occurs with several conditions may be positional—that is, it is increased or decreased by changes in the patient's position. Patients with micrognathia (Fig. 7–6) (e.g., Pierre Robin syndrome) generally have increased stridor and distress in the supine position, presumably because gravity pulls the posteriorly placed tongue farther into the compromised airway. The same effect occurs in macroglossia. Glossoptosis usually accompanies both macroglossia and micrognathia. Stridor also tends to be increased by the supine position in infants with laryngomalacia and in older children with enlargement of the tonsils and adenoids. With supraglottic cysts, associated inspiratory stridor may increase or decrease with changes in the patient's position, probably because the cysts move in position with respect to the airway.

Patients with certain conditions tend to adopt positions that evidently lessen the degree of airway obstruction or discomfort. Patients with a vascular ring and those with a retropharyngeal abscess tend to keep their heads extended, often adopting a position of opisthotonos. This position can be a valuable clue in identifying cases of vascular ring and in distinguishing epiglottitis from retropharyngeal abscess, which can otherwise closely resemble epiglottitis clinically; the different and distinctive posture in epiglottitis is described later in this chapter. Nasopharyngeal tumors frequently present with chronic nasal discharge, sinusitis, and epistaxis. In a teenage boy, a nasopharyngeal mass is most commonly a juvenile nasopharyngeal angiofibroma, which may present not only with nasal obstruction and epistaxis but also with

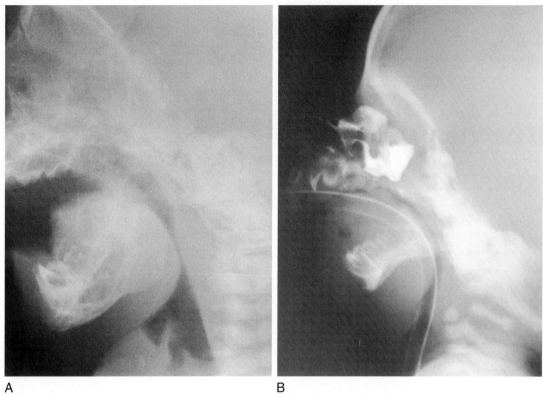

A   B

Figure 7–6
Two infants with micrognathia. *A,* Pierre Robin syndrome. *B,* Treacher Collins syndrome; contrast material in the nose demonstrates choanal atresia. The small mandible carries the tongue posteriorly, partially obstructing the upper airway. Obstruction is more severe in the supine than in the prone position.

symptoms of intracranial involvement and distortion of the palate or face because of its aggressive behavior.

Approximately half of infants whose stridor results from a subglottic hemangioma have at least one hemangioma on the skin, most frequently on the head or neck. A salmon-colored rash often accompanies episodes of airway obstruction in hereditary angioneurotic edema; a family history and a history of previous attacks are also helpful diagnostically.

The clinical history is particularly important in several other settings as well. A history of the child's putting an object into the mouth shortly before the onset of stridor suggests a foreign body in the esophagus or airway. A history of neonatal difficulties requiring endotracheal intubation suggests acquired subglottic stricture or, occasionally, a subglottic cyst[45] as a possible cause of the findings. Older children who underwent neonatal repair of esophageal anomalies (e.g., tracheoesophageal fistula or esophageal atresia) may develop subsequent esophageal stricture and obstruction causing respiratory symptoms; even if the history is not available, surgical scars or radiographic findings of distorted ribs or surgical clips can suggest the probable diagnosis.

On occasion with upper airway obstruction, respiratory symptoms are severe enough that stridor and other signs of proximal airway obstruction are masked or overlooked or

the findings can suggest primary disease of other organ systems. For example, infants with failure to thrive have been cured by the removal of very large and presumably chronically obstructing tonsils and adenoids.[50] Such chronically obstructing lesions may cause marked cardiomegaly with or without apparent pulmonary venous hypertension, and the findings may suggest a primary cardiac lesion. The mechanism is presumably related to increased pulmonary vascular resistance secondary to hypoxia. Cor pulmonale has also been described in laryngomalacia, Pierre Robin syndrome, Crouzon's disease, and other conditions.

Acute pulmonary edema, usually without cardiomegaly, can accompany acute airway obstruction. This finding is reversible when the obstruction is relieved. Pulmonary edema has been observed with croup, epiglottitis, and an aspirated foreign body. The radiologist, who may encounter the chest radiograph before the upper airway lesion is suspected, should be familiar with these manifestations of upper airway obstructions. Other manifestations of upper airway obstruction on the chest film include (1) a tendency toward normal or diminished aeration, as opposed to the hyperinflation seen with most other causes of respiratory distress; (2) a narrowed portion of the airway; and (3) a distended hypopharynx, if that area is included on the film.[8]

Certain children, most commonly adolescents, may suffer psychogenic or "hysterical" stridor. This condition is primarily a diagnosis of exclusion, although psychological and laboratory clues to the condition exist.[29]

NORMAL RADIOGRAPHIC ANATOMY AND ARTIFACTS OF THE PROXIMAL AIRWAY

Adequate radiography of a child's neck usually requires only two views, a lateral and a frontal, but the radiographic technique must be excellent if the important structures are to be evaluated adequately. Hair braids, necklaces, ties on hospital gowns, and other external objects should be removed from the beam. The lateral view, particularly, must be a nonrotated examination to avoid extraneous structures, such as an earlobe, being cast over the airway and to ensure that the epiglottis does not appear abnormally wide because of rotation. The filming technique is one that is routinely used for soft tissues and appropriate to the thickness of the patient's neck. The film is exposed in the inspiratory cycle near the end of an inspiration.

With the important exception of cases of possible epiglottitis, it is very important that the patient's head be extended as fully as possible. An older child can produce this extension on demand; with younger children and infants, adequate extension is easily obtained by placing the patient in a supine position with the head hanging backward over a bolster or rolled towel. This extension is necessary because the redundant prevertebral soft tissues in infants and young children tend to thicken markedly with neck flexion, simulating a retropharyngeal mass. Occasionally, pressure may be required on the front of the neck to resolve such a pseudo-mass (Fig. 7–7), but with adequate extension this is usually not necessary.

The anteroposterior film of the neck employs a filtered, high-kilovoltage beam to permit clear delineation of the cervical and upper thoracic airway against the bony background

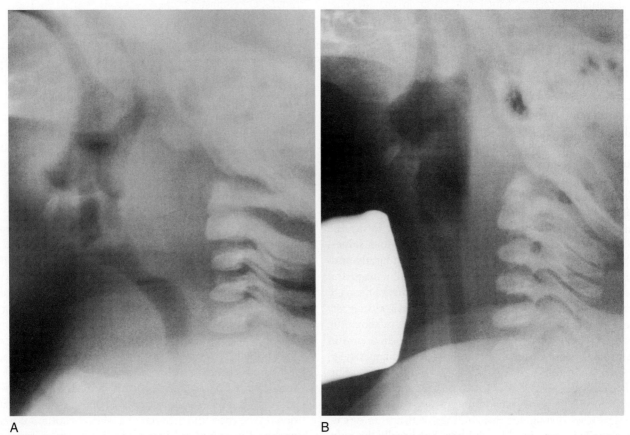

A   B

Figure 7–7
False-positive identification of a retropharyngeal mass. *A,* An examination with poor head extension suggests a retropharyngeal mass. *B,* A repeat examination with better head extension and pressure applied to the anterior neck with a gloved finger; the retropharyngeal soft tissues are normal. Intervention with a gloved finger is seldom necessary if the film is repeated in full extension and inspiration.

of the spine. A peak kilovoltage of 130 to 150 kVp is used with a 1-mm brass filter. This technique, which is routine in most active pediatric radiology services, has been described in detail elsewhere.[21] The anteroposterior view, like the lateral view, is exposed near the end of an inspiration. If a small-focal-spot x-ray tube is available, the views of the neck may be done with magnification radiography, which may provide slightly more information. Views of the neck in expiration are seldom helpful.

It is important to know the normal radiographic anatomy of the neck if abnormalities are to be diagnosed. Examples of normal neck radiographic anatomy are presented in Figures 7–8 through 7–16. Structures and regions that are normally visible include the base of the tongue, valleculae, epiglottis, aryepiglottic folds, pyriform sinuses, body and wings of the hyoid bone, subglottic airway and cervical trachea, and prevertebral (retropharyngeal) soft tissues. The true and false cords and laryngeal ventricle (see Fig. 7–15) are often, but not invariably, discernible. With proper technique, enough may usually be seen of these regions to permit an adequate judgment of, at the very least, whether they are normal or abnormal.

An important variation of normal is a result of the laxity of the infant's trachea, which can result in considerable buckling of the airway in the subglottic and cervical regions (see Fig. 7–14). This finding is not a cause for alarm, as long as the tracheal walls are smooth and approximately parallel. Lack of parallelism usually represents edema or an impinging mass (Fig. 7–17), and focal defects in the air column suggest intrinsic tracheal lesions. Another important artifact is swallowing, which some nervous children do frequently. A film exposed during swallowing can produce an unnerving picture that suggests total ablation of the airway (Fig. 7–18), although the presence of swallowed air in the proximal esophagus is often a useful clue, as is familiarity with the phenomenon. The film is then simply repeated. Findings that occupy a borderline area between normal and abnormal are enlarged tonsils and adenoids (Fig. 7–19). It is well known that these can be associated with stridor and, sometimes, with severe symptoms, but very large tonsils and adenoids are frequently noted as incidental findings on skull films made for unrelated reasons. The decision as to whether these structures are of symptomatic importance is made on the basis of clinical findings, not radiographic evidence. Large adenoids are frequently associated with allergic rhinitis, which may be manifested radiographically by swollen turbinates (Fig. 7–20).

In adults, cartilages of the neck may calcify, forming densities that may be radiographically confusing when a foreign body is sought.[27] Such normal calcifications may occasionally be seen in older children, but usually the only structure calcified in a child's neck is the cervical spine and the body and wings of the hyoid bone. Any other radiopaque structure is usually pathologic.

IMAGING EVALUATION OF STRIDOR: GENERAL CONSIDERATIONS

The essential radiographic evaluation of a patient with stridor begins and may end with plain radiographs. These include two views of the chest, usually together with a frontal and lateral view of the neck, as discussed earlier. A barium esophagram is often a useful adjunct to plain radiographs. Additionally, with an experienced operator, airway fluoroscopy often defines the site of obstruction and provides a helpful adjunct to bronchoscopy.[35] Further evaluation is dictated by the results of these studies, by the most likely lesions causing the findings, and by considerations of both economics and common sense. Commonly, further evaluation is not required. If the cause of stridor does require further delineation, more complex (and typically more expensive) modalities may be indicated. Helical computed tomography (CT), especially multiplanar reconstruction, permits accurate evaluation and three-dimensional visualization of the airway and associated vascular structures.[42] Indeed, CT reconstructions can permit "virtual endoscopy," whereby software manipulation permits the observer to examine the upper airway in a manner that visually suggests bronchoscopy.[6] Magnetic resonance imaging (MRI) has a definite role in characterizing vascular lesions and probably in other causes of airway obstruction as well.[2] Cine MRI permits real-time visualization of airway obstructive lesions without the drawback of ionizing radiation.[15]

IMPORTANT CONDITIONS CAUSING STRIDOR

The following sections describe four conditions that are, because of their frequency and severity, the most important diseases causing stridor in general pediatric practice. These conditions are croup, epiglottitis, vascular lesions, and upper airway foreign body. For all of these, radiographic evaluation is the cornerstone of accurate diagnosis.

CROUP

Clinical Features Croup is also known as *laryngotracheitis* or, if there is associated bronchitis, *laryngotracheobronchitis*. Other than specifying the anatomic regions involved, these sesquipedal terms add little to an understanding or discussion of the condition; thus, the word *croup*, which has been used medically since 1765, will be used here.

Text continued on page 264

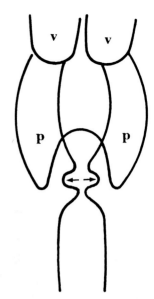

Figure 7–8
Frontal airway: diagrammatic representation. The valleculae (v) and pyriform sinuses (p) are paired structures. When the pyriform sinuses are distended with air, their inferior border marks the approximate location of the true cords. The laryngeal ventricle *(arrows),* often visible radiographically on the lateral view, is defined by the false cords above and the true cords below. Note that the subglottic region has symmetrically rounded, convex borders.

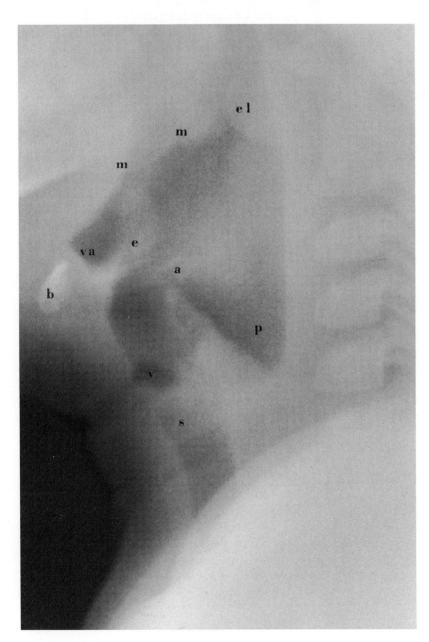

Figure 7–9
Normal structures of the upper airway as seen radiographically. a, Ala of the hyoid; b, body of the hyoid; e, epiglottis; el, ear lobe; m, mandible; p, pyriform sinuses; s, subglottic trachea; v, laryngeal ventricle; va, valleculae.

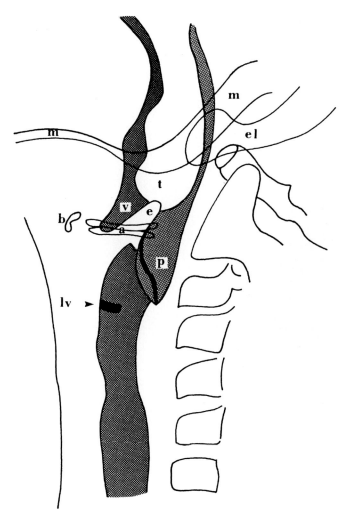

Figure 7–10
Normal airway: diagrammatic representation of the lateral radiograph. a, Ala of hyoid; b, body of hyoid; e, epiglottis, el, ear lobe; lv, laryngeal ventricle; m, mandible; p, pyriform sinuses; t, tonsil; v, valleculae.

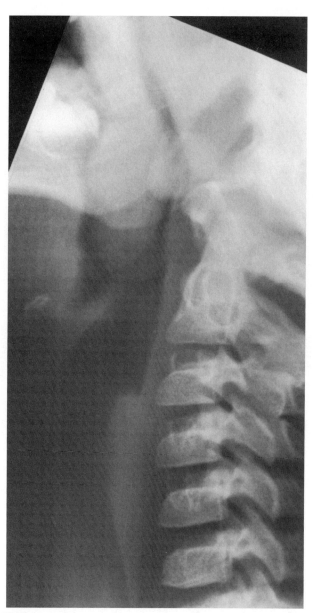

Figure 7–11
Lateral radiograph of a normal airway; refer to Figure 7–10.

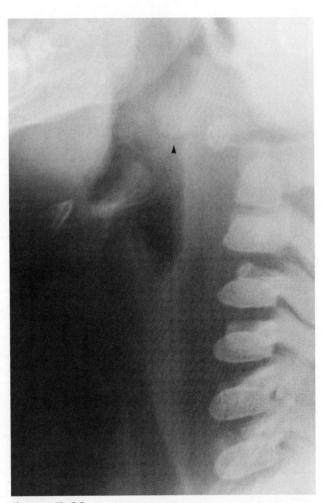

Figure 7–12
Normal airway. Dense shadow superimposed over the posterior oropharynx is an ear lobe *(arrowhead)*.

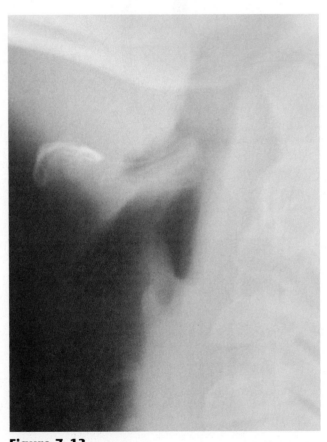

Figure 7–13
Normal airway. Slight angulation of the beam superiorly projects the bases of the pyriform sinuses at different levels.

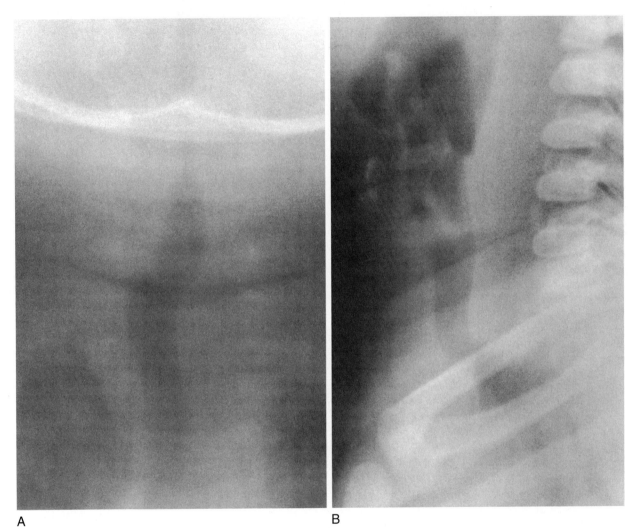

A   B

Figure 7–14
Normal tracheal buckling. Radiographs of a 6-month-old child demonstrate tracheal buckling, a normal occurrence when the film is exposed during flexion and/or expiration. *A,* In the frontal projection, normal tracheal buckling occurs rightward, away from the aortic arch. Note the occiput superimposed on the supraglottic airway. *B,* Anterior buckling is evident on the lateral projection. This normal anterior tracheal displacement frequently causes confusion because it simulates a retropharyngeal mass. Note the shape of the normal epiglottis when viewed with a slight degree of obliquity.

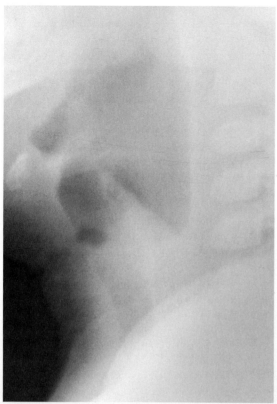

Figure 7–15
Normal airway with slight distention of the pyriform sinuses. Note the well-defined laryngeal ventricle.

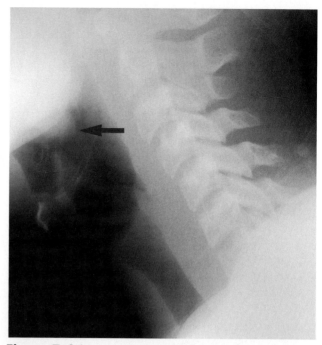

Figure 7–16
Normal airway. Note the lingual tonsils *(arrow)* superior to the tip of the epiglottis.

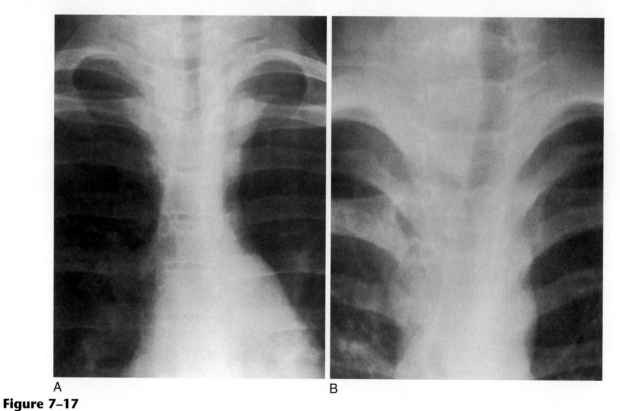

A   B

Figure 7–17
Extrinsic mass impressing the trachea. Two patients are shown, each with an abnormal thyroid gland producing tracheal compression. *A*, A 10-year-old girl with tracheal compression from an enlarged thyroid gland (Graves' disease). *B*, A 14-year-old boy with focal indentation of the trachea by a thyroid carcinoma.

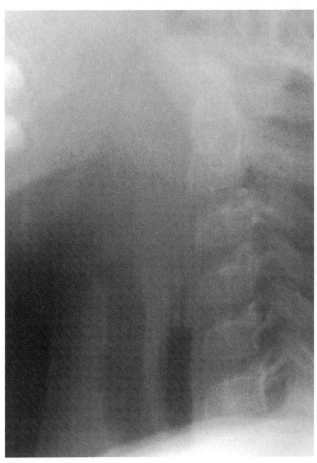

Figure 7–18
Swallowing artifact. The supraglottic airway is completely effaced, and swallowed gas is seen in the proximal esophagus.

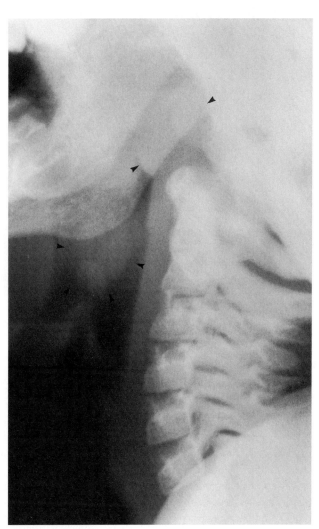

Figure 7–19
Large tonsils and adenoids. Radiograph of a 2-year-old child with enlarged adenoids that fill much of the nasopharynx *(upper arrowheads)* and with large tonsils as well *(lower arrowheads)*.

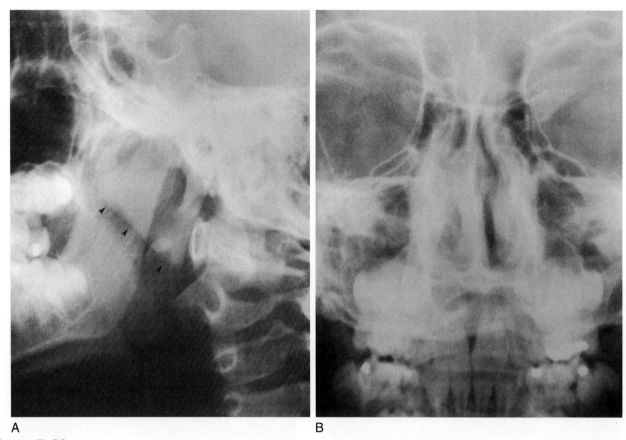

A   B

Figure 7–20
Large adenoids and swollen turbinates. *A,* Large adenoids in an 8-year-old girl, with chronic allergic rhinitis manifested radiographically by swollen turbinates *(B).*

Because the presence or absence of associated bronchitis is of relatively little clinical significance and because many authors ignore the distinction, it is difficult and possibly irrelevant to choose among laryngotracheitis, laryngotracheobronchitis, and even laryngotracheobronchiolitis.

Croup is most commonly caused by a viral infection. The major viruses responsible are myxoviruses: parainfluenza type 1 and influenza type A.[49] Outbreaks of these viruses within communities tend to occur between autumn and spring, most frequently in the last 3 months of the year. Although croup is a disease of preschool children, an older school-age child is the most common carrier of viruses to susceptible individuals in the family. The age range for children with croup is 6 months to 5 years, but most cases occur in children between 1 and 3 years of age.

Although the onset of croup may be abrupt, it usually follows several days of an upper respiratory infection. Coughing intensifies and assumes croup's typical "barking" sound, the voice often becomes hoarse, and inspiratory stridor occurs. With severe croup, stridor may become biphasic. Croup tends to become worse at night, with increased stridor, and remits during the day, with nocturnal

resurgences during the next several nights. The usual course of the disease from onset to full recovery is 4 to 10 days. Usually croup is a relatively mild disease, but occasionally the airway obstruction is sufficiently severe that intubation or tracheostomy is required.

Croup is associated with a low-grade fever (usually less than 102°F). On physical examination, the typical cough is usually apparent, together with inspiratory stridor and wheezes. Retractions in the intercostal spaces and supraclavicular regions are common. The pharynx is usually only slightly or moderately inflamed. Children with croup tend to be restless and anxious; with prolonged obstruction, children tire and sleep briefly and fitfully. A state of restless exhaustion, or biphasic stridor, may indicate approaching asphyxia and suggests the need for endotracheal intubation. The leukocyte count is usually mildly elevated, generally not above 10,000/mm³, and lymphocytosis is often evident. Frequently, blood gas evidence of hypoxia and carbon dioxide retention is found, but overt cyanosis is an unusual and ominous sign.

Bacterial croup (tracheitis) is uncommon but warrants discussion because of its relatively severe nature and unusual radiographic appearance. Bacterial croup is usually secondary to hemolytic *Staphylococcus aureus* or *Haemophilus influenzae* infection of the larynx and trachea.[12] It affects children predominantly in the same age range as those affected by viral croup but is relatively more common in children in older age groups, up to 9 years old.[18,32] Clinically, the condition resembles viral croup with exaggerated severity: the fever is higher, and greater "toxicity," greater leukocytosis, and a diminished response to racemic epinephrine are present. About half of the affected children have an associated pneumonia. Dyspnea is frequently increased by the occurrence of adherent or semiadherent mucopurulent membranes ("membranous croup") in the subglottic airway and upper trachea; distress may be lessened by the removal of these membranes.

In any case of stridor, the radiographic task is twofold: to identify the location of the obstruction and to identify as precisely as possible the pathophysiologic nature of the obstructing lesion. In the clinical setting of croup, however, the most essential question is: "Does the patient have epiglottitis?" There are several interrelated reasons for this question. First, in the acute clinical setting, croup and epiglottitis can resemble each other surprisingly closely. Second, direct visualization of the epiglottis can be hazardous in patients with epiglottitis; a simple tongue blade injudiciously or carelessly applied can be a life-threatening instrument, at least in circumstances in which an emergency airway cannot be established immediately. Third, radiography can provide the distinction quickly, simply, and relatively safely. Finally, the diagnostic distinction between the two diseases is important, because management and therapy differ considerably.

When epiglottitis is excluded by laryngoscopy or by identification of a normal epiglottis on a lateral radiograph, the next step is to identify the cause of stridor. This is necessary not merely to reassure the pediatrician that the child indeed has croup, but also, more importantly, to ensure that the child has *only* croup and not some other lesion. It must then be determined whether there is associated pneumonitis that would require additional therapy. Finally, some authorities, pointing to cases of subglottic stenosis and other lesions that have been obscured by intercurrent croup, suggest re-evaluation of the airway when the croup has resolved. With complete resolution of stridor and other findings, this would not seem to be necessary for most straightforward cases of croup.

Radiographic Evaluation In general, the initial decision to be made in the radiographic assessment of stridor is whether the probable site of obstruction is the pharynx or the laryngeal or sublaryngeal region. In patients with suspected croup, the symptoms clearly indicate a lesion in the larynx or below. The initial radiograph is therefore a radiograph of the neck, and because the epiglottis is best seen in the lateral projection, the lateral view is done first. If epiglottitis is present, immediate measures are taken to ensure the safety of the patient's airway, and all further radiographic studies are abandoned. If the epiglottis is normal, an anteroposterior view of the neck and frontal and lateral chest films are done to provide supplementary information about the lungs and lower airway.

If results of all plain radiograph studies are normal, a barium examination of the pharynx and esophagus is indicated to exclude foreign body and vascular causes of obstruction. Depending on the findings, either more elaborate radiographic studies such as CT may be undertaken or radiographic efforts may be abandoned in favor of direct visualization. The choice of the next best diagnostic step depends on several factors, including the patient's condition, the nature of the most probable lesions, the skill of the pediatric endoscopist, and the necessity of further delineating the lesion's location, pathologic character, and vascular supply.

For the initial lateral film, it is helpful if the patient's neck is extended, but when positioning the patient, it must be recalled that children with epiglottitis may suffer complete airway occlusion if excited or forced into a supine position. Ideally, the patient is placed in a supine position with the head hanging backward over a bolster or rolled towel; however, a lateral view, performed with the patient seated and upright and with the neck extended only as much as the patient tolerates, is acceptable and even desirable in patients with possible epiglottitis. If epiglottitis is not present and a retropharyngeal abscess appears possible, the examination may be repeated with greater neck extension.

Radiographic Findings It must be emphasized that in croup, the epiglottis and aryepiglottic folds are normal. If the epiglottis is swollen, the patient has epiglottitis, even though other findings suggest croup.

On the lateral view of the neck, distention or "ballooning" of the hypopharynx is usually present. Such distention is a very useful sign of upper airway obstruction from any cause and suggests that the obstruction is significant. Hypopharyngeal ballooning is evidently a neurogenic response[25] that probably serves to reduce overall airway resistance; it is not related to pressure differentials or to the physical characteristics of labored respiration.

Croup produces subglottic narrowing of the airway. On the lateral view, the narrowing may be mild. The subglottic airway is often nearly normal in caliber but generally has fuzzy margins with indistinctness of the airway. On the frontal view, the narrowing is much more apparent, because in croup, the inspiratory collapse occurs primarily laterally. Instead of the normal parallel walls ("stovepipe" appearance) of the subglottic airway, there is a tapered narrowing that has been likened to a pencil, funnel, or steeple (Fig. 7–21). This appearance is considerably less marked in expiration, indicating that the inspiratory collapse is not fixed as it is in the similar-appearing condition of subglottic stenosis. The cords generally appear thickened, with fuzzy margins.

The radiographic findings in "membranous croup"[18] are very similar except that in many patients mucosal irregularity of the subglottic airway is evident, and often the appearance

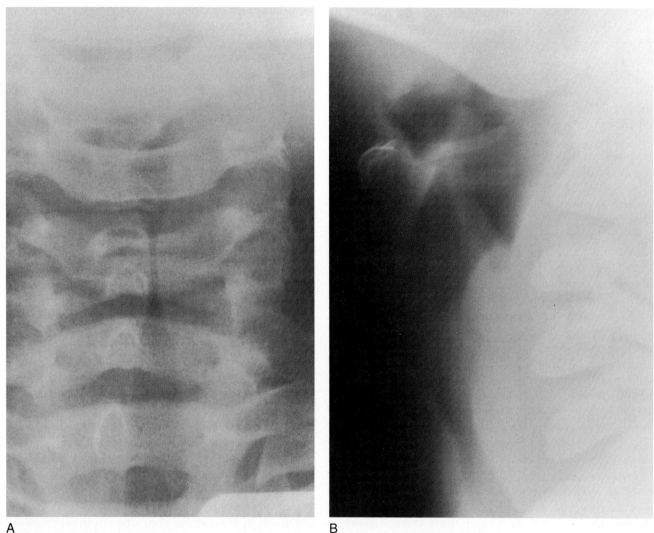

A   B

Figure 7–21
Croup. The characteristic subglottic "penciling" of croup is always best and sometimes solely evident on the frontal view. *A,* A frontal view of the same patient demonstrates moderately severe subglotic "penciling." Frontal chest radiographs often demonstrate this finding in patients with croup. *B,* A lateral view of a 5-year-old boy with croup demonstrates mild subglottic narrowing. The value of the lateral film is not to diagnose croup but to exclude epiglottitis as a cause of stridor. Note the sharply defined and normal epiglottis.

of loose membranes in the airway can erroneously suggest foreign bodies. These loose membranes may change in position in serial films.

EPIGLOTTITIS

Clinical Features Acute epiglottitis is a bacterial infection of the epiglottis and aryepiglottic folds. The organism responsible is almost always *H. influenzae* type B, which can be recovered not only from the larynx but also from the blood in the vast majority of patients.[9] The disease is slightly more common during the winter months, but community outbreaks of epiglottitis do not occur. The age range is larger

than that for croup, occurring primarily in children between 1 and 9 years old; most cases occur in children 3 to 6 years of age. Occasionally, epiglottitis affects adults. As with most causes of stridor, there is a small male preponderance. Since vaccination against *H. influenzae* has become widespread, the incidence of epiglottitis appears to have diminished,[51] but the disorder will probably remain important as a life-threatening cause of airway obstruction for at least the next decade and perhaps longer.

Unlike croup, epiglottitis generally has a very rapid onset, usually within a day or even a few hours. Epiglottitis begins with a sore throat that rapidly progresses to an inability to swallow and resultant drooling. A somewhat fluttering inspiratory stridor appears, with marked respiratory distress

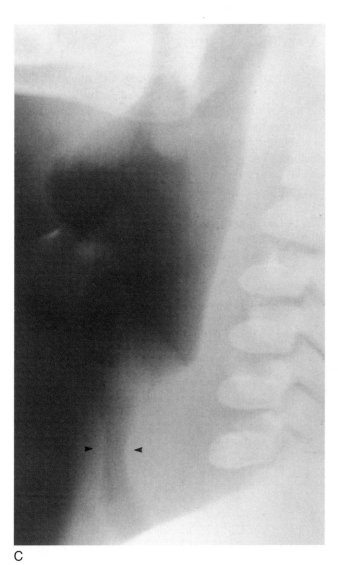

C

Figure 7–21—cont'd

C, A lateral view of a 4-year-old boy with croup shows mild airway narrowing in the subglottic region *(arrowheads)* and hypopharyngeal distention.

and restlessness. The voice may be muffled or normal. The child sits upright, braced in a "tripod position," with the head forward and the tongue frequently protruding, accompanied by drooling. The symptoms are so alarming that emergency medical care is almost invariably sought.

Epiglottitis is usually associated with a high fever (often 105°F). Patients appear pale and "toxic." Extensive cervical adenopathy is usually present. Peripheral blood usually shows considerable leukocytosis (more than 10,000/mm³) with many immature polymorphonuclear leukocytes. If the epiglottis is visualized directly, it is seen to be markedly swollen and bright red. However, casual (tongue blade) attempts to visualize the epiglottis are vigorously discouraged, because such attempts may precipitate complete and catastrophic closure of the airway.

If left untreated, the frequent course of epiglottitis is progressive toxicity, prostration, air hunger, and death. It must be emphasized that children with epiglottitis are in mortal danger; sudden death is not uncommon and may follow any maneuvers that excite or frighten them or make it harder for them to breathe. For this reason, such children should never be left unattended and should always be accompanied by an individual with the skills and apparatus necessary to establish an emergency airway. In extreme situations in which complete airway closure occurs, vigorous oxygen ventilation with a mask and bag or mouth-to-mouth resuscitation can force gas past the obstruction and may be lifesaving.

Radiographic evaluation should be considered only after the child with probable or suspected epiglottitis has been stabilized and is accompanied by personnel prepared to establish an emergency airway. In many institutions, laryngoscopy by experienced individuals who are prepared to establish an emergency airway is a safe method of diagnosis,[23,46] and radiography is not required. However, when such facilities are lacking or if the diagnosis is uncertain, radiography offers a noninvasive substitute for direct visualization of the epiglottis, to confirm the suspected presence of the disease and to exclude other diagnostic possibilities. Important conditions that could simulate epiglottitis clinically are croup, retropharyngeal abscess, and laryngeal foreign body. The radiographic examination should provide this distinction quickly and relatively safely. If, inadvertently or deliberately, an inflamed epiglottis has been seen during physical examination, the radiographic examination is unwarranted.

Radiographic Evaluation Again, it must be emphasized that children with epiglottitis are in life-threatening danger. Their radiographic examinations should be treated as emergency procedures, and the patients should never be left unattended. They should be treated with great care to avoid disturbing or alarming them, and they should never be forced to move against their will during radiographic positioning. It is safest to radiograph children in the position they assume, which is generally seated upright. A single soft tissue lateral view of the neck is exposed, timing the exposure to the latter portion of inspiration. The film is examined immediately, and if epiglottitis is present, no further radiographic studies are indicated. Chest radiography is deferred until the patient has a stable airway. If the epiglottis is normal, the radiographic examination proceeds with a filtered high-kilovoltage anteroposterior view of the neck, a chest radiograph, and whatever additional studies are required to establish the etiology of the stridor.

Radiographic Findings The essential radiographic findings in epiglottitis are seen on the lateral neck film, which is the reason this is the first and, if positive, the only film exposed. In the lateral projection, the epiglottis can be identified by following the upper surface of the tongue backward and down to the vallecula; the epiglottis lies just posterior to the vallecula. Another method is to look posterior and slightly cephalad to the body of the hyoid bone. The normal epiglottis presents a slender shadow that has proportions suggesting those of a finger (Figs. 7–22 and 7–23A). With epiglottitis (Figs. 7–23B–D, and 7–24), the epiglottis becomes swollen and rounded. Associated swelling and thickening of the aryepiglottic folds are present, which may cause the folds to become convex superiorly. The degree of swelling may be mild, or there may be extensive supraglottic edema that effaces the pyriform sinuses and vallecula, so that the normal structural definition is replaced by a nondescript mass of abnormal tissue.

Distention ("ballooning") of the hypopharynx is commonly present with epiglottitis, as it is with most upper airway obstructions. The subglottic airway may be normal, but in about one fourth of cases, associated subglottic edema suggestive of croup is evident. For this reason, the diagnosis of croup should never be made without examining the epiglottis; if any swelling of the epiglottis or aryepiglottic folds is present, the diagnosis is epiglottitis.

Swelling of the epiglottis can occasionally occur in conditions other than infectious epiglottitis. These include angioneurotic edema, irritation by a foreign body, chronic epiglottitis, and trauma.[48] Usually such conditions can be distinguished from acute epiglottitis by the clinical findings, although the radiographic appearance may be similar.

VASCULAR LESIONS

Clinical Features Vascular rings and slings are aberrant segments of the embryonic aortic arch that compress the trachea, the esophagus, or both (Figs. 7–25 and 7–26). Such anomalies account for about 1% to 4% of cases of stridor in children[24] and approximately 15% of cases of congenital stridor.[22] The most common of these anomalies is compression or indentation of the anterior trachea by a somewhat distally placed innominate artery or a common trunk of the innominate and left carotid arteries. Although an indentation in the anterior tracheal wall above the carina may be related to the innominate artery, this finding is commonly seen in lateral radiographs of infants, and it is unusual for such an indentation to cause significant symptoms. Unless it is persistent, very marked, and associated with symptoms (i.e., apnea or stridor), it should be considered a normal variant.

The most severe vascular lesion (i.e., that causing the greatest airway compression) is a right or left double aortic arch that surrounds both the trachea and the esophagus, forming a true vascular ring. Several other types of anomalies produce rings and cause symptoms but are relatively rare and usually milder in their manifestations.[43] Occasionally, even rings that are "open" may cause symptoms late in childhood.

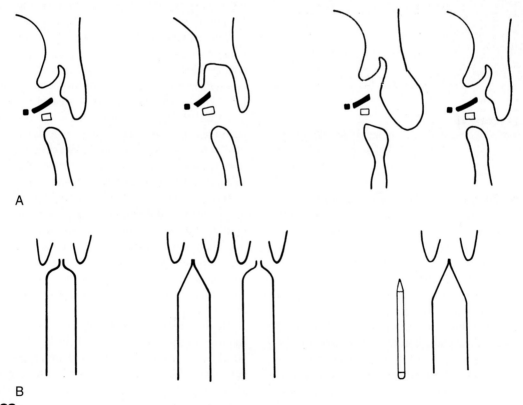

A

B

Figure 7–22
Diagrammatic representation of the normal airway and the airway with epiglottitis and croup. *A,* Lateral view. *B,* Frontal view.

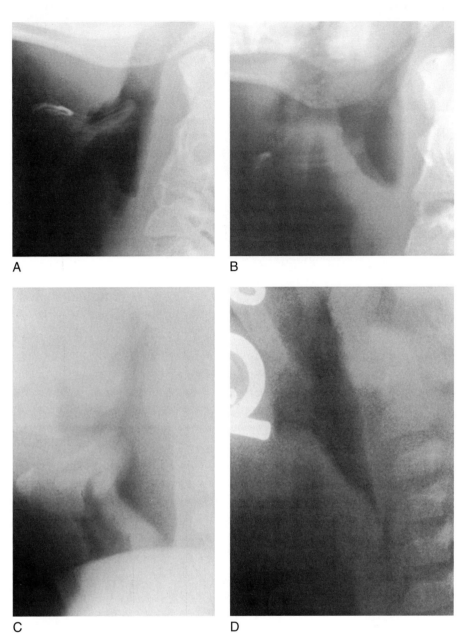

A

B

C

D

Figure 7–23

Epiglottitis. In the lateral projection the shadow of the epiglottis loses its distinct digital shape and appears rounded, blunted, and enlarged. Secondary signs include swelling of the aryepiglottic folds and partial or complete obliteration of the valleculae and anterior portion of the pyriform sinuses. The frontal view, which is not necessary or recommended if the lateral view shows epiglottitis, is usually normal, but one fifth of patients show subglottic narrowing (identical to croup), indicating infraglottic involvement. *A,* Normal epiglottis, shown for comparison. *B,* Epiglottitis in a 5-year-old boy. *C,* Epiglottitis in a 3-year-old girl. *D,* Severe epiglottitis in a 2-year-old child. Marked swelling and edema make definition of the epiglottis difficult, obliterate the valleculae, and deform the pyriform sinuses.

The so-called "vascular sling" (or pulmonary artery sling) is seen less often than the double aortic arch but is nonetheless a relatively common cause of vessel-related symptoms. In this lesion, the left pulmonary artery arises from the right pulmonary artery and crosses to the left lung between the trachea and the esophagus just above the carina.

Significant vascular malformations generally are detected during the first 6 months of life. The more severe the airway obstruction, the earlier the lesions are manifested. The progressive character of the symptoms suggests that vascular rings do not grow as fast as the rest of the patient. The earliest sign of a vascular ring may be expiratory stridor, which is often present from birth. The stridor tends to increase with time and, because the lesion is relatively "fixed" in terms of airway

caliber, to become biphasic (inspiratory and expiratory). Feeding problems occur and may be related both to esophageal compression and to increased respiratory efforts with feeding, involving increased stridor, cyanotic episodes, and frequent regurgitation; dysphagia, however, is uncommon. Patients often have a history of recurrent respiratory tract infections.[47] A barking, brassy, or bitonal cough frequently accompanies respiratory difficulties. With severe obstruction, patients assume an opisthotonic position, and flexion of the neck increases the dyspnea. With milder obstructions, the nonspecificity of findings and symptoms often results in considerable diagnostic delay.[33]

With the exception of upper airway noises, the physical examination of infants with significant vascular malformations

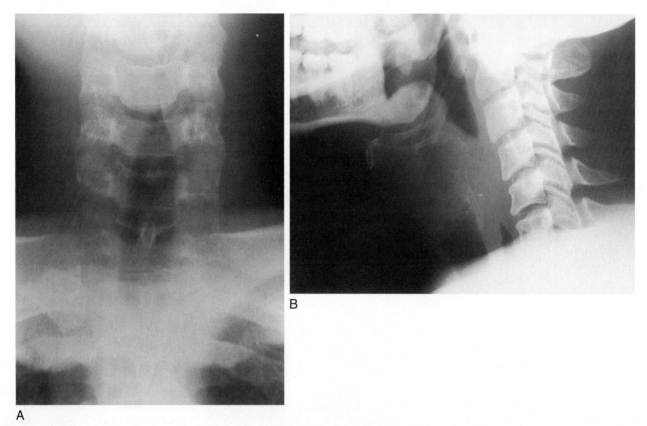

Figure 7–24

Stridor in a 22-year-old man. *A,* Frontal view. *B,* Lateral view. Note the swollen epiglottis and swallowed air in the esophagus. *Haemophilus influenzae* type B was recovered from blood cultures. The diagnosis of epiglottitis is sometimes missed in adults because it is not considered.

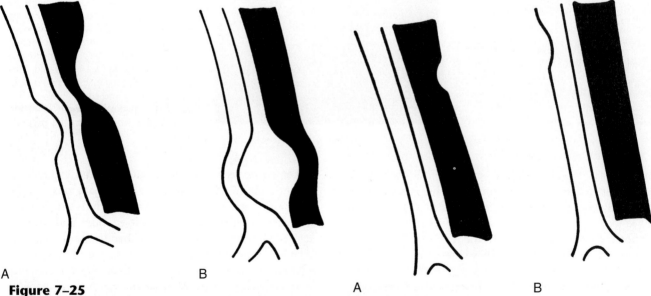

Figure 7–25

Important vascular malformations: diagrammatic representation. The esophagus is depicted in black and the airway in white; the two are seen in a lateral view. *A,* Representation of a double aortic arch, with indentation of the anterior trachea and the posterior esophagus. *B,* Depiction of the findings seen with a pulmonary artery sling or a mediastinal mass (usually a bronchogenic cyst) between the esophagus and airway.

Figure 7–26

Insignificant vascular malformations: diagrammatic representation. *A,* A posterior esophageal indentation is most commonly due to an aberrant subclavian artery, which is almost always an incidental finding. *B,* The innominate artery may sometimes cause an anterior tracheal impression, the importance of which has been controversial. Most authorities believe it to be of no significance.

is usually normal. Lung sounds are unremarkable, and a cardiac murmur is rare. Bronchoscopy reveals bulges in the tracheal wall, and compression of these bulges with the bronchoscope will diminish radial and temporal pulses; however, bronchoscopy has intrinsic risks and generally adds little to the much less invasive radiographic examination.

By the time radiographic consultation is requested, there usually is strong clinical suspicion that the patient has a vascular malformation causing stridor. Lack of signs of infection points away from croup and other infectious diseases, and the child is frequently too young to suggest foreign body obstruction as a plausible diagnosis. Nonetheless, the patient's symptoms may have been increased by an intercurrent infection, so the first step is confirmation of the presence of a vascular malformation. The second, and possibly more important, step is to determine the character of the malformation—that is, whether it is a type requiring surgery and, if so, what sort of surgery is needed. A final step, and one that is usually unnecessary for the more common lesions, is to determine the exact vascular morphology as revealed by MRI or CT.

Radiographic Evaluation If the likelihood of a vascular malformation is very high, it may be reasonable to forgo films of the neck, but if foreign bodies or other intracervical lesions are a possibility, radiographs of the neck, as previously described, are obtained. A frontal and lateral chest film of good technical quality is mandatory. This is followed by a barium esophagram. The esophagus is studied by the radiologist using fluoroscopy; having a technologist do a blind "cardiac series" can result in missed lesions. The child (who should be hungry at the time of examination) is given barium to drink, and spot films are made of the filled esophagus in the frontal, lateral, and oblique projections. If the patient does not drink sufficiently to fill the esophagus, barium can be injected into the esophagus through a feeding tube. Watching indentations on the esophagus fluoroscopically to see if they pulsate, in hopes of distinguishing a vascular impression from a mediastinal mass, can be a tedious and radiation-laden pursuit, especially because of the tendency for solid masses to transmit vascular pulsations.

With the more common lesions, diagnostic morphology is adequately demonstrated by plain chest films and the esophagram. Occasionally, however, surgeons desire a more detailed evaluation of the vascular anatomy. At some centers, this necessitates plain or digital subtraction angiography. In interpreting such angiograms, it must be kept in mind that a significant segment of many vascular rings is the ligamentum arteriosum, which is not opacified during the angiogram. Both CT (Fig. 7–28), using bolus contrast material injection and mediastinal windows, and MRI (Fig. 7–29) reveal needed vascular anatomy. Color Doppler flow mapping is another potentially useful imaging modality.[17]

Radiographic Findings The presence of a vascular ring or sling may frequently be suggested from the plain chest film, and this may be a very helpful observation in a child in whom the lesion is not yet suspected. The possibility of a vascular ring, as well as other extracardiac and intracardiac anomalies, should be considered when a right-sided aortic arch is identified. In an infant, this is usually manifested by the trachea lying slightly left of midline. The lateral film is scrutinized to see whether tracheal narrowing in the vicinity of the aortic arch is indicated; if so, the presence of a vascular ring is strongly suggested. Findings of a vascular sling are more subtle; on the frontal film, one may see a right-sided compression of the trachea in the immediate supracarinal area and narrowing of this region on the lateral view.

The diagnosis may essentially be confirmed by the esophagram (Fig. 7–30). The various patterns of abnormalities seen in esophagrams of patients with vascular malformations are described in detail elsewhere.[4,43] A tight vascular ring caused by a double aortic arch produces quite distinctive findings.

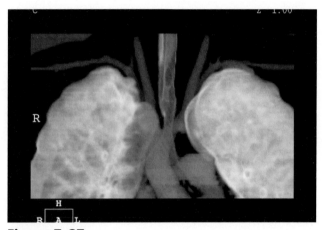

Figure 7–27
Double aortic arch.

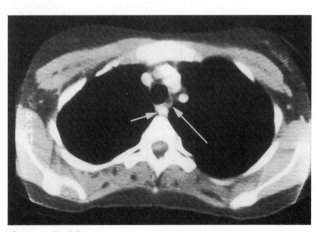

Figure 7–28
Aberrant right subclavian artery: computered tomography. This postinfusion scan demonstrates a vascular structure (*short arrow*) posterior to the trachea and esophagus. The esophagus (*long arrow*) has a small amount of gas within its lumen.

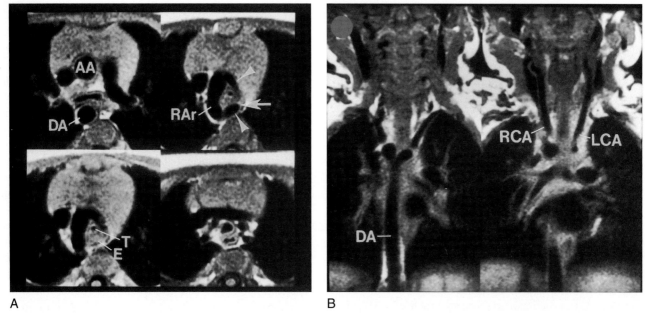

A   B

Figure 7–29

Double aortic arch with an atretic segment located between the origin of the left subclavian artery and the left carotid artery. Magnetic resonance imaging is the technique of choice for defining the precise anatomy of congenital vascular malformations of the aortic arch. *A,* Multiple transaxial scans through the upper thorax reveal a right aortic arch (RAr). Anterior and posterior branches of the left aortic arch are indicated with an *arrowhead*. A discrete, focal area of atresia is noted between the two limbs of the left aortic arch *(arrow)*. AA, Ascending aorta; D*A,* descending aorta; E, esophagus; T, trachea. *B,* Two T1-weighted images reveal posterior anastomosis of the two arches as they form the descending aorta. LCA, Left carotid artery; RCA, right carotid artery.
(From Bisset GS III. Magnetic resonance imaging of the pediatric thorax: Semin Ultrasound CT MR 12 :429–447, 1991.)

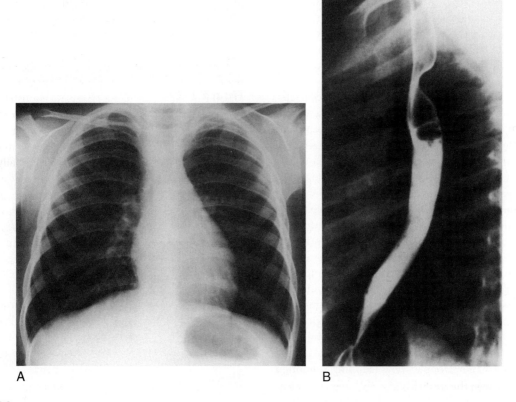

A   B

Figure 7–30

Right aortic arch and vascular ring in a 3-year-old boy who presented with dysphagia and mild chronic stridor. *A,* A posteroanterior view of the chest shows a right aortic arch. *B,* An esophagram in the lateral projection demonstrates a single prominent indentation in the posterior esophagus.

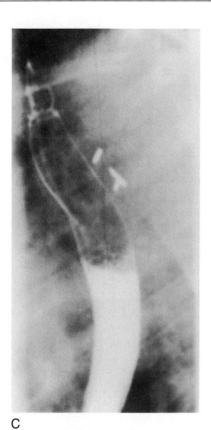

C

Figure 7–30—cont'd
C, A normal esophagram obtained after surgical opening of a vascular ring made up of the right arch, an aberrant left subclavian artery, and the ligamentum arteriosum.

With such a ring, the posterior portion of the divided aorta is usually superior to and larger than the anterior portion. Thus, on the lateral view, a large indentation is seen on the posterior wall of the barium-filled esophagus. Frequently, an anterior indentation on the barium column, generally slightly lower and smaller than the posterior compression, is also present. Importantly, the tracheal air column, also usually best evaluated on the lateral view, is compressed anteriorly and often deviated posteriorly by the anterior element of the double aorta. Other modalities may be employed to confirm the lesion and to obtain more details of the vascular anatomy, but many surgeons do not believe additional studies are necessary if the characteristic findings are present with less invasive methods. CT or MRI may obviate the need for angiography in many patients by providing increased vascular anatomic detail and excluding the relatively remote possibility of an encircling mass.

A vascular sling also presents a very characteristic picture on an esophagram (Fig. 7–31). The aberrant left pulmonary artery courses between the trachea and esophagus, compressing and separating these structures in the region just above the carina. On frontal plain films, the sling occasionally may be seen to "tug" the supracarinal trachea to the left and

elevate the proximal right main bronchus. Pulmonary angiography, although it can diagnose the lesion, usually can be obviated by CT or MRI, both of which can also exclude the possibility that the esophagus and trachea are separated by a bronchogenic cyst.

UPPER AIRWAY FOREIGN BODY

Clinical Features Aspirated foreign bodies cause at least 2000 deaths each year in children in the United States, along with considerable additional morbidity. The majority of deaths are in boys 5 years of age and younger. Ninety percent of foreign body aspirations occur in toddlers (children 1 to 4 years of age). Children in this age group have the mobility to encounter a variety of objects and the inclination to put appropriate-size objects in their mouths. A noteworthy characteristic of foreign body aspiration is that the history is often lacking or misleading because the incident may not have been observed and because the acute cough, gagging, and respiratory distress that immediately follow aspiration may subside to a relatively asymptomatic state.[11] The continuing symptoms depend on the site at which the foreign body lodges. Approximately 80% of aspirated foreign bodies lodge in the bronchial tree, and the most common symptoms are cough, wheezing, and dyspnea; stridor is relatively uncommon. Foreign bodies at the bronchial level are discussed in Chapter 8. Stridor, as well as cough and dyspnea, is much more commonly seen with laryngotracheal or esophageal foreign bodies.[5]

Objects in the laryngotracheal area cause symptoms by their irritative effect and by direct obstruction to gas flow. Objects impacted in the esophagus may obstruct the airway because of physical deformation, erode into the airway, or embed in the esophageal wall, forming a foreign body granuloma. There may be considerable delay in the diagnosis of esophageal foreign bodies; children, especially those in the age groups in which liquid, soft, or pureed foods form the bulk of the diet, may have no suggestive dysphagia, and a history of occasional vomiting, drooling, choking, or difficulty in eating may be masked by or ignored because of respiratory symptoms. Such patients may have recurrent pneumonias because of repeated aspiration due to the partial esophageal obstruction. The most common impacted esophageal foreign body is a coin (Fig. 7–32).

The majority of aspirated foreign bodies are foods, especially peanuts (the most common aspirated foreign body[31]), sunflower seeds, and material related to foods, such as eggshells, fruit skins, bones, and seeds; thus, most foreign bodies are radiolucent. Foreign bodies that are firm and irregular, such as eggshells, frequently become impacted in the larynx, whereas smoother objects often pass the larynx and reach the trachea. Objects within the trachea, if they do not reach the bronchi, may rest against the tracheal wall, which causes

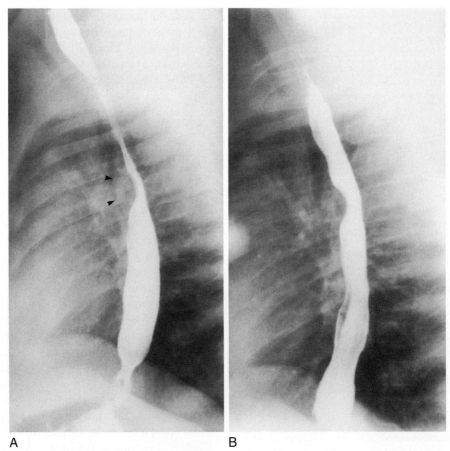

Figure 7–31
Aberrant left pulmonary artery: esophagram. *A,* A mass *(arrowheads)* is seen interposed between the distal trachea and the esophagus of a 3-year-old child. *B,* Full distention of the esophagus better defines the size of the lesion. An aberrant left pulmonary artery or a bronchogenic cyst are two diagnostic possibilities at this age.

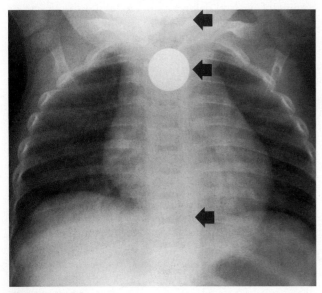

Figure 7–32
Three common sites of esophageal foreign bodies. *A,* Cricopharyngeus muscle. *B,* Aortic arch. *C,* Gastroesophageal junction.

subsidence of symptoms; others may be blown about, producing more vigorous and paroxysmal symptoms. Airway obstruction results not only from the foreign body itself, but also from the associated edema and inflammation. A child who has stridor with a foreign body frequently demonstrates a barking or croupy cough, wheezing, hoarseness, hemoptysis, and respiratory distress. Laryngeal foreign bodies may produce aphonia. Unlike children with viral croup, children with foreign body aspiration are usually entirely healthy before the onset of symptoms.

The most lethal aspirated foreign body is a rubber toy balloon, which accounted for 121 reported deaths during 1973 to 1988.[36] Because such balloons are radiotransparent, radiographs may not be helpful; however, the radiologist may play an important role merely by suggesting the possibility of a foreign body. One case at our institution involved an infant who was found cyanotic; despite endotracheal intubation, extraordinarily high ventilator pressures were required to move air. The radiologist insisted that a foreign body must be involved, because nothing else accounted for the findings. The radiologist's persistence was rewarded by the appearance in his office of a surgeon, in full surgical regalia, who dropped a damp balloon on his desk. This foreign body, apparently a gift from an older sibling, had been found resting on the infant's carina.

A pharyngeal foreign body generally causes less obstruction and less difficulty in diagnosis and management than an airway foreign body, but special note must be made of sharp objects in the pharynx. Not infrequently, such objects cause abscesses, and abscesses may form after the object has been identified and removed (Figs. 7–33 and 7–34). A retropharyngeal abscess in children older than 1 year of age is related most commonly to a sharp foreign body,[26] and children should be carefully monitored for this complication after a tack or pin has been removed.

Radiographic Evaluation A clinical history of a suspected foreign body may be helpful in tailoring the radiographic study; for example, the radiologist might suggest careful examination of the larynx in several projections to try to demonstrate a bit of eggshell on edge. Sometimes, however, the history may be misleading, as when a parent suggests a metallic foreign body when actually a nonmetallic object has been aspirated. Absence of a metallic object should not terminate the search for the source of symptoms.

As noted earlier, most foreign bodies, including foods, most plastics, and aluminum, are radiolucent. Nonetheless, many such objects may be identified either directly, by the air contrast produced by the object itself in the airway (Fig. 7–35), or indirectly, by the associated edema. Even if no object is identified, the examination may be useful in excluding other causes of stridor, such as viral croup. Few more difficult tasks exist in radiology than identification of a loose radiolucent foreign body in the upper airway, but it can be done surprisingly often if impeccable technique is employed; indeed, the diagnosis can be at least suggested by findings on neck films in the great majority of patients.[14]

The radiographic examination begins with films of the neck and chest; the high-kilovoltage anteroposterior film is of particular importance in this setting to permit visualization of the airway "through" the bones of the cervical spine. A similar view of the intrathoracic airway may also be useful, as may routine chest radiographs. If these studies are inconclusive, it is important to proceed with an esophagram to exclude an occult foreign body in the esophagus. The use of barium-soaked cotton pledgets or barium capsules is seldom necessary in children and may complicate the problem.

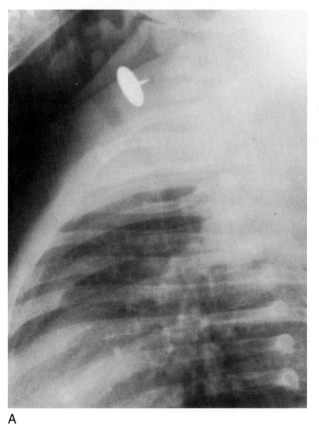
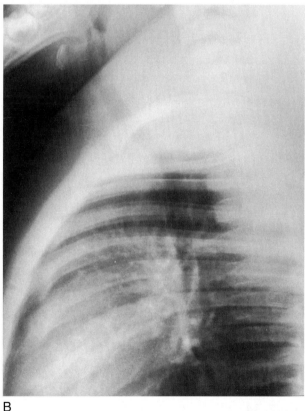

A

B

Figure 7–33

Retropharyngeal abscess following a foreign body. *A,* A 1-year-old girl with a thumbtack in the hypopharynx. The thumbtack was removed. *B,* One month later a chest radiograph was exposed to evaluate "wheezing." Retropharyngeal swelling was noted but no action was taken.

Continued

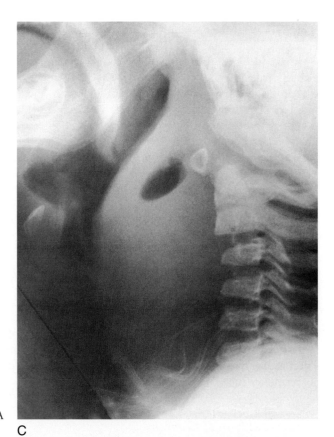

Figure 7–33—cont'd
C, Two months later the patient presented with severe stridor and fever. A large retropharyngeal abscess was present with an air-fluid level.

C

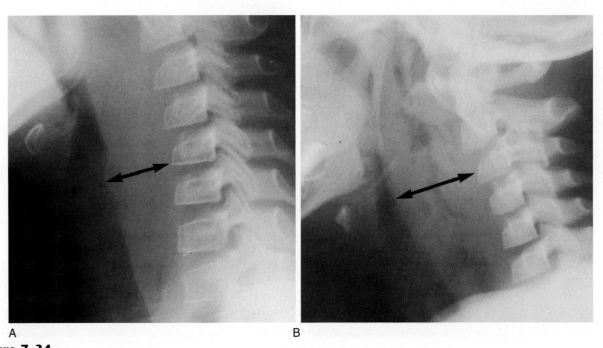

A   B

Figure 7–34
Two patients with retropharyngeal abscess formation. Note the markedly increased soft tissue density between the airway and spine, extending from the first cervical vertebral body to the thoracic inlet *(arrows)*. The cervical spine is bowed away from the area of inflammation, and the posterior pharyngeal fat stripe is no longer visible. *A,* A 5-year-old girl with fever and pain on swallowing. *B,* A 3-year-old boy with a history of falling with a lollipop stick in his mouth.

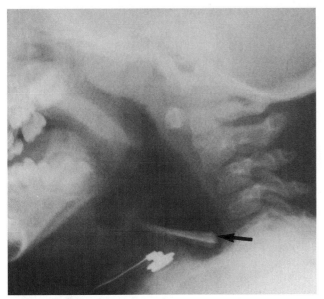

Figure 7–35
An apple peel lodged in the base of the pyriform sinus *(arrow)*. Foreign bodies in the upper airway often induce choking and vomiting.

Although instances have been described in which small chicken and fish bones have been completely obscured by ordinary barium examination, these foreign bodies are much more frequent in adults than in children. Furthermore, adults have considerably more calcified structures in the neck than do children; in children, small bones are usually much easier to identify. Despite advice to the contrary, the use of water-soluble ionic contrast material has virtually no place in the investigation of esophageal foreign bodies because of the hazard of aspiration.

In suspected foreign body aspiration, as in other causes of stridor (with the exception of acute epiglottitis), at least two views of every area should be obtained. This is necessary because, for example, a single frontal view of the chest, showing a coin in the esophagus, can conceal the fact that actually two or more coins are overlying each other, and an impacted eggshell may be invisible unless positioned edge-on to the beam.

In certain circumstances, an esophageal foreign body may be removed without subjecting the child to endoscopy.[7] Such circumstances involve a foreign body that is smooth, such as a coin, and one that has been ingested within 24 hours, before a significant mucosal reaction has occurred; the appearance of an associated mass, reflecting edema, is a contraindication to the maneuver. The technique is described in more detail elsewhere.[37] Essentially, a balloon catheter is passed through the mouth, and the balloon is inflated with air or contrast material. The inflated balloon is used to pull the object into the pharynx, from which it may easily be removed. Alternatively, the balloon may be used to push the object into the stomach, from which objects such as coins pass readily. A drawback to this technique is the possibility that the retrieved object in the pharynx will be aspirated into the airway; although this possibility appears to be more theoretical than real, catheter manipulations are done only in the presence of emergency apparatus and by someone experienced in the technique.

Finally, it must be noted that stridor, although usually connoting an upper airway lesion, may also occur with endobronchial foreign bodies; in addition, foreign bodies may be multiple. Thus a lower airway foreign body should be considered and radiographically excluded; this is discussed in Chapter 8.

Radiographic Findings A radiopaque foreign body is easily localized. A problem can arise when multiple foreign bodies overlie each other, as with stacked coins, but filming in two projections elucidates this. Objects that are radiopaque but nearly planar, such as eggshells, may be visible only when the beam is parallel to the object's plane; this is particularly important, because eggshells commonly become impacted in infants' larynges. Other calcified objects, particularly bones, may be "lost" in the cervical spine and in calcified cartilages. In infants, the only neck structures normally calcified, other than the spine, are the body and wings of the hyoid bone. With increasing age, however, laryngeal structures may calcify, and it is necessary to know the normal anatomy of these structures[27] so that foreign bodies may be recognized.

Aluminum is a common metal that is almost radiolucent, although, like eggshells, planar aluminum objects sometimes are visible edge-on. The most common aluminum object is a removable pop-top tab from soft drink and beer cans; this may lodge in the esophagus when swallowed. Fortunately, the use of these tabs is diminishing. Foreign coins are commonly made of aluminum and are thus virtually radiolucent, but current United States coins are radiopaque and easily seen. It has often been noted that on a frontal film an esophageal coin is face up (Fig. 7–36), whereas an endotracheal coin is edge-on. When a lateral view is lacking, this would seem to be a useful rule, except that endotracheal coins are so uncommon that many pediatric radiologists have never encountered one.

Objects that are completely radiolucent (i.e., of water density), such as most food materials, are, unfortunately, the most common foreign bodies aspirated. Surprisingly often, however, these may be seen by the contrast afforded by the surrounding airway; they appear as focal filling defects in the gas column (Fig. 7–37). Objects that are fixed in place tend to evoke a local inflammatory response that occurs very rapidly with vegetable materials such as peanuts; the local inflammation causes swelling that is often visible radiographically, even if the object itself is not. A foreign body in the larynx may produce enough swelling to suggest a primary inflammatory disease, and correct diagnosis requires a lack of infectious symptoms and laboratory findings, preferably with a suggestive history.

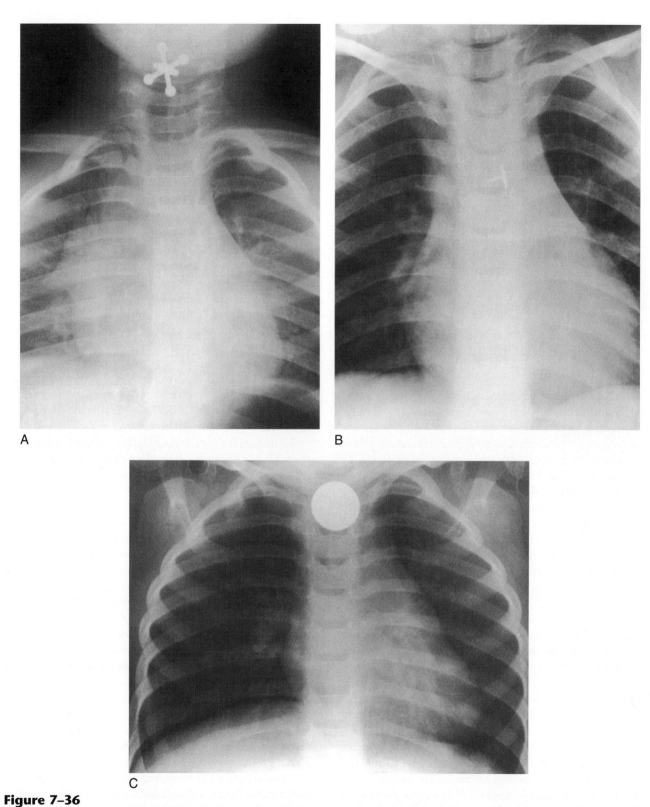

A

B

C

Figure 7–36
Radiopaque esophageal foreign bodies. *A*, A 2-year-old boy with a foreign body (a jack) at the level of the cricopharyngeal muscle. This normal chest was radiographed during expiration, thus falsely suggesting cardiac failure. *B*, A 1-year-old girl with an esophageal coin at the level of the aortic arch. *C*, An esophageal foreign body (a tack) in another common site of lodgment, near the crossing of the aorta and left main bronchus in a 6-year-old boy. The tack was subsequently passed spontaneously.

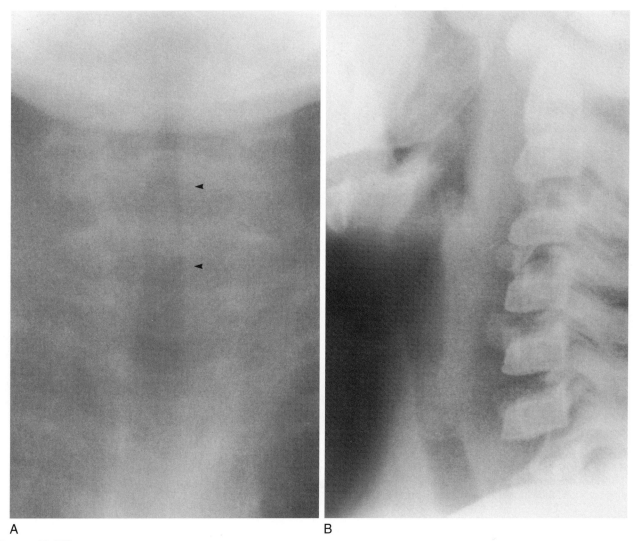

A   B

Figure 7–37
Aspirated tracheal foreign body. Frontal *(A)* and lateral *(B)* views of the neck in a 2-year-old girl show a filling defect *(arrows)* in the tracheal air column. This was an aspirated sunflower seed, rendered visible by contrast with the surrounding air.

Distention of the hypopharynx, which is itself a nonspecific sign of upper airway obstruction, can be a useful indicator that genuine obstruction is present, even if the obstruction itself is unseen.

Radiolucent objects in the esophagus may appear as a mass seen on the lateral view as impinging on the posterior airway and deviating it forward. The mass may be composed not only of the foreign body itself, but also of inflammatory tissue and food materials that have been unable to pass the object. Most impacted foreign bodies tend to lodge at areas of normal narrowing (see Fig. 7–36): the cricopharyngeal muscle, the thoracic inlet, the crossing of the left main bronchus and the aorta, and (less commonly in children than in adults) the gastroesophageal junction. A foreign body lodged at another area should raise the question of whether underlying esophageal disease is present. Strictures related to

previous surgery are common following repair of esophageal atresia and tracheoesophageal fistula, and surgical clips may alert the radiologist to this possibility, even if the history is lacking (Fig. 7–38).

With esophageal foreign bodies, the esophagram usually demonstrates the foreign body as a filling defect in the barium column. The defect, if the object is small, may be seen on only one of the four projections. Filling defects of associated food will also frequently be seen, as is inflammatory swelling. If the impaction is in an unusual location, a repeat esophagram is done after the object has been removed and the edema (Fig. 7–39) has subsided to investigate a possible underlying stricture. A foreign body that has been impacted for a considerable length of time may itself also produce a stricture, requiring subsequent radiographic examination and possible surgical correction. It is not routinely

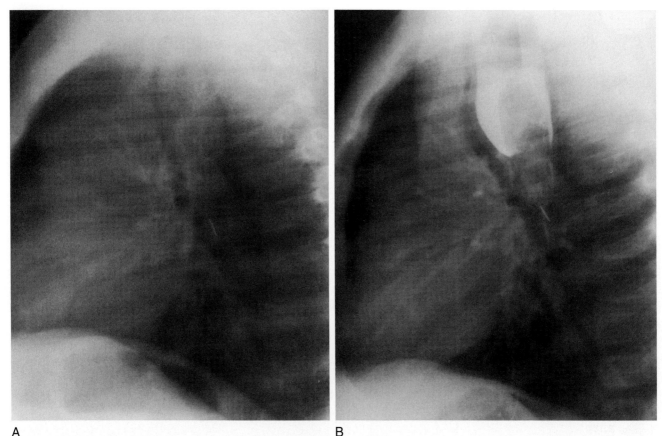

A

B

Figure 7–38
Esophageal obstruction secondary to stricture in a 2-year-old child who had undergone repair of a tracheoesophageal fistula in infancy. *A,* This lateral chest film shows a mass deviating the airway anteriorly. A surgical clip is present, providing a helpful diagnostic clue. *B,* An esophagram shows food impacted above the stricture.

necessary to reexamine a patient in whom foreign body lodgment is in an expected area and in whom symptoms subside following removal of the object.

SUMMARY

Stridor is noisy breathing. Because it almost always indicates some degree of airway obstruction, it must be regarded as a serious and potentially life-threatening finding. Stridor may be produced by a variety of entities, reflecting the many anatomic regions in which obstruction may occur. Such entities may be congenital, producing symptoms from or shortly after birth, or acquired. Noninflammatory acquired lesions, such as slow-growing tumors, usually produce stridor that is chronic, whereas inflammatory lesions and foreign bodies tend to produce stridor with acute onset. Acute stridor presents as a medical emergency demanding immediate diagnosis and therapy more frequently than does chronic stridor, which can often be evaluated at relative leisure.

Certain characteristics of stridor may be diagnostically helpful. For example, stridor produced by lesions above the thoracic inlet tends to be loudest with inspiration, whereas lesions within the thorax more frequently produce expiratory stridor. Lesions with which the stridor is biphasic (both inspiratory and expiratory) tend to be more occlusive than lesions producing stridor that is purely inspiratory or expiratory. Stridor accompanied by vocal changes suggests an abnormality affecting the glottis. Cough tends to be a prominent feature of lesions in the subglottic region. Stridor associated with feeding difficulties should suggest lesions that affect both the airway and the swallowing process. Of course, many exceptions to these rules exist, and clinical impressions based on such rules must be substantiated by more concrete evidence. Such evidence may be provided by an adequate radiographic evaluation. In many patients, endoscopy will ultimately be required, but even in these patients, the radiographic evaluation is helpful in guiding the endoscopist and excluding other lesions.

The essential radiographic tasks are, first, to demonstrate the location of the obstruction and, second, to obtain as much information as possible about the pathophysiologic nature of the lesion in a manner that is as noninvasive as possible. In its simplest form, the radiographic evaluation is

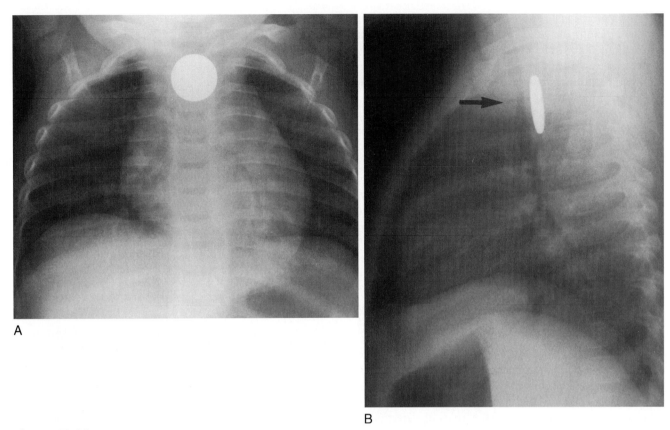

Figure 7–39
An impacted coin in the esophagus at the level of the aortic arch, causing edema with significant tracheal narrowing (*arrow*). *A*, Frontal view. *B*, Lateral view.

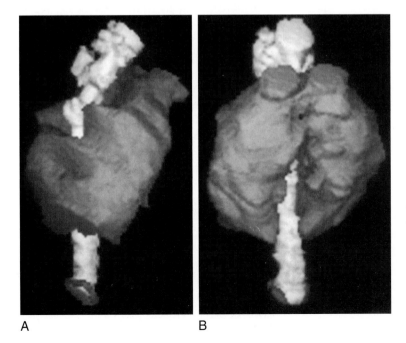

Figure 7–40
Three-dimensional computed tomography reconstruction: a neonate with stridor caused by a goitrous thyroid encircling the airway. Left anterior oblique *(A)* and left posterior oblique *(B)* views demonstrate severe glandular hypertrophy compressing the airway. The stridor resolved with exogenous thyroxine administration in this hypothyroid infant.
(From Optican RJ, White KS, Effmann EL. Goitrous cretinism manifesting as newborn stridor: CT evaluation. AJR Am J Roentgenol 157:557–558, 1991.)

merely a bidirectional view of the entire upper airway, using the airway's intrinsic gas as a contrast medium to outline obstructions, followed by a similar view of the upper alimentary tract, using barium as a contrast medium. This evaluation requires nothing more than conventional radiographic apparatus, modified with a filter for the frontal neck view, plus a sound knowledge of normal radiographic anatomy. With these tools, the majority of significant lesions can be located and, to a considerable extent, characterized.

For many lesions, it is desirable to employ secondary radiographic techniques. Such techniques can be selected only after a specific lesion is located or strongly suspected by simpler techniques. Angiography, for example, may be needed to characterize a vascular malformation or to investigate the vascular supply of a tumor. Neck masses that lie on either side or in front of the airway may be investigated by ultrasonography to obtain information about the masses' solid and cystic characteristics and their spatial relationships with other structures. Masses that contain functional thyroid tissue may be imaged with radionuclide scans. Lesions anywhere in the body may be examined by CT; CT, with tailored injections of contrast material, can be used to examine vascular anatomy in detail and to separate vascular from solid masses, which may obviate angiography in the evaluation of vascular rings and slings. CT is also extremely sensitive to slight differences in radiographic density, permitting detection of subtle calcifications. Similarly, MRI will probably play an increasing role in characterizing lesions that produce stridor; already it has an important role in evaluating neck and chest tumors as well as vascular malformations. Both CT and MRI permit three-dimensional reconstructions that can be quite helpful in delineation of mass lesions and in surgical planning (Fig. 7–40).

REFERENCES

1. Arthurton MW. Stridor in a paediatric department. Proc R Soc Med 63:712–714, 1970.
2. Auringer ST, Bisset GS 3rd, Myer CM 3rd. Magnetic resonance imaging of the pediatric airway. Compared with findings at surgery and/or endoscopy. Pediatr Radiol 21:329–332, 1991.
3. Azizkhan RG, Dudgeon DL, Buck JR, et al. Life-threatening airway obstruction as a complication to the management of mediastinal masses in children. J Pediatr Surg 20:816–822, 1985.
4. Berdon WE, Baker DH. Vascular anomalies and the infant lung: Rings, slings, and other things. Semin Roentgenol 7:39–64, 1972.
5. Blazer S, Naveh Y, Friedman A. Foreign body in the airway. A review of 200 cases. Am J Dis Child 134:68–71, 1980.
6. Burke AJ, Vining DJ, McGuirt WF Jr, et al. Evaluation of airway obstruction using virtual endoscopy. Laryngoscope 110:23–29, 2000.
7. Campbell JB, Condon VR. Catheter removal of blunt esophageal foreign bodies. Survey of the Society for Pediatric Radiology. Pediatr Radiol 19:6–7, 1989.
8. Capitano MA, Kirkpatrick JA. Obstructions of the upper airway in children as reflected on the chest radiograph. Radiology 107:15 9–161, 1973.
9. Cohen SR, Chai J. Epiglottitis. Twenty-year study with tracheostomy. Ann Otol Rhinol Laryngol 87:461–467, 1978.
10. de Marie S, Tjon A Tham RT, Van der Mey AG, Meerdink G, van Furth R, van der Meer JW. Clinical infections and nonsurgical treatment of parapharyngeal space infections complicating throat infection. Rev Infect Dis 11:975–982, 1989.
11. Di Marco CJ, Mauer TP, Reinhard RN. Airway foreign bodies: A diagnostic challenge. J Am Osteopath Assoc 91:481–486, 1991.
12. Donnelly BW, McMillan JA, Weiner LB. Bacterial tracheitis: Report of eight new cases and review. Rev Infect Dis 12:729–735, 1990.
13. Dunbar JS. Upper respiratory tract obstruction in infants and children. AJR Am J Roentgenol 109:227–246, 1970.
14. Esclamado RM, Richardson MA. Laryngotracheal foreign bodies in children. A comparison with bronchial foreign bodies. Am J Dis Child 141:259–262, 1987.
15. Faust RA, Rimell FL, Remley KB. Cine magnetic resonance imaging for evaluation of focal tracheomalacia: innominate artery compression syndrome. Int J Pediatr Otorhinolaryngol 65:27–33, 2002.
16. Friedman EM, Vastola AP, McGill TJ, Healy GB. Chronic pediatric stridor: Etiology and outcome. Laryngoscope 100:277–280, 1990.
17. Gnanapragasam JP, Houston AB, Jamieson MP. Pulmonary artery sling: Definitive diagnosis by colour Doppler flow mapping avoiding cardiac catheterization. Br Heart J 63:251–252, 1990.
18. Han BK, Dunbar JS, Striker TW. Membranous laryngotracheobronchitis (membranous croup). AJR Am J Roentgenol 133:53–58, 1979.
19. Holinger LD. Etiology of stridor in the neonate, infant and child. Ann Otol Rhinol Laryngol 89:397–400, 1980.
20. Holinger PH. Foreign bodies in the air and food passages. Trans Am Acad Ophthalmol Otolaryngol 66:193–210, 1962.
21. Joseph PM, Berdon WE, Baker DH, Slovis TL, Haller JO. Upper airway obstruction in infants and small children. Improved radiographic diagnosis by combining filtration, high kilovoltage, and magnification. Radiology 121:143–148, 1976.
22. Kahn A, Baran D, Spehl M, Dab I, Blum D. Congenital stridor in infancy. Clinical lessons derived from a survey of 31 instances. Clin Pediatr 16:19–26, 1977.
23. Mauro RD, Pool SR, Lcokhart CH. Differentiation of epiglottitis from laryngotracheitis in the child with stridor. Am J Dis Child 142:679–682, 1988.
24. Maze A, Bloch E. Stridor in pediatric patients. Anesthesiology 50:132–145, 1979.
25. Meine FJ, Lorenzo RL, Lynch PF, Capitanio MA, Kirkpatrick JA. Pharyngeal distention associated with upper airway obstruction. Experimental observations in dogs. Radiology 111:395–398, 1974.
26. Morrison JE Jr, Pashley NR. Retropharyngeal abscesses in children: A ten-year review. Pediatr Emerg Care 4:9–11, 1988.
27. Muroff LR, Seaman WB. Normal anatomy of the larynx and pharynx and the differential diagnosis of foreign bodies. Semin Roentgenol 9:267–272, 1974.
28. Nowlin JH, Zalzal GH. The stridorous infant. Ear Nose Throat J 70:84–88, 1991.
29. Ophir D, Katz Y, Tavori I, Aladjem M. Functional upper airway obstruction in adolescents. Arch Otolaryngol Head Neck Surg 116:1208–1209, 1990.
30. Pelton DA, Whalen JS. Airway obstruction in infants and children. Int Anesthesiol Clin 10:123–150, 1972.
31. Puhakka H, Svedstrom E, Kero P, Valli P, Iisalo E. Tracheobronchial foreign bodies. A persistent problem in pediatric patients. Am J Dis Child 143:543–545, 1989.
32. Rabie I, McShane D, Warde D. Bacterial tracheitis. J Laryngol Otol 103:1059–1062, 1989.
33. Rivilla F, Utrilla JG, Alvarez F. Surgical management and follow-up of vascular rings. Z Kinderchir 44:199–202, 1989.

34. Rosenfield NS, Peck DR, Lowman RM. Xeroradiography in the evaluation of acquired airway abnormalities in children. Am J Dis Child 132:1177–1180, 1978.

35. Rudman DT, Elmaraghy CA, Shiels WE, Weit GJ. The role of airway fluoroscopy in the evaluation of stridor in children. Arch Otolaryngol Head Neck Surg 129:305-309, 2003.

36. Ryan CA, Yacoub W, Paton T, Avard D. Childhood deaths from toy balloons. Am J Dis Child 144:1221–1224, 1990.

37. Shakelford GD, McAlister WH, Robertson CL. The use of a Foley catheter for removal of blunt esophageal foreign bodies from children. Radiology 105:455–456, 1972.

38. Simpson I, Campbell PE. Mediastinal masses in childhood: A review from a paediatric pathologist's point of view. Prog Pediatr Surg 27:92–126, 1991.

39. Singer JI, McCabe JB. Epiglottitis at the extremes of age. Am J Emerg Med 6:228–231, 1988.

40. Sivan Y, Deakers TW, Newth CJ. Thoracoabdominal asynchrony in acute upper airway obstruction in small children. Am Rev Respir Dis 142:540–544, 1990.

41. Slawinski EB, Jamieson DG. Studies of respiratory stridor in young children: Acoustical analyses and tests of a theoretical model. Int J Pediatr Otorhinolaryngol 19:205–222, 1990.

42. Sorantin E, Geiger B, Lindbichler F, Eber E, Schimpl G. CT-based tracheobronchoscopy in children—Comparison with axial CT and multiplanar reconstruction: preliminary results. Pediatr Radiol 32:8–15, 2002.

43. Swischuk LE. Plain Film Interpretation in Congenital Heart Disease. 2nd ed. Baltimore: Williams & Wilkins, 1979, pp 205–226.

44. Swischuk LE, Smith PC, Fagan CJ. Abnormalities of the pharynx and larynx in childhood. Semin Roentgenol 9:283–300, 1974.

45. Toriumi DM, Miller DR, Holinger LD. Acquired subglottic cysts in premature infants. Int J Pediatr Otorhinolaryngol 14:151–160, 1987.

46. Trollfors B, Nylen O, Strangert K. Acute epiglottitis in children and adults in Sweden 1981–3. Arch Dis Child 65:491–494, 1990.

47. van Aalderen WM, Hoekstra MO, Hess J, Gerritsen J, Knol K. Respiratory infections and vascular rings. Acta Paediatr Scand 79:477–480, 1990.

48. Watts FB Jr, Slovis TL. The enlarged epiglottis. Pediatr Radiol 5:133–136, 1977.

49. Wenner HA. Airway obstruction: Acute infections and hypersensitivity reactions. In Jazbi B, ed. Pediatric Otorhinolaryngology: A Review of Ear, Nose and Throat Problems in Children. New York: Appleton-Century-Crofts, 1980, pp 183–191.

50. Williams EF III, Woo P, Miller R, Kellman RM. The effects of adenotonsillectomy on growth in young children. Otolaryngol Head Neck Surg 104:509–516, 1991.

51. Wilson N, Wenger J, Mansoor O, Baker M, Martin D. The beneficial impact of Hib vaccine on disease rates in New Zealand children. N Z Med J 115:U122, 2002.

ADDITIONAL READING

Baines PB, Sarginson RE. Upper airway obstruction. Hosp Med 65:108–111, 2004.

Hammer J. Acquired upper airway obstruction. Paediatr Respir Rev 5:25–33, 2004.

Klass P. Croup—The bark is worse than the bite. N Engl J Med. 351:1283–1284, 2004.

Kussman BD, Geva T, McGowan FX. Cardiovascular causes of airway compression. Paediatr Anaesth 14:60–74, 2004.

Leung AK, Kellner JD, Johnson DW. Viral croup: A current perspective. J Pediatr Health Care 18:297–301, 2004.

Ozanne A, Marsot-Dupuch K, Ducreux D, Meyer B, Lasjaunias P. Acute epiglottitis: MRI. Neuroradiology. 46:153–155, 2004.

THE CHILD WHO WHEEZES

Outline

David K. Edwards, III, MD

CHAPTER 8

THE CHILD WHO WHEEZES

DEFINITION OF WHEEZING

Wheezing, like stridor, is an abnormal sound made in the process of breathing. Stridor is generally understood to mean noisy breathing that is audible to the unaided ear; wheezing, although it may be heard by the physician at a distance from the patient or by patients themselves, is usually considered to be a stethoscopic finding. In attempting to describe wheezing with more exactitude, one enters the confused and confusing realm of lung sound terminology, wherein rales, rhonchi, crepitations, and crackles abound amid a welter of colorful descriptive adjectives.[12] In an effort to bring sense to this welter, the American College of Chest Physicians and the American Thoracic Society suggested restricting the terms used to *rhonchus* and *rale* or, alternatively and synonymously, *wheeze* and *crackle*.[1] However, this advice has not been widely followed. In this chapter, the word *wheeze* is used in preference to *rhonchus*. A wheeze is a lung sound that has perceptible duration—that is, it is not one of the very brief sounds that in aggregate result in a crackle. Generally, wheezes are musical in character and are high pitched, with a dominant frequency of 400 Hz or more.[42] They are heard predominantly but not exclusively in expiration. The medical prototype of a wheeze is the sound produced by an asthmatic patient during an acute attack, and auscultation of such a patient is preferable to any amount of descriptive prose.

SIGNIFICANCE OF WHEEZING

Wheezing is an important symptom or finding because, like stridor, it reflects airway obstruction. The sound is produced by a turbulent flow of gas past one or many obstructions. Generally speaking, with wheezing, the sites of obstruction are more distal in the airway than those that produce stridor; the usual level is beyond the carina, somewhere between the main bronchi and the bronchioles.[59] Admitting that there are many exceptions, such as in severe asthma or infantile bronchiolitis, wheezing is of less immediate life-threatening importance than stridor. Furthermore, most causes of wheezing respond at least partially to medical (bronchodilator) therapy, so emergency measures to diagnose the exact nature of the obstruction are seldom necessary, permitting diagnosis to progress at a relatively methodical pace. It must be noted that the convenient separation of stridor and wheezing is much easier in a textbook than it is at the bedside. Lesions that "ought" to produce stridor (upper airway obstructions) may in fact exhibit wheezing as a prominent feature. Despite its relatively benign character, wheezing may reflect a wide variety of diseases in which an accurate diagnosis is imperative for providing appropriate treatment and maximizing patient prognosis. These diseases include chronic, inexorably fatal, diseases such as cystic fibrosis, acute viral infections and their sequelae, and one-time treatable conditions such as foreign body aspiration. Radiographic imaging often is only a small part of the diagnostic effort that may be required, but it is a very important part, particularly in the initial presentation of disease. The intent of this chapter is to expedite diagnosis by making radiographic evaluation of patients with wheezing as efficient and useful as possible.

The material in this chapter considerably overlaps in content with the material in Chapters 7 (The Child With Stridor) and 9 (The Child With Cough and Fever). This is because there is great intrinsic overlap in the diseases that produce stridor, cough and fever, and wheezing; the ironclad separation demanded by written description is not honored by a child with an intrathoracic disease. Ideally, for the thorough evaluation of such a child, all three chapters should be reviewed as a unit.

DIFFERENTIAL DIAGNOSIS OF WHEEZING IN CHILDHOOD

MAJOR CAUSES OF WHEEZING IN CHILDREN

Wheezing is a nonspecific finding. Indeed, it is difficult to imagine any significant intrathoracic disease that could never produce wheezing as a clinical manifestation. Fortunately the number of diseases in which wheezing is common or predominant is finite (Table 8–1).[26,57] One useful way of reducing this list to a more manageable size is considering whether the wheezing encountered in a particular patient is acute, chronic, or recurrent. For the most part, congenital and developmental lesions (e.g., familial diseases,

asthma, and cardiac conditions) produce chronic or recurrent wheezing. Acute, nonrecurring wheezing is more suggestive of infection, foreign body aspiration, and traumatic or allergic causes. Of course, all of the chronic causes have an initial manifestation, at which time the condition is, for all practical purposes, acute.

IMPORTANT CAUSES OF WHEEZING AT DIFFERENT AGES

As with virtually all pediatric symptoms, the patient's age is an extremely helpful clue in narrowing the list of diagnostic possibilities in wheezing (Table 8–2). In the immediate newborn period, the causes of wheezing are relatively limited. Strong consideration must be given to congenital abnormalities that impinge on the major airways; these are discussed in more detail in Chapter 7. The newborn aspiration syndromes, particularly meconium aspiration syndrome, as well as neonatal pneumonias and retained fetal lung fluid, can produce air trapping and wheezes. Consideration must also be given to severe morphologic abnormalities of the heart, particularly those that produce left-sided obstruction, such as the hypoplastic left heart variants and total anomalous pulmonary venous return with obstruction.

Although congenital causes remain important during the first year of life, pulmonary infections predominate, particularly viral infections and especially those caused by respiratory syncytial virus (RSV). So-called "cardiac asthma," which is usually secondary to acyanotic left-to-right shunts with pulmonary venous hypertension, commonly appears during the first year of life. Wheezing from chronic aspiration caused by gastroesophageal reflux is most frequent in children in this age group. Although asthma is commonly believed to be a disease of older children, a substantial number of children with asthma present during the first year of life.[37] Recurrent pneumonias in patients of this age group may lead to the diagnosis of cystic fibrosis or, much less commonly, one of the various immunodeficiency diseases.

Viral infections continue to be important causes of wheezing in children between the ages of 1 and 2 years, but the RSV is relatively less prevalent in this age group than in younger children.[6,27] This organism remains the most common cause of infectious wheezing during the first 5 years of life.[27] As children become independently mobile, foreign bodies are encountered and aspirated; this is the age group (1 to 2 years) in which foreign body aspiration most often occurs. Asthma, cystic fibrosis, and immunodeficiency states are commonly first diagnosed at this age. Gastroesophageal reflux and congenital causes of wheezing for the most part are diagnosed earlier, but some instances of these are still encountered in children 1 to 2 years old.

TABLE 8-1 Major Causes of Wheezing in Children

Congenital and Developmental Causes (see Chapter 7)

Upper airway
  Laryngomalacia
  Laryngeal web
  Chondromalacia
  Hemangioma
  Polyps
Tracheal and bronchial anomalies
  Tracheomalacia; tracheobronchomalacia
  Tracheal stenosis
  Tracheal web
  Tracheoesophageal fistula
  Laryngotracheoesophageal cleft
  Congenital lobar emphysema
  Bronchostenosis
Great vessel anomalies
  Vascular ring
  Pulmonary sling
Lung bud anomalies
  Cystic adenomatoid malformation
  Pulmonary sequestration
  Bronchogenic cyst

Familial Diseases (see Chapter 9)

Cystic fibrosis
Various immunodeficiency diseases
Alpha$_1$-antitrypsin deficiency
Immotile cilia syndrome
Bronchial cartilage deficiency (Williams-Campbell
  syndrome)

Infections (see Chapter 9)

Viral (bronchitis/bronchiolitis)
Mycoplasma infection
Bacterial pneumonia
Fungal infection
Tuberculosis
Parasitic disease
Bronchiolitis obliterans

Mechanical Obstruction

Intrinsic lesions
  Airway foreign body

Esophageal foreign body
Endobronchial tumor
Endobronchial granuloma
Mucous plug
Extrinsic lesions
  Tumors, cysts
  Enlarged lymph nodes
  Mediastinal mass (leukemia, lymphoma, thymoma,
    teratoma, etc.)
  Pneumothorax
  Pleural effusion

Traumatic

Chemical vapor and hydrocarbon inhalation
Smoke/fire-product inhalation
Near-drowning
Episodic aspiration (e.g., following seizure, surgery, etc.)
Bronchopulmonary dysplasia

Airway Hyperreactivity

Atopic asthma
Allergic reactions
  Foods
  Drugs (including radiographic contrast agents)
  Insect stings

Secondary to Other Diseases

Gastroesophageal reflux; achalasia
Obstructing gastrointestinal lesions that promote
  aspiration (e.g., esophageal stricture)
Choanal atresia, cleft palate, or disturbances of
  swallowing that may lead to aspiration
Cardiogenic diseases ("cardiac asthma")
  Ventricular septal defect
  Patent ductus arteriosus
  Cardiomyopathy
  Enlarged heart compressing bronchus
  Left ventricular failure from any cause
Pulmonary edema from any cause
Organophosphate poisoning

Asthma and foreign body aspiration dominate the causes of wheezing in children between the ages of 2 and 5 years. Viral infections, although still common in these children, have less significance than in younger age groups. A substantial number of cases of cystic fibrosis are diagnosed at this age; indeed, the clinical variability of cystic fibrosis is such that some cases are not diagnosed until adulthood.

In school-age children, chronic wheezing is most commonly caused by asthma. *Mycoplasma pneumoniae* pneumonia is the predominant infectious cause.[27] As children become increasingly independent, leaving home without direct supervision, various acute pulmonary insults that produce wheezing (e.g., near-drowning and hydrocarbon aspiration) are more frequently encountered.

TABLE 8-2 IMPORTANT CAUSES OF WHEEZING AT DIFFERENT AGES*

Immediate Newborn Period
Newborn aspiration syndromes
Congenital or perinatally acquired lung infections
Congenital and developmental causes
Severe cardiac malformations
First Year of Life
Viral infections (bronchitis/bronchiolitis)
    Respiratory syncytial virus
    Parainfluenza virus types 1 and 3
    Adenovirus
Left-to-right shunts ("cardiac asthma")
Gastroesophageal reflux
Congenital and developmental causes
Cystic fibrosis
1 to 2 Years
Viral infections
    Respiratory syncytial virus
    Adenovirus
    Parainfluenza virus types 1 and 3
    Influenza
Foreign body, airway or esophagus
Asthma
Cystic fibrosis
Gastroesophageal reflux
Nonviral lung infections

Congenital and developmental causes
Immunodeficiency diseases
"Cardiac asthma"
2 to 5 Years
Asthma
Foreign body, airway or esophagus
Viral infections
    Adenovirus
    Parainfluenza virus types 1 and 3
    Respiratory syncytial virus
    Influenza
Nonviral lung infections
Cystic fibrosis
Traumatic causes (hydrocarbon ingestion, etc.)
School Age
Mycoplasma pneumoniae pneumonia
Asthma
Allergic reactions
Cystic fibrosis
Traumatic causes
Viral infections
    Influenza
    Parainfluenza
Bronchiolitis obliterans
Mediastinal tumors, adenopathy

*Where categories of diseases are listed, such as "Congenital and developmental causes," refer to Table 8–1.

AUSCULTATORY ASPECTS OF WHEEZING FROM DIFFERENT CAUSES

Certain auscultatory features of wheezing may provide helpful diagnostic clues. For example, global wheezing that is heard equally over both sides of the thorax is suggestive of widespread airflow obstruction, such as that occurring in asthma. A fixed, monophonal wheeze of constant pitch that is heard asymmetrically is suggestive of partial occlusion of a major bronchus,[42] indicating an intrinsic or extrinsic bronchial lesion. A harsh or low-pitched wheezing sound should arouse suspicion of an obstruction of the trachea or major bronchus. In general, certain etiologies of wheezing are suggested by symmetric and diffuse wheezing, whereas other conditions tend to cause local or asymmetric findings (Table 8–3). Wheezing that is asymmetric, suggesting a focal lesion, is easier to diagnose than symmetric, global wheezing, because sometimes lesions that are unequivocally focal, such as an aspirated foreign body, may elicit widespread bronchospasm that may convincingly simulate asthma; indeed, such lesions respond at least partially to bronchodilators. Similarly, lesions of the upper airway that would be expected to produce stridor may instead produce wheezing. Sometimes this occurs because the transmitted quality of the stridor is sufficiently high pitched to simulate wheezing, but occasionally there is genuine bronchospasm as well. The reasons that such "false" wheezing occurs are complex and poorly understood, involving a wide variety of neural and hormonal factors that may affect the smooth muscle of the distal airways.[11] A description of the known details of these pathways is beyond the scope of this chapter; it is sufficient to note that sometimes a focal obstruction in a bronchus or even the upper airway can produce global bronchospasm and wheezing.

RADIOGRAPHIC EVALUATION OF WHEEZING

Radiographic evaluation plays a relatively small role in the diagnosis of many important conditions that cause wheezing. Asthma, for example, is diagnosed by clinical history, immunologic maneuvers, and airway challenges. Cystic fibrosis,

TABLE 8-3 DIFFERENTIAL DIAGNOSIS OF
WHEEZING BY AUSCULTATORY FINDINGS

Wheezing That Is Symmetric or Diffuse
Upper airway and tracheal causes
Vascular ring
Bronchogenic cyst
Familial diseases
Bronchitis/bronchiolitis
Esophageal foreign body
Mediastinal mass or enlarged nodes
Traumatic causes
Asthma
Allergic reactions
Gastroesophageal reflux
Ventricular septal defect, patent ductus arteriosus
Pulmonary edema
Organophosphate poisoning (occasionally, lesions listed
    below)
Wheezing That Is Asymmetric or Local
Congenital lobar emphysema
Bronchostenosis
Pulmonary sling
Cystic adenomatoid malformation
Pulmonary sequestration
Focal pneumonias and infections
Bronchiolitis obliterans
Airway foreign body
Endobronchial lesions; mucous plug
Tumors, cysts
Pneumothorax
Pleural effusion
Enlarged heart compressing the bronchus

which is often suggested by a history of recurrent pneumonias, is diagnosed by the sweat chloride test. Immunodeficiency states also are diagnosed and characterized by laboratory methods, whereas bronchitis is primarily diagnosed clinically. In all such conditions, radiographic techniques are ancillary at best and useful mostly for identifying complicating conditions. Even in conditions in which radiographic techniques have revealed a focal lesion, the final diagnosis is usually provided by the bronchoscopist and pathologist.

It remains true, especially considering the wide variety of conditions that can cause wheezing (see Table 8–1), that at least a plain chest film should be obtained when a child first presents with wheezing. The only exception might be a child with classic and mild bronchitis encountered in the setting of a family with viral respiratory infections. A chest film is absolutely mandatory when the clinician encounters wheezing

whose etiology is not obvious or that is asymmetric or focal, because the provoking lesions are frequently surgical rather than medical in nature (see Table 8–3). In this section, the radiographic modalities available for diagnosis in such settings are discussed; which modality is selected depends largely on the nature of the lesion that has most likely been encountered.

PLAIN CHEST RADIOGRAPHS

The basic radiographic study in the evaluation of wheezing is the plain chest film. This study forms the basis for all subsequent radiographic investigations and, to a large extent, determines which studies should be undertaken next. Subsequent studies are tailored in type and in location as a result of the findings on the plain chest film. The plain chest study is actually two films: a frontal and a lateral view; the study is incomplete in the absence of either of these. In extreme emergencies *only*, the frontal view alone may suffice (Fig. 8–1). In infants, young children, and older children who are too ill to stand, the frontal view is exposed anteroposterior with the patient lying in a supine position; the lateral view is taken in the same position, using a horizontal beam. The films are exposed during quiet breathing, *not* during crying; if at all possible, a crying child should be soothed or offered a pacifier. In children who are old enough and well enough to cooperate, the frontal view is exposed posteroanterior with the patient standing; the lateral view is also done standing, and both views are filmed with the child holding a full inspiration. For the lateral view, care must be taken to keep the child's arms well above the head so that they do not obscure the intrathoracic airway and the anterior superior mediastinum.

Details of plain chest film interpretation are given in Chapter 9.

EXPIRATORY RADIOGRAPHS

Expiratory radiographs are generally undesirable but may be extremely useful in identifying focal air trapping, most commonly in the setting of a possible endobronchial foreign body. An expiratory film is also useful in showing a small pneumothorax that is equivocal on a plain film. In older children who can cooperate, expiratory radiographs are exposed just as are plain chest films, except that the child holds a breath at full expiration. In infants and young children, bilateral decubitus views can be done; the dependent lung is taken to be expiratory.[14] This technique is suboptimal because it involves two exposures and does not clearly delineate a mediastinal shift; a better technique for obtaining full expiration on a single anteroposterior film is the assisted expiratory view (see Chapter 9).[77]

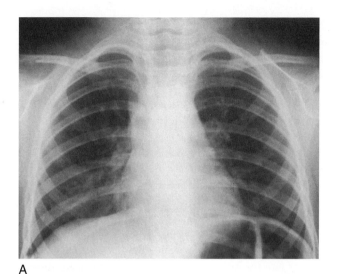

A

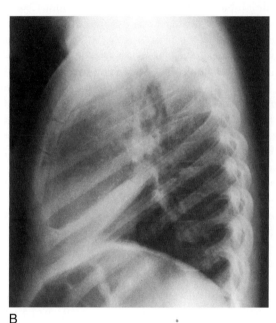

B

Figure 8–1
Radiographs demonstrating the utility of the lateral view. *A,* Frontal chest film of a 2-year-old child with wheezing showing only minimal obscuration of the right heart border. *B,* The accompanying lateral view adds considerable information, as it often does: the right middle lobe is completely collapsed.

DECUBITUS VIEWS

Decubitus views are exposed with the patient lying on the side, using a horizontal (or "lateral") beam. The side of the patient that is down (the side for which the view is named; e.g., a left lateral decubitus film is exposed with the patient lying on the left side) depends on the radiographic question being addressed. With a small or equivocal pleural effusion, the side in question is placed down. The decubitus view is also useful, especially in infants, in identifying small pneumothoraces; in this setting, the side in question is placed up,

so that the lung falls downward with the ectopic gas rising to outline the lung edge. In the setting of wheezing that may be secondary to an ill-defined pulmonary infiltrate, lung detail, especially in the retrocardiac area, which is difficult to see, may be enhanced using a decubitus view with the suspicious side uppermost.[21]

HIGH-KILOVOLTAGE RADIOGRAPHY

The usefulness of the technique of "washing out" the overlying shadows of bones from the airway shadows is discussed in Chapter 7. With this technique, lesions of the upper airway that may cause wheezing (see Table 8–1) are often revealed. Lower in the chest, the technique is helpful in delineating masses in and impinging on the larger bronchi, as well as for defining the presence and extent of bronchiectasis.

UPPER GASTROINTESTINAL SERIES

In wheezing of uncertain cause, the importance of the upper gastrointestinal series, especially the esophagram portion of the study, cannot be overemphasized. The most important lesions that may be revealed or elucidated are gastroesophageal reflux, tracheoesophageal fistula, obstructing gastrointestinal tract lesions contributing to reflux aspiration, vascular rings and slings, and occult foreign bodies impacted in the esophagus.[28,69] The last cause is of considerable importance because it is often overlooked, leading to substantial delays in diagnosis.[51,68]

Details of performing the upper gastrointestinal series are presented in Chapter 13. For virtually all examinations used in the evaluation of wheezing, barium is an adequate contrast material. Water-soluble ionic agents should be avoided because of their pulmonary toxicity if aspirated.

COMPUTED TOMOGRAPHY

Computed tomography (CT) can be extremely helpful in the further evaluation of masses seen on plain films, that is, masses that may be mediastinal or in the lung. Possibly a greater use for CT is in the evaluation of vascular malformations impinging on the airway.

IMPORTANT CONDITIONS CAUSING WHEEZING

Of the numerous causes of wheezing in children, the four selected for detailed discussion—endobronchial foreign body, cardiogenic wheezing, bronchitis/bronchiolitis, and asthma—were chosen because they are relatively common and serious. Cystic fibrosis, a very important disease that frequently presents with wheezing, is discussed in Chapter 9, as are familial causes of wheezing such as the immotile cilia syndrome and alpha$_1$-antitrypsin deficiency. Endobronchial foreign body is also discussed in Chapter 9, but from the somewhat different standpoint of recurrent pneumonia.

LOWER AIRWAY FOREIGN BODY ASPIRATION

Foreign body aspiration into the lower airway is a serious and occasionally lethal accident that may result in chronic symptoms and irreversible lung damage if not diagnosed and treated promptly.[20,39,40,48] Although in most children aspiration of foreign bodies is diagnosed correctly within a few days, an appreciable diagnostic delay of weeks to months occurs in as many as one third of patients.[4,9] One reason for this delay is that the child's parents do not seek medical attention immediately. This situation is particularly common when the aspiration is not witnessed or is uneventful enough that it is recalled only in retrospect. Another reason is that physicians often forget foreign body aspiration as a possible cause of wheezing and other respiratory symptoms; this "forgetfulness" is reversible with education.[58] With a high index of suspicion, most aspirated foreign bodies are gratifyingly easy to diagnose and treat. In Chapter 7, upper airway foreign bodies, supracarinal obstructions that generally produce stridor as a more striking finding than wheezing, are discussed. In Chapter 9, "missed" foreign bodies as an important cause of recurrent pneumonias are discussed. In this chapter, lower airway foreign bodies are considered from the standpoint of their major symptom: wheezing.

Pathogenetic Features

The epidemiology of foreign body aspiration is primarily age dependent and is discussed in Chapter 7. Essentially, foreign body aspiration occurs in young children who are becoming independently mobile, crawling and toddling about, and thus encountering objects that can be put in the mouth. The peak incidence occurs in children between 1 and 2 years old, with only about 10% of cases occurring in those younger than 1 year or older than 4 years.[9] Aspiration has a strong male preponderance.

The usual foreign material inhaled by children is food, most commonly a peanut.[9] Miscellaneous household objects and toys are much less frequently aspirated, although safety pins are commonly aspirated by infants. A tooth or tooth fragment may be aspirated as a result of an accident.

The most common site of lodgment is a main bronchus, right and left approximately equally, followed in frequency by the trachea, larynx, and a lobar bronchus. Occasionally multiple foreign bodies may be inhaled, but this is unusual.

Following lodgment, the foreign body itself acts as an irritating obstruction, producing reduced or obliterated gas flow and wheezing, which is caused partly by the obstruction itself and partly by neural reflex mechanisms that may result in widespread wheezing. The foreign body aspiration also evokes a local inflammatory response whose severity is determined by the object's composition; the most marked inflammation results from peanuts and other vegetable materials. Local swelling further impedes gas flow. Local hypoxemia produces local vasoconstriction in the portion of the lung distal to the foreign body. In most cases, at least during the first few days after foreign body aspiration, the tendency of the elastic airways to expand during inspiration permits gas to flow past the foreign body during the inspiratory phase of respiration but impedes flow during expiration. This results in air trapping (obstructive emphysema) distal to the foreign body. If the object is blown farther into the airway or if increasing local edema blocks passage, complete obstruction with distal atelectasis occurs; this takes place in one tenth to one fourth of patients. The completely obstructed portion becomes a nidus for pneumonia and, ultimately, bronchiectasis (Fig. 8–2). As an emphatic aside, mention must be made of a foreign body impacted in the esophagus. A radiolucent foreign body in this location can definitely cause wheezing,[51] presumably from aspiration pneumonitis, and may also become a very deceptive cause of recurrent pneumonias.[68] This is particularly true in infants and young children, whose diet of soft or liquid foods permits the respiratory symptoms to mask any associated dysphagia.

Clinical Features

Immediately following foreign body aspiration, there is a paroxysm of violent coughing, gasping, choking, and often vomiting. If this paroxysm is witnessed by parents—especially if an object that the child was holding is noted to be missing—it is of diagnostic benefit. Unfortunately, such episodes are often not observed or noted, and the immediate paroxysm very frequently and for no known reason (but presumably because of adaptation of sensory receptors) subsides to a relatively asymptomatic state. During this latent period, there may be chronic symptoms, primarily cough, episodic wheezing, and recurrent pneumonias. At physical examination, the findings in a child who has a foreign body in the lower airway vary with the duration of the condition; in the immediate hours following aspiration, there may be cough, wheezing, dyspnea, and cyanosis. The wheezing is usually, but not invariably, asymmetric or unilateral, often with localized rales or a region of decreased breath sounds.[9,41] Close examination may reveal unilateral thoracic overexpansion. A patient seen after the immediate postaspiration period may have signs and symptoms of acute pneumonia,

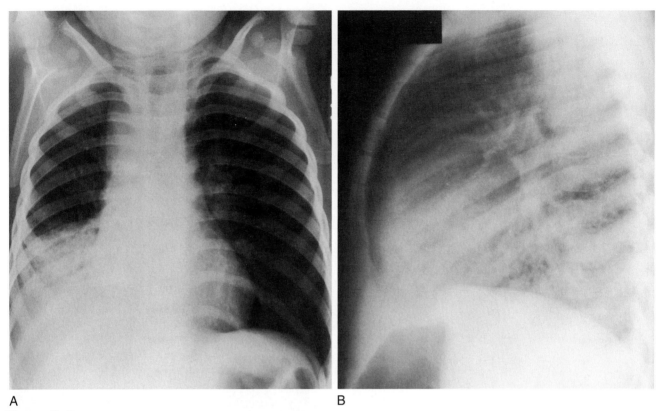

Figure 8–2
Chronically impacted foreign body in a 9-year-old boy who presented with recurring pneumonias. *A,* The right lower lobe is collapsed, with a mediastinal shift reflecting volume loss and ill-defined lucencies within the collapsed region. *B,* Lateral view showing the ill-defined lucencies to better advantage; these represented bronchiectasis distal to an impacted and forgotten peanut.

with cough and fever. Hemoptysis is not uncommon with foreign bodies that have become "chronic."[4]

Laboratory examination is seldom revealing. Of course, if the child has an acute pneumonia, then the leukocyte count will be elevated and blood cultures may be positive.

Radiographic Evaluation and Findings

The initial radiographic examination in the child with a suspected lower airway foreign body is a plain chest film, both frontal and lateral views. In a minority of the cases in which the foreign body is radiopaque, the radiologist's task is completed after informing the bronchoscopist about the bronchus of interest. Unfortunately, in most cases, the foreign body is radiotransparent. When a radiotransparent foreign body has caused complete obstruction, distal atelectasis or pneumonia is the result. These findings are indistinguishable from those of any other occluding bronchial lesion, such as a granuloma. In this setting, a high-kilovoltage view of the airway in the expected region of the obstruction may reveal the proximal part of the foreign body outlined by air. This indicates that the lesion clearly requires bronchoscopy. Often, the greatest service the radiologist may provide is

suggesting that a recalcitrant "pneumonia" is in fact a foreign body, a possibility that may not have been considered.[74]

The findings involving a radiotransparent foreign body that has not produced complete obstruction are variable. In as many as 16% of patients, the radiograph is normal.[9] In rare patients in whom several food particles have been aspirated, a multiplicity of tiny densities suggesting miliary disease may be seen.[32] More commonly noted is focal hyperlucency or evidence of focal hyperinflation (e.g., a shifted mediastinum or fissures or unilaterally wide intercostal spaces) (Fig. 8–3), but because radiographs are conventionally exposed during inspiration, such findings may be vague or almost imperceptible (Fig. 8–4). Sometimes focal hyperlucency may be overlooked and the secondary compressive changes that affect the rest of the lung may be misinterpreted as pneumonia (Fig. 8–5).

The most significant aspect of the radiographic diagnosis of partially obstructing foreign bodies is the expiratory view. With full expiration, the nonobstructed portions of the lung empty much of their contained air, causing them to have substantially increased radiodensity. The obstructed portion of the lung remains filled with gas and generally contrasts

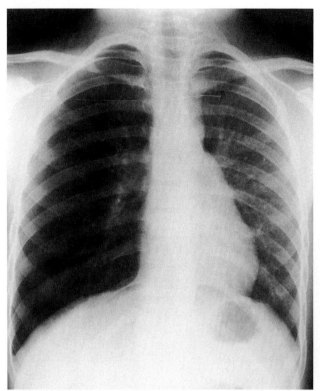

Figure 8–3
Hyperlucent right lung secondary to a foreign body (a piece of carrot) in the right main bronchus. There is mediastinal shift, as well as mild plethora of the left lung, possibly secondary to shunting of blood away from the hypoxic right lung.

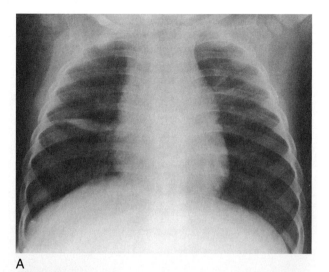

A

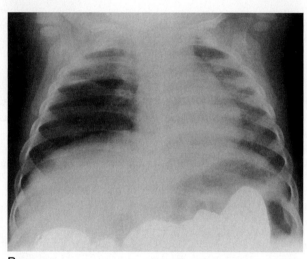

B

Figure 8–4
Radiographic view of an 18-month-old boy who presented with wheezing. He was treated for 6 days with bronchodilators, which resolved all of the wheezing except for faint, residual sounds on the right. *A,* The admission chest film reveals a patch of platelike atelectasis on the right. *B,* An assisted expiratory radiograph taken 6 days later showing a mediastinal shift to the left and virtually complete collapse of the lungs except for the right middle and lower lobes (the metallic density across the abdomen is the author's gloved fist). A piece of bean was removed from the bronchus intermedius.

markedly with the normal regions. The method by which an expiratory film is obtained depends largely on the age of the patient. In older, cooperative children, the expiratory film is exposed in exactly the same manner as the inspiratory film except that the child is asked to blow out all air and hold it for the exposure.

In infants and young children, obtaining an expiratory film is more challenging. Attempting to time the radiographic exposure to coincide with expiration is difficult and frustrating. A better technique is to obtain bilateral decubitus films of the chest, interpreting the dependent hemithorax as the expiratory examination.[14] However, this method has several disadvantages: it requires two separate radiographs, the degree of expiration on the dependent side is seldom profound, and the mediastinal shift is difficult to evaluate.

The best method of obtaining an expiratory view in an infant or young child is assisted expiratory chest radiography.[13,77] This is accomplished by immobilizing the child in a supine position for an anteroposterior chest radiograph and placing one gloved hand on the child's head (to prevent it from sliding off the table) and a gloved fist in the epigastrium. At the end of the child's ordinary expiration or cry, gentle but vigorous pressure should be applied cephalad and

inward to the epigastrium, forcing the diaphragm upward and providing near-maximum expiration. The film, exposed at the end of this maneuver, clearly reveals air trapping by the sharp contrast between the lucent, abnormal region and the opaque normal areas, as well as by a mediastinal shift away from the abnormal region (Figs. 8–6 and 8–7). No important complications have been described.

If assisted expiratory radiography is unrevealing, it is possible, although unlikely, that chest fluoroscopy may significantly aid in the diagnosis. Although fluoroscopy is widely touted to show a mediastinal shift and air trapping in this

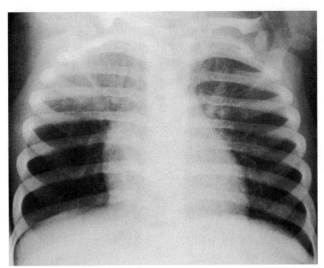

Figure 8–5
Foreign body in the bronchus intermedius. The hyperlucency at the right base was not recognized, and the initial diagnosis was right upper lobe pneumonia because of the increased density in this lobe from compressive atelectasis.

setting, it is a procedure that tends to become extended and radiation-laden if findings are not immediately apparent. This is especially true with younger patients, in whom the resting diaphragmatic excursion is low. When this is the case, provoking such patients to cry may facilitate observation.

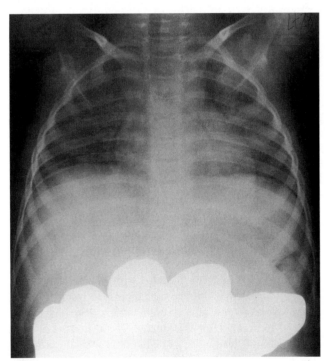

Figure 8–6
Normal assisted expiratory view. No focal air trapping (hyperlucency) is seen, the lungs are symmetrically collapsed, and the mediastinal structures remain midline.

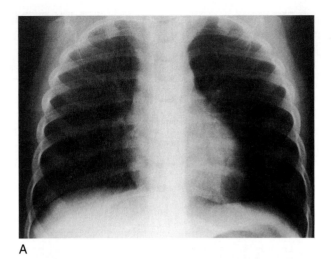

A

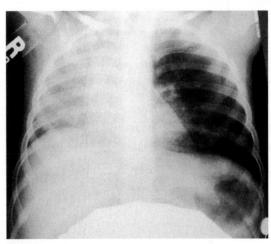

B

Figure 8–7
A foreign body in the left main bronchus. *A,* The plain frontal view of the chest is essentially normal; the faint hyperlucency of the left lung might easily be overlooked. *B,* An assisted expiratory view revealing air trapping in the left lung, with considerable mediastinal shift. An almond was recovered from the left main bronchus.

Although no study has been done in which chest fluoroscopy and assisted expiratory radiography are compared in the setting of foreign body aspiration, the latter is suggested to be the more preferable examination because of its simplicity, brevity, and clarity of results. Furthermore, the assisted expiratory examination can be successfully performed by a trained technologist, so the radiologist's presence is not mandatory.

Because regions of the lung that are distal to partially obstructing foreign bodies are relatively underperfused, radionuclide lung scanning has been proposed as an appropriate diagnostic technique. Such lesions can indeed be seen by lung scanning, but it has not been shown that this technique is more reliable or safer than adequate expiratory techniques. In an unusual patient whose history overwhelmingly suggests foreign body aspiration but whose other studies have been negative, a lung scan might be a sensible next step; for the most part, however, radionuclide lung scans have no significant role in the evaluation of a patient who has aspirated a foreign body.

At present, experience with CT remains too limited to assess its utility in diagnosing aspirated foreign bodies. CT offers a theoretical advantage in its ability to discern faint differences in radiodensity, thus possibly allowing a distinction between, for example, lung tissue and a peanut. However, most children with foreign body aspiration are so young that high-quality CT scans of the chest are difficult to obtain.

CARDIOGENIC WHEEZING

Although cardiogenic wheezing ("cardiac asthma") is a well-known entity, the significant cardiopulmonary disease that it reflects is frequently ignored in infants and children who have cardiac abnormalities. There is a tendency, which is easily understood, to treat children who present with wheezing, hyperinflation, atelectasis, and recurrent pneumonias as if they have primary pulmonary disease, when in fact the pulmonary symptoms are merely manifestations of the heart lesion. This distinction is important as it suggests a major difference in therapeutic approaches.

Pathogenesis

The simplistic way to understand the pathogenesis of cardiogenic wheezing is to recall that the thorax is a space with limited volume. The major components of this volume are gas, tissue, and fluid (mostly blood). A marked increase in the volume of any of these components occurs at the expense of the other components. Thus, the ectopic gas of a large pneumothorax may exert sufficient "tension" (i.e., positive intrapleural pressure) to impede venous filling of the heart ("air block"). Similarly, excessive blood in the lungs from a significant left-to-right shunt limits the volume of air space available for gas exchange, so pulmonary side effects should not be surprising findings. Pulmonary obstructive abnormalities do not accompany lesions that reduce pulmonary blood flow.[3]

Although this explanation may be useful, the actual abnormalities that produce cardiogenic wheezing are more complex. These abnormalities require much consideration to understand the pulmonary phenomena that occur in affected children. First, one should recall the anatomy of the heart, great vessels, and proximal airways. These lie in the center of the chest in close proximity to one another. Specifically, the left main bronchus lies just above the left atrium and the central pulmonary veins. Proximally, the left pulmonary artery lies just anterior to the left main bronchus and then swings downward behind the left upper lobe bronchus. The left main bronchus is thus effectively surrounded by the left pulmonary artery, the pulmonary

veins, and the left atrium.[15] The left lower lobe bronchus also lies in close proximity to the left atrium. Considering these relationships, it is understandable that left atrial enlargement or generalized cardiomegaly—the left atrium is the most posterior portion of the heart—tends to compromise the airways on the left, specifically the left lower lobe bronchus and the left main bronchus.

In infants and young children, the lesions most likely to cause left atrial enlargement are ventricular septal defect and patent ductus arteriosus; generalized cardiomegaly may result from any decompensated lesion, but of the possible lesions, cardiomyopathy seems most likely to compress the left-sided airways. In adults, similar airway compression can occur as a result of any condition that produces elevated left atrial pressure; mitral insufficiency is one of the more common conditions.[17]

The airway most sensitive to left atrial enlargement seems to be the left lower lobe bronchus; certainly, collapse of the left lower lobe is more commonly seen in this setting than is collapse of the entire left lung, although this occurs not infrequently. In infants and young children who have left lower lobe collapse from this cause, the atelectasis becomes increasingly difficult to reverse with increasing duration of collapse; bronchoscopy is generally futile, because the cause of obstruction is not endobronchial. The collapsed lung may become a nidus of infection, leading to recurrent pneumonias.

Other sites of purely mechanical compression of the airways are seen primarily in cases of fixed pulmonary arterial hypertension; these are the bronchus intermedius, from the enlarged right lower lobe artery just above it, and the trachea, from a distended left pulmonary artery that pushes the aorta against it.[17] These sites do not seem to be of much importance in infants and children.

Factors other than mechanical compression of the central airways are also involved in cardiogenic wheezing. The second most common area of cardiogenic atelectasis, after the left lower lobe bronchus, is the right upper lobe.[54] This location is difficult to understand, because the bronchus is not usually compressed by vascular structures. One possible explanation is redistribution of the arterial flow, with blood shunted away from the relatively hypoxic left lung and flowing preferentially to the right. The excessive flow to the right upper lobe may render it more vulnerable to airway narrowing.[54]

Diffuse hyperinflation, together with wheezing and other signs of obstructive lung disease, appears to result from left heart failure of any cause. Several mechanisms have been invoked to account for this, including an increase in peribronchial fluid, leading to increased resistance to gas flow in the small, soft airways of infants; edema of the bronchial wall itself, from increased systemic and pulmonary venous pressure; and reflex bronchoconstriction.[29] Of these, the first seems most plausible, but at present the question remains unanswered, and all three of these factors, as well as others, may be involved.

Another relevant mechanism in cardiogenic wheezing results from pulmonary compliance that is markedly diminished because of excessive blood in the lungs or, more likely, increased pulmonary artery pressure.[3] The diminished compliance demands considerable effort to move gas in and, especially, out of the lungs; the result of this is that intrapleural pressure is positive during expiration. This increased pressure leads to collapse of the pliable airways, a collapse that radiographically is most dramatically noted in the intrathoracic trachea.[15] The symptoms thus provoked suggest bronchiolitis.

The fact that all of these pulmonary abnormalities are a result of cardiac lesions is confirmed by autopsy evidence[17] and by the fact that the lungs become clear and symptoms resolve following corrective surgery.[29,54] Indeed, one reason recognition of cardiogenic wheezing is important is because it suggests the need for corrective surgery rather than for temporizing.[29] A second reason is that recognition of the lesion will ensure that efforts are directed toward improving the patient's cardiovascular status (i.e., through digitalis and diuretics) rather than toward managing an infectious process that often does not exist or is secondary to the heart abnormality.

Clinical Features

On unusual occasions, a child with congenital heart disease initially presents with wheezing and "bronchiolitis." In such a setting, the wheeze may mask the murmur, and the chest radiograph may provide the first clue to the true diagnosis. Much more commonly, cardiogenic wheezing appears in an infant or child who is known to have a cardiac lesion, most often ventricular septal defect, patent ductus arteriosus, or cardiomyopathy.

Compared with patients who have heart lesions without airway problems, patients who have heart lesions and cardiogenic wheezing tend to be younger at presentation and to have larger left-to-right shunts and higher pulmonary artery pressures.[53] When such patients present with signs of obstructive lung disease, they usually have congestive heart failure with tachypnea, tachycardia, and hepatomegaly; however, the pulmonary findings tend to dominate the clinical picture.[29] Wheezing is seen in virtually all such patients.

Laboratory evaluation generally reveals no evidence of infection except in those patients whose chronic atelectasis has led to pneumonitis, which may be recurrent or chronic.[54] Arterial blood gas analysis reveals hypercapnia in most patients.[29] The routine evaluation should include chest radiography as well as electrocardiography, echocardiography, and, if needed, cardiac catheterization.

Cardiogenic wheezing is a strong indication for prompt corrective surgery. Following successful surgery, the symptoms of airway disease disappear over a variable period of time, often quite rapidly.[29,53] If correction is delayed, the lung disease may become chronic and debilitating.[54]

Radiographic Findings

The basic form of radiographic evaluation in cardiogenic wheezing is the plain chest film. The essential finding is cardiovascular disease, specifically a left-to-right shunt or cardiomyopathy. Thus, expected findings include a variable degree of cardiomegaly, with engorged "shunt" vessels in the hilar and perihilar regions in patients with left-to-right shunt alone (Fig. 8–8). Patients who have cardiomyopathy exhibit cardiomegaly as the most notable feature, with varying degrees of vascular plethora. In common shunt lesions, the main pulmonary artery is often enlarged. In infants and young children, the "double density" of an enlarged left atrium is an unreliable sign that occurs in normal children; a more reliable sign of left atrial enlargement is elevation and posterior displacement of the left main bronchus. The two important shunt lesions that cause cardiogenic wheezing, ventricular septal defect (VSD) and patent ductus arteriosus (PDA), can frequently be distinguished on plain film by the fact that the aorta is enlarged in PDA but not in VSD.

Patients who have cardiogenic wheezing exhibit other abnormalities, superimposed on the findings of the underlying cardiac lesion, that are radiographic reflections of the lung disease perceived clinically. The most striking and consistent of these is overinflation, which may be quite marked. Overinflation is manifested by hemidiaphragms that project below the ninth posterior rib on the frontal view and by flat or inverted hemidiaphragms and increased upper chest dimension on the lateral view. Usually, the hyperinflation is diffuse, but in some instances, lobar emphysema can be seen.[29] Atelectasis, which may be subsegmental, bilateral, and scattered or focal, is also common. Focal collapse most commonly involves the left lower lobe (Fig. 8–9), but the right upper lobe and the entire left lung are also frequently involved.[54]

The entire picture, except for the abnormal cardiovascular structures, strongly suggests bronchitis/bronchiolitis. The clue to the correct diagnosis is the abnormal heart and vessels. Of course, such patients are not immune to pulmonary infections, and these may be superimposed; indeed, the abnormal pulmonary bed in this setting is prone to infection, and chronic foci of pneumonia and bronchiolitis have been observed at lung biopsy in patients who have diffuse lung abnormalities and cardiogenic wheezing.[54] Nonetheless, the fundamental lesion is cardiac, and primary attention should be so directed.

With correction of the heart lesion, radiographic clearing occurs. Normal inflation is seen in most patients after 1 month,[53] but full resolution of the radiographic abnormalities may require months to years. If subsequent wheezing or radiographic worsening occurs, either another lesion or imperfect repair should be suspected.

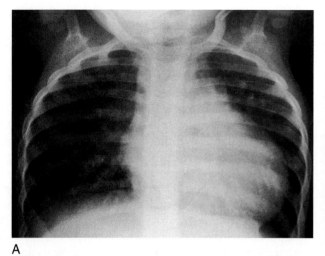

A

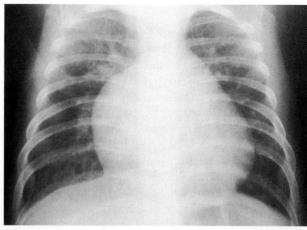

B

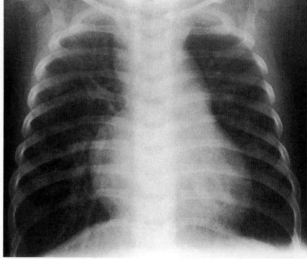

C

Figure 8–8
Three patients with cardiogenic wheezing. All show cardiomegaly, engorged central arteries ("shunt vessels"), and hyperexpansion. The patients whose radiographs are shown in *A* (patent ductus arteriosus) and *B* (endocardial cushion defect) were known to have cardiovascular disease when they presented with wheezing; nevertheless, the initial diagnosis was superimposed bronchiolitis. The patient whose radiograph is shown in *C* (ventricular septal defect) was not known to have cardiovascular disease before radiographic examination. Note the marked hyperinflation seen in this patient, who has low, flat hemidiaphragms.

BRONCHITIS/BRONCHIOLITIS

In the absence of a pathologic specimen, the clinical and radiographic distinction among bronchitis, bronchiolitis, and even viral pneumonia can be very difficult to make.[19,36,45] For the purpose of this discussion, this spectrum of pulmonary infections is referred to as *bronchiolitis*, recognizing that this is an imprecise abbreviation only; these related conditions have also been lumped together and referred to as *wheezing-associated respiratory infections*,[27] which is more correct but wordy.

Epidemiologic and Pathologic Features
The clinical syndrome of bronchiolitis is caused by viral infection, most commonly the RSV, although other viruses may also be responsible (see Table 8–2). It most often affects infants and children younger than 2 years of age. The viral infections that cause bronchiolitis tend to occur in well-defined epidemics with seasonal preponderance, a tendency

that can be very helpful diagnostically when a wheezing infant is encountered in a setting of viral illness in a community.[6,27]

In infants and young children, viral infections of the respiratory tract tend to affect the small airways. The clinical and radiographic manifestations of bronchiolitis have been explained by differences between the small airways of infants and those of adults.[71] Several factors seem to be involved. First, the small airways of infants are disproportionately narrow. Viral infections, which produce peribronchial cellular infiltration, edema, and spasm, as well as intraluminal sloughed cells and debris, are thus able to produce substantially more obstruction to gas flow than would occur with a similar infection in an adult.

Clinical Features
Elastic recoil, or the tendency of tissues to recover their shape after deformation, is relatively deficient in the airways of infants, which predisposes them to easy airway closure.

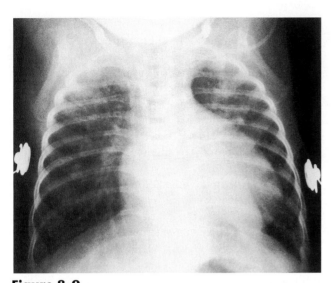

Figure 8–9
Chronic left lower lobe collapse secondary to cardiomegaly. The collapsed lobe is seen as a triangular area of increased radiodensity behind the heart. The patient has cardiomegaly secondary to cor pulmonale in bronchopulmonary dysplasia. The lung disease accounts for much of the hyperinflation seen.

Inflammation of these pliable airways thus leads to increased airway closure at higher lung volumes, producing a significant disturbance in gas exchange and obstruction that is greatest during expiration, that contributes to both air trapping and the expiratory character of the wheeze. In addition, the pores of Kohn and the canals of Lambert, both pathways of collateral gas flow, seem to be reduced in both size and number in infants. This feature, combined with the somewhat tenacious mucus in infants, tends to cause patches of atelectasis distal to the obstructed airways. These resultant twin tendencies, air trapping and focal lung collapse, produce considerable derangement in gas exchange. The ensuing respiratory distress may be compounded by the infant's relatively weak diaphragm and soft thoracic cage.[71]

Wheezing of infectious origin in older children is most commonly caused by *M. pneumoniae*, not by viruses.[27]

Although sporadic cases of bronchiolitis occur throughout the year, most cases appear during periodic epidemics in the colder months. Most patients who suffer from bronchiolitis are younger than 5 years of age, and the majority of these are younger than 2 years; the peak incidence occurs at age 6 months. As with most causes of wheezing, there is a slight male preponderance, both in the number of cases and in the severity of the illness.

The disease usually originates as a "cold," with rhinorrhea, cough, and low fever. After 1 to 3 days, tachypnea and expiratory wheezing appear. The wheezing is frequently loud and symmetric, and the degree of respiratory distress varies from mild to very severe. With severe airway obstruction, a reduction in wheezing is suggestive of almost complete absence of gas flow, a very serious sign. Substantial and intercostal

retractions are common in infants. Unless there is bacterial superinfection, the fever seldom exceeds 38°C.

In the immediate stages of the illness, laboratory studies are seldom helpful. With severe bronchiolitis, arterial blood gas analysis often reveals hypoxia and hypercarbia. The white blood cell count is usually modestly elevated and seldom helpful, although marked leukocytosis suggests concomitant or superimposed bacterial infection. Definitive diagnosis requires a positive viral culture from the nasopharynx or trachea; however, the delay required by viral cultures is such that their utility in a given patient is primarily academic.

Most patients improve over a period of 4 days to 1 week and are essentially well within 2 weeks. In as many as one in five infants, however, wheezing may persist for days or even weeks. Surprisingly, most such infants tolerate their extended course of respiratory symptoms quite well; these "happy wheezers" are active, with good appetites and normal development.[71]

It is likely that patients whose bronchiolitis becomes worse, generally in the second week of illness, with markedly increased symptoms and usually a high fever, have bacterial superinfection. This relatively unusual complication seems to be more common in children with marginal or poor nutritional status.[6] The possibility of superinfection with an antibiotic-resistant organism is one of the major reasons for avoiding hospitalization of children who have bronchiolitis, if this is possible.

Following an acute attack of bronchiolitis, most children remain symptom free. However, chronic sequelae to bronchiolitis are not uncommon; more than half of the survivors have airway hyperreactivity as measured by methacholine challenge,[25] and abnormal pulmonary function is noted years after infantile bronchiolitis.[70] Recurrent episodes of wheezing are also common.[70] It appears that bronchiolitis produces some degree of lung damage that is long-lived and possibly permanent in some patients; it has even been speculated that bronchiolitis predisposes patients to chronic obstructive pulmonary disease in adulthood.[25]

There may also be a predisposition to asthma caused by bronchiolitis, or, alternatively, children who have a genetic predisposition to asthma may be likely to develop bronchiolitis.[33] The relationship among bronchiolitis, allergy, and asthma is not clear, but it seems almost certain that a relationship does exist. It is plausible that the viral infection damages airway receptors, thereby producing hyperreactive airways; but it can be argued with equal plausibility that the airways were already hyperreactive. In any case, because attacks of genuine viral bronchiolitis are seldom recurrent, infants who have three or more attacks of "bronchiolitis" should be considered to have asthma.[71]

A more obvious sequela of bronchiolitis is bronchiolitis obliterans, leading to the unilateral hyperlucent lung syndrome, with recurrent pneumonias, dyspnea, exercise intolerance, and sometimes death. This condition is usually a result of adenovirus bronchiolitis and is most common in genetically susceptible populations such as Samoans and North American Indians.

Radiographic Evaluation and Findings

It may be argued that a mild and "classic" case of bronchiolitis that occurs in the clinical setting of a local epidemic does not require a radiographic examination. However, considering the wide variety of lesions that can cause wheezing, some of which may be unmasked by concurrent infection, elimination of this method of evaluation may be potentially hazardous. It is a sound and safe rule of thumb to obtain a plain chest radiograph with any first episode of wheezing, although this policy has been disputed.[23]

The plain chest film (anteroposterior and lateral views) constitutes the essential radiographic evaluation in bronchiolitis. The primary purpose of the film is to confirm that the infection is indeed bronchiolitis and not some other condition. Secondary purposes are to distinguish the unusual cases of bacterial pneumonia in which the patient presents with wheezing, to identify patients in whom bacterial superinfection has occurred, and to identify such distinctly unusual but occasional complications as pneumothorax.

The major radiographic differences between viral and bacterial lower respiratory infections are discussed in Chapter 9. The most important radiographic findings in bronchiolitis are hyperinflation along with streaks of abnormal density that represent areas of atelectasis. This paradoxic combination of overaeration with focal regions of underaeration is strongly suggestive of bronchiolitis and is nearly pathognomonic in the appropriate clinical setting.

Hyperinflation is manifested by an increased radiolucency of the lungs and downward displacement of the diaphragm (to the posterior ninth rib or lower), sometimes severe enough to reverse the normal upward bowing of the hemidiaphragms. Flattening of the hemidiaphragms is often best recognized on the lateral projection, as is an increased retrosternal clear space. The pulmonary vessels may appear normal or attenuated.

In patients with mild bronchiolitis, hyperinflation may be the only finding that is present (Fig. 8–10). Usually, however, streaky densities representing atelectasis are scattered about the lungs in nonsegmental distribution; sometimes these become coalescent enough to be suggestive of pneumonia (Fig. 8–11).[55] A film that is accidentally obtained in full expiration suggests that the patient does not have bronchiolitis, because full expiration is usually prevented by the associated air trapping of bronchiolitis.

On close inspection, bronchial wall thickening, producing perihilar linear streaks and ring shadows, is usually revealed. Overall, the lungs appear "dirty," with considerable abnormal high-frequency shadows that may represent small foci of atelectasis, peribronchial thickening, and combinations and summation shadows of these. The major abnormalities appear most markedly centrally and are interstitial, rather than having the alveolar pattern of most bacterial pneumonias (Fig. 8–12). Hilar adenopathy is distinctly uncommon, although the hila may appear somewhat bulky and indistinct

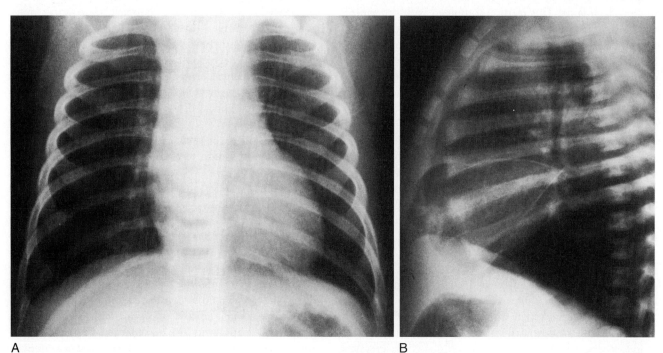

A   B

Figure 8–10
A and *B* show bronchiolitis in an infant whose only radiographic abnormality is hyperinflation.

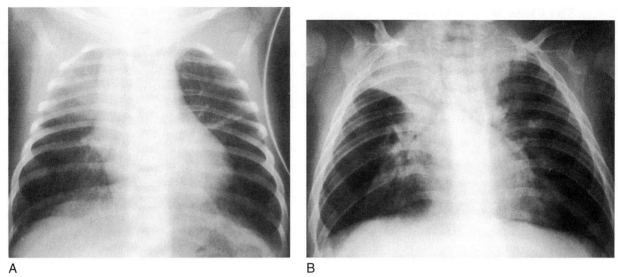

A   B

Figure 8–11
Severe bronchitis and bronchiolitis in two infants who have respiratory syncytial virus infection. *A,* Hyperinflation with scattered densities reflecting atelectasis; the beginning collapse of the right upper lobe misleadingly suggests pneumonia in that region. *B,* Another infant in whom there is complete right upper lobe collapse on a background of hyperinflation and scattered patches of atelectasis. Focal collapse suggests the possibility of bacterial infection, which neither of these patients had.

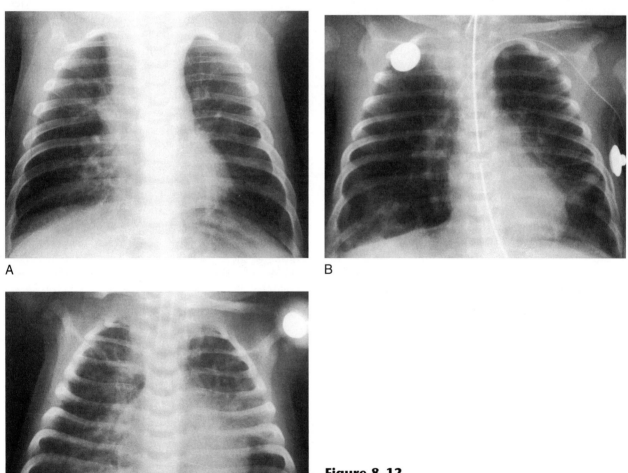

A   B

C

Figure 8–12
Spectrum of bronchitis and bronchiolitis. The patients whose radiographs are shown in *A* and *B* have typical findings of hyperinflation, with the somewhat paradoxical feature of scattered areas of atelectasis on a background of increased interstitial markings. *C,* A more severely affected infant with confluent densities that could represent bacterial bronchopneumonia but in fact were due to viral infection.

on the lateral view because of the central predominance of the abnormalities.[55] Pleural effusion is also unusual in bronchiolitis, and the observation of either adenopathy or effusion is suggestive of bacterial pneumonia, either as a primary process or as a superinfection.

For most patients with bronchiolitis, the initial chest radiograph is sufficient for radiographic evaluation; following the disease with serial chest films to document complete radiographic clearing, a process that often requires several weeks, is pointless in patients with uncomplicated disease. However, repeat radiographs are certainly indicated if the patient experiences unexplained clinical deterioration or if the initial findings are uncertain or equivocal. Repeat radiographs are also indicated in children with adenovirus infections, particularly those of susceptible races, to detect the possible appearance of bronchiolitis obliterans.

Asthma

Epidemiologic Features

The American Thoracic Society has defined asthma as "... a disease characterized by an increased responsiveness of the trachea and bronchi to various stimuli and manifested by a widespread narrowing of the airways that changes in severity either spontaneously or as a result of therapy."[2] This definition, although it is broad enough to be satisfactory, does not suggest the great heterogeneity of the disease. The "various stimuli" can be as disparate as lung infection, vigorous exercise, cold air, cigarette smoke, air pollutants, aspirin, and animal danders, to name a few of the more common provokers of asthma attacks. The severity of the disorder varies widely among patients, ranging from benign episodic wheezing in mildly affected patients to a serious, debilitating, and sometimes life-threatening respiratory handicap in severely affected patients. In addition, the severity of the disorder varies markedly within individual patients, with a notable tendency for largely unpredictable remissions and relapses, and a given patient may be sensitive to different provoking stimuli at different times in his life. Considering this great variability in the disease, it is understandable why the basic etiology of asthma remains a mystery, despite its prevalence (up to 18% of school children).[16]

Asthma is largely a disease of temperate climates and industrial nations.[66] There is a distinct male preponderance, both of asthma generally and especially of severe asthma.[78] The genetics of asthma are unclear, but genetic factors are certainly involved in the disease; the inheritance may be polygenic or multifactorial.[16,62] Genetic factors are most convincingly suggested by the tendency for cases to cluster in families and by the definite association of asthma with allergy. Families of those with asthma seem to have a general tendency toward developing atopic diseases, and atopic children have an increased likelihood of developing asthma;

for example, approximately 60% of the children who have atopic eczema develop either asthma or some other allergic state, and 5% to 10% of the children who have allergic rhinitis develop asthma.[38]

As noted in the previous section, the relationship among acute viral bronchiolitis, chronic bronchitis, and asthma is unclear; causal relationships may exist, but their exact nature is unknown. Certainly it is common for a child's first asthmatic attack to occur in the setting of infectious bronchiolitis. In the setting of acute wheezing, particularly in the first year of life, asthma and bronchiolitis can be extremely difficult to differentiate.[72] Certainly asthma may develop very early in life; more than half of the children who have asthma experience the onset of wheezing during the first 2 years of life, and 25% of these present before 1 year of age.[44] "Chronic bronchitis" in children, a common diagnosis, considerably overlaps with asthma pathophysiologically and in clinical manifestations and treatment, and, indeed, it may simply be a manifestation of asthma.[73]

Another condition with characteristics that considerably overlap those of asthma is gastroesophageal reflux. Indeed, it has been suggested that in some instances gastroesophageal reflux is a cause of asthma, particularly nocturnal asthma, which appears during sleep.[7] However, this has been disputed, and the association, if any, between the two conditions is unclear.[30] Neither wheezing as a result of low-grade aspiration pneumonias nor reflux in a patient whose intra-abdominal pressure is increased by the work of breathing is unexpected.

Cystic fibrosis and asthma share many common features, not least among which is an overlap in radiographic appearances (Fig. 8–13A and B). Several clinical manifestations are also common to both, including chronic airway disease, frequent nasal polyps, and increased viscosity of the respiratory mucus with mucous plugging. More than half of patients with cystic fibrosis also show increased airway reactivity.[47] Although these similarities do not imply anything about the etiology of either condition, they emphasize the necessity of excluding the diagnosis of cystic fibrosis in an asthmatic child.

Much emphasis has been placed on the emotional components of asthma, and it is well known that emotional stresses can trigger asthma attacks. However, asthma is not a psychosomatic disease. Asthmatic children have been shown to differ from unaffected children in temperament, but this is to be expected in those with a chronic and often debilitating disease.[34]

Pathogenetic Factors

Asthma is a chronic disease of the terminal airways. These airways, even in normal children, are reactive to exogenous stimuli; in asthma, the reactivity, which tends to close the airways, is exaggerated. Hence the concept of bronchial hyperreactivity, which is sometimes used as a synonym for asthma. With exposure to a wide and idiosyncratic variety of

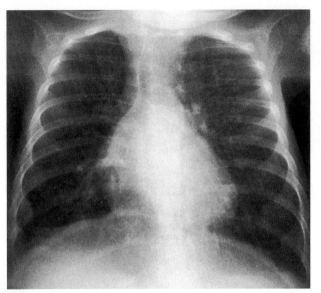
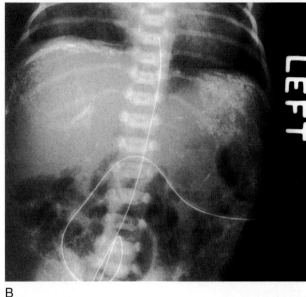

A   B

Figure 8–13
Cystic fibrosis. *A,* Radiograph of a 4-month-old child who was thought to have recurrent bronchiolitis and who showed persistent hyperinflation and increased interstitial markings on her chest films. *B,* Cystic fibrosis. Newborn infant with incidental finding of extensive calcification throughout the peritoneal cavity but more concentrated around the liver. Meconium peritonitis, unique to the newborn age group, is produced by antenatal perforation of the bowel with plaque formation. More than half of newborns with meconium peritonitis will have cystic fibrosis.

agents, the airways "hyperreact," bronchoconstriction occurs, and the small airways become sufficiently narrow to cause dyspnea and wheezing. The excessive contraction of airway smooth muscle may lead to muscular hyperplasia and hypertrophy, which may exacerbate the air trapping and produce chronic hyperinflation.

In addition to the mechanisms that involve smooth muscle hyperreactivity, the tracheobronchial mucus and mucociliary function are also involved in the pathogenesis of asthma.[76] In response to an offending agent, excessive mucus is secreted from hypertrophied mucous glands. The physical properties of the mucus may be abnormal, but this is uncertain. The respiratory epithelium of asthmatics also contains relatively few cilia. The excessive mucus, often mixed with cellular material, including eosinophils, is poorly cleared by the deficient cilia. The overall result of this is diminished air flow, increasing the air trapping caused by bronchospasm and, thus, clinical symptoms (Fig. 8–14).

Clinical Features

Patient age at onset of asthma is highly variable, with some patients presenting in the first months of life and others presenting well into adulthood. The majority of children who have severe asthma develop it early in life, most before the age of 3 years; children who have relatively mild asthma tend to develop it later.[44] The initial presentation is often in the setting of viral bronchiolitis; in asthmatic children, the disease generally clears slowly, and there may be repeated attacks. As previously noted, recurrent bronchiolitis, chronic bronchitis, and asthma are difficult to differentiate in young children.

Allergic factors may not be prominent in the first years of asthma but may become manifest as the disease progresses. The affected child frequently has a history of other manifestations of atopy, such as eczema or allergic rhinitis, and a family history of atopic disease is common.

The major symptoms of an acute asthmatic attack are cough, dyspnea, and wheezing.[50,52,60] Cough, which in asthmatics may be chronic, is frequently unrecognized as an important symptom of asthma; indeed, there is a subpopulation of asthmatic children in whom cough rather than wheezing so dominates the clinical picture that the correct diagnosis is delayed, sometimes for years.[35] The symptom most distressing to the patient is dyspnea, which is widely described as "tightness" of the chest or "like trying to breathe through a soda-straw." The dyspnea accounts for the marked anxiety children frequently exhibit during acute attacks.

On physical examination, the most notable finding is wheezing, which is generally symmetric and polyphonic and may be both inspiratory and expiratory, with the expiratory component being more prominent. The severity of wheezing varies from terminal expiratory wheezing, to entire expiratory wheezing, to inspiratory and expiratory wheezing heard without a stethoscope, and to absence of wheezing[5]; the last,

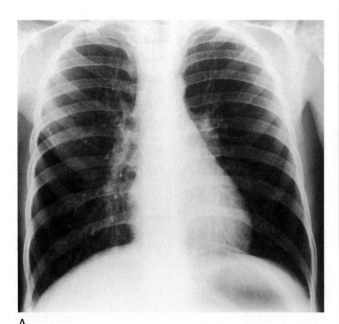

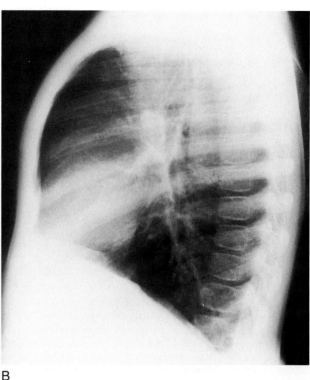

A   B

Figure 8–14
Asthma. *A,* Fairly typical findings in a 9-year-old child. There is slight overinflation and abnormal accentuation of the peribronchial markings. *B,* Lateral view showing hyperinflation with fairly flat hemidiaphragms and an increased anteroposterior diameter superiorly.

which implies that the airway obstruction is so severe that air velocity is too low to produce sounds, is very ominous and represents an unequivocal medical emergency. Other signs of respiratory distress, such as retractions, nasal flaring, and the use of accessory muscles of respiration, are variable. In very severe attacks, there may be circumoral cyanosis. Patients who have long-standing disease may have enlarged chests from chronic hyperinflation. The condition of status asthmaticus, in which the symptoms respond only poorly to medication, probably reflects widespread mucous plugging of the smaller airways; intensive therapy and hydration are required to loosen and clear them.

In the setting of an acute attack, laboratory examinations are seldom useful, although in very severe attacks arterial blood gas determinations may help to direct therapy. Clinical improvement following administration of epinephrine or a beta₂-agonist is expected with asthma but also occurs with most other causes of wheezing and thus, although suggestive, is diagnostically nonspecific. A delayed response to such agents may be seen when there is widespread mucous plugging of the airways. Other suggestive but nonspecific findings include blood or sputum eosinophilia, elevated immunoglobulin E (IgE) levels, and skin or airway hyperreactivity to various antigens. Nasal polyps and thickened sinus soft tissues ("allergic sinusitis") are also common findings in asthmatic patients.

There is no single test by which asthma can conclusively be identified; the diagnosis is made presumptively on the basis of a variety of studies. The clinical history of repeated, characteristic attacks is very suggestive. A negative sweat chloride test excludes the possibility of cystic fibrosis, and this important examination should not be overlooked in a child who wheezes. Pulmonary function testing is expected to reveal obstructive lung disease that is at least partly reversed by an adrenergic drug and that responds in a hyperreactive manner when a challenging agent such as methacholine or histamine is administered.

The natural history of childhood asthma can be extremely variable. Between acute attacks, the child is often completely asymptomatic, but abnormalities such as hyperinflation, leading to lung damage in the form of reduced elastic recoil that is chronic and may be permanent, may persist during such periods in as many as two thirds of the patients.[37] Asthmatic children are also relatively subject to recurrent pulmonary infections, which may cause wheezing in the absence of other provoking factors.[18]

There is a well-known tendency for asthma to improve during adolescence,[43] but despite this inclination, it is unwarranted to assure the parents of affected children that "they will grow out of it." Certain risk factors for disease that continues into adulthood are known, including severity of the asthma at onset,[8] bottle rather than breastfeeding, the presence of another atopic condition, atopy in a close relative, and nasal polyps.[38] Still, the prognosis in a given patient is difficult to assess. Overall, approximately half of patients who have childhood asthma are free of the disease as adults[8,38]; the remainder have continuing symptoms of varying frequency and severity.

Radiographic Evaluation and Findings

Typical Radiographic Findings Considering the wide variability of the severity of asthma in children, it is difficult to discuss the findings on a "typical" chest film because there is no such thing. In some patients who have mild to moderate asthma, the chest film is entirely normal between or even during attacks. Nevertheless, there exist certain radiographic findings that, when encountered, strongly suggest asthma.

The most common radiographic abnormality is bronchial wall thickening. This thickening is manifested in several ways. In its mildest form, there is an accentuation of lung markings centrally, so that the lung appears "busy" or "dirty." With more marked wall thickening or peribronchial thickening, abnormal parallel lines, which represent the walls of the proximal lobar or segmental bronchi, are visible; when seen on end, these form ring shadows (Fig. 8–14). Hyperinflation (or hyperaeration) is a less common finding. On the frontal view, the hemidiaphragms may be abnormally low, flat, or even inverted, with exposure of diaphragmatic muscular slips in the costophrenic angles. The lungs appear hyperlucent. The lateral view is more sensitive in detecting hyperinflation; with mild degrees of hyperinflation, the hemidiaphragms, particularly posteriorly, lose their normal cephalic doming and become flat (see Fig. 8–14B). The lateral view may also reveal excessive gas in the retrosternal and retrocardiac spaces. With chronic hyperinflation, bony changes, particularly sternal bowing and kyphosis, may occur, but these findings are relatively uncommon in childhood asthma. Radiographic microcardia is frequently seen when there is hyperinflation.

The hilar shadows are often disproportionately prominent in asthmatic patients; the reason for this is uncertain. No convincing evidence has been published that confirms that asthmatic children have pulmonary arterial hypertension, so it is doubtful that the prominent hila represent dilated arteries from this cause. Chronic, low-grade infection with secondary adenopathy may contribute to the finding.

It must be emphasized that these findings are not specific for asthma. Essentially identical findings may be seen in early or mild cystic fibrosis; indeed, there is considerable overlap between the radiographic findings in this condition and those in asthma. Similar findings may also be seen in acute viral infections of nonasthmatic children and in a number of chronic conditions such as immunodeficiency disease and gastroesophageal reflux.

The Radiograph in Acute Asthmatic Attacks In acute asthmatic attacks, the chest radiograph may reveal any of the several complications of asthma that are discussed in this section. More pertinent is the question of whether a chest radiograph should be obtained in the setting of an acute attack. Several studies have addressed this question, with the modestly surprising result that in this setting no chest radiograph is warranted.[23,24,61] It has been noted, for example, that the degree of hyperinflation seen on the film view has no relationship to the clinical severity of the asthmatic attack.[24] Furthermore, in a large series of patients, the chest radiograph did not provide information that led to changes in the treatment plan.[61] It seems that in known asthmatics, a chest radiograph is not routinely indicated in acute attacks.

A more difficult question is the role of chest radiography in a patient's *first* asthma attack. It seems prudent, considering that "all that wheezes is not asthma" (see Table 8–1), to examine a child radiographically at the first episode of wheezing, even if such examination is not necessary during subsequent attacks. However, this conclusion was not supported in a study of 371 children who were consecutively seen and evaluated at their first attack of asthma.[23] In this series, 94% of the children exhibited only the expected findings of asthma: hyperinflation, peribronchial thickening, and minimal subsegmental atelectasis. The remaining patients with "positive" films had pneumonia, segmental atelectasis, or pneumomediastinum, or combinations of these; furthermore, most of these patients were predicted to have complicated wheezing on clinical grounds alone (tachypnea, tachycardia, fever, and asymmetric breath sounds). No foreign bodies or cardiac lesions were encountered, and only patients who were older than 1 year were studied.

It remains to be seen whether these results will be confirmed by other investigators and whether such results are valid for children who are younger than 1 year of age. In the meantime, I (and this is a very personal, subjective "I") continue to recommend a chest radiograph at the first presentation of every child who is wheezing because of the seemingly substantial number of nonasthmatic wheezers I have encountered; however, time and subsequent studies may reveal this procedure to be unproductive.

Complications and Associations

Atelectasis and Pneumonia Areas of linear or platelike subsegmental atelectasis are very commonly seen in asthmatic patients, during both asymptomatic periods and acute attacks (Fig. 8–15). Segmental atelectasis is less commonly encountered. Atelectasis in this setting usually reflects mucous plugging of a bronchus. Sometimes it is difficult to distinguish atelectasis from the consolidation produced by pneumonia. However, distinguishing features include the following: atelectasis produces volume loss, reflected by a change in the position of fissures, the mediastinum, or the hemidiaphragms; atelectasis may be evanescent, appearing and disappearing from film to film; and

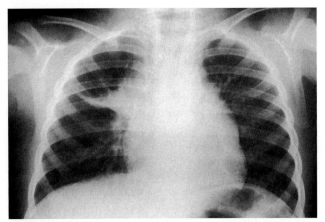

Figure 8–15
Asthma complicated by a mucous plug and distal atelectasis (right perihilar region). This appearance is difficult to distinguish from a bacterial pneumonia. In this infant, the radiographic findings promptly became normal following chest percussion and drainage.

atelectasis, unlike consolidation, rarely contains an air bronchogram.

Children who have asthma are prone to recurring pulmonary infections. Viral infections are generally manifested by an exaggeration of the features of the underlying asthma: increased hyperinflation, subsegmental or segmental atelectasis, and peribronchial thickening. Bacterial pneumonias resemble their counterparts in nonasthmatic children, although the infiltrates are superimposed on the underlying asthmatic abnormalities.

Pneumomediastinum Pneumomediastinum occasionally occurs in asthmatics, virtually always in the setting of an acute attack; pneumothorax is very rare. The radiographic findings are streaky, largely linear lucencies in and just adjacent to the shadows of the mediastinal structure, usually seen most clearly amid the vascular structures on the left (Fig. 8–16).

In older children, the gas frequently dissects into the neck and the soft tissues of the upper neck and occasionally down into the retroperitoneum. The ectopic gas seldom requires drainage but is significant because it may cause chest pain and increased anxiety. A finding that may occasionally be confused with a pneumomediastinum is an optical illusion called the *Mach effect,* in which the eye creates a spurious line of blackness between the light and dark shadows of the mediastinum and lung.

Mucous Plugs Mucoid impaction of a bronchus is a common phenomenon in asthma and is usually of note because of the distal atelectasis that it provokes. Mucous plugs can be the cause of considerable confusion on chest radiographs, especially in patients whose asthmatic history is unknown or has been overlooked. These plugs have several confusing aspects. First, they frequently result in distal atelectasis, suggesting infiltrate or more ominous causes of bronchial obstruction. When they move from place to place,

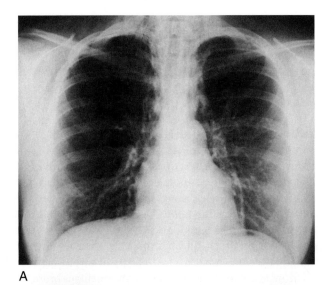

A

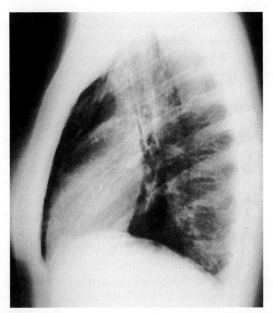

B

Figure 8–16
Asthma complicated by a pneumomediastinum. *A,* Frontal view revealing ectopic gas outlining the mediastinum and dissecting upward into the neck. *B,* Lateral view showing hyperlucency in the retrosternal area and an outlined thymus superiorly.

the fleeting areas of atelectasis may be suggestive of Loeffler's syndrome.[10,31] If the obstruction is partial, the distal overdistended area of the lung may be suggestive of a cyst, a foreign body, or an abscess. The plugs themselves may be visible as solitary pulmonary nodules mimicking cancer, tuberculosis, vascular malformations, round pneumonias, or other focal pulmonary lesions.[22,31] Mucous plugs have been the cause of unnecessary surgical resection in patients in whom the true diagnosis was not determined preoperatively.

When mucous plugs are suspected radiographically, vigorous medical therapy and chest physiotherapy may often dislodge the plugs; if these methods are unsuccessful, many plugs are within reach of a fiberoptic bronchoscope. Such plugs should be removed, because they may produce focal bronchiectasis at their site of impaction and because distal atelectasis (or hyperexpansion) may ultimately cause irreversible lung damage.

In a young child who has asthma, the finding of a mucous plug should raise the question of cystic fibrosis, a disease whose early manifestations may closely mimic those of asthma; mucous plugs that are radiographically apparent are much more common in cystic fibrosis than in asthma. This is important in terms of genetic counseling of the parents, as well as therapy and prognosis for the affected child. It is generally a good idea to keep in mind the possibility of cystic fibrosis in all children who have wheezing until a sweat chloride test has excluded the possibility of this diagnosis.

Allergic Bronchopulmonary Aspergillosis Allergic bronchopulmonary aspergillosis (ABPA) is being recognized with increased frequency in children. A history of asthma is present in almost all affected patients. The condition is an important one to diagnose because it is treatable; if left untreated, it may progress to severe, irreversible lung damage with bronchiectasis and pulmonary fibrosis. The diagnosis involves several criteria that are primarily immunologic but include radiographic findings; indeed, the chest radiograph often provides the first clue to the presence of the disease.[65] In children, the average age at diagnosis is about 15 years, but ABPA has also been reported in children as young as 6 years.[75]

Radiographically, ABPA is manifested by large, central mucous plugs that produce a tubular or branching "gloved fingers" appearance.[46] These plugs may cause distal atelectasis that is variably fleeting. The plugs, with their contained fungi, produce an important manifestation of ABPA, which is marked, central, cylindrical bronchiectasis with relative sparing of the peripheral airways. All of these manifestations tend to be more prominent in the upper lobe. It has been reported that bronchography shows the extent of the bronchiectasis and that this extent determines prognosis; however, in virtually all cases, this information should be obtainable with much more benign procedures such as high-kilovoltage radiography or tomography.

Upper Airway Abnormalities Nasal polyps are much more common in asthmatic than in nonasthmatic children; it is likely that they result from chronic allergic rhinitis. Their significance is not only that they produce additional airway obstruction, but also that they are associated with asthma that is relatively severe and has a poor long-term prognosis.[38]

It has been known for many years that there is an association between sinusitis and asthma, but the exact nature of this association remains uncertain. In some patients, surgical drainage or lavage of infected sinuses has ameliorated asthma, suggesting a causal relationship. Certainly, infected sinuses may be a cause of recurrent or chronic pneumonia, but opaque sinuses seen radiographically in asthmatic patients are not necessarily infected; "allergic sinusitis" with soft tissue thickening and mucous retention cysts is a well-known phenomenon that is possibly another manifestation of upper airway atopy. Radiographic investigation of asymptomatic sinuses of all patients who have asthma is not warranted.

SUMMARY

Wheezing is an abnormal lung sound that reflects airway obstruction, usually, but not invariably, of the smaller air passages. Wheezing as a symptom or finding considerably overlaps with stridor (Chapter 7) and cough with fever (Chapter 9). Airway obstructions at any site, including upper airway and unilateral bronchial obstructions, may provoke diffuse wheezing from neural reflex mechanisms, as can pneumonia. The causes of wheezing are numerous, but the most common are bronchiolitis in infants and asthma in older children. The differential diagnosis can be approached from the standpoint of the age of the patient, expecting entities such as congenital abnormalities and bronchiolitis in infants and asthma and *Mycoplasma* pneumonia in older children. Another approach is to determine whether the wheezing is acute (e.g., an aspirated foreign body) or chronic or recurrent (e.g., cystic fibrosis or asthma). Finally, causes of wheezing can be divided according to auscultatory characteristics: symmetric wheezing usually reflects a global or systemic problem, whereas asymmetric wheezing is more common with a focal obstruction.

In comparison with its role in many entities that are discussed in this text, radiography plays a relatively small role in the diagnosis of the causes of wheezing. The basic modality used is the plain chest radiograph (frontal and lateral views). Ancillary studies may be indicated by the clinical findings or by findings on the plain radiograph; the most important of such studies are expiratory radiographs, decubitus views, high-kilovoltage radiographs, and the upper gastrointestinal series. Radiographic techniques are generally more useful in patients with asymmetric wheezing, such as occurs with focal obstructions, than in those with symmetric wheezing, which usually results from systemic disease or infection.

There are five conditions in which wheezing is the major finding:

1. H-type gastroesophageal fistula, which can be surgically corrected (Fig. 8–17).
2. Foreign body aspiration, a condition that is readily amenable to treatment but is often overlooked as a cause of wheezing.
3. Cardiogenic wheezing, which is usually secondary to an acyanotic left-to-right shunt with heart failure. Such wheezing may incorrectly suggest lung infection,

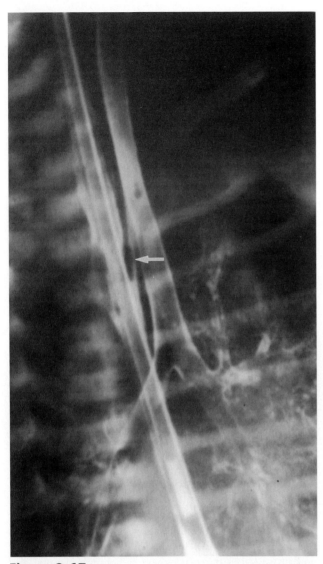

Figure 8–17
H-type gastroesophageal fistula. This malformation is an exceedingly rare cause of wheezing. Symptoms of choking and coughing are present at birth and mimic gastroesophageal reflux. Endoscopy or upper gastrointestinal examination is usually diagnostic. The *arrow* indicates the narrow connection between the trachea and the esophagus. There is a moderate amount of aspiration in the left upper lobe.

when in fact it is an indication for prompt medical therapy for heart failure, followed by corrective surgery, which halts the pulmonary manifestations.
4. Bronchitis/bronchiolitis, a viral infection of infants that is related in obscure ways to asthma.
5. Asthma, which is important for several reasons, not least of which is its large number of children affected.
Asthma and bronchitis, although they respond well to supportive care, are unlike aspirated foreign body and cardiogenic wheezing, because they have no specific cure;

however, bronchiolitis is generally self-limited, and asthma has an unpredictable tendency to remit.

REFERENCES

1. American College of Chest Physicians-American Thoracic Society. Pulmonary terms and symbols. Chest 67:583–593, 1975.
2. American Thoracic Society. Definitions and classifications of chronic bronchitis, asthma, and pulmonary emphysema. Am Rev Respir Dis 86:762, 1962.
3. Bancalari E, Jesse MJ, Gelband H, et al. Lung mechanics in congenital heart disease with increased and decreased pulmonary blood flow. J Pediatr 90:192–195, 1977.
4. Banks W, Potsic WP. Elusive unsuspected foreign bodies in the tracheobronchial tree. A nidus for infections that may be quiet for long periods of time. Clin Pediatr (Phila) 16:31–35, 1977.
5. Ben-Zvi Z, Lam C, Hoffman J, Teets-Grimm KC, Kattan M. An evaluation of the initial treatment of acute asthma. Pediatrics 70:348–353, 1982.
6. Berman S, Duenas A, Bedoya A, et al. Acute lower respiratory tract illnesses in Cali, Columbia: A two-year ambulatory study. Pediatrics 71:210–218, 1983.
7. Berquist WE, Rachelefsky GS, Kadden M, et al. Gastroesophageal reflux-associated recurrent pneumonia and chronic asthma in children. Pediatrics 68:29–35, 1981.
8. Blair H. Natural history of childhood asthma. 20-year follow-up. Arch Dis Child 52:613–619, 1977.
9. Blazer S, Naveh Y, Friedman A. Foreign body in the airway. A review of 200 cases. Am J Dis Child 134:68–71, 1980.
10. Blue JA. Rare complications of bronchial asthma. J Asthma Res 10:109–116, 1972.
11. Boushey HA, Holtzman MJ, Sheller JR, Nadel JA. Bronchial hyperreactivity. Am Rev Respir Dis 121:389–413, 1980.
12. Bunin NJ, Loudon RG. Lung sound terminology in case reports. Chest 76:690–692, 1979.
13. Caglayan S, Erkin S, Coteli I, Oniz H. Bronchial foreign body vs asthma. Chest 96:509–511, 1989.
14. Capitanio MA, Kirkpatrick JA. The lateral decubitus film. An aid in determining air-trapping in children. Radiology 103:460–462, 1972.
15. Cochran ST, Gyepes MT, Smith LE. Obstruction of the airways by the heart and pulmonary vessels in infants. Pediatr Radiol 6:81–87, 1977.
16. Cox DW, Talamo RC. Genetic aspects of pediatric lung disease. Pediatr Clin North Am 26:467–480, 1979.
17. Edwards JE, Burchell HB. Effects of pulmonary hypertension of (*sic*) the tracheobronchial tree. Dis Chest 38:272–284, 1960.
18. Eigen H, Laughlin JJ, Homrighausen J. Recurrent pneumonia in children and its relationship to bronchial hyperreactivity. Pediatrics 70:698–704, 1982.
19. Eisenklam EJ. Primary varicella pneumonia in a three-year-old-girl. J Pediatr 69:452–454, 1966.
20. Esclamado RM, Richardson MA. Laryngotracheal foreign bodies in children. A comparison with bronchial foreign bodies. Am J Dis Child 141:259–262, 1987.
21. Faerber EN, Darling DB, Leonidas JC. Diagnosis of ill-defined pulmonary infiltrates by lateral decubitus chest radiography. Pediatrics 71:192–195, 1983.
22. Fanburg BL, Kushner DC, Kim SH, et al. Clinicopathological exercise 49–1981. N Engl J Med 305:1398, 1981.
23. Gershel JC, Goldman HS, Stein REK, Shelov SP, Ziprkowski M. The usefulness of chest radiographs in first asthma attacks. N Engl J Med 309:336–339, 1983.
24. Gillies JD, Reed MH, Simons FER. Radiologic assessment of severity of acute asthma in children. J Can Assoc Radiol 31:45–47, 1980.

25. Gurwitz D, Mindorff C, Levison H. Increased incidence of bronchial reactivity in children with a history of bronchiolitis. J Pediatr 98:551–555, 1981.

26. Halken S, Host A, Husby S, Hansen LG, Osterballe O, Nyboe J. Recurrent wheezing in relation to environmental risk factors in infancy: A prospective study of 276 infants. Allergy 46:507–514, 1991.

27. Henderson FW, Clyde WA Jr, Collier AM, et al. The etiology and epidemiologic spectrum of bronchiolitis in pediatric practice. J Pediatr 95:183–190, 1979.

28. Heyman S. Esophageal scintigraphy (milk scans) in infants and children with gastroesophageal reflux. Radiology 144:891–893, 1982.

29. Hordof AJ, Mellins RB, Gersony WM, Steeg CN. Reversibility of chronic obstructive lung disease in infants following repair of ventricular septal defect. J Pediatr 90:187–191, 1977.

30. Hughes DM, Spier S, Rivlin J, et al. Gastroesophageal reflux during sleep in asthmatic patients. J Pediatr 102:666–672, 1983.

31. Irwin RS, Thomas HM III. Mucoid impaction of the bronchus. Diagnosis and treatment. Am Rev Respir Dis 108:955–959, 1973.

32. Kaplan SL, Gnepp DR, Katzenstein AL, Feigin RD. Miliary pulmonary nodules due to aspirated vegetable particles. J Pediatr 92:448–450, 1978.

33. Kattan M. Long-term sequelae of respiratory illness in infancy and childhood. Pediatr Clin North Am 26:525–535, 1979.

34. Kim SP, Ferrara A, Chess S. Temperament of asthmatic children. A preliminary study. J Pediatr 97:483–486, 1980.

35. Konig P. Hidden asthma in childhood. Am J Dis Child 135:1053–1055, 1981.

36. Korppi M, Leinonen M, Koskela M, Makela PH, Saikku P, Launiala K. Bacterial infection in under school age children with expiratory difficulty. Pediatr Pulmonol 10:254–259, 1991.

37. Kraemer R, Meister B, Schaad UB, Rossi E. Reversibility of lung function abnormalities in children with perennial asthma. J Pediatr 102:347–350, 1983.

38. Kuzemko JA. Natural history of childhood asthma. J Pediatr 97:886–892, 1980.

39. Leonidas JC, Stuber JL, Rudavsky AZ, Abramson AL. Radionuclide lung scanning in the diagnosis of endobronchial foreign bodies in children. J Pediatr 83:628–631, 1973.

40. Losek JD. Diagnostic difficulties of foreign body aspiration in children. Am J Emerg Med 8:348–350, 1990.

41. Majd NS, Mofenson HC, Greensher J. Lower airway foreign body aspiration in children. An analysis of 13 cases. Clin Pediatr (Phila) 16:13–16, 1977.

42. Mak H, Metz SJ, Stokes DC, Moser RL, Wang KP, Turner CS. Recurrent wheezing and massive atelectasis in an adolescent. J Pediatr 102:955–962, 1983.

43. Martin AJ, McLennan LA, Landau LI, Phelan PD. The natural history of childhood asthma to adult life. Br Med J 4:1397–1400, 1980.

44. McNicol KN, Williams HB. Spectrum of asthma in children. I. Clinical and physiological components. Br Med J 4:7–11, 1973.

45. Mertsola J, Ziegler T, Ruuskanen O, Vanto T, Koivikko A, Halonen P. Recurrent wheezy bronchitis and viral respiratory infections. Arch Dis Child 66(l):124–129, 1991.

46. Mintzer RA, Rogers LF, Kruglik GD, Rosenberg M, Neiman HL, Patterson R. The spectrum of radiologic findings in allergic bronchopulmonary aspergillosis. Radiology 127:301–307, 1978.

47. Mitchell I, Corey M, Woenne R, Krastins IR, Levison H. Bronchial hyperreactivity in cystic fibrosis and asthma. J Pediatr 93:744–748, 1978.

48. Mu L, He P, Sun D. Inhalation of foreign bodies in Chinese children: A review of 400 cases. Laryngoscope 101(6, Pt 1):657–660, 1991.

49. Murphy CM, Coonce SL, Simon PA. Treatment of asthma in children. Clin Pharm 10:685–703, 1991.

50. Muth D, Schafermeyer RW. All that wheezes. Pediatr Emerg Care 6:110–112, 1990.

51. Newman DE. The radiolucent esophageal foreign body: An often-forgotten cause of respiratory symptoms. J Pediatr 92:60–63, 1978.

52. O'Connell EJ, Rojas AR, Sachs MI. Cough-type asthma: A review. Ann Allergy 66:278–282, 285, 1991.

53. Oh KS, Park SC, Galvis AG, Young LW, Neches WH, Zuberbuhler JR. Pulmonary hyperinflation in ventricular septal defect. J Thorac Cardiovasc Surg 76:706–709, 1978.

54. Oh KS, Bowen A, Park SC, Galvis AG, Young LW: Patent ductus arteriosus: Its occurrence with unequal pulmonary vascularity and hyperlucent left lung. Am J Dis Child 135:637–639, 1981.

55. Osborne D. Radiologic appearance of viral disease of the lower respiratory tract in infants and children. AJR Am J Roentgenol 130:29–33, 1978.

56. Penketh AR, Wise A, Mearns MB, Hodson ME, Batten JC. Cystic fibrosis in adolescents and adults. Thorax 41:526–532, 1987.

57. Poole SR, Mauro RD, Fan LL, Brooks J. The child with simultaneous stridor and wheezing. Pediatr Emerg Care 6:33–37, 1990.

58. Puterman M, Gorodischer R, Leiberman A. Tracheobronchial foreign bodies: The impact of a postgraduate educational program on diagnosis, morbidity, and treatment. Pediatrics 70:96–98, 1982.

59. Rheuban KS, Ayres N, Still JG, et al. Pulmonary artery sling: A new diagnostic tool and clinical review. Pediatrics 69:472–475, 1982.

60. Ros SP. Emergency management of childhood bronchial asthma: A multicenter survey. Ann Allergy 66:231–234, 1991.

61. Rushton AR. The role of the chest radiograph in the management of childhood asthma. Clin Pediatr 21:325–328, 1982.

62. Schatz M, Zeiger RS, Hoffman CP, Saun ders BS, Harden FM, Forsythe AB. Increased transient tachypnea of the newborn in infants of asthmatic mothers. Am J Dis Child 145:156–158, 1991.

63. Schreier L, Cutler RM, Saigal V. Vomiting as a dominant symptom of asthma. Ann Allergy 58:118–120, 1987.

64. Schroeckenstein DC, Busse WW. Viral "bronchitis" in childhood: Relationship to asthma and obstructive lung disease. Semin Respir Infect 3:40–48, 1988.

65. Schuyler MR. Allergic bronchopulmonary aspergillosis. Clin Chest Med 4:15–22, 1983.

66. Sennhauser FH, Guntert BJ. Prevalence of bronchial asthma in childhood in Switzerland: Significance of symptoms and diagnosis. Schweiz Med Wochenschr 122:189–193, 1992.

67. Slovis TL. Noninvasive evaluation of the pediatric airway: A recent advance. Pediatrics 59:872–880, 1977.

68. Smith PC, Swischuk LE, Fagan CJ. An elusive and often unsuspected cause of stridor or pneumonia (the esophageal foreign body). Am J Roentgenol Radium Ther Nucl Med 122:80–89, 1974.

69. Sterling CE, Jolley SG, Besser AS, Matteson KM. Nursing responsibility in the diagnosis, care, and treatment of the child with gastroesophageal reflux. J Pediatr Nurs 6:435–441, 1991.

70. Stokes GM, Milner AD, Hodges IGC, Groggins RC. Lung function abnormalities after acute bronchiolitis. J Pediatr 98:871–874, 1981.

71. Tabachnik E, Levison H. Infantile bronchial asthma. J Allergy Clin Immunol 67:339–347, 1981.

72. Tal A, Bavilski C, Yohai D, Bearmen JE, Gorodischer R, Moses SW. Dexamethasone and salbutamol in the treatment of acute wheezing in infants. Pediatrics 71:13–18, 1983.

73. Taussig LM, Smith SM, Blumenfeld R. Chronic bronchitis in childhood: What is it? Pediatrics 67:1–5, 1981.

74. Vane DW, Pritchard J, Colville CW, West KW, Eigen H, Grosfeld JL. Bronchoscopy for aspirated foreign bodies in children. Experience in 131 cases. Arch Surg 123:885–888, 1988.

75. Wang JLF, Patterson R, Mintzer R, Roberts M, Rosenberg M. Allergic bronchopulmonary aspergillosis in pediatric practice. J Pediatr 94:376–381, 1979.

76. Wanner A. Tracheobronchial mucus: Abnormalities related to asthma and its treatment. J Asthma 18:27–29, 1981.

77. Wesenberg RL, Blumhagen JD. Assisted expiratory chest radiography: An effective technique for the diagnosis of foreign-body aspiration. Radiology 130:538–539, 1979.

78. Williams HE, McNicol KN. The spectrum of asthma in children. Pediatr Clin North Am 22:43–52, 1975.

ADDITIONAL READING

Amirav I, Balanov I, Gorenberg M, Luder AS, Newhouse MT, Groshar D. Beta-agonist aerosol distribution in respiratory syncytial virus bronchiolitis in infants. J Nucl Med. 43:487–491, 2002.

Guill MF. Asthma update: Clinical aspects and management. Pediatr Rev 25:335–344, 2004.

Krost WS. Pediatric pulmonary emergencies. Emerg Med Serv 33:71–77, 2004.

Piippo-Savolainen E, Remes S, Kannisto S, Korhonen K, Korppi M. Asthma and lung function 20 years after wheezing in infancy: Results from a prospective follow-up study. Arch Pediatr Adolesc Med 158:1070–1076, 2004.

Sahni JK, Mathur NN, Kansal Y, Rana I. Bronchial foreign body presenting as an accidental radiological finding. Int J Pediatr Otorhinolaryngol 64:229–232, 2002.

Smart BA, Slavin RG. Rhinosinusitis and pediatric asthma. Immunol Allergy Clin North Am 25:67–82, 2005.

Tsai S, Crain EF, Silver EJ. What can we learn from chest radiographs in hypoxemic asthmatics? Pediatr Radiol 32:498–504, 2002.

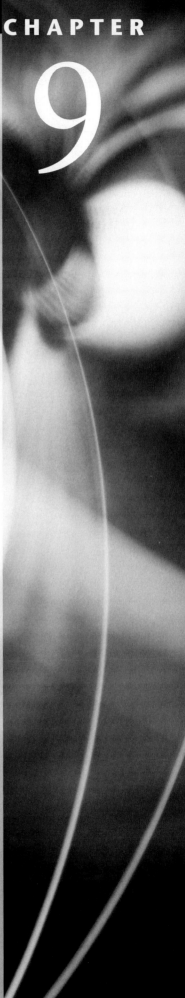

THE CHILD WITH COUGH AND FEVER

Outline

CHAPTER

9

Richard L. Wesenberg, MD,
Maria S. Figarola, MD, and
Benjamin Estrada, MD

THE CHILD WITH COUGH AND FEVER

Cough and fever are two of the most common symptoms of illness in the pediatric age group and suggest respiratory pathogenesis, particularly pneumonia. A rational approach to the evaluation of pneumonias requires good communication between the pediatrician and the radiologist.

The most important function of the chest film is that it enables the radiologist to determine whether pneumonia or other pulmonary disease is present. This fundamental decision requires technically excellent films. The chest radiograph has a high sensitivity for detecting pneumonia, but only mediocre specificity for determining etiology.[30,31,54,66,91] Radiographic findings in combination with clinical evaluation are vital in deciding whether treatment with antibiotics or further studies are indicated.

If false-negative radiographic results are obtained, there is the possibility of missed, and therefore potentially progressive, pulmonary disease.[22,58] A false-positive interpretation may result in unwarranted or inappropriate antibiotic therapy. The primary physician may believe the cause of the fever has been determined. This may result in a delay in, or may even prevent, a search for infection in other sites that may be the actual source of the fever. The important causes of false-positive evaluations are discussed later in this chapter.

The character of the pneumonia that is revealed radiographically, in combination with the clinical pattern of the disease, assists the physician in deciding whether antibiotics are indicated. In addition, the radiographic character of the pneumonia is often useful in determining the type of responsible organism, which aids in the immediate management, including correct selection of antibiotics until culture results are available. For example, a bilateral, perihilar infiltrate is consistent with viral pneumonia. This finding, in combination with an appropriate clinical setting, suggests withholding antibiotics and treating symptomatically until the results of laboratory studies are obtained.

Despite numerous advances in pediatric care and imaging modalities, the plain chest radiograph remains the most valuable tool available for evaluating the airway and the lungs and for assessing the site and gross character of pulmonary disease. In the following sections, the symptoms of cough and fever are discussed primarily from an etiologic standpoint. Etiologic findings direct the course of therapy, but the fundamental orientation is radiographic, founded primarily on the plain chest radiograph and the pathologic abnormalities revealed.

DIFFERENTIAL DIAGNOSIS OF COUGH AND FEVER

In considering the multiple entities that cause cough and fever in the pediatric age group, two approaches to differential diagnosis are available. The first is based on the clinical character of the symptoms, specifically acute illness versus illness that is chronic or recurrent. The second approach is based on the age of the patient, because there are distinct age predilections of agents that cause cough and fever in children. These approaches are not only equally valid but also complementary and mutually instructive. Both are discussed in this chapter.

DIFFERENTIAL DIAGNOSIS ACCORDING TO CLINICAL CHARACTER OF ILLNESS

Acute Pneumonias

The three main causes of acute community-acquired pneumonias (CAPs) in pediatric patients are (1) viral, (2) atypical, and (3) bacterial.

The most common cause of cough and fever in the pediatric age group is viral infection. Cough and fever are generally acute and self-limited, may or may not be responsive

to specific therapy, and require a minimum of radiographic examination and laboratory investigation.

As a group, viruses account for approximately 65% of all pneumonias that occur in pediatric patients.[49] Of the viral agents, respiratory syncytial virus (RSV) is the responsible organism in approximately 50% of cases. Metapneumovirus, a recently recognized virus, accounts for approximately 10% to 20% of cases, particularly in infants.[18,19,33,70,96] The exact incidence is, as yet, unknown.[19] Parainfluenza virus types 1, 2, and 3 are causal in 25% of cases.[53] The relative incidence of the different etiologic agents varies significantly according to the age of the patient. The respiratory viruses as a group account for approximately 90% of the agents recovered from children younger than 4 years of age.

The most common specific agent that produces demonstrable pneumonia in the pediatric age group is a bacterium, *Mycoplasma pneumoniae*, formerly classified as a near-virus, which causes approximately 30% of all childhood pneumonias.[5,32,36,49] *M. pneumoniae* infection is most prevalent in school-age children. It is one of the main causes of atypical pneumonia.[6,13,84,92] In children who are younger than 5 years of age, the incidence of *Mycoplasma* pneumonitis drops to 20%, and in children who are younger than 4 years of age, the incidence drops to approximately 5%.

Another recently classified bacterium, *Chlamydia pneumoniae*, is increasingly being recognized as a pathogen in school-age children. *C. pneumoniae* causes an atypical pneumonia virtually indistinguishable from that caused by *Mycoplasma*. Clinically, sore throat and hoarseness are more common with *C. pneumoniae*.[12,23,34,40,57] *C. pneumoniae* has risen in importance as a common pathogen in school-age children to be second only to *Mycoplasma* (15%).

The epidemic and seasonal occurrence of pneumonias and lower respiratory tract infections in children is a well-known phenomenon. In preschool children, RSV and metapneumovirus are responsible for yearly outbreaks of pneumonia during the winter and early spring. Influenza A viral epidemics often occur concomitantly with RSV epidemics.[82] Parainfluenza virus types 1 and 3 sporadically induce epidemics that are usually temporally separated by at least 1 month from the predictable annual occurrence of RSV epidemics.

The pattern of epidemic occurrence for school-age children (4 to 18 years) is distinctly different from that for preschool children. In school-age children, epidemics are relatively less marked, primarily because the *Mycoplasma* infections common in this age group are endemic. Most (approximately 75%) *Mycoplasma* pneumonias occur from September to January.[46,49,51,82,83]

Other bacterial agents are much less common causes of cough and fever in children, probably representing fewer than 5% of the total. It is important to establish the etiologic agent, however, because specific antimicrobial agents exist. The most common cause of other bacterial pneumonia in the pediatric age group is *Streptococcus pneumoniae.*[27,43,87,89,90] In addition, there has been a recent increase in the prevalence of pneumonias caused by community-acquired methicillin-resistant *Staphylococcus aureus* (MRSA).[69,72] Less common causative bacteria are *Streptococcus pyogenes, Klebsiella* species, and gram-negative organisms.[24,99]

DIFFERENTIAL DIAGNOSIS ACCORDING TO AGE

Infants (1 Month to 1 Year)

The primary type of infantile pneumonia is viral (Table 9–1).[87] RSV is the most common cause of these pneumonias, accounting for approximately 33% of cases.[22,58] This organism not only produces pneumonias in infants, but it is also the single most important cause of bronchiolitis in this age group. Metapneumovirus is another common cause of infantile pneumonia and bronchiolitis.[19] As a group, influenza virus types A and B and parainfluenza virus types

---

TABLE 9-1 CAUSES OF PNEUMONIAS IN INFANTS (1 MONTH TO 1 YEAR)

Acute Pneumonias
Common
Viral
    Respiratory syncytial virus (26%)
    Metapneumovirus (in 25%)
    Influenza A and B (20%)
    Parainfluenza types 1 and 3 (20%)
    Adenovirus (15%)
Atypical pneumonia
    Chlamydia trachomatis
Bacterial
    Streptococcus pneumoniae (pneumococcus)
    Streptococcus pyogenes (group A and group B)
    Staphylococcus aureus
Acute aspiration pneumonias
    Aspiration of formula, milk, or gastric contents
        because of gastroesophageal reflux, gastrointestinal
        dysfunction, or obstruction
Chronic or Recurrent Pneumonias
Common
Aspiration pneumonia
Cystic fibrosis
Uncommon
Immotile cilia syndrome, congenital pulmonary
    abnormalities, Heiner's syndrome, primary tuberculosis
    (TB), syphilis, fungal disease, foreign body aspiration,
    immunodeficiency states, chronic interstitial
    pneumonia, cat-scratch fever

---

1 and 3 are the next most common viruses causing infantile pneumonia and tend to occur in well-defined epidemics. Together all these viruses account for at least 80% of pneumonias in infants.

Adenovirus infection accounts for approximately 20% of infections in infants, causing a high incidence of chronic pulmonary sequelae: bronchiectasis, Swyer-James syndrome (bronchiolitis obliterans), and recurrent pneumonias, particularly in genetically susceptible populations (e.g., Native Americans).[35,77]

Chlamydia trachomatis pneumonia tends to become symptomatic when the infant is between 2 and 12 weeks of age and is commonly accompanied by conjunctivitis, a whooping cough, and eosinophilia, frequently without fever.[12]

Superimposed bacterial infection may complicate any of the previously mentioned viral agents, usually during the second week of illness. Responsible bacteria are usually gram-positive cocci such as *S. pneumoniae, S. pyogenes,* and *S. aureus.*

Young Children (1 to 5 Years)

The primary causes of pneumonias in young children are listed in Table 9–2. As in infants, viruses predominate. RSV causes 50% of the pneumonias in children between the ages of 1 and 3 years and 25% of those in children between the ages of 3 and 5 years.[87] Metapneumovirus is the next most likely etiologic agent, with clinical findings virtually identical to those with RSV. Parainfluenza virus types 1 and 3 cause 28% of the pneumonias in children between the ages of 1 and 5 years. *Mycoplasma* causes approximately 10% of pneumonias in this age group. Any of the viral infections can be complicated by bacterial superinfections (5%), the most common of which are caused by *Streptococcus* species.[24,78,99]

Older Children (5 to 18 Years)

Table 9–3 lists the common causes of pneumonias in older children. The most important of these, *C. pneumoniae* (28%) and *Mycoplasma pneumoniae* (27%), account for the majority of pneumonias in this age group.[7,23,36,47] This large number has important implications because *Mycoplasma* and *Chlamydia* respond to macrolide therapy. Parainfluenza virus types 1 and 3 account for only approximately 10% of all infections in older children, with RSV, metapneumovirus, and adenovirus together accounting for less than 10%.

Bacterial superinfection in *Mycoplasma* pneumonia or *Chlamydia* infection is unusual. Of course, older children may acquire acute bacterial infections, usually with common organisms (*S. pneumoniae* and *S. pyogenes*). *Staphylococcus* is unusual, but its MRSA form is increasing as a cause of CAP. Gram-negative bacilli are rarely encountered in this age group.

Chronic and recurrent pneumonias in older children seldom manifest as diagnostic problems, because most causes have been identified earlier in life.

TABLE 9-2 CAUSES OF PNEUMONIAS IN YOUNG CHILDREN (1 TO 5 YEARS)

Acute Pneumonias
Common
Viral
  Respiratory syncytial virus
  Metapneumovirus
  Parainfluenza types 1 and 3
  Influenza A and B
  Adenovirus
Bacterial
  S. pneumoniae (pneumococcus)
  Streptococcus pyogenes (group A)
Foreign body aspiration
Hydrocarbon ingestion
Uncommon
Atypical
  Mycoplasma pneumoniae
  Chlamydia pneumoniae
Bacterial
  Staphylococcus and other gram-positive bacteria
  Bartonella henselae
Other agents
  Chemical aspiration, respiratory burns and smoke inhalation, acute hypersensitivity alveolitis and near-drowning
Chronic or Recurrent Pneumonias
Common
Undetected foreign body aspiration
Cystic fibrosis
Uncommon
TB, fungal disease, congenital pulmonary abnormalities, idiopathic pulmonary hemosiderosis, alpha$_1$ antitrypsin deficiency, chronic lipoid pneumonia, pulmonary abscess, eosinophilic (Löffler's) pneumonia, hypersensitivity alveolitis

TABLE 9-3 CAUSES OF PNEUMONIAS IN OLDER CHILDREN AND TEENAGERS (5 TO 18 YEARS)

Acute Pneumonias
Common
Atypical
  M. pneumoniae
  C. pneumoniae
Bacterial
  S. pneumoniae (pneumococcus)
  Streptococcus pyogenes (group A)
  Staphylococcus (MRSA)
Uncommon
Viral
  Influenza and parainfluenza viruses, adenovirus, respiratory syncytial virus, metapneumovirus, coronavirus, rhinovirus
Bacterial
  Staphylococcus aureus, gram-negative bacilli, *B. henselae*
Other agents
  Chemical aspiration (including hydrocarbon from gasoline siphonage), respiratory burns and smoke inhalation, acute hypersensitivity alveolitis
Chronic and Recurrent Pneumonias
Common
Cystic fibrosis
Asthma
Uncommon
Alpha$_1$-antitrypsin deficiency (especially in cigarette or marijuana smokers), chronic bronchiectasis, TB, fungal disease, allergic bronchopulmonary aspergillosis, human immunodeficiency virus (HIV)/acquired immunodeficiency syndrome (AIDS), pulmonary abscess, chronic interstitial pneumonias

RADIOGRAPHIC EVALUATION AND TECHNIQUE

Various imaging techniques are available for examining the internal morphology of the chest. These range in complexity (and cost) from plain chest radiographs to elaborate, technically sophisticated modalities such as computed tomography (CT), magnetic resonance imaging (MRI) and positron emission tomography (PET)-CT scanning. In this section, several of these techniques are discussed, with emphasis on the simpler modalities, which in most instances are entirely adequate for satisfactory diagnostic evaluation.

PLAIN CHEST RADIOGRAPH

The most essential imaging modality and the initial radiographic examination used for all the symptoms discussed in this chapter is a frontal and lateral radiograph of the chest. In infants and in children who are too young or too ill to cooperate, the frontal view is exposed anteroposteriorly, with the patient in a supine position; the lateral view is a supine, horizontal-beam (cross-table) exposure.[93] In children who can cooperate, the frontal view is exposed posteroanteriorly and is taken while the patient is sitting in a device such as a Pigg-O-Stat. The lateral view, without which the examination is incomplete, must never be considered optional; only in emergencies is a single view acceptable. Single anteroposterior or posteroanterior films are acceptable for follow-up examinations.

DECUBITUS FILMS

Decubitus films are useful in evaluating the presence and quantity of free-flowing pleural fluid. These films are exposed anteroposteriorly with a horizontal beam while the patient is reclining with the side of interest directed downward. Free fluid flows along the lateral aspect of the chest, where it is radiographically apparent. A decubitus film may occasionally be useful when a small pneumothorax is suspected in an infant or young child; in this setting the suspicious side is placed upward rather than downward.[93,94]

ULTRASOUND, COMPUTED TOMOGRAPHY, MAGNETIC RESONANCE, AND POSITRON EMISSION TOMOGRAPHY-COMPUTED TOMOGRAPHY IMAGING

Ultrasound may be of value in evaluating the opaque hemithorax.[52] Small to large amounts of pleural effusion are easily evaluated. Air is essentially impenetrable to ultrasonic waves, however, and, thus, evaluation of aerated lungs is worthless.

CT may be very helpful in patients with complicated pneumonia, pulmonary abscess or masses, and mediastinal lesions impinging on the airway.[11,15,42,65,76] High-resolution CT (HRCT) of the chest (slice thickness 1 mm or less) is useful in evaluating chronic or recurrent pneumonias in children (see Figs. 9–20, 9–28, and 9–34).[3,10,41,61,85] Diffuse lung disease is also best evaluated with this modality (see Figs. 9–8 and 9–39).[56,100] In the last decade, HRCT of the lungs in children has become more widely used. Despite this trend, there is still no consensus on when or how to use HRCT, even with common diseases such as asthma, cystic fibrosis (CF), bronchopulmonary dysphasia (BPD), and infection. It can be agreed, however, that low-dose CT techniques including low milliamperes, high peak kilowatt voltage, small field of view, and short scan times are desirable. Some of the more common indications for HRCT in children are (1) an abnormal yet nonspecific chest radiograph, (2) detection of bronchiectasis, (3) detection of the sequelae of infection, (4) staging and therapeutic evaluation in cystic fibrosis, and (5) evaluation of the severity of BPD.

An overview of the more common airway and parenchymal lung disorders with their associated HRCT patterns is presented in Table 9–4.[56]

MRI is the modality of choice for detailed anatomic delineation of cardiac and vascular anomalies and can be very helpful in defining pulmonary hemosiderosis.[16,95]

TABLE 9-4 HIGH-RESOLUTION COMPUTED TOMOGRAPHY PATTERNS OF AIRWAY AND LUNG DISORDERS

SIGNS/PATTERNS	ETIOLOGIES
Bronchiectasis Bronchus larger than accompanying vessel	Cystic fibrosis, ciliary dyskinesia, allergic bronchopulmonary aspergillosis bronchiolitis obliterans, foreign body, Williams-Campbell syndrome
Diffuse air trapping	Asthma, bronchiolitis
Focal air trapping and mosaic perfusion pattern	Asthma with superimposed infection, obliterative bronchiolitis
Ground glass opacities Increased lung attenuation with preserved underlying parenchymal detail	Acute respiratory distress syndrome, hemorrhage, exudates, edema, lymphoid interstitial pneumonitis (LIP), pulmonary alveolar proteinosis, interstitial pneumonitis
Smooth septal thickening Reticular pattern	Fluid overload, lymphangiectasia, pulmonary vein atresia or obstruction
Nodular septal thickening Irregular bronchovascular bundle thickening	Metastatic sarcomas, lymphoma, and, rarely, neuroblastoma
Pulmonary nodules Small, ill-defined centrilobular	Hypersensitivity pneumonia, LIP, capillary hemangiomatosis, hemosiderosis
Small soft tissue	Metastatic disease, miliary TB, granulomatous and fungal infection, Langerhans' cell histiocytosis, hemosiderosis
Larger nodules/masses	Metastases, lymphoma, fungal, infectious bronchiolitis obliterans–organizing pneumonia, vasculitis, septic emboli, arteriovenous malformations, artery aneurysms

Data from Kuhn JP; Brody AS: High-resolution CT of pediatric lung disease. Radiol Clin North Am 40:89–110, 2002. Please refer to this reference for a more detailed discussion of these imaging patterns and techniques.

Fast echo-planar MRI can be used for pulmonary function studies, including ventilation/perfusion MRI for pulmonary embolus.[17,37,38] MRI is rarely used to evaluate pneumonia, owing to the expense of the study. However, pneumonia is occasionally noted incidentally on chest, abdominal, or thoracic spine MRI (see Fig. 9–22).

A dynamic new imaging modality is PET-CT, which merges the molecular imaging of PET with the cross-sectional anatomic imaging of CT. These studies utilize a radioisotope, [18F]fluorodeoxyglucose (FDG), which acts at the metabolic level. [18F]FDG is highly sensitive in identifying areas of "up-regulated" glucose metabolism that typically occur in lymphoid tissue positive for infection or certain malignancies.[64] The use of PET-CT is increasing in pediatric patients, owing to its high sensitivity in Hodgkin's lymphoma. Therefore, although its primary use has mainly been in diagnosis and staging of cancers, pneumonias, as well as other infections involving the chest, have incidentally been discovered (see Fig. 9–19). At this time, the indications for using PET-CT in children are limited due to the lack of support by the Centers for Medicare & Medicaid Services. However, the use of PET-CT has great promise for increased understanding of the pathophysiology of pediatric disease.[50]

ARTIFACTS AND PSEUDOPNEUMONIAS

Pseudopneumonias are factitious infiltrates that may appear on chest films for a variety of reasons. Familiarity with these various phony infiltrates aids in the prevention of false-positive diagnoses of pneumonia and unwarranted treatment.

An infiltrate in the right middle lobe is the most common misdiagnosed pneumonia. The asymmetry produced by normal right-sided hilar and infrahilar vascular structures is often thought to be an infiltrate. An attempt to define the infiltrate on the lateral view reveals it to be nonexistent. Conversely, left lower lobe pneumonia is most commonly missed owing to "hiding behind the heart." These errors are made most often with radiographs of infants or young children.

Of the several technical factors that influence the translucency of the lungs, the most important in pediatric patients is the stage of respiration at the time of the radiographic exposure. On an adequate basal respiratory (noncrying) anteroposterior film, the dome of a neonate's right hemidiaphragm is approximately at the level of the posterior right eighth rib. By 6 months of age, with progressive lung development, the hemidiaphragm is at the level of the eighth posterior intercostal space, increasing to the right ninth rib by the age of 1 year. By the end of the tenth year of life, the dome of the right hemidiaphragm projects approximately at the tenth rib with an adequate inspiratory effort. Hypoaeration is seen when the dome of the right hemidiaphragm projects one interspace or more superiorly.

On the anteroposterior projection, these levels must be correlated with the configuration of the posterior aspect of the diaphragm on the lateral projection, which normally reveals a smooth cephalic convexity. With underaeration, the lateral projection reveals increased cephalic doming of the diaphragm. The most common cause of underaeration in the pediatric age group is filming during expiration. An obvious clue to this problem is a diffuse infiltrate seen on the frontal but not the lateral view or vice versa. If the findings are questionable, it is best to repeat the examination rather than to try to interpret a technically unsatisfactory film.

Hyperaeration, which is a nonspecific response of the pediatric lung to virtually any foreign substance (e.g., blood, pus, or edema fluid), is seen when the dome of the right hemidiaphragm projects at least one interspace inferior to the rib indices listed. The lateral view shows flattening of the hemidiaphragms. This is the most frequent abnormality of aeration associated with the pneumonias of childhood. Diseases with associated bronchospasm (bronchiolitis, bronchitis, and asthma) generally have the most striking hyperaeration.[21,77,93]

Rotation of the patient may result in geometric distortion, superimposing normal structures such as rib ends and sternal ossification centers on the lungs. These can be misinterpreted as infiltrates.

The thymus gland often contributes significantly to the borders and width of the anterior mediastinum until approximately 3 years of age, after which it usually involutes to such a degree that it is rarely a problem. A normal thymus may still contribute to the mediastinal width, however, particularly on chest CT, until the early teens. There is marked variability in the size and shape of the thymus. A large thymus is most commonly misinterpreted as cardiomegaly or a mediastinal mass. When the thymus has a triangular ("sail") configuration, it may be thought to represent an area of pneumonia or atelectasis (Fig. 9–1). The fact that the mass is of thymic origin can be deduced in several ways. First, the lateral view often reveals the thymus in the anterior mediastinum. Second, mild indentations are produced by the anterior ribs, resulting in a wavy outline on the frontal projection. Third, if cardiomegaly is erroneously diagnosed, the lateral view will show the heart to be of normal size.

Artifacts such as film defects (e.g., poor film-screen contact or processing artifacts), overlying clothing, hair braids, breast buds in pubertal girls, and jewelry are usually correctly identified when two projections are obtained, because the density is usually either seen on one projection and not the other or is seen "in" the chest on one projection and superficial to the chest on the other (Fig. 9–2).

The use of a Pigg-O-Stat restraining device in infants and young children may produce areas of increased density over the lungs from the plastic chest holders. These Pigg-O-Stat "pneumonias" are usually seen on the frontal view, whereas the lateral view is clear (Fig. 9–3).

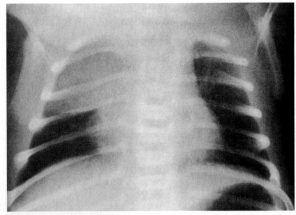

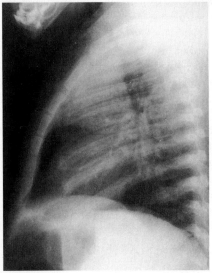

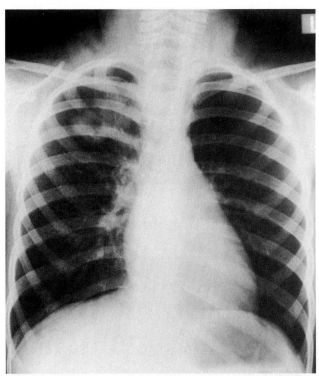

Figure 9–2

Pseudopneumonia due to a hair braid. This frontal view of a 14-year-old girl with a positive tuberculin test shows a density in the right upper lobe that has an apparent central lucency. An erroneous diagnosis of "active, cavitating pulmonary tuberculosis" was made. The abnormality was caused by overlying hair braids, which can faintly be seen in the supraclavicular regions bilaterally

Figure 9–1

Pseudopneumonia due to a large thymus gland in an infant with mild cough and fever. *A,* The anteroposterior (AP) film reveals opacification of the right upper lung. This "infiltrate" has a lateral margin that is slightly lobulated and does not quite extend to the pleural surface. The patient is rotated toward the right. *B,* A lateral chest radiograph. An increased density in the anterior mediastinum tapers inferiorly in the immediate substernal region. Posteriorly, the chest is clear. The right upper lung density is characteristic of a prominent right lobe of the thymus. There is a subtle "thymic wave" sign on the frontal projection (the lobulated lateral margin). In infants, either lobe of the thymus may be this prominent; indeed, the lobes may extend to the diaphragm.

PHYSIOLOGIC CONSIDERATIONS

Accurate interpretation of pediatric chest films also requires a basic understanding of the physiologic and anatomic differences among adults, neonates, and infants (for an excellent explanation of these differences, the reader is referred to articles by Griscom[28–30] and for similar details for chest film interpretation of newborn infants to an article by Wesenberg[93]). The most important differences include the following: (1) the peripheral airways of infants are relatively smaller than those of adults, and collateral pathways of ventilation are less developed; (2) the airways of infants are more prone to collapse in response to pressure changes than are those of adults; and (3) infants also have relatively more mucous glands and greater mucous production. For these reasons, the peripheral airways of infants are more susceptible to inflammatory narrowing than are adult airways.

In older children and adults, respiratory infections most commonly involve the interstitium and alveoli. Lower respiratory infections in infants, on the other hand, manifest their primary effects in the smaller airways, producing peripheral mucous obstruction and disproportionately severe respiratory distress. This is revealed on chest films by generalized hyperaeration (air trapping) with focal irregularities of aeration that reflect atelectasis from mucous plugging. True consolidative (alveolar) pneumonia is a much less frequent occurrence.[29]

CHARACTERIZATION OF PULMONARY INFILTRATES

Characterization of pulmonary infiltrates is important, because patterns of abnormality suggest specific organisms and etiologies. The three basic kinds of infiltrates are

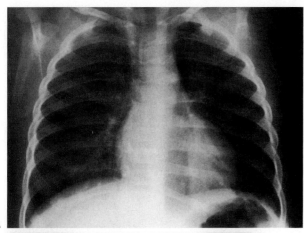

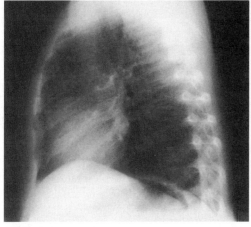

Figure 9–3
Pseudopneumonia due to a Pigg-O-Stat in a 1-year-old boy with cough and mild fever. *A*, A frontal chest film, showing an area of increased density in the left lung base medially, seen through the left heart. This "pneumonia" ends medially in a vertical straight line that does not correspond to any anatomic boundary. It is typical of an artifact produced by the cylindrical restraining device known as a Pigg-O-Stat, which is commonly used in North America to restrain children in an upright position for chest films. The diagnostic clue for Pigg-O-Stat pseudopneumonia is the straight vertical boundary medially, which may be projected over either hemithorax. *B*, The lateral view is normal. If the apparent infiltrate on the frontal projection were genuine, it would be in the lower lobe, causing increased density posteriorly on the lateral projection.

(1) interstitial, (2) alveolar, and (3) mixed. These patterns are discussed here to provide an overview of findings that will permit an intelligent approach to the radiographic interpretation of films of children who have cough and fever.

Interstitial Infiltrates

The interstitial pattern has been described with a variety of confusing radiographic terms. When mild, an interstitial infiltrate is characterized by a stringy collection of densities that fan out from the hila, seen on the lateral projection as apparent enlargement and poor (fuzzy) definition of the hila.

This is classical perihilar pneumonia. When the pneumonia is severe, the pattern shows a diffuse, bilateral, sharply defined reticular (stringy) infiltrate (Figs. 9–4 and 9–5). There are no air-bronchograms and no associated pleural effusion.

Alveolar Infiltrates

Alveolar (air-space) disease is characterized by a plethora of descriptive names.[13] The typical alveolar infiltrate is a smooth, homogeneous increase in density (whiteness) of the lungs or portion of the lungs (see Figs. 9–14, 9–16, and 9–17). The most common alveolar infiltrate is well defined, dense, homogenous lobar or segmental consolidation, with an air bronchogram within it (see Figs. 9–12 and 9–15). There is commonly associated pleural effusion.

Mixed Infiltrates

Mixed infiltrates, not surprisingly, have features of both alveolar and interstitial patterns. If an unknown pulmonary infiltrate cannot comfortably be classified as either alveolar or interstitial, it is considered to have the mixed pattern. The prototype of a mixed infiltrate is an ill-defined area of mildly increased density (segmental) containing finely dilated air bronchioles (see Fig. 9–10). A perihilar interstitial infiltrate at age 4 and older also falls into this class. There is usually no significant pleural effusion.

PATTERNS OF THE THREE COMMON CAUSES OF PNEUMONIA

Acute *viral* pneumonias are typically *interstitial* (usually perihilar) in appearance (see Fig. 9–4). *Atypical (Mycoplasma or Chlamydia)* pneumonias are *mixed* (see Fig. 9–10). Most acute *bacterial* pneumonias are *alveolar* (see Fig. 9–16). Finer distinctions are noted in the discussions of the individual pneumonias.

EVALUATION OF THE MOST IMPORTANT CAUSES OF COUGH AND FEVER

VIRAL PNEUMONIAS

Respiratory Syncytial Virus

Epidemiology and Pathophysiology RSV is the major cause of cough and fever resulting from pneumonia among infants. It is also the single most common cause of bronchiolitis in children younger than 2 years, accounting for at least one third of cases.[30]

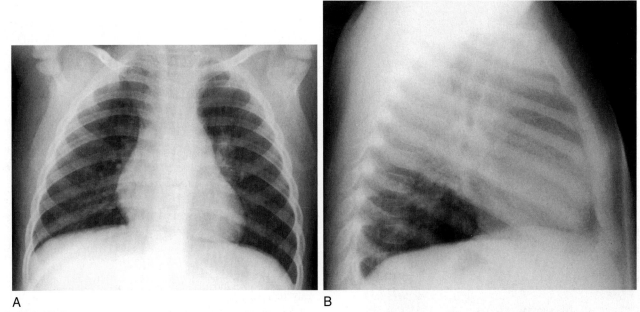

A   B

Figure 9–4
Respiratory syncytial virus (RSV) bronchiolitis in a 22-month-old child with fever, cough, and wheezing. *A,* The AP radiograph demonstrates prominent and indistinct hila secondary to a perihilar interstitial infiltrate. *B,* These findings are confirmed on the lateral radiograph, which shows dense, enlarged hilar markings centrally.

The striking aspects of RSV pneumonia are its age predilection (i.e., children younger than 7 years, including neonates and infants) and its predictable annual epidemics, which last 4 or 5 months, usually beginning in December and continuing through early spring. Transplacentally transmitted RSV antibody, although universal, appears to have no protective effect in newborns and infants, thus explaining the high attack rates. Affected infants develop rhinitis and pharyngitis, usually with fever. Bronchiolitis, bronchitis, and viral pneumonia occur in 20% to 40% of patients. Bronchiolitis, which overlaps clinically with RSV pneumonia, is the most common diagnosis in infants hospitalized with RSV infection.[25,45,88]

Clinical Findings The incubation period for RSV infection is approximately 3 to 5 days. The first signs of RSV infection in an infant are mild rhinorrhea and low-grade fever, followed by cough. Wheezing begins shortly after the cough develops. Rhinorrhea and intermittent fever usually persist throughout the illness. In some infants and most young children, RSV pneumonia follows a course more suggestive of pneumonia than bronchitis, with dyspnea, cyanosis, loss of appetite, and listlessness following a minimum of wheezing. Fever is variably present.

Routine hematologic tests are not particularly helpful. Definitive diagnosis of RSV infection requires viral culture; unfortunately, the results are usually not available until 2 to 3 days after the sample is collected. Much earlier diagnosis can be achieved by examining nasoepithelial secretions using rapid tests, which can produce diagnostic results in a few hours.[86]

The mortality rate for infants hospitalized with RSV infection is approximately 2%. The prognosis is worse for infants with congenital heart disease or BPD. Recurrent wheezing occurs in one third to one half of children who have RSV bronchiolitis in infancy.

Radiographic Findings The radiographic findings in RSV bronchiolitis are predominantly those of hyperaeration of the lungs with a variable degree of perihilar interstitial infiltrate.[4,57] Usually the lungs are clear peripherally (see Fig. 9–4). Typically the bilateral, perihilar interstitial infiltrate is suggestive of mild to moderate hilar enlargement that is indistinct on both projections. A more widespread interstitial infiltrate occurs in more severe infections, and areas of subsegmental atelectasis are common, reflecting mucous plugging (Fig. 9–6).

The lungs in RSV pneumonia commonly are also hyperaerated but generally less so than in RSV bronchiolitis. Radiographic clearing is not as rapid as clinical recovery, and complete clearing may take as long as 2 to 5 months.

Metapneumovirus

Epidemiology Metapneumovirus (MPV), a newly described paramyxovirus has been found to be a significant cause of upper and lower respiratory infections, especially among infants.[18,96] In the Northern Hemisphere, the incidence of infection from this agent peaks during late winter and early spring. In some studies, MPV has been detected by reverse transcription–polymerase chain reaction in up to 20% of respiratory specimens of infants with pneumonia.[19,33]

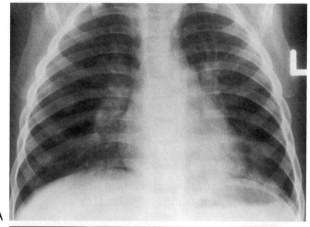

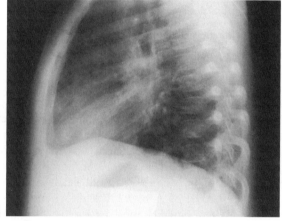

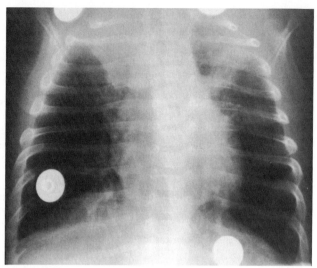

Figure 9–6
Severe viral pneumonitis: RSV pneumonia in a 2-month-old boy with severe respiratory distress and mild cyanosis. Partial atelectasis of the right upper lobe is secondary to mucous plugging; subsegmental atelectasis also involves the left upper lobe, with smaller patches of wedge-shaped, subsegmental atelectasis in both lower lobes. Despite extensive atelectasis, the chest demonstrates significant hyperaeration. Multiple areas of atelectasis caused by mucous plugging are common in moderate and severe RSV pneumonia.

Figure 9–5
Severe viral pneumonitis: parainfluenza type 3 pneumonia in an 18-month-old boy who presented after 1 day of progressive, severe cough with low-grade fever. A, Bilateral, perihilar infiltrate extends into both lower lobes. In addition, there is a diffuse pattern of interstitial infiltrate. Air bronchograms are seen in the lower lobes, most notably on the left. B, The lateral view shows enlarged, ill-defined hila with only mild hyperaeration. The pattern of perihilar and diffuse interstitial disease is typically viral. Superimposed consolidation suggests bacterial superinfection, which most commonly occurs during the second week of viral pneumonia and is usually preceded by a striking increase in fever and clinical symptoms. In this case, the alveolar infiltrate was present on the initial films and was caused by parainfluenza virus; there was no clinical suggestion of bacterial superinfection.

The clinical presentation of infections with MPV resembles that of infection with RSV.[19] Cough, coryza, and fever are the most common symptoms, followed by irritability, anorexia, and wheezing.

Radiographic Findings Radiographic findings in MPV pneumonia and bronchiolitis are very similar to those observed in RSV infection and include perihilar infiltrates and hyperinflation (see Fig. 9–4).

Parainfluenza Viruses

Epidemiology Parainfluenza virus types 1 and 3 account for approximately 20% of all childhood pneumonias.

They most commonly occur in children 5 years of age or younger. In addition, parainfluenza viruses account for about 50% of cases of croup and 15% of cases of bronchiolitis and bronchitis. Parainfluenza virus type 1 infections occur predominantly in the late summer and fall; parainfluenza virus type 3 has no predictable seasonal pattern.[53]

Radiographic Findings The radiographic findings in parainfluenza pneumonia are nonspecific. Perihilar interstitial infiltrates are common.[21] Patchy pulmonary infiltrates (subsegmental atelectasis) are seen in slightly more than 50% of patients (see Fig. 9–5).

Adenovirus

Epidemiology and Pathophysiology Adenoviruses cause approximately 5% to 8% of acute respiratory disease in infants and children and are most common in those younger than 5 years.

In addition to pneumonia, these viruses produce fever and pharyngoconjunctivitis, epidemic keratoconjunctivitis, and follicular conjunctivitis. There is also a high association between adenoviral infection and exudative tonsillitis.

Clinical Findings Most adenoviral infections are characterized by rhinitis, pharyngitis, and pneumonitis, with or without conjunctivitis. Of the protean clinical syndromes produced by adenovirus infection, pharyngoconjunctival fever, commonly called *pink eye,* is the symptom most specific for adenoviral infection.

An important aspect of adenoviral pneumonia is its high incidence of complications and sequelae.[35] Epidemics of adenovirus types 3, 4, 7, and 21 can cause pulmonary disease that is devastating to infants. The incidence of chronic pulmonary disease following adenoviral pneumonia varies from 53% to 87%. The incidence of chronic lung disease is considerably higher in children younger than 2 years (64%) than in older children. Certain racial groups (e.g., Native Americans) are at increased risk of acquiring adenoviral pneumonia and experiencing its complications. One of the most common complications is necrotizing bronchiolitis, progressing to obliterative bronchiolitis and the "unilateral hyperlucent lung syndrome" (Swyer-James or MacLeod's syndrome).[100] In other patients, bronchiectasis, interstitial fibrosis, or both can be seen.[58]

Radiographic Findings The initial radiographic findings in adenoviral pneumonia are nonspecific and are shared with the other viral pneumonias.[35] The most common manifestation is a bilateral, perihilar interstitial infiltrate (Figs. 9–7 and 9–8).

The pulmonary sequelae of adenovirus pneumonia are usually evident on follow-up films. A mild form of adenoviral pneumonia is chronic pneumonitis, with associated fibrosis and mild bronchiectasis (see Fig. 9–7). In severe disease, necrotizing bronchiolitis progresses to obliterative bronchiolitis, which leads to unilateral hyperlucent lung (Swyer-James syndrome), with or without areas of associated bronchiectasis and chronic atelectasis (Fig. 9–9). Bronchiectasis is best imaged with HRCT of the chest (see Fig. 9–34).

Influenza Virus Influenza virus can also cause interstital infiltrates. Occasionally, influenza can lead to findings consistent with ARDS (adult respiratory distress syndrome), as is the case with the recently described outbreaks of avian influenza (H5N1) in Southeast Asia (see additional reference 4).

ATYPICAL PNEUMONIAS

Mycoplasma pneumoniae

Epidemiology and Pathophysiology *Mycoplasma pneumoniae*, a bacterium, is the most common organism producing pneumonia in the school-age child (4 to 18 years), with a peak incidence occurring between 10 and 15 years of age. Infection occurs in children younger than 4 years, but it is usually asymptomatic. *Mycoplasma* infections are generally mild, but may be severe in children who have sickle cell anemia.[92]

Mycoplasma infections most commonly occur from September to January (75%). Epidemics of *Mycoplasma* infection tend to be long-lasting and occur at irregular intervals. Usually, several members of a patient's family are also infected but are considered to have "colds."

Clinical Findings The incubation period for *Mycoplasma* infection is approximately 1 to 3 weeks.

The onset of cough and fever is gradual, with accompanying headache, malaise, and sore throat; rhinitis and diarrhea rarely occur. Bullous myringitis and a maculopapular rash may occur.

Nonrespiratory sites of involvement include the skin (rash), heart (myopericarditis), blood (thrombocytopenia), joints (arthritis and arthralgia), and central nervous system (meningitis). Patients who have *Mycoplasma* infections seldom require hospitalization, and fatal illnesses are rare. The complication of a superimposed bacterial infection is distinctly unusual.

The routine hematologic indices are usually unrevealing. The diagnosis is established by cold hemagglutinins or specific antibodies obtained from acute-phase serum, followed by a repeat convalescent serum analysis 10 days to 3 weeks later; a specific increase in antibodies confirms *Mycoplasma* infection.

Radiographic Findings The radiographic pattern produced by *M. pneumoniae* (Fig. 9–10) is most commonly an ill-defined, mildly increased density segmental or lobar consolidation with involvement that is usually in the lower lobes. Acutely, a perihilar interstitial pattern is present. Typically, there are areas of bronchiolar and acinar dilatation, commonly within the consolidation, that suggest mild microcyst formation. A patchy, alveolar bronchopneumonic pattern may occasionally be seen. There is usually no pleural effusion.[7,47,84] Because of its high incidence, pneumonia in school-age children should be considered to be *Mycoplasma* pneumonia until proven otherwise.

Chlamydia Pneumoniae

C. pneumoniae, an organism identified in 1986, causes CAP that is quite indistinguishable from *Mycoplasma* pneumonia. Sore throat and hoarseness are more common in *Chlamydia* pneumonia. Radiologically, the pneumonia is virtually identical to that caused by *Mycoplasma,* but minimal pleural effusion is seen in 25% of patients. The diagnosis is made by serologic analysis, which is not widely available.[23,41]

Chlamydia Trachomatis

Epidemiology and Pathophysiology *Chlamydia* organisms, long considered large viruses, more recently have been classified as bacteria. *Chlamydia* organisms thrive in crowded and unsanitary living conditions. *C. trachomatis* pneumonia in newborns and infants is thought to be acquired by passage through an infected birth canal. Some 2% to 6% of all infants acquire chlamydial infection, causing conjunctivitis, pneumonia, or both.

Clinical Findings *C. trachomatis* pneumonia is usually detected when an infant is between 2 and 12 weeks of age and most commonly at about 1 month. Conjunctivitis or a history of conjunctivitis is noted in half of patients. Striking findings include tachypnea with a cough that characteristically occurs in staccato paroxysms (parapertussis).

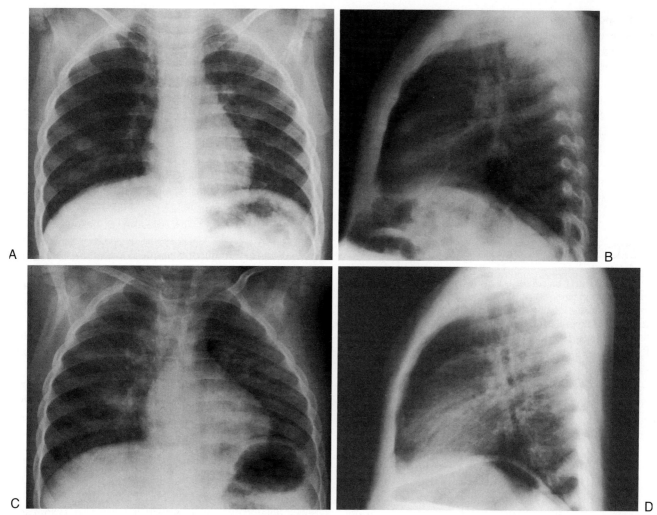

Figure 9–7

Adenovirus pneumonia in a 2-year-old Native American girl with a 2-day history of moderately severe cough, mild dyspnea, and low-grade fever. *A,* The frontal view shows a bilateral, perihilar infiltrate, slightly more marked on the left than on the right. *B,* The lateral view shows prominent, ill-defined hila. These findings, combined with the frontal film findings, are consistent with any viral pneumonia. *C,* Two months later, the patient continued to have a cough that was worse at night. As seen on this radiograph, the bilateral perihilar pattern had persisted, with ill-defined nodules in the right middle and left lower lobes. *D,* The lateral view shows mild hyperaeration; the chronic perihilar infiltrate is again evident. The tendency for acute adenoviral pneumonia to become chronic is common, particularly in susceptible populations. Radiographic clearing occurred in this patient 6 months after the initial infection.

Usually there is no fever. Poor weight gain, minimal malaise, and secretory otitis media may be evident. Peripheral eosinophilia occurs in 71% of patients. Serum immunoglobulin levels, particularly immunoglobulin (Ig) M, are elevated. The diagnosis can be established with special cultures of nasopharyngeal secretions or by serum antibody measures.

Radiographic Findings Patients who have *C. trachomatis* pneumonia have a fairly typical bilateral, perihilar interstitial pattern of infiltrate (Fig. 9–11).[51] Patchy, fluffy-appearing alveolar infiltrates are usually bilaterally superimposed on this pattern, and the radiographic findings are often more severe than clinical symptoms. When this pattern occurs in a 2- to 12-week-old infant, the radiographic

pattern is characteristic enough to suggest the diagnosis of *C. trachomatis* pneumonia.

BACTERIAL PNEUMONIAS

Bacterial pneumonias constitute only 3% to 5% of all childhood pneumonias. Most childhood pneumonias are viral or atypical. In general, bacterial pneumonias have a sudden onset.

Clinical Findings A viral respiratory infection commonly precedes the bacterial pneumonia by several days to a week. In infants and younger children, cough and fever

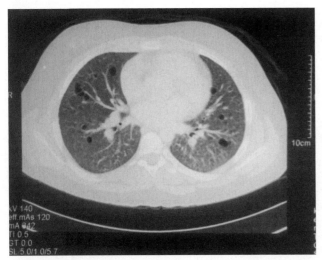

Figure 9–8
A 16-year-old with Langerhans' cell histiocytosis (LCH) and super-imposed viral pneumonia. A chest computed tomography (CT) axial image at the lung bases demonstrates prominent reticular, interstitial markings that extend into the periphery as well as intra-pulmonary cysts. LCH is the most common cause of acquired diffuse cystic lung disease in children.

may be minimal, and the physical examination may reveal little. In older children who have bacterial pneumonia, the more typical clinical pattern often includes shaking chills, high fever, productive cough (which is occasionally bloody), and pleuritic pain. Myalgia is not usually a prominent feature of bacterial pneumonias, as it is of viral pneumonias.

The white blood cell count in bacterial pneumonia is usually elevated, with a shift toward neutrophilia. Unfortunately, there is much overlap with viral pneumonia in this regard, particularly in infants. Blood cultures, when positive, may be of value in establishing the diagnosis. Sputum cultures or cultures obtained during bronchoalveolar lavage may also be helpful.

Radiographic Findings Radiologically, bacterial pneumonias usually cause dense lobar or segmental consolidation that frequently contains an air bronchogram. Patchy bronchopneumonia is the second most common pattern. When present, ancillary findings that suggest bacterial rather than viral pneumonia include significant pleural effusion, abscess, and pneumatocele formation within the pneumonic infiltrates.[31,66] Early pneumatocele formation (1 to 2 days) is highly suggestive of MRSA pneumonia.

Streptococcus Pneumoniae (Pneumococcus)

S. pneumoniae is a gram-positive bacterium usually seen in pairs or in short chains microscopically. The incidence of

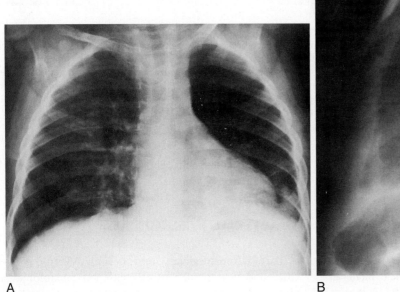

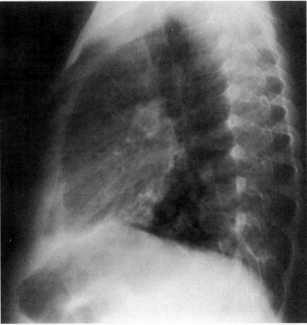

A   B

Figure 9–9
Viral pneumonitis with chronic sequelae in a 5-year-old Native American boy with severe adenovirus infection lasting several months. *A*, One year after the initial infection, there is bronchiectasis with chronic infiltrate in the left lower lobe. Mild perihilar and basilar infiltrates are also seen. *B*, The lateral view shows multiple irregularly dilated bronchi, particularly in the retrocardiac area, consistent with extensive bronchiectasis. Chronic pulmonary disease follows 50% to 80% of adenoviral pneumonias in susceptible populations.

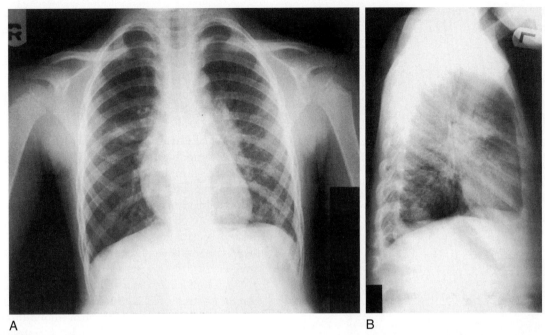

A   B

Figure 9–10
A 4-year-old boy with *Mycoplasma* pneumonia. There was a history of cough and fever for 1 week. Both the frontal *(A)* and lateral *(B)* radiographs show hilar prominence and interstitial infiltrates radiating out from the hila. Early alveolar (airspace) consolidation is also seen in the anterior segment of the right upper lobe. This is not as dense as the consolidation seen with bilateral pneumonia.

S. pneumoniae pneumonia is highest in late winter and early spring, when viral respiratory infections are most common.[87] Epidemics of pneumococcal pneumonia have been noted immediately following viral epidemics.[74] The incidence of *S. pneumoniae* pneumonia is decreasing with widespread use of a polyvalent vaccine.[20]

Children are particularly susceptible to *S. pneumoniae* pneumonia if they have sickle cell disease, leukemia, or diabetes and congenital asplenia complement deficiencies, or if they have undergone surgical removal of the spleen.[68,73]

Clinical Findings Clinical findings in older children and teenagers generally include high fever, cough, chest pains, and shaking chills. In infants and young children, there is more commonly an initial mild upper respiratory tract infection (a "cold"), followed several days later by an abrupt onset of high fever, respiratory distress, restlessness, and apprehension. There may be significant air hunger and cyanosis. Severe respiratory distress is manifested by tachypnea, grunting, nasal flaring, and chest wall and neck retractions. Cough is not prominent initially but appears later in the course of the disease.

In younger patients, the physical findings are often confusing. Lower lobe pneumonias may manifest with referred abdominal pain. When accompanied by abnormal abdominal findings, the pneumonia may be confused with acute appendicitis. This occurs often enough that many institutions require a "three-way abdomen" (an anteroposterior supine view and left lateral decubitus or upright view of the abdomen, with an anteroposterior view of the chest) to avoid unnecessary abdominal surgery. The leukocyte count is significantly elevated, with a marked shift to the left. The diagnosis is established by culture from lung aspiration, tracheal aspiration, blood, or pleural fluid.

Radiographic Findings Typically *S. pneumoniae* pneumonia manifests as a dense, homogeneous, alveolar lobar or segmental consolidation of lung parenchyma (Figs. 9–12 and 9–13). The consolidation begins in the peripheral air spaces and thus almost invariably abuts a pleural surface.[33] The consolidation usually has an air bronchogram and a well-defined border. Pleural effusion or empyema is common. Infants and younger children may have a patchy bronchopneumonic pattern.

S. pneumoniae is one of the common organisms that produce a so-called "round" pneumonia (Fig. 9–14). The round pneumonia is seen almost exclusively in children, usually in the superior segment of one of the lower lobes, abutting a pleural surface. Occasionally its appearance may be mistaken for a neoplasm. Round pneumonias may be caused by other organisms, such as *S. pyogenes, Klebsiella* (Fig. 9–15), or, rarely, *Staphylococcus*. A round pulmonary lesion associated with the clinical findings of pneumonia should suggest antibiotic therapy rather than evaluation for neoplasm. With appropriate therapy, radiographic clearing usually occurs within 10 to 14 days. Pneumatoceles may form during resolution and are considered a favorable prognostic sign (see Fig. 9–17).

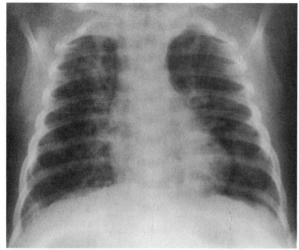

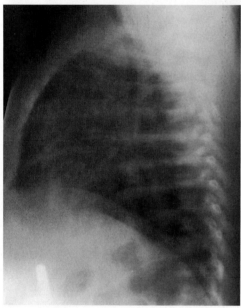

Figure 9–11

Chlamydia trachomatis pneumonia in a 1-month-old boy who had persistent conjunctivitis since birth and a dry, hacking cough for 2 days. *A,* Bilateral, ill-defined interstitial infiltrate and alveolar, fluffy-appearing patches of pneumonic consolidation in both upper lobes and the left lower lobe. *B,* The lateral view, shows mild hyperaeration and fluffy, ill-defined infiltrates. Usually the radiographic findings demonstrate greater severity than would be indicated by the patient's symptoms. These radiographic findings, although not pathognomonic, are characteristic of *C. trachomatis* pneumonia in patients who are 2 to 12 weeks of age. Concomitant clinical findings of conjunctivitis and eosinophilia further suggest the diagnosis.

Streptococcus Pyogenes

S. pyogenes (group A *Streptococcus*) is a gram-positive organism that on blood agar produces beta hemolysis surrounding rapidly growing colonies.[87] Group A streptococcal infections are most commonly limited to the upper respiratory tract. Certain viral infections, particularly the epidemic influenzas, predispose certain patients to streptococcal pneumonia and croup, most commonly children between the ages of 3 and 5 years and occasionally infants. Group A streptococcal pneumonia is a severe, diffuse necrotizing pneumonia that is most common in school-age children and adolescents. The incidence of this infection has increased markedly in the past decade, not only in infants but also in children who have chronic lung disease and viral respiratory infections.

Clinical Findings Group A beta-hemolytic streptococci most commonly infect the respiratory tract, soft tissues (erysipelas), skin (impetigo), and blood. Sequelae of untreated or inappropriately treated streptococcal infection include glomerulonephritis and rheumatic fever. Acutely affected patients have cough, chills, dyspnea, and (in severe disease) marked prostration. Chest pain is common. Occasionally there is an insidious onset, with cough, low-grade fever, and mild illness.

Significant leukocytosis with a shift to the left is common. Group A streptococcal infection may be suspected by obtaining a culture of the organism from a throat swab or sputum. However, definitive diagnosis requires demonstration of the organism on a smear or culture of lung aspirate, pleural fluid, blood, or bronchial washings.

Radiographic Findings Group A streptococcal pneumonia has radiographic findings that are indistinguishable from those of *S. pneumoniae* pneumonia. Lobar or segmental dense homogeneous or patchy consolidation commonly involves the lower lobes and may be bilateral (Figs. 9–14, 9–16, and 9–17). Pleural effusion, empyema, or both are common. An air bronchogram within the consolidation is frequent. Bilateral patchy bronchopneumonia may occur but is unusual, as are lung abscesses or pneumatoceles within areas of consolidation. Culture-proven group A streptococcal pneumonia may follow tonsillopharyngitis or sinusitis.

Staphylococcus Aureus

S. aureus is a gram-positive organism that is seen on smear in clumps or in groups. Culture on blood agar reveals gold and yellow colonies that are surrounded by hemolysis.

Clinical Findings Pneumonia caused by *S. aureus* is devastating to children. Since the late 1990s, there has been a resurgence in the incidence of superficial and invasive infections caused by community-acquired MRSA among previously healthy individuals.[69,72] According to different reports, *S. aureus* pneumonias account for a significant number of cases of invasive *S. aureus* infection.[69] As with other pyogenic bacterial infections, when staphylococcal pneumonia occurs, it tends to complicate viral infections, particularly influenza. The clinical symptoms and physical and laboratory findings are indistinguishable from those of other bacterial pneumonias.

Radiographic Findings The radiographic findings are indistinguishable from those of other bacterial pneumonias (Figs. 9–17 and 9–18). There is a tendency, however, for staphylococcal pneumonia to manifest initially as a patchy bronchopneumonia, with dense alveolar consolidation developing very rapidly, and usually involving a whole lobe or multiple lobes.[62]

Pleural effusion (or empyema) occurs in more than 90% of cases,[87] and pneumatoceles occur in 40% to 60% of cases (Figs. 9–17 and 9–18).[66] It is believed that pneumatoceles result from a ball valve obstruction of a communication between a bronchial lumen and a peribronchial abscess, resulting in

thin-walled cystic spaces that may become enormous, shifting the heart and mediastinum, and that often contain air-fluid levels.[39,44,87] Usually, pneumatoceles appear late in the first week of pneumonia and disappear spontaneously, generally within 6 weeks. The pneumatoceles may "rupture" with a resultant incidence of pneumothorax of up to 70%. The MRSA form can be suspected by early (1 to 2 days) development of abscesses, "a necrotizing pneumonia."[14]

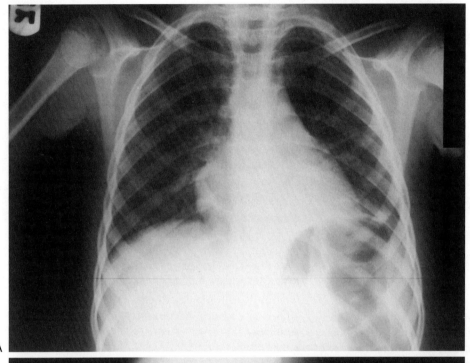

A

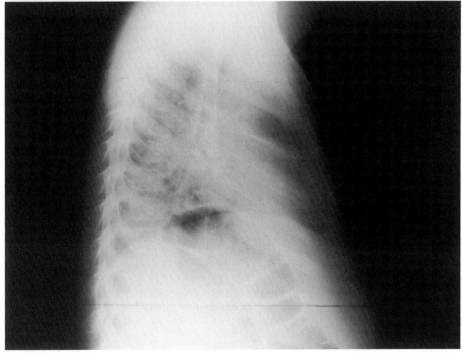

B

Figure 9–12

A 5-year-old with left lower lobe *Streptococcus pneumoniae* pneumonia. *A,* The frontal radiograph reveals a dense, homogeneous alveolar opacity in the left retrocardiac region. Note that the left hemidiaphragm medially is obscured by this consolidation. *B,* The lateral radiograph reveals a positive "spine sign." *C,* A CT scan in mediastinal windows shows the dense alveolar disease with associated air bronchograms.

Continued

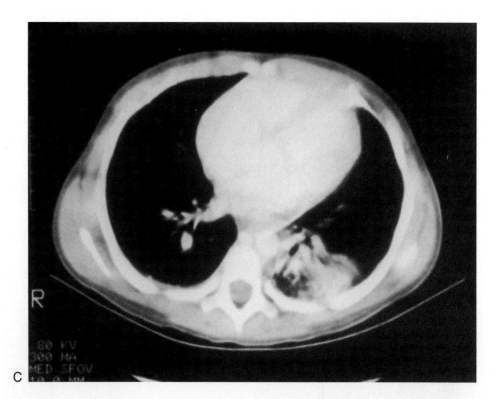

Figure 9–12—cont'd   C

Gram-Negative Bacteria

Haemophilus influenzae B was once the predominant organism in this group. However, with widespread inoculation for the bacterium, infection with *H. influenzae* has become nearly extinct in industrialized countries. During the past few decades, considerable progress in the antibiotic treatment of gram-positive bacteria has resulted in a decreased overall incidence of infections with gram-positive organisms. This decrease has permitted gram-negative bacilli to emerge as important pathogens, particularly in hospital environments. The widespread use and overuse of penicillin and broad-spectrum antibiotics have favored the proliferation of these more resistant organisms.[78]

The use of steroids and immunosuppressive agents, by decreasing host-defense mechanisms, has increased certain patients' susceptibility to gram-negative bacilli. Nosocomial (hospital-acquired) infections develop in 3% to 15% of patients, and most of these infections are caused by gram-negative organisms[78] (Fig. 9–19).

Cat-Scratch Disease

Cat-scratch disease most commonly presents as a regional lymphadenitis. However, it can also be a multiorgan infection. The causative agent is *Bartonella henselae* in most cases. This is a slow-growing, pleomorphic, gram-negative organism. Although it is relatively rare for cat-scratch disease to have pulmonary features, such cases do occur (Fig. 9–20). Typically, lung findings develop 1 to 5 weeks after

lymphadenopathy. Systemic signs of infection, including fever, are usually present. Chest wall abscesses have also been known to occur.[1,60] *B. henselae* is sensitive to a variety of antibiotics.

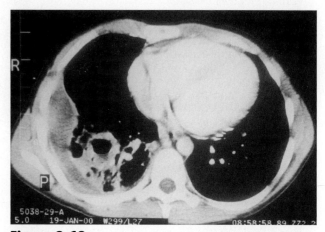

Figure 9–13

An 8-year-old girl with *S. pneumoniae* pneumonia and empyema. Contrast-enhanced CT (CECT) image at the level of the lung bases demonstrates a dense bronchopneumonia involving the posterior basal segment of the right lower lobe. A lung abscess is present with a thick, shaggy wall and an air-fluid level. In addition, there is a contrast enhancing, loculated empyema with the anterior aspect having the classic biconvex shape. *S. pneumoniae* is the most frequent bacterial organism to cause an empyema.

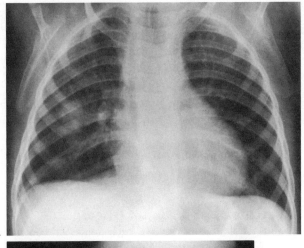

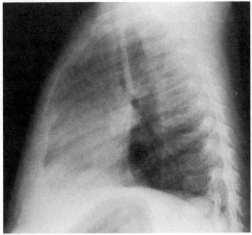

Figure 9–14

Bacterial pneumonia: "round" pneumonia (*S. pneumoniae*) in an 11-month-old girl with a 2-day history of cough and spiking fever. There was leukocytosis with a shift to the left. *A*, The AP view shows a round, nodular area of consolidation in the right midlung. *B*, On the lateral projection, the "nodule" lying in the right middle lobe appears somewhat triangular. Such round pneumonias are usually caused by one of the common bacterial pathogens and are most commonly located in the superior segment of a lower lobe. Confusion with a metastatic lesion is possible, but the clinical findings are those of pneumonia. An important radiographic clue is that the consolidation typically appears round on the frontal projection, a shape that does not persist on the lateral view. (Here the infiltrate appears triangular.)

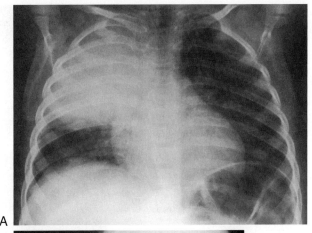

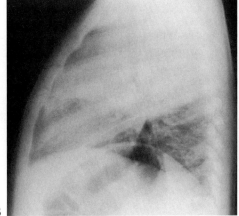

Figure 9–15

Bacterial pneumonia: *Klebsiella* pneumonia in an 18-month-old child with a 3-day history of severe cough, moderate dyspnea, and high fever. *A*, A dense pneumonic consolidation is seen in the right upper lobe, with minimal right pleural effusion. *B*, The lateral view also shows dense alveolar consolidation in the right upper lobe. The pneumonia expands the volume of the right upper lobe, bulging both the major and minor fissures inferiorly. This expansile, lobar infiltrate is the most common appearance of *Klebsiella* pneumonia, but occasionally it may also be seen with other bacterial pathogens, particularly MRSA staphylococcal pneumonia. *Klebsiella* also has a predilection for rapid development of abscesses within the pneumonia, similar to MRSA.

Acute Chest Syndrome

Acute chest syndrome (ACS) in sickle cell disease (SCD) is a complex pulmonary illness. It is defined as a *new* infiltrate on chest radiograph with the onset of one or more *new* symptoms such as fever, cough, sputum production, dyspnea, or hypoxia.[48,71]

Radiographic and clinical findings in ACS resemble those of pneumonia. However, the etiologies are felt to be multifactorial, including infection, infarction, and fat emboli. Infarction is caused by capillary occlusion with the sickled hemoglobin S red blood cells that have become deoxygenated. Fat embolization is due to bone marrow infarcts.[55]

ACS is often precipitated by an infectious process, particularly in the younger child. *Mycoplasma* is the most common pathogen, followed by viral and bacterial disease. Radiologic alveolar consolidation (air-space disease) can be multilobar with a predominance for the lower lobes (Figs. 9–21 and 9–22).[55] At present, thin-section CT of the lungs has shown chronic fibrotic changes or, in the subacute phase, a mosaic attenuation pattern.[56] However, its sensitivity in differentiating

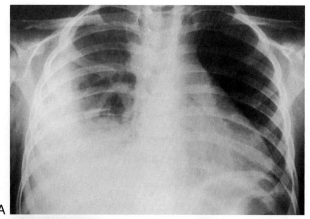

A

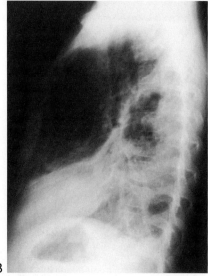

B

Figure 9–16
Bacterial pneumonia, empyema, and pneumatoceles in a 5-year-old boy with a 1-week history of "cold" symptoms, followed by the sudden onset of increased cough and high, spiking fever. *A*, A dense pneumonic consolidation in the right lower and middle lobes "silhouettes out" the right hemidiaphragm and a portion of the heart border. A large right pleural effusion extends to the apex of the right lung. Multiple air-filled pneumatoceles lie in the right mid-lung. Mild pneumonic consolidation is also present in the left lower lobe. *B*, The lateral view shows that the pneumatoceles are in the superior segment of the right lower lobe. The left upper lobe is hyperaerated anteriorly. The combination of dense pneumonic consolidation with pneumatocele formation and empyema is characteristic of bacterial infection; pleural effusion permits diagnostic thoracentesis for bacteriologic identification.

between infection, infarction, and embolism has not been established.

Other findings of SCD that can be typically seen on plain radiographs include cardiomegaly and vascular congestion due to anemia and chronic interstitial infiltrates in the lung bases. Osteonecrosis of bone with "H-shaped" vertebral bodies and sclerotic long bone infarcts, cholelithiasis, and splenomegaly and autoinfarction of the spleen, with an "absent spleen" sign also are common.

Most often, there is no identifiable etiology for ACS. In some studies, patients with fat emboli tended to be older and more hypoxic with a predilection for upper lobe infiltrates. Patients with infarction were also older and commonly had long bone and delayed chest radiographic findings 2 to 3 days after onset of chest pain.[56]

Therapy includes broad-spectrum antibiotics (including a macrolide), bronchodilators, and transfusions for patients with significant anemia.

GRANULOMATOUS PNEUMONIAS

Tuberculosis and Fungal Disease

Considerable progress has been made in controlling tuberculosis (TB) in most industrialized societies. During the last decade there has been a significant decrease in the number of cases of tuberculosis in the United States. Between 1993 and 2002, the average year-to-year decrease in the rate of tuberculosis in the United States was 6.8%.[9] In 2003, a total of 14,871 cases were reported, representing a decline of 1.9% over the previous year. A significant number of these cases occurred in foreign-born individuals.[9] Primary fungal infections as well as sarcoidosis have much in common with primary TB and therefore are discussed here. The most common mycotic infections affecting children in North America are histoplasmosis (endemic in the Mississippi River Valley), coccidioidomycosis (endemic in the southwestern United States), and blastomycosis (endemic in the south central United States and in Central and South America). Less common mycotic infections include cryptococcosis, mucormycosis, sporotrichosis, and aspergillosis.

TB is most commonly transmitted to infants and children by an adult member of the family who has cavitary TB. Primary fungal infections result from inhalation of spores and spherules in earth and dust particles within the various endemic areas; person-to-person transmission is rare. Sarcoidosis most commonly occurs in blacks in the southeastern United States.

Clinical Findings In most patients who have primary TB or primary fungal disease, infection is asymptomatic.[63] Symptoms, when they do occur, are nonspecific and are frequently attributed to a "cold." Low-grade fever may be present for a few days to a few weeks. Cough, when present, is mild. There may be minimal weight loss, anorexia, irritability, and malaise, and the patient may easily become fatigued. Primary histoplasmosis is clinically indistinguishable from primary tuberculosis. Primary coccidioidomycosis produces symptoms of influenza in 40% of patients, with malaise, chills, and fever. Sarcoidosis also mimics primary TB, but commonly has accompanying hepatomegaly, skin lesions, and uveitis or iritis.

Anorexia and night sweats are common in these diseases.[63] A sore throat and persistent dry cough may be

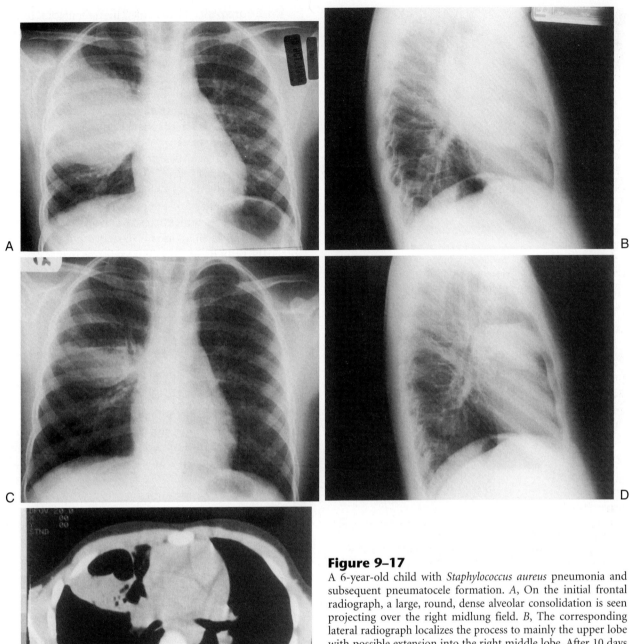

Figure 9–17

A 6-year-old child with *Staphylococcus aureus* pneumonia and subsequent pneumatocele formation. *A,* On the initial frontal radiograph, a large, round, dense alveolar consolidation is seen projecting over the right midlung field. *B,* The corresponding lateral radiograph localizes the process to mainly the upper lobe with possible extension into the right middle lobe. After 10 days of antibiotic therapy, frontal *(C)* and lateral *(D)* radiographs demonstrate formation of a pseudocyst with an air-fluid level in the right upper lobe. Pneumatoceles are characteristic of *Staphylococcus* pneumonia. *E,* A CECT image just below the carina confirms the pneumatocele, which is differentiated from a lung abscess by its thin, smooth wall.

present. Other variable findings include headache, backache, chest pain, and a generalized, fine macular erythematous rash. Arthritis, conjunctivitis, and painful pleurisy occur occasionally. It must be emphasized, however, that most patients are asymptomatic.

On rare occasions, TB or mycotic infections may spread hematogenously to virtually any organ in the body. This is usually a striking event clinically, with rapid onset of profound illness. Common findings include high fever with progressive dyspnea, cyanosis, and hepatosplenomegaly.

The diagnosis can usually be established by skin testing. In anergic patients, sputum and gastric aspirates are confirmatory for TB. Serologic testing may be performed to establish the diagnosis of fungal infections.[63]

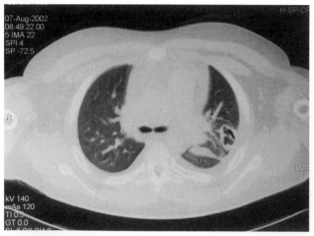

Figure 9–18
A 12-year-old child with *Staphylococcus* septicemia and lung abscesses. A single CECT image in the lung windows at the carina demonstrates two adjacent pleural-based "embolic" abscesses in the left upper lobe. Note the thick, irregular walls characteristic of a lung abscess. Early (1 to 2 days) development of lung abscesses is highly suggestive of MRSA pneumonia.

Radiographic Findings The radiographic findings in primary TB, sarcoidosis, and fungal diseases are virtually indistinguishable from one another. These findings include a primary focus of infection that appears as a variable-sized area of alveolar consolidation limited to a *single* lobe.[2,66] Unilateral hilar lymphadenopathy involves the nodes draining the lobe, with ipsilateral small to moderate pleural effusion; this is the classic triad of consolidation, lymphadenopathy, and pleural effusion (Figs. 9–23 and 9–24).[2] Rarely, endobronchial spread with varying degrees of bilateral alveolar consolidation may occur. Just as rarely, hematogenous spread occurs, with bilateral miliary infiltrates superimposed on the pattern of the primary infection (Fig. 9–25). With adequate treatment, resolution of the infiltrates in these diseases is slow, usually taking months. Healing of either the primary or disseminated forms may leave calcific residuals that are relatively common findings on adult chest films.

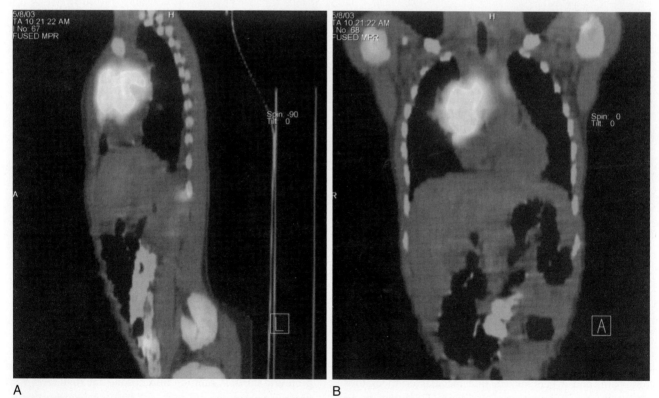

A   B

Figure 9–19
A 17-year-old adolescent girl with history of fever and CT findings of a perihilar mass that extends into the chest wall. Sagittal *(A)* and coronal *(B)* fusion images from positron emission tomography–CT demonstrate abnormal hypermetabolic activity throughout the mass and adjacent chest wall musculature. The remaining activity is normal physiologic uptake of fluorodeoxyglucose. A subsequent biopsy confirmed infection with *Fusobacterium necrophorum*, a rare gram-negative bacteria most often originating from the normal oral flora.

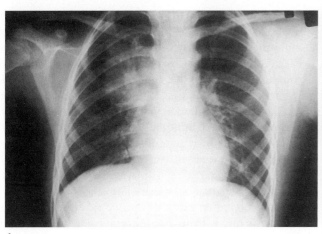
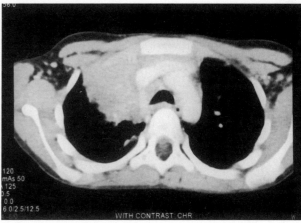

A   B

Figure 9–20
A 7-year-old child with cat-scratch disease (CSD). *A*, A frontal view of the chest shows focal alveolar opacity with air bronchograms adjacent to the right hilum and suprahilar region. *B*, A CECT image at the level of the carina demonstrates dense alveolar consolidation in the anterior segment of the right upper lobe. This intraparenchymal extension of CSD is extremely rare.

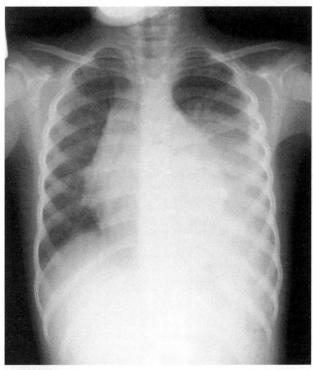

Figure 9–21
A 3-year-old girl with known hemoglobin SS sickle cell disease and numerous admissions for acute chest syndrome (ACS). She presented with fever and cough. This frontal view of the chest shows typical features of ACS, including cardiomegaly and extensive opacification of the left lung with sparing of the apex, as well as a left pleural effusion.

ALLERGIC BRONCHOPULMONARY ASPERGILLOSIS

Allergic bronchopulmonary aspergillosis (ABPA) is increasingly recognized among individuals with asthma in North America.[66,91] Clinical criteria for the diagnosis of ABPA include (1) asthma, (2) eosinophilia, (3) immediate skin reactivity to *Aspergillus*, (4) precipitating antibodies against *Aspergillus*, (5) elevated serum IgE level, (6) central bronchiectasis, and (7) pulmonary infiltrates (transient or fixed).

Chest radiographs show centrally located bronchiectatic changes with multiple mucoid impactions (Fig. 9–26). There is a mild predilection for upper lobe involvement. In addition, there are commonly bilateral, perihilar infiltrates simulating adenopathy. Air-fluid levels may be present within the dilated, partially obstructed bronchi. Chronic mucoid impactions are common. Recurrent episodes of consolidation occur and may resolve. More common is residual damage to the larger bronchi.

ASPIRATION PNEUMONIAS

Transglottic Aspiration

Acute aspirations in infants are characterized by cough and variable degrees of respiratory distress; fever may not occur in the immediate newborn period. After the first few hours of life, acute aspiration pneumonia usually reflects gastrointestinal tract dysfunction or obstruction that produces aspiration of milk, formula, or gastric contents. Aspiration of gastric fluid with a pH less than 2.4 acutely produces pulmonary edema in areas in which the aspirated

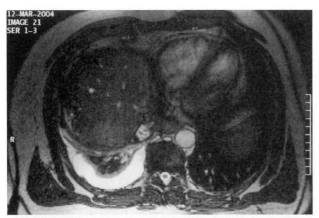

Figure 9–22
A 17-year-old adolescent girl with a history of sickle cell disease. The patient underwent magnetic resonance cholangiopancreatography to further evaluate her acute biliary obstruction as seen on a recent ultrasound examination. This image from an axial T2-weighted sequence incidentally shows pneumonic consolidation of the posterior segment of the right lower lobe with an adjacent parapneumonic effusion.

fluid is distributed. This is often followed by an intense inflammatory response and a necrotizing chemical pneumonitis. The latter may be complicated by a superimposed bacterial infection. In the supine position, aspiration most commonly involves the right upper lobe, the superior segment of the right lower lobe, or the left perihilar region.

Chronic mild aspiration in infants may result in a bilateral, perihilar, interstitial infiltrate with hyperaeration (Figs. 9–27 and 9–28). This may progress to diffuse interstitial pneumonitis. It is speculated that repeated, low-level aspiration from gastroesophageal reflux may be a primary causal factor in diffuse interstitial pulmonary fibrosis.

Evaluation of unexplained chronic or recurrent pneumonias in infants with feeding difficulties includes an upper gastrointestinal series to determine the presence of gastroesophageal reflux (the most common cause of chronic vomiting and aspiration). This series also evaluates swallowing function, motility, and any obstructive lesions.

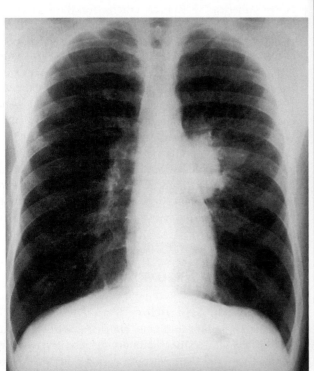
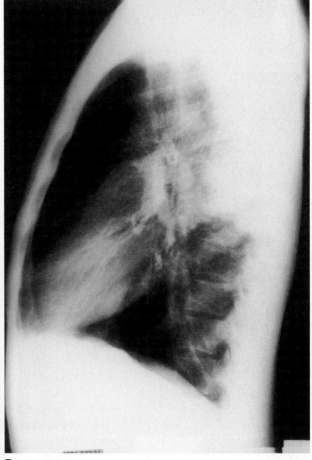

A   B

Figure 9–23
A 14-year-old child with proven primary tuberculosis. Frontal *(A)* and lateral *(B)* views of the chest show hyperinflation, prominent left hilar lymphadenopathy, and alveolar consolidation involving the posterior segment of the left upper lobe as well as the superior segment of the left lower lobe.

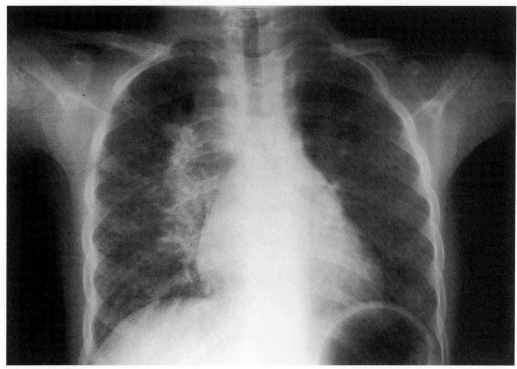

Figure 9–24

An 8-year-old child with a history of cough. A single frontal view of the chest shows marked right hilar and paratracheal lymphadenopathy with alveolar disease involving the right mid and lower lung fields. This was also a case of primary tuberculosis.

Endobronchial Foreign Body Aspiration

Most foreign body aspirations manifest acutely, causing little, if any, fever. Foreign bodies in the upper airways are discussed in Chapter 7. Smaller foreign bodies, such as nuts, buttons, and small toys, often pass beyond the larynx and trachea to lodge in a bronchus, producing the so-called "ball valve obstruction," with focal air trapping that is most easily diagnosed with an expiratory chest film.[94] If the foreign body lodges in and completely obstructs a bronchus, then lobar or segmental atelectasis, a less common occurrence, takes place, involving the lung distal to the obstructed bronchus.

In about one third of patients, the initial choking and coughing episode is not observed by the parents or care-givers; thus, a significant number of patients present initially with unexplained respiratory distress. An atelectatic lobe or segment distal to a complete obstruction becomes a focus for chronic or recurrent pneumonia. The correct diagnosis may not be suspected radiographically, because atelectasis is a very nonspecific finding. Even with ball valve air trapping, the lesion may be overlooked, as the assisted expiratory technique has a 5% rate of false-negative findings.[59,94] Bronchoscopy also is not a panacea. Foreign bodies, especially nuts, may be deliberately or accidentally crushed during removal and the fragments retained (fortunately, this occurs in fewer than 5% of all foreign body aspirations).

"Missed" foreign body aspiration usually produces chronic or recurrent cough and low-grade fever. Physical examination may elicit findings of atelectasis as well as wheezing that, because of reflex bronchospasm, may be global instead of focal. There may be mild elevation of the leukocyte count and an elevated sedimentation rate. In general, the clinical findings are nonspecific.

The most accurate technique for diagnosing bronchial foreign body with ball valve obstruction is expiratory chest radiography. However, most "missed" or chronic foreign bodies produce significant inflammation of the airway, leading to complete atelectasis.

The findings in foreign body aspiration with endo-bronchial impaction are lobar or subsegmental atelectasis, with superimposed episodes of pneumonia recurring in the same site (Figs. 9–29 and 9–30). During acute infections, empyema may occur. Commonly, there is ipsilateral hilar lymphadenopathy as a result of lymphadenitis. After endo-bronchial obstruction has been established, bronchoscopy is indicated. Complications of unsuccessful or incomplete removal of foreign bodies include air trapping, bronchiectasis, lung abscess, and septicemia.

Toxic Chemical Inhalation

Acute respiratory distress may follow thermal and chemical injury to the lungs, particularly inhalation of carbon

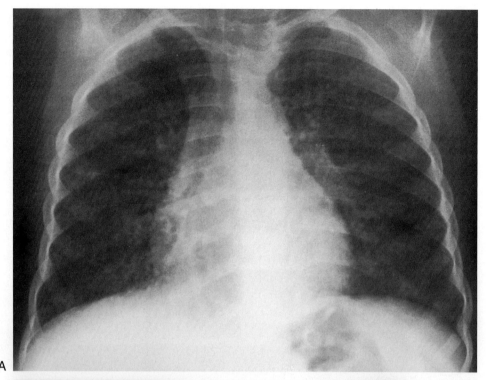

A

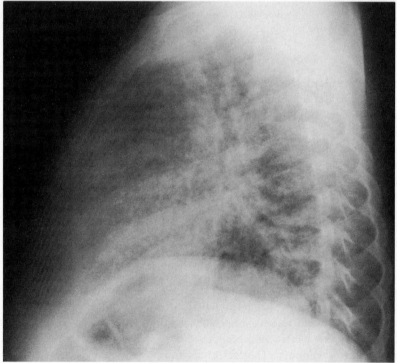

B

Figure 9–25

Miliary tuberculosis in a $2^1/_2$-year-old child with a 5-month history of chronic mild cough, low-grade fever, and severe failure to thrive. *A*, There is a diffuse interstitial pattern with a miliary component. *B*, Neither hyperaeration nor lymphadenopathy is seen. These findings are not specific for tuberculosis; a similar pattern is seen with idiopathic lymphoid hyperplasia and lymphoid interstitial pneumonitis in human immunodeficiency virus (HIV)/acquired immunodeficiency syndrome (AIDS).

monoxide with concomitant asphyxia after exposure to fire and smoke. A variety of noxious inhalants may be generated by fires; these include nitrogen and sulfur oxides, hydrochloric acid, acetaldehyde, corrosive acids and alkalies, and fine particles of soot.[19] Any of these noxious inhalants may produce diffuse alveolar edema and alveolitis.

Hydrocarbon Pneumonitis

Hydrocarbon pneumonia results from drinking fluids such as gasoline, kerosene, charcoal lighter fluid, and furniture polish. Pneumonia is caused by direct aspiration of the fluid into the lungs, inducing edema, inflammation, and hemorrhage. Initially, there is usually coughing and

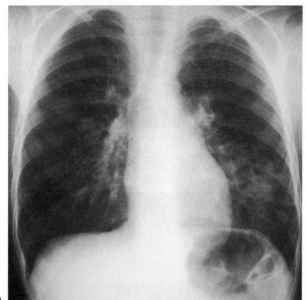
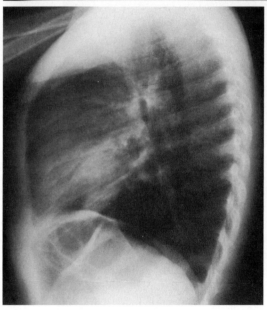

Figure 9–26
Asthmatic patient with allergic bronchopulmonary aspergillosis (ABPA). This 3-year-old child had recurrent episodes of asthma, then became febrile and acutely worse before these films were taken. *A*, Dense nodular foci are seen in the right mid-lung and left lower lung. *B*, The lungs are hyperaerated, with chronic infiltrates in the lingula and left lower lobe and centrally dilated bronchi. The nodular areas represent foci of mucoid impaction. Such centrally located bronchiectasis is characteristic of ABPA. The patient responded well to steroid therapy.

vomiting and, within hours, fever. With mild aspiration, the symptoms and radiographic findings may not be evident for 12 to 24 hours.

Radiographic findings typically consist of bilateral, basilar, ill-defined alveolar infiltrates (Fig. 9–31). In severe conditions, clinical clearing requires 2 to 5 days, usually with a delay in

radiographic clearing. During the healing phase, pneumatoceles often form within the areas of infiltration, generally after the first week. Complications, which are unusual, include superimposed bacterial infection, pneumothorax, pleural effusion, and empyema. Bacterial superinfection is likely if there is a recurrence of or a striking increase in fever during recovery. This is usually accompanied by increased infiltrate on chest films. In general, patient prognosis is excellent.

GENETIC DISEASES OF THE LUNGS

Cystic Fibrosis

Cystic fibrosis is the most common lethal genetic abnormality in North America. The condition is inherited as an autosomal recessive trait whose basic genetic defect remains undefined. Approximately 5% of whites are carriers (heterozygotes) of the cystic fibrosis gene. The incidence of homozygotes (patients who may have cystic fibrosis) is between approximately 1 in 1500 and 1 in 2000 live births. In contrast, the incidence in African-Americans is only 1 in 17,000 live births.[22]

Clinical Findings The major clinical manifestations of cystic fibrosis include chronic pulmonary disease, pancreatic exocrine insufficiency, and high sweat electrolyte concentrations. Abnormal secretions may accumulate and dilate any of the mucus-producing glands in the body. Absence or partial involvement of any of the various body systems leads to great heterogeneity in the clinical findings and in the severity of the disease.[63] At one end of the spectrum, the pulmonary disease may be manifested in infancy and progress rapidly to unrelenting recurrent and chronic pneumonias, bronchiectasis, cor pulmonale, and death before the child has reached the age of 6 years. At the other end, are the milder cases, seen in patients who are discovered to have pulmonary disease while in their late teens or even young adulthood.[58]

Chronic pulmonary disease affects most patients who have cystic fibrosis sooner or later, although the time of onset ranges from weeks to years after birth. The manifestation is commonly subtle: often a dry, nonproductive cough followed by an acute respiratory infection, either bacterial or viral, with variable degrees of respiratory distress and fever. This cycle tends to be repeated, with one respiratory tract infection following another. These pulmonary events are due to abnormally viscous mucus in the bronchial tree, producing bronchial and bronchiolar obstruction with secondary atelectasis. An atelectatic lung is readily infected. Successive infections progressively damage the bronchial walls, producing bronchiectasis. Once irreversible bronchiectasis occurs, there is continuous pooling of secretions, forming foci for perpetual or recurrent infection.

As a result of aggressive antibiotic therapy in affected patients, *P. aeruginosa*, *Burkholderia cepacia*, and

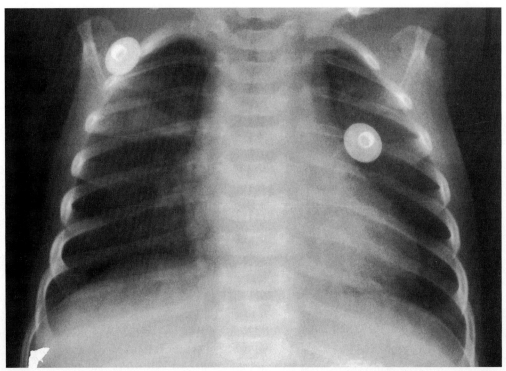

Figure 9–27
Transglottic aspiration of gastric contents: moderately severe chronic aspiration pneumonia. This 3-month-old child had gross gastroesophageal reflux that was resistant to medical management. The AP film reveals a patch of alveolar consolidation in the right upper lobe and also in the left lower lobe. Gastroesophageal reflux usually resolves by 1 year of age. If the reflux causes failure to thrive or recurrent pulmonary infiltrates, an antireflux procedure (Nissen fundoplication) is often curative.

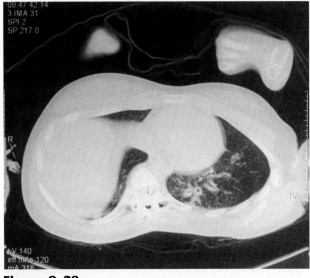

Figure 9–28
A 15-year-old patient with cerebral palsy who had bronchiectasis due to chronic aspiration. A CT scan in lung windows reveals the classic signet-ring sign in the left posterior basilar segment. There is peribronchial thickening and dilatation of the segmental bronchi, which are larger than their accompanying arteries.

Stenotrophomonas maltophilia have become the predominant organisms causing acute pneumonias in cystic fibrosis. Other organisms are identified much less frequently. Chronic *Pseudomonas* infections in patients with cystic fibrosis has become commonplace and, interestingly, seems to be surprisingly well tolerated. Such infections can be suppressed but not eradicated by treatment. This situation is the opposite of *Pseudomonas* infection in burn or immunosuppressed patients, in whom such infection is fulminant and commonly lethal.[22]

Radiographic Findings If a newborn presents with meconium ileus, the diagnosis of cystic fibrosis is certain. In the absence of meconium ileus, another finding that is highly suggestive of cystic fibrosis is persistent, unexplained, and often striking hyperaeration of the lungs, particularly when accompanied by recurring episodes of segmental or lobar atelectasis, most frequently in the upper lobes.[93] These findings are definite indications for a sweat test or genetic testing.

Most cases are not diagnosed until infancy (1 month to 2 years of age), when the pattern of recurrent or persistent respiratory tract infections is noted (Fig. 9–32). Almost all patients have or develop chronic sinusitis, and nasal polyps occur in 65% to 70% of these.

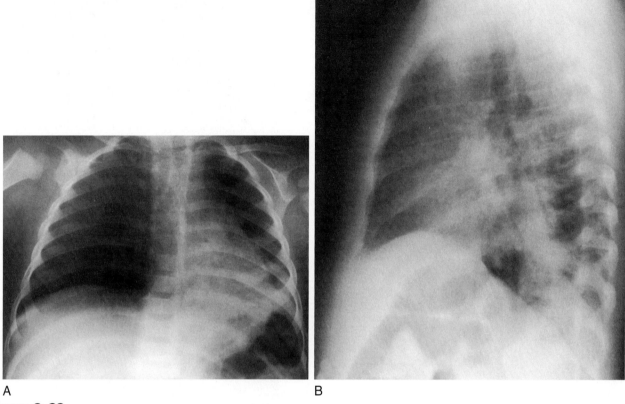

A   B

Figure 9–29
Endobronchial foreign body aspiration in an 18-month-old boy with recurrent left lower lobe pneumonias. *A*, Atelectasis of the left lower lobe is confirmed by a shift of the mediastinum toward the left and compensatory emphysema of the right lung. *B*, The lateral view shows dense atelectasis and pneumonia in the left lower lobe. An air bronchogram lies within the consolidation. Bronchoscopy revealed a peanut in the left mainstem bronchus.

The initial atelectasis and pneumonia in cystic fibrosis tend to involve the upper lobes more than the lower, but the disease very rapidly becomes diffuse (Fig. 9–33). Chronic bilateral pneumonia accompanies progressive bronchiectasis (Fig. 9–34). The hila are commonly enlarged, reflecting chronic lymphadenitis along with pulmonary hypertension in the later stages of the disease. The lungs become progressively hyperaerated and emphysematous, with flat hemidiaphragms and generally increased radiolucency (Fig. 9–33). Complications include pneumothorax and single or multiple lung abscesses. Unilateral or bilateral alveolar infiltrates in association with hemoptysis represent pulmonary hemorrhage and may be easily identified radiographically. Rarely, empyema may be a complication in infants.

Immotile Cilia Syndrome

Recognition of the immotile cilia syndrome is an outgrowth of investigations of Kartagener's syndrome, which involves situs inversus, bronchiectasis, and sinusitis. After specific ciliary abnormalities of respiratory epithelial cells were recognized, a genetic disorder of variable expression was defined. This syndrome also frequently includes chronic or recurrent otitis media, rhinitis, and nasal polyps. The *term immotile cilia syndrome* is used to describe the spectrum of this disorder.[58]

The incidence of immotile cilia syndrome has been estimated to be approximately 1 in 12,500 persons.[58] By way of comparison, the incidence of situs inversus is approximately 1 in 10,000 persons.

Clinical Findings The basic finding in the immotile cilia syndrome is impaired mucous clearance from the lungs by defective cilia. Chronic and recurrent episodes of upper respiratory tract infection and bronchitis are common. Untreated or inadequately treated bronchitis results in bronchiectasis.

The diagnosis of immotile cilia syndrome may be suspected when chronic or recurrent respiratory tract infections occur within a kinship that has a history of situs inversus. Definitive diagnosis requires electron microscopic examination of nasal or bronchial mucosa to evaluate ciliary morphology.[61]

Radiographic Evaluation and Findings The radiologic diagnosis of immotile cilia syndrome is apparent when Kartagener's triad of dextrocardia, sinusitis, and

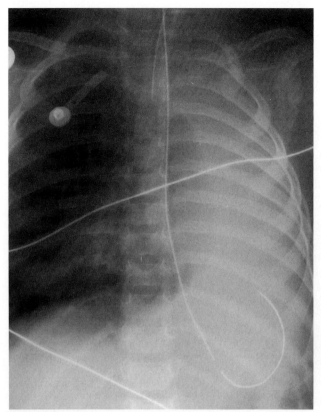

Figure 9–30

Endobronchial foreign body aspiration in a 4-year-old girl with gradual onset of fevers and respiratory distress. This frontal film reveals complete atelectasis of the left lung with herniation of the right lung across the midline. Also note the infiltrate in the region of the right hilum. Mild edema and inflammation of the right mainstem bronchus with complete occlusion of the left mainstem bronchus were seen at bronchoscopy. The plastic base of a Christmas tree light was tightly lodged in the left mainstem bronchus. Notably absent was any history of choking during the Christmas holidays, which had occurred 12 weeks earlier.

bronchiectasis is present. If Kartagener's triad is not present and immotile cilia syndrome is suspected, previous chest films of family members should be reviewed for situs inversus.

In milder cases of immotile cilia syndrome, nonspecific recurrent atelectasis or pneumonia, commonly with hyperaeration during acute illness, is often seen (Fig. 9–35). Complications include bronchiectasis (initially cylindrical, progressing to cystic), most commonly in the lower lobes, middle lobe, and lingula.

PNEUMONIAS IN THE COMPROMISED HOST

Human Immunodeficiency Virus/Acquired Immunodeficiency Syndrome

A condition distinct from other recognized immunodeficiency states was first described by Gottlieb et al. in 1981,

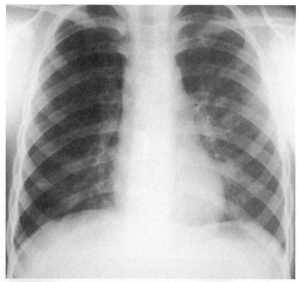

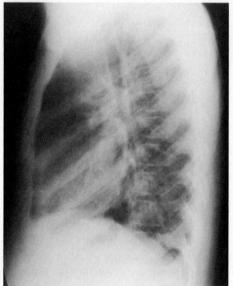

Figure 9–31

Acute hydrocarbon aspiration pneumonia in a 6-year-old boy who drank gasoline (stored in a soda bottle) 6 hours before presentation. *A,* Bilateral, ill-defined alveolar infiltrates are seen in the bases. *B,* The positive "spine sign" reflects infiltrate in the lower lobes. Note the sparing of the upper lobes, which is typical of hydrocarbon ingestion. Two weeks later, the patient was well but had asymptomatic pneumatoceles; these cleared in another 2 weeks.

in four homosexual patients who manifested mucosal candidiasis, recurrent cytomegalovirus (CMV) or *Pneumocystis jiroveci (*formerly *Pneumocystis carinii)* pneumonia, lymphopenia, and an absence of lymphocyte proliferation in response to antigens. This condition, known as acquired immunodeficiency syndrome (AIDS), has occurred in epidemic proportions, not only in the larger cities of the United States,

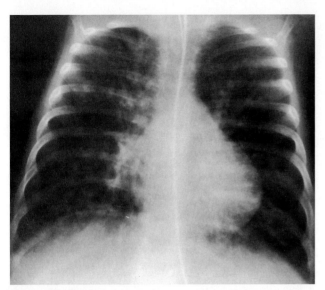

Figure 9–32
Cystic fibrosis with *Pseudomonas* pneumonia. This 3-month-old girl presented with mild tachypnea and unexplained hyperaeration of the lungs; a sweat test was positive. A bilateral, patchy bronchopneumonia is present. Tracheal washings grew *Pseudomonas*, the most common pathogen in cystic fibrosis.[98]

but also in Africa, India, South America, and some portions of Europe.

By the end 2001, an estimated 11.8 million people aged 15 to 24 were living with AIDS. During 2001, 800,000 new pediatric human immunodeficiency virus (HIV) infections were reported. During the same year 14 million children were orphaned by AIDS worldwide.[98]

HIV has been isolated from most tissues and secretions, including human semen, blood, urine, tears, saliva, cerebrospinal fluid (CSF), stool, cervix, lymph nodes, bone marrow, and brain tissue.

At the time of seroconversion, the patient may experience a mononucleosis-like syndrome, sometimes accompanied by aseptic meningitis. HIV can be isolated from CSF at that time. Asymptomatic carriers may remain so for a variable length of time, with some even surviving for a decade without symptoms. When the disease recurs, it is often with generalized adenopathy with or without constitutional symptoms of fatigue, weight loss, and gastrointestinal symptoms. Symptoms from HIV infections are mainly caused by involvement of the respiratory or gastrointestinal systems and, often, the central nervous system.

Initially, infected pediatric patients consisted of those who needed blood transfusion, most commonly for hemophilia. Most of these patients have since died or developed seropositivity or clinical symptoms of the disease. The other large group in whom HIV infection occurs are neonates born to infected mothers; the perinatal infection rate if the mother does not receive antiretroviral therapy during pregnancy is between 30% and 50%. With the use of antiretroviral therapy during pregnancy and immediately after birth in industrialized countries, the rate of perinatally acquired HIV infection has significantly decreased during the last decade. Unfortunately, that is not the case in developing countries where antiretroviral therapy is not widely available. In the United States there has been a recent increase in the rate of HIV infection among adolescents who engage in high-risk behaviors.[8,9] Currently, maternal infection is most commonly caused by sexual transmission or direct inoculation from contaminated needles shared among drug addicts.

Infected children may present initially with lymphoid interstitial pneumonitis composed of lymphocytes, plasma cells, and immunoblasts. At the time of this typical pulmonary alteration, the patient is usually asymptomatic. The radiographic appearance of this disease is identical to that of miliary tuberculosis,[26] and differentiation can usually be made clinically or by seropositivity (Figs. 9–36 and 9–37). Although lymphoid interstitial pneumonitis is predominantly seen in children, it has also been identified in adults.[75,79]

Pediatric acquired AIDS has nonspecific clinical manifestations, including failure to thrive, along with enteropathy and malabsorption, chronic diarrhea, persistent oral candidiasis, lymphadenopathy, and hepatosplenomegaly. Some children have the unusual symptom of parotid swelling.

Pulmonary disease is the major cause of morbidity and mortality in the pediatric and adult population. *P. jiroveci* and CMV are the most common infectious causes,[80] followed by *Mycobacterium avium*, *Mycobacterium kansasii*, *Cryptosporidium* species, and *Nocardia asteroides*. The appearance of pulmonary infections in children with AIDS is no different from that in immunodeficiency from other causes.

Other Opportunistic Pneumonias

Opportunistic pneumonias are caused by ordinary, nonpathogenic organisms that infect children with impaired host resistance. In the broad sense, opportunistic infection also includes unusual infections caused by ordinary pathogens and heightened susceptibility to ordinary pathogens; indeed, about half of the primary pneumonias in compromised hosts are caused by common pathogens rather than opportunistic organisms.[80] There are at least five general conditions that alter host defenses against pulmonary infection and thus predispose the host to opportunistic pneumonias (Table 9–5).

The three major modes of defense against pulmonary infection available to the host are (1) mechanical barriers in the upper and lower respiratory system that promote aerodynamic filtration of organisms; (2) successful phagocytosis and destruction of organisms by macrophages and leukocytes through interaction with serum proteins, and (3) the mucociliary transport system, including an intact cough mechanism and functional lymphatics, to remove organisms from the lung.[25]

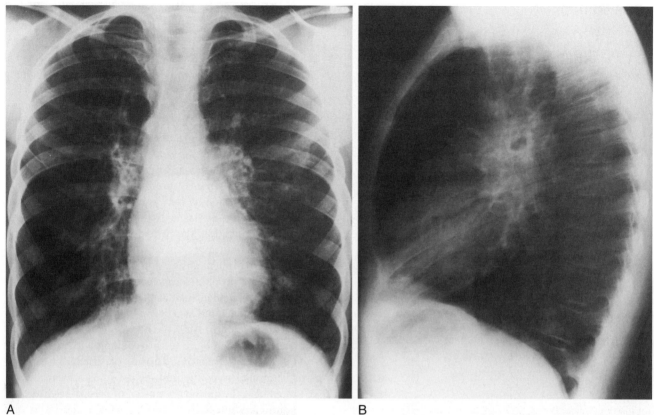

A   B

Figure 9–33
Severe, chronic changes of cystic fibrosis in a 14-year-old boy who had had numerous previous pneumonias, emphysema, and early clubbing of the fingers. *A*, Bilateral, perihilar pneumonia and fibrosis involve the upper and lower lobes. Bronchiectasis is seen in both lower lobes. *B*, The lateral view shows increased anteroposterior diameter and flattening of the hemidiaphragms. The hila are prominent because of a combination of chronic lymphadenitis and early pulmonary arterial changes of pulmonary hypertension.

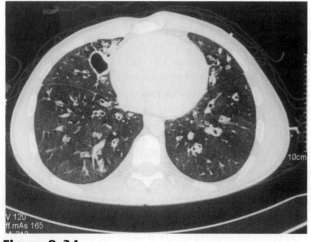

Figure 9–34
High-resolution CT in a 12-year-old with cystic fibrosis. Numerous areas of bronchiectasis are revealed in both lung bases. A particularly large cystic dilatation is seen in the right middle lobe.

Any of the innumerable factors and agents that may derange any aspect of host defenses can lead to opportunistic infection.

Clinical Findings The clinical findings of opportunistic pneumonias are as varied as the conditions listed in Table 9–5. The possibility of an opportunistic pneumonia should be strongly considered when pneumonia occurs in a child whose host defenses are known to be compromised. A greater challenge is pneumonia in a compromised child who has not yet been identified as such. Generally, immunodeficiency diseases are suggested by either an unusual response to normally benign infectious agents or infections with unusual organisms. Important organisms encountered in immunodeficient patients are *P. jiroveci*, CMV, rubeola virus, and varicella virus.[80] A patient who develops a pneumonia from any of these agents can reasonably be assumed to be immunosuppressed and requires an appropriate evaluation. The following are suggestive of immunodeficiency in general: *P. jiroveci* pneumonia, intractable diarrhea, intractable eczema, "ulcerative colitis" in children younger than 1 year of age, severe seborrheic dermatitis (Leiner's disease), and recurrent pyogenic infections.[80]

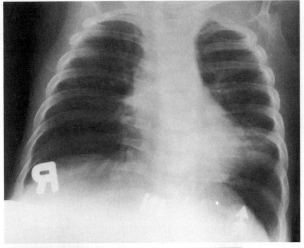

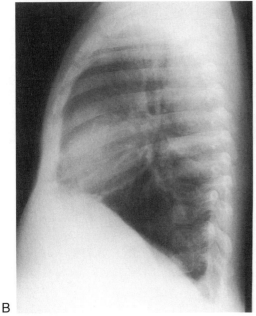

Figure 9–35
Immotile cilia syndrome in an 8-month-old boy who was a sibling of a patient with Kartagener's syndrome. The child had recurrent pneumonias, chronic sinusitis, and chronic otitis media. *A,* Acute pneumonia is seen in the superior segment of the right lower lobe and the lingula. *B,* The hemidiaphragms are flattened, confirming hyperaeration. The infiltrates in the superior segment of the right lower lobe and lingula are evident. The patient responded to antibiotic therapy.

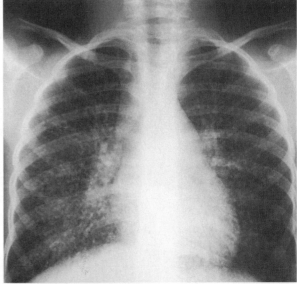

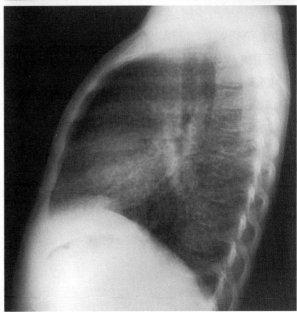

Figure 9–36
HIV infection. Frontal *(A)* and lateral *(B)* radiographs of a 14-year-old boy with hemophilia who was HIV-positive but asymptomatic. Note the diffuse, tiny nodules evenly distributed throughout the lungs. The boy was prophylactically treated with aerosolized pentamidine when he developed his first *Pneumocystis jiroveci* infection 6 months after these radiographs were taken but succumbed to overwhelming *P. jiroveci* pneumonia 3 years later.

Radiographic Findings The radiologic findings of bacterial pneumonia in compromised hosts are similar to those in normal children: usually lobar or segmental dense consolidation, with or without air bronchograms, or a patchy, bronchopneumonic pattern. The common pathogenic viral pneumonias occur with considerable frequency in compromised hosts, with radiographic findings of perihilar and interstitial disease identical to those in noncompromised children.[67,97] Certain specific infections display patterns that are somewhat more distinctive; these are described in the next section.

Although radiographic patterns of disease may assist in distinguishing these entities (see Figs. 9–36 and 9–37), lung biopsy (percutaneous or open) may be required, especially in cases in which progression is rapid.

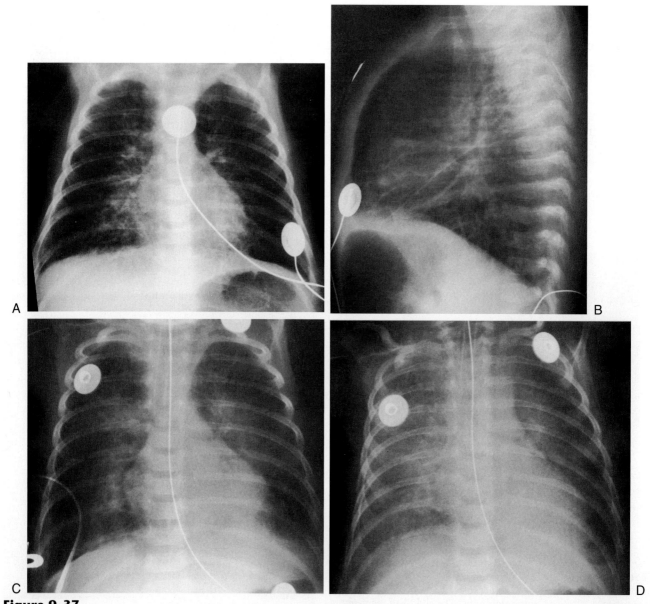

Figure 9–37
Opportunistic infection: *P. jiroveci* pneumonia in a 1-month-old girl who was treated with total parenteral nutrition. She was acutely tachypneic and mildly cyanotic. *A*, Bilateral interstitial infiltrates fan out from the hila. *B*, Lung hyperaeration and a diffuse interstitial infiltrate are evident. *C*, Eight hours after presentation, the pattern has become a bilateral alveolar process with a "bat wing" appearance. A small pneumomediastinum is present. The extreme periphery of the lungs is clear. *D*, Ten hours after presentation, the diffuse alveolar process is approaching complete opacity. This very rapid progression of diffuse interstitial infiltrates to an extensive alveolar process is typical for *P. jiroveci* pneumonia in a patient who is immunosuppressed for any reason. The pattern in *A* and *B* is also very suggestive of cytomegalovirus (CMV) infection in a compromised child. With CMV pneumonia, however, this interstitial pattern usually persists.

Specific Organisms Causing Opportunistic Pneumonias *P. jiroveci* pneumonia is currently the most common opportunistic pneumonia seen in immunocompromised children. It is particularly common in patients with T-cell deficiency, as well as in patients receiving chronic steroid therapy, immunosuppressive therapy, cytotoxic chemotherapy, and irradiation. Patients tend to be clustered, particularly in pediatric oncology wards. *Pneumocystis*

pneumonia may have either a fulminant or an insidious (subacute) onset. The fulminant form is characterized by a sudden onset of cough, fever, and tachypnea and rapid development of cyanosis. The respiratory symptoms progress out of proportion to the auscultatory and radiologic findings. Dyspnea, the most prominent symptom, occurs in more than 90% of patients.[63] The subacute form has a protracted course with gradually progressive symptoms over a 1- to

TABLE 9-5 DIAGNOSIS OF PATHOGENS IN THE COMPROMISED HOST

HOST DEFECT	EXAMPLE OF DISORDER	LIKELY PATHOGENS
Defective neutrophils	Chronic granulomatous disease *Neutropenia*	Gram-negative bacteria *S. aureus, Aspergillus spp*
Defective complement pathways	Congenital and collagen-vascular diease	*S. pneumoniae, H. influenzae*
Cell-mediated Immunodeficiency (T-cell)	HIV infection, chemotherapy corticosteroid therapy	Mycobacteria, HSC, CMV *P. jiroveci. Cryptococcus* *T. gondii, Nocardia spp* *Candida albicans*
Humoral immunodeficiency (B-cell)	agammaglobulinemia Multiple myeloma Selective IgA deficiency	*S. pneumoniae, H. influenzae* *S. aureus*

2-month period. In one fourth of patients with *Pneumocystis* pneumonia, other concurrent infections (e.g., CMV infection) exist.

The initial radiographic findings are bilateral, ill-defined, perihilar infiltrates that may extend to the periphery of the lung in an interstitial pattern (Fig. 9–37). The radiographic findings are rarely as striking as the very rapid clinical deterioration. In the fulminant form, a bilateral alveolar pattern appears, within 6 to 12 hours, with central density fanning out from the hila (Fig. 9–37C and D). Severe disease may progress to diffuse alveolar "whiteout" of the lungs (Fig. 9–38). The chronic form of *Pneumocystis* pneumonia may originate with a localized consolidated area or nodular foci.[80] Minimal amounts of pleural effusion may be seen.

Cytomegalovirus CMV pneumonia, like many opportunistic infections, varies in severity with the degree of host

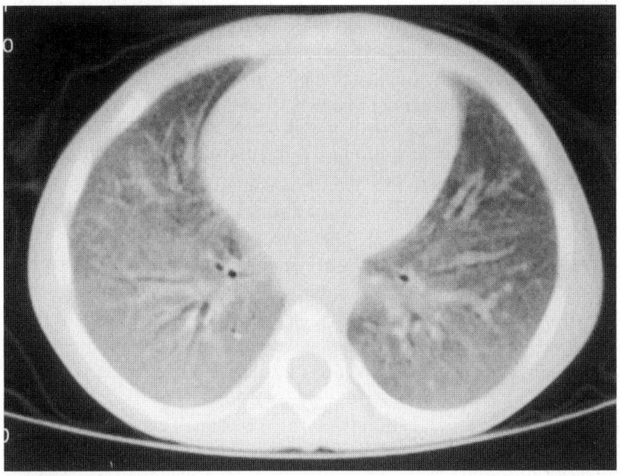

Figure 9–38
A 3-year-old child with HIV infection and *P. jiroveci* pneumonia. On this CT image, there is diffuse interstitial as well as alveolar disease involving both lung bases. This patient had severe symptoms of pneumonia.

immunosuppression. In addition, CMV pneumonia further impairs both cellular and humoral defenses against infection, and, therefore, severe superinfection, especially by gram-negative bacilli and *Pneumocystis*, is common.

Viruses of note found in immunodeficient patients are influenza, herpes simplex, and varicella zoster.[61] These commonly produce diffuse, bilateral, perihilar infiltrates, with superimposed micromiliary nodules or diffuse acinar densities. Persistent infection with RSV has been associated with severe combined immunodeficiency.

Toxoplasmosis simulates the radiographic pattern of *P. jiroveci* infection, progressing rapidly from early mild perihilar infiltrates to rapid alveolar filling.

Another group of pneumonias include those caused by atypical mycobacteria of which *M. avium* complex (MAC) is the prototype. MAC is a common cause of pulmonary infection especially among immunocompromised individuals with T-cell deficiencies such as advanced HIV infection (Fig. 9–39).[1,81]

SUMMARY

Cough and fever are important symptoms in children and frequently indicate pneumonia. Most pneumonias in preschool children are viral in nature; in school-age children most are atypical. The differential diagnosis of pneumonias may be based on the patient's age or the character of the illness (acute or chronic and recurring). By combining the two approaches, an intelligent assessment can be made of the organisms or causative agents that are most likely to be responsible. Such assessment is particularly important early in the course of pneumonia, before microbiologic techniques have established the diagnosis with certainty, because specific antibiotic therapy may thereby be instituted.

When a child who has cough and fever is evaluated, the most basic and essential radiographic procedure is technically

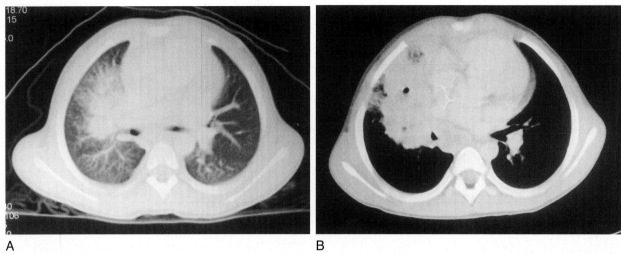

A   B

Figure 9–39
A 5-year-old child with HIV infection and *Mycobacterium avium* complex (MAC) pneumonia. *A*, The initial CT image in the lung windows demonstrates right middle lobe consolidation and right hilar adenopathy. *B*, A CT image in the mediastinal windows from the same patient at the lung bases reveals extensive infrahilar lymphadenopathy and alveolar consolidation of the right middle lobe.

adequate frontal and lateral chest films. Ancillary radiographic techniques may be suggested by the findings on these films or by clinical evaluation of specific entities. The chest film provides the essential immediate information, namely, a strong suggestion as to whether the agent encountered is most apt to be viral, specific atypical, or other bacterial, in which case antimicrobial drugs are required. This information is most pertinent in the acute situation. Certain more or less characteristic radiographic features of various infections permit probability estimates of the most likely etiologies, but it must be recalled that the radiograph is no substitute for bacteriologic tests, and pneumonias of many different causes may look alike during imaging. It is crucial that the radiographic findings be interpreted in light of the clinical features.

REFERENCES

1. Abbassi S, Chesney PJ. Pulmonary manifestations of cat-scratch disease: A case report and review of the literature. Pediatry Infect Dis J 14:547–548, 1995.
2. Agrons GA, Markowitz RL, Kramer SS. Pulmonary tuberculosis in infants and children. Semin Roentgenol 28:158–172, 1993.
3. Ambrosino MM, Roche KJ, Genieser NB, Kaul A, Lawrence RM. Application of thin-section low-dose chest CT (TSCT) in the management of pediatric AIDS. Pediatr Radiol 25:393–400, 1995.
4. Bachur R, Perry H, Harper MB. Occult pneumonias: Empiric chest radiographs in febrile children with leukocytosis. Ann Emerg Med 33:166–173, 1999.
5. Block S, Hedrick J, Hammerschlag MR, Cassell GH, Craft JC. *Mycoplasma pneumoniae* and *Chlamydia* pneumonias in pediatric community-acquired pneumonia: Comparative efficacy and safety of clarithromycin vs. erythromycin ethylsuccinate. Pediatr Infect Dis J 14:471–477, 1995.
6. Buck GE, Eid NS. Diagnosis of *Mycoplasma pneumoniae* pneumonia in pediatric patients by polymerase chain reaction (PCR). Pediatr Pulmonol 20:297–300, 1995.
7. Castriota-Scanderbeg A, Popolizio T, Sacco M, Coppo M, Scarale MG, Cammisa M. Diagnosis of *Mycoplasma* pneumonia in children: Which is the role of thoracic radiography? Radiol Med (Torino) 89:782–786, 1995.
8. Centers for Disease Control and Prevention (CDC). Heterosexual transmission of HIV—29 states 1999–2002. MMWR Morb Mortal Wkly Rep 53:125–129, 2004.
9. Centers for Disease Control and Prevention (CDC). Trend in tuberculosis—United States 1998–2003. MMWR Morb Mortal Wkly Rep 53:209–214, 2004.
10. Copley SJ, Coren M, Nicholson AG, Rubens MB, Bush A, Hansell DM. Diagnostic accuracy of thin-section CT and chest radiography of pediatric interstitial lung disease. AJR Am J Roentgenol 174:549–554, 2000.
11. Coren ME, Ng V, Rubens M, Rosenthal M, Bush A. The value of ultrafast computed tomography in the investigation of pediatric chest disease. Pediatr Pulmonol 26:389–395, 1998.
12. Darvill T. *Chlamydia*. Pediatr Rev 19:85–91, 1988.
13. Davis SF, Sutter RW, Strebel PM, et al. Concurrent outbreaks of pertussis and *Mycoplasma pneumoniae* infection: Clinical and epidemiological characteristics of illness manifested by cough. Clin Infect Dis 20:621–628, 1995.
14. Donnelly LF, Klosterman LA. Pneumonia in children: Decreased parenchymal contrast enhancement-CT sign of intense illness and impending cavitary necrosis. Radiology 205:817–820, 1997.
15. Donnelly LF, Klosterman LA. The yield of CT of children who have complicated pneumonia and noncontributory chest radiography. AJR Am J Roentgenol 170:1627–1631, 1998.
16. Donnelly LF, Strife JL, Bisset GS. The spectrum of extrinsic lower airway compression in children: MR imaging. AJR Am J Roentgenol 168:59–62, 1997.
17. Edelman RR; Hatabu H, Tadamura E, Li W, Prasad PV. Noninvasive assessment of regional ventilation in the human lung using oxygen-enhanced magnetic resonance imaging. Nat Med 2:1236–1239, 1996.
18. Estrada B. A new human paramyxovirus on the horizon. Infect Med 20:7, 2003.

19. Estrada B. Human metapneumovirus: What have we learned? Infect Med 21 :59, 2004.

20. Estrada B. Pediatric bulletin: Preventing pneumococcal disease in young children. Infect Med 17:318–319, 2000.

21. Evans ED, Kramer SS, Kravitz RM. Pediatric diseases of the lower airways. Semin Roentgenol 33:136–150, 1998.

22. Feigin RD, Cherry J, Demmler G, et al. Textbook of Pediatric Infectious Diseases. 4th ed. Philadelphia: WB Saunders; 2003.

23. File TM, Jan JS. *Chlamydia pneumoniae* pneumonia, Semin Respir Crit Care Med 21:285–294, 2000.

24. Gendrel D, Raymond J, Moulin F, et al. Etiology and response to antibiotic therapy of community-acquired pneumonia in French children. Eur J Clin Microbiol Infect Dis 16; 388–391, 1997.

25. Glezen WP, Taber LH, Frank AL, Kasel JA. Risk of primary infection and reinfection with respiratory syncytial virus. Am J Dis Child 140:543–546, 1996.

26. Gonzalez Dominguez I, Sabata Diaz J, Lopez Barrio A, Leon Leal JA, Lucena de Lucena E. Clinico-radiological correlation of pulmonary complications of pediatric HIV infection. Rev Clin Esp 199:496–502, 1999.

27. Gordon RC. Community-acquired pneumonia in adolescents. Adolesc Med 11:681–695, 2000.

28. Griscom NT. Caldwell lecture. Respiratory problems of early life now allowing survival into adulthood: Concepts of radiologists. AJR Am J Roentgenol 158:1–8, 1992.

29. Griscom NT. Diseases of the trachea, bronchi and smaller airways. Radiol Clin North Am 31:605–615, 1993.

30. Griscom NT. Pneumonia in children and some of its variants. Radiology 167:297–302, 1998.

31. Grossman LK, Caplan SE. Clinical, laboratory, and radiological information in the diagnosis of pneumonia in children. Ann Emerg Med 17:43–46, 1998.

32. Guckel C, Benz-Bohm G. Widemann B. Mycoplasmal pneumonias in childhood: Roentgen features, differential diagnosis and review of literature. Pediatr Radiol 19:499–503, 1989.

33. Hamelin M, Abed Y, Boivin G. Human metapneumovirus: A new player among respiratory viruses. Clin Infect Dis 38:983–990, 2004.

34. Hammerschlag MR: *Chlamydia pneumoniae* and the lung. Eur Respir J 16:1001–1007, 2000.

35. Han BK, Son JA, Yoon HK, Lee SI. Epidemic adenoviral lower respiratory tract infection in pediatric patients: Radiographic and clinical characteristics. AJR Am J Roentgenol 170:1077–1080,1998.

36. Harris JA, Kolokathis A, Campbell M, Cassel GH, Hammerschlag MR. Safety and efficacy of azithromycin in the treatment of community-acquired pneumonia in children. Pediatr Infect Dis J 17:865–871, 1998.

37. Hatabu H, Chen Q, Stock KW, Gefter WB, Itoh H. Fast magnetic resonance imaging of the lung. Eur J Radiol 29:114–132, 1999.

38. Hatabu H, Stock KW, Sher S, et al. Magnetic resonance imaging of the thorax: Past, present, and future. Clin Chest Med 20:775–803, 1999.

39. Hedlund GL, Navoy JF, Galliani CA, Johnson WH Jr. Aggressive manifestations of inflammatory pulmonary pseudotumor in children. Pediatr Radiol 29:112–116, 1999.

40. Heiskanen-Kosma T, Korppi M, Laurila A, Jokinen C, Kleemola M, Saikku P. *Chlamydia pneumoniae* is an important cause of community-acquired pneumonia in school-age children: Serological results of prospective, population-based study. Scand J Infect Dis 31:255–259, 1999.

41. Helbich TH, Heinz-Peer G, Eichler I, et al. Cystic fibrosis: CT assessment of lung involvement in children and adults. Radiology 213:537–544, 1999.

42. Heller RM, Hernanz-Schulman M. Applications of new imaging modalities to the evaluation of common pediatric conditions. J Pediatr 135:632–639, 1999.

43. Hickey RW, Bowman MJ, Smith GA. Utility of blood cultures in pediatric patients found to have pneumonia in the emergency department. Ann Emerg Med 27:721–725, 1996.

44. Hoffer FA, Bloom DA, Colin AA, Fishman SJ. Lung abscess versus necrotizing pneumonia: Implications for interventional therapy. Pediatr Radiol 29:87–91, 1999.

45. Howard TS, Hoffman LH, Stang PE, Simoes EA. Respiratory syncytial viral pneumonia in the hospital setting: Length of stay, charges, and mortality. J Pediatr 137:227–232, 2000.

46. Jadavji T, Law B, Lebel MH, Kennedy WA, Gold R, Wang EE. A practical guide for the diagnosis and treatment of pediatric pneumonia. CMAJ 156:703–711, 1997.

47. John SD, Ramanathan J, Swischuk LE. Spectrum of clinical and radiographic findings in pediatric mycoplasma pneumonia. Radiographics 21:121–131, 2001.

48. Johnson CS: Sickle cell disease: The acute chest syndrome, 1995. Available at http://sickle.bwh.harvard.edu/acutechest.html.

49. Juven T, Mertsola J, Waris M, et al. Etiology of community-acquired pneumonia in 254 hospitalized children. Pediatr Infect Dis J 19:293–298, 2000.

50. Kaste SC: Issues specific to implementing PET-CT for pediatric oncology: What we have learned along the way. Pediatr Radiol 34:205–215, 2004.

51. Kiekara O, Korppi M, Tanska S, Soimakallio S. Radiological diagnosis of pneumonia in children. Ann Med 28:69–72, 1996.

52. Kim OH, Kim WS, Kim MJ, Jung JY, Suh JH. US in the diagnosis of pediatric chest disease. Radiographics 20:653–671, 2000.

53. Knott AM, Long CE, Hall CB. Parainfluenza viral infections in pediatric outpatients: Seasonal patterns and clinical characteristics. Pediatr Infec Dis J 13:269–273, 1994.

54. Korppi M. Kiekara O, Heiskanen-Kosma T, Soimakallio S. Comparison of radiological findings and microbial aetieology of childhood pneumonia. Acta Pediatr 82:360–363, 1993.

55. Kuhn JP. Disorders of pulmonary circulation. In Kuhn JP, Slovis TL, Haller JO, eds. Caffey's Pediatric Diagnostic Imaging. 10th ed. Philadelphia: Mosby, 2004, pp 1086–1088.

56. Kuhn JP, Brody AS: High-resolution CT of pediatric lung disease. Radiol Clin North Am 40 :89–110, 2003.

57. Latham-Sadler BA, Morell VW. Viral and atypical pneumonias. Prim Care 23:837–848, 1996.

58. Long SS, Pickering LK, Prober CG, et al. Principles and Practice of Pediatric Infectious Diseases. 2nd ed. London: Churchill Livingstone, 2002.

59. Lucaya J, Garcia-Peña P, Herrera L, Enriquez G, Piqueras J. Expiratory chest CT in children, AJR Am J Roentgenol 174:235–241, 2000.

60. Lundstrom K, Allen GC, Colman JA, et al., eds. Catscratch Disease. eMedicine.com, Inc., 2005.

61. Lynch DA, Hay T, Newell JD, Jr. Divgi VD, Fan LL. Pediatric diffuse lung disease: Diagnosis and classification using high-resolution CT. AJR Am J Roentgenol 173:713–718, 1999.

62. Macfarlane J, Rose D. Radiographic features of staphylococcal pneumonia in adults and children. Thorax 51:539–540, 1996.

63. Maldonado YA, Arantha RG, Hersh AL. *Pneumocystis carinii* pneumonia prophylaxis and early clinical manifestations of severe perinatal human immunodeficiency virus type 1 infection. Northern California Pediatric HIV Consortium. Pediatr Infect Dis J 17:398–402, 1998.

64. Mancao M, Manci E, Figarola MS. Fusobacterium necrophorum infection presenting as an anterior chest wall mass in a child. Clin Pediatr 44:73–75, 2005.

65. Manson D, Reid B, Dalal I, Roidman CM. Clinical utility of high-resolution pulmonary computed tomography in children with antibody deficiency disorders. Pediatr Radiol 27:794–798, 1997.

66. Markowitz RI, Ruchelli E. Pneumonia in infants and children: Radiological-pathological correlation. Semin Roentgenol 33:151–162, 1998.

67. Marks MJ, Haney PJ, McDermott MP, White CS, Vennos AD. Thoracic disease in children with AIDS. RadioGraphics 16:1349–1362, 1996.

68. Marrie TJ. Pneumococcal pneumonias: Epidemiology and clinical features. Semin Respir Infect 1:227–236, 1999.

69. Martinez-Aguilar G, Hammerman WA, Mason EO Jr, Kaplan SL. Clindamycin treatment of invasive infections caused by community-acquired, methicillin-resistant and methicillin-susceptible Staphylococcus aureus in children. Pediatr Infect Dis J 22:593–598, 2003.

70. McIntosh K, Mc Adam AJ. Human metapneumovirus—An important new respiratory virus. N Engl J Med 350:431–435, 2004.

71. Miller ST, Hammerschlag MR, Chirgwin K, et al. Role of Chlamydia pneumoniae in acute chest syndrome of sickle cell disease. J Pediatr 118:30–33, 1991.

72. Mongkolrattanothai K, Boyle S, Kahana MD, Daum RS. Severe Staphylococcus aureus infections caused by clonally related community-acquired methicillin-susceptible and methicillin-resistant isolates. Clin Infect Dis 37:1050–1058, 2003.

73. Mufson MA, Stanek RJ. Bacteremic pneumococcal pneumonia in one American city: A 20-year longitudinal study, 1978–1997. Am J Med 107:34S-43S, 1999.

74. O'Brien KL, Walters MI, Sellman J, et al. Severe pneumococcal pneumonia in previously healthy children: The role of preceding influenza infection. Clin Infect Dis 30:784–789, 2000.

75. Oh YW, Effmann EL, Godwin JD. Pulmonary infections in immunocompromised hosts: The importance of correlating the conventional radiologic appearance with the clinical setting. Radiology 217:647–656, 2000.

76. Oppenheim C, Mamou-Mani T, Sayegh N, de Blic J, Scheinmann P, Lallemand D. Bronchopulmonary dysplasia: Value of CT in identifying pulmonary sequelae. AJR 163:169–172, 1994.

77. Owayed AF, Campbell DM, Wang EE. Underlying causes of recurrent pneumonia in children. Arch Pediatr Adolesc Med 154:190–194, 2000.

78. Patel JC, Mollitt DL, Pieper P, Tepas JJ 3rd. Nosocomial pneumonia in the pediatric trauma patient: A single center's experience. Crit Care Med 28:3530–3533, 2000.

79. Pennington DJ, Lonergan GJ, Benya EC. Pulmonary disease in the immunocompromised child. J Thorac Imaging 14:37–50, 1999.

80. Perez Mato, Van Dyke RB. Pulmonary infections in children with HIV infection. Semin Respir Infect 17:33–46, 2002.

81. Phongsamart W, Chokephaibulkit K, Chaiprasert A, vanprapa N, chearskul S, Lolekha R. Mycobacterium avium complex in HIV infected Thai children. J Med Assoc Thai 85(Suppl 2):S682–S689, 2002.

82. Prevention and control of influenza: Recommendations of the Advisory Committee on Immunization Practices (ACIP). MMWR 46:1–25, 1997.

83. Ruuskanen O, Mertsola J. Childhood community-acquired pneumonia. Semin Respir Infect 14:163–172, 1999.

84. Saez-Llorens X, Castano E, Wubbel L, et al. Importance of Mycoplasma pneumoniae and Chlamydia pneumoniae in children with community-acquired pneumonia. Rev Med Panama 23:27–33, 1998.

85. Seely JM, Effmann EL, Muller NL. High-resolution CT of pediatric lung disease: Imaging findings. AJR Am J Roentgenol 168:1269–1275, 1977.

86. Stark JM. Lung infection in children. Curr Opin Pediatr 5:273–280, 1993.

87. Steele RW, Thomas MP, Kolls JK. Current management of community-acquired pneumonia in children: An algorithmic guideline recommendation. Infect Med 16:46–54, 1999.

88. Tristram DA, Miller RW, McMillan JA, Weiner LB. Simultaneous infection with respiratory syncytial virus and other respiratory pathogens. Am J Dis Child 142:834–836, 1988.

89. Tuomanen EI, Austrian R, Masure HR. Pathogenesis of pneumococcal infection. N Engl J Med 332:1280–1284, 1995.

90. Vuori E, Peltola H, Kallio MJ, Leinonen M, Hedman K. Etiology of pneumonia and other common childhood infections requiring hospitalization and parenteral antimicrobial therapy. Clin Infect Dis 27:566–572, 1998.

91. Wahlgren H, Mortensson W, Eriksson M, Finkel Y, Forsgren M, Leinonen M. Radiographic patterns and viral studies in childhood pneumonia at various ages. Pediatr Radiol 25:627–630, 1995.

92. Waris ME, Toikka P, Saarinen T, et al. Diagnosis of Mycoplasma pneumoniae pneumonia in children. J Clin Microbiol 36:3155–3159, 1998.

93. Wesenberg RL. The Newborn Chest. Hagerstown, MD: Harper & Row, 1973.

94. Wesenberg RL, Blumhagen JD. Assisted expiratory chest radiography. Radiology 130:538, 1979.

95. White CS. Magnetic resonance imaging of the chest. Resp Care 46:922–931, 2001.

96. Williams JV, Harris PA, Tollefson SJ, et al. Human metapneumovirus and lower respiration tract disease in otherwise healthy infants and children. N Eng J Med 350 :443–450, 2004.

97. Winer-Muram HT, Archeart KL, Jennings SG, et al. Pulmonary complications in children with hematologic malignancies: Accuracy of diagnosis with chest radiography and CT. Radiology 204:643–649, 1997.

98. World Health Organization: Children and young people are at the center of the HIV epidemic, 2004. Available at http://www.who.int/child-adolescent-health/HIV/HIV_epidemic.htm.

99. Wubbel L, Muniz L, Ahmed A, et al. Etiology and treatment of community-acquired pneumonia in ambulatory children. Pediatr Infect Dis J 18:98–104, 1999.

100. Zhang L, Irion K, da Silva Porto N, Abreu e Silva F. High-resolution computed tomography in pediatric patients with postinfectious bronchiolitis obliterans. J Thorac Imaging 14:85–89, 1999.

ADDITIONAL READING

Andronikou S, Joseph E, Lucas S, et al. CT scanning for the detection of tuberculosis mediastinal and hilar lymphadenopathy in children. Pediatr Radiol 34:232–236, 2004.

Andronikou S, Wieselthaler N. Modern imaging of tuberculosis in children: Thoracic, central nervous system and abdominal tuberculosis. Pediatr Radiol 34:861–875, 2004

Babyn PS, Gahunia HK, Massicotte P. Pulmonary thromboembolism in children. Pediatr Radiol 35:258–n274, 2005.

Chokephailbvilkit K, et al. A child with Avian Influenza A (H5N1) infection. The Pediatric Infectious Diseases Journal 24:162–166, 2005.

Hammerschlag MR. Chlamydia pneumoniae and the heart: Impact of diagnostic methods. Curr Clin Top Infect Dis 22:24–41, 2002.

Klig JE. Current challenges in lower respiratory infections in children. Curr Opin Pediatr 16:107–112, 2004.

McGraw EP, Kane JM, Kleinman MB, Scherer LR, Cervical abscess and mediastinal adenopathy: An unusual presentation of childhood histoplasmosis. Pediatr Radiol 32:862–864, 2002.

Michelow IC, Olsen K, Lozano J, et al. Epidemiology and clinical characteristics of community-acquired pneumonia in hospitalized children. Pediatrics. 113:701–707, 2004.

Monagle P, Adams M, Mahoney M, et al. Outcome of pediatric thromboembolism disease: A report from the Canadian Childhood Thrombophilia Registry. Pediatr Res 47:763-766, 2000.

Moon WK, Kim WS, Kim I-O, et al. Complicated pleural tuberculosis in children: CT evaluation. Pediatr Radiol 29:153–157, 1999.

Neu N, Saiman L, San Gabriel P, et al. Diagnosis of pediatric TB in the modern era. Pediatr Infect Dis J 18:122–126, 1999.

Salazar GE, Schmitz TL, Cama R, et al. Pulmonary tuberculosis in children in a developing country. Pediatrics 108:448–453, 2001.

Schlegel N. Thromboembolic risks and complications in nephritic children. Semin Thromb Hemost 23:271–280, 1997.

Swischuk LE. Vomiting, diarrhea and—oh! oh! what is that? Pediatr Emerg Care 20:54–56, 2004.

Tormente D, Simioni P, Prandoni P, et al. The incidence of venous thromboembolism in thrombophilic children: A prospective cohort study. Blood 100:2403–2405, 2002.

Ulloa-Gutierrez R, Skippen P, Synnes A, et al. Life-threatening human metapneumovirus pneumonia requiring extracorporeal membrane oxygenation in a preterm infant. Pediatrics. 114:e517-e519, 2004.

van Ommen CH, Heijboer H, Buller HR, Hirasing RA, Heijmans HS, Peters M. Venous thromboembolism in childhood: A prospective two-year registry in The Netherlands. J Pediatr 139:676-681, 2001.

Vargas SO, Kozakewich HP, Perez-Atayde AR, McAdam AJ. Pathology of human metapneumovirus infection: Insights into the pathogenesis of a newly identified respiratory virus. Pediatr Dev Pathol 7:478–486, 2004.

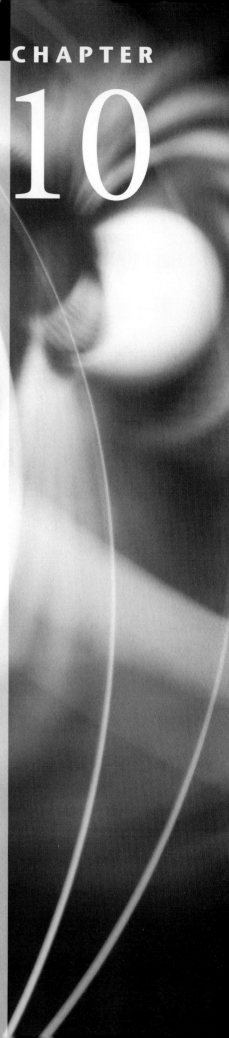

THE CHILD WITH ABDOMINAL TRAUMA

Outline

Marilyn J. Siegel, MD

THE CHILD WITH ABDOMINAL TRAUMA

Trauma accounts for about 10% of all childhood deaths[18] and is the leading cause of death among children ages 1 to 14 years. Blunt trauma causes more than one half of trauma-related deaths and injuries and is usually due to motor vehicle accidents.[18] Other causes of blunt trauma include bicycle, skateboard, all-terrain vehicle, or motorcycle accidents; falls; and assaults.[7] The remaining trauma-related deaths and injuries are due to gunshot or stabbing incidents, burns, drowning, and child abuse.

Multisystem injury is typical of blunt trauma, and the common sites of injury are the musculoskeletal system and head and neck followed by the abdomen and thorax. Abdominal injuries occur in approximately 8% of children with major trauma.[18] The majority of such injuries are hepatic, splenic, or renal. Pancreatic, intestinal, and mesenteric injuries occur far less commonly. The detection or confident exclusion of these injuries is a challenging problem. In this chapter the value of diagnostic imaging studies, particularly computed tomography (CT), in assessing intra-abdominal organs after trauma and in effecting patient management is discussed.

GENERAL CLINICAL CONSIDERATIONS

PRIMARY ASSESSMENT

The initial and essential goal in the management of children with major or multisystem injuries is recognition and treatment of potentially life-threatening injuries.[18,33,44] Most preventable deaths in children with blunt trauma are caused by (1) acute respiratory failure resulting from airway obstruction, tension pneumothorax, or hemothorax; (2) massive hemorrhage, producing shock; and (3) severe intracranial injuries. Details of acute hemodynamic and respiratory resuscitation are beyond the scope of this text.

Once the patient is stable, an orderly, system-oriented physical examination; laboratory studies; diagnostic imaging; and other diagnostic or therapeutic procedures, such as peritoneal lavage or chest tube placement, are appropriate.[10,44] The diagnosis of abdominal injuries can be difficult in children with altered mental status and in young children who are unable to accurately localize the sites of injury.[95] Signs and symptoms of abdominal injury include abdominal tenderness, ecchymosis, abrasion, and distention. Laboratory results suggesting intra-abdominal trauma include elevation of liver enzyme levels, substantial hematuria, and dropping or low hematocrit levels.[33,129] When there is a strong history or external signs of abdominal trauma or abnormal laboratory tests, abdominal CT examination is indicated, but only if the patient is clinically and hemodynamically stable.[126,129] Patients who have unreliable physical examinations because of young age or impaired neurologic status also are candidates for CT imaging. Neurologic impairment without signs referable to the abdomen is a low-yield indication for CT.[4,125]

ASSOCIATED INJURIES

The distribution of traumatic injuries, by organ system, is as follows: head or spine, 79%; musculoskeletal, 36%; thoracic, 24%; abdominal, 17%; and soft tissue, 11%.[10,18] (Percentages total more than 100% because of multisystem injuries.) When compared with adults, children tend to have relatively more diffuse cerebral edema and fewer intracranial hemorrhages.[44] When hemorrhagic lesions occur, they are usually intracerebral hematomas or, uncommonly, subdural or epidural hematomas.[10]

The most common chest injuries are pulmonary contusion (49% to 65%), pneumothorax or hemothorax (34% to 35%), and rib fractures (35% to 70%).[18,44,79,115,121] Parenchymal lacerations, great vessel trauma, pneumopericardium, airway or esophageal rupture, and sternal injuries are less frequent.

Fractures of the femur, tibia, and humerus are common extremity injuries. These injuries are not life threatening, but they must be recognized to make the patient comfortable and to preserve limb function.

IMAGING EVALUATION

GENERAL IMAGING CONSIDERATIONS

Once the patient has been stabilized and a thorough physical examination has been performed, cross-table lateral cervical spine and anteroposterior chest radiographs are obtained, usually with the patient immobilized on a stretcher or backboard. If these do not demonstrate abnormalities that require immediate treatment, standard radiographs of the cervical spine should be performed, as fractures of the odontoid process, C1–C2 rotary injuries, and C7 injuries may be occult on the lateral view alone.[96] Next, radiographs of the skull,

face, thoracolumbar spine, abdomen, and extremities are obtained if clinically indicated. A head CT scan is needed in children with signs of intracranial injury. As noted earlier, abdominal CT is indicated when evaluation of the abdomen is unreliable. CT is also indicated to confirm suspected solid organ or hollow viscera injuries. Patients who are in shock or have life-threatening head, chest, or abdominal injuries and unstable vital signs require urgent surgical intervention without the delay implicit with an abdominal CT scan.

CT has virtually replaced all other imaging studies in the evaluation of blunt and penetrating abdominal trauma because of its noninvasive nature and excellent sensitivity (95%).[40,56,102] It permits rapid identification of patients needing surgical treatment and allows for more confident nonoperative management of children with relatively minor injuries.[40,51,57,76,77,80,93–95,129,130,132]

Grading of the severity of hepatic and splenic injury has been suggested in an attempt to predict which patients can be managed conservatively and in which patients nonoperative management is more likely to fail (Tables 10–1 and 10–2).[76] These systems evaluate the size of the injury, integrity of the capsule, involvement of the hilar and segmental vessels, and extent of nonperfused parenchyma. As expected, the incidence of operation increases with increasing severity of injury. However, grading systems are not infallible, and some patients with extensive splenic parenchymal injuries and a large hemoperitoneum can be managed nonoperatively. The grading system for the severity of pancreatic injury is based on the extent of parenchymal injury and ductal disruption (Table 10–3).[77] Unlike solid organ injuries, which generally are managed more conservatively, hollow viscus injury usually is an indication for prompt surgery.

Before the advent of CT, abdominal sonography and scintigraphy had been widely used to image children following abdominal trauma. However, the sonographic examination is often impaired by abdominal tenderness and the ileus associated with trauma. Moreover, the spleen may be difficult to evaluate because of a gas-filled stomach. The main value of sonography in patients with blunt abdominal trauma is in detecting hemoperitoneum.[8,15,50,59,70–72] The sonographic finding of fluid indicates solid or hollow viscus injury. When sonography demonstrates peritoneal fluid in a hemodynamically stable patient, CT is indicated to detect the presence and extent of intra-abdominal injury. In the unstable patient, clinical judgment will determine the need for exploratory laparotomy or CT. Scintigraphy is no longer utilized in abdominal trauma because it is insensitive and organ specific.

CT has also replaced peritoneal lavage in the assessment of hemodynamically stable children with suspected abdominal injury. Peritoneal lavage has a sensitivity of greater than 95% for detecting abdominal injuries, but it also has a number of limitations, including overestimation of the severity of injury, nonspecificity, and invasiveness.[52] Lavage detects only intraperitoneal injuries, not those in the retroperitoneum.

TABLE 10-1 SPLEEN INJURY SCALE

GRADE	INJURY DESCRIPTION	
I	Hematoma	Subcapsular, <10% surface area
	Laceration	Capsular tear, <1 cm parenchymal depth
II	Hematoma	Subcapsular, 10%–50% surface area: intraparenchymal, <5 cm in diameter
	Laceration	1–3 cm parenchymal depth that does not involve a trabecular vessel
III	Hematoma	Subcapsular, >50% surface area or expanding; ruptured subcapsular or parenchymal hematoma; intraparenchymal hematoma >5 cm or expanding
	Laceration	<3 cm parenchymal depth or involving trabecular vessels
IV	Laceration	Laceration involving segmental or hilar vessels producing major devascularization (>25% of spleen)
V	Laceration	Completely shattered spleen
	Vascular	Hilar vascular injury which devascularizes spleen

From Moore EE, Cogbill TH, Jurkovich GJ, Shackford SR, Malangoni MA, Champion HR. Organ injury scaling: spleen and liver (1994 revision). *J Trauma* 323–324, 1995.

TABLE 10-2 LIVER INJURY SCALE

GRADE	INJURY DESCRIPTION	
I	Hematoma	Subcapsular, <10% surface area
	Laceration	Capsular tear, <1 cm parenchymal depth
II	Hematoma	Subcapsular, 10%–50% surface area: intraparenchymal, <10 cm in diameter
	Laceration	1–3 cm parenchymal depth, <10 cm in length
III	Hematoma	Subcapsular, >50% surface area or expanding; ruptured subcapsular or parenchymal hematoma; intraparenchymal hematoma >10 cm or expanding
	Laceration	>3 cm parenchymal depth
IV	Laceration	Parenchymal disruption involving 25%–75% of hepatic lobe or 1–3 Couinaud's segments within a single lobe
V	Laceration	Parenchymal disruption involving >75% of hepatic lobe or >3 Couinaud's segments within a single lobe
	Vascular	Juxtahepatic venous injuries; i.e., retrohepatic vena cava/central major hepatic veins

From Moore EE, Cogbill TH, Jurkovich GJ, Shackford SR, Malangoni MA, Champion HR. Organ injury scaling: spleen and liver (1994 revision). *J Trauma* 323–324, 1995.

TABLE 10-3 PANCREATIC INJURY SEVERITY SCALE

GRADE	INJURY DESCRIPTION
I	Minor contusion or superficial laceration without duct injury
II	Major contusion or laceration without duct injury or tissue loss
III	Distal transection or parenchymal injury with duct injury
IV	Proximal transection or parenchymal injury involving ampulla
V	Massive disruption of pancreatic head

From Moore EE, Cogbill TH, Malangoni MA, et al. Organ injury scaling: pancreas, duodenum, small bowel, colon, and rectum. *J Trauma* 30:1427–1429, 1990.

If the decision to operate is based only on lavage demonstration of hemoperitoneum, then up to 85% of children with positive peritoneal lavage results will undergo unnecessary laparotomies.[129] Indications for peritoneal lavage include evaluation of the child who is hemodynamically unstable or who has a severe head injury and is unable to undergo abdominal CT and confirmation of suspected bowel perforation.

TECHNICAL ASPECTS OF COMPUTED TOMOGRAPHIC IMAGING

Identification of abdominal visceral injuries requires the use of intravenous contrast medium to improve differentiation between normal and pathologic parenchyma.[58,100,101,102]

Parenchymal injuries are hypovascular and easily recognized as low-attenuation areas compared with the adjacent enhancing parenchyma. The diagnosis of active arterial hemorrhage and leakage of contrast-opacified urine is also facilitated by vascular opacification.[46,58,99] Non–contrast-enhanced scans add little if any useful clinical information in the evaluation of blunt abdominal trauma.

The use of oral contrast medium is controversial. The risk of a potential delay in diagnosis and lack of substantial added benefit for detection of bowel and mesenteric injury have been stated as reasons to eliminate the use of oral contrast material in the CT evaluation of abdominal trauma.[2,29,41,124] The use of multidetector CT, with its ability to acquire thinner sections with higher resolution, appears to allow improved detection of distal small bowel, colonic, and mesenteric injuries without the use of oral contrast material.[124] The benefit of the use of oral contrast material may be in the improved detection of duodenal and proximal jejunal injuries. Thus, when possible, hemodynamically stable patients without neurologic injury should receive oral contrast medium to ensure opacification of proximal small bowel loops. In neurologically impaired patients with absent gag or cough reflexes, all remaining oral contrast medium in the stomach at the conclusion of the CT examination should be withdrawn via the nasogastric tube to minimize the risk of aspiration. The remaining oral contrast medium is usually not withdrawn from the stomach in neurologically intact children because the risk of aspiration is extremely low.

Sedation has little role in the setting of acute abdominal injuries. It is contraindicated in children with significant head injury or those who are vomiting and at risk for aspiration.

Technique

Intravenous contrast medium can be administered by mechanical or hand injection. The former type of administration should be performed if a 22-gauge or larger cannula can be placed into an antecubital vein. The injection rate for the contrast medium is determined by the caliber of the intravenous catheter. Contrast medium is infused at 1.5 to 2.5 mL/sec for a 22-gauge catheter and at 3.0 to 4.0 mL/sec for a 20-gauge catheter. The site of injection is closely monitored during the initial injection of contrast medium to minimize the risk of contrast medium extravasation. The contrast medium should be administered by a hand injection using a bolus technique if intravenous access is through a peripheral access line or a smaller caliber antecubital catheter.

For most abdominal trama CT scans, the scan delay time between the start of contrast medium administration and scan initiation is 55 to 60 seconds. CT angiography is used in the evaluation of suspected great vessel injuries. The time delay for an arterial phase acquisition is 20 to 25 seconds. Delayed images through the abdomen and pelvis should be obtained after the arterial phase imaging. The venous phase images are acquired 55 to 60 seconds after the start of contrast medium administration.[100]

Strategies that minimize radiation dose are mandatory for CT examinations in children. The milliamperage needs to be the lowest possible that maintains image quality.[39] A peak kilovoltage of 80 kVp should be considered for patients weighing less than 50 kg. In larger patients, a higher peak kilovoltage (100–120 kVp) should be used to compensate for the higher noise.[106]

CT examinations should be performed with scan times of 1 second or less. Detector collimation and pitch will vary depending on the type of scanner used. For a four-row detector scanner, 2.5-mm collimation with a pitch of 1.5 to 2.0 is adequate for routine scanning. For a 16-row detector, 1.25- to 1.5-mm collimation with a pitch of 1.0 to 1.5 suffices. For a 64-row detector, 0.6- to 1.25-mm collimation and a pitch of 1.0 to 1.5 suffices (See Protocol 10–1).

CT examinations are performed with breath-holding at suspended inspiration in cooperative patients, usually children older than 5 to 6 years of age. Scans are obtained during quiet respiration in children who are unable to cooperate with breath-holding instructions and in patients who are sedated.

Before the examination, all extraneous tubes, catheters, and electrocardiograph monitor leads should be removed from the field of view. The tip of a nasogastric tube should be withdrawn into the esophagus to minimize streak artifacts. The patient's arms are routinely extended above the head whenever possible to decrease streak artifacts from dense cortical bone and to provide an accessible route for intravenous injection. The upper extremities can be restrained by sandbags, adhesive tape, or Velcro straps.

The CT images are viewed at standard soft tissue window (level, 40 Hounsfeld units [HU]; width, 350 HU). In addition to soft-tissue windows, images of the lower thorax and upper abdomen should be viewed at lung windows (level, −500 to −600 HU; width, 1500 to 2000 HU) to increase detection of small pneumothoraces and free intraabdominal air. The CT scans should also be viewed with bone window settings (level, 400 HU; width, 1500 HU) if vertebral or pelvic fractures are suspected.

IMPORTANT CONDITIONS ASSOCIATED WITH ABDOMINAL TRAUMA

HEMOPERITONEUM

The mesenteric attachments and peritoneal compartments largely determine the spread and site of intraperitoneal fluid and blood. Knowledge of these anatomic compartments, which have been elegantly described by Meyers,[73,74] will

PROTOCOL 10–1

INDICATION	ABDOMEN/PELVIS SURVEY
Extent	Diaphragm to pubic symphysis
Scanner settings	kVp: 80 for patients weighing <50 kg; higher kVp for larger patient
	mA: lowest possible based on patient weight
Detector collimation	4-row: 2.5 mm
	16-row: 1.25–1.5 mm
	64-row: 0.6–1.25 mm
Pitch	4-row: 1.5–2.0
	16-row: 1.0–1.5
	64-row: 1.0–1.5
Slice reconstruction thickness	3–5 mm for viewing
Oral contrast medium	Water-soluble contrast material given 45–60 minutes before scan. Additional volume given 15 minutes before scan.
	Oral contrast medium should be used with caution if patient has a depressed level of consciousness.
Intravenous contrast volume	2 mL/kg (maximum of 4 Ml/kg or 125 mL)
Contrast injection rate	Hand injection: rapid bolus administration
	Power injector:
	22 gauge: 1.5 –2.5 mL/sec
	20 gauge: 3.0–4.0 mL/sec
Scan delay	55–60 seconds after onset of contrast injection (i.e., scan in portal venous phase of enhancement)
Miscellaneous	1. Arterial phase images should be acquired if vascular injury is suspected.
	2. Delayed images are helpful if an abnormality of the bladder or renal collecting system is suspected.

facilitate recognition of free fluid and intraperitoneal blood.

The peritoneal cavity is divided into the upper abdomen and pelvis. The transverse mesocolon divides the abdominal cavity into supra- and inframesocolic compartments. The supramesocolic peritoneal cavity is divided into right and left spaces by the falciform ligament. The right peritoneal compartment contains the perihepatic space, which consists of a subphrenic space, subhepatic space, and the lesser sac. The left peritoneal space is divided into the anterior and posterior perihepatic spaces and the anterior and posterior subphrenic spaces. The right subhepatic space is continuous inferiorly with the right pericolic gutter. In contrast, the left subphrenic space is divided from the left pericolic gutter by the phrenicocolic ligament.

Small amounts of blood from hepatic injuries generally pool in the right subhepatic space, or Morison's pouch, because of its dependent posterior position. Larger amounts spill over into the right subphrenic space and the right pericolic gutter and from there to the pelvis. Once in the pelvis, fluid may extend into the left pericolic gutter. Blood from splenic injuries initially collects in the left subphrenic area; it may then flow across the midline into Morison's pouch.

Flow down the left pericolic gutter is limited by the phrenicocolic ligament.[73,74] In the pelvis, blood preferentially accumulates in the posterior cul-de-sac and the paravesical fossae of the pelvis (Fig. 10–1).

Freshly extravasated intraperitoneal blood has the same attenuation value as unenhanced circulating blood (30 to 45 HU).[63] A lower attenuation value may indicate underlying anemia, prior peritoneal lavage resulting in dilution of the hemorrhage, or a delay or 24 hours or more between the time of trauma and the CT examination. Within hours of the acute injury, clot formation begins and the attenuation value of the blood increases, reaching 50 to 100 HU. Very densely clotted blood may have an attenuation value exceeding 100 HU. Within several days, clot lysis begins, and the attenuation value of the blood starts to decrease. After 2 to 3 weeks, lysed blood usually has attenuation values close to those of water (0 to 20 HU). In some patients, the resolving blood may show a hematocrit effect with layering of the lighter, low-attenuation supernatant serum on the heavier, high-attenuation sedimented erythrocytes and clot. The presence of a large amount of peritoneal blood suggests that severe abdominal trauma has occurred and is associated with an increased need for laparotomy[114] and blood

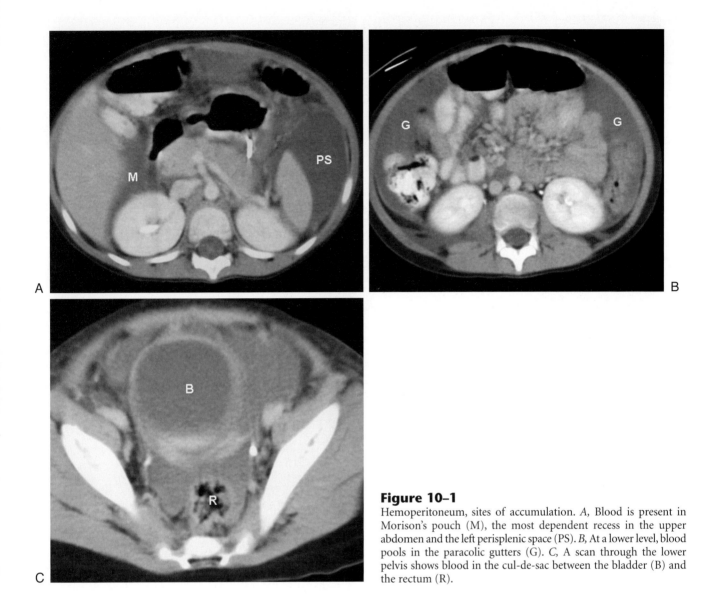

Figure 10–1

Hemoperitoneum, sites of accumulation. *A*, Blood is present in Morison's pouch (M), the most dependent recess in the upper abdomen and the left perisplenic space (PS). *B*, At a lower level, blood pools in the paracolic gutters (G). *C*, A scan through the lower pelvis shows blood in the cul-de-sac between the bladder (B) and the rectum (R).

transfusion. It does not necessarily reflect active hemorrhage. Hemoperitoneum is most commonly associated with hepatic and splenic injuries.

Hemoperitoneum usually shows substantial clearing or resolution by 7 days. Hemoperitoneum that remains unchanged or increases in volume 3 to 7 days after injury should raise concern for ongoing intraperitoneal bleeding.

HYPOVOLEMIC SHOCK

Visceral injuries producing large volumes of intraperitoneal blood and large losses of fluid into the gastrointestinal tract may result in significant loss of circulatory volume (hypovolemia) and hypovolemic shock. As noted previously, patients who are hemodynamically unstable and demonstrate signs of hypovolemic shock require surgery rather than radiologic evaluation. Occasionally, the severity of blood loss is not clinically obvious, and a CT scan is done because of suspected abdominal injury.

The CT findings of hypovolemia are a flattened inferior vena cava and renal veins and sometimes a small aorta. The CT findings indicating systemic hypotension and hypovolemic shock consist of diffuse dilatation of bowel with fluid; abnormally intense contrast enhancement of the bowel wall, mesentery, and kidneys; diminished size of the inferior

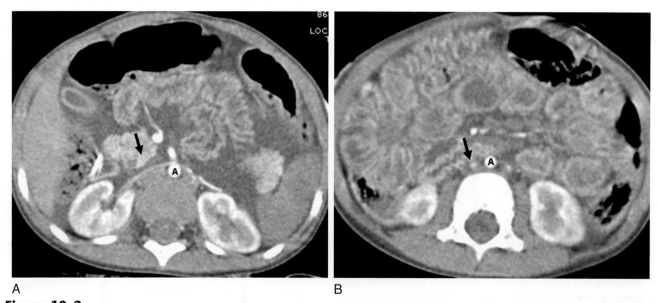

A   B

Figure 10–2
Hypovolemic shock. A and B, Two contrast-enhanced computed tomography (CT) scans show dilated small bowel with intensely enhancing walls and a small aorta *(A)* and inferior vena cava *(arrow)*. Blood is noted in Morison's pouch and in the mesentery.

vena cava and abdominal aorta; and large hemoperitoneum (Fig. 10–2).[47,113,128]

In some patients with hypovolemia and massive intraperitoneal hemorrhage, a focal collection of extravasated contrast material may be noted at the site of active bleeding.[46,99,112,131] This finding usually indicates hemodynamic instability and should suggest immediate surgical intervention. The freshly extravasated blood has an attenuation value similar to that of the abdominal aorta and its branches. It often is surrounded by low-attenuation hematoma (Fig. 10–3).

HEPATIC INJURIES

The liver is the most commonly injured organ, accounting for approximately 40% of blunt abdominal injuries.[55,56,132] Affected children typically present with abdominal pain and tenderness and elevated hepatic enzyme levels.[42,83] Although these tests of liver function can identify children with hepatic injury, they cannot reliably determine the severity of injury. The extent of injury and amount of hemoperitoneum are accurately depicted by CT.[137]

Imaging Appearance
Hepatic injuries are characterized according to site of involvement and type of injury. The right hepatic lobe is injured in about 80% of pediatric patients, the left lobe in approximately 20%, and the caudate lobe in 1 to 2%. Multiple hepatic segments are injured in approximately 35% of patients. Of right lobe injuries, two-thirds occur in the

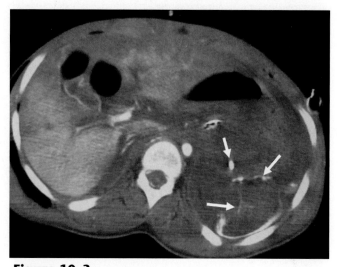

Figure 10–3
Active arterial extravasation. A CT scan through the upper abdomen shows high-attenuation areas of extravasated contrast-enhanced blood *(arrows)* in the splenic parenchyma, which is nonenhancing. Avulsion of the splenic vascular pedicle with active bleeding was confirmed at surgery.

posterior segment, and the remainder occur in the dome and in the anterior segment. Left lobe injuries are evenly divided between the medial and lateral segments.[120]

The spectrum of hepatic injuries includes subcapsular and parenchymal hematomas, lacerations, and fractures.[120]

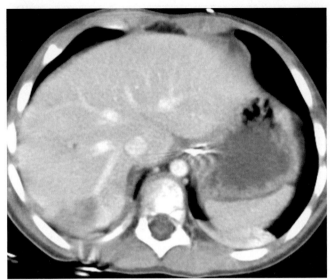

Figure 10–4
Intrahepatic hematoma. A contrast-enhanced CT scan demonstrates a low-attenuation hematoma in the posterior aspect of the right hepatic lobe.

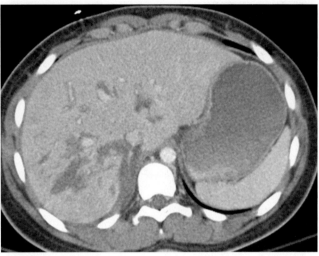

Figure 10–6
Complex hepatic laceration. Note the branching pattern of multiple low-attenuation lacerations.

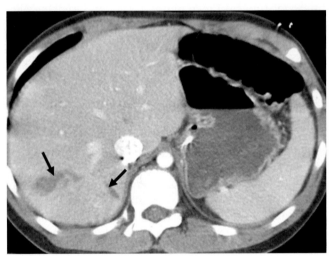

Figure 10–5
Simple hepatic laceration. A linear low-attenuation laceration *(arrows)* is seen in the parenchyma of the right hepatic lobe.

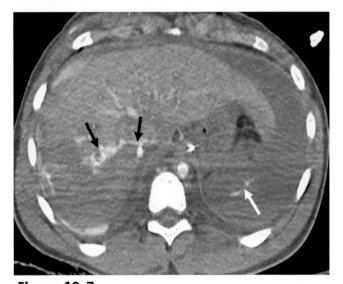

Figure 10–7
Hepatic fracture. A deep parenchymal laceration extends through the right hepatic lobe posteriorly, resulting in an avulsed, nonperfused segment. Linear area of high attenuation indicates active bleeding *(black arrows)*. An area of arterial bleeding is also noted in the perisplenic space *(white arrow)*, resulting from an associated splenic injury. Also noted is a hemoperitoneum.

Subcapsular hematomas appear as low-attenuation lenticular fluid collections that flatten the lateral hepatic margin. Most occur along the anterolateral margin of the right hepatic lobe. Intrahepatic hematomas appear as either oval or rounded collections of blood with either well-defined or irregular margins (Fig. 10–4), whereas lacerations appear as linear or branching areas within the hepatic parenchyma. Well-defined, linear lacerations are referred to as *simple lesions* (Fig. 10–5), whereas poorly defined, disorganized lacerations with a branching or stellate appearance are termed *complex lesions* or *intrahepatic burst injuries* (Fig. 10–6). Hepatic fractures extend completely through the parenchyma, dividing it into two or more separate fragments (Fig. 10–7). In general, right lobe injuries tend to be hematomas or simple lacerations, and left lobe injuries are more often complex lesions.[120]

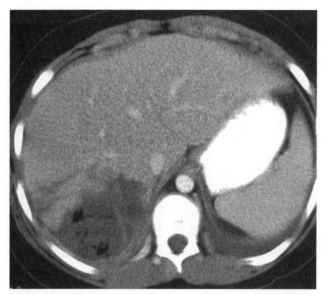

Figure 10–8
Intraparenchymal gas. A CT scan 2 days after blunt abdominal trauma demonstrates an intrahepatic hematoma posteriorly containing small bubbles of gas, representing tissue ischemia and necrosis. The gas and hematoma progressively decreased in size and resolved with conservative management.

After a bolus injection of intravenous contrast medium, the normal liver increases in density; hepatic hematomas and lacerations do not enhance and appear hypodense. Rarely, they are hyperdense compared with normal liver if there is active hemorrhage at the site of laceration.[138]

Other findings associated with hepatic injuries include intraparenchymal or subcapsular gas, presumably related to hepatic necrosis,[1,86] and low-attenuation areas surrounding portal structures, referred to as *periportal tracking*.[69,88,98,104,116] Intraparenchymal or subcapsular gas usually occurs 1 to 2 days after blunt trauma (Fig. 10–8). Periportal tracking of blood or lymph has been demonstrated in 50% of patients with hepatic injuries. Two thirds of patients with periportal tracking have either hepatic lacerations or fractures; in the remaining patients, periportal tracking is the only sign of injury (Fig. 10–9). Periportal edema is attributed to increased central venous pressure secondary to tension pneumothorax, pericardial tamponade, or vigorous administration of intravenous fluids.

Parenchymal injuries are frequently associated with hemoperitoneum. The amount of hemoperitoneum is variable; it may be small and limited to the right subphrenic and subhepatic spaces or when more marked, filling the pericolic gutters and pelvis.

Imaging Pitfalls

Potential pitfalls relate to beam-hardening artifacts from adjacent ribs and streak artifacts from gastric air-fluid levels.

Ideally, the stomach should be deflated or at least not overdistended with air. Streak artifacts tend to be linear, whereas lacerations and fractures are irregular.

Clinical Management

Approximately two thirds of children with hepatic injuries evident on CT have associated abdominal or thoracic injuries. Right hepatic injuries are more often associated with rib fractures, pneumothorax, lung contusions, and ipsilateral renal injuries. Left hepatic lobe trauma is more usually associated with pancreatic and duodenal injuries.[120]

Acute hepatic injury does not represent a surgical emergency in most children. Most patients with blunt hepatic injuries are treated conservatively, especially when an isolated subcapsular or intrahepatic lesion with little or no hemoperitoneum is demonstrated by CT.[9,21,38,43,84] Indeed, most patients with hepatic fractures, capsular disruptions, and relatively large amounts of hemoperitoneum can be successfully managed conservatively unless there is continuous massive bleeding or extrahepatic injuries that require operation. The leading cause of death is exsanguination, usually from laceration of major hepatic vessels or the inferior vena cava.[84]

Hepatic hematomas and lacerations characteristically undergo an orderly progression of resolution, beginning with resorption of the hematoma and intraperitoneal blood during the first 10 to 14 days after injury.[15,34] Occasionally, an early increase in the size of the lesion may be noted, probably as a result of coalescence of lacerations. Complete healing usually occurs by 6 months.[21] Persistent or increasing hemoperitoneum or progression of any parenchymal lesion over several examinations suggests an unstable lesion with ongoing hemorrhage.[34]

Sonography has also been used in the follow-up evaluation of hepatic injuries.[21,137] Hepatic injuries have a variable sonographic appearance related to the age of the hematoma. Acute parenchymal or subcapsular blood appears hyperechoic or nearly isoechoic with normal liver because of the presence of fibrin or clot formation. Within 2 to 3 days, the hematoma becomes more hypoechoic and cystic as the blood undergoes liquefaction with resorption of hemoglobin.

Complications

Complications occur in about 10% of patients with hepatic injuries and include biloma, hepatic abscess, aneurysm, pseudoaneurysm, and hemobilia.[68,83,84,120] Bilomas may be intrahepatic or located within the peritoneal cavity. They appear as well-defined, water-attenuation masses on CT and as anechoic masses with enhanced sound transmission on sonography. Occasionally, they contain debris and a few septations. Hepatic abscesses may appear either as unilocular masses or as complex masses with internal septations. On CT, they appear as low-attenuation lesions with enhancing walls. On sonography, they range from hypo- to hyperechoic lesions. Percutaneous needle aspiration is the method

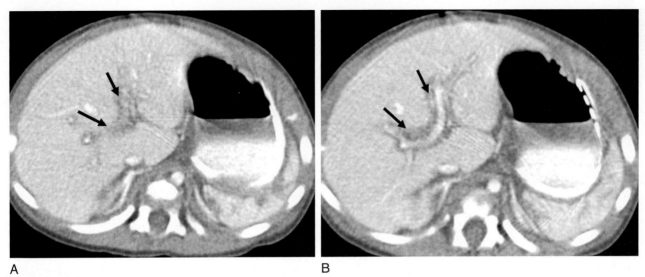

Figure 10–9
Periportal low attenuation. *A* and *B,* Two CT scans demonstrate low attenuation areas *(arrows)* surrounding the enhanced portal vasculature. There was no CT evidence of an overt hepatic injury. In this case, the periportal low attenuation was attributed to lymphedema secondary to elevated central venous pressure following vigorous intravenous fluid resuscitation. The splenic heterogeneity is normal and is related to early acquisition of images following administration of intravenous contrast material.

of choice to distinguish between biloma and abscess and is often therapeutic. Post-traumatic hepatic aneurysms and pseudoaneurysms demonstrate color signals on Doppler sonography and show enhancement after administration of intravenous contrast material. Such lesions require either angiographic embolization or surgery. Hemobilia, or hemorrhage from the biliary tree, appears as a high-attenuation focus in the gallbladder on CT and as echogenic debris on sonography. Blood within the gallbladder resulting from biliary ductal trauma should be distinguished from primary gallbladder injury. The CT findings of blunt injuries to the gallbladder include intraluminal and pericholecystic hematoma, a collapsed gallbladder lumen or thickened wall, and peritoneal fluid owing to blood or bile leakage.[48]

SPLENIC INJURIES

The spleen is the second most frequently injured intraperitoneal organ in children with blunt abdominal trauma, accounting for approximately 20% of abdominal injuries.[18,55] The two most common clinical findings indicating splenic injury are a low or decreasing hematocrit level and localized peritoneal irritation in the left upper quadrant.

Imaging Appearance

The sensitivity of CT for diagnosing splenic injury is close to 100%.[4,56,61,130] The spectrum of splenic injuries seen on CT ranges from small intraparenchymal and subcapsular hematomas to large, complex lacerations or fractures with capsular disruption and splenic pedicle injuries.[30] Splenic hematomas and lacerations do not enhance and appear hypodense on contrast-enhanced CT scans. Splenic hematomas appear as round or oval lesions with smooth or irregular margins. Subcapsular hematomas are crescentic lowattenuation lesions flattening the lateral contour of the splenic parenchyma (Fig. 10–10). Lacerations generally produce indistinct splenic margins and linear or branching areas of low attenuation on contrast-enhanced CT scans (Fig. 10–11). Splenic fractures are deep lacerations that traverse the splenic parenchyma and divide the spleen into two parts (Fig. 10–12). Splenic injuries usually are associated with hemoperitoneum, which may be small and limited to the perisplenic area or larger and identifiable in Morison's pouch and the pelvis. Perisplenic hematoma is present in more than 85% of splenic lacerations, and occasionally it is the only CT abnormality.[85] Splenic injury occasionally results in extraperitoneal hemorrhage that tracks into the anterior pararenal space.[110]

Splenic pedicle injuries include both avulsion of the splenic artery and occlusion resulting from intimal dissection. The CT appearance of avulsion is that of marked hemoperitoneum and nonenhancement of the spleen (see Fig. 10–3); occasionally, however, the upper pole of the spleen may show perfusion via short gastric arteries. Traumatic occlusion of the splenic artery also produces a nonperfused normal-size spleen, but because of the occlusion of the splenic artery, there is little hemoperitoneum.

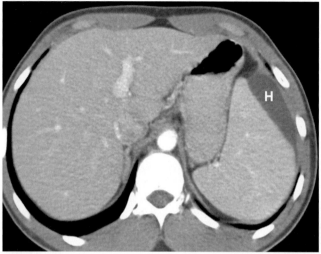

Figure 10–10
Subcapsular splenic hematoma. A low-attenuation lenticular-shaped subcapsular hematoma (H) flattens the lateral splenic contour.

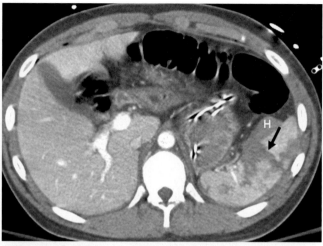

Figure 10–12
Splenic fracture. A deep laceration (arrow) extends through the splenic parenchyma from the medial to lateral surface, consistent with fracture. Blood fills the fracture line. Several smaller lacerations are noted in the posterior part of the spleen, and there is an associated perisplenic hematoma (H).

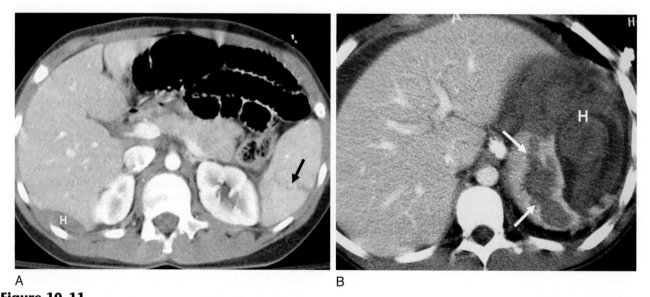

A   B

Figure 10–11
Splenic laceration. A, A contrast-enhanced CT scan demonstrates a linear low-attenuation laceration (arrow) extending to the splenic margin laterally. Also noted a small subcapsular hepatic hematoma (H). B, A contrast-enhanced CT scan in another patient shows a low attenuation splenic laceration (arrows) and hematoma (H) along the anterolateral splenic margin.

As mentioned previously, sonography has a limited role in evaluating the acutely traumatized patient, but because of its ease of performance, sonography may be the screening procedure of choice in patients with relatively minor trauma in whom an isolated splenic injury is suspected.[31] As with other organs, the echogenicity of the hemorrhage varies with age. Acute hematoma appears either hyper- or isoechoic relative to normal splenic parenchyma. At this stage, the lesions may be indistinguishable from normal splenic tissue. With time, as the protein and hemoglobin are resorbed, the hematoma becomes complex or hypoechoic relative to adjacent spleen.

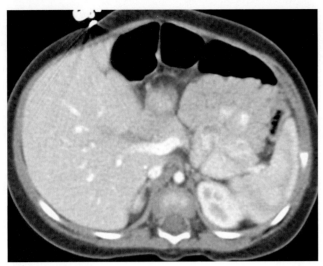

Figure 10–13
Splenic heterogeneity. Note the normal serpentine pattern of parenchymal enhancement, reflecting variable blood flow through the splenic sinusoids. This heterogeneity is transient. The absence of perisplenic clot and hemoperitoneum supports the diagnosis of a normal spleen.

Imaging Pitfalls

A congenital cleft may lead to a false-positive diagnosis of splenic laceration. Clefts, however, usually lie along the medial aspect of the spleen and are not associated with perisplenic or intraperitoneal blood, whereas splenic lacerations generally involve the lateral surface of the spleen and are frequently associated with hemoperitoneum.[30] A patchy pattern of splenic parenchymal enhancement is a normal phenomenon on CT scans seen immediately after a bolus injection of contrast material.[22,101,102] This pattern simulates fragments of splenic parenchyma (see Figs. 10–9 and 10–13). This early heterogeneity is transient and on scans in the portal venous phase of enhancement, the normal spleen exhibits a homogeneous appearance, whereas a true splenic injury often remains visible and is associated with a perisplenic clot and hemoperitoneum. Occasionally, postinjection hypoperfusion of the splenic parenchyma can be found in hypotensive patients and may be misinterpreted as a vascular pedicle injury. The precise mechanism of this decreased perfusion is unclear, but it may result from arterial vasoconstriction from sympathetic stimulation. The presence of hypovolemic shock should suggest the correct diagnosis. Finally, streak artifacts may produce a heterogeneous appearance of the splenic parenchyma, distinguishable from lacerations by the absence of perisplenic clot or hemoperitoneum.

Clinical Management

Nearly all children with splenic injuries are managed nonoperatively.[9,22,90] Nonoperative management is preferred, not only because of the risk of surgery and anesthesia but also because of the lifelong risk of postsplenectomy septicemia.[95] Children who require surgery usually need it for massive or ongoing hemorrhage. The mortality rate for splenic trauma is about 1% and is generally related to delayed rupture or significant extra-abdominal injuries. Delayed splenic rupture (rupture after an asymptomatic period of 48 hours) may result from sudden expansion of an intrasplenic hematoma[87] or from rupture of a perisplenic or subcapsular hematoma into the peritoneal cavity.[133]

CT or sonography can be used to monitor the condition of the spleen during nonoperative management.[27] Splenic enlargement greater than 10% is common in patients with either splenic or hepatic injuries and usually is not a sign of deterioration or bleeding. It probably represents a return of the spleen to normal size after physiologic contraction in response to volume depletion at the time of injury.[37]

In general, hemoperitoneum resolves within 4 weeks.[27,67,90] Intrasplenic hematomas and lacerations decrease in attenuation and become sharply circumscribed as they mature. Splenic injuries may resolve with no sequela or leave a deformed splenic margin.

Complications

The major complication of splenic injury in children is septicemia following splenectomy. This risk has encouraged nonoperative therapy of splenic injuries. Occasional complications are post-traumatic pseudocyst and pseudoaneurysm.[23]

RENAL INJURIES

Renal injuries account for approximately 15% to 40% of abnormalities in children with blunt abdominal trauma.[40,54,55,130] Children with marked hematuria (>50 red blood cells per high power field) or shock are more likely to have renal injuries, whereas those with minimal hematuria (<50 red blood cells per high power field) rarely have renal damage.[32,119,127]

Based on clinical and radiographic findings, renal injuries are classified into four groups.[57,89] Category I lesions, which account for 75% to 85% of all injuries, consist of hematomas and small corticomedullary lacerations that do not extend into the collecting system. Category II lesions, comprising about 10% of injuries, include lacerations that extend into the renal collecting system and fractures that separate the kidney into two parts. Category III lesions, occurring in 5% of all injuries, consist of shattered kidneys and injuries to the renal vascular pedicle, either arterial occlusion or avulsion. Lesions in category IV are rare and include avulsion of the ureteropelvic junction and laceration of the renal pelvis.

Imaging Appearance

On contrast-enhanced CT, renal hematomas and superficial lacerations appear as focal areas of low attenuation

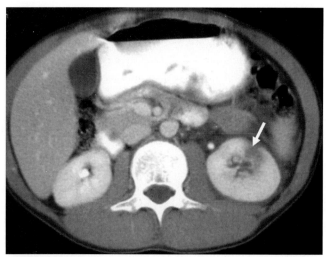

Figure 10–14
Renal hematoma (category I injury). A CT scan shows a low attenuation area *(arrow)* in the cortex of the lower pole of the left kidney. The hematoma did not extend into the collecting system.

within normally enhancing parenchyma.[28] Renal hematomas are round or oval lesions with smooth or irregular margins, whereas lacerations are linear and irregular in configuration (Figs. 10–14 and 10–15). Renal fractures typically occur in an axial plane and often parallel segmental arteries and veins. Deep lacerations and fractures may result in segmental infarcts related to occlusion or compromise of segmental vessels (Fig. 10–16).

Subcapsular or perirenal hematomas frequently accompany parenchymal injuries. Subcapsular hematomas, located between the renal parenchyma and the renal capsule, are usually small and flatten the renal parenchyma. The relatively inelastic capsule also leads to a lenticular configuration, characteristic of a subcapsular hematoma. Perirenal hematomas occur within the perinephric (Gerota's) fascia and typically gravitate dorsolaterally, displacing the kidney anteriorly, medially, and superiorly. Acute subcapsular and perirenal hematomas have lower attenuation values relative to enhancing parenchyma following the administration of intravenous contrast material. On delayed scans, the attenuation value of the fluid may increase because of leakage of opacified urine into the fluid. Both may be associated with fascial thickening. With significant disruption of fascial planes, collections of blood or urine may not be limited to the perirenal space. Extension may occur to four sites: (1) along the ureter, (2) within the interfascial space or intraconal fascia, (3) into the anterior pararenal space, and (4) into the psoas compartment. The presence of fluid in the last three spaces appears to be associated with more severe injuries.[103]

The most severe renal injuries include shattered kidneys and renal pedicle injuries. CT findings of shattered kidney are multiple, perfused or nonperfused renal fragments, which are nearly always accompanied by large perirenal urinoma/hematomas. Renal artery occlusion or avulsion results in absence of contrast enhancement in the injured kidney.

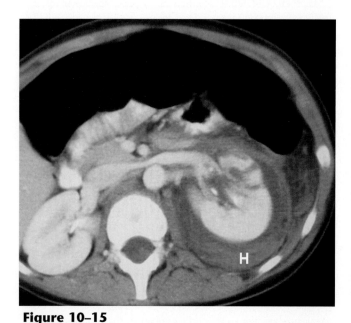

Figure 10–15
Deep cortical lacerations (category II lesion). A contrast-enhanced CT scan demonstrates several lacerations in the mid-pole of the left kidney. These extended into the renal sinus. An associated perirenal hematoma (H) confined by Gerota's fascia is also evident. A follow-up CT scan 6 months later showed focal cortical scarring.

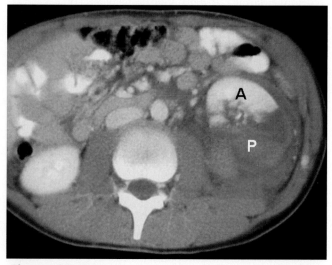

Figure 10–16
Renal fracture (category II injury). A contrast-enhanced CT scan shows a fracture in the mid-pole of the left kidney. The fracture divides the kidney into two parts. The anterior part (A) is perfused; the posterior part (P) is avulsed and avascular. Blood is present in the perirenal space.

In some instances, peripheral or medullary enhancement can be seen as a result of perfusion by capsular or periureteral collaterals, respectively.[28,66,82] Other findings include abrupt termination of the renal artery and retrograde filling of the renal vein.[89] Partial or total avulsion of the renal artery characteristically results in extensive perirenal hemorrhage. Renal artery occlusion is not associated with perirenal hematoma, because arterial flow is completely obstructed (Fig. 10–17).

CT findings of ureteropelvic junction avulsion and renal pelvis laceration include intact renal parenchyma, absent opacification of the ipsilateral ureter distal to the disruption, and contrast medium leakage, which may be confined to the medial perirenal space or extend into the periureteral and anterior pararenal spaces.[60,103,134]

Myoglobinuria due to rhabdomyolysis is a rare cause of renal failure and a prolonged nephrogram on CT.[78] Iodinated contrast agents should be administered with caution if myoglobinuria is suspected clinically because of their potential to initiate or worsen actual renal failure. The discrepancy between the dark color of the urine, the positive Hematest, and the absence of significant hematuria on microscopic examination should suggest the diagnosis of myoglobinuria.

Sonography is capable of detecting renal and perirenal hematoma and can assess the integrity of the renal vasculature.[31] However, sonography is often difficult to perform because of abdominal tenderness and paralytic ileus, and it is inferior to CT in depicting other associated abdominal injuries.

Imaging Pitfalls

Potential pitfalls in the interpretation of renal injuries include renal pseudofracture and pseudosubcapsular hematoma.[28] Pseudosubcapsular hematoma appears as a lenticular, low-attenuation area around the kidney that simulates subcapsular hematoma. The artifact is due to respiratory motion of the kidney during the scan cycle. The absence of the "lesion" on repeat or adjacent scans provides the correct diagnosis.

About 5% of children with renal trauma have an underlying renal abnormality predisposing to injury. The most common abnormalities are hydronephrotic kidney, Wilms' tumor, horseshoe kidney, and renal cystic disease.[36,91] An underlying malformation or a mass should be suspected if CT demonstrates an unusual appearance of an injured kidney.[91]

Clinical Management

Patients with category I and II trauma, including patients with renal fractures, can be managed conservatively if they are hemodynamically stable.[64] Patients with catastrophic injuries generally require urgent surgery. Revascularization of arterial occlusion or avulsion is required within 12 hours if renal function is to be preserved.

Complications

Minor injuries usually resolve without sequelae, whereas major injuries often result in focal or polar atrophy or calcification. A potential risk of renal trauma is hypertension. Clinical surveillance is important, as post-traumatic hypertension can develop years after the injury.[142]

BLADDER INJURIES

The spectrum of bladder injuries includes rupture and hematoma. Contrast-enhanced CT is as sensitive for detecting bladder injuries as contrast cystography if the bladder is adequately distended.[53,65,107,135] Delayed scans and CT cystography can increase detection of bladder injury.

Extraperitoneal rupture of the bladder is more common than intraperitoneal rupture. Extraperitoneal bladder rupture may result from several mechanisms: penetration of the bladder wall by a bone fragment when the pelvis is fractured, a direct blow to a distended bladder, or a shearing injury of the bladder base against the pelvic ring. CT findings include leakage of contrast material from the bladder into the pre- or perivesical spaces and displacement of the bladder posteriorly. Large collections may extend downward into the inguinal canal, thigh, or scrotum or upward into the posterior pararenal space.[19,53,65] Extraperitoneal bladder injury usually can be treated with transurethral catheter drainage and antibiotic therapy. Surgery is preferred if it is suspected that a bony spicule from a pelvic fracture has penetrated the bladder.

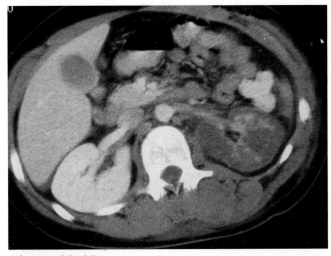

Figure 10–17
Vascular pedicle injury, traumatic renal artery occlusion. A contrast-enhanced CT scan obtained 7 days after a motor vehicle accident shows absent perfusion of the cortex of the left kidney. There is some enhancement of the medulla. Note the absence of extrarenal fluid collection.

Intraperitoneal bladder rupture usually results from a direct blow to a distended bladder. CT demonstrates high-density contrast medium in the peritoneal spaces and recesses, outlining the bowel loops and displacing the urinary bladder inferiorly, but not posteriorly (Fig. 10–18).[3] Intraperitoneal injury requires operative repair. Bladder hematoma results in focal or diffuse wall thickening without contrast medium leakage.[65]

ADRENAL HEMORRHAGE

Adrenal hemorrhage occurs in approximately 3% of children who sustain blunt abdominal trauma. Clinical signs and symptoms are nonspecific, and most children present with abdominal tenderness and hematuria.[111] Adrenal hemorrhage is usually unilateral, is commonly seen on the right side, and is often associated with ipsilateral intraabdominal and intrathoracic injuries. CT findings are an enlarged oval or triangular gland.[140] Associated findings include increased attenuation of the periadrenal fat, intra- and retroperitoneal blood, and thickening of the ipsilateral diaphragmatic crus.[111]

PANCREATIC INJURIES

Blunt trauma to the pancreas is rare, accounting for only 5% of all abdominal injuries in children.[130] Bicycle injuries are the most common cause of pancreatic trauma in children.

Injuries of the pancreatic head are common when the vector of force is to the right of the spine, whereas the body and tail of the pancreas are injured in left-sided trauma. Transection of the junction between the body and tail of the pancreas results when the force of impact is midline, compressing the pancreas against the lumbar vertebrae.[24,136]

Pancreatic injury is difficult to diagnose from physical examination alone, as there usually are no localizing signs and peritoneal irritation is often absent because of the retroperitoneal position of the pancreas. Therefore, the diagnosis of pancreatic injury requires a high index of clinical suspicion and should be considered in patients who have sustained a blow to the upper abdomen and have epigastric pain, tenderness, bilious vomiting, and hyperamylasemia. Cutaneous linear ecchymosis also may be present from a seat belt injury.[117]

Serum amylase levels are elevated in most patients with pancreatic trauma. However, amylase levels may be normal immediately after trauma, and false-positive values may occur with salivary gland contusion or bowel injury. Moreover, serum amylase levels do not vary in proportion to the severity of pancreatic injury and may be higher in patients with pancreatic contusions than in those with pancreatic fractures.

Imaging Appearance

CT is the primary imaging study for the initial evaluation of suspected pancreatic injury in children. Abdominal sonography is useful in the follow-up of peripancreatic fluid collections that may evolve into pseudocysts.[49,50,105]

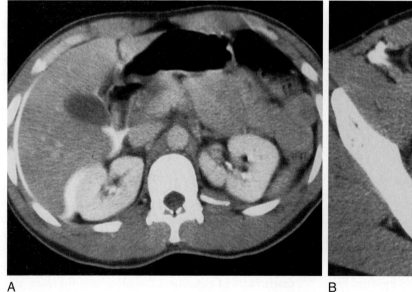
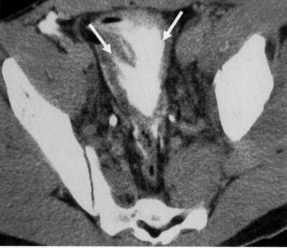

A   B

Figure 10–18
Intraperitoneal bladder rupture. *A,* A CT scan through the upper abdomen demonstrates contrast-opacified urine in Morison's pouch and the perihepatic space. *B,* A scan through the pelvis demonstrates high-attenuation urine in the perivesical space *(arrows).*

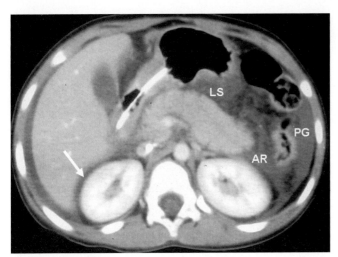

Figure 10–19
Traumatic pancreatitis. A CT scan demonstrates a mildly enlarged pancreas and fluid in the lesser sac (LS), anterior pararenal space (AR), Morison's pouch *(arrow)*, perihepatic space, and the left paracolic gutter (PG).

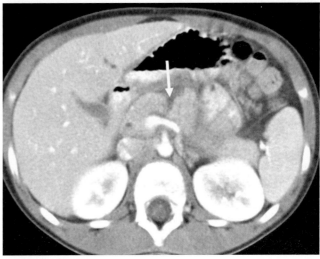

Figure 10–20
Pancreatic fracture. A CT scan through the upper abdomen demonstrates a low-attenuation fracture line *(arrow)* at the junction of the pancreatic body and neck.

Endoscopic retrograde cholangiopancreatography or magnetic resonance cholangiopancreatography is selectively performed to delineate pancreatic ductal integrity in patients who are undergoing surgical exploration or who have failed percutaneous drainage.

Pancreatic injuries may involve the parenchyma alone or the parenchyma and duct. The integrity of the pancreatic duct is an important factor in morbidity and mortality. The spectrum of pancreatic injuries ranges from pancreatitis and hematoma with an intact capsule and duct to deep lacerations and fractures with extensive parenchymal and ductal disruption.[24] The CT changes of acute traumatic pancreatitis include focal or diffuse pancreatic enlargement, parenchymal heterogeneity, irregular contour of the gland, and increased attenuation of the peripancreatic fat with thickening of Gerota's fascia (Fig. 10–19). Pancreatic secretions often break through the connective tissue surrounding the gland. Common sites of extrapancreatic fluid collections include the anterior pararenal space, lesser sac, lateroconal fascia, and small bowel mesentery. In the setting of trauma, fluid in the anterior pararenal space or lesser sac in the absence of other visceral injury is highly suspicious for pancreatic injury.[105,108,109] In a patient with blunt abdominal trauma, the presence of unexplained peripancreatic fluid in the anterior pararenal space or lesser sac in the absence of other visceral injury should be considered as highly suspicious for pancreatic injury.

Pancreatic hematoma appears as a poorly marginated low-attenuation area in the pancreatic parenchyma.[24] Pancreatic lacerations and fractures appear as linear clefts of decreased attenuation (Fig. 10–20). These injuries usually involve the pancreatic neck and are perpendicular to the long axis of the gland.[24,136] In pancreatic fracture, the two ends of the gland are separated by a variable amount of low-attenuation fluid. Edema of the peripancreatic fat and thickening of the left anterior pararenal and Gerota's fasciae are common associated findings.

Imaging Pitfalls

False-positive diagnoses of pancreatic fracture or laceration can result when streak artifacts from gastric air-fluid levels or physiologic thinning of the pancreatic neck are misinterpreted as a parenchymal injury. Additionally, unopacified jejunal loops adjacent to the pancreatic tail may be mistaken for focal pancreatic swelling. Most of these pitfalls can be avoided by careful scrutiny of contiguous CT sections. False-negative diagnosis may result if scans are obtained soon after pancreatic trauma, when peripancreatic inflammation may be minimal. As intra- and peripancreatic edema and inflammation develop over time, the diagnosis of pancreatic injury becomes more evident.

Clinical Management

The treatment for pancreatic injuries is based on the extent of parenchymal injury and ductal disruption. Pancreatitis is treated conservatively. The treatment for laceration or fracture is laparotomy and drainage or partial pancreatectomy, depending on the severity of injury.[118,122,141] The principal determinant of outcome is the integrity of the main pancreatic duct. Ductal disruption results in an increased frequency of pseudocyst formation, severe pancreatitis, pancreatic necrosis, and sepsis.[122]

Complications

Late sequelae of pancreatic injury include pseudocyst formation and abscess formation. The CT appearance of a pseudocyst is that of a low-attenuation fluid collection with a well-defined wall (Fig. 10–21). The contents of the pseudocyst may be anechoic or hypoechoic on sonography. Pancreatic abscess also appears as a fluid-filled mass with thick walls. A specific diagnosis of abscess can be made if the mass contains an air-fluid level. In the absence of an air-fluid level, percutaneous aspiration may be of value both to diagnose and to treat pancreatic abscess.

GASTROINTESTINAL INJURIES

Gastrointestinal injuries account for 5% to 15% of blunt abdominal injuries in children[26] and commonly result from seat belts, bicycle handlebars, or child abuse. Clinically, patients present with abdominal pain, tenderness, or vomiting, with symptoms often simulating those of intestinal obstruction. Massive bleeding is infrequent, although minimal hematemesis or melena is not unusual. Linear ecchymoses, owing to a seat belt, may be noted on physical examination and are associated with a high incidence of morbidity.[117,123]

Blunt injury to the intestine can result from several mechanisms: a crush injury, in which the bowel is compressed between the anterior abdominal wall and the spine; a shearing injury causing disruption of the small bowel and mesentery at sites of ligamentous attachment; and a direct blow to the abdomen causing a sudden increase in pressure within

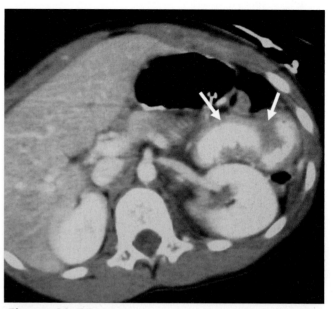

Figure 10–22
Jejunal hematoma. A CT scan through the upper abdomen demonstrates circumferential thickening of the jejunal walls *(arrows)*, consistent with intramural hematoma.

a bowel loop and perforation.[139] The segments of bowel most susceptible to blunt injury are the duodenum, proximal small bowel, and distal ileum. The duodenum is retroperitoneal and therefore relatively immobile anterior to the spine, the proximal jejunum is fixed by the ligament of Treitz, and the distal ileum is immobilized by its cecal attachment. Colon and gastric injuries occur, but they are less common than small bowel injuries. Bowel injuries may be classified as hematomas, lacerations, perforations, or complete transections.

Imaging Appearance

The combination of plain abdominal radiography, contrast studies, and CT has been used to evaluate suspected bowel injury. The diagnosis of intestinal injury on plain radiography is based on demonstration of pneumoperitoneum, intramural air, and scoliosis (splinting), but unfortunately these findings are found in fewer than 50% of small bowel lacerations.[26,92] Conventional contrast examinations of bowel are useful for diagnosing duodenal hematomas but have limited value in distal small bowel injuries. CT has become the study of choice for detecting bowel injury.[16,26,92,123]

Intramural hematoma produces thickening of the mucosal folds or a mass that narrows the bowel lumen (Figs. 10–22 and 10–23).[62,81] The CT density of intramural hematoma is relatively high initially but decreases as the hematoma ages.

Retroperitoneal duodenal laceration or rupture should be suspected when there is evidence of extraluminal gas or contrast in the right paraduodenal and pararenal

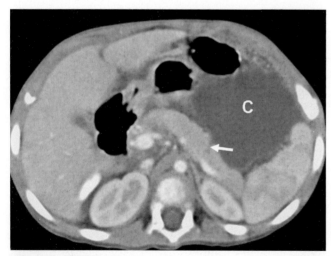

Figure 10–21
Pancreatic pseudocyst. A CT scan immediately following blunt abdominal trauma had shown a fracture at the junction of the pancreatic body and neck. A follow-up CT scan 1 month later again demonstrates the fracture line *(arrow)* along with a low-attenuation pseudocyst (C).

spaces (Fig. 10–24).[62] Gas may be noted also in other retroperitoneal spaces or in the peritoneal spaces when there is significant disruption of fascial planes around the duodenum.[45]

CT findings indicating distal small bowel and colonic lacerations and perforations include extraluminal collections of gas or contrast medium, free peritoneal air or fluid, focal areas of bowel wall thickening, and high-attenuation clot adjacent to bowel (the "sentinel sign").[11,13,17,20,45,75,85,92,112,124] The clotted hematoma or sentinel sign is believed to localize the site of injury. Free intraperitoneal air may be found anteriorly in the midabdomen or over the peritoneal surface of the liver. In some patients, small collections of air may be better visualized on wide CT windows (lung windows) than on standard soft tissue windows.

Free peritoneal fluid due to viscus rupture accumulates in the interloop compartment and has a triangular appearance. Extravasated fluid from the bowel lumen is usually of low attenuation, <20 HU.[11,75] Extraluminal oral contrast material has an attenuation value higher than that of small bowel contents and blood. Extravasation of oral contrast material from the bowel lumen is specific for bowel perforation.

The mesentery is also susceptible to injury, and in some series mesenteric injury is more common than intrinsic bowel injuries. Mesenteric injuries may be classified as hematomas or lacerations. CT findings of mesenteric hematoma include high-attenuation clot in the mesentery (Fig. 10–25), streaky soft-tissue infiltration of the mesenteric fat, and intermediate- to high-attenuation intra-abdominal fluid. Mesenteric lacerations are more difficult to diagnose than hematomas. CT findings suggesting laceration of the superior mesenteric artery or vein include hemoperitoneum, absence of hepatic or splenic injury, and high-attenuation clot in the mesentery. The presence of moderate or large amounts of free intra-abdominal blood in the absence of CT evidence of other hollow or solid organ injury should raise suspicion of mesenteric laceration.

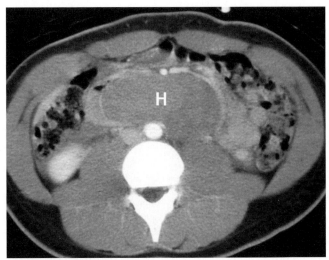

Figure 10–23
Duodenal hematoma. A contrast-enhanced CT scan demonstrates a large intramural hematoma (H) arising in the wall of the transverse duodenum, obstructing the lumen which contains a faint amount of oral contrast material peripherally.

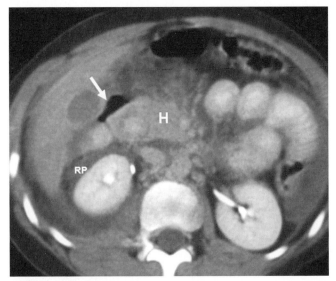

Figure 10–24
Duodenal perforation. A CT scan demonstrates a high-attenuation hematoma (H) in the transverse duodenum and air in the right paraduodenal area *(arrow)*. There also is air and fluid in the right pararenal space (RP).

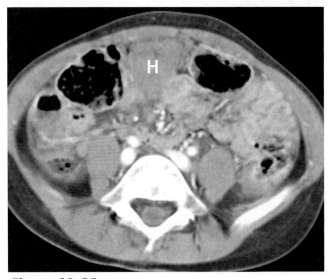

Figure 10–25
Mesenteric hematoma. A CT scan shows a large hematoma (H) in the small bowel mesentery.

Imaging Pitfalls

Although intestinal perforations have been recognized by CT, the diagnosis often is difficult to establish because the findings can be subtle. Normal CT scans have been reported in the presence of small bowel perforations, presumably because the CT examination was done immediately after the injury, before significant bleeding or accumulation of extraluminal air or fluid had occurred.

Clinical Management

Isolated intestinal or mesenteric hematomas are usually treated nonoperatively. The presence of bowel perforation, manifested by pneumoperitoneum, extraluminal gas, or leakage of oral contrast medium, is an indication for immediate surgery.

Complications

Complications of blunt injury to the bowel or mesentery include ischemia, infarction, and stricture.[97] Adhesions resulting from perforation and peritonitis are other complications.

SUMMARY

Contrast-enhanced CT is the initial imaging method of choice when hemodynamically stable patients with a history of severe blunt abdominal or pelvic trauma are evaluated. CT can readily define the location and extent of injury, assess the amount of associated hemoperitoneum, and identify other intra-abdominal injuries. This diagnostic information can be valuable in determining the need for laparotomy and in diagnosing post-traumatic complications.

REFERENCES

1. Abramson SJ, Berdon WE, Kaufman RA, Ruzal-Shapiro C. Hepatic parenchymal and subcapsular gas after hepatic laceration caused by blunt abdominal trauma. AJR Am J Roentgenol 153:1031–1032, 1989.
2. Allen TL, Mueller MT, Bonk R, Harker CP, Duffy OH, Stevens MH. Computed tomographic scanning without oral contrast solution for blunt bowel and mesenteric injuries in abdominal trauma. J Trauma 56:314–322, 2004.
3. Auh YH, Rubenstein WA, Markisz JA, Zirinsky K, Whalen JP, Kazam E. Intraperitoneal paravesical spaces: CT delineation with US correlation. Radiology 159:311–317, 1986.
4. Beaver BL, Colombani PM, Fal A, et al. The efficacy of computed tomography in evaluating abdominal injuries in children with major head trauma. J Pediatr Surg 22:1117–1122, 1987.
5. Benya EC, Lim-Dunham JE, Landrum O, Stratter M. Abdominal sonography in examination of children with blunt abdominal trauma. AJR Am J Roentgenol 174:1613–1616, 2000.
6. Bhalla S, Siegel MJ. Multislice computed tomography in pediatrics. In Silverman PM, ed. Multislice Computed Tomography: A Practical Approach to Clinical Protocols. Philadelphia: Lippincott Williams & Wilkins, 2002, pp 231–282.
7. Bhutta ST, Greenberg SB, Fitch SJ, Parnell D. All-terrain vehicle injuries in children: Injury patterns and prognostic implications. Pediatr Radiol 34:130–133, 2004.
8. Bode PJ, Niezen RA, van Vugt AB, Schipper J. Abdominal ultrasound as a reliable indicator for conclusive laparotomy in blunt abdominal trauma. J Trauma 34:27–31, 1993.
9. Bond SJ, Eichelberger MR, Gotschall CS, Sivit CJ, Randolph JG. Nonoperative management of blunt hepatic and splenic injury in children. Ann Surg 223:286–289, 1996.
10. Breaux CW Jr, Smith G, Georgeson KE. The first two years' experience with major trauma at a pediatric trauma center. J Trauma 30:37–43, 1990.
11. Breen DJ, Janzen DL, Zwirewich CV, Nagy AG. Blunt bowel and mesenteric injury: Diagnostic performance of CT signs. J Comput Assist Tomogr 21:706–712, 1997.
12. Bretan PN, McAninch JW, Federle MP, Jeffrey RB. Computerized tomographic staging of renal trauma: 85 consecutive cases. J Urol 136:561–565, 1986.
13. Brody JM, Leighton DB, Murphy BL, et al. CT of blunt trauma bowel and mesenteric injury: Typical findings and pitfalls in diagnosis. RadioGraphics 20:1525–1536, 2000.
14. Brown MA, Casola G, Sirlin CB, Patel NY, Hoyt DB. Blunt abdominal trauma: Screening US in 2,693 patients. Radiology 218:352–358, 2001.
15. Bulas DI, Eichelberger MR, Sivit CJ, Wright CJ, Gotschall CS. Hepatic injury from blunt trauma in children: Follow-up evaluation with CT. AJR Am J Roentgenol 160:347–351, 1993.
16. Bulas DI, Taylor GA, Eichelberger MR. The value of CT in detecting bowel perforation in children after blunt abdominal trauma. AJR Am J Roentgenol 153:561–564, 1989.
17. Butela ST, Federle MP, Chang PJ, et al. Performance of CT in detection of bowel injury. AJR Am J Roentgenol 176:129–135, 2001.
18. Cooper A, Barlow B, DiScala C, String D. Mortality and truncal injury: The pediatric perspective. J Pediatr Surg 29:33–38, 1994.
19. Corriere JN Jr, Sandler CM. Mechanisms of injury, patterns of extravasation and management of extraperitoneal bladder rupture due to blunt trauma. J Urol 139:43–44, 1988.
20. Cox TD, Kuhn JP. CT scan of bowel trauma in the pediatric patient. Radiol Clin North Am 34:807–818, 1996.
21. Cywes S, Rode H, Millar AJW. Blunt liver trauma in children: Nonoperative management. J Pediatr Surg 20:14–18, 1985.
22. Delius RE, Frankel W, Coran AG. A comparison between operative and nonoperative management of blunt injuries to the liver and spleen in adult and pediatric patients. Surgery 106:788–792, 1989.
23. Do HM, Cronan JJ. CT appearance of splenic injuries managed nonoperatively. AJR Am J Roentgenol 157:757–760, 1991.
24. Dodds WJ, Taylor AJ, Erickson SC, Lawson TL. Traumatic fracture of the pancreas: CT characteristics. J Comput Assist Tomogr 14:375–378, 1990.
25. Donnelly LF, Foss JN, Frush DP, Bisset GS III. Heterogeneous splenic enhancement patterns on spiral CT images in children: Minimizing misinterpretation. 210:493–497, 1999.
26. Donohue JH, Federle MP, Griffiths BG, Trunkey DD. Computed tomography in the diagnosis of blunt intestinal and mesenteric injuries. J Trauma 27:11–17, 1987.
27. Emery KH, Babcock DS, Borgman AD, Garcia VF. Splenic injury diagnosed with CT: US follow-up and healing rate in children and adolescents. Radiology 212:515–518, 1999.
28. Fanney DR, Casillas J, Murphy BJ. CT in the diagnosis of renal trauma. RadioGraphics 19:29–40, 1990.
29. Federle MP. Diagnosis of intestinal injuries by computed tomography and the use of oral contrast medium. Ann Emerg Med 31:769–771,1998.
30. Federle MP, Griffiths B, Minagi H, Jeffrey RB. Splenic trauma: Evaluation with CT. Radiology 162(1 Pt 1):69–71, 1987.
31. Filiatrault D, Longpre D, Patriquin H, et al. Investigation of childhood blunt abdominal trauma: A practical approach using ultrasound as the initial diagnostic modality. Pediatr Radiol 17:373–379, 1987.

32. Fleisher G. Prospective evaluation of selective criteria for imaging among children with suspected blunt renal trauma. Pediatr Emerg Care 5:8–11, 1989.

33. Foglia RP, Winthrop AL. Abdominal trauma. In Olham KT, Colombani PM, Foglia RP, eds. Surgery of Infants and Children: Principles and Practice. Philadelphia: Lippincott-Raven, 1997, p. 463.

34. Foley WD, Cates JD, Kellman GM, et al. Treatment of blunt hepatic injuries: Role of CT. Radiology 164:635—638, 1987.

35. Frush DP, Donnelly LF, Bisset GS. Effect of scan delay on hepatic enhancement for pediatric abdominal multislice helical CT. AJR Am J Roentgenol 176:1559–1561, 2001.

36. Gary R, Cass AS, Johnson CF. Computed tomography diagnosis of traumatic rupture of congenital hydronephrotic renal pelvis. Urology 32:65–66, 1988.

37. Goodman LR, Aprahamian C. Changes in splenic size after abdominal trauma. Radiology 176:629–632, 1990.

38. Gross M, Lynch F, Canty T, Peterson B, Spear R. Management of pediatric liver injuries: A 13-year experience at a pediatric trauma center. J Pediatr Surg 34:811–816, 1999.

39. Haaga JR. Commentary. Radiation dose management weighing risk versus benefit. AJR Am J Roentgenol 177:289–291; 2001.

40. Haftel AJ, Lev R, Mahour GH, Senac M, Akhtar Shah SI. Abdominal CT scanning in pediatric blunt trauma. Ann Emerg Med 17:684–689, 1988.

41. Hanks, PW, Brody JM. Blunt injury to the mesentery and small bowel: CT evaluation. Radiol Clin North Am 41:1171–1182, 2003.

42. Hennes HM, Smith DS, Schneider K, Hegenbarth MA, Duma MA, Jona JZ. Elevated liver transaminase levels in children with blunt abdominal trauma: A predictor of liver injury. Pediatrics 86:87–90, 1990.

43. Hiatt JR, Harrier HD, Koenig BV, Ransom KJ. Nonoperative management of major blunt liver injury with hemoperitoneum. Arch Surg 125:101–103, 1990.

44. Jaffe D, Wesson D. Emergency management of blunt trauma in children. N Engl J Med 324:1477–1482, 1991.

45. Jamieson DH, Babyn PS, Pearl R. Imaging gastrointestinal perforation in pediatric blunt abdominal trauma. Pediatr Radiol 26:188–194, 1996.

46. Jeffrey RB Jr, Cardoza JD, Olcott EW. Detection of active intraabdominal arterial hemorrhage: Value of dynamic contrast-enhanced CT. AJR Am J Roentgenol 156:725–729, 1991.

47. Jeffrey RB Jr, Federle MP. The collapsed inferior vena cava: CT evidence of hypovolemia. AJR Am J Roentgenol 150:431–432, 1988.

48. Jeffrey RB, Federle MP, Laing FC, Wing VW. Computed tomography of blunt trauma to the gallbladder. J Comput Assist Tomogr 10:756–758, 1986.

49. Jeffrey RB, Laing FC, Wing VW. Ultrasound in acute pancreatic trauma. Gastrointest Radiol 11:44–46, 1986.

50. Jehle D, Guarino J, Karamanoukian H. Emergency department ultrasound in the evaluation of blunt abdominal trauma. Am J Emerg Med 11:342–346, 1991.

51. Kane NM, Cronan JJ, Dorfman GS, DeLuca F. Pediatric abdominal trauma: Evaluation by computed tomography. Pediatrics 82:11–15, 1988.

52. Kane NM, Dorfman GS, Cronan JJ. Efficacy of CT following peritoneal lavage in abdominal trauma. J Comput Assist Tomogr 6:998–1002, 1987.

53. Kane NM, Francis IR, Ellis JH. The value of CT in the detection of bladder and posterior urethral injuries. AJR Am J Roentgenol 153:1243–1246, 1989.

54. Karp MP, Jewett TC Jr, Kuhn JP, Allen JE, Dokler ML, Cooney DR. The impact of computed tomography scanning on the child with renal trauma. J Pediatr Surg 21:617–623, 1986.

55. Kaufman RA. CT of blunt abdominal trauma in children: A five-year experience. In Siegel MJ, ed. Pediatric Body CT. New York: Churchill Livingstone, 1986, p 313.

56. Kaufman RA, Towbin R, Babcock DS, et al. Upper abdominal trauma in children: Imaging evaluation. AJR Am J Roentgenol 142:449–460, 1984.

57. Kawashima A, Sandler CM, Corl FM, et al. Imaging of renal trauma: A comprehensive reivew. RadioGraphics 21:557–574, 2001.

58. Kelly J, Raptopoulos V, Davidoff A, Waite R, Norton P. The value of non-contrast-enhanced CT in blunt abdominal trauma. AJR Am J Roentgenol 152:41–48, 1989.

59. Kennedy C, Kempf J. FAST exams in pediatric abdominal trauma. Acad Emerg Med 9:519; 2002.

60. Kenney PJ, Panicek DM, Witanowski LS. Computed tomography of ureteral disruption. J Comput Assist Tomogr 11:480–484, 1987.

61. Kohn JS, Clark DE, Isler RJ, Pope CF. Is computed tomographic grading of splenic injury useful in the nonsurgical management of blunt trauma? J Trauma 36:385–390, 1994.

62. Kunin JR, Korobkin M, Ellis JH, Francis IR, Kane NM, Siegel SE. Duodenal injuries caused by blunt abdominal trauma: Value of CT in differentiating perforation from hematoma. AJR Am J Roentgenol 160:1221–1223, 1993.

63. Levine CD, Patel UJ, Silverman PM, Wachsberg RH. Low attenuation of acute traumatic hemoperitoneum on CT scans. AJR Am J Roentgenol 166:1089–1093, 1996.

64. Levy JB, Baskin LS, Ewalt DH, et al. Nonoperative management of blunt pediatric major renal trauma. Urology 42:418–424, 1993.

65. Lis LE, Cohen AJ. CT cystography in the evaluation of bladder trauma. J Comput Assist Tomogr 14:386, 1990.

66. Lupetin AR, Mainwaring BL, Daffner RH. CT diagnosis of renal artery injury caused by blunt abdominal trauma. AJR Am J Roentgenol 153:1065–1068, 1989.

67. Lynch JM, Meza MP, Newman V, Gardner MJ, Albanese CT. Computed tomography of splenic injury is predictive of the time required for radiographic healing. J Pediatr Surg 32:1093–1095, 1997.

68. MacGillivray DC, Valentine RJ. Nonoperative management of blunt pediatric liver injury—late complications: Case report. J Trauma 29:251–254, 1989.

69. Macrander SJ, Lawson TL, Foley WD, Dodds WJ, Erickson S, Quiroz FA. Periportal tracking in hepatic trauma: CT features. J Comput Assist Tomogr 13:952–957, 1989.

70. McGahan JP, Rose J, Coates TL, Wisner DH, Newberry P. Use of ultrasonography in the patient with acute abdominal trauma. J Ultrasound Med 16:653–662, 1997.

71. McGahan JP, Richards J, Gillen M: The focused abdominal sonography for trauma scan: Pearls and pitfalls. J Ultrasound Med 21:789–800, 2002.

72. McKenney M, Lentz K, Nunez D, et al. Can ultrasound replace diagnostic peritoneal lavage in the assessment of blunt trauma? J Trauma 37:439–441, 1994.

73. Meyers MA. Dynamic Radiology of the Abdomen: Normal and Pathologic Anatomy. 4th ed. New York: Springer-Verlag, 1994.

74. Meyers MA, Oliphant M, Berne AS, Feldberg MAM. The peritoneal ligaments and mesenteries: Pathways of intraabdominal spread of disease. Radiology 163:593–604, 1987.

75. Mirvis SE, Gens DR, Shanmuganathan K. Rupture of the bowel after blunt abdominal trauma: Diagnosis with CT. AJR Am J Roentgenol 159:1217–1221, 1992.

76. Moore EE, Cogbill TH, Jurkovich GJ, Shackford SR, Malangoni MA, Champion HR. Organ injury scaling: Spleen and liver (1994 revision). J Trauma 323–324, 1995.

77. Moore EE, Cogbill TH, Malangoni MA, et al. Organ injury scaling: Pancreas, duodenum, small bowel, colon, and rectum. J Trauma 30:1427–1429, 1990.

78. Mukherji SK, Siegel MJ. Rhabdomyolysis and renal failure in child abuse. AJR Am J Roentgenol 148:1203, 1987.

79. Nakayama DK, Ramenofsky ML, Rowe MI. Chest injuries in childhood. Ann Surg 210:770–775, 1989.

80. Neish AS, Taylor GA, Lund DP, Atkinson CC. Effect of CT information on the diagnosis and management of acute abdominal injury in children. Radiology 206:327–331, 1998.
81. Nghiem HV, Jeffrey RB Jr, Mindelzun RE. CT of blunt trauma to the bowel and mesentery. AJR Am J Roentgenol 160:53–58, 1993.
82. Nunez D Jr, Becerra JL, Fuentes D, Pagson S. Traumatic occlusion of the renal artery: Helical CT diagnosis. AJR Am J Roentgenol 167:777–780, 1996.
83. Oldham KT, Guice KS, Kaufman RA, Martin LW, Noseworthy J. Blunt hepatic injury and elevated hepatic enzymes: A clinical correlation in children. J Pediatr Surg 19:457–461, 1984.
84. Oldham KT, Guice KS, Ryckman F, Kaufman RA, Martin LW, Noseworthy J. Blunt liver injury in childhood: Evolution of therapy and current perspective. Surgery 100:542–549, 1986.
85. Orwig D, Federle MP. Localized clotted blood as evidence of visceral trauma on CT: The sentinel clot sign. AJR Am J Roentgenol 153:747–749, 1989.
86. Panicek DM, Paquet DJ, Clark KG, Urrutia EJ, Brinsko RE. Hepatic parenchymal gas after blunt trauma. Radiology 159:343–344, 1986.
87. Pappas D, Mirvis SE, Crepps JT. Splenic trauma: False-negative CT diagnosis in cases of delayed rupture. AJR Am J Roentgenol 149:727–728, 1987.
88. Patrick LE, Ball TI, Atkinson GO, Winn KJ. Pediatric blunt abdominal trauma: Periportal tracking at CT. Radiology 183:689–691, 1992.
89. Pollack HM, Wein AJ. Imaging of renal trauma. Radiology;172:297–308, 1989.
90. Pranikoff T, Hirschl RB, Schlesinger AE, Polley TZ, Coran AG. Resolution of splenic injury after nonoperative management. J Pediatr Surg 29:1366–1369, 1994.
91. Rhyner P, Federle MP, Jeffrey RB. CT of trauma to the abnormal kidney. AJR Am J Roentgenol 142:747–750, 1984.
92. Rizzo MJ, Federle MP, Griffiths BG. Bowel and mesenteric injury following blunt abdominal trauma: Evaluation with CT. Radiology 173:143–n148, 1989.
93. Ruess L, Sivit CJ, Eichelberger MR, Gotschall CS, Taylor GA. Blunt abdominal trauma in children: Impact of CT on operative and nonoperative management. AJR Am J Roentgenol 169:1011–1014, 1997.
94. Ruess L, Sivit CJ, Eichelberger MR, Taylor GA, Bond SJ. Blunt hepatic and splenic trauma in children: Correlation of a CT injury severity scale with clinical outcome. *Pediatr Radiol* 25:321–325, 1995.
95. Schiffman MA. Nonoperative management of blunt abdominal trauma in pediatrics. Emerg Med Clin North Am 7:519–535, 1989.
96. Shaffer MA, Doris PE. Limitation of the cross table lateral view in detecting cervical spine injuries: A retrospective analysis. Ann Emerg Med 10:508–513, 1981.
97. Shalaby-Rana E, Eichelberger M, Kerzner B, Kapur S. Intestinal stricture due to lap-belt injury. AJR Am J Roentgenol 158:63–64, 1992.
98. Shanmuganathan K, Mirvis SE, Amoroso M. Periportal low density on CT in patients with blunt trauma: Association with elevated venous pressure. AJR Am J Roentgenol 160:279–283, 1993.
99. Shanmuganathan K, Mirvis SE, Sover ER. Value of contrast-enhanced CT in detecting active hemorrhage in patients with blunt abdominal or pelvic trauma. AJR Am J Roentgenol 161:65–69, 1993.
100. Siegel MJ, Pediatric applications of computed body tomography. IN: Lee JKT, Sagel SS, Stanley RJ, Heiken JP, eds. Computed Body Tomography with MRI Correlation. Philadelphia: Lippincott Williams and Wilkins, 2006: xxx.
101. Siegel MJ. Techniques. In Siegel MJ, ed. Pediatric Body CT. Philadelphia: Lippincott Williams & Wilkins, 1999.
102. Siegel MJ. Thoracoabdominal trauma. In Siegel MJ, ed. Pediatric Body CT. Philadelphia: Lippincott Williams & Wilkins, 1999, p 346.
103. Siegel MJ, Balfe DM. Blunt renal and ureteral trauma in childhood: CT patterns of fluid collections. AJR Am J Roentgenol 152:1043–1047, 1989.
104. Siegel MJ, Herman TE. Periportal low attenuation at CT in childhood. Radiology 183:685–688, 1992.
105. Siegel MJ, Sivit CJ. Pancreatic emergencies. Radiol Clin North Am 35:815–830, 1997.
106. Siegel MJ, Suess C, Schmidt B, Bradley D, Hildebolt C. Radiation dose and image quality in pediatric CT: Effect of technical factors and phantom size and shape. Radiology 233:515–522, 2004.
107. Sivit CJ, Cutting JP, Eichelberger MR. CT diagnosis and localization of rupture of the bladder in children with blunt abdominal trauma: Significance of contrast material extravasation in the pelvis. AJR Am J Roentgenol 164:1243–1246, 1995.
108. Sivit CJ, Eichelberger MR. CT diagnosis of pancreatic injury in children: Significance of fluid separating the splenic vein and the pancreas. AJR Am J Roentgenol 165:921–924, 1995.
109. Sivit CJ, Eichelberger MR, Taylor GA, Bulas DI, Gotschall CS, Kushner DC. Blunt pancreatic trauma in children: CT diagnosis. AJR Am J Roentgenol 158:1097–1100, 1992.
110. Sivit CJ, Frazier AA, Eichelberger MR. Prevalence and distribution of extraperitoneal hemorrhage associated with splenic injury in infants and children. AJR Am J Roentgenol 172:1015–1017, 1999.
111. Sivit CJ, Ingram JD, Taylor GA, Bulas DI, Kushner DC, Eichelberger MR. Posttraumatic adrenal hemorrhage in children: CT findings in 34 patients. AJR Am J Roentgenol 158:1299–1302, 1992.
112. Sivit CJ, Peclet MH, Taylor GA. Life-threatening intraperitoneal bleeding: Demonstration with CT. Radiology 171:430, 1989.
113. Sivit CJ, Taylor GA, Bulas DI, Kushner DC, Potter BM, Eichelberger MR. Posttraumatic shock in children: CT findings associated with hemodynamic instability. Radiology 182:723–726, 1992.
114. Sivit CJ, Taylor GA, Bulas DJ, Bowman LM, Eichelberger MR. Blunt trauma in children: Significance of peritoneal fluid. Radiology 178:185–188, 1991.
115. Sivit CJ, Taylor GA, Eichelberger MR. Chest injury in children with blunt abdominal trauma: Evaluation with CT. Radiology 171:815, 1989.
116. Sivit CJ, Taylor GA, Eichelberger MR, Bulas DI, Gotschall CS, Kushner DC. Significance of periportal low-attenuation zones following blunt trauma in children. Pediatr Radiol 23:388–390, 1993.
117. Sivit CJ, Taylor GA, Newman KD, et al. Safety-belt injuries in children with lap-belt ecchymosis: CT findings in 61 patients. AJR Am J Roentgenol 157:111–114, 1991.
118. Smego DR, Richardson JD, Flint LM. Determinants of outcome in pancreatic trauma. J Trauma 25:771–776, 1985.
119. Stalker HP, Kaufman RA, Stedje K. The significance of hematuria in children after blunt abdominal trauma. AJR Am J Roentgenol 154:569–571, 1990.
120. Stalker HP, Kaufman RA, Towbin R. Patterns of liver injury in childhood: CT analysis. AJR Am J Roentgenol 147:1199–1205, 1986.
121. Stark P. Radiology of thoracic trauma. Invest Radiol 25:1265–1275, 1990.
122. van Steenbergen W, Samain H, Pouillon M, et al. Transection of the pancreas demonstrated by ultrasound and computed tomography. Gastrointest Radiol 12:128–130, 1987.
123. Strouse PJ, Close BJ, Marshall KW, Cywes R. CT of bowel and mesenteric trauma in children. RadioGraphics 19:1237–1250, 1999.
124. Stuhlfaut JW, Soto JA, Lucey BC, et al. Blunt abdominal trauma: Performance of CT without oral contrast material. Radiology 233:689–694, 2004.

125. Taylor GA, Eichelberger MR. Abdominal CT in children with neurologic impairment following blunt trauma. Ann Surg 210:229–233, 1989.

126. Taylor GA, Eichelberger MR, O'Donnell R, Bowman L. Indications for computed tomography in children with blunt abdominal trauma. *Ann Surg* 213:212, 1991.

127. Taylor GA, Eichelberger MR, Potter BM. Hematuria. A marker of abdominal injury in children after blunt trauma. Ann Surg 208:688–693, 1988.

128. Taylor GA, Fallat ME, Eichelberger MR. Hypovolemic shock in children: Abdominal CT manifestations. Radiology 164:479–481, 1987.

129. Taylor GA, Fallat ME, Potter BM, Eichelberger MR. The role of computed tomography in blunt abdominal trauma in children. J Trauma 28:1660–1664, 1988.

130. Taylor GA, Guion CJ, Potter BM, Eichelberger MR. CT of blunt abdominal trauma in children. AJR Am J Roentgenol 153:555–559, 1989.

131. Taylor GA, Kaufman RA, Sivit CJ. Active hemorrhage in children after thoracoabdominal trauma: Clinical and CT features. AJR Am J Roentgenol 162:401–404, 1994.

132. Taylor GA, O'Donnell R, Sivit CJ, Eichelberger MR. Abdominal injury score: A clinical score for the assignment of risk in children after blunt trauma. Radiology 190:689–694, 1994.

133. Taylor CR, Rosenfield AT. Limitations of computed tomography in the recognition of delayed splenic rupture. J Comput Assist Tomogr 8:1205–1207, 1984.

134. Townsend M, DeFalco AJ. Absence of ureteral opacification below ureteral disruption: A sentinel CT finding. AJR Am J Roentgenol 164:253–254, 1995.

135. Vaccaro JP, Brody JM. CT cystography in the evaluation of major bladder trauma RadioGraphics 20:1373–1381, 2000.

136. Van Steenbergen W, Samain H, Pouillon M, et al. Transection of the pancreas demonstrated by ultrasound and computed tomography. Gastrointest Radiol 12:128–130, 1987.

137. Vock P, Kehrer B, Tschaeppeler H. Blunt liver trauma in children: The role of computed tomography in diagnosis and treatment. J Pediatr Surg 21:413–418, 1986.

138. Whitten C, Grimes C, Isler R, Curci M, Dibbins A. CT of an actively-hemorrhaging liver laceration in a 9-year-old child. Pediatr Radiol 20:558–559, 1990.

139. Williams RD, Sargent FT. The mechanism of intestinal injury in trauma. J Trauma 3:288–294, 1963.

140. Wilms G, Marchal G, Baert A, Adisoejoso B, Mangkuwerdojo S. CT and ultrasound features of post-traumatic adrenal hemorrhage. J Comput Assist Tomogr 11:112–115, 1987.

141. Wong Y-C, Wang L-J, Lin B-C, Chen C-J, Lim K-E, Chen R-J. CT grading of blunt pancreatic injuries: Prediction of ductal disruption and surgical correlation. J Comput Assist Tomogr 21:246–250, 1997.

142. Yale-Loehr AJ, Kramer SS, Quinlan DM, La France ND, Mitchell SE, Gearhart JP. CT of severe renal trauma in children: Evaluation and course of healing with conservative therapy. AJR Am J Roentgenol 152:109–113, 1989.

ADDITIONAL READING

Ali M, Safriel Y, Sclafani SJ, Schulze R. CT signs of urethral injury. RadioGraphics 23:951–966, 2003.

Coley BD, Mutabagani KH, Martin LC, et al. Focused abdominal sonography for trauma (FAST) in children with blunt abdominal trauma. J Trauma 48:902–906, 2000.

Durbin DR, Arbogast KB, Moll EK. Seat belt syndrome in children: A case report and review of the literature. Pediatr Emerg Care 17:474–477, 2001.

Harris AC, Zwirewich CV, Lyburn ID, Torreggiani WC, Marchinkow LO. CT findings in blunt renal trauma. RadioGraphics 21:S201–S214, 2001.

Hollingsworth CL, Bisset GS. CT evaluation of pediatric abdominal trauma: Pitfalls and quandaries. Emerg Radiol 8:67–74, 2001.

Hewett JJ, Freed KS, Sheafor DH, Vaslef SN, Kliewer MA. The spectrum of abdominal venous CT findings in blunt trauma. AJR Am J Roentgenol 176: 955–958, 2001.

Kawashima A, Sandler CM, Corl FM, West OC, Tamm EP, Fishman EK, Goldman SM. Imaging of renal trauma: A comprehensive review. RadioGraphics 21:557–574, 2001.

Kawashima A, Sandler CM, Corl FM, West OC, Tamm EP, Fishman EK, Goldman SM. Imaging evaluation of posttraumatic renal injuries. Abdom Imaging 27:199–213, 2003.

Larici AR, Gotway MB, Litt HI, et al. Helical CT with sagittal and coronal reconstructions: Accuracy for detection of diaphragmatic injury. AJR Am J Roentgenol 179:451–457, 2002.

Minarik L, Slim M, Rachlin S, Brudnicki A: Diagnostic imaging in the follow-up of nonoperative management of splenic trauma in children. Pediatr Surg Int 18:429–431, 2002.

Morgan DE, Nallamala LK, Kenney PJ, Mayo MS, Rue LW III. CT cystography: Radiographic and clinical predictors of bladder rupture. AJR Am J Roentgenol 174:89–95, 2000.

Nance ML, Mahboubi S, Wickstrom M, Prendergast F, Stafford CW. Pattern of abdominal free fluid following isolated blunt spleen or liver injury in the pediatric patient. J Trauma 52:85–87, 2002.

Navarro O, Babyn PS, Pearl RH: The value of routine follow-up imaging in pediatric blunt liver trauma. Pediatr Radiol 30:546–550, 2000.

Novelline RA, Rhea JT, Rao PM, Stuk JL. Helical CT in emergency radiology. Radiology 213:321–339, 1999.

Scaglione M, Pinto F, Lassandro F, Romano L, Pinto A, Grassi R. Value of contrast-enhanced CT for managing mesenteric injuries after blunt trauma: Review of five-year experience. Emerg Radiol 9:26–31, 2002.

Vaccaro MJ, Brody JM. CT cystography in the evaluation of major bladder trauma. RadioGraphics 20:1373–1381, 2000.

Vasile M, Bellin MF, Helenon O, Mourey I, Cluzel P. Imaging evaluation of renal trauma. Abdom Imaging 25:424–430, 2000.

Willmann JK, Roos JE, Platz A, et al: Multidetector CT: Detection of active hemorrhage in patients with blunt abdominal trauma. AJR Am J Roentgenol 179:437–444, 2002.

Yao DC, Jeffrey RB Jr, Mirvis SE, et al. Using contrast-enhanced helical CT to visualize arterial extravasation after blunt abdominal trauma: Incidence and organ distribution. AJR Am J Roentgenol 178:17–20, 2002.

THE CHILD WITH BLOODY STOOLS

Outline

Saskia VON *Waldenburg Hilton, MD*

THE CHILD WITH BLOODY STOOLS

Rectal bleeding is a relatively common occurrence in children. It is a symptom that almost invariably causes considerable parental alarm and prompt solicitation of medical help. Fortunately, causes of rectal bleeding in children usually can be readily diagnosed and treated. Unlike in adults, malignant causes of rectal bleeding in children are very rare, and usually the extent of bleeding is not life threatening. In this chapter, an approach to rectal bleeding is presented that in almost all instances will permit timely diagnosis and therapy.

DIFFERENTIAL DIAGNOSIS OF RECTAL BLEEDING

The diagnostic approach to children with rectal bleeding primarily depends on establishing the most likely diagnosis as defined by the clinical findings. In a given patient, the most likely causes of bleeding can be accurately predicted by the following general features: the character of the bleeding, the volume of blood loss, the presence of specific physical signs and symptoms, and patient age. The most important factor in the differential diagnosis of rectal bleeding is the patient's age.

CHARACTER OF THE BLEEDING

Bright red blood that coats stool rather than being mixed with stool implies anorectal bleeding, which is most commonly due to an anal fissure. Blood mixed with stool and mucus, forming the so-called "currant-jelly stools," results from colonic irritation coupled with lymphatic and vascular congestion, which typically occurs with intussusception. Melena usually implies an upper gastrointestinal bleeding source but occasionally is associated with a distal source if the patient is constipated or the volume of blood loss is small. The most accurate way to assess whether bleeding is from an upper or lower source is by passing a nasogastric tube into the stomach and examining the gastric aspirate for the presence of blood.

VOLUME OF BLOOD LOSS

Estimating the volume of blood loss is also helpful in determining the cause of rectal bleeding in children. Occult blood loss manifesting itself as chronic anemia is rare in children; it occurs most commonly with juvenile polyps. Minimal overt bleeding is frequently produced by anal fissures and juvenile polyps, whereas moderate to severe hemorrhage occurs with most Meckel's diverticula, peptic ulcers, stress ulcers, and esophageal varices.

SPECIFIC SIGNS AND SYMPTOMS

Clinical signs and symptoms often suggest a specific diagnosis; for example, painless bleeding is most commonly associated with Meckel's diverticulum; paroxysmal pain with an abdominal mass suggests an intussusception; and splenomegaly may reflect portal hypertension and, thus, variceal bleeding. Major hemorrhage in a trauma or burn victim most likely arises from a stress ulcer.

PATIENT AGE

The causes of gastrointestinal bleeding in children are largely related to age. For example, necrotizing enterocolitis is not commonly encountered other than in hospitalized, premature infants, although rarely a term infant or older child may be affected. In neonates, most instances of bleeding occur from idiopathic and self-limited causes. Intussusceptions and most Meckel's diverticula present by 2 years of age. By age 5 years, idiopathic intussusceptions are rarely seen, and intussusceptions that do occur usually have a "lead point," or a pathologic mass that initiates the intussusception; these include a Meckel's diverticulum, lymphoma, or lymphosarcoma. The peak age for juvenile polyps is 5 years; they occur very rarely before 1 year or after 14 years of age. Similarly, bleeding from varices is not seen before the age of 1 year and becomes more common with advancing age. Inflammatory bowel disease and peptic ulcers are also most common in older children. In the remainder of this section, the most common causes of bleeding as a function of the patient's age are discussed in greater detail.

Neonates (Birth to 1 Month)
Necrotizing enterocolitis is a disease seen almost exclusively in premature neonates, who frequently have complications

of respiratory distress syndrome such as intracranial bleeding and cardiac compromise from a patent ductus arteriosus. Gross or occult blood in the stool, abdominal distention, and retained feedings are frequent clinical findings. Plain radiographs may reveal persistently dilated loops of bowel, pneumatosis, air-fluid levels, ascites, portal venous air, or free intraperitoneal air. In an intensive care nursery, necrotizing enterocolitis usually is quickly suspected and easily confirmed. After an infant is released from the hospital, this disease rarely occurs.

Full-term newborn infants may have considerable blood loss from hematemesis, hematochezia, or both. Because there is a favorable prognosis for spontaneous resolution in this group of patients and because surgical causes are exceedingly rare, radiographic investigations are seldom indicated.[21] In a study of 98 neonates with neonatal gastrointestinal bleeding, Sherman and Clatworthy[47] noted the following etiologies: swallowed maternal blood, anorectal trauma with anal fissure, hemorrhagic disease of the newborn with hypoproteinemia, colitis (allergic, infectious, or related to Hirschsprung's disease), congenital heart disease with intestinal hypoperfusion, hypoglycemia, and unexplained bleeding with spontaneous cessation (50%). The last group probably contained many infants with stress ulcers (Table 11–1).

A small percentage of neonates with Hirschsprung's disease initially present with bloody stools from enterocolitis. Because Hirschsprung's disease is notoriously difficult to diagnose in neonates, contrast enema examination and suction biopsy should be carried out in infants with a functional distal small bowel obstruction and with a history of delayed passage of meconium (95% of infants with Hirschsprung's

TABLE 11-1 CAUSES OF RECTAL BLEEDING IN NEONATES (BIRTH TO 1 MONTH)

Common
Idiopathic
Anorectal trauma
Swallowed maternal blood
Necrotizing enterocolitis (premature infants)
Rare
Hemorrhagic disease of newborn
Congenital heart disease
Hypoglycemia
Hirschsprung's disease
Midgut volvulus
Stress ulcer
Intestinal duplication
Neonatal appendicitis
Hemangiomatosis
Infectious colitis
Neonatal hepatic necrosis

disease pass no meconium by 48 hours, whereas 95% of normal infants do).

Swallowed maternal blood, hemorrhagic disease of the newborn, and hypoglycemia can be diagnosed by laboratory tests. Bedside proctoscopic examination of infants readily reveals anal fissures or colitis. As noted previously, rectal bleeding in a term newborn infant stops spontaneously in most cases, and thus patient prognosis is excellent. Therefore, radiographic investigation is seldom required in most newborns for whom the cause is unknown, and no associated signs or symptoms are evident. A definite exception to this "watch-and-wait" approach is a neonate who has bloody stools accompanied by bile-stained vomiting. The possibility of a midgut volvulus must be excluded by an upper gastrointestinal (UGI) examination, even when plain films in such patients are normal.

Infants (1 Month to 2 Years)

The most common causes of rectal bleeding in infants are anal fissure, intussusception, stress ulcer, and Meckel's diverticulum. The differential diagnosis can be further narrowed by subdividing the lesions into those resulting in mild bleeding and those causing more extensive blood loss. In this age group, many causes of rectal bleeding are lesions that require surgery; thus, aggressive diagnostic efforts are often mandatory.

Minimal bleeding is seen with anal fissure, intussusception, intestinal ischemia, and inflammation, whereas moderate to severe rectal bleeding is caused by stress ulcer and Meckel's diverticulum. Anal fissures are readily diagnosed by inspection. Intussusception is rarely a diagnostic problem because of the typical features of paroxysmal pain, currant-jelly stools, and a palpable abdominal mass. Plain films may show a mass with or without evidence of bowel obstruction. If a nonobstructive gas pattern is present, hydrostatic reduction should be attempted. If radiographs reveal a distal small bowel obstruction suggesting vascular compromise, a lead point, or both, a diagnostic enema (with no attempt to reduce the lesion) is indicated (Table 11–2).

Any possibility of vascular compromise causing bloody stools must be vigorously pursued, because almost all these conditions are life-threatening surgical lesions. Midgut volvulus or trauma (frequently from unrecognized child abuse) are the usual causes of vascular compromise. The major clinical signs are pain, abdominal distention, mildly bloody stools, and shock. In midgut volvulus, the superior mesenteric artery is occluded as the mesentery becomes twisted. In child abuse, forceful blows to the abdomen cause mesenteric tears and avulsion of major vessels.

Bloody diarrhea without fever suggests colitis due to milk protein or soybean allergy. If fever is present, an infectious cause is more likely (usually *Campylobacter, Salmonella*, or *Yersinia* species). Endoscopy is an excellent method for revealing inflammation, and stool cultures will usually identify the

organism responsible for the infection. Note that stool cultures should be obtained before barium studies are done, because barium may inhibit the growth of many diarrhea-producing organisms.

Young (2 to 5 Years) and Older Children

Juvenile polyps, varices, stress ulcers, and inflammatory bowel diseases are common causes of rectal bleeding in young (2 to 5 years) and older children, whereas idiopathic intussusception without a pathologic lead point is rare (Table 11–3). As in infants, many of the most common causes of rectal bleeding are amenable to specific treatment; thus, diagnostic studies should be pursued vigorously. Again, the specific diagnostic maneuvers are dictated by the most likely causes as indicated by the presenting clinical features.

Mild Bleeding   Blood-streaked stool or mild bleeding is the usual presentation of juvenile polyps. Proctosigmoidoscopy is diagnostic and therapeutic in most children in whom a single polyp is located within 10 cm of the anus and, therefore, can be snared. An air-contrast barium enema may be indicated (1) when findings from sigmoidoscopy are negative, (2) when a second episode of bleeding follows polypectomy, or (3) if the resected polyp histologically is not a juvenile polyp.

Hemolytic-uremic syndrome is the most common cause of renal failure in young children (Fig. 11–1). The micropathic hemolytic anemia can be triggered by a multitude of causes including verotoxin-producing strains of *Escherichia coli*,

---

TABLE 11-2 CAUSES OF RECTAL BLEEDING IN INFANTS (1 MONTH TO 2 YEARS)

Common
Anorectal trauma
Intussusception
Meckel's diverticulum
Colitis
Swallowed blood
Rare
Stress ulcer
Midgut volvulus
Ischemia secondary to trauma (tearing of mesentery with avulsion of vessels)
Gastroesophageal reflux
Hemophilia
Hemolytic-uremic syndrome
Gastritis (drug-induced)
Gastric outlet obstruction (pyloric stenosis)
Duplication cyst with ectopic gastric mucosa
Parasitic infestation
Varices
Foreign bodies

TABLE 11-3 CAUSES OF RECTAL BLEEDING IN
YOUNG (2 TO 5 YEARS) AND OLDER
CHILDREN

Common
Anorectal trauma
Juvenile polyps
Varices
Swallowed blood
Inflammatory bowel disease
Infectious colitis
Duodenal ulcers
Rare
Stress ulcer
Gastritis
Henoch-Schönlein purpura
Meckel's diverticulum
Intussusception with lead point
Hemophilia
Peutz-Jeghers syndrome
Osler-Weber-Rendu disease
Vascular malformations
Klippel-Trenaunay-Weber syndrome
Parasitic infestation
Duodenal ulcers

Salmonella, or *Shigella* or endotoxemia. Only the prodrome of this disease causes diagnostic confusion. The earliest symptoms are those of gastroenteritis or an upper respiratory infection, Diarrhea, which is often bloody, fever, vomiting, and abdominal pain appear 5 to 10 days before the onset of the classic symptoms of pallor, oligemia, irritability, and weakness. The average age of onset is before 4 years of age.

Infectious colitis is another important cause of mild, bloody diarrhea in young and older children. Diarrhea is almost always the dominant symptom. Diagnosis is identical to that in the younger age groups. Inflammatory bowel disease may present with bloody stools in older children, but more common symptoms are weight loss, abdominal pain, fever, and anemia. An air-contrast barium enema is the examination of choice for suspected inflammatory bowel disease. Both inflammatory bowel disease and infectious colitis are discussed in detail in Chapter 15.

Moderate to Severe Bleeding In young and older children, massive bleeding may be divided into lower and upper bleeding. The presence of blood in the gastric aspirate suggests that the cause is esophageal varices, gastritis, or gastric or duodenal ulcers. In this setting, endoscopy is an appropriate diagnostic maneuver. Stress ulcers are a secondary complication seen in children after trauma or burns and in those with severe central nervous system disorders; pain is

usually absent, and the initial sign is gastrointestinal bleeding. Esophageal varices result from portal hypertension and generally are accompanied by splenomegaly; chronic liver disease, which normally has been previously diagnosed, is a common cause. In the absence of known liver disease, portal vein obstruction and, rarely, undiagnosed cystic fibrosis are likely possibilities.

Massive bleeding that does not produce any blood in the gastric aspirate is most commonly due to Meckel's diverticulum; only rarely does a duodenal ulcer bleed significantly without producing gastric blood. Henoch-Schönlein purpura may present with rectal bleeding preceding the onset of skin purpura and hematuria by several days. Likewise, the passage of rectal blood may be the dominant primary symptom of the hemolytic-uremic syndrome.

EVALUATION OF THE MOST IMPORTANT CONDITIONS CAUSING RECTAL BLEEDING

In the following sections the most common entities responsible for rectal bleeding in children are discussed. The diseases were selected not only because they occur frequently, but also because radiology plays an important role in their diagnosis and management (with the exception of anal fissures). The entities discussed are anal fissures, intussusception, Meckel's diverticulum, and juvenile polyps.

ANAL FISSURES

The leading cause of rectal bleeding in young children is anal fissures. The history and physical examination of the patient will indicate the diagnosis of this frequent condition in almost all cases. In the history, only a small amount of red blood is usually described; it most often appears as a stripe on the outside of the stool of an otherwise healthy child. A drop of bright red blood may follow the passage of the stool and may discolor the toilet tissue or diaper. Bleeding is almost never profuse. There is often a history of constipation and passage of a large or hard stool, accompanied by discomfort and frank pain.

Anal fissures are most frequently found in children between the ages of 4 months and 3 years. An acute fissure is usually a fresh crack or abrasion in the anal mucosa, caused by trauma from a hard, large stool; fissures may be multiple. Chronic fissures may develop from untreated acute fissures or may result from diarrhea with secondary infection of anal glands and crypts. The predominant symptom is pain, especially with defecation; however, blood on a diaper or on

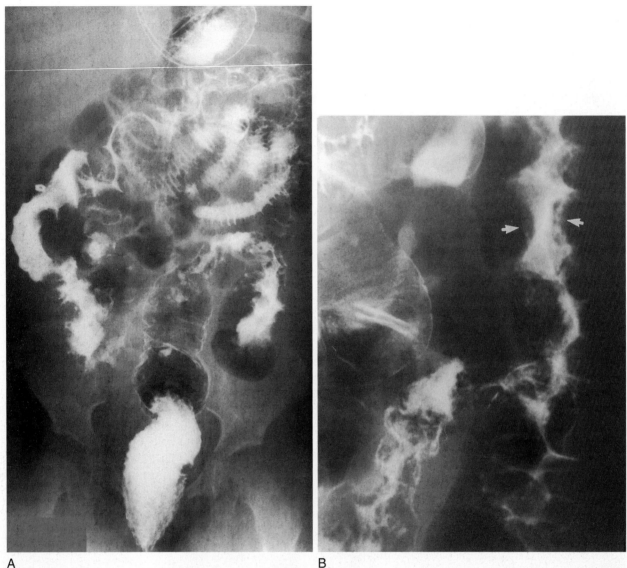

A   B

Figure 11–1
Hemolytic-uremic syndrome. *A,* A barium enema and upper gastrointestinal examination revealed diffuse effacement and distortion of the colon. The remaining visible bowel showed mild fold thickening that involved even the stomach and rectum. Diffuse submucosal bleeding caused the abnormal bowel pattern. Clinical signs of hemolytic-uremic syndrome were preceded by bloody stools in this 3-year-old girl. *B,* Large submucosal defects *(arrows)* indenting the colonic lumen are evident on this spot film of the descending colon.

the outside of the stool may be the only sign. Conscious withholding of stool because of fear of painful defecation may produce cyclic constipation, producing harder stools that cause more pain and bleeding.

If the child's anus is examined with adequate illumination, most fissures can be seen without use of instruments. If the patient can strain, the fissures may be seen even more readily. Acute fissures appear as longitudinal slits in the anal mucosa below the pectinate line. Chronic fissures are indurated ulcers with edematous skin tags distally and hypertrophied anal papillae proximally.

The treatment goal is to break the cycle of hard stools, fissures, pain, reflex spasm, and withholding of stool.

Radiographic studies are neither appropriate nor diagnostic; thus, before a barium enema for rectal bleeding is performed, the possibility of anal fissures must be excluded.

INTUSSUSCEPTION

During the last decade the diagnosis and treatment options for intussusception of childhood have expanded greatly. Ultrasound is now being used to diagnose and treat the disease.

Prompt diagnosis of intussusception and early reduction considerably decrease the morbidity and mortality rates in

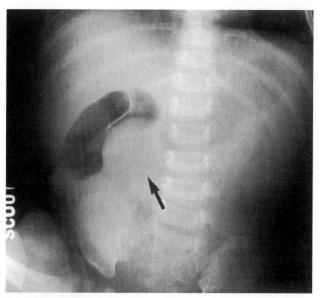

Figure 11–2
Intussusception: abdominal mass in a 6-month-old boy with a paucity of abdominal gas. The mass of the intussusception *(arrow)* is easily defined. No obstructive gas pattern is present. This lesion was easily reduced.

this potentially fatal disease. The most important challenge confronting the clinician is suggesting this diagnosis in children with atypical presentations. The radiologist, however, is faced with two problems: first, if reduction is indicated, and second, if it is indicated, how to successfully and safely accomplish the reduction (Figs. 11–2, 11–3, and 11–4).

Pathoanatomy

Intussusception is a invagination of the proximal bowel into its distal lumen. The invaginating portion is termed the *intussusceptum*, and the recipient bowel is called the *intussuscipiens*. Approximately 90% of intussusceptions are ileocolic, with the remaining 10% being ileoileal and colocolic.

Ileoileal intussusceptions are most frequently seen in postoperative patients and are thought to result from abnormal peristalsis during resolution of an ileus. Ileocolic and colocolic intussusceptions (the latter of which is rare) may be divided into two groups: those that have a definable lead point and

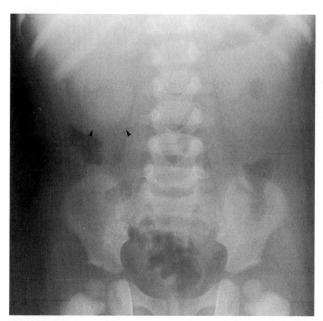

Figure 11–3
Intussusception: abdominal mass. A 10-month-old girl presented with bloody stools as the sole abnormality. This supine radiograph demonstrated a well-defined mass at the hepatic flexure *(arrowheads)*. There is no evidence of bowel obstruction. The intussusception was easily reduced with a therapeutic enema. Once hydrostatic reduction has been decided on, delays should be kept to a minimum.

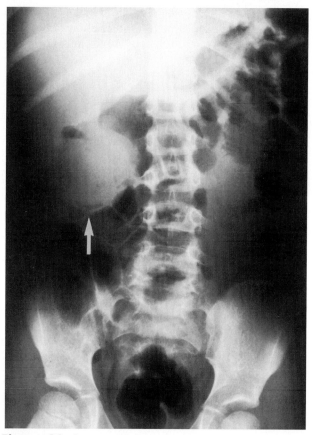

Figure 11–4
Intussusception: abdominal mass in a 4-year-old boy with abdominal pain and bloody stools. A mass in the right upper quadrant *(arrow)*, indenting the transverse colon, is clearly defined. Radiographic signs of obstruction are absent. Despite the older age of the patient, this mass was reduced without difficulty.

those that do not. Lead points include Meckel's diverticulum, submucosal hemorrhage, lymphoma or lymphosarcoma, polyps, and bowel duplications.

Idiopathic intussusceptions (i.e., those without a lead point) account for 95% of all those that occur in the peak incidence age of 5 to 9 months. Proposed causes include lymphoid hyperplasia in the terminal ileum, hyperperistalsis due to viral infections, and a greater disproportion of size between the ileocecal valve and the ileum in infants compared with that in older children. At present, the cause remains unknown.

Among intussusceptions caused by a lead point, the nature of the lead point depends on the patient's age. In children younger than 2 years, the most common lead point is a Meckel's diverticulum, whereas in the child 5 years old or older, the most common cause is lymphoma or lymphosarcoma. Neonates, who rarely suffer from intussusception, most frequently have a bowel duplication as a lead point. Less common lead points include polyps; intramural hematoma, as seen in Henoch-Schönlein purpura or the hemolytic-uremic syndrome; and, rarely, a normal appendix.

Whatever the cause of the intussusception, the resulting pathophysiologic process is similar (Fig. 11–5). As the bowel invaginates into the distal lumen, compression causes variable degrees of venous occlusion. Unless the intussusception reduces spontaneously, bowel swelling occurs, with concurrent arterial compromise. Bowel ischemia results in loss of mucosal integrity, with resultant oozing of blood and mucus from mucosal surfaces. Progressive bowel edema eventually causes complete vascular occlusion, local ischemic necrosis, and bowel infarction. Perforation then leads to peritonitis.

Clinical Presentation

The overall incidence of intussusception is between 1.9 and 4.0 per 1000 births. The incidence varies according to geographic location and season, being most common in winter and spring. The male-to-female ratio is 3:2. Sixty percent of the cases occur during the first year of life, and 90% occur by the end of the second year. The highest incidence is in those infants between 5 and 9 months of age.

The most prominent clinical symptoms of idiopathic intussusception are intermittent abdominal pain (94%), vomiting (91%), bloody stools (66%), and a palpable abdominal mass (59%).[29] Twenty percent of affected children have an upper respiratory infection at presentation, and 10% have had diarrhea before onset of the disease. Fever is common. In the absence of bloody stools, the major differential diagnostic consideration is viral gastroenteritis. Typical currant-jelly stools usually appear within 24 hours of onset, but infrequently they may appear as much as 2 days later.

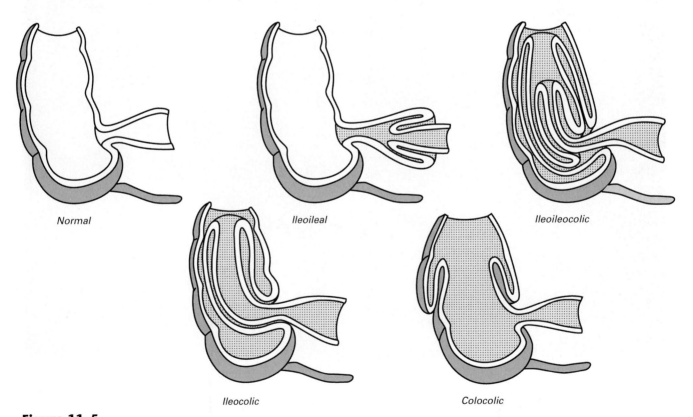

Normal   *Ileoileal*   *Ileoileocolic*

Ileocolic   *Colocolic*

Figure 11–5
Diagrammatic representation of intussusception. From PRACTICAL PEDIATRIC IMAGING, Second Edition, Page 880, Fig. 7-162, 1991, Little Brown and Company.

The pain is often characteristically colicky, severe, and intermittent. The paroxysms of pain are frequently accompanied by straining efforts, and initially the child may appear and act perfectly normal between the paroxysms. Vomiting of gastric contents is common; vomitus may later consist of bile-stained fluid, introducing the possibility of acute midgut volvulus. As the disease continues, increasing pain, elevated temperature, and signs of circulatory collapse may become evident.

On physical examination, the most consistent and helpful sign is the presence of a palpable, tubular mass, most frequently found in the right upper quadrant, although sometimes it may be hidden beneath the costal margin. The mass may be ill defined and tender. The presence of such a mass in children who have clinical signs of intussusception virtually ensures the diagnosis (Figs. 11–6 and 11–7).

More than 50% of patients older than 5 years of age will have a lead point causing their intussusception.[45] The most common lead point is a Meckel's diverticulum, which occurs in almost half of these patients.[15] The second most frequent lead point is lymphoma, which is present in 17% of children.[17] Patients with lymphoma are often more chronically ill, with pain of longer duration (weeks to months), weight loss, and an abdominal mass.

Radiographic Evaluation

Intussusception is potentially a surgical disease; thus, all patients are treated as preoperative candidates. Vascular access is obtained, blood is typed and crossmatched, and operating room personnel are notified. Most importantly, all decisions are made jointly with the pediatric surgical consultant in attendance. Reduction of an intussusception obviates the morbidity of anesthesia and surgery in those children with both viable bowel and absence of a lead point. When selecting candidates for safe reduction, therefore, the clinician must consider factors that help predict bowel viability and the presence of a lead point. Young children are not likely to have a lead point. However, in those patients who do have a lead point (most commonly a Meckel's diverticulum), there is a high incidence of complete bowel obstruction, and reduction is less likely, even when vigorously attempted. By the age of 2 years, a child's chance of having a lead point increases, and by 5 years more than 50% of intussusceptions are caused by a lead point.

Many authors advocate sonography for an initial screening of patients suspected of having intussusception.[42,51] Two patterns are described as typical: (1) multiple, concentric, echogenic rings alternating with hypoechoic regions resembling a doughnut and (2) a fusiform, hypoechoic mass with

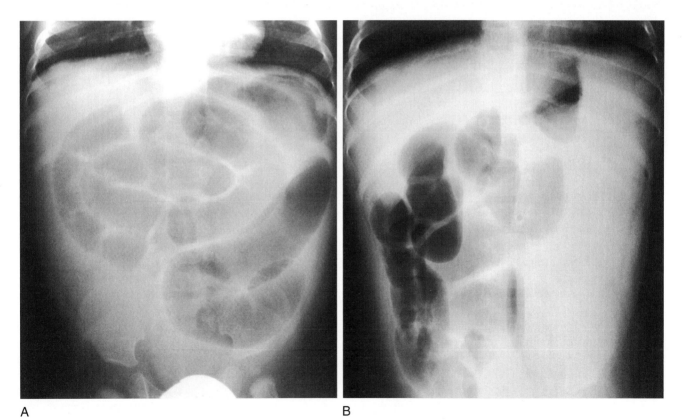

A   B

Figure 11–6

Intussusception. *A,* Supine view of a 6-month-old boy with paroxysmal pain and vomiting of 8 hours' duration. This plain film reveals dilated small bowel with no colonic gas visible. *B,* This left lateral decubitus (left-side-down decubitus) view demonstrates multiple air-fluid levels and the absence of free intraperitoneal air. Hydrostatic reduction was attempted but failed. The intussusception was easily reduced surgically, and the bowel was viable.

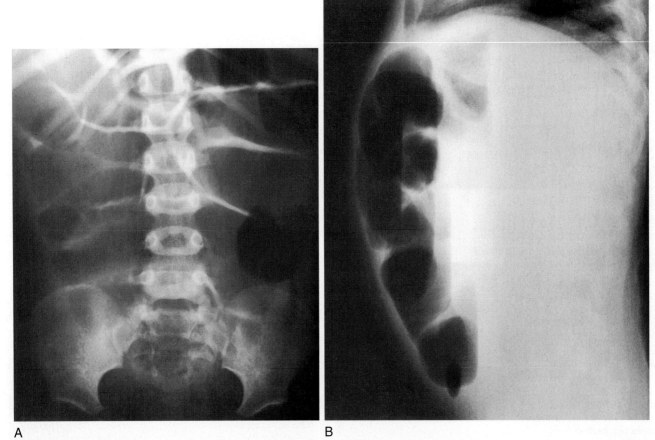

A   B

Figure 11–7
Intussusception: supine plain radiograph. *A,* A supine abdominal radiograph of an 18-month-old girl with abdominal distention, bloody stools, and vomiting. This frontal plain film reveals multiple dilated small bowel loops, indicating a mechanical obstruction. *B,* This cross-table lateral view of the same patient demonstrated multiple air-fluid levels, confirming a mechanical bowel obstruction. A diagnostic enema demonstrated an intussusception in the transverse colon. Partial bowel resection was necessary because of ischemic and necrotic bowel.

a central echogenic focus that has a pseudokidney appearance. The multiple concentric rings represent interfaces of bowel wall. This finding is comparable to the target sign identified on plain films.[39]

It is important to recognize the sonographic appearance of intussusception, as this may be the initial examination performed in an older patient who presents with a mass and atypical clinical findings. The sonographic findings are suggestive but not diagnostic unless multiple concentric rings are identified.[5] Tumor and inflammatory bowel disease may have a pseudokidney sign.

The initial radiographic evaluation includes a supine radiograph and at least one horizontal-beam film.[3] Contraindications for radiographic reduction include hypovolemic shock, peritonitis, and evidence of perforation. Thus, free air on the decubitus examination or evidence of peritoneal fluid is a sign of a surgical abdomen and a contraindication for therapeutic reduction of the intussusception.

Supine plain radiographs may be normal in 25% of patients with the disease. In about half of patients with an intussusception, the plain film reveals a soft tissue mass or an abnormal bowel pattern.[55] Twenty-five percent of patients demonstrate evidence of a distal small bowel obstruction. It is important to remember that although the diagnosis of intussusception can be suggested on plain films, a normal examination does not exclude the diagnosis[3] (Fig. 11–8).

Diagnostic Enema At times it is not possible or desirable to reduce an intussusception; these instances include intussusceptions in a patient older than 5 years, who is likely to have a lead point, and in some patients with severe, prolonged bowel obstruction. In these patients, it is desirable to perform an enema and diagnose an intussusception with certainty, because a child with a medical cause of rectal bleeding is not a candidate for surgery (Figs. 11–9 and 11–10). Common medical causes that may be confused with an intussusception include infectious colitis, hemolytic-uremic

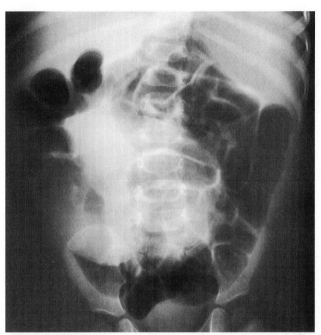

Figure 11–8

Intussusception plain film: Supine radiograph of an 8-month-old girl who presented with mild rectal bleeding of 48 hours' duration. The physical examination revealed a large, easily palpable mass in the midabdomen. This radiograph shows a large soft tissue mass displacing the small bowel. Moderate bowel dilatation is evident, and a decubitus view (not shown) demonstrated multiple air-fluid levels, indicating that the intussusception had produced a mechanical bowel obstruction.

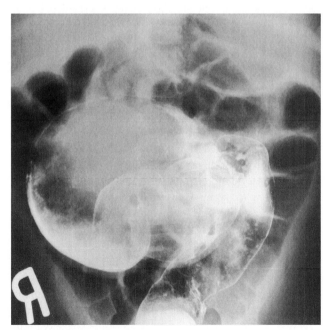

Figure 11–9

Intussusception: barium enema. This diagnostic enema revealed a large intussusception in the sigmoid colon. Hydrostatic reduction was unsuccessful. Surgical exploration revealed a large, gangrenous intussusception. The patient recovered uneventfully.

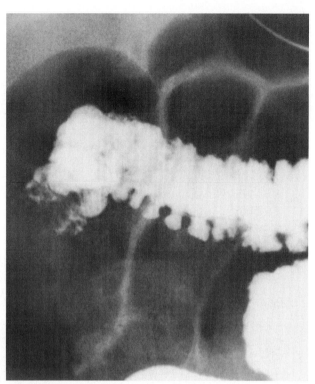

Figure 11–10

Intussusception: diagnostic enema using barium. In a diagnostic enema, a single spot film is sufficient to make the diagnosis of intussusception. As soon as the obstruction is encountered, no further contrast material is introduced. This minimizes the possibility of perforation. Radiographically, the typical "coiled spring" appearance is seldom seen, because contrast does not insinuate itself between the intussusceptum and the intussuscipiens. Note the lack of distention of the distal colon, the absence of the coiled spring appearance, and dilated small bowel loops.

syndrome, and Henoch-Schönlein purpura. A diagnostic enema is a simple, rapid procedure that confirms the presence of a surgical abdomen; it is modified as follows:

1. Barium or diatrizoate meglumine–diatrizoate sodium (Hypaque) (diluted to serum osmolality) is used as the contrast material.
2. A small-caliber rather than a large-caliber rubber catheter is used so that filling of the colon is slow.
3. As soon as an intussusception is encountered, influx of contrast material is stopped, and a single spot film is taken for documentation.
4. Rectal decompression is achieved by retaining the tube.
5. *If colitis or other causes are evident, the colon is examined, and a postevacuation film is obtained. If mucosal detail is diagnostically insufficient with diatrizoate meglumine–diatrizoate sodium, then the colon is drained, and the examination is repeated with barium.*
   Therapeutic Enema

Once the diagnosis of intussusception has been suggested by clinical findings, plain radiographs, or sonography, a contrast enema is performed unless the patient has physical signs of a surgical abdomen (Fig. 11–11). Prolonged symptoms of small bowel obstruction and older age are relative contraindications for the conservative pediatric radiologist, as intussusceptions in such patients are rarely reduced. However, studies show that although patients with small bowel obstruction or longer duration of symptoms have a decreased rate of successful reduction, they do not have an increased rate of complications[4,6,34,49] (Figs. 11–12 and 11–13).

Before the reduction is started, the following are performed:

1. A surgeon is consulted to verify the absence of signs of perforation or peritonitis and agree that a reduction is indicated.
2. Intravenous access is obtained and hydration is begun.
3. Analgesic premedication is given if indicated (i.e., in a child with moderate agitation or crying).[30] Crying or straining induces the Valsalva maneuver, which increases intra-abdominal pressure and makes reduction of the intussusception more difficult.

A double-blind study showed that the use of glucagon was of no value in the reduction of intussusception.[22]

Contrast Agents   A number of different contrast agents are currently used for the reduction of intussusceptions. The primary agents are barium, water-soluble media, and air.

Barium traditionally has been the contrast agent of choice because it gives superb detail of abnormalities and is inexpensive and iso-osmolar. This excellent detail is very helpful if the cause of bloody stools is medical (e.g., infectious colitis, Henoch-Schönlein purpura, or hemolytic-uremic syndrome). The main disadvantage of barium is the inflammatory reaction that can result in cases of bowel perforation and with spillage of contrast into the peritoneum.

Water-soluble contrast media are inexpensive and less hazardous in patients with bowel perforation. However, mucosal detail may be insufficient to diagnose other causes of bloody stools.

Air theoretically is the ideal contrast agent because it provides sufficient visibility to reduce the intussusception and causes no harm in cases of perforation. However, air cannot define other medical causes of bloody stools because of the lack of sufficient mucosal contrast. Air has been used successfully in several large pediatric centers in the United States without major complications.

Campbell[6] surveyed pediatric radiologists in children's hospitals in North America to determine the contrast media of choice. Eighty-five percent always used barium and an additional 7.5% almost always use barium. The principles of barium enema reduction were initially described by Ravitch[44] and have changed very little.

A large-bore, unlubricated, end-hole soft rubber catheter is placed high in the rectum. Most pediatric radiologists tape the buttocks tightly together to prevent the catheter from being pushed out. The airtight seal achieved with a Foley catheter

balloon is thought to increase the possibility of bowel perforation, and, therefore, its use is discouraged. A safe approach to the reduction is as follows:

1. The barium bag is suspended 3 feet above the table.
2. Three attempts at reduction are made.
3. Three minutes of prolonged pressure are allowed per attempt.

The aim of the therapeutic enema is to achieve a constant, nonfluctuating, safe level of intraluminal pressure that will push back the intussusceptum. Maneuvers such as clamping the tube, milking the tube, or palpating the abdomen are contraindicated, as they may raise the pressure to unpredictably high levels. Clamping the tube after the procedure has begun creates a closed system in which high pressures can be generated when the infant strains or cries. Milking the tube or palpating the child's abdomen may similarly and dangerously elevate pressure.

Reduction of the intussusception usually proceeds at variable and uneven rates; frequently, a considerable delay is encountered at the cecum. If no reduction is achieved after 3 minutes in one location, the child is permitted to evacuate, which frequently aids in moving the intussusceptum. We usually make two additional attempts to fill, followed by evacuation, before abandoning the procedure in favor of surgical reduction.

As contrast material flows into the colon, a temporary halt occurs as the intussusception is encountered. This may be located anywhere from the rectum to the cecum. The more distally the intussusception is encountered, the lower the rate of reduction.[49] When the intussusception is met in the ascending colon, a 75% reduction rate can be expected; however, only 25% of intussusceptions met in the rectum can be reduced. As the intraluminal pressure rises, barium insinuates itself between the intussusceptum and intussuscipiens, outlining the mucosa and producing a "coiled spring" appearance. Reduction occurs at uneven rates with a usual delay at the cecum.

Spot films are taken for documentation when the intussusception is first encountered and when reflux into the terminal ileum is achieved. An overhead radiograph at the end of the procedure documents reduction and verifies filling of several feet of ileum. A postevacuation film also identifies the few intussusceptions that recur with evacuation. During the procedure, fluoroscopic visualization is used sparingly and intermittently.

To reduce an intussusception successfully, reflux is obtained into several feet of ileum. If there is no reflux into the terminal ileum, the child must be considered to have an irreducible intussusception. Once irreducibility is established, complete draining of barium is advisable. Leaving the rectal tube in place ensures decompression, rendering perforation unlikely. Surgical reduction is then performed as soon as possible.

Residual edema of the ileocecal valve and ileum is common and should not be mistaken for a pathologic mass.[14,55]

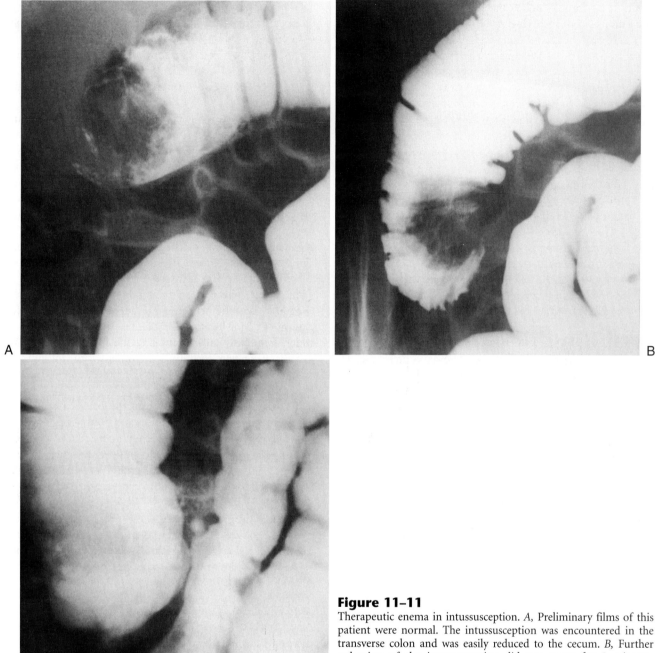

A

B

C

Figure 11–11

Therapeutic enema in intussusception. *A,* Preliminary films of this patient were normal. The intussusception was encountered in the transverse colon and was easily reduced to the cecum. *B,* Further reduction of the intussusception did not occur for 5 minutes. Evacuation and refilling are sometimes helpful in permitting continued reduction when the head of the intussusception remains in one location for a prolonged period of time. A delay in reduction at the ileocecal valve is common. *C,* This spot film documents the fact that reduction into the terminal ileum has taken place.

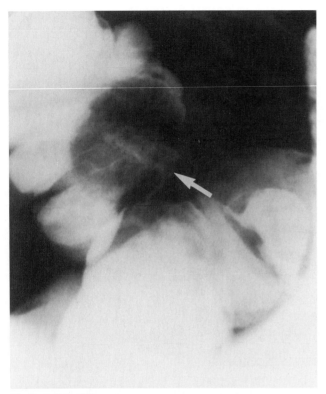

Figure 11–12
Complication: mass effect of ileocecal valve. Although this is usually of no consequence, it may become a complication if the edematous ileocecal valve is mistaken for a nonreduced intussusception. The location of the mass, its well-defined roundness and central contrast material *(arrow)*, and reflux into the terminal ileum make differentiation of edematous ileocecal valve from intussusception easy.

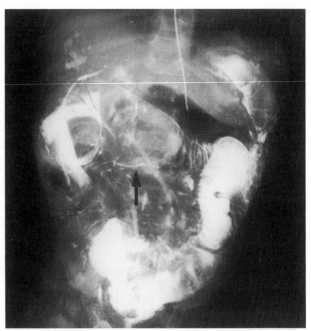

Figure 11–13
Complication: perforation. This is a preoperative plain film showing barium perforation with intussusception. The mass of the intussusceptum is seen in the transverse colon *(arrow)*. Barium is seen within the peritoneal cavity. The child was taken immediately to surgery, where the peritoneal cavity was lavaged and ischemic bowel resected. This patient had no complications from the barium spillage.

A residual intraluminal filling defect in the barium column after adequate flooding of the terminal ileum indicates a lead point and represents an indication for laparotomy.

Proponents of water-soluble contrast media suggest that the adverse effects of leakage of this agent into the peritoneal space are fewer than if barium were to be spilled into the peritoneum. Cochran et al.[7] experimentally demonstrated that the combination of barium and feces was more harmful than either substance alone. More recent data presented by Hernandez-Schulman revealed the following when a median lethal dose (LD_{50}) solution of feces mixed with 40 mL of different contrast agents was injected into the peritoneum of guinea pigs: survival rate at 36 hours: barium sulfate, 0%; iothalamate meglumine 30 (Conray 30), 30%; iothalamate meglumine 15 (Conray 15), 90%; saline, 100%; air, 100%. The incidence of perforation in children is extremely low (0.39%).[6] In more than 14,000 patients with intussusception studied by Campbell,[6] there were only 55 perforations. Most of these perforations occurred with barium and were well tolerated; there was only one death. Blane et al.[4] similarly reported no increased mortality or morbidity in patients

with perforation during attempted barium enema reduction of intussusception.

Pneumatic reduction of intussusceptions has become the standard in the United States (Fig. 11–14). The technique was first used in China and Canada.[27,28,58] The major advantages of this method are (1) faster reduction, (2) a significant decrease in radiation dose, and (3) no contrast spill into the peritoneal cavity should bowel perforation occur. Potential problems include a possible tension pneumoperitoneum with perforation, failure to identify the intussusception because of excess gas in the bowel, failure to recognize complete reduction, and failure to identify a lead point.[3] The success rate with pneumatic reduction is 80% to 98%. Stringer and Ein[50] recommended that air enemas not be used in patients older than 4 years of age, as the incidence of lead points is higher.

The air insufflation method uses a simple Y connector that is attached to a pressure monitor.[3,48] A bulb syringe and blood pressure manometer are attached through the Y connector to an end-hole rubber catheter, which is inserted into the rectum. Also available is a specifically designed single-piece, aneroid-gauge bulb insufflator that allows operation of the equipment with one hand.

When air reduction is performed, a pressure of 80 to 120 mm Hg is optimal and safe. One pitfall of this method is that it is possible to produce extensive reflux of gas into the

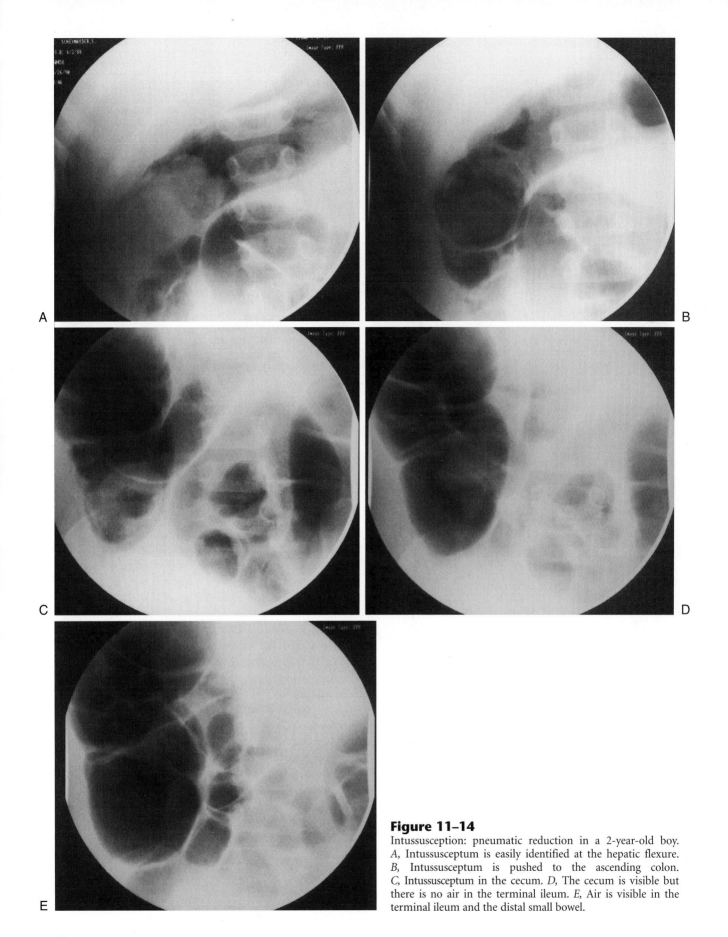

Figure 11–14

Intussusception: pneumatic reduction in a 2-year-old boy. *A*, Intussusceptum is easily identified at the hepatic flexure. *B*, Intussusceptum is pushed to the ascending colon. *C*, Intussusceptum in the cecum. *D*, The cecum is visible but there is no air in the terminal ileum. *E*, Air is visible in the terminal ileum and the distal small bowel.

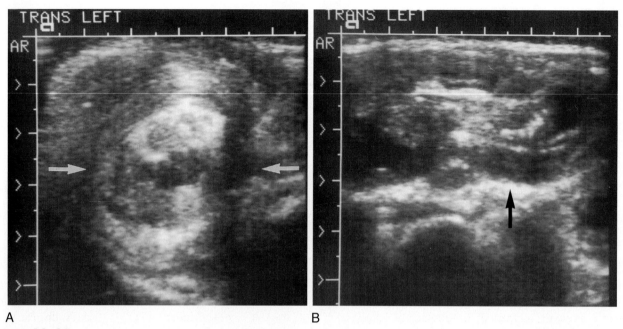

A   B

Figure 11–15
Sonographic diagnosis of intussusception: transverse *(A) (white arrows)* and longitudinal *(B) (black arrow)* images of a palpable mass in the right upper quadrant of a 10-month-old boy. Note the alternating bands of hyperechoic and hypoechoic tissue. The longitudinal image has a "pseudokidney" appearance.

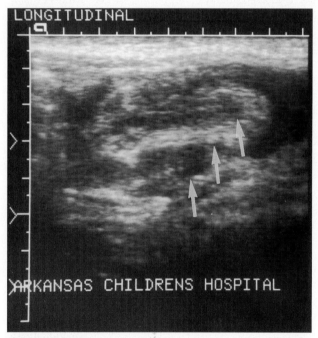

Figure 11–16
Sonographic diagnosis of intussusception in a 4-month-old boy with plain film findings of small bowel obstruction. Abdominal sonography demonstrates multiple concentric rings *(arrows)* of alternating increased and decreased echogenicity. This finding represents a longitudinal view of the intussusception. The lesion could not be reduced. Although sonography is not the primary imaging modality for intussusception, it is important to recognize the sonographic appearance of this disease, as sonography is often the first form of diagnostic imaging performed in children with an abdominal mass or an acute abdomen.

distal small bowel without reducing the intussusception when pressures of 30 to 50 mm Hg are used. In such situations reduction occurs when pressures are elevated to 80 to 120 mm Hg. Most likely there is incomplete obstruction of the bowel lumen, and the gas passes through the intussusceptum at low pressures (Fig. 11–15).

Almost all patients are observed for 24 hours after successful reduction to detect possible recurrence or other complications. The rate of recurrent intussusception is 3.5% to 10%.[3] It is safe and desirable to repeat the reduction in children who are in the typical age range for idiopathic intussusception (5 to 9 months) and are therefore unlikely to have a lead point. Finally, intussusceptions are not static events; surveillance with real time ultrasound has show that the process is spontaneously reversible in symptomatic and asymptomatic patients (Fig. 11–16).

Safe hydrostatic or pneumatic reduction of an intussusception is a relatively easy procedure that needs to be done with great care and attention to detail; however, few radiographic emergencies are as gratifying for the radiologist. Although there are several valid approaches to reducing an intussusception, we have found the technique described here to be simple, safe, and almost always successful.

MECKEL'S DIVERTICULUM

Anatomy and Pathophysiology
Meckel's diverticulum is the most common congenital malformation of the gastrointestinal tract; it is found in 2%

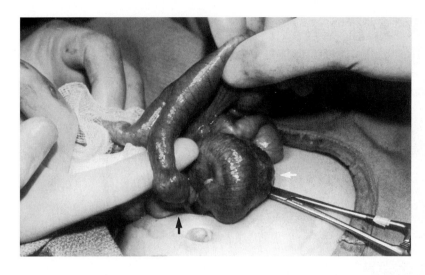

Figure 11–17
Meckel's diverticulum. A Meckel's diverticulum *(black arrow)* is demonstrated on the antimesenteric border of the distal ileum. Bleeding from ectopic gastric mucosa has caused distention of the distal bowel *(white arrow)*.

of routine autopsies. It is a true diverticulum containing mucosal, submucosal, muscularis and serosal layers. The diverticulum is a vestigial remnant of the omphalomesenteric duct that arises along the antimesenteric border approximately 70 cm proximal to the terminal ileum. About half of the diverticula contain heterotopic tissue, most commonly ectopic gastric mucosa and, less often, pancreatic, jejunal, or colonic mucosa. The most frequent complications are peptic ulceration, perforation, intussusception, and acute or chronic blood loss. Mechanical difficulties may also occur, especially if the omphalomesenteric duct remnant persists as a cord between the tip of the diverticulum and the umbilicus. Twenty five percent of Meckel's diverticula are attached to the umbilicus with a fibrous band, and 75% are free. A loop of bowel twisting around this cord may cause small bowel volvulus and total mechanical bowel obstruction. Local inflammation from diverticulitis, stone formation, or a foreign body may cause matting of adjacent bowel loops. Meckel's diverticulitis may mimic appendicitis. Bowel obstruction may also occur in neonates with large diverticula and in those with incarceration of the diverticulum in an inguinal hernia (i.e., Littre's hernia).

The presence of a Meckel's diverticulum does not invariably cause clinical symptoms. The two groups at risk for symptoms are patients with ectopic gastric mucosa, which may cause peptic complication, and those who have a persistent omphalomesenteric band that may cause mechanical obstruction (Fig. 11–17).

Clinical Presentation

Although omphalomesenteric duct malformations have an equal sex incidence, a significantly greater number of males have complications. The male predominance is most pronounced in peptic ulceration with a male-to-female ratio of 4.7:1. Meckel's diverticulum has several clinical presentations. If rectal bleeding is considered to be the key symptom, the differential diagnosis is limited essentially to peptic complications that result in blood loss. Bleeding may

be noted at any time but most commonly occurs within the first 2 years of life. Painless rectal bleeding is the most important clinical indicator of a Meckel's diverticulum. Bleeding is usually recurrent and may be severe. Blood is often passed without stool and is usually dark red; with more forceful bleeding, it becomes bright red. Infrequently, abdominal pain may result from the inflammation caused by peptic ulceration; more commonly, however, pain is notably absent.

Diagnostic Evaluation

If a Meckel's diverticulum is suspected clinically, contrast studies (UGI examination, small bowel series, and contrast enema) are not the primary diagnostic modalities because they result in few positive studies and because retained barium interferes with more successful diagnostic modalities (scintigraphy). UGI examination may be indicated if the results of a good-quality scintigram are normal. Rarely, the abdominal plain film shows calcification within the diverticulum, and sometimes the diverticulum itself may fill on small bowel examination. The newer technique of enteroclysis has slightly increased the positive yield of filling the diverticulum.[36]

When inflammatory complications are associated with bleeding, secondary changes may be seen in the colon. Localized perforation causes marked irregularity and spasm of portions of the sigmoid colon. This finding can be helpful in suggesting the correct diagnosis when a barium enema is performed to rule out the possibility of appendicitis or inflammatory bowel disease (Fig. 11–18).

Although a Meckel's diverticulum may occasionally be seen or its presence inferred from barium studies, the initial examination of choice is a sodium pertechnetate Tc 99m scintigram of the abdomen to identify ectopic gastric mucosa. Scintigraphic evaluation precedes proctoscopic examination because even the mild trauma during proctosigmoidoscopy may result in localized hyperemia, a potential cause of a false-positive scan. Barium should not be administered until

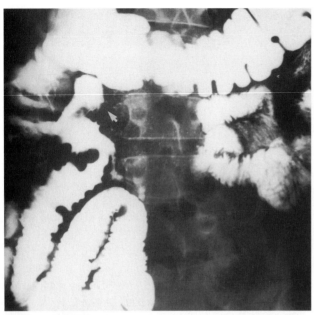

Figure 11–18
Meckel's diverticulum with peptic disease. A Meckel's diverticulum is filled with barium *(arrow)*, and extensive inflammatory changes are present in the distal ileum. This 17-year-old boy presented with abdominal pain and heme-positive stools.

a technically satisfactory scan has been obtained, as barium sulfate attenuates the 140-keV photons of technetium and limits the reliability of the scan. Currently the overall accuracy of sodium pertechnetate Tc 99m scanning for a bleeding Meckel's diverticulum is approximately 98%; lower figures reflect earlier studies that may have been hindered by suboptimal equipment and technique and by clinicians' limited experience in interpreting results from a new procedure.

Virtually all Meckel's diverticula complicated by blood loss contain gastric mucosa. Sodium pertechnetate Tc 99m localizes in the surface mucous cells of both orthotopic and ectopic gastric mucosa, where injected tracer is accumulated and secreted. Meckel's diverticula and intestinal duplications with gastric mucosa usually accumulate enough to allow detection (Figs. 11–19 through 11–22).

Diagnosis of a Meckel's diverticulum is made by demonstration of appearance of activity in an ectopic site other than the body of the stomach. Activity should appear simultaneously in the stomach and in the diverticulum.[8,12]

Most false-positive examinations are due to urinary tract abnormalities (ectopic kidney, extrarenal pelvis, ureteropelvic junction obstruction, and vesicoureteral reflux), lesions with an increased blood pool (localized hyperemia from peptic ulceration, Crohn's disease, or abscess), or vascular lesions (hemangioma, carcinoid, or aneurysm).

The diagnostic accuracy of the examination is greater than 90%.[24,47] Resection of the diverticulum is a simple and curative procedure.

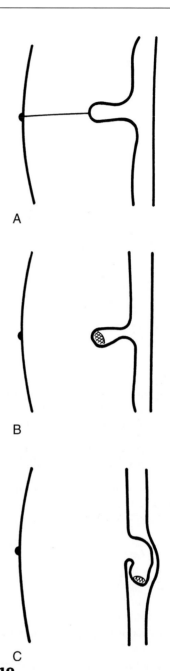

Figure 11–19
Complication of Meckel's diverticulum: diagrammatic representation. *A,* Omphalomesenteric duct remnant. *B,* Ectopic gastric mucosa with peptic complications. *C,* Intussusception.

JUVENILE POLYPS

Anatomy and Pathophysiology

Juvenile polyps (retention, inflammatory, or cystic polyps) account for 90% of all polyps in children younger than 10 years of age. These polyps range in diameter from a few millimeters to several centimeters and are almost always pedunculated. Although the stalk is covered by normal colonic mucosa, the surface of the polyp is often denuded and partially ulcerated.

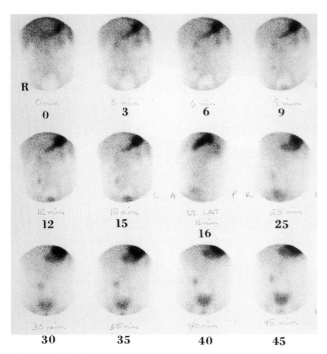

Figure 11–20
Meckel's diverticulum. Intramuscular glucagon was administered to this 2-year-old boy 10 minutes before injection of sodium pertechnetate Tc 99m. *Top row,* 0-, 3-, 6-, and 9-minute images. Hepatic, splenic, and renal blood pools are seen on the 0-minute image. Slight gastric activity is present. Note the clear definition of renal position by pelvocalyceal isotope on the 3-, 6-, and 9-minute images. Bladder activity first appears at 6 minutes. *Middle row,* 12-, 15-, 16-, and 25-minute images. Persistent focal tracer in the right lower quadrant is typical of Meckel's diverticulum. Note the further increase in gastric activity and the progressive decrease in pelvocalyceal activity bilaterally. *Bottom row,* 30-, 35-, 40-, and 45-minute images. There is continued clear definition of Meckel's diverticulum in the right lower quadrant.

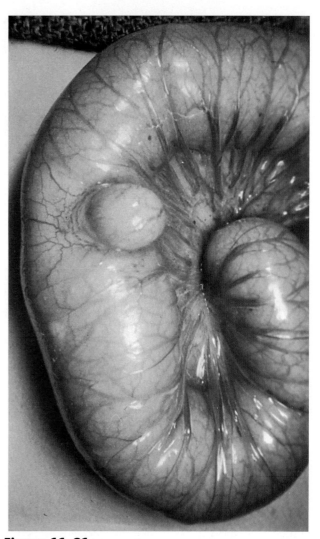

Figure 11–21
Jejunal duplication in Figure 11–22 evident at surgical exploration. Note that duplication is not located at the mesenteric side of the bowel, where mesenteric cysts are usually seen.

The etiology of juvenile polyps is thought to be localized obstruction and inflammation of glands in the colonic mucosa. Histologically, the polyps are filled with cystic spaces that contain a large amount of mucus, nuclear debris, and polynuclear leukocytes.

Juvenile polyps are the most common tumor of the colon in children. With the use of colonoscopy, at least one half of patients with one juvenile polyp have been found to have multiple polyps. Twenty-five percent to 60% of the polyps are proximal to the sigmoid colon.[11,37] Rarely, the colon is diffusely involved with juvenile polyps. There is a definite familial tendency for multiple juvenile polyps, but the exact mode of inheritance is unknown.

In the past juvenile polyps were thought to be universally benign; however, new studies have urged the adoption of a more cautious attitude for the risk of malignant transformation in later life.

Clinical Presentation

The peak incidence of juvenile polyps in children occurs between 4 and 5 years of age. They are rarely seen in patients younger than 1 year or older than 14 years. The most common presentation is rectal bleeding (90% of patients). Bleeding is usually minimal and intermittent and is manifested by streaks of fresh blood on the outside of formed stool. Less frequent symptoms include prolapse of the polyp through the rectum (35%), pain and diarrhea (25%), and autoamputation with passage of the polyps in the stool (10%).

Physical examination is normal, and routine laboratory values may indicate only a mild anemia. The major differential diagnostic consideration is painless bleeding from a Meckel's diverticulum. However, Meckel's diverticulum tends to occur in patients younger than 2 years, and the volume of bleeding

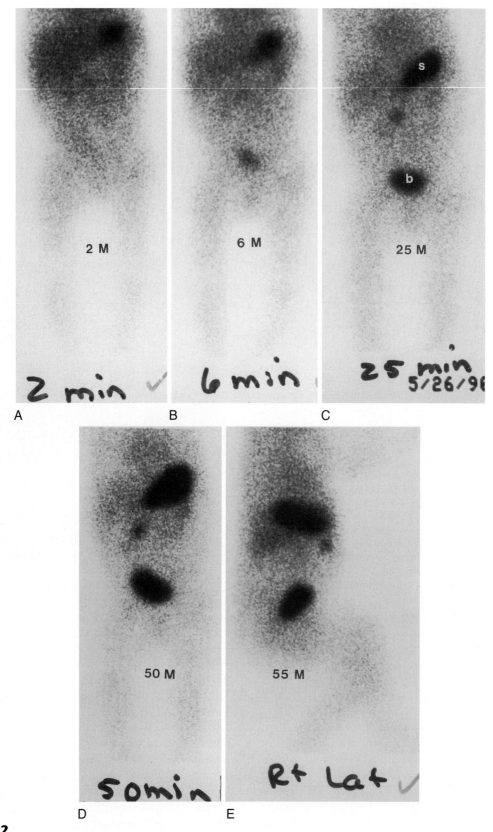

A   B   C

D   E

Figure 11–22

Jejunal duplication with ectopic gastric mucosa: sodium pertechnetate Tc 99m scan of a 2-year-old boy. *A,* At 2 minutes, activity is seen only in the gastric fundus. *B,* Initial visualization of isotope in the midepigastrium is seen at 6 minutes and persists throughout the study. *C,* Note the well-defined, rounded appearance of isotope uptake in the midepigastrium. If this were isotope secreted from the stomach and in the intestine, a tubular shape would be more likely. b, Bladder; s, stomach. *E,* The right lateral view shows rounded uptake anteriorly, which excludes renal and duodenal uptake.

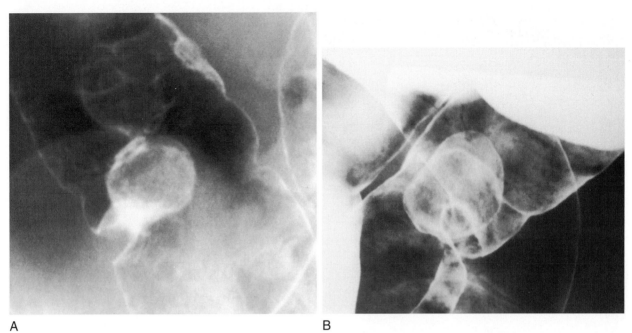

A   B

Figure 11–23
Juvenile polyp: air-contrast barium enema. *A,* Juvenile polyp on a stalk in the descending colon. *B,* Juvenile polyp on a broad-based stalk in the ascending colon.

is usually greater than that typically seen with juvenile polyps (Fig. 11–23).

Radiographic Evaluation

Radiographic evaluation is needed in only a few children with juvenile polyps because endoscopy is both diagnostic and therapeutic. Air-contrast barium enema is the radiographic examination of choice for detection of polyps. Adequate preparation of the colon is essential to eliminate stool that may be mistaken for polyps. We request a clear liquid diet for 3 days before the examination in addition to administration of suppositories, enemas, and milk of magnesia. It is a very difficult task for young children to maintain a clear liquid diet for 3 days. The compliance rate is higher if both parent and child are thoroughly instructed on the importance of adhering to the diet (Fig. 11–24).

Air-contrast enemas are highly accurate for detecting small colonic lesions, because the entire mucosal surface is coated with barium and the colon is distended with air. The technique begins with the patient prone, followed by the introduction of barium into the rectum to slightly beyond the splenic flexure. The barium is then drained, the patient is turned into the right decubitus position, and air is introduced. This permits the barium to coat the transverse and ascending colon and allows air to distend the sigmoid and descending colon. Next, the head of the table is elevated to allow air to rise and distend the transverse colon. The patient is then turned into the left decubitus position to allow air to distend the ascending colon.

An alternative method is to fill almost the entire colon with contrast agent, permit the child to evacuate, and then introduce the desired amount of air. Liquid Polibar is diluted with water in a ratio of 1000:350 mL and is introduced to the level of the splenic flexure, as is done in a solid-column colon examination. The child is then asked to evacuate, and without delay the desired amount of air is introduced, under fluoroscopic control, through a soft rectal tube. Routine filming is then performed. The advantage of this method is that it makes patients more maneuverable and lessens their discomfort.[3]

Multiple spot films are taken of all abnormalities. Spot films of the flexures are obtained with the patient upright. Overhead films include the following sequence: posteroanterior, right lateral decubitus, supine, and postevacuation views. If there is residual stool, evacuation after distention of the colon will frequently result in a clean colon.

The radiographic findings in a patient with a juvenile polyp include (1) a pedunculated oval or round filling defect and (2) limited movement. Movement of a true polyp is limited by its stalk, whereas stool is freely movable.

The detection of juvenile polyps is a time-consuming but relatively simple procedure. Radiographic examination provides precise information about the location and multiplicity of polyps that lie beyond the reach of the sigmoidoscope. Removal of juvenile polyps is desirable to relieve the symptoms of bleeding, occasional pain, and diarrhea; histologic evaluation is important to ensure that the polyp is of the juvenile type and hence is benign.

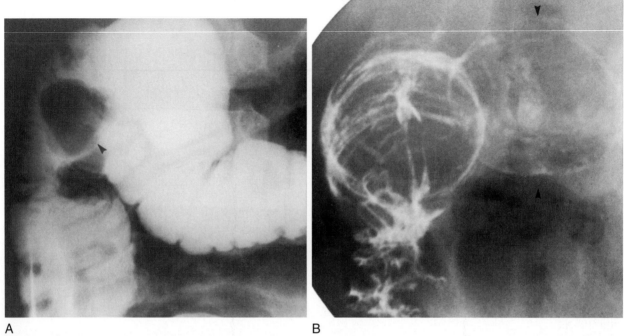

A   B

Figure 11-24

Intussuscepting polyp. *A*, A large pedunculated polyp is identified *(arrowhead)* in the ascending colon. *B*, During the examination, the polyp was seen to intermittently act as a lead point, causing a colocolic intussusception. Note the polyp *(arrowheads)* and the characteristic appearance of intussusception in the distal ascending colon.

▌SUMMARY

Rectal bleeding is a common problem in clinical pediatrics. It almost never signifies malignant disease and rarely is the bleeding severe enough to be life threatening. During the neonatal period, this problem is usually self-limiting and benign; thus, extensive investigation is usually unnecessary. Beyond the first month of life and into adolescence, diagnostic investigation is directed toward a specific, likely diagnosis. The most probable cause of bleeding generally can be narrowed down to one or two diagnostic possibilities, depending on the age of the patient, the severity of the bleeding, and associated symptoms. Definitive diagnosis is desirable, as many of these lesions are amenable to surgical or medical management. The prognosis for most children is excellent. Although there are many correct ways of approaching the problem of bloody stools in children, the specific approach that we have outlined is both simple and safe.

REFERENCES

1. Alavi A, Dann RW, Baum S, Biery DN. Scintigraphic detection of acute gastrointestinal bleeding. Radiology 124:753–756, 1977.
2. Armstrong EA, Dunbar JS, Graviss ER, Martin L, Rosenkrantz J. Intussusception complicated by distal perforation of the colon. Radiology 136:77–81, 1980.
3. Bissett GS III, Kirks DR. Intussusception in infants and children: Diagnosis and therapy. Radiology 168:141–145, 1988.
4. Blane CE, DiPietro ME, White SJ, Klein ME, Coran AG, Wesley JR. An analysis of bowel perforation in patients with intussusception. Assoc Radiol 35:113–115, 1984.
5. Bowerman RA, Silver TM, Jaffe MH. Real-time ultrasound diagnosis of intussusception in children. Radiology 143:527–529, 1982.
6. Campbell JB. Contrast media in intussusception. Pediatr Radiol 19:293–296, 1989.
7. Cochran DQ, Almond CH, Shucart WA. An experimental study of the effects of barium and intestinal contents in the peritoneal cavity. AJR Am J Roentgenol 89:883–887, 1963.
8. Conway JJ. Radionuclide diagnosis of Meckel's diverticulum. Gastrointest Radiol 5:209–213, 1980.
9. Cooney DR, Duszynski DO, Camboa E, Karp MP, Jewett TC Jr. et al. The abdominal technetium scan (a decade of experience). J Pediatr Surg 17:611–619, 1982.
10. Cross VF, Wendth AJ, Phelan JJ, Goussous HG, Moriarty DJ. Giant Meckel's diverticulum in a premature infant. AJR Am J Roentgenol 108:591–597, 1971.
11. Cynamon HA, Milov DE, Andres JM. Diagnosis and management of colonic polyps in children. J Pediatr 114:593–596, 1989.
12. Dalinka MK, Wunder JF. Meckel's diverticulum and its complications, with emphasis on roentgenologic demonstration. Radiology 106:295–298, 1973.
13. Datz FL, Christian PE, Hutson WR, Moore JG, Morton KA. Physiological and pharmacological interventions in radionuclde imaging of the tubular gastrointestinal tract. Semin Nucl Med 21:140–152, 1991.
14. Devred PH, Faure F, Padovani J. Pseudotumoral cecum after hydrostratic reduction of intussusception. Pediatr Radiol 14:295–298, 1984.

15. Ein SH. Leading points in childhood intussusception. J Pediatr Surg 11:209–211, 1976.

16. Ein SH, Shandling B, Reilly BJ, Stringer DA. Hydrostatic reduction of intussusceptions caused by lead points. J Pediatr Surg 21:883–886, 1986.

17. Ein SH, Stephens CA, Shandlin B, Filler RM. Intussusception due to lymphoma. J Pediatr Surg 21:786–788, 1986.

18. Erbe RW. Inherited gastrointestinal-polyposis syndromes. N Engl J Med 294:1101–1104, 1976.

19. Euler AR, Seibert JJ. The role of sigmoidoscopy, radiographs, and colonoscopy in the diagnostic evaluation of pediatric age patients with suspected juvenile polyps. J Pediatr Surg 16:500–502, 1981.

20. Fitch SJ, Magill HL, Benator RM, Parvey LS, Hixson SD. Pseudoreduction of intussusception: Is ileal reflux the end point? Gastrointest Radiol 10:181–183, 1985.

21. Franken EA Jr. Gastrointestinal Imaging in Pediatrics. 2nd ed. New York: Harper & Row, 1982.

22. Franken EA, Smith WL, Chernish SM, Campbell JB, Fletcher BD, Goldman HS. The use of glucagon in hydrostatic reduction of intussusception. A double blind study of 28 patients. Radiology 146:687–689, 1983.

23. Fries M, Mortensson W, Robertson B. Technetium pertechnetate scintigraphy to detect ectopic gastric mucosa in Meckel's diverticulum. Acta Radiol (Diagn) 25:417–422, 1984.

24. Gierup J, Jorulf H, Livaditis A. Management of intussusception in infants and children: A survey based on 288 consecutive cases. Pediatrics 50:535–546, 1972.

25. Girdany BR, Bass LW, Sieber WK. Roentgenologic aspects of hydrostatic reduction of ileocolic intussusception. AJR Am J Roentgenol 82:455–461, 1959.

26. Goldberger LE. Barium enema techniques. Gastrointest Endosc 26:12S–14S, 1980.

27. Gu L, Alton DJ, Daneman A, et al. Intussusception reduction in children by rectal insufflation of air. AJR Am J Roentgenol 150:1345–1348, 1988.

28. Guo J, Ma X, Zhou Q. Results of air pressure enema reduction of intussusception: 6,396 cases in 13 years. J Pediatr Surg 21:1201–1203, 1986.

29. Hedlund GL, Johnson JF, Strife JL. Ileocolic intussusception: Extensive reflux of air proceeding pneumatic reduction. Radiology 174:187–189, 1990.

30. Hubert BC. Analgesic premedication in the management of ileocolic intussusception. Pediatrics 79:432–433, 1987.

31. Johnson JF, Woisard KK. Ileocolic intussusception: New sign on the supine cross-table lateral radiograph. Radiology 170:483–486, 1989.

32. Junzhe Z, Yenxia W, Linchi W. Rectal inflation reduction of intussusception in infants. J Pediatr Surg 21:30–32, 1986.

33. Kuhns LR, Holt JF. Use of isotonic water soluble contrast and low kilovoltage in neonatal gastrointestinal exams in neonates. Presented at the 23rd Annual Meeting of the Society of Pediatric Radiology, Salt Lake City, UT, 1980.

34. Leonidas JC. Treatment of intussusception with small bowel obstruction: Application of decision analysis. AJR Am J Roentgenol 145:665–669, 1985.

35. LeVine M, Schwartz S, Katz I, Burko H, Rabinowitz J. Plain film findings in intussusception. Br J Radiol 37:678–681, 1964.

36. Maglinte DT, Elmore MF, Isenberg M, Dolan PA. Meckel diverticulum: Radiologic demonstration by enteroclysis. AJR Am J Roentgenol 134:925–932, 1980.

37. Mestre JR. The changing pattern of juvenile polyps. Am J Gastroenterol 81:312–314, 1986.

38. Parienty RA, Lepreux JF, Gruson B. Sonographic and CT features of ileocolic intussusception. AJR Am J Roentgenol 136:608–610, 1981.

39. Patcliffe JF, Fong S, Cheong I, O'Connell P. Plain film diagnosis of intussusception: Prevalence of target sign. AJR Am J Roentgenol 158:619–621, 1992.

40. Petrokubi RJ, Baum S, Rohrer GV. Cimetidine administration resulting in improved pertechnetate imaging of Meckel's diverticulum. Clin Nucl Med 3:385–388, 1978.

41. Powsner R, Royal H, Parker A. Gravity-aided Meckel's scan. Interesting images. Clin Nucl Med 8:654–655, 1987.

42. Pracros JP, Tran–Minh VA, Morin de Finfe CH, Defrenne-Pracros P, Louis D, Basset T. Acute intestinal intussusception in children. Contribution of ultrasonography (145 cases). Ann Radiol (Paris) 30:525–530, 1987.

43. Priebe CJ, Marsden S, Lazarevic B. The use of 99m technetium pertechnetate to detect transplanted gastric mucosa in the dog. J Pediatr Surg 9:605–613, 1974.

44. Ravitch MM. Pediatric Surgery. 3rd ed. Chicago: Year Book Medical, 1979, pp 1079–1082.

45. Reijnen JAM, Josten HJM, Festen C. Intussusception in children 5–15 years of age. Br J Surg 74:692–693, 1987.

46. Sfakianakis GN, Gentili A, Buckner DM, Oiticica C. The use of glucagon to improve Tc99m-pertechnetate (TcP) abdominal scintigraphy for ectopic gastric mucosa: Clinical experience [Abstract]. J Nucl Med 17:1034–1035, 1986.

47. Sherman NJ, Clatworthy HW Jr. Gastrointestinal bleeding in neonates: A study of 94 cases. Surgery 62:614–619, 1967.

48. Shiels WE II, Bisset GS III, Kirks DR. Simple device for air reduction of intussusception. Pediatr Radiol 30:472–474, 1990.

49. Stephenson CA, Seibert JJ, Strain JD, Glasier CM, Leithiser RE Jr, Iqbal V. Intussusception: Clinical and radiographic factors influencing reducibility. Pediatr Radiol 20:57–60, 1989.

50. Stringer DA, Ein SH. Pneumatic reduction: Advantages, risks and indications. Pediatr Radiol 20:475–477, 1990.

51. Swischuk LE, Hayden CK, Boulden T. Intussusception: Indications for ultrasonography and an explanation of the doughnut and pseudokidney signs. Pediatr Radiol 15:388–391, 1985.

52. Treves S, Grand RJ, Erakis AJ. Pentagastrin simulation of technetium 99m uptake by ectopic gastric mucosa in Meckel's diverticulum. Radiology 128:711–712, 1978.

53. Wayne ER, Campbell JB, Burrington JD, Davis WS. Management of 344 children with intussusception. Radiology 107:597–601, 1973.

54. Wayne ER, Campbell JB, Kosloske AM, Burrington JD. Intussusception in the older child—Suspect lymphosarcoma. J Pediatr Surg 11:789–794, 1976.

55. White SJ, Blane CE. Intussusception: Additional observations on the plain radiograph. AJR Am J Roentgenol 139:511–513, 1982.

56. Wilton G, Froelich JW. The "false–negative" Meckel's scan. Clin Nucl Med 7:441–443, 1982.

57. Winzelberg GG, McKusick KA, Strauss HW, et al. Evaluation of gastrointestinal bleeding by red blood cells labeled in vivo with technetium-99m. J Nucl Med 20:1080–1086, 1979.

58. Ya–Xiong S. Treatment of intestinal intussusception with particular emphasis on reduction by coinsufflation. Report on 5110 cases. Chir Pediatr 23:373–378, 1982.

ADDITIONAL READING

Brazowski E, Rozen P, Misonzhnick-Bedny F, Gitstein G. Characteristics of familial juvenile polyps expressing cyclooxygenase-2. Am J Gastroenterol 100:130–138, 2005.

Henrikson S, Blane CE, Koujok K, Strouse PJ, DiPietro MA, Goodsitt MM. The effect of screening sonography on the positive rate of enemas for intussusception. Pediatr Radiol 33:190–193, 2003.

Kornecki A, Daneman A, Navarro O, Connolly B, Manson D, Alton DJ. Spontaneous reduction of intussusception: Clinical spectrum, management and outcome. Pediatr Radiol 30:58–63, 2000.

Meyer JS, Dangman BC, Buonomo C, et al. Air and liquid contrast agents in the management of intussusception: A controlled, randomized trial. Radiology 188: 507–511, 1993.

Navarro OM, Daneman A, Chae A: Intussusception: The use of delayed, repeated reduction attempts and the management of intussusceptions due to pathologic lead points in pediatric patients. AJR Am J Roentgenol 182:1169–1176, 2004.

Ojha S, Menon P, Rao KL. Meckel's diverticulum with segmental dilatation of the ileum: Radiographic diagnosis in a neonate. Pediatr Radiol 34:649–651, 2004.

Oktar SO, Yucel C, Ozdemir H, Uluturk A, Isik S. Comparison of conventional sonography, real-time compound sonography, tissue harmonic sonography, and tissue harmonic compound sonography of abdominal and pelvic lesions. AJR Am J Roentgenol 181:1341–1347, 2004.

Strouse PJ, DiPietro MA, Saez F. Transient small-bowel intussusception in children on CT. Pediatr Radiol 33:316–320, 2003.

THE CHILD WITH AN ABDOMINAL MASS

Outline

Sandra L. Wootton-Gorges, MD

THE CHILD WITH AN ABDOMINAL MASS

Radiologic evaluation of an infant or child with an abdominal mass includes (1) confirming the presence of a mass; (2) demonstrating its precise extent; (3) providing the specific pathologic diagnosis, when possible; and (4) documenting tumor spread.[108] Although the possible causes of an abdominal mass in an infant or child are numerous (Tables 12–1 and 12–2), only a few lesions comprise the vast majority. The radiographic data, combined with the age of the child and the clinical information, usually allow a specific diagnosis or markedly decrease the differential diagnosis list. This chapter discusses only the relatively common neoplastic causes of abdominal masses in children; less common causes may be explored using the extensive reference list.

DIFFERENTIAL DIAGNOSIS ACCORDING TO AGE

NEONATES (BIRTH TO 1 MONTH)

An abdominal mass in a neonate is most commonly benign and of renal origin.[81,123,147] Neonatal hydronephrosis is the most common cause at this age and may be due to ureteropelvic junction obstruction, ureterovesical reflux, posterior urethral valves, ectopic ureterocele, ureterovesical junction obstruction, and prune-belly syndrome (Fig. 12–1).[108] The most common cause of hydronephrosis resulting in a palpable mass is a severe ureteropelvic junction obstruction.[112] Multicystic dysplastic kidney is more common than any single type of hydronephrosis[88] (Figs. 12–2 and 12–3). Renal neoplasms are unusual in this age group, although mesoblastic nephroma sometimes occurs. A flank mass in a neonate with hematuria and a history of dehydration, sepsis, or maternal diabetes usually represents renal vein thrombosis. Bilateral flank masses

TABLE 12-1 POSSIBLE CAUSES OF AN ABDOMINAL MASS IN THE NEONATE (BIRTH TO 1 MONTH)

Renal (55%)
Hydronephrosis
   Ureteropelvic junction obstruction
   Posterior urethral valves
   Vesicoureteral reflux
   Ectopic ureterocele
   Prune-belly syndrome
   Ureterovesical junction obstruction
Multicystic dysplastic kidney
Renal ectopia
Polycystic kidney disease
   Autosomal recessive
   Autosomal dominant
Renal vein thrombosis
Mesoblastic nephroma
Wilms' tumor
Abscess
Genital (15%)
Hydrometrocolpos
Ovarian mass
   Simple cyst
   Torsion
   Teratoma
Gastrointestinal (15%)
Duplication
Volvulus
Complicated meconium ileus
Mesenteric/omental cyst
Bowel atresia with proximal cystic dilatation
Hypertrophic pyloric stenosis
Gastric teratoma
Nonrenal retroperitoneal (10%)
Adrenal hemorrhage
Neuroblastoma
Teratoma
Rhabdomyosarcoma
Lymphangioma
Hemangioma
Lipoma
Anterior meningocele
Hepatobiliary masses (5%)
Metastases
Hemangioendothelioma
Hepatoblastoma
Mesenchymal hamartoma
Simple cyst of the liver
Hematoma of the liver
Choledochal cyst
Hydrops of gallbladder

Data from Refs. 33, 60, 81, 108, and 179.

TABLE 12-2 POSSIBLE CAUSES OF ABDOMINAL MASS IN INFANTS AND CHILDREN (1 MONTH TO 18 YEARS)

Renal (55%)
Wilms' tumor
Hydronephrosis
Cystic disease
Congenital malformation
Perinephric abscess
Renal vein thrombosis
Hematoma
Leukemic infiltration
Renal cell carcinoma
Multilocular cystic nephroma
Rhabdoid tumor
Clear cell sarcoma
Nonrenal retroperitoneal (23%)
Neuroblastoma
Rhabdomyosarcoma
Teratoma
Lymphoma
Lymphangioma
Hemangioma
Lipoma
Gastrointestinal and hepatopancreaticosplenobiliary (18%)
Appendiceal abscess
Intussusception
Gastrointestinal duplication
Functional constipation
Hirschsprung's disease
Mesenteric/omental cyst
Lymphoma
Teratoma
Hepatoblastoma
Hepatocellular carcinoma
Adenoma
Hamartoma
Fibronodular hyperplasia
Choledochal cyst
Simple cyst
Hematoma
Pancreatic pseudocyst
Pancreatic neoplasm
Genital (4%)
Ovarian mass
   Cyst
   Torsion
   Teratoma
Hydrometrocolpos
Neoplasm or torsion in undescended testis

Data from Refs. 33, 60, and 108.

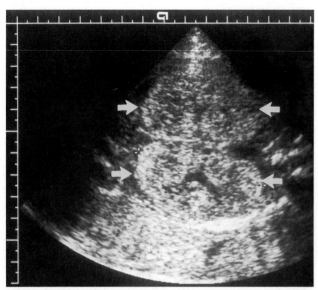

Figure 12–1
Prenatal diagnosis: bilateral renal enlargement. This coronal image of a fetal abdomen at 26 weeks of gestation reveals markedly enlarged and echogenic kidneys (arrows). The fetus also had an occipital encephalocele. At birth, the infant had bilateral abdominal masses caused by the renal enlargement. The diagnosis of Meckel-Gruber syndrome was made; the infant died.

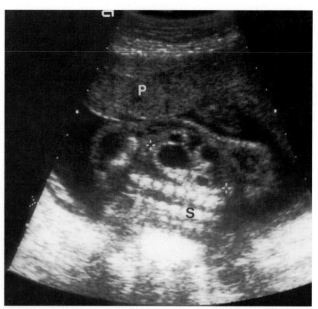

Figure 12–2
Prenatal diagnosis: unilateral multicystic dysplastic kidney. This coronal image of a right kidney shows cysts of variable size that do not communicate. The contralateral kidney was normal. At birth, the infant had a right-sided abdominal mass that proved to be a multicystic dysplastic kidney. P, Placenta; S, spine.

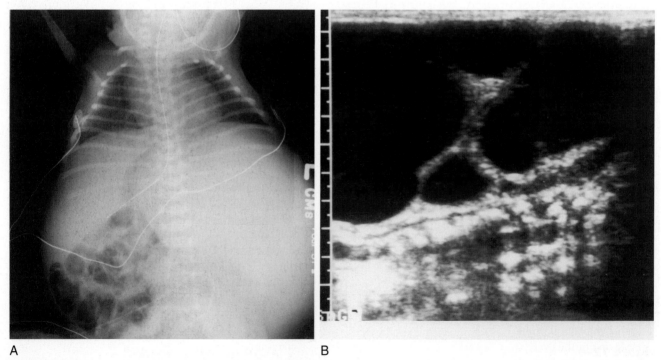

A   B

Figure 12–3
Multicystic dysplastic kidney. Images of a newborn with a left-sided abdominal mass. The large abdominal girth necessitated cesarean delivery. A, Abdominal radiograph showing the large, noncalcified, left abdominal mass. B, Longitudinal sonogram through the left renal fossa showing the multicystic dysplastic kidney, with multiple noncommunicating cysts of varying size.

suggest polycystic renal disease, bilateral hydronephrosis, or nephroblastomatosis (Fig. 12–4).

An upper abdominal mass in neonates with a history of anoxia, septicemia, congenital syphilis, maternal diabetes, or low platelet count may be an adrenal hemorrhage. Such infants are often anemic and jaundiced (from hemolysis). Seventy percent of adrenal hemorrhages occur on the right,[123] and about 10% are bilateral (Fig. 12–5). Early adrenal hemorrhage may appear solid and may be differentiated from congenital neuroblastoma sonographically: no vessels are present within a hemorrhage.[47] Cystic neuroblastoma is more difficult to differentiate from an adrenal hemorrhage; however, hematoma has a characteristic sonographic course of involution and a distinctive pattern of calcification on plain films.

If intestinal obstruction is associated with an abdominal mass, the etiology is probably gastrointestinal.[81] Masses arising outside the gastrointestinal tract, even if large, rarely obstruct the bowel. The most common gastrointestinal mass in the neonate is a bowel duplication, usually arising from the terminal ileum. These masses may cause volvulus or intussusception.[117] Cystic meconium peritonitis also presents as an abdominal mass at the time of birth.

With the exclusion of an enlarged bladder, the most common cause of a fixed midline abdominal mass arising from the neonatal female pelvis is hydrometrocolpos. A mobile anterior mass in a girl is usually an ovarian cyst (Fig. 12–6).

Sacrococcygeal teratoma is the most common neoplasm in newborns.[174] This tumor is usually mostly external, but is occasionally exclusively intrapelvic.[103] About 90% are benign at birth. Teratoma may invade or displace pelvic structures, and neurologic deficit may result from intraspinal extension.

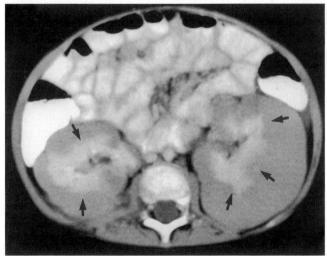

Figure 12–4
Nephroblastomatosis. This enhanced computed tomography (CT) image of a newborn with an abdominal mass shows bilateral diffuse nephroblastomatosis surrounding the normally enhancing renal parenchyma *(arrows)*.

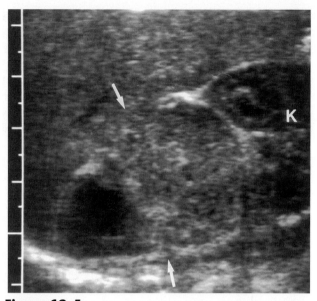

Figure 12–5
Adrenal hemorrhage. Image of a newborn with an acute right adrenal hemorrhage. This longitudinal sonogram through the right adrenal gland and kidney shows the adrenal hemorrhage *(arrows)*, with solid and cystic components, indenting the upper pole of the right kidney (K).

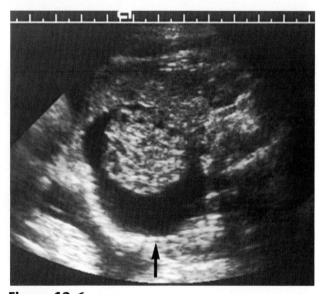

Figure 12–6
Prenatal diagnosis: ovarian torsion. Image of a third-trimester fetus reveals a large, complex pelvic mass *(arrow)* with solid and cystic internal components. Surgery performed shortly after birth revealed an ovarian torsion

INFANTS AND YOUNG CHILDREN (1 MONTH TO 5 YEARS)

Abdominal masses in infants and young children (excepting hepatosplenomegaly, which usually reflects a hematologic disorder such as leukemia[122]) are predominantly retroperitoneal in origin.[118] The incidence of malignancy, notably Wilms' tumor and neuroblastoma, increases greatly in later infancy and childhood.[108]

Appendiceal abscess is the most common cause of a gastrointestinal mass in infants and children.[108,123] A palpable mass in a patient between the ages of 5 months and 2 years with crampy abdominal pain and bloody stools is likely to be an intussusception (Fig. 12–7). Metastases to the liver are more common than primary hepatic masses, and two thirds of primary hepatic masses are also malignant. Choledochal cysts, which probably result from reflux of pancreatic secretions into the biliary tree,[123] are rare. Half of choledochal cysts, producing jaundice, an abdominal mass, and abdominal pain, are found by 10 years of age (Fig. 12–8). Primary gastrointestinal malignancies are rare in children, but Burkitt's lymphoma of the small bowel is occasionally seen. Pancreatic and splenic neoplasms are extremely rare.

Genital masses are uncommon; because of the small size of the bony pelvis in children, these usually present as an abdominal mass. Almost all pediatric genital masses are ovarian with most arising from germ cells. Benign teratomas are the most common ovarian tumor; the peak age for presentation is 6–11 years (Fig. 12–9).[123,175] Granulosa–theca cell tumors are rare, benign tumors. However, because these tumors are hormonally active, patients present with isosexual precocious puberty.[123]

Rhabdomyosarcoma, most commonly seen in the paranasal sinuses, may arise in the genitourinary tract or retroperitoneum. Most patients with bladder rhabdomyosarcoma present within the first 3 years of life.[123] Teratomas are uncommon; their most common location is presacral.[108] Unlike in neonates, about 70% of teratomas in children older than 4 months are malignant.

Lymphangiomas most frequently arise in the small bowel mesentery; other sites of origin include the mesocolon, omentum, and retroperitoneum.[172] Most affected children are asymptomatic and have a doughy abdominal mass. Complications include infection, hemorrhage, and bowel obstruction.

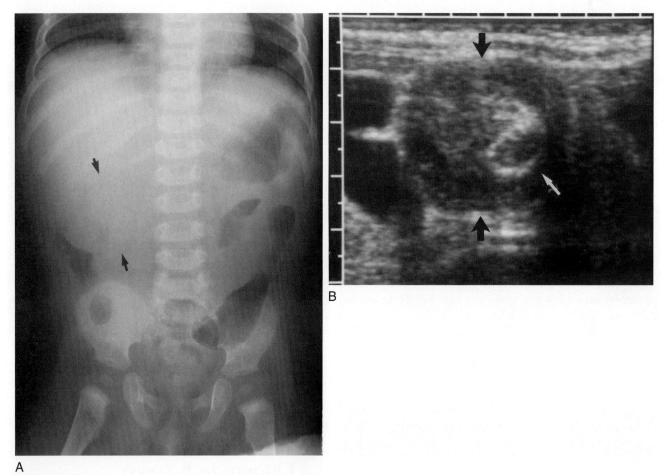

Figure 12–7
Ileocolic intussusception. Images of an 8-month-old infant with an abdominal mass and bloody stools. *A,* An abdominal radiograph shows a right upper quadrant mass *(arrows)*. *B,* A transverse ultrasound image through the right upper quadrant mass *(black arrows)* shows the typical "target sign" *(white arrow)* of an intussusception.

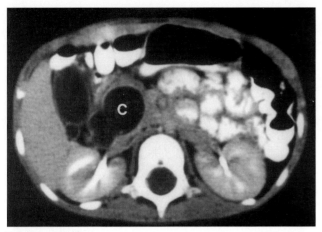

Figure 12–8
Choledochal cyst. Image of a 5-year-old child with a choledochal cyst (C). This enhanced CT image shows the cyst medial to the gallbladder and extending into the head of the pancreas.

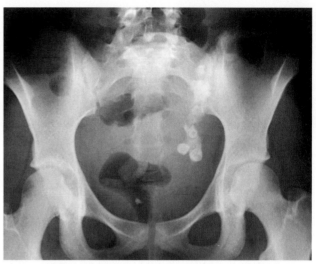

Figure 12–9
Ovarian cystic teratoma. Radiograph of a 13-year-old girl with a left ovarian cystic teratoma. This 12-cm mass contained several teeth.

IMPORTANT CONDITIONS PRESENTING AS AN ABDOMINAL MASS

WILMS' TUMOR

Epidemiology

Wilms' tumor (nephroblastoma)[187,190] is both the most common renal tumor and the most common intra-abdominal tumor of childhood. It accounts for one fourth of all renal masses in children older than 1 year[98] and for about 10% of all childhood malignancies.[52] Approximately 350 to 500 new cases of Wilms' tumor are diagnosed in the United States each year; the overall incidence is about 7 per 1 million children under age 16 years.[194] The disease is seen with equal frequency in boys and girls, and there is no racial predilection. The peak age at diagnosis is 2 to 3 years; about 80% of patients present at between 1 and 5 years of age. Wilms' tumor is unusual in the first year of life.

Clinical Evaluation

In 70% of patients with Wilms' tumors the initial finding is an asymptomatic abdominal mass discovered by the pediatrician or parent. Hypertension resulting from increased renin production is present in 25% to 50% of patients. Other findings, each seen in about 25% of patients, include malaise, abdominal pain, and hematuria. A new left varicocele may be the initial finding in boys with a left Wilms' tumor that has invaded the renal vein.

Congenital anomalies accompany Wilms' tumor in 15% of patients. The tumor develops in about one third of patients with sporadic aniridia.[131] The incidence is also increased in patients with hemihypertrophy (3%), Beckwith-Wiedemann syndrome, Sotos syndrome (cerebral gigantism), Perlman's syndrome (fetal gigantism),[176] malformations of the genitourinary system (cryptorchidism, hypospadias, gonadal dysgenesis, and horseshoe kidney,[127] and neurofibromatosis.[52] The triad of Wilms' tumor, glomerulopathy, and pseudohermaphroditism comprises the Drash syndrome.[76] Both the diffuse and the multifocal forms of nephroblastomatosis are associated with Wilms' tumor.[133] One percent of children with Wilms' tumor have an affected relative, usually a cousin or sibling.[42] In familial cases, the incidence of bilaterality is about 30%.[25,107]

The genetics of Wilms' tumor is complicated. Recent research has defined two tumor suppressor genes, *WT1* and *WT2*, at 11p13 and 11p15 on chromosome 11.[125,145] The former is associated with aniridia and the latter with Beckwith-Wiedemann syndrome. Loss or mutation of these tumor suppressor genes may permit the development of Wilms' tumor. Some patients with Wilms' tumor also have abnormalities of the long arm of chromosomes 16, 1, and 8.[113] There are no specific hematologic markers in Wilms' tumor.[42]

Physical examination typically reveals a nontender mass confined to one side of the abdomen. Distended superficial abdominal veins suggest extension into the inferior vena cava.

Radiologic Evaluation

Precise preoperative diagnosis and evaluation of tumor extension is imperative for planning the surgical approach. Imaging traditionally begins with plain radiographs of the abdomen; these usually reveal the mass displacing adjacent bowel. Calcification is visible in only 5% of patients and tends to be curvilinear or amorphous.[99,107]

Abdominal sonography is useful in excluding other diagnoses and defining the intrarenal location of the mass.[44,178] Wilms' tumors are usually hyperechoic compared with normal renal or hepatic parenchyma (Fig. 12–10).[96] Areas of necrosis and cysts, if present, are hypoechoic. The renal vein and inferior vena cava are carefully assessed to exclude vascular extension of tumor: the renal vein is involved in 15% of patients[136,163] and the inferior vena cava in 5% to 10%. Tumor extension into the right atrium is a potentially lethal complication present up to 1%.[185,162] Sonography is more sensitive than computed tomography (CT) in evaluating vascular tumor extension. The involved vessels are focally enlarged and contain echogenic tumor (Figs. 12–11 and 12–12). Fixation of the tumor thrombus to the vascular wall suggests invasion. It may be helpful to scan the patient upright to distend the inferior vena cava.[180] Adenopathy is also assessed; normal abdominal lymph nodes are seldom visualized by sonography in children.[159] Enlarged nodes may be reactive or infiltrated by tumor. The opposite kidney is examined, because 5% of tumors are bilateral; two thirds of these are synchronous, and one third are metachronous.[16] The liver is evaluated for metastases.

Unenhanced CT demonstrates a round, well-defined, intrarenal mass that is less dense than the normal renal parenchyma.[63,148,105] The mass distorts the renal parenchyma and the collecting system. Calcification is noted in up to 15% of patients. Areas of fat,[61] necrosis, hemorrhage, and cyst formation may be evident.[79,137] Enhancement is inhomogeneous and always less than the normal renal parenchyma (see Fig. 12–10).[148] A central nonenhancing collection suggests necrosis or hemorrhage. The margin of the tumor is well defined because of a pseudocapsule of compressed

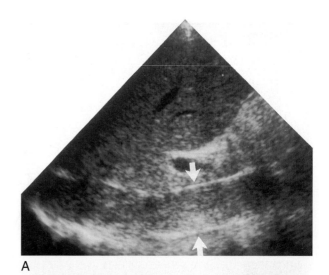

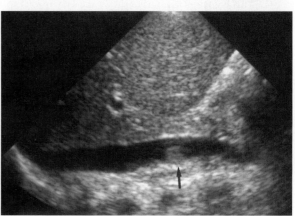

B

Figure 12–11
Tumor thrombus. *A,* Image of a 10-year-old child. This longitudinal sonogram through the inferior vena cava shows it to be enlarged and completely filled with echogenic tumor thrombus *(arrows)*. The thrombus extended into the right atrium. *B,* Image of an 8-year-old child with a left Wilms' tumor. Echogenic tumor thrombus *(arrow)* is seen extending just into the inferior vena cava.

renal parenchyma. CT is superior to sonography in the detection of perirenal extension, lymphadenopathy, and contralateral tumors.[148] Plaque-like or nodular thickening of the peritoneum, mesentery, and omentum may reflect neoplastic involvement following tumor rupture.[161] CT evaluation of the chest may be performed simultaneously; 8% to 15% of patients have pulmonary metastases at presentation (Fig. 12–13).[33,123]

Nonenhanced magnetic resonance imaging (MRI) is equal to or better than CT in the evaluation of the renal mass[15] (Figs. 12–14 and 12–15), perinephric extension, the contralateral kidney, and hepatic metastases[36]; further, MRI detects intravascular extension more easily than CT.[185] The mass enhances inhomogeneously with gadolinium[8] and less than the normal renal parenchyma.[72] MRI is less sensitive than CT in detecting pulmonary metastases.[36]

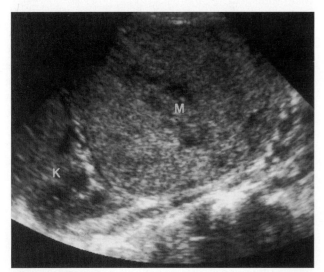

Figure 12–10
Wilms' tumor. Image of a 3-year-old child. This longitudinal sonogram through the right kidney shows the hyperechoic mass (M) involving all but the right upper pole (K).

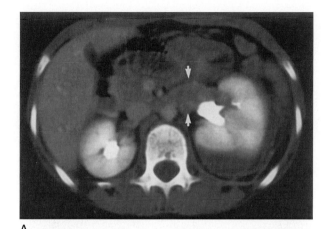

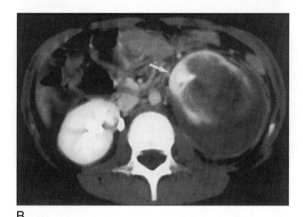

Figure 12–12
Wilms' tumor. CT scans of an 8-year-old child. *A,* This enhanced CT image shows a large left mass originating from renal tissue *(arrow)* and enhancing less than the normal renal parenchyma. *B,* A second enhanced CT image shows tumor thrombus filling the left renal vein *(arrows).*

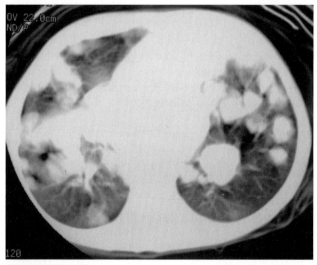

Figure 12–13
Wilms' tumor. Image of a 5-year-old child. This CT scan of the chest photographed at the lung windows shows multiple pulmonary metastases.

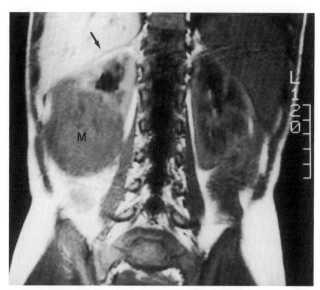

Figure 12–14
Wilms' tumor. Image of a 3-year-old child with an abdominal mass. This T1-weighted coronal magnetic resonance (MR) image shows a tumor (M) that is lower in signal intensity than the normal upper pole parenchyma *(arrow).*

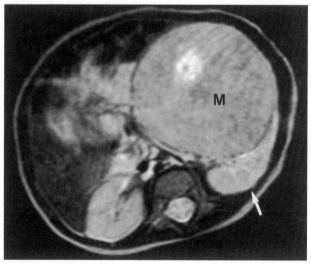

Figure 12–15
Wilms' tumor. Image of an 8-month-old infant. This T2-weighted axial MR image shows a well-circumscribed tumor (M). Areas of necrosis are seen within it. Note the residual renal tissue *(arrow).*

Pathology and Staging

Stage I Wilms' tumors are limited to the kidney and are completely resected.[35] In stage II, tumor extends into the perirenal soft tissues, periaortic lymph nodes, or veins, but resection is complete. Intravascular extension, if removed at surgery, does not worsen the prognosis.[149]

In stage III, residual tumor remains after resection. This may be caused by tumor rupture during surgery, peritoneal implants, nonresected nodes beyond the periaortic chain, or local tumor invasion of vital structures. In stage IV, hematogenous metastases are present. Distant metastases are usually pulmonary, less frequently hepatic, and rarely osseous or intracranial. In stage V, both kidneys are involved, at the time of diagnosis or subsequently (Table 12–3).

The tumors usually contain epithelial, blastemal, and stromal elements.[12,14] The derivation from primitive metanephric blastema accounts for the rare occurrence of fat, skeletal muscle, cartilage, and squamous epithelium within the tumor.[22] Epithelial, blastemal, and stromal elements with variable maturation are labeled as "favorable histology,"[12] with the expectation of an excellent prognosis (Fig. 12–16).

Approximately 10% of tumors exhibit foci of extreme anaplasia or nuclear atypia. These are described as "unfavorable histology" and are often resistant to therapy, especially with extension beyond the renal capsule. Sixty percent of deaths from Wilms' tumor occur in children with unfavorable histology. Multifocal nephroblastomatosis is present in the affected kidney in approximately 25% of perinatal postmortem examinations with unilateral Wilms' tumor[25,126] as opposed to only 1% of random perinatal postmortem examinations; it is present in all patients with bilateral tumors.

Treatment and Prognosis

Treatment involves surgical removal of the tumor, chemotherapy, and occasionally radiation therapy.[42,126] Prognosis depends on both tumor stage and histology. For children with favorable histology, the prognosis is excellent: the 2-year relapse-free survival rate for those with stage I and II tumors is 90%, for stage III tumors is 80%, and for stage IV tumors is 63%. Patients with unfavorable histology and stage II or higher tumors have a poorer prognosis: the 2-year relapse-free survival rate for all stages is approximately 63%.[42] Development of a metachronous tumor reduces the survival rate to 39%.[126]

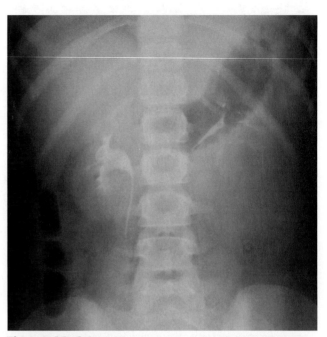

Figure 12–16
Wilms' tumor. Image of a 9-year-old child. This 15-minute film from an excretory urogram shows the left lower pole mass and distortion of the left collecting system.

Surveillance of patients after treatment for Wilms' tumor includes periodic evaluation of the tumor bed for local recurrence using ultrasonography, CT, or MRI. A new soft tissue mass in the renal fossa and enlargement of the ipsilateral psoas muscle suggest recurrence.[159] The opposite kidney is carefully evaluated for the development of a metachronous tumor, especially if the removed kidney contained nephroblastomatosis. Another complication is susceptibility of the remaining kidney to hyperfiltration injury, suggested by increasing parenchymal echogenicity over time.[180]

Chest radiographs and/or CT scans permit a search for metastatic disease. Ninety-six percent of metastases develop within 2 years of diagnosis.[17] Second malignant neoplasms develop with a standardized incidence ratio of 8.4, with leukemia and lymphoma being the most common.[27]

Differential Diagnosis

Wilms' tumor is by far the most common intrarenal neoplasm of childhood. Occasionally, neuroblastoma may invade the kidney; careful evaluation for vascular encasement and intraspinal extension of the tumor will facilitate correct diagnosis. Other, rarer solid tumors include renal cell carcinoma (Fig. 12–17), rhabdomyosarcoma, multilocular cystic nephroma (Fig. 12–18), rhabdoid tumor, clear cell sarcoma, lymphoma (Fig. 12–19), and teratoma. Rarely, a renal hematoma caused by trauma may simulate a tumor (Fig. 12–20).[181] In children younger than 1 year, mesoblastic nephroma is more common than Wilms' tumor.

STAGE	TUMOR CHARACTERISTICS	RESECTION
I	Tumor limited to kidney	Complete
II	Tumor extends into the perirenal soft tissues, periaortic lymph nodes, or veins	Complete
III	Residual tumor present at resection	
IV	Hematogenous metastases present	
V	Both kidneys involved, either at time of diagnosis or subsequently	

TABLE 12-3 WILMS' TUMOR STAGING

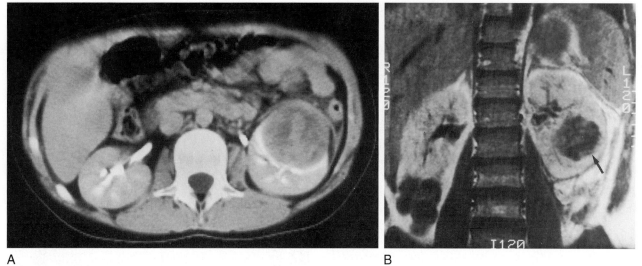

Figure 12–17
Renal cell carcinoma. Images of an 11-year-old child. *A,* An enhanced CT image shows a well-circumscribed left intrarenal mass that enhances less than the normal renal parenchyma. *B,* A gadolinium-enhanced T1-weighted coronal MR image also shows the mass enhancing less than the normal kidney.

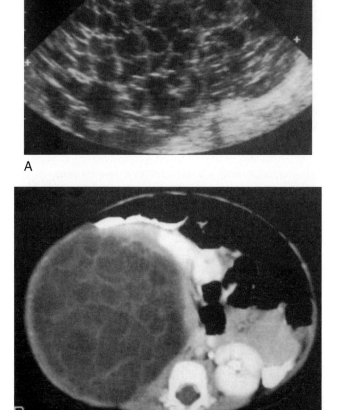

Figure 12–18
Multilocular cystic nephroma. Images of a 1-year-old infant. *A,* A longitudinal sonogram shows multiple septated cysts. *B,* An enhanced CT scan shows multiple cysts replacing the kidney.

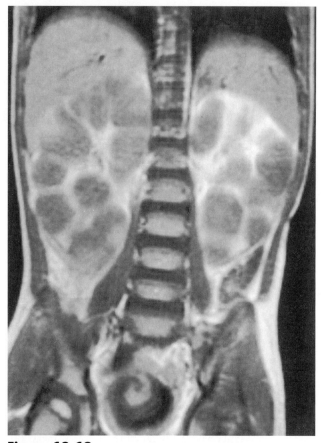

Figure 12–19
Burkitt's lymphoma. Image of a 3-year-old child. This gadolinium-enhanced coronal T1-weighted MR image shows multiple masses within both kidneys.

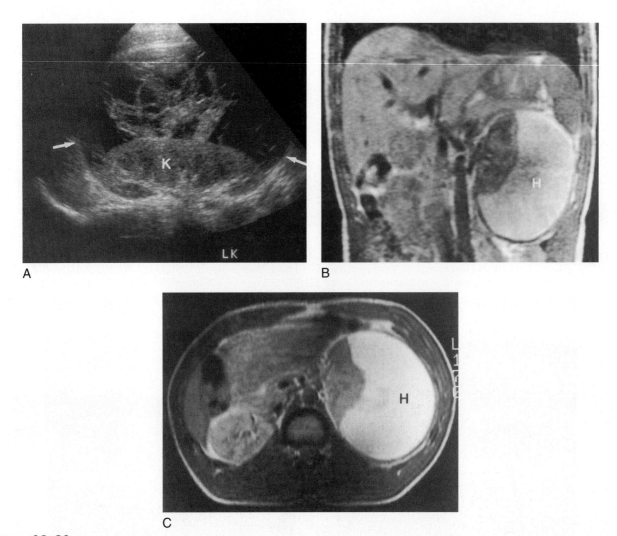

Figure 12–20
Perinephric hematoma. Images of a teenager with a left perirenal hematoma. *A*, A longitudinal sonogram reveals a complex mass *(arrows)* arising from the lateral border of the kidney (K). *B*, A T1-weighted coronal MR image shows the subacute, high-signal, left perinephric hemorrhage (H) distorting the lateral border of the kidney. *C*, A T2-weighted axial MR image with subacute, high-signal hemorrhage (H).

CONGENITAL MESOBLASTIC NEPHROMA

Epidemiology

The spectrum of congenital mesoblastic nephroma (fetal renal hamartoma) ranges from the classic benign lesion, through atypical or cellular congenital mesoblastic nephroma, to malignant spindle cell sarcoma.[11] This tumor is histologically distinct from Wilms' tumor.[21,192] Congenital mesoblastic nephroma is the most common renal tumor in neonates and accounts for about 3% of all renal neoplasms.

Clinical Evaluation

Affected infants have a nontender abdominal mass; the mean age at presentation is 3 months,[90] but the tumor has been detected in utero.[93] Findings include hematuria (20% of patients), hypertension (4%), and anemia.

Congenital mesoblastic nephroma is the most common renal tumor in children who present with hypercalcemia.[22] About 14% of patients have associated abnormalities including polyhydramnios,[193] gastrointestinal tract malformations, neuroblastoma,[84] and genitourinary tract anomalies.[32]

Radiologic Evaluation

Plain radiographs of the abdomen typically show a large, noncalcified, soft-tissue mass (Fig. 12–21). Sonography typically demonstrates a well-defined hypoechoic mass. The presence of concentric echogenic and hypoechoic rings is a helpful diagnostic feature.[32] A more complex pattern follows hemorrhage, cyst formation, and necrosis. CT demonstrates the intrarenal location of the mass. The attenuation pattern is nonspecific, and the mass may be homogeneous or inhomogeneous. Enhancement following administration of

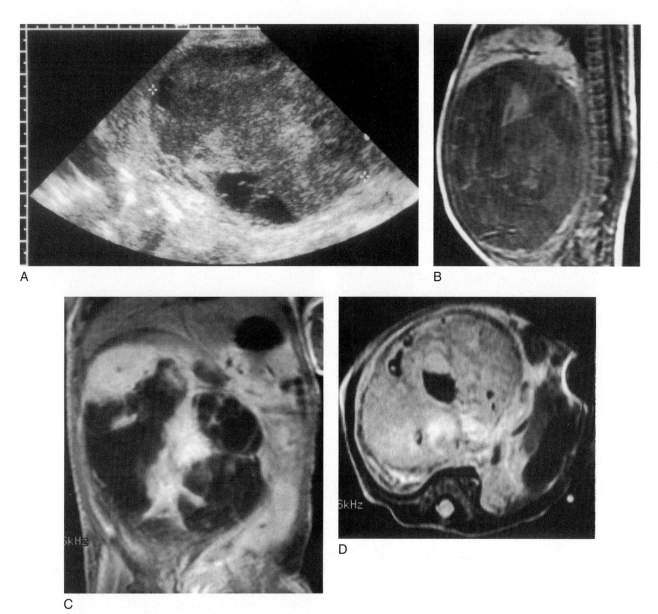

Figure 12–21

Congenital mesoblastic nephroma in a newborn infant. *A,* A longitudinal sonogram reveals a complex mass *(cursors)* replacing the right kidney and filling the abdomen. *B,* A sagittal T1-weighted MR image shows an inhomogeneous mass with areas of hemorrhage. *C,* A coronal T1-weighted gadolinium-enhanced image shows inhomogeneous areas and nonenhancing cyst formation and necrosis. *D,* An axial T2-weighted image reveals a high-signal mass with areas of necrosis and hemorrhage.

contrast material may be due to nephrons trapped within the neoplasm or to high vascularity.[106] Similarly, the tumor is variable in signal and enhancement with MRI.[146]

Congenital mesoblastic nephroma is the only pediatric renal neoplasm that evokes significant scintigraphic uptake on renal scans.[54,106,153]

Pathology

The tumor is a solid, firm, unencapsulated mass, whose cut surface has a whorled appearance similar to that of a uterine leiomyoma. Hemorrhage, cysts, and necrosis are occasionally seen.[32] Histopathologically, the tumor is composed of bundles of spindle cells. Foci of cystic, dysplastic, or immature renal tubules are seen within the mesoblastic substance.[22]

Treatment

The tumor is resected with a wide surgical margin, because tumor is microscopically infiltrative.[13]

Complete excision obviates further treatment.[84] Tumor cells at the surgical margin requires re-exploration for removal of residual disease. Chemotherapy is occasionally used for microscopic residual disease and in instances of tumor rupture. Treatment of tumor recurrence or metastases, which are infrequent, includes surgical resection and chemotherapy.[77]

ABDOMINAL NEUROBLASTOMA

Epidemiology

Neuroblastoma is the most common extracranial solid tumor of childhood[24,41,85] and the most common malignant tumor in infancy.[41] It accounts for 10% of pediatric neoplasms and for 15% of all deaths from cancer in children.[24] The median age at diagnosis is 2 years,[85] and the tumor is unusual in children older than 10 years (Table 12–6). It is slightly more common in boys.[182] Neuroblastoma arising in the abdomen accounts for 37% of all tumors diagnosed before 1 year of age and for 55% of all tumors in older children[51,85] (Figs. 12–22 and 12–23).

Clinical Evaluation

The tumor is usually clinically silent until it invades or compresses adjacent structures, or metastasizes, or causes a paraneoplastic syndrome.[24] Nearly half of patients present with an abdominal mass.[51] Tumor compression of veins may cause edema of the legs. Stretching or compression of the renal vessels may evoke hypertension. If the tumor arises in the pelvis, the patient may have constipation or oliguria. Extension into the spinal canal can be silent[75,142] or may lead to spinal cord compression,[24] manifested by paraplegia, extremity weakness, a change in bowel or bladder habits, or radicular pain. Other symptoms include fever, weight loss, irritability, and generalized pain.[24,85]

Half of infants and about two thirds of children have tumor beyond the primary site at presentation.[24,85,123] Metastases to the liver, seen in one third of children and in half of infants,

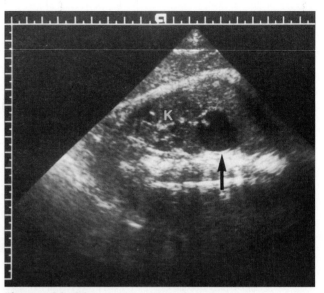

Figure 12–22
Prenatal diagnosis: neuroblastoma. Semi-coronal image of a term fetal right kidney (K) with a cystic mass in the region of the adrenal *(arrow)*. A stage I neuroblastoma was removed at surgery, and the child was disease free when last seen at 3 years of age.

can cause hepatomegaly, sometimes severe enough to hamper respiration. Metastases to the bones or marrow may cause pain, limping, or a pathologic fracture. Orbital metastases can result in ecchymosis or proptosis. Skin metastases,

TABLE 12-4 ABDOMINAL NEUROBLASTOMA: EVANS STAGING SYSTEM		
STAGE	**TUMOR CHARACTERISTICS**	**% OF TUMORS**
I	Tumor confined to organ of origin	13.5
II	Tumor extends beyond organ of origin, but not across midline	11
III	Tumor extends beyond midline; regional lymph nodes may be involved on one or both sides of body	8
IV	Primary tumor with distant disease	44
IV-S	Includes patients who would be stage I or II except for distant disease to skin, liver, or bone marrow	9

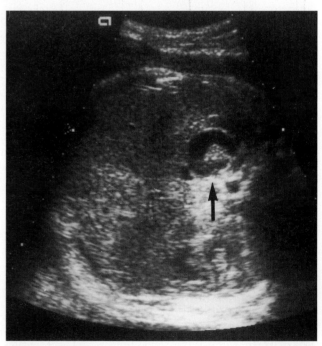

Figure 12–23
Prenatal diagnosis: congenital neuroblastoma. An axial image of a 38-week fetus shows a complex adrenal mass *(arrow)*. A stage I neuroblastoma was resected shortly after birth.

more commonly seen in infants, are nontender, bluish, mobile skin nodules.

Children with neuroblastoma or ganglioneuroblastoma may develop a paraneoplastic syndrome, of which there are two types.[9,24,85] The first is opsoclonus-myoclonus syndrome, or myoclonic encephalopathy of infancy ("dancing eyes, dancing feet"); these patients exhibit irregular eye movements,[184] jerky truncal and limb movements, and cerebellar ataxia. Patients with neuroblastoma and myoclonic encephalopathy have a mean age at presentation of 17 months; girls are affected more frequently than boys. The tumor is found in the posterior mediastinum in 50% of patients and in the abdomen or pelvis in 40%.[9,100] This syndrome has not been explained, but theories include viral infection, antitumor antibody production cross-reaction with the central nervous system, and a neurotoxic substance produced by the tumor.

The second paraneoplastic syndrome associated with neuroblastoma is the constellation of intractable watery diarrhea, hypokalemia, and achlorhydria. This is seen in 7% of patients with neuroblastoma and results from excess vasoactive intestinal peptide production by the tumor.[24]

Physical examination of abdominal or pelvic neuroblastoma reveals a firm, irregular, slightly tender mass that, unlike Wilms' tumor, often crosses the midline.[24,85] Eighty percent to 90% of children with neuroblastoma have increased 24-hour urinary levels of catecholamine metabolites,[24,85] although only 10% of children are hypertensive. These metabolites include vanillylmandelic acid, homovanillic acid, norepinephrine, dopamine, and vanillacetic acid. The presence of vanillacetic acid implies a poorer prognosis. A rise or fall in the levels of these metabolites after therapy parallels growth or regression of the tumor.

Radiologic Evaluation

An abdominal plain film often reveals a soft tissue mass. Calcification within it, demonstrable in about half of patients,[4,5,24,34] may be mottled, dense, or rim-like (Fig. 12–24). Hepatomegaly suggests liver metastases. Widening of the interpediculate distance or erosion of pedicles suggests extradural, intraspinal tumor extension, a finding more commonly seen with intrathoracic tumors.[55,89] Skeletal metastases are permeative and lytic and often show periosteal reaction[24,34,85] (Fig. 12–25).

Abdominal sonography reveals the tumor to be an inhomogeneous, echogenic, poorly defined extrarenal mass that is often large[1,24,34,45,101,159,188] (Figs. 12–26 and 12–27) Hypoechoic regions may reflect hemorrhage, necrosis, or cyst formation. Areas of calcification are hyperechoic. A characteristic well-defined echogenic lobule, described in 40% of larger neuroblastomas,[3] has been related to aggregates of uniform tumor cells surrounded by collagen. Aggressive tumors can invade the kidney and thus may erroneously suggest an exophytic Wilms' tumor.

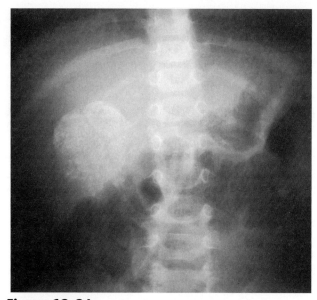

Figure 12–24
Right adrenal neuroblastoma. This abdominal radiographs shows mottled calcification.

The primary tumor or retroperitoneal adenopathy often encases the great vessels, displacing them anteriorly and across the midline.[45,179] Tumor encasement may also involve the celiac axis and superior mesenteric artery. Hepatic metastases may be identified sonographically as focal, discrete, hypoechoic masses or diffuse, ill-defined hyperechogenicity.[24] Rarely neuroblastoma may invade the great veins.[43] The extent of metastatic spreading of the disease to the liver may be underestimated by ultrasonography, especially in younger children with diffuse hepatic infiltration.[1] CT is more sensitive than sonography for hepatic metastases.[67] Although the tumor may invade the pancreas, it is rare to see ductal obstruction or vascular compromise.[179] Before ossification of the posterior elements, intraspinal extension can be assessed by sonography.

CT is a superb modality for detection and delineation of primary neuroblastomas[7,20,24,41,91,170] (Figs. 12–28 through 12–31). It accurately stages 82% of tumors; when combined with bone marrow biopsy, this increases to 94%.[170] Its ability to demonstrate the primary tumor, contiguous spread, vascular encasement, intraspinal extension,[91] retroperitoneal adenopathy, and liver metastases makes it extremely valuable. Pulmonary metastases, seen in about 3% of patients with stage IV neuroblastoma at diagnosis, may be detected as noncalcified nodules.[97] CT is also useful in detecting occult tumors in patients with opsomyoclonus.[58]

Noncontrast-enhanced CT images show pleomorphic calcification in 50% to 90% of abdominal neuroblastomas.[1,5,7,24,34,41,170] Contrast-enhanced CT is preferred for staging.[7,68] The neuroblastoma appears as an irregularly shaped, lobulated, unencapsulated, inhomogeneous tumor,

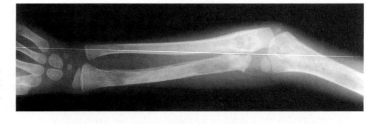

Figure 12–25
Osseous metastatic neuroblastoma. Image of a 3-year-old child with metastatic neuroblastoma. This radiograph of the right forearm shows permeative and lytic metastases with periosteal reaction of the radius, ulna, and humerus.

often with central low density reflecting necrosis.[57] If adrenal in origin, the mass displaces the kidney inferiorly. Adjacent lymph node involvement and direct tumor spread may separate the aorta and inferior vena cava and displace them anterolaterally.[34] The tumor often encases other vessels, such as the celiac axis and superior mesenteric artery, by spreading along the subperitoneal space.[139,140] Renal invasion occurs in up to 10% of tumors.[34] Features that help distinguish neuroblastoma with renal invasion from a Wilms' tumor include renal displacement of the kidney by a predominant suprarenal mass, growth across the midline, multifocal calcification within the mass, and displacement of the great vessels.[144] Neuroblastoma may also metastasize to the kidney.[62] Bilateral primary neuroblastoma is very rare.[111]

MRI is accurate in neuroblastoma[41,51,66,83,166] and represents the imaging modality of choice (Figs. 12–32, 12–33, and 12–34). It is equal to CT in depicting the primary tumor but is superior in imaging adenopathy, vascular involvement, and bone marrow metastases.[36,37] Neuroblastoma tends to show uniform signal intensity and well-defined margins,[65,155] and its internal structure is more homogeneous than that of Wilms' tumor.[36]

Imaging in the coronal[50,51,164] plane best evaluates the tumor in relation to the kidney and great vessels and assesses the intraspinal extension that is present in up to 15% of

patients.[41,160] Coronal and sagittal T1-weighted images evaluate marrow metastases well[51]; cranial dural metastases are best seen on T2-weighted images. Axial images can best demonstrate vascular encasement of the celiac axis and superior mesenteric artery.

Scintigraphy with technetium Tc 99m methylene diphosphonate (Tc-MDP) is the modality of choice for identification of bony metastases, because it detects 50% to 70% more sites than a radiographic skeletal survey[24,34] (Fig. 12–35). Seventy percent to 100% of osseous metastases have increased uptake of radiotracer,[24,69,70] but decreased uptake is seen rarely.[38] Most commonly, metastases involve the metaphyseal region of long bones and the cranium. During bone scanning, the primary tumor is identified in 60 to 70% of cases. Tracer uptake does not correlate with the amount of calcification within the tumor but is more common in larger tumors.[119,158]

Radioactive iodine I 123 and 131 metaiodobenzylguanidine (MIBG) is transported and stored by chromaffin cells in

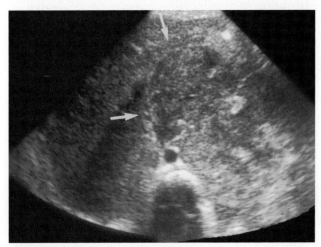

Figure 12–26
Neuroblastoma. Image of a 3-year-old child with neuroblastoma. This transverse upper abdominal sonogram reveals a large, left-sided hyperechoic inhomogeneous mass crossing the midline *(arrows)*.

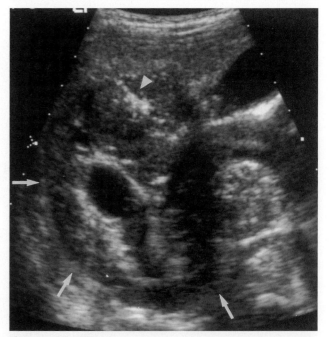

Figure 12–27
Neuroblastoma. Image of a 1-year-old infant with right adrenal neuroblastoma. This transverse sonogram shows the right adrenal mass *(arrows)* with areas of fine calcifications *(arrowhead)* and necrosis.

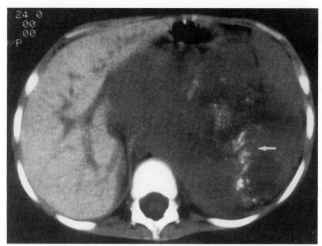

Figure 12–28
Neuroblastoma. Unenhanced CT image of a 3-year-old child with neuroblastoma shows a large, left-sided, low-density mass with mottled calcification *(arrow)*. The mass crosses the midline.

adrenergic secretory tissues.[41,85,95] I 123 MIBG exhibits better image resolution and lower radiation dose, but has a much shorter half-life than I 131. High detection rates for both primary (86%) and metastatic (71%) neuroblastomas have been found.[85,95] Because of discordance between MIBG examinations and bone scintigraphy in 20% of those with disseminated disease, some authors[143] suggested that both studies should be performed at diagnosis. Cortical uptake

cannot be differentiated from marrow uptake by MIBG imaging.[1]

Positron emission tomography (PET) is useful in the evaluation and staging of neuroblastoma. Tumor cells accumulate fluoro-2-deoxy-D-glucose[156] and [11C]hydroxyephedrine.[157] These agents may be especially useful in tumors that do not concentrate MIBG.

Pathology and Staging

Neuroblastoma arises from primitive neuroblasts of the embryonic neural crest,[24,85] the adrenal medulla, and sympathetic ganglia. Microscopic rests of these neuroblasts ("neuroblastoma in situ") are normally seen in about 1% of infants younger than 3 months of age and are present in almost all fetuses between 17 and 20 weeks' gestation.[85] Undifferentiated tumors of neural crest cells are seen in neuroblastoma, whereas more mature cells are present in ganglioneuromas.

Cytogenetic abnormalities are noted in 80% of patients with neuroblastoma.[85] The most common abnormality is partial 1p monosomy with deletion of the region between 1p32 and 1p36, evidently resulting in loss of tumor suppressor gene(s).[125] The proto-oncogene N-*myc* is located on the short arm of chromosome 2, and the number of copies of N-*myc* is amplified in half of children with disseminated neuroblastoma. In localized tumor, N-*myc* amplification is rare.[85]

There are several different, widely used staging systems for neuroblastoma.[35,85] In the Evans staging system, stage I

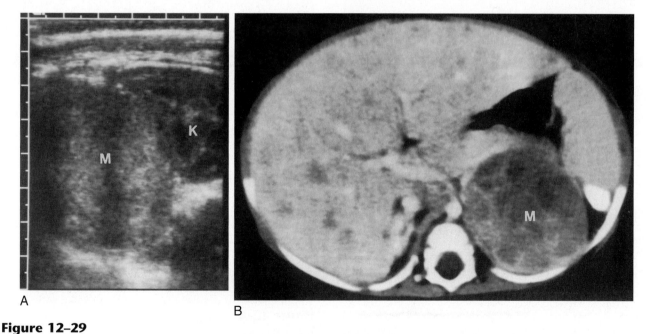

A
B

Figure 12–29
Hepatic metastatic neuroblastoma. Images of a 6-month-old infant with neuroblastoma. *A,* Longitudinal sonogram shows the left suprarenal mass (M) indenting the upper pole of the kidney (K). *B,* An enhanced CT image shows the left-sided adrenal primary tumor and multiple liver metastases.

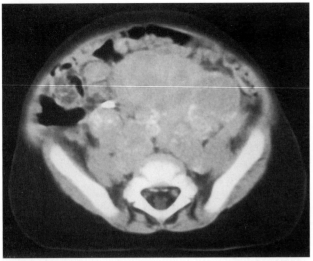

Figure 12–30

Pelvic neuroblastoma. Image of a 1-year-old infant with neuroblastoma. This enhanced CT scan shows the calcified, lobulated, pelvic tumor with central areas of low density representing necrosis.

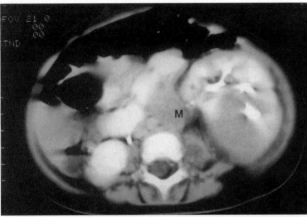

A

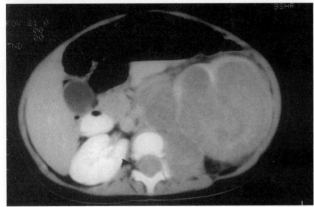

B

Figure 12–31

Spinal tumor extension. Images of a 1-year-old infant with neuroblastoma. *A,* An enhanced CT image shows a lobulated paraspinal mass (M) that displaces and partially encases the aorta. The mass invades the left psoas muscle and left kidney. *B,* A second enhanced CT image shows the left neuroblastoma, with extension into the spinal canal *(arrows).*

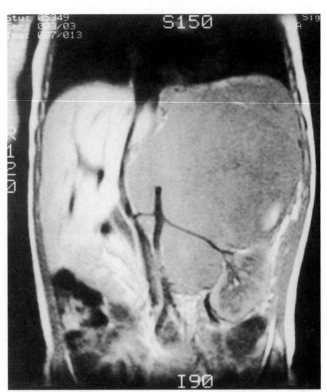

Figure 12–32

Neuroblastoma. MR scan of a 3-year-old child with neuroblastoma. A coronal T1-weighted image shows the large, left-sided tumor. There is encasement of the aorta, and tumor grows between the aorta and inferior vena cava. The left kidney is displaced inferiorly by the mass.

tumor (14%[24]) is confined to the organ of origin; stage II tumor (11%) extends beyond the organ of origin but does not cross the midline; stage III tumor (8%) extends beyond the midline, and regional lymph nodes may be involved on one or both sides of the body; stage IV tumor (44%) includes distant disease; stage IV-S (9%) includes tumors that would be stage I or II except for distant disease confined to the skin, liver, or bone marrow. In 14% of tumors, the organ of origin cannot be determined (Table 12–4).

The Pediatric Oncology Group (POG), now part of the Children's Oncology Group, prefers another staging system[138] in which stage A indicates complete resection of primary tumor and any adherent lymph nodes; intracavitary lymph nodes and the liver are normal. In stage B, primary tumor resection is incomplete, but the lymph nodes and liver are normal. In stage C, the tumor may be completely or incompletely resected; the intracavitary lymph nodes are involved, but the liver is normal. Stage D indicates disseminated disease (Table 12–5).

The more recently developed INSS (International Neuroblastoma Staging System)[28,29] includes radiologic findings, lymph node involvement, bone marrow involvement, and surgical resectability of the tumor. Stage 1 tumors are

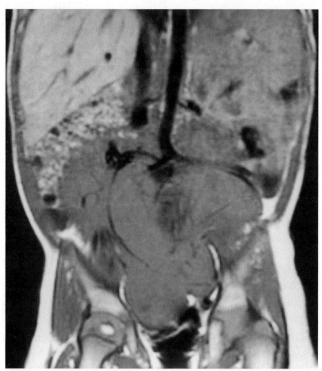

Figure 12–33
Neuroblastoma. Image of an 11-month-old infant with neuroblastoma arising from the organ of Zuckerkandl. A plain radiograph of the abdomen showed a large noncalcified mass in the lower abdomen displacing the bowel superiorly. A coronal T1-weighted image shows the tumor mass elevating the aortic bifurcation.

confined to the area of origin, are completely grossly resected, and have no nodal involvement. Stage 2A tumors are localized but incompletely resected, with benign nodes. Stage 2B tumors are unilateral and may be completely or incompletely resected. There are positive ipsilateral but negative contralateral nodes. Stage 3 tumors include those crossing the midline,

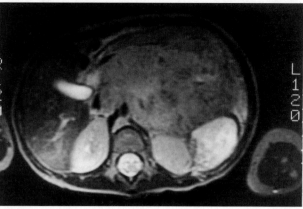

Figure 12–34
Neuroblastoma. MR scan of a 3-year-old child with neuroblastoma. This T2-weighted image shows the large, left-sided mass, which is higher in signal intensity than the liver. The tumor encases the aorta and extends between the aorta and the inferior vena cava.

unilateral tumors with contralateral positive nodes, or midline tumors with bilateral nodal involvement. Stage 4 includes disseminated tumor. Stage 4S disease includes a localized primary tumor (stage 1, 2A, or 2B) with dissemination limited to the skin, liver, or bone marrow in infants younger than 1 year of age.

Treatment and Prognosis

Complete surgical resection is the goal, but this may be precluded by vascular encasement. Resection may become possible after preoperative chemotherapy. Surgical resection alone is the preferred treatment in Evans stage I and II and POG stage A lesions.

Multiagent chemotherapy is usually curative in patients with localized unresected disease and in infants with disseminated disease.[85] In older children with advanced disease, the

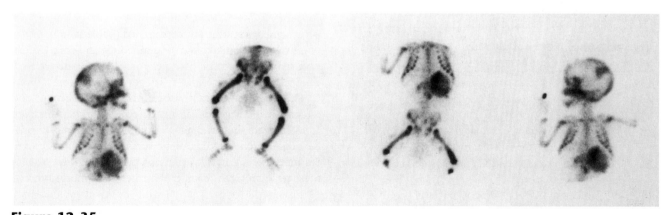

Figure 12–35
Osseous metastatic neuroblastoma. Image of a 1-year-old infant with metastatic neuroblastoma. This technetium Tc 99m methylene diphosphonate (Tc-MDP) bone scan shows that the left adrenal primary tumor is Tc-MDP avid. Multiple metastases are revealed involving the right iliac bone, both femurs, both tibias, and the posterior dura.

TABLE 12-5	ABDOMINAL NEUROBLASTOMA: PEDIATRIC ONCOLOGY GROUP STAGING SYSTEM	

STAGE	TUMOR CHARACTERISTICS
A	Complete resection of primary tumor and any adherent lymph node; intracavitary lymph nodes normal; normal liver
B	Incomplete primary tumor resection; intracavitary lymph nodes normal; normal liver
C	Complete or incomplete tumor resection; intracavitary lymph nodes involved; normal liver
D	Disseminated disease

response to chemotherapy is 70%, but overall survival is unaffected.[24]

Radiation therapy is mostly used for local tumor control. Indications include cord compression, loss of vision as a result of orbital metastases, and painful skeletal metastases. It may also be used as adjuvant therapy in POG stage C or D tumors.

Prognosis depends on age, stage, and location of the primary tumor.[24] The single most important factor at diagnosis is age[41]; prognosis worsens with increasing age. Children with tumors in the abdomen have a poorer prognosis than those with extra-abdominal tumors; children with primary adrenal neuroblastomas have the highest mortality rate. The overall survival rate for patients with a thoracic primary tumor is 61%, but for those with an adrenal primary tumor it is only 20%.[24] The 8-year survival rate for older than 1 year with POG stage A tumors is 100%; with stage B tumors is 80%, with stage C tumors is 30%, and with stage D tumors

TABLE 12-6	ABDOMINAL NEUROBLASTOMA

International Neuroblastoma Staging System

STAGE	TUMOR CHARACTERISTICS
1	Confined to area of origin, completely resected
2A	Incompletely resected localized tumor. Negative nodes
2B	Unilateral tumor, completely or incompletely resected. Positive ipsilateral nodes
3	Tumors crossing midline Midline tumors Unilateral tumors with contralateral positive nodes
4	Disseminated tumor
4S	Infant < 1 year with stage 1, 2A, or 2B plus dissemination limited to skin, liver, marrow

is 15%.[85] Although patients with opsomyoclonus tend to have a better prognosis, neurologic sequelae (cerebellar signs and mental retardation) are seen in approximately 80%. Miscellaneous other adverse prognostic signs exist.[2]

Appropriate imaging of children during and after the completion of treatment for neuroblastoma depends on the initial site, stage, and extent of tumor. CT is very useful in gauging response to treatment and identifying tumor recurrence, with accuracy rates reported at 94% and 85%, respectively.[169] The false-positive rate of CT evaluation for recurrence is 3%. However, in one study,[30] 91% of patients had a recurrence between the surveillance imaging intervals, which was detected clinically before radiographic confirmation.

With response to chemotherapy, the tumor usually shrinks and further calcifies. MRI is useful in assessing the response to therapy[51] and in evaluating its complications. Gadolinium-enhanced imaging may be useful in evaluating residual masses, surgical scars, and inactive, organized fibrous residual disease.[1]

Recent work[53,121] suggests a relationship between neuroblastoma treated in young infants and subsequent development of renal cell carcinoma. These secondary tumors developed between 2 and more than 30 years after the neuroblastoma and did not appear to be associated with prior radiation therapy or chemotherapy. This suggests a genetic association, now recognized because of improved survival of patients treated for high-stage neuroblastoma.[64] Other malignant neoplasms have developed in patients treated for neuroblastoma, including bone and soft tissue sarcomas, leukemia and lymphoma, and others.[120]

Differential Diagnosis

A solid adrenal mass detected by prenatal sonography is most likely a congenital neuroblastoma. A cystic mass in the suprarenal region of a fetus may represent obstruction of the upper pole of a duplex kidney, an adrenal hemorrhage, or a cystic congenital neuroblastoma. Hemorrhage also occurs in cystic neuroblastoma, which results in a complex sonographic appearance. Therefore, when a suprarenal mass suggests an adrenal hemorrhage, liquefaction and contraction of the putative hematoma must be verified over several weeks. Failure to regress should suggest that the true diagnosis is congenital neuroblastoma.

The imaging characteristics described earlier in this section are highly specific for abdominal neuroblastoma in a child beyond the neonatal period. Other adrenal masses, including adrenocortical carcinoma and pheochromocytoma, are rare in children.[1] Adrenocortical carcinoma usually presents in children younger than 5 years, is more common in girls, and is associated with Beckwith-Wiedemann syndrome and hemihypertrophy. These are typically large (>6 cm) at presentation[23] and are inhomogeneous with irregular contrast enhancement. They are locally aggressive and may invade the inferior vena cava.[74]

Pheochromocytoma is another tumor of neural crest origin. These are multiple in one third of patients, and are usually located in the adrenal gland.[1] They are associated with neurofibromatosis, von Hippel-Lindau disease, Sturge-Weber syndrome, and multiple endocrine neoplasia. These tumors are best imaged by MRI,[1] and also show avid MIBG uptake.[71]

HEPATOBLASTOMA

Epidemiology

Primary tumors of the liver account for 15% of abdominal neoplasms and about 1% of all neoplasms in children.[86] Approximately 60% of these are malignant, with an incidence of 1.6 per 1 million children. Hepatoblastoma[191] is the most common primary pediatric hepatic tumor,[87] with an incidence of 0.9 per 1 million children. It is more common in boys and in patients younger than 3 years old;[18] half of these tumors are diagnosed before 18 months of age.

Clinical Evaluation

Most children with hepatoblastoma present with an asymptomatic abdominal mass or abdominal enlargement.[73,80] Anorexia, weight loss, and pain are noted in about one third of patients; jaundice, vomiting, or fracture due to metastatic disease or osteopenia are presenting symptoms in one tenth. Rarely, children present with an acute abdominal crisis provoked by rupture of the tumor. Three percent of hepatoblastomas cause isosexual precocious puberty.[80] Hepatoblastoma has been associated with Beckwith-Wiedemann syndrome, hemihypertrophy, fetal alcohol syndrome, biliary atresia, and maternal ingestion of oral contraceptives and gonadotropin. An increased incidence has also been described in patients with familial polyposis and Gardner syndrome.[171]

Physical examination reveals abdominal distention and hepatic enlargement; a discrete mass may be palpable.[80] Splenomegaly is occasionally present. Half of patients are anemic, with leukocytosis in 20%. Alpha-fetoprotein levels are elevated in 66% to 90% of patients,[80] transaminase levels are elevated in 33%, and bilirubin levels in 15%.

Radiologic Evaluation

Plain films of the abdomen reveal hepatomegaly or a soft tissue mass in the right upper quadrant.[42] Calcification is present in up to half of patients.[40,42,189] Chest radiographs often show elevation of the right hemidiaphragm, and pulmonary metastases are noted in 10% of children at initial diagnosis (Fig. 12–36).

Sonography correctly depicts the extent of hepatoblastoma in 72% of patients. Typically, the lesion is a large (>10 cm), well-defined, intrahepatic mass,[42,46] typically septated with a lobulated outline.[42,177] Foci of hypoechogenicity may be cysts,[128] necrosis, hemorrhage, or extramedullary hematopoiesis.[42]

Imaging features useful in determining the intrahepatic origin of a large upper abdominal mass include displacement of the hepatic vascular radicles, external bulging of the liver capsule, and posterior displacement of the inferior vena cava.[78] Extrahepatic masses, by contrast, show internal invagination of the liver capsule, discontinuity of the liver capsule, a triangular retroperitoneal fat wedge, anterior displacement of the right kidney, and an anterior and medial shift of the inferior vena cava.

Amputation or invasion of one or more branches of the portal vein[10] or hepatic veins[31,177] is an important sonographic predictor of malignancy. High-velocity flow in the hepatic artery has been associated with neovascularity in hepatoblastoma. Ascites is rarely seen but is suggestive of metastasis when present.[42]

CT is superior to sonography for determining the presence and extent of masses within the liver.[19,94,110] Hepatoblastoma appears as a well-defined, often inhomogeneous, lobulated intrahepatic mass with lower attenuation and enhancement than normal liver. Fibrous bands are seen in 20% of tumors after contrast material administration. Calcification is coarse and dense instead of fine and granular, as seen in hemangioendothelioma, and areas of hemorrhage or cyst formation may be noted. However, CT cannot determine respectability of hepatoblastoma, because scans may over- or underestimate the tumor's extent.[104]

Unenhanced MRI and CT are equally effective in defining the intrahepatic mass, although MRI may be more sensitive than CT in the detection of recurrent tumor postoperatively.[19] Gadolinium-enhanced magnetic resonance angiography may be useful in defining the vascular anatomy before resection[82]; angiography is seldom required.

The preoperative evaluation must define the extent of the primary tumor and metastatic disease. Local spread commonly occurs into the porta hepatis. Metastases most frequently affect the lungs but may also occur in the abdominal lymph nodes, viscera, central nervous system, bone, and bone marrow.

Pathology and Staging

Histologically, two types of hepatoblastoma are recognized: the epithelial type (with fetal or embryonal cells), accounting for 70%, and the mixed type (with mesenchymal components in addition to epithelial components), accounting for 30%.[26,85] Extramedullary hematopoiesis is associated with the fetal epithelial type of tumor.[19] Calcification resulting from osteoid formation is frequent in the mixed type of tumor.[85] The epithelial component is the most important histologic predictor of prognosis,[85] with the fetal type having a better prognosis.

Treatment and Prognosis

Cure requires complete tumor resection. Preoperative chemotherapy may reduce tumor bulk and facilitate resection.

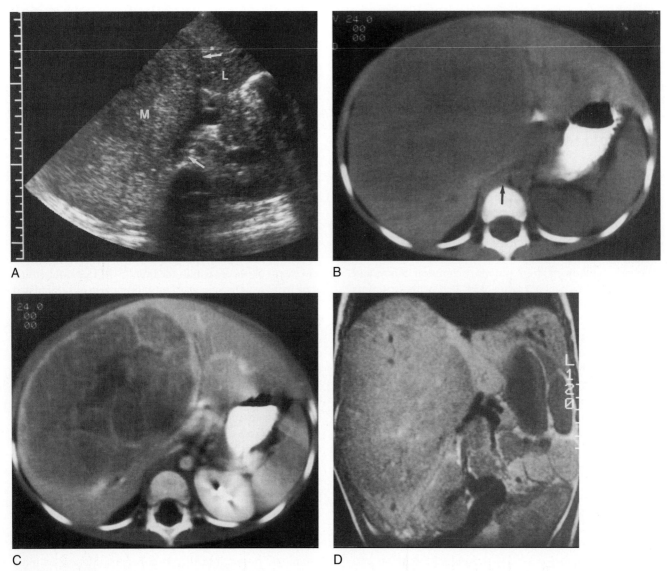

Figure 12–36

Hepatoblastoma. Images of a 3-year-old child with hepatoblastoma. *A*, A transverse abdominal sonogram shows the hyperechoic tumor (M) replacing and expanding the right lobe and medial segment of the left lobe of the liver *(arrows)*. Compare the normal echotexture of the left lobe (L). *B*, A nonenhanced CT image shows the large, slightly inhomogeneous, hypodense mass involving all but the lateral segment of the left lobe of the liver. There is also an enlarged retrocrural lymph node *(arrow)*. *C*, An enhanced CT image shows the mass enhancing less than the normal liver. Fine septa within the mass are seen to enhance. *D*, A coronal T1-weighted MR image shows that the mass is slightly lower in signal intensity than the normal liver. The tiny, high-signal foci are areas of hemorrhage. The mass displaces the right kidney inferiorly.

Complete excision is possible in 50% to 60% of patients. Adjuvant chemotherapy is beneficial. Children with unresectable tumor may undergo intrahepatic chemoembolization of their tumor, followed by orthotopic liver transplant.[6] Radiation therapy has a limited role in the treatment of hepatoblastoma.

Differential Diagnosis

The differential diagnosis mainly includes metastases to the liver, inflammatory disease, and, rarely, other primary liver tumors. Hepatic metastases (commonly from Wilms' tumor, neuroblastoma, or lymphoma) are more frequent than primary hepatic neoplasms. Hepatic abscesses tend to occur in immunocompromised children and may be solitary or multiple. Rhabdomyosarcoma of the biliary tree may present as an intrahepatic mass. Embryonal sarcoma is another rare primary hepatic tumor (Fig. 12–37). Infantile hemangioma and mesenchymal hamartoma are discussed later in this chapter. Differentiation of hepatoblastoma from hemangioendothelioma may be difficult in the very young neonate.[92,183]

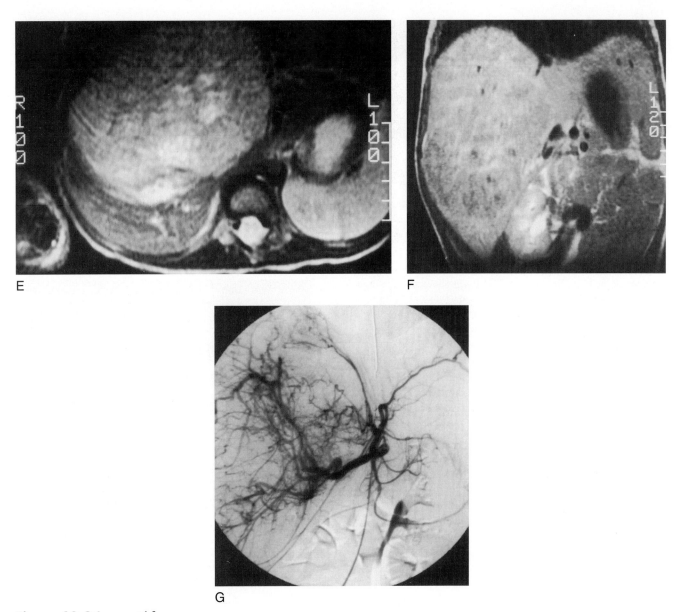

Figure 12–36—cont'd
E, An axial T2-weighted MR image shows the high-signal mass with areas of hemorrhage within it. *F,* A gadolinium-enhanced coronal T1-weighted image shows inhomogeneous enhancement of the tumor. *G,* A subtracted angiographic image of a selective common hepatic injection shows neovascularity within the hepatoblastoma. The lateral segment of the left lobe of the liver is spared, and shunting is absent.

HEPATOCELLULAR CARCINOMA

Epidemiology

Hepatocellular carcinoma is much less common than hepatoblastoma in patients younger than 5 years old. The peak age for diagnosis in children is 12 to 15 years; it is slightly more common in boys.

Clinical Evaluation

Children with hepatocellular carcinoma usually present with an abdominal mass or an enlarging abdomen.

Abdominal pain, anorexia, weight loss, and jaundice occur in about 20% of patients,[56] whereas vomiting and fever are found in 10%. Because of the severity of these symptoms, their duration before presentation is often only 1 or 2 months. Hepatocellular carcinoma in childhood has been associated with exposure to hepatitis B virus before or after birth, hereditary tyrosinemia (in which it is the leading cause of death), biliary cirrhosis caused by extrahepatic biliary atresia, and multiple other conditions.

Physical examination reveals abdominal distention and a right upper quadrant mass. Nearly half of these children

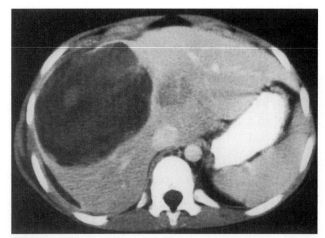

Figure 12–37
Embryonal sarcoma. Image of a 10-year-old child with an embryonal sarcoma of the liver. This enhanced CT image shows that the mass enhances much less than the normal liver. It is lobulated and involves the right lobe and medial segment of the left lobe of the liver.

are anemic,[56] but occasionally extrarenal erythropoietin production causes polycythemia. Thrombocytosis may occur. Transaminase and alkaline phosphatase levels are commonly elevated. Alpha-fetoprotein levels are elevated in 50% of patients and bilirubin levels in 25%.[56] Paraneoplastic phenomena include hypoglycemia, osteomalacia, male precocious puberty, feminization, hyperlipidemia, hypercalcemia, and cystathioninuria.[19] Children with hepatocellular carcinoma should be screened for hepatitis B exposure.

Radiologic Evaluation

Abdominal radiographs of children with hepatocellular carcinoma usually demonstrate a right upper quadrant mass or hepatomegaly, with punctate calcifications in 10% to 25%. Sonography clearly defines the presence, site, and extent of the abdominal mass, which tends to be large when diagnosed (Fig. 12–38). Both lobes of the liver are involved in nearly half of patients, and one third of tumors are multicentric. Diffuse hepatic involvement should be suspected if the sonogram reveals a diffusely inhomogeneous echogenicity, sometimes with distortion of the vascular anatomy.[177] Focal masses are predominantly hyperechoic,[129] although necrosis and hemorrhage are hypoechoic.

CT shows the extent of the tumor[165] better than sonography. Hepatocellular carcinoma is lower in attenuation than normal liver[110] and enhances inhomogeneously.[129] Ring enhancement and dynamic peripheral-to-central enhancement may be seen. Pseudoencapsulation is less evident than with hepatoblastoma.

With MRI, hepatocellular carcinoma shows a high signal on T2-weighted images[19,134] and is better seen on such images.[152,186] A Chemical shift artifact, owing to fatty infiltration or higher triglyceride content of the tumor, is seen in

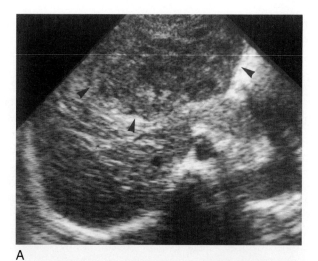

A

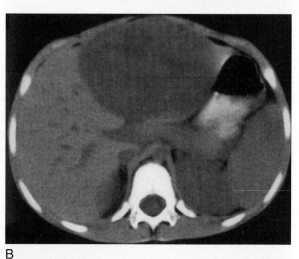

B

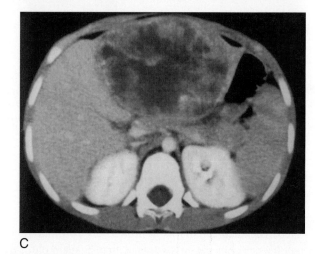

C

Figure 12–38
Hepatocellular carcinoma. Images of a 6-year-old child with hepatocellular carcinoma. *A,* A transverse sonogram of the liver shows the inhomogeneous mass in the left lobe of the liver *(arrowheads)*. *B,* A nonenhanced CT image shows that the mass is hypodense when compared with the normal hepatic parenchyma. *C,* An enhanced CT scan shows peripheral tumor enhancement.

about half of patient.[170] A pseudocapsule is seen in 25% of patients and peritumoral edema (on T2-weighted images) in 30%. These features are diagnostically useful, because metastases to the liver do not show encapsulation, and only malignant lesions have peritumoral edema. MRI defines the internal architecture of the tumor well[150] and seems to be better than CT in detecting postoperative tumor recurrence.[19] Gadolinium-enhanced images may improve the detectability of small lesions, as well as diffuse involvement of the liver with tumor.[87]

The preoperative evaluation must accurately define local extent and distant spread of the tumor as well as exact hepatic segmental involvement. Local spread may occur into the nodes in the porta hepatis. Distant metastases occur most frequently in the lungs[85] and less commonly in skeleton and brain.

Pathology and Staging

The resected tumor, which is usually extensive and often multicentric, may show foci of hemorrhage and necrosis, but no hematopoiesis. Microscopy shows enlarged hepatocytes, nuclear pleomorphism, prominent nucleoli, and tumor giant cells. A recently defined subset, the fibrolamellar type, is typically seen in older children and young adults and has a better patient prognosis than the more typical hepatocellular carcinoma.

Staging is based on the extent of tumor and the completeness of surgical resection. Group I tumors are completely resected as the initial treatment. Group II tumors have microscopic residual disease after surgery. In group III, there is gross residual disease, nodal involvement, or spilled tumor. Patients with group IV tumors have distant metastases.

Treatment and Prognosis

Cure requires complete tumor resection, which can be accomplished in only about 30% of patients.[85] Preoperative chemotherapy may make an inoperable tumor resectable. Even after complete resection, only one third of patients are long-term survivors, although the 5-year survival rate for those with the fibrolamellar subset is as high as 62%. Chemotherapy may lead to partial remission, but it is usually temporary. Radiation therapy offers little.

INFANTILE HEMANGIOMA

Epidemiology

Benign tumors account for approximately one third of all primary neoplasms of the liver. Infantile hemangioma, also known as capillary hemangioma and infantile hemangioendothelioma, accounts for one half to three fourths[115] of these benign lesions (Fig. 12–39). The condition is twice as common in girls as in boys,[39] and 85% of patients present before 6 months of age.[94]

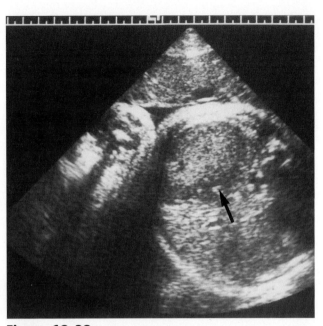

Figure 12–39
Prenatal diagnosis. Hepatic hemangioma. A semiaxial image of a fetus near term shows a solid hepatic mass (arrow). Surgical removal after delivery revealed a hemangioma.

Clinical Evaluation

Presenting symptoms vary from none to florid congestive heart failure.[115,167] Seventy percent of patients have an abdominal mass or hepatic enlargement.[109] About 50% have congestive heart failure of variable severity.[109,115] Cutaneous hemangiomas are noted in about 45%.[114] Intraperitoneal rupture of the tumor is a rare but life-threatening presentation.[173] Other presenting features include jaundice or platelet consumption coagulopathy (Kasabach-Merritt syndrome).[39,115,173]

Results of liver function studies are typically normal. Alpha-fetoprotein levels are elevated in about half of these children.[115]

Radiologic Evaluation

Abdominal radiographs show a right upper quadrant mass or enlargement of the liver, with fine calcification in about one third of patients.[173] Cardiomegaly and pulmonary edema may also be noted.

Sonography will localize the tumor to the liver. The tumor is predominantly solid and may be single or multifocal, large or small.[109,130] It is more often discrete than ill-defined[173] and may be hypoechoic or hyperechoic.[12,39,109] Echogenic stroma and septa may be seen within it.[12,109]

Dilatation of the proximal aorta, an abrupt decrease in the caliber of the aorta below the celiac axis, enlargement of the celiac artery and hepatic artery, and dilatation of the hepatic veins are all important signs of shunting through this vascular tumor[2,39,173] (Fig. 12–40). Arteriovenous shunting is typically not seen in hepatoblastoma, the lesion with which

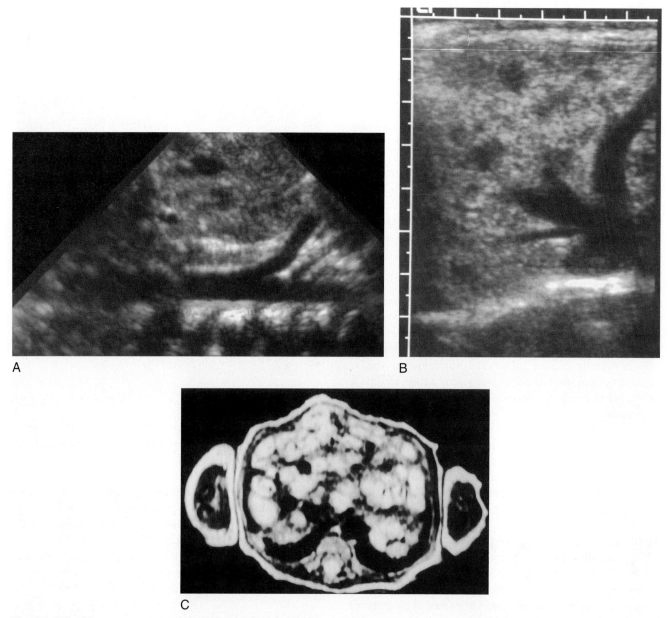

Figure 12–40
Infantile hemangioma. Images of a 6-month-old infant. *A,* A longitudinal sonogram of the aorta shows a markedly enlarged celiac artery and abrupt tapering of the aorta just below the celiac axis. *B,* A transverse sonogram of the liver shows markedly enlarged hepatic veins. The hemangioma is seen as multiple hypoechoic masses within the liver. *C,* A T2-weighed image shows multiple round, high-signal masses throughout the hepatic parenchyma.

it is most likely confused.[2] Doppler sonography shows flow in 60% of these tumors,[109] but the pattern is variable and overlaps with characteristics seen with malignant tumors.[141]

The tumor is usually round or oval, well circumscribed, homogeneous, and hypodense on nonenhanced CT.[39,94,114] Calcification is seen in about 40% of tumors[173] (Fig. 12–41). With bolus contrast agent administration and dynamic imaging, half of the hemangiomas show early peripheral enhancement, followed over 20 to 30 minutes by progressive

central enhancement.[94,114] A persistent central nonenhancing cleft may be seen.[102] Smaller tumors may enhance homogeneously and densely. Nonenhancement reflects areas of necrosis or thrombosis.[173] Delayed images of the multifocal or diffuse form of the tumor show it to become isodense with normal liver.[114]

MRI is as good as CT in defining the extent of tumor.[19] It is also as accurate as CT in predicting benignity, but not accurate enough to obviate biopsy.[19]

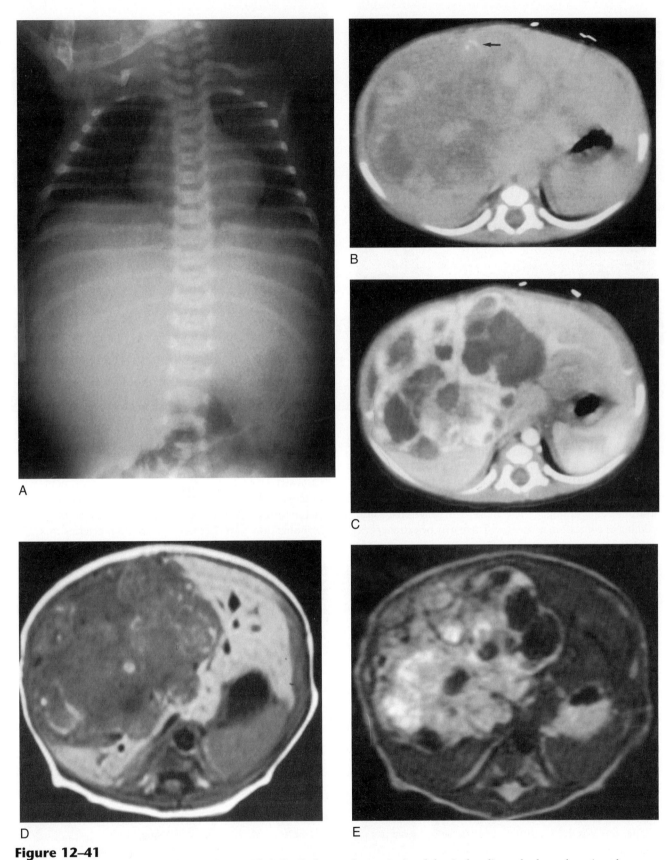

Figure 12–41

Infantile hemangioma. Images of a newborn with infantile hemangioma. *A,* An abdominal radiograph shows hepatic enlargement. *B,* A nonenhanced CT image shows the inhomogeneous, hypodense liver mass with peripheral calcification *(arrow). C,* An enhanced CT image shows marked inhomogeneous enhancement of the mass. *D,* An axial T1-weighted MR image shows the inhomogeneous, predominantly low signal mass. Multiple vessels are seen within. *E,* A T2-weighted axial image shows the inhomogeneous, mixed-signal nature of the mass. The varying signal likely represents a mixture of tissue, hemorrhage, necrosis, and fibrosis. Multiple vessels are again seen.

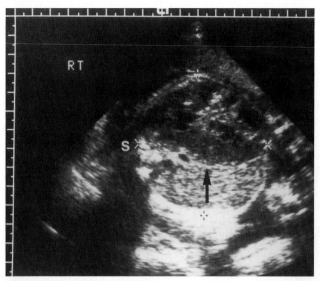

Figure 12–42

Prenatal diagnosis: hemangioendothelioma. This axial image of a 26-week twin fetus reveals a large, heterogeneous, solid hepatic mass (*arrow*). The fetus died in utero, and necropsy revealed a hemangioendothelioma. S, Spine.

Angiography is reserved for diagnostically difficult tumors and for patients in whom ligation of the hepatic artery or embolization is considered. Typically, the hepatic artery is enlarged, the aortic diameter lessens abruptly immediately below the celiac axis, and there is early venous filling from intratumoral shunting.[115] The mass is hypervascular, and puddling of contrast may be seen.[2] There may be extrahepatic

collaterals from the superior mesenteric, intercostal, phrenic, adrenal, and internal mammary arteries.[2,59] Portal vein connections may be inferred from late reopacification of the hepatic mass.[59]

Pathology

Infantile hemangiomas may be round or multilobular, and although they lack a capsule, they tend to be well demarcated by compression of normal liver due to their rapid growth (Fig. 12–42). One popular histologic classification describes two subtypes[48]: type I hemangiomas have vascular spaces of variable size lined by immature, endothelial cells supported on a reticulin network, whereas type II hemangiomas have a more aggressive pattern of pleomorphic cells with hyperchromatic nuclei. Mulliken and Glowacki[135] showed that early in their development, infantile hemangiomas are hypercellular because of endothelial multiplication. During their later involution, the endothelium ceases to proliferate, and fibrous tissue grows between the vascular spaces.

Treatment and Prognosis

The natural history of infantile hemangioma is growth for 6 months to 1 year and then involution.[173] No treatment is necessary in asymptomatic individuals. Congestive heart failure may be managed with diuretics and digitalis. The Kasabach-Merritt syndrome may require treatment with aminocaproic acid or cryoprecipitate.[115] Systemic steroid therapy and interferon-alpha may accelerate involution. Embolization[59] or ligation of feeding arteries may be

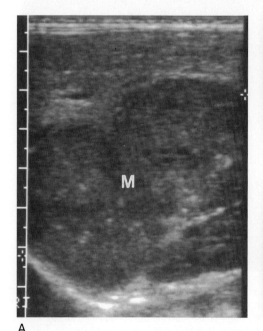

A

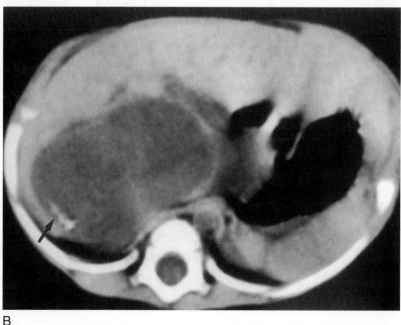

B

Figure 12–43

Mesenchymal hamartoma. Images of a 2-month-old infant. *A,* A transverse ultrasound image shows a mildly hypoechoic mass in the right lobe of the liver. *B,* A nonenhanced CT image shows peripheral calcification (*arrow*) within the hypodense mass.   *Continued*

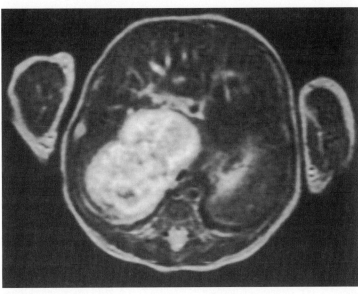

C

Figure 12–43—cont'd
C, a T2-weighted axial MR image shows the well-defined mass, which has high signal intensity when compared with the normal liver.

necessary. Other treatment options include radiation and chemotherapy. Resection is limited to medical failures and instances of tumor rupture. This treatment strategy leads to a survival rate of more than 90%.[115]

Differential Diagnosis

The major differential diagnostic consideration in infantile hemangioma is hepatoblastoma. Mesenchymal hamartoma is the second most common benign liver mass in infancy (Fig. 12–43); 80% are found within the first 2 years of life and patients usually come to medical attention because of an abdominal mass or respiratory distress. Mesenchymal hamartoma characteristically is a multiseptate cystic mass.[168] Other diagnostic considerations include metastases (usually from neuroblastoma or Wilms' tumor, with the primary site almost always being obvious), focal nodular hyperplasia, abscess, and simple cysts of the liver.[114]

REFERENCES

1. Abramson SJ. Adrenal neoplasms in children. Radiol Clin North Am 35:1415–1153, 1997.
2. Abramson SJ, Lack EE, Teele RL. Benign vascular tumors of the liver in infants: Sonographic appearance. AJR Am J Roentgenol 138:629–632, 1982.
3. Amundson GM, Trevenen CL, Mueller DL, Rubin SZ, Wesenberg RL. Neuroblastoma: A specific sonographic tissue pattern. AJR Am J Roentgenol 148:943–945, 1987.
4. Andresen J, Madsen B, Steenskov V. Radiological and clinical evaluation of 20 neuroblastomas. Clin Radiol 32:191–198, 1981.
5. Araki T, Itai Y, Iio M. CT features of calcification in abdominal neuroblastoma. J Comput Assist Tomogr 6:789–791, 1982.
6. Arcement CM, Towbin B, Meza MP, et al. Intrahepatic chemoembolization in unresectable pediatric liver malignancies. Pediatr Radiol 30:779–785, 2000.
7. Armstrong EA, Harwood-Nash DCF, Fitz CR, Chaung S, Pettersson H. CT of neuroblastomas and ganglioneuromas in children. AJR Am J Roentgenol 139:571–576, 1982.
8. Babyn P, Owens C, Gyepes M, D'Angio GJ. Imaging patients with Wilms tumor. Hematol Oncol Clin North Am 9:1217–1252, 1995.
9. Baker ME, Kirks DR, Korobkin M, Bowie JD, Filston HC. The association of neuroblastoma and myoclonic encephalopathy: An imaging approach. Pediatr Radiol 15:184–190, 1985.
10. Bates SM, Keller MS, Ramos IM, Carter D, Taylor KJ. Hepatoblastoma: Detection of tumor vascularity with duplex Doppler US. Radiology 176:505–507, 1990.
11. Beckwith JB. Mesenchymal renal neoplasms of infancy revisited [Editorial]. J Pediatr Surg 9:803–805, 1974.
12. Beckwith JB. Wilms' tumor and other renal tumors of childhood. A selective review from the National Wilms' Tumor Study Pathology Center. Hum Pathol 14:481–492, 1983.
13. Beckwith JB. Wilms tumor and other renal tumors of childhood: An update. J Urol 136:320–324, 1986.
14. Beckwith JB, Palmer NF. Histopathology and prognosis of Wilms' tumors. Results from the National Wilms' Tumor Study. Cancer 41:1937–1948, 1978.
15. Belt TG, Cohen MD, Smith JA, Cory DA, McKenna S, Weetman R. MRI of Wilms' tumor: Promise as the primary imaging method. AJR Am J Roentgenol 146:955–961, 1986.
16. Bishop HC, Tefft M, Evans AE, D'Angio GJ. Survival in bilateral Wilms' tumor—Review of 30 National Wilms' Tumor Study cases. J Pediatr Surg 12:631–638, 1977.
17. Bissett GS, Strife JL, Kirks DR. Genitourinary tract. In Kirks DR, ed. Practical Pediatric Imaging. 2nd ed. Boston: Little, Brown, 1991, pp 994–1010.
18. Boechat MI, Kangarloo H, Gilsanz V. Hepatic masses in children. Semin Roentgenol 23:185–193, 1988.
19. Boechat MI, Kangarloo H, Ortega J, et al. Primary liver tumors in children: Comparison of CT and MR imaging. Radiology 169:727–732, 1988.
20. Boechat MI, Ortega J, Hoffman AD, Cleveland RH, Kangerloo H, Gilsanz V. Computed tomography in stage III neuroblastoma. AJR Am J Roentgenol 145:1283–1287, 1985.
21. Bogdan R, Taylor DEM, Mostofi FK. Leiomyomatous hamartoma of the kidney: A clinical and pathologic analysis of 20 cases from the Kidney Tumor Registry. Cancer 31:462–467, 1973.

22. Bolande RP, Brough AJ, Izant RJ Jr. Congenital mesoblastic nephroma of infancy. Pediatrics 40:272–278, 1967.
23. Boothroyd A, Dicks-Mireau C, Malone M. Adrenal cortical tumors in children. Eur J Radiol 18:199–204, 1994.
24. Bousvaros A, Kirks DR, Grossman H. Imaging of neuroblastoma: An overview. Pediatr Radiol 16:89–106, 1986.
25. Bove KE. Pathology of selected abdominal masses in children. Semin Roentgenol 23:147–160, 1988.
26. Breslow NE, Churchill G, Nesmith B, et al. Clinicopathologic features and prognosis for Wilms' tumor patients with metastases at diagnosis. Cancer 58:2501–2511, 1986.
27. Breslow NE, Takashima JR, Whitton JA, Moksness J, D'Angio GJ, Green DM. Second malignant neoplasms following treatment for Wilms' tumor: A report from the National Wilms' Tumor Study Group J Clin Oncol 13:1851–1859, 1995.
28. Brodeur GM, Pritchard J, Berthold F, et al. Revisions of the international criteria for neuroblastoma diagnosis, staging, and response to treatment. J Clin Oncol 11:1466–1477, 1993.
29. Brodeur GM, Seeger RC, Barrett A, et al. International criteria for diagnosis, staging and response to treatment in patients with neuroblastoma. J Clin Oncol 6:1874–1881, 1988.
30. Bruggers CS, Bolinger C. Efficacy of surveillance radiographic imaging in detecting progressive disease in children with advanced stage neuroblastoma. J Pediatr Hematol Oncol 29(2):104–107, 1988.
31. Brunelle F, Chaumont P. Hepatic tumors in children: Ultrasonic differentiation of malignant from benign lesions. Radiology 150:695–699, 1984.
32. Chan HSL, Cheng MY, Mancer K, et al. Congenital mesoblastic nephroma: A clinicoradiologic study of 17 cases representing the pathologic spectrum of the disease. J Pediatr 111:64–70, 1987.
33. Cohen MD. Commentary: Imaging and staging on Wilms tumors: Problems and controversies. Pediatr Radiol 26:307–311, 1996.
34. Cohen MD. Radiology of pediatric abdominal masses. In Poznanski AK, Kirkpatrick JA, eds. Syllabus: A Categorical Course in Diagnostic Radiology, Pediatric Radiology. Oak Brook, IL: RSNA Publications, 1989, pp 197–211.
35. Cohen MD, Bugaieski EM, Haliloglu M, Faught P, Siddiqui AR. Visual presentation of the staging of pediatric solid tumors. Radiographics 16:523–545, 1996.
36. Cohen MD, Weetman RM, Provisor AJ, et al. Efficacy of magnetic resonance imaging in 139 children with tumors. Arch Surg 121:522–529, 1986.
37. Cohen MD, Weetman RM, Provisor AJ, et al. Magnetic resonance imaging of neuroblastoma with a 0.15-T magnet. AJR Am J Roentgenol 143:1241–1248, 1984.
38. Cook AM, Waller S, Loken MK. Multiple "cold" areas demonstrated on bone scintigraphy in a patient with neuroblastoma. Clin Nucl Med 7:21–24, 1982.
39. Dachman AH, Lichtenstein JE, Friedman AC, et al. Infantile hemangioendothelioma of the liver: A radiographic-pathologic-clinical correlation. AJR Am J Roentgenol 140:1091–1096, 1983.
40. Dachman AH, Pakter RL, Ros PR, Hartman DS. Hepatoblastoma: Radiologic-pathologic correlation in 50 cases. Radiology 164:15–19, 1987.
41. Daneman A. Adrenal neoplasms in children. Semin Roentgenol 23:205–215, 1988.
42. D'Angio GJ, Beckwith JB, Breslow N, et al. Wilms' tumor (nephroblastoma, renal embryoma). In Pizzo PA, Poplack DG, eds. Principles and Practice of Pediatric Oncology. Philadelphia: JB Lippincott, 1989, pp 583–606.
43. Day DL, Johnson R, Cohen MD. Abdominal neuroblastoma with inferior vena caval tumor thrombus: Report of three cases (one with right atrial extension). Pediatr Radiol 21:205–207, 1991.
44. deCampo JF. Ultrasound of Wilms' tumor. Pediatr Radiol 16:21–24, 1986.
45. De Campo M. Ultrasound diagnosis of abdomino-pelvic neuroblastoma. Pediatr Radiol 15:324–328, 1985.
46. deCampo M, deCampo JF. Ultrasound of primary hepatic tumours in childhood. Pediatr Radiol 19:19–24, 1988.
47. Deeg KH, Bettendorf U, Hofmann V. Differential diagnosis of neonatal adrenal hemorrhage and congenital neuroblastoma by colour coded Doppler sonography and power Doppler sonography. Eur J Pediatr 157: 294–297, 1998.
48. Dehner LP, Ishak KG. Vascular tumors or the liver in infants and children. Arch Pathol 92:101–111, 1971.
49. Diament MJ, Parvey LS, Tonkin ILD, Johnson KD, Bernstein R, Webber B. Hepatoblastoma: Technetium sulfur colloid uptake simulating focal nodular hyperplasia. AJR Am J Roentgenol 139:168–171, 1982.
50. Dietrich RB, Kangarloo H. Retroperitoneal mass with intradural extension: Value of magnetic resonance imaging in neuroblastoma. AJR Am J Roentgenol 146:251–254, 1986.
51. Dietrich RB, Kangarloo H, Lenarsky C, Feig SA. Neuroblastoma: The role of MR imaging. AJR Am J Roentgenol 148:937–942, 1987.
52. Donaldson JS, Shkolnik A. Pediatric renal masses. Semin Roentgenol 23:194–204, 1988.
53. Donnelly LF, Rencken IO, Shardell K, et al. Renal cell carcinoma after therapy for neuroblastoma. AJR Am J Roentgenol 167:915–917, 1996.
54. Drubach KA, Connolly LP, Chung T, Treves ST. Four and 24-hour imaging of mesoblastic nephroma with Tc-99 DMSA. Clin Nucl Med 22:797, 1997.
55. Eklof O, Galatius-Jensen F, Damgaard-Pedersen K. Malignant versus benign paravertebral widening in children. Pediatr Radiol 11:193–201, 1981.
56. Exelby PR, Filler RM, Grosfeld JL. Liver tumors in children in the particular reference to hepatoblastoma and hepatocellular carcinoma: American Academy of Pediatrics Surgical Section Survey 1974. J Pediatr Surg 10:329–337, 1975.
57. Faerber EN, Carter BL, Sarno RC, Leonidas JC. Computed tomography of neuroblastic tumors in children. Clin Pediatr 23:17–21, 1984.
58. Farrelly C, Daneman A, Chan HSL, Martin DJ. Occult neuroblastoma presenting with opsomyoclonus: Utility of computed tomography. AJR Am J Roentgenol 142:807–810, 1984.
59. Fellows KE, Hoffer FA, Markowitz RI, O'Neill JA Jr. Multiple collaterals to hepatic infantile hemangioendotheliomas and arteriovenous malformations: Effect on embolization. Radiology 181:813–818, 1991.
60. Felson B, Reeder MM. Gamuts in Radiology. Cincinnati, OH: Audiovisual Radiology of Cincinnati, 1987.
61. Fernbach SK, Donaldson JS, Gonzalez-Crussi F, Sherman JO. Fatty Wilms' tumor simulating teratoma; Occurrence in a child with horseshoe kidney. Pediatr Radiol 18:424–426, 1988.
62. Filiatrault D, Hoyoux C, Benoit P, Garel L, Esseltine D. Renal metastases from neuroblastoma: Report of two cases. Pediatr Radiol 17:137–138, 1987.
63. Fishman EK, Hartman DS, Goldman SM, Siegelman SS. The CT appearance of Wilms' tumor. J Comput Assist Tomogr 7:659–665, 1983.
64. Fleitz JL, Wootton-Gorges SL, Wyatt-Ashmead J, et al. Renal cell carcinoma following treatment of advanced stage neuroblastoma in early childhood. Pediatr Radiol 33:540–545, 2003.
65. Fletcher BD, Kopiwoda SY, Strandjord SE, Nelson AD, Pickering SP. Abdominal neuroblastoma: Magnetic resonance imaging and tissue characterization. Radiology 155:699–703, 1985.
66. Foglia RP, Fonkalsrud EW, Feig SA, Moss TJ. Accuracy of diagnostic imaging as determined by delayed operative intervention for advanced neuroblastoma. J Pediatr Surg 24:708–711, 1989.
67. Forman HP, Leonidas JC, Berdon WE, Slovis TL, Wood BP, Samudrala R. Congenital neuroblastoma: Evaluation with multimodality imaging. Radiology 175:365–368, 1990.

68. Fujioka M, Saiki N, Aihara T, Yamamoto K. Imaging evaluation of infants with neuroblastoma detected by VMA screening spot test. Pediatr Radiol 18:479–483, 1988.

69. Garty I, Friedman A, Sandler MP, Keder A. Neuroblastoma: Imaging evaluation by sequential Tc-99m MDP, I-131 MIBG, and Ga-67 citrate studies. Clin Nucl Med 14:515–522, 1989.

70. Garty I, Koren A, Goshen Y, Siplovich L. The complementary role of sequential 99mTc-MDP and 67Ga-citrate scanning in the diagnosis and follow-up of neuroblastoma. Eur J Nucl Med 11:224–229, 1985.

71. Gelfand M. Meta-iodobenzylguanidine in children. Semin Nucl Med 23:237–242, 1983.

72. Geller E, Smergel EM, Lowry PA. Renal neoplasms of childhood. Radiol Clin North Am 35:1391–1413, 1997.

73. Giacomantonio M, Ein SH, Mancer K, Stephens CA. Thirty years of experience with pediatric primary malignant liver tumors. J Pediatr Surg 19:523–526, 1984.

74. Godine L, Berdon W, Brasch R, Leonidas JC. Adrenocortical carcinoma with extension into inferior vena cava and right atrium: Report of three cases in children. Pediatr Radiol 20:166–168, 1990.

75. Golding SJ, McElwain TJ, Husband JE. The role of computed tomography in the management of children with advanced neuroblastoma. Br J Radiol 57:661–666, 1984.

76. Goldman SM, Garfinkel DJ, Oh KS, Dorst JP. The Drash syndrome: Male pseudohermaphroditism, nephritis, and Wilms' tumor. Radiology 141:87–91, 1981.

77. Gormley TS, Skoog SJ, Jones RV, Maybee D. Cellular congenital mesoblastic nephroma: What are the options. J Urol 142:479–483, 1989.

78. Graif M, Manor A, Itzchak Y. Sonographic differentiation of extra- and intrahepatic masses. AJR Am J Roentgenol 141:553–556, 1983.

79. Gray GG, Amodio JB, Wood BP. Multilocular cystic Wilms tumor: Radiological case of the month. Arch Pediatr Adolesc Med 152:705–706, 1998.

80. Greenberg M, Filler RM. Hepatic tumors. In Pizzo PA, Poplack DG, eds. Principles and Practice of Pediatric Oncology. Philadelphia: JB Lippincott, 1989.

81. Griscom NT. The roentgenology of neonatal abdominal masses. AJR Am J Roentgenol 93:447–463, 1965.

82. Haliloglu M, Hoffer FA, Gronemeyer SA, Furman WL, Shochat SJ. 3D gadolinium-enhanced MRA: Evaluation of hepatic vasculature in children with hepatoblastoma. J Magn Reson Imaging 11:65–68, 2000.

83. Hall-Craggs MA, Finn JP, Malone M, Steward C. 4-S neuroblastoma on high field MR. Pediatr Radiol 20:124–125, 1989.

84. Hartman DS, Lesar MSL, Madewell JE, Lichtenstein JE, Davis CJ Jr. Mesoblastic nephroma: Radiologic-pathologic correlation of 20 cases. AJR Am J Roentgenol 136:69–74, 1981.

85. Hayes FA, Smith EI. Neuroblastoma. In Pizzo PA, Poplack DG, eds. Principles and Practice of Pediatric Oncology. Philadelphia: JB Lippincott, 1989, pp 607–622.

86. Heiken JP, Lee JKT, Glazer HS, Ling D. Hepatic metastases studied with MR and CT. Radiology 156:423–427, 1985.

87. Helmberger TK, Ros PR, Mergo PJ, Tomczak R, Feiser MF. Pediatric liver neoplasms: A radiologic-pathologic correlation. Eur Radiol 9:1339–1347, 1999.

88. Hendren WH. Abdominal masses in newborn infants. Am J Surg 107:502–510, 1964.

89. Holgersen LO, Santulli TV, Schullinger JN, Berdon WE. Neuroblastoma with intraspinal (dumbbell) extension. J Pediatr Surg 18:406–411, 1983.

90. Howell CG, Othersen HB, Kiviat NE, Norkool P, Beckwith JB, D'Angio GJ. Therapy and outcome in 51 children with mesoblastic nephroma: A report of the National Wilms' Tumor Study. J Pediatr Surg 17:826–831, 1982.

91. Hugosson C, Nyman R, Horulf H, et al. Imaging of abdominal neuroblastoma in children. Acta Radiol 40:534–542, 1999.

92. Ingram JD, Yerushalmi B, Connell J, Karrer FM, Tyson RW, Sokol RJ. Hepatoblastoma in a neonate: A hypervascular presentation mimicking hemangioendothelioma. Pediatr Radiol 30:794–797, 2000.

93. Irsutti M, Puget C, Baunin C, Duga I, Sarramon MF, Guitard J. Mesoblastic nephroma: Prenatal ultrasonographic and MRI features. Pediatr Radiol 30:147–150, 2000.

94. Jabra AA, Fishman EK, Taylor GA. Hepatic masses in infants and children: CT evaluation. AJR Am J Roentgenol 158:143–149, 1992.

95. Jacobs A, Delree M, Desprechins B, et al. Consolidating the role of *I-MIBG-scintigraphy in childhood neuroblastoma: Five years of clinical experience. Pediatr Radiol 20:157–159, 1990.

96. Jaffe MH, White SJ, Silver TM, Heidelberger KP. Wilms' tumor: Ultrasonic features, pathologic correlation, and diagnostic pitfalls. Radiology 140:147–152, 1981.

97. Kammen BF, Matthay KK, Pacharn P, Gerbing R, Brasch RC, Gooding CA. Pulmonary metastases at diagnosis of neuroblastoma in pediatric patients: CT findings and prognosis. AJR Am J Roentgenol 176:755–759, 2001.

98. Kasper TE, Osborne RW Jr, Semerdjian HS, Miller HC. Urologic abdominal masses in infants and children. J Urol 116:629–633, 1976.

99. Kaufman RA, Holt JF, Heidelberger KP. Calcification in primary and metastatic Wilms' tumor. AJR Am J Roentgenol 130:783–785, 1978.

100. Kinast M, Levin HS, Rothner AD, Erenberg G, Wacksman J, Judge J. Cerebellar ataxia, opsoclonus and occult neural crest tumor: Abdominal computerized tomography in diagnosis. Am J Dis Child 134:1057–1059, 1980.

101. Keller MS, Buckley PJ. Sonographic tissue pattern in neuroblastoma. AJR Am J Roentgenol 150:693, 1988.

102. Keslar PJ, Buck JL, Selby DM. Infantile hemangioendothelioma of the liver revisited. RadioGraphics 13:657–670, 1993.

103. Keslar PJ, Buck JL, Suarez ES. Germ cell tumors of the sacrococcygeal region: Radiologic-pathologic correlation. RadioGraphics 14:607–620, 1994.

104. King SJ, Babyn PS, Greenberg ML, Phillips MJ, Filler RM. Value of CT in determining the respectability of hepatoblastoma before and after chemotherapy. AJR Am J Roentgenol 160:793–798, 1993.

105. Kirks DR. Pediatric imaging: Body computed tomography. Curr Probl Pediatr 14:1–63, 1984.

106. Kirks DR, Kaufman RA. Function within mesoblastic nephroma: Imaging-pathologic correlation. Pediatr Radiol 19:136–139, 1989.

107. Kirks DR, Kaufman RA, Babcock DS. Renal neoplasms in infants and children. Semin Roentgenol 22:292–302, 1987.

108. Kirks DR, Merten DF, Grossman H, Bowie JD. Diagnostic imaging of pediatric abdominal masses: An overview. Radiol Clin North Am 19:527–545, 1981.

109. Klein MA, Slovis TL, Chang CH, Jacobs IG. Sonographic and Doppler features of infantile hepatic hemangiomas with pathologic correlation. J Ultrasound Med 9:619–624, 1990.

110. Korobkin M, Kirks DR, Sullivan DC, Mills SR, Bowie JD. Computed tomography of primary liver tumors in children. Radiology 139:431–435, 1981.

111. Kramer SA, Bradford WD, Anderson EE. Bilateral adrenal neuroblastoma. Cancer 45:2208–2212, 1980.

112. Lebowitz RL, Griscom NT. Neonatal hydronephrosis: 146 cases. Radiol Clin North Am 15:49–59, 1977.

113. Lowe LH, Isuani BH, Heller RM, et al. Pediatric renal masses: Wilms' tumor and beyond. RadioGraphics 20:1585–1603, 2000.

114. Lucaya J, Enriquez G, Amat L, Gonzalez-Rivero MA. Computed tomography of infantile hepatic hemangioendothelioma. AJR Am J Roentgenol 144:821–826, 1985.

115. Luks FI, Yazbeck S, Brandt ML, Bensoussan AL, Brochu P, Blanchard H. Benign liver tumors in children: A 25-year experience. J Pediatr Surg 11:1326–1330, 1991.

116. MacManus M. The diagnosis and staging of neuroblastoma. Clin Radiol 34:523–527, 1983.

117. Macpherson RI. Gastrointestinal tract duplications: Clinical, pathologic, etiologic and radiologic considerations. RadioGraphics 13:1063–1080, 1993.

118. Mahaffey SM, Ryckman FC, Martin LW. Clinical aspects of abdominal masses in children. Semin Roentgenol 23:161–174, 1988.

119. Martin-Simmerman P, Cohen MD, Siddiqui A, Mirkin D, Provisor A. Calcification and uptake of Tc-99m diphosphonates in neuroblastomas: Concise communication. J Nucl Med 25:656–660, 1984.

120. Meadows AT, Baum E, Fossati-Bellani F, et al. Second malignant neoplasms in children: An update from the late effects study group. J Clin Oncol 3:532–538, 1985.

121. Medieros LJ, Palmedo G, Krigman HR, Kovacs G, Beckwith JB. Oncocytoid renal cell carcinoma after neuroblastoma: A report of four cases of a distinct clinicopathologic entity. Am J Surg Path 23:772–780, 1999.

122. Melicow MM, Uson AC. Palpable abdominal masses in infants and children: A report based on a review of 653 cases. J Urol 81:705–710, 1959.

123. Merten DF, Kirks DR. Diagnostic imaging of pediatric abdominal masses. Pediatr Clin North Am 32:1397–1425, 1985.

124. Mertens F, Heim S. Clonal karyotypic evolution in a pediatric neurofibrosarcoma. Cancer Genet Cytogenet 81:135–138, 1995.

125. Mertens F, Mandahl N, Mitelman J, Heim S. Cytogenetic analysis in the examination of solid tumors in children. Pediatr Hematol Oncol 11:361–377, 1994.

126. Mesrobian HGJ. Wilms' tumor: Past, present, future. J Urol 140:231–238, 1988.

127. Mesrobian HGJ, Kelalis PP, Hrabovsky E, Othersen HB Jr, deLorimier A, Nesmith B. Wilms' tumor in horseshoe kidneys: A report from the National Wilms' Tumor Study. J Urol 133:1002–1003, 1985.

128. Miller JH. The ultrasonographic appearance of cystic hepatoblastoma. Radiology 138:141–143, 1981.

129. Miller JH, Greenspan BS. Integrated imaging of hepatic tumors in childhood, part I: Malignant lesions (primary and metastatic). Radiology 154:83–90, 1985.

130. Miller JH, Greenspan BS. Integrated imaging of hepatic tumors in childhood, part II: Benign lesions, congenital, reparative, and inflammatory. Radiology 154:91–100, 1985.

131. Miller RW, Fraumeni JF, Manning MD. Association of Wilms' tumor with aniridia, hemihypertrophy and other congenital malformations. N Engl J Med 270:922–927, 1964.

132. Mohd TBH, Yip CH. Cystic neuroblastoma with colonic fistula. Pediatr Radiol 18:406, 1988.

133. Montgomery P, Kuhn JP, Berger PE, Fisher J. Multifocal nephroblastomatosis: Clinical significance and imaging. Pediatr Radiol 14:392–395, 1984.

134. Moss AA, Goldberg HI, Stark DB, et al. Hepatic tumors: Magnetic resonance and CT appearance. Radiology 150:141–147, 1984.

135. Mulliken JB, Glowacki J. Hemangiomas and vascular malformations in infants and children: A classification based on endothelial characteristics. Plast Reconstr Surg 69:412–422, 1982.

136. Nakayama DK, Ortega W, D'Angio GJ. The nonopacified kidney with Wilms' tumor. J Pediatr Surg 23:152–155, 1988.

137. Navoy JF, Royal SA, Vaid YN, Mroczek-Muslman EC. Wilms' tumor: Unusual manifestations. Pediatr Radiol 25:S76–S86, 1995.

138. Nitschke R, Smith EI, Shochat S, et al. Localized neuroblastoma treated by surgery: A Pediatric Oncology Group Study. J Clin Oncol 6:1271–1279, 1988.

139. Oliphant M, Berne AS. Mechanism of direct spread of abdominal neuroblastoma: CT demonstration and clinical implications. Gastrointest Radiol 12:59–66, 1987.

140. Oliphant M, Berne AS. Aggressive neuroblastoma simulating Wilms' tumor. Radiology 167:878, 1988.

141. Paltiel HJ, Patriquin HB, Keller MS, babcock DS, Leithiser RE Jr. Infantile hepatic hemangioma: Doppler US. Radiology 182:735–742, 1992.

142. Payne J, Wolfson P, Northrup BE. Dumbbell neuroblastoma presenting without spinal cord findings. J Pediatr Surg 21:995–996, 1986.

143. Perel Y, Conway J, Kletzel M, et al. Clinical impact and prognostic value of metaiodobenzylguanidine imaging in children with metastatic neuroblastoma J Pediatr Hematol Oncol 21:13–18, 1999.

144. Peretz GS, Lam AH. Distinguishing neuroblastoma from Wilms' tumor by computed tomography. J Comput Assist Tomogr 9:889–893, 1985.

145. Petruzzi MJ, Green DM. Wilms' tumor. Pediatric oncology. 44:939–952, 1997.

146. Puvaneswary M, Roy GT. Congenital mesoblastic nephroma: Other magnetic resonance imaging findings. Australas Radiol 43:532–534, 1999.

147. Raffensperger J, Abousleiman A. Abdominal masses in children under one year of age. Surgery 63:514–521, 1968.

148. Reiman TA, Siegel MJ, Shackelford GD. Wilms' tumor in children: Abdominal CT and US evaluation. Radiology 160:501–505, 1986.

149. Ritchey ML, Kelalis PP, Breslow N, Offord KP, Shochat SJ, D'Angio GJ. Intracaval and atrial involvement with nephroblastoma: Review of National Wilms' Tumor Study 3. J Urol 140:1113–1118, 1988.

150. Rosenfield NS, Leonidas JC, Barwick KW. Aggressive neuroblastoma simulating Wilms' tumor. Radiology 166:165–167, 1988.

151. Roshkow JE, Haller JO, Berdon WE, Sane SM. Hirschsprung's disease, Ondine's curse, and neuroblastoma—manifestations of neurocristopathy. Pediatr Radiol 19:45–49, 1988.

152. Rummeny E, Weissleder R, Stark DD, et al. Primary liver tumors: Diagnosis by MR imaging. AJR Am J Roentgenol 152:63–72, 1989.

153. Sacks G, Mitchell M, Fleischer AC, Sandler M. Scintigraphic and sonographic diagnosis of neonatal mesoblastic nephroma. Clin Nucl Med 8:252–253, 1983.

154. Saeki M, Hagane K, Nakano M. Radiologic evaluation of surgical resectability in abdominal neuroblastoma. J Pediatr Surg 24:378–381, 1989.

155. Schultz CL, Haaga JR, Fletcher BD, Alfidi RJ, Schultz MA. Magnetic resonance imaging of the adrenal glands: A comparison with computed tomography. AJR Am J Roentgenol 143:1235–1240, 1984.

156. Shulkin BL, Hutchinson RJ, Castle VP, Yanik GA, Shapiro B, Sisson JC. Neuroblastoma: Positron emission tomography with 2-(fluorine-18)-fluoro-2-deoxy-D-glucose compared with metaiodobenzylguanidine scintigraphy. Radiology 199:743–750, 1996.

157. Shulkin BL, Wieland DM, Baro ME, et al. PET hydroxyephedrine imaging of neuroblastoma. J Nucl Med 37:16–21, 1996.

158. Siddiqui AR, Cohen M, Moran DP. Abdominal masses in children: Multiorgan imaging with 99mTc methylene diphosphonate. AJR Am J Roentgenol 139:35–38, 1982.

159. Siegel MJ. Pediatric Sonography. New York: Raven Press, 1991, pp 124–160, 275–278.

160. Siegel MJ, Jamroz GA, Glazer HS, Abramson CL. MR imaging of intraspinal extension of neuroblastoma. J Comput Assist Tomogr 10:593–595, 1986.

161. Slasky BS, Bar-Ziv J, Freeman AI, Peylan-Ramu N. CT appearances of involvement of the peritoneum, mesentery and omentum in Wilms tumor. Pediatr Radiol 27:14–17, 1997.

162. Slovis TL, Cushing B, Reilly BJ, et al. Wilms' tumor to the heart: Clinical and radiographic evaluation. AJR Am J Roentgenol 131:263–266, 1978.

163. Slovis TL, Philippart AI, Cushing B, et al. Evaluation of the inferior vena cava by sonography and venography in children with renal and hepatic tumors. Radiology 140:767–772, 1981.

164. Smith FW, Cherryman GR, Redpath TW, Crosher G. The nuclear magnetic resonance appearance of neuroblastoma. Pediatr Radiol 15:329–332, 1985.
165. Snow JH Jr, Goldstein HM, Wallace S. Comparison of scintigraphy, sonography and computed tomography in the evaluation of hepatic neoplasms. AJR Am J Roentgenol 132:915–918, 1979.
166. Sofka CM, Semelka RC, Kelekis NL, et al. Magnetic resonance imaging of neuroblastoma using current techniques. Magnetic Resonance Imaging 17:193–198, 1999.
167. Stanley P, Gates GF, Eto RT, Miller SW. Hepatic cavernous hemangiomas and hemangioendotheliomas in infancy. AJR Am J Roentgenol 129:317–321, 1977.
168. Stanley P, Hall TR, Woolley MM, Diament MJ, Gilsanz V, Miller JH. Mesenchymal hamartomas of the liver in childhood: Sonographic and CT findings. AJR Am J Roentgenol 1986; 147:1035–9.
169. Stark DD, Brasch RC, Moss AA, et al. Recurrent neuroblastoma: The role of CT and alternative imaging tests. Radiology 148:107–112, 1983.
170. Stark DD, Moss AA, Brasch RC, et al. Neuroblastoma: Diagnostic imaging and staging. Radiology 148:101–105, 1983.
171. Stoupis C, Ros PR. Imaging findings in hepatoblastoma associated with Gardner's syndrome. AJR Am J Roentgenol 161:593–594, 1993.
172. Stoupis C, Ros PR, Abbitt PL, Burton SS, Gauger J. Bubbles in the belly: Imaging of cystic mesenteric or omental masses. RadioGraphics 14:729–737, 1994.
173. Stringer DA. Pediatric Gastrointestinal Imaging. Toronto, Canada: BC Decker, 1989, pp 527–534.
174. Sty JR, Wells RG. Other abdominal and pelvic masses in children. Semin Roentgenol 23:216–231, 1988.
175. Surratt JT, Siegel MJ. Imaging of pediatric ovarian masses. RadioGraphics 11:533–548, 1991.
176. Taybi H, Lackman RS. Radiology of Syndromes, Metabolic Disorders and Skeletal Dysplasias. 3rd ed. Chicago: Year Book Medical Publishers, 1990, pp 46–47, 145, 211–212, 362, 432–433.
177. Taylor KJW, Ramos I, Morse SS, Fortune KL, Hammers L, Taylor CR. Focal liver masses: Differential diagnosis with pulsed Doppler US. Radiology 164:643–647, 1987.
178. Teele RL, Henschke CI. Ultrasonography in the evaluation of 482 children with an abdominal mass. Clin Diag Ultrasound 14:141–165, 1984.
179. Teele RL, Share JC. The abdominal mass in the neonate. Semin Roentgenol 23:175–184, 1988.
180. Teele RL, Share JC. Ultrasonography of Infants and Children. Philadelphia: WB Saunders, 1991, pp 252–255, 269–271.
181. Thyss A, Taviere V, Quintana E, et al. Spontaneous hematoma of the kidney simulating a nephroblastoma. Am J Pediatr Hematol Oncol 12:355–358, 1990.
182. Triche TJ, Askin FB. Neuroblastoma and the differential diagnosis of small-, round-, blue-cell tumors. Hum Pathol 14:569–595, 1983.
183. von Schweinitz D, Gluer S, Midenberger H. Liver tumors in neonates and very young infants: Diagnostic pitfalls and therapeutic problems. Eu J Pediatr Surg 5:72–76, 1995.
184. Warrier RP, Kini R, Besser A, Wiatrak B, Raju U. Opsomyoclonus and neuroblastoma. Clin Pediatr 24:32–34, 1985.
185. Weese DL, Applebaum H, Taber P. Mapping intravascular extension of Wilms' tumor with magnetic resonance imaging. J Pediatr Surg 26:64–67, 1991.
186. Weinreb JC, Cohen JM, Armstrong E, Smith T. Imaging the pediatric liver: MRI and CT. AJR Am J Roentgenol 147:785–790, 1986.
187. White KS, Grossman H. Wilms' and associated renal tumors of childhood. Pediatr Radiol 21:81–88, 1991.
188. White SJ, Stuck KJ, Blane CE, Silver TM. Sonography of neuroblastoma. AJR Am J Roentgenol 141:465–468, 1983.
189. Wolfson BJ, Gainey MA, Faerber EN, Capitanio MA. Renal masses in children. An integrated imaging approach to diagnosis. Urol Clin North Am 12:755–769, 1985.
190. Wootton SL. Wilms' tumor. Contemp Diagn Radiol 15:1–5, 1992.
191. Wootton SL. Hepatoblastoma. Contemp Diagn Radiol. 16:1–5, 1993.
192. Wootton SL, Rowen SJ, Griscom NT. Pediatric case of the day: Mesoblastic nephroma. RadioGraphics 11:719–721, 1991.
193. Yazaki T, Akimoto M, Tsuboi N, Kawai H, Miyamoto M, Suzuki T. Congenital mesoblastic nephroma. Urology 20:446–450, 1982.
194. Young JL, Miller RW. Incidence of malignant tumors in U.S. children. J Pediatr 86:254–258, 1975.

ADDITIONAL READING

Alobaidi M, Shirkhoda A. Malignant cystic and necrotic liver lesions: A pattern approach to discrimination. Curr Probl Diagn Radiol 33:254–268, 2004.
Bell MG, Goodman TR. Perinephric cystic mesoblastic nephroma complicated by hepatic metastases: A case report. Pediatr Radiol 32:829–831, 2002.
Burrows PE, Dubois J, Kassarjian A. Pediatric hepatic vascular anomalies. Pediatr Radiol 2001; 31:533–545.
Chen CC, Kong MS, Yang CP, Hung IJ. Hepatic hemangioendothelioma in children: Analysis of thirteen cases. Acta Paediatr Tw 2003; 44:8-13, 2003.
Daw NC, Kauffman WM, Bodner SM, Bratt CB, Hoffer FA. Patterns of abdominal relapse and role of sonography in Wilms tumor. Pediatr Hematol Oncol 19:107–115, 2002.
Dighe MK, Parnell S, Yeh MM, Lalani T. Hepatic epithelioid hemangioendothelioma: Multiphase CT appearance and correlation with pathology. Crit Rev Comput Tomogr 45:343-354, 2004.
Elsayes KM, Mukundan G, Narra VR, Lewis JS, Shirkhoda A, Farooki AM, Brown JJ. Adrenal masses: MR imaging features with pathologic correlation. RadioGraphics 24:S73–S86, 2004.
Gunther P, Schenk JP, Wunsch R, Troger J, Waag KL. Abdominal tumours in children: 3-D visualization and surgical planning. Eur J Pediatr Surg 14:316–321, 2004.
Kushner BH. Neuroblastoma: A disease requiring a multitude of imaging studies. J Nucl Med 45:1172–1188, 2004.
Laffan EE, O'Connor R, Ryan SP, Donoghue VB. Whole-body magnetic resonance imaging: A useful additional sequence in paediatric imaging. Pediatr Radiol 34:472–480, 2004.
Meyer JS, Harty MP, Khademian Z. Imaging of neuroblastoma and Wilms' tumor. Magn Reson Imaging Clin North Am 10:275–302, 2002.
Ozturk A, Haliloglu M, Akpinar E, Tekgul S. Cellular congenital mesoblastic nephroma with contralateral medullary nephrocalcinosis. Br J Radiol 77:436–437, 2004.
Riccabona M. Imaging of renal tumours in infancy and childhood. Eur Radiol 13 (Suppl 4): L116–L129, 2003.
Riebel T, Kebelmann-Betzing C, Sarioglu N, Wit J, Seeger K. Unusual mesoblastic nephroma in a young child. Pediatr Radiol 33:62–65, 2003.
von Schweinitz D. Neonatal liver tumours. Semin Neonatol 8:403–410, 2003.

THE CHILD WITH VOMITING

Outline

Saskia von Waldenburg Hilton, MD

THE CHILD WITH VOMITING

Vomiting is a common symptom in infants and children that is difficult to ignore and can be extremely distressing. However, vomiting is a nonspecific symptom and often is induced by disorders in systems other than the gastrointestinal tract. For example, vomiting may be incited by diverse conditions such as otitis media, urinary tract infection, appendicitis, and viral gastroenteritis, as well as by formula intolerance and overfeeding, anatomic obstruction, and lesions of the central nervous system.

In older children, vomiting per se is rarely sufficiently prolonged or severe enough to cause complications; aspiration of vomitus and esophageal tears are extremely rare in children. In infants, however, prolonged vomiting can produce dehydration and electrolyte imbalance. These complications are most frequently encountered with gastrointestinal obstruction such as pyloric stenosis, but they may also occur in infants with viral gastroenteritis. In fact, it is the degree of dehydration that is usually the decisive factor in deciding whether a vomiting child should be hospitalized.

The major role of imaging in infants and children who vomit is to exclude or document the cause of the obstruction. In 95% of cases the cause is due to pyloric stenosis, cogenital obstructing lesion, and midgut volvulus. Almost all of these conditions can be identified and treated.

DIFFERENTIAL DIAGNOSIS OF VOMITING

The incidence of abnormalities that cause vomiting varies greatly according to the age of the patient. Thus, when considering differential diagnostic possibilities, the initial and essential factor is the patient's age. In this section, the differential diagnosis of vomiting is discussed as it pertains to major pediatric age groups, recognizing that considerable overlap exists. The diagnostic possibilities are listed as common and uncommon, a somewhat arbitrary categorization but one that is helpful in the rational planning of diagnostic maneuvers.

NEONATES (BIRTH TO 1 MONTH)

The important causes of vomiting in newborn infants are listed in Table 13–1. Vomiting, or regurgitation, is common in neonates, and, in most instances, it represents benign gastroesophageal reflux ("spitting up") rather than serious disease. Benign regurgitation is most common in the first days of life and usually occurs following feeding, particularly overfeeding. The vomited material is milk, which wells up in the infant's mouth, without "projectile" or forceful emission. When infants take feedings normally and gain weight (after the first 2 or 3 days), it is unlikely that disease is responsible for such regurgitation.

Neonatal sepsis can present with a multiplicity of symptoms, including vomiting. Sepsis should be considered in infants who are lethargic or drowsy, who fail to demand feedings, or in whom other signs or predisposing factors are present.

Congenital atresias and severe stenoses are relatively less common lesions that almost invariably present with vomiting. Vomiting from proximal atresias generally occurs early; the first manifestation is often polyhydramnios, which alerts the radiologist to carefully examine the fetus and exclude proximal bowel atresia and other anomalies. The possibility of trisomy 21 should be excluded prenatally in a fetus with atresia of the second portion of the duodenum. Esophageal atresia may be suspected at birth when there is failure to pass a stomach catheter, excessive saliva and mucus are seen in the infant's mouth, and choking and vomiting occur with feeding. Duodenal atresia often presents with repeated vomiting in the absence of abdominal distention. Both of these lesions can usually be identified with certainty on plain radiographs. Esophageal atresia is seen as a blind pouch in the upper thorax, into which a catheter may be placed to show the extent. The presence of air in the intestine permits inferences about associated tracheoesophageal fistulae. Duodenal atresia causes the "double bubble" sign, with the distal bubble indicating the site of obstruction (Fig. 13–1).

More distal atresias usually involve the ileum and present with abdominal distention. With distal atresias, the site of obstruction can be estimated by evaluating the number of air-filled, dilated loops seen on the plain abdominal radiograph. In proximal atresia, only a few loops are seen, whereas in distal atresia, many loops are seen. In cases of distal bowel obstruction, a contrast examination of the colon is used to differentiate anatomic from functional obstruction. This permits differential diagnosis of ileal atresia (common) and colonic atresia (uncommon) from functional obstruction such as Hirschsprung's disease (distal aganglionosis), neonatal small left colon syndrome (relative obstruction at the splenic flexure), meconium ileus (inspissated meconium in cystic fibrosis), and meconium plug.

TABLE 13-1 CAUSES OF VOMITING IN NEONATES (BIRTH TO 1 MONTH)

Common
Gastroesophageal reflux, especially following overfeeding
Neonatal sepsis
Necrotizing enterocolitis (premature infants)
Hypertrophic pyloric stenosis
Uncommon
Congenital atresias or stenoses (esophagus to anus)
Functional obstruction due to Hirschsprung's disease
Functional obstruction due to meconium ileus or plug
Malrotation with midgut volvulus
Functional obstruction due to neonatal small left colon syndrome
Sucking or swallowing difficulties
Lactobezoar
Drugs and toxic agents
Kernicterus
Cerebral causes, including subdural fluid
Renal causes
Metabolic disorders
Neonatal appendicitis

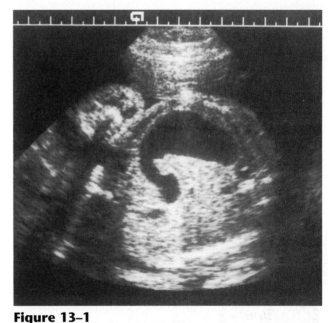

Figure 13–1
Prenatal diagnosis: duodenal atresia. This axial image of the fetal abdomen at 32 weeks of gestation shows gastric and proximal duodenal dilatation. Duodenal atresia was proven. The infant did not have trisomy 21.

Neonatal necrotizing enterocolitis may present with vomiting, usually with concomitant abdominal distention and plainly bloody or guaiac-positive stools. A variety of radiographic signs may suggest necrotizing enterocolitis, but the diagnosis can be made with absolute confidence only when gas is noted in the bowel wall or in the peritoneum. Necrotizing enterocolitis is usually a disease of premature infants and, as such, is beyond the scope of this book.

Volvulus due to intestinal malrotation will be discussed as a separate entity. Volvulus is important, not because it is common, but because it is often lethal if unrecognized. The important clinical hallmark of midgut volvulus is bile-stained (green) vomitus. Bilious vomiting must be distinguished from yellow colostrum or vomitus containing meconium. It is important to remember that bilious vomiting in the neonate is due to either sepsis or obstruction. This symptom in an infant constitutes a radiologic emergency; it is not safe to temporize when one is faced with a possible midgut volvulus.

In summary, vomiting, although a common problem in newborn infants, is usually of benign etiology. Relatively rarely, it results from atresias or other obstructions, and, in such instances, radiographic examination is usually simple and diagnostic.

INFANTS (1 MONTH TO 2 YEARS)

The major causes of vomiting in infants after the newborn period are listed in Table 13–2. The most common causes are gastroesophageal reflux, formula intolerance, viral gastroenteritis, and infections of other organ systems. Gastroesophageal reflux may be diagnosed radiographically, by monitoring the acidity of the esophagus, or by other techniques; however, the condition is usually obvious from a thorough medical history or simply by watching the infant feed. Gastroesophageal reflux does not usually require surgery for treatment and cure. Formula intolerance may also be suspected from the history and may be treated by dietary manipulations.

Viral gastroenteritis is usually diagnosed presumptively, based on its epidemic nature, sudden onset, mild fever, and relatively short duration. Systemic infections that cause fever, which is believed to incite vomiting, are common and usually are readily diagnosed by physical examination and laboratory evaluation, suggesting the organ system involved. Urosepsis and appendicitis are common but may be elusive.

A frequent obstructive cause of vomiting in infants is pyloric stenosis, which is discussed in a later section. Pyloric stenosis has a specific time of onset, a feature that, together with typical projectile vomiting and the presence of the characteristic abdominal mass ("olive") makes the entity easy to diagnose in most infants. Occasionally, it may be confused with gastroesophageal reflux.

TABLE 13-2 CAUSES OF VOMITING IN INFANTS (1 MONTH TO 2 YEARS)

Common
Gastroesophageal reflux (chalasia)
Formula intolerance
Infection (urinary tract infection, pneumonia, otitis media, meningitis)
Viral gastroenteritis
Hypertrophic pyloric stenosis
Intussusception
Uncommon
Appendicitis
Increased intracranial pressure (trauma, tumors)
Drugs and toxic agents
Whooping cough
Midgut volvulus
Metabolic disorders (phenylketonuria, maple syrup urine disease, galactosemia, diabetes, methylmalonic acidemia, adrenocortical hyperplasia)
Diencephalic syndrome

Intussusception usually manifests itself by crampy abdominal pain and mildly bloody stools. However, vomiting may be the initial symptom.

Less common causes of vomiting in infants generally present with other symptoms that suggest the correct diagnosis. For example, increased intracranial pressure almost invariably is associated with neurologic signs and symptoms. Gastroesophageal reflux remains by far the most common cause of vomiting in infants.

YOUNG CHILDREN (2 TO 5 YEARS)

The most common causes of vomiting in young children ages 2 to 5 years are listed in Table 13–3. With increasing age, there is a greater frequency of vomiting related to systems other than the gastrointestinal system. Pyloric stenosis is rare in children older than 6 months, and most cases of gastroesophageal reflux resolve by 1 year of age. Psychologic causes, although rare, become increasingly important. Intussusception and appendicitis also become important considerations simply because they are common diseases in the young child. Virtually all the significant causes of vomiting in this age group have associated symptoms that suggest the correct diagnosis.

OLDER CHILDREN (5 TO 18 YEARS)

The common causes of vomiting in children older than 5 years of age are listed in Table 13–4. Obstructive lesions of

TABLE 13-3 CAUSES OF VOMITING IN YOUNG CHILDREN (2 TO 5 YEARS)

Common
Infection (otitis media, urinary tract, pneumonia, meningitis)
Viral gastroenteritis
Intussusception
Appendicitis
Uncommon
Celiac disease
Increased intracranial pressure
Achalasia
Psychogenic (excitement, anxiety, self-induced vomiting)
Antral stricture due to ingestion of caustic substance
Ingestion of drugs, nonfood materials (including lead)

the gastrointestinal tract are uncommon (Figs. 13–2 and 13–3). Previous abdominal surgery may result in adhesions in this and all other age groups, but the most frequent cause of vomiting is gastroenteritis. Psychogenic causes, especially cyclic vomiting, are relatively unusual in this age group but are more common than in younger patients. Eating disorders become important in adolescent girls; although self-induced vomiting after overeating is common, vomiting is done in secret and is almost never a presenting complaint. Peptic ulcer disease, although much less common in older children than in adults, is seen with increasing frequency. Achalasia, or failure of relaxation of the lower esophageal sphincter, sometimes occurs. With achalasia, vomiting almost always

TABLE 13-4 CAUSES OF VOMITING IN OLDER CHILDREN (5 TO 18 YEARS)

Common
Viral gastroenteritis
Food poisoning
Cyclic vomiting (psychogenic)
Other psychogenic causes
Uncommon
Appendicitis
Achalasia
Ulcer disease
Crohn's disease, causing gastric outlet obstruction
Increased intracranial pressure (including pseudotumor cerebri)
Renal colic
Migraine
Drugs and toxic agents
Testicular torsion

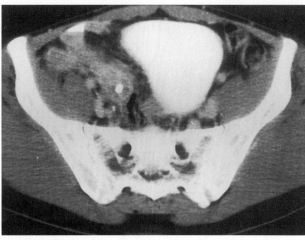

Figure 13–2
Appendicitis in a 15-year-old boy who presented with vomiting. This axial computed tomography scan at the level of the terminal ileum reveals a periappendiceal mass with an appendicolith. Mass effect and inflammation have caused minimal displacement and indentation on the bladder.

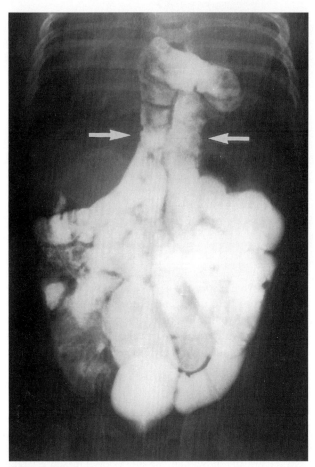

Figure 13–3
Morgagni hernia in a 3-year-old boy who presented with vomiting. Herniation of the transverse colon through an anteromedial diaphragmatic defect *(arrows)* has resulted in a mild bowel obstruction.

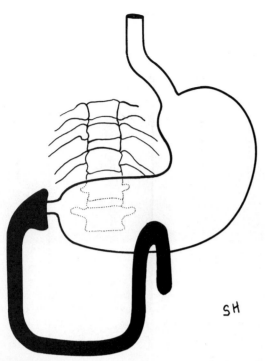

Figure 13–4
Normal duodenojejunal junction. The normal duodenojejunal junction, or ligament of Treitz, is at the same level as the duodenal bulb. On barium examination, this location is the most reliable way of ensuring that the ligament of Treitz is normally situated, thus excluding malrotation.

occurs at night and represents regurgitation of esophageal contents that have not reached the stomach (Fig. 13–4).

IMPORTANT CONDITIONS CAUSING VOMITING

In the following sections, a detailed analysis of three important conditions that produce vomiting in children—midgut volvulus, hypertrophic pyloric stenosis, and gastroesophageal reflux—is presented. These particular entities were selected for detailed discussion because imaging plays a crucial role in their diagnosis.

MIDGUT VOLVULUS

Anatomy and Pathophysiology

In the normal individual, the small bowel mesentery fans out from its origin in the retroperitoneum along a line extending from the left upper quadrant to the right lower quadrant. Fixation of the small bowel in this manner prevents twisting of the bowel on its pedicle when one portion is

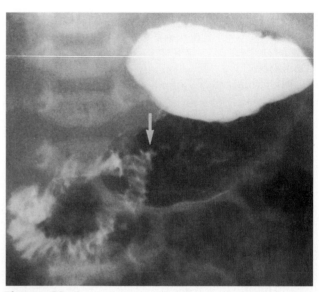

Figure 13–5
Normal position of the ligament of Treitz *(arrow)*. This spot film was performed during routine study of a vomiting infant. Note that the first pass of contrast material through the duodenum is photographed so that the position of the ligament of Treitz (duodenojejunal junction) can be accurately determined. Once the proximal small bowel fills, it is impossible to determine the position of this important landmark.

distended by the passage of liquid or gas. In children with malrotation, the line of fixation extends only a short distance. The upper fixation point is below the normal position of the ligament of Treitz, and usually the cecum is not located normally in the right lower quadrant (Fig. 13–5). Identifying the ligament of Treitz in an abnormal location establishes the diagnosis of malrotation (Fig. 13–6). Short mesenteric fixation is seen consistently, not only in errors of rotation, but also in children with omphalocele, gastroschisis, congenital left diaphragmatic hernia, and the asplenia and polysplenia syndromes.

Short mesenteric insertions do not lead invariably to midgut volvulus, and it is unknown why some are predisposed to twisting and others remain asymptomatic and are noted as incidental findings on studies done for other reasons (Fig. 13–7). When volvulus of the bowel occurs, the superior mesenteric artery, vein, and lymphatics run at right angles to the direction of the twist. As the twisting of the bowel becomes tighter, there is not only obstruction of the bowel lumen, but also obstruction of the arterial, venous, and lymphatic flow. Both the clinical presentation and the radiographic findings are influenced by the fact that the degree of twisting varies and may occur intermittently (Figs. 13–8 and 13–9).

Abnormal mesenteric fixation is often accompanied by congenital peritoneal bands, or Ladd's bands, which most commonly originate from the malpositioned cecum and attach to the right lateral peritoneal wall (Fig. 13–10).

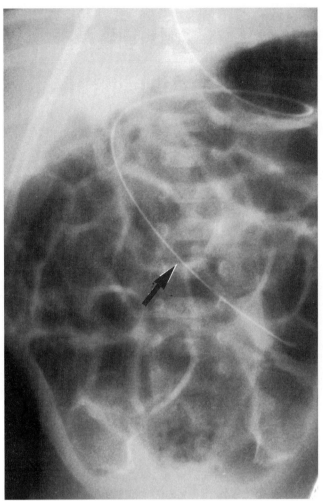

Figure 13–6
Feeding tubes *(arrow)* can normally displace the ligament of Treitz during infancy. After the age of 4 years, the ligament is no longer mobile.

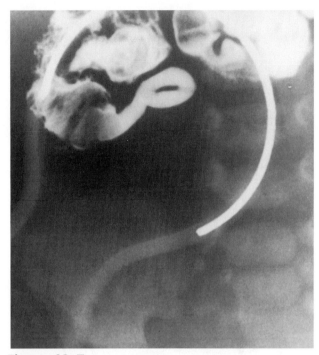

Figure 13–7
Abnormal position of the cecum in a normal neonate: note that the terminal ileum is elevated. In some normal children, the cecum is attached to a long mesentery and therefore is mobile, whereas in other normal neonates the cecum has not yet descended into the right lower quadrant. Either position may erroneously suggest the diagnosis of malrotation.

Although their origin and insertion may vary, they often cause compression of the duodenum and are sometimes the sole cause of mechanical obstruction.

Children who are prone to volvulus also have an increased incidence of intrinsic duodenal anomalies, such as duodenal webs and duodenal stenosis. Although surgery is indicated in obstruction regardless of the cause, a combination of these abnormalities may lead to two important errors: (1) failure to recognize that mechanical obstruction of the duodenum may be associated with vascular compromise, with a resultant delay in surgery; and (2) at the time of operation, failure to note that, in addition to midgut volvulus and peritoneal bands, there may be an incomplete, nonpalpable duodenal diaphragm.[17] Radiographic evaluation prior to surgery, along with recognition that this association occurs, avoids these errors.

Clinical Presentation

Midgut volvulus may present with a variety of symptoms that are more easily understood when one remembers that the basic problem of this entity is twisting of the bowel around its vascular pedicle. Thus, there may be mechanical bowel obstruction, ischemia or infarction, and lymphatic obstruction. In addition, because spontaneous untwisting may occur occasionally, symptoms may be intermittent and protracted.

Onset of symptoms in 70% of patients with midgut volvulus occurs during the first 3 weeks of life. Initial manifestations are most commonly those of mechanical obstruction, followed by symptoms of vascular compromise. Because the mechanical obstruction occurs distal to the papilla of Vater, bile-stained vomiting is typical and is the clinical hallmark of this anomaly. Bilious vomiting in an infant must be regarded as a serious symptom and should be considered indicative of midgut volvulus until proved otherwise.

Most infants with malrotation have a history of repeated episodes of vomiting, indicating the presence of intermittent torsion or relatively low-grade obstruction from external compression by peritoneal bands (Fig. 13–11). In many other infants, however, an abrupt change in feeding pattern occurs,

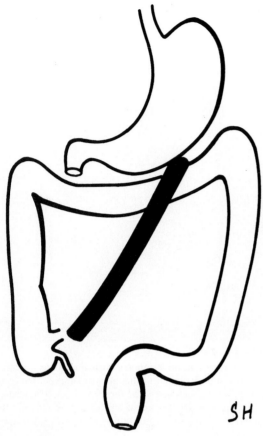

Figure 13–8

Normal small bowel mesenteric attachment. The normal attachment of the small bowel mesentery extends from the ligament of Treitz to the ileocecal valve.

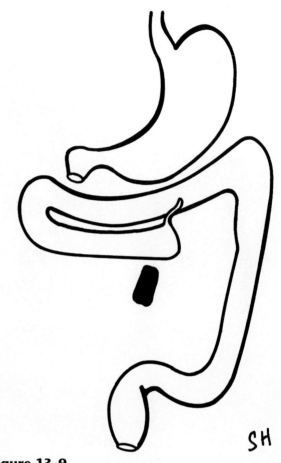

Figure 13–9

Abnormal small bowel mesenteric attachment. The upper extent of the mesenteric attachment lies inferior and medial to the normal ligament of Treitz, whereas the lower extent lies superior and medial to the normal cecal position. The resulting attachment is thus abnormally short, more readily permitting volvulus of the midgut.

from a normal feeding pattern to pernicious vomiting with irritability. Abdominal distention may occur, depending on the degree of vascular compromise and whether gastric decompression has occurred through vomiting. The presence of marked distention suggests vascular compromise. The presence or absence of peristaltic sounds in infants younger than 2 months of age is not diagnostically helpful in evaluating infants with this disease (Fig. 13–12).

Constipation is a frequent concomitant problem and presumably is due to the decrease in fluid intake, particularly in infants with acute or, more commonly, intermittent partial obstruction.

The bile-stained vomitus initially may contain gastric contents but subsequently becomes feculent. When vascular compromise is evident, melena or "currant-jelly stools" may be the presenting symptom. By the time blood appears in the stools, signs of vascular collapse, such as tachycardia, pallor, and other indications of shock, are usually present. The mesenteric arterial and venous obstructions are followed by

thrombosis of the vessels and perforation of the bowel wall with peritonitis. Because the superior mesenteric artery supplies the gut from the ligament of Treitz to the midtransverse colon, infarction of this large extent of bowel can be expected.

In patients in whom volvulus is not constant, the presenting symptoms often include intermittent vomiting or cyclic abdominal pain. This occurs most commonly in older patients, and frequently the erroneous diagnosis of a psychosomatic disorder is made.

Occasionally, a mild twist of the narrow pedicle may cause subacute mesenteric venous obstruction, as well as lymphatic obstruction. Children with such obstructions may present with chronic bloody stools. If lymphatic obstruction predominates, there may be signs of intestinal malabsorption, with loose, bulky stools and failure to thrive. These children have chronic congestion of the midgut with dilated lymphatics and enlarged mesenteric lymph nodes. Occasionally, chylous ascitic fluid is also present.

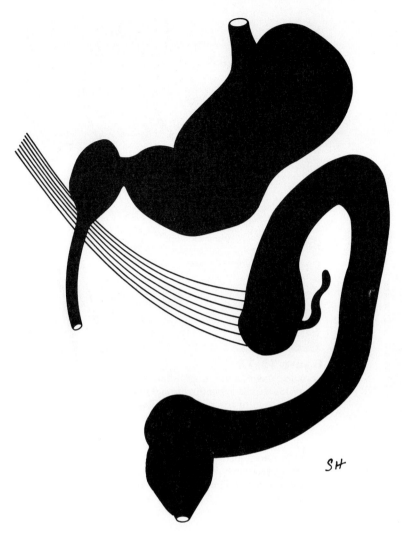

SH

Figure 13–10
Ladd's bands: diagrammatic representation. Ladd's bands originate from the malpositioned cecum and usually attach to the right lateral peritoneal wall. Although their origin and insertion may vary, they almost always cause a transverse compression of the duodenum and are sometimes the sole cause of mechanical duodenal obstruction.

In summary, the majority of children with malrotation and midgut volvulus present during infancy with a mechanical bowel obstruction, which progresses, if it remains uncorrected, to bowel infarction (Fig. 13–13). Unusual manifestations include intermittent abdominal pain or vomiting, malabsorption, and chylous ascites.

Radiographic Evaluation

In a child with vomiting, the major question that must be answered by the radiologist is whether a mechanical obstruction is present. In a child whose vomiting is bilious, the emergency situation of a midgut volvulus must be excluded. The first management decision made for a child who may have a midgut volvulus is whether radiographic contrast studies are safe or the child's condition requires immediate surgery. A child with an acute abdomen (i.e., signs of peritonitis, perforation, or shock) needs immediate surgical intervention. However, even in very ill patients, plain abdominal films may be helpful and can be performed quickly and safely.

The supine film is supplemented with a left-side-down decubitus film (left lateral decubitus) to determine whether bowel perforation has occurred (Fig. 13–14).

In patients who can tolerate contrast examination, the first examination of choice is the upper gastrointestinal (UGI) series.

Formerly, the barium enema was considered to be the procedure of choice; this is still true at some medical centers. However, for several anatomic and technical reasons, in patients with midgut volvulus, the UGI is the examination of choice.[45] The justification for performing a contrast enema is to identify a malrotation (and, by inference, midgut volvulus) by demonstrating an abnormal position of the cecum. However, in a few normal neonates, the cecum may not be located in the right lower quadrant. This may be because the cecum has not yet descended to its final position or because it is attached to an abnormally long mesentery. Thus, the barium enema cannot distinguish among a normal child with a high-positioned cecum, a child with

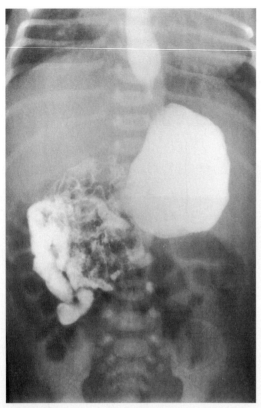

Figure 13–11
Complete malrotation. The proximal small bowel is located in the right side of the abdomen, and the duodenojejunal junction is not in its normal location. This was an incidental finding in this 3-week-old girl with complex congenital heart disease and gastroesophageal reflux. She was studied for "vomiting" of several days' duration. If a contrast enema had been performed, the cause of vomiting might have erroneously been ascribed to malrotation with secondary volvulus instead of gastroesophageal reflux.

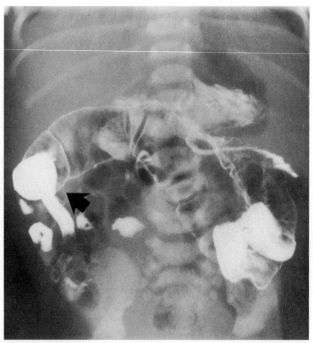

Figure 13–12
Complete malrotation: delayed film of the same patient shown in Figure 13–11. The appendix *(arrow)* is located in the right midabdomen instead of the right lower quadrant. Identification of the appendix reliably indicates cecal position. Unfortunately, a high cecal position is not pathognomonic for malrotation; it may also be seen in normal children whose cecum has not yet descended into the right lower quadrant and in children who have a long cecal mesentery. Very rarely, infants with midgut volvulus have a normally located cecum. Cecal position is therefore an unreliable marker for midgut volvulus.

malrotation who has symptoms for reasons other than a midgut volvulus, and a child with genuine malrotation with a midgut volvulus.

Even experienced personnel cannot always confidently identify the neonatal cecum by contrast enema (Figs. 13–15 through 13–20). The most helpful indicator for identifying the cecum is the appendix, but this structure often does not fill with contrast in infants. Cecal identification may be made by a reflux of contrast barium into the small bowel, but often this is difficult to accomplish and is hampered by the inability to differentiate small bowel from large bowel in neonates.

For these reasons, the UGI series is the examination of choice. If perforation is diagnosed or strongly suspected, then surgery, rather than any contrast examination, is indicated. When performing a UGI series on a neonate or young child with possible obstruction, it is often helpful to insert a nasogastric tube to empty any secretions from the stomach.

Even a child who has not been fed and has recently vomited may have considerable gastric residual. Contrast can be introduced through this tube and also can be aspirated through the same tube at the end of the examination. Passing a nasogastric tube may seem to be an unnecessary bother, but it is well worth the effort, as it permits precise control of the quantity and rapidity of administration of the contrast material. It also results in radiographs of better quality because of improved mucosal coating in the absence of fluid in the stomach.

Radiographic Findings

Detailed descriptions of the embryology of malrotation and descriptions of the several types of rotational errors that may occur are not included in this book, because clinically the subdivision of various forms appears to have little practical utility. Specifically, these subdivisions do not predict which patients are at greatest risk for midgut volvulus.

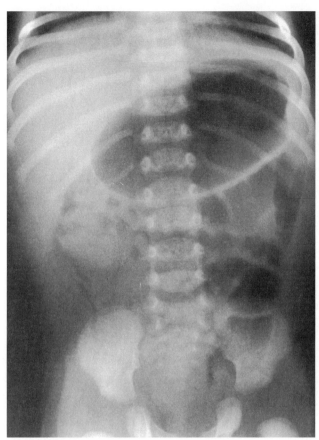

Figure 13–13
Normal neonatal abdomen. Note that gastric air is round or oval but not bilobed.

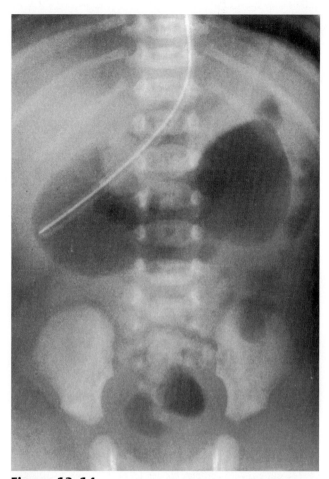

Figure 13–14
Midgut volvulus: typical plain film. Supine abdominal radiograph of a 4-day-old infant with bile-stained vomiting. There is marked dilatation of the duodenum with a paucity of intestinal gas distally. The stomach is decompressed. A "double bubble" suggestive of duodenal atresia may be seen in the midgut volvulus. Proximal duodenal dilatation with little gas distally is the most common plain film presentation of a midgut volvulus.

The major radiographic findings in malrotation (not necessarily with volvulus) are as follows:

1. The ligament of Treitz (duodenojejunal junction) lies inferior to the duodenal bulb and usually does not lie to the left of the spine. The assessment of the position of the ligament of Treitz is best made on a UGI series by watching the first bolus of contrast that traverses the duodenum. It is important to make this assessment before the jejunum is filled with barium. This assessment should be made as a routine part of every UGI series done on children. Malposition of the ligament of Treitz is the most accurate, but also the most subtle, sign of malrotation (Figs. 13–21 and 13–22).
2. Small bowel situated on the right of the midline.
3. Ascending colon located in the left side of the abdomen.
4. Cecum or appendix not in the right lower quadrant but high and directed transversely.
5. An abnormal position of a nasogastric tube on plain films (tube passing downward into an abnormally

right-sided jejunum) does not necessarily imply malrotation, as there is considerable mobility of the ligament of Treitz early in life.

The duodenojejunal flexure can be readily displaced to the right of the spine in more than two thirds of infants when manually manipulated under fluoroscopic control.[32] Thus, displacement of the ligament by a feeding tube is a normal phenomenon during the neonatal period. Moderate mobility is present until 4 years of age; after this age the duodenojejunal flexure is no longer mobile.[31,32]

If any question remains as to whether the patient has malrotation after the UGI series is performed, a delayed film, which will sometimes show the position of the cecum or the appendix, can be obtained.

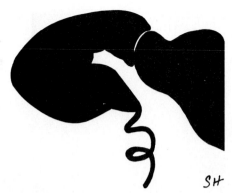

Figure 13–15
Midgut volvulus: diagrammatic representation of incomplete obstruction. Note the dilatation of the duodenal bulb and proximal duodenum, terminating in a cone-shaped narrowing. Also shown is the "corkscrew" pattern of the proximal small bowel, an appearance that is pathognomonic of an acute midgut volvulus.

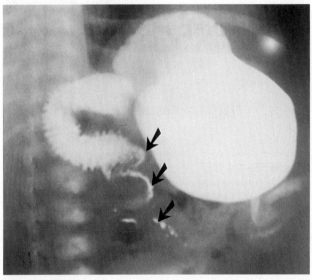

Figure 13–16
Midgut volvulus: upper gastrointestinal (UGI) series. The obstruction is incomplete, with moderate dilatation of the duodenal bulb and proximal duodenum. The corkscrew pattern of the proximal and small bowel (arrows) is pathognomonic of a midgut volvulus.

The plain film findings in midgut volvulus include the following:
1. Normal, or nonspecific, abdomen
2. A prominent, air-filled duodenal bulb, forming an air-fluid level on decubitus films ("double bubble" sign)
3. A variable degree of gastric distention, depending on whether the infant has recently vomited
4. A generalized paucity of gas distal to the obstruction
5. Distention of gas-filled distal bowel, probably related to vascular compromise
6. Rarely, pneumatosis, pneumoperitoneum, or both

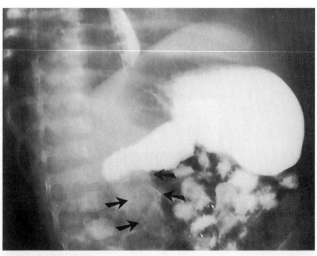

Figure 13–17
Midgut volvulus: UGI series in a 6-week-old infant with bile-stained vomiting. In this patient, the obstruction is incomplete. The small bowel folds are thickened (white arrows), reflecting vascular compromise and edema. The corkscrew pattern of a volvulus (black arrows) is evident.

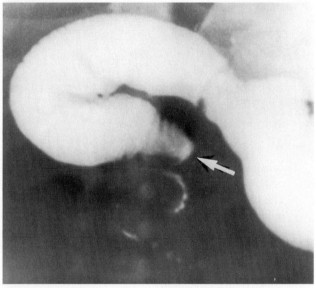

Figure 13–18
Midgut volvulus: UGI series. In this patient, the mechanical obstruction is almost complete. A small amount of barium has passed beyond the obstruction. The dilated distal antrum and proximal duodenum terminate in a characteristic cone-shaped configuration (arrow).

In most patients, the partial duodenal obstruction produces the most important plain film findings. It must be stressed that normal, or nonspecific, plain films are often seen and should not dissuade the clinician from the diagnosis of midgut volvulus. The plain film in this situation serves as a prelude to the UGI contrast examination and identifies lesions that

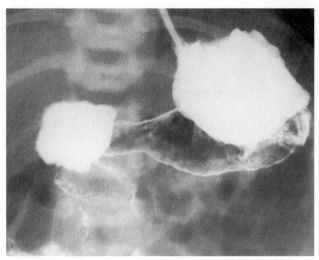

Figure 13–19
Midgut volvulus: UGI series in a 2-week-old infant with acute onset of bile-stained vomiting. The characteristic corkscrew pattern of the proximal small bowel is apparent.

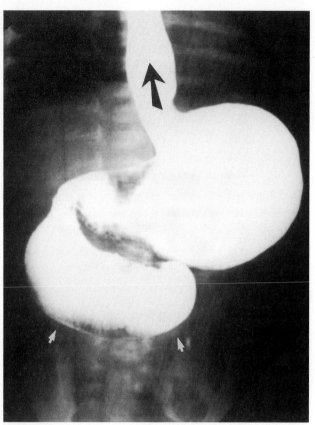

Figure 13–21
Midgut volvulus: UGI series. Severe dilatation of the proximal duodenum exists, but in this frontal view, the diagnosis of a midgut volvulus cannot be established because the contrast-filled duodenum *(white arrows)* conceals the point of obstruction. Gastroesophageal reflux is present, as it commonly is in this setting, but should not be assumed to explain the symptom of vomiting without complete examination of the distal antrum and duodenum.

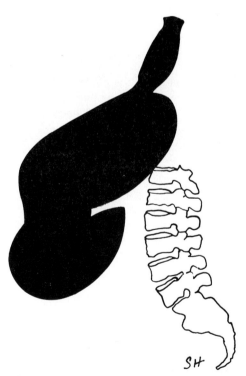

Figure 13–20
Midgut volvulus: diagrammatic representation of complete obstruction. The cone-shaped termination of the barium column is more rounded than that seen with incomplete obstruction. Gastroesophageal reflux is a frequent concomitant finding in children with mechanical obstruction.

require immediate surgical attention such as bowel perforation (Fig. 13–23).

The following are the most important radiographic findings seen on UGI series in patients with midgut volvulus:

1. Persistent dilatation of the duodenal bulb and proximal duodenum, terminating in a distinctive conical shape. Because of the overlying duodenal dilatation, the cone may be hidden and apparent only in straight lateral or oblique projections.
2. A corkscrew pattern of the contrast material that passes beyond the point of obstruction.
3. Thickened folds, caused by vascular obstruction and lymphatic engorgement, may be seen in the corkscrew bowel segment. Because of the small amount of contrast material that passes the obstruction and because of the mucosal edema, the corkscrew bowel segment may be difficult to see (see Fig. 13–17) and may not be appreciated unless it is sought with a watchful eye.

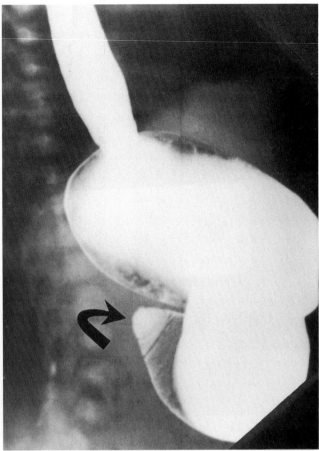

Figure 13-22
Midgut volvulus: UGI series in the same patient shown in Figure 13–21. Rotation of the patient into a near-lateral projection clearly reveals the characteristic cone-shaped obstruction of a midgut volvulus *(arrow)*.

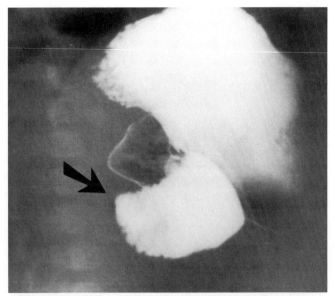

Figure 13-23
Midgut volvulus: UGI series in a 3-week-old infant with bile-stained vomiting. The lateral projection reveals the cone-shaped obstruction diagnostic of the condition *(arrow)*. Note that complete obstruction is accompanied by relatively pronounced proximal dilatation. This patient had no visible small bowel gas on preliminary plain film.

4. If tight Ladd's bands are evident, then the termination of the contrast column will often form an oblique line. It is sometimes impossible to differentiate an obstruction from an entirely extrinsic peritoneal band or an intrinsic duodenal obstruction from the cone classically seen in volvulus.

5. Gastroesophageal reflux is a frequent, unimportant associated finding.

Abdominal sonography may be the initial examination performed in the infant in whom the clinical signs of midgut volvulus are unclear or who is thought to have pyloric stenosis.[24,26,36] A retrospective study showed that the relative position of the superior mesenteric artery and vein was visible in 74% of children examined for pyloric stenosis with sonography. In 5 of 337 infants, the superior mesenteric vein was located to the left of the artery, and all 5 had intestinal malrotation.[53] Sonographic assessment of mesenteric vessel orientation must be performed with great care, and there are a number of pitfalls.[53] Although sonography should not be used to exclude the presence of a midgut volvulus, the determination of mesenteric vessel orientation may be useful when the vomiting infant is shown to have a normal pyloric muscle.

In summary, the UGI series will accurately identify the presence of malrotation if the position of the ligament of Treitz is assessed correctly during fluoroscopy. If there is an acute volvulus, the contrast study will delineate the proximal morphology of the obstruction. If the typical cone-shaped narrowing or the classic corkscrew pattern is present, the diagnosis of midgut volvulus is straightforward. If complete obstruction is seen in the second or third portion of the duodenum without the presence of distinguishing morphologic characteristics, the patient must be assumed to have a midgut volvulus and must be prepared for surgery immediately (Figs. 13–24, 13–25, and 13–26). Such patients most commonly have severely obstructing peritoneal bands and may or may not have an accompanying volvulus.

HYPERTROPHIC PYLORIC STENOSIS

Epidemiology, Anatomy, and Pathophysiology

Hypertrophic pyloric stenosis is a very common disease, with an incidence of 1 per 500 live births. It is the second most common disease requiring surgical intervention in infancy in the United States (herniorrhaphy is the most common surgical procedure in infancy). Male infants are affected four to five times more frequently than are female infants, and the disease is much less common in blacks than in whites. Although at one time it was thought that first-born males had the highest incidence of the disease, this is not true. Genetic studies indicate that hypertrophic pyloric stenosis is inherited as a dominant polygenic trait.[23,28] Women must carry a greater number of genes than men for the genes to be expressed, and once a woman is affected, she has a much

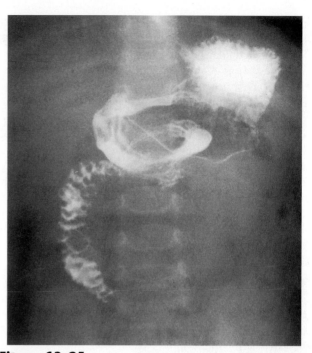

Figure 13–25
Recurrence of a midgut volvulus after surgical repair. A 6-week-old boy presented with bile-stained vomiting after uneventful repair of a midgut volvulus. The mother returned with her infant and announced that the disease had recurred. Although rare, this complication does exist.

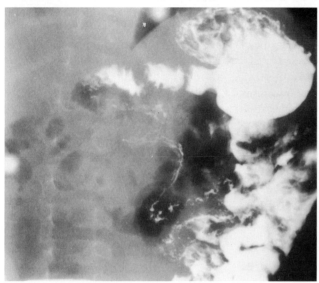

Figure 13–24
Chronic midgut volvulus: UGI series in a 16-month-old girl with chronic diarrhea, weight loss, and malnutrition. Lymphatic obstruction results in malabsorption, loose and bulky stools, and failure to thrive. Chylous ascites or bloody stools may be rare presenting symptoms of a chronic midgut volvulus.

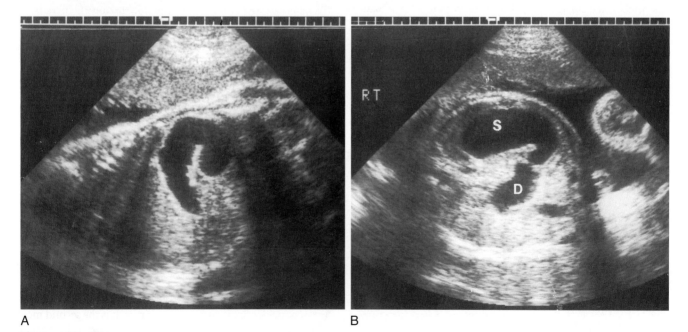

A   B

Figure 13–26
Prenatal diagnosis: midgut volvulus. *A*, Image of a 32-week twin fetus with a single dilated loop of bowel that was contiguous with the stomach. *B*, Axial image revealed a dilated stomach (S) and proximal duodenum (D). Surgery immediately after birth revealed a midgut volvulus with a viable small bowel. The infant survived and has done well.

higher probability of producing affected offspring. Although much work has been done to elucidate the cause of this disease, the etiology remains unknown (Fig. 13–27).

The usual age at onset of pyloric stenosis is 2 to 6 weeks. However, a few patients may present before 2 weeks or as late as 3 or more months of age. The age of onset in premature infants is the same as that in term infants. The basic anatomic problem in hypertrophic pyloric stenosis is hypertrophy of the pyloric musculature. The hypertrophied muscle forms a circumferential mass around the pylorus, eventually causing the lumen of the pylorus to become too narrow to permit adequate passage of gastric contents. This muscle mass is responsible for the signs that make pyloric stenosis a relatively easy radiographic diagnosis. Spasm of the pylorus, although often said to be confusing, produces none of the radiographic signs of a pyloric mass (Fig. 13–28).

The need for imaging of the neonate with vomiting who is suspected of having pyloric stenosis varies greatly with the experience and expertise of the pediatrician and surgeon who are caring for the child. Patients who have clear-cut clinical symptoms as well as typical findings on physical examination usually need no diagnostic imaging. However, patients in whom the diagnosis is in doubt should be imaged to establish a firm diagnosis preoperatively, identify other causes of obstruction, or confirm the absence of a mechanical cause of vomiting.

Once the diagnosis of pyloric stenosis is made, the infant is rehydrated, and any electrolyte disturbances are corrected prior to surgery. Pyloromyotomy is the treatment of choice in North America. Medical management, with its prolonged hospitalization, is the less conservative treatment in typical cases of pyloric stenosis.

Figure 13–27
Morbid anatomic changes with hypertrophic pyloric stenosis. *A*, A normal stomach in a 4-week-old infant. Note that the pyloric muscle is slightly thicker than that of the body of the stomach. *B*, Marked thickening of the pyloric muscle is seen secondary to the hypertrophy of the circular muscle fibers. This thickened muscle is elongated and projecting into the more proximal portion of the stomach. The pyloric canal is elongated and constricted, and the pyloric muscle also bulges into the base of the duodenal cap.

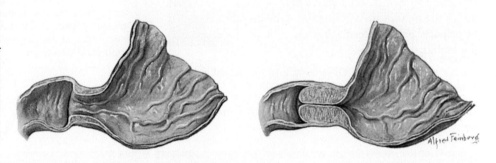

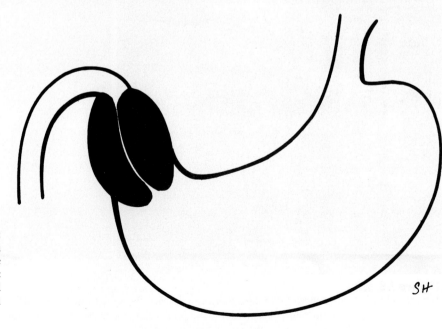

Figure 13–28 Pyloric muscle mass: diagrammatic representation. The diagram shows hypertrophied pyloric musculature encircling and largely obstructing the gastric outlet. The numerous radiographic and sonographic "signs" of pyloric stenosis can readily be deduced from this drawing.

Clinical Presentation

The hallmark of pyloric stenosis is nonbilious vomiting, which commences between the second and sixth weeks of life. Vomiting initially begins with regurgitation and over time becomes more forceful and more frequent. It may be lessened in severity by glucose and water feedings but is not affected by changes in formula. The vomitus generally contains sour formula or clear gastric contents but almost never bile. As the obstruction progresses, loss of weight becomes a conspicuous feature. Constipation and scant urine output occur as the gastric outlet obstruction becomes more complete. Many patients have a metabolic alkalosis of varying severity with potassium depletion. Indirect-reacting hyperbilirubinemia is seen occasionally, a finding that remains unexplained.

On physical examination, the infant, although malnourished, is alert, irritable, and eager to eat, drinking fluids ravenously. When the stomach is filled, peristaltic waves can be seen traveling across the left upper quadrant to the right and terminating beyond the midline. The forcefulness of the peristaltic waves increases until the patient vomits. A small, firm mass ("olive"), representing the pseudotumor of the hypertrophied pyloric musculature, is palpated most effectively when the stomach is empty. Usually it is located just to the right of the midline above the umbilicus but may be palpated high, under the liver edge, or low, at the level of the umbilicus (Fig. 13–29).

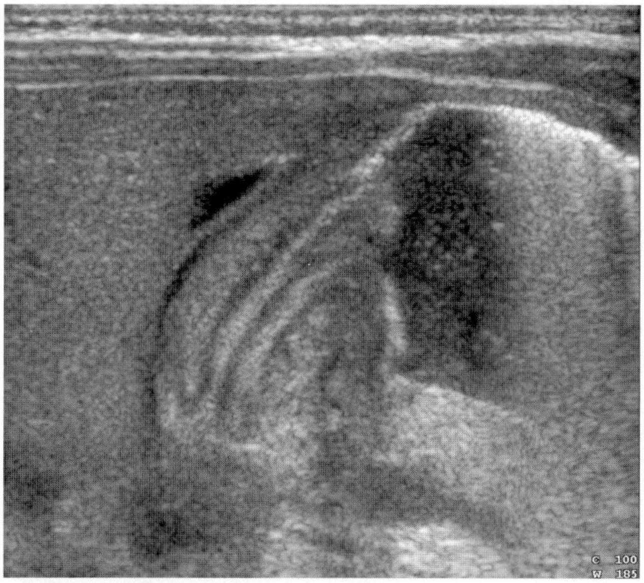

Imaging of the Neonate With Pyloric Stenosis

The role of imaging studies in cases of neonatal vomiting is to determine whether a mechanical obstruction exists and to define its cause. The most common etiology is pyloric stenosis, but sometimes another, rare form of mechanical obstruction such as partial obstruction from a duodenal diaphragm or Ladd's bands may be identified. The major differential diagnostic consideration of a nonsurgical cause is gastroesophageal reflux. A patient who is clinically believed to have gastroesophageal reflux is generally treated by medical management and is referred for radiographic examination only if the symptoms fail to respond or progress. Pyloric stenosis is rarely confused with midgut volvulus because of the absence of bile-stained vomitus in pyloric stenosis (Fig. 13–30).

During the 1980s the sonographic diagnosis of hypertrophic pyloric stenosis was popularized and refined. Although initially described in 1977 by Teele and Smith,[51] it was

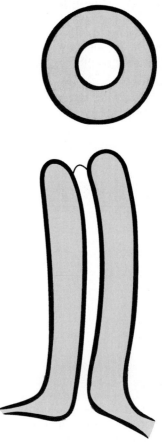

Figure 13–30
Hypertrophic pyloric stenosis: diagrammatic representation.

Figure 13–29
Hypertrophic pyloric stenosis. Ultrasound images display the bulging muscle mass compressing the pyloric canal.

Blumhagen et al.[9] who proved in a large prospective study that pyloric stenosis could be confidently diagnosed without false-positive results and with a false-negative rate of 13% when strictly adhering to a 4-mm width of pyloric musculature. Since that time, additional studies have further refined other measurements to include the length of the elongated pyloric canal and the length of the pyloric musculature.[7,18,25,37,52,55] Sonography has become the modality of choice to diagnose pyloric stenosis in all pediatric hospitals and in most other centers. Performance of the examination is technically demanding and requires considerable experience; however, despite these obstacles, it is currently being adopted by general radiologists.

A number of factors enter into the decision of whether to commence the evaluation of the vomiting infant with sonography or traditional upper intestinal barium examination. If technically qualified personnel are available, the most reasonable approach is to start with sonography in those patients who are likely to have pyloric stenosis and with upper gastrointestinal examination in those who are unlikely to have the disease (Figs. 13–31, 13–32, and 13–33).

The following criteria can be used alone or in combination to determine the probability of the presence of the disease:

1. Clinical findings. Was there a questionable pyloric mass or could none be found by an experienced examiner?
2. Age (typically 2 to 6 weeks).
3. Sex (male-to-female ratio, 5:1).
4. Race (uncommon in blacks).
5. Family history (very likely in male offspring of an affected mother).
6. Gastric residual. One study states an 89% accuracy rate in differentiating infants with and without pyloric stenosis based on the volume of aspirated gastric residual. Infants with a gastric residual greater than 10 mL were likely to have pyloric stenosis, whereas those with less than 10 mL were unlikely to have the disease.[20]

Thus, a black girl who presents at 12 weeks of age without a palpable mass is very unlikely to have pyloric stenosis, whereas a 4-week-old white boy with a palpable olive has a high probability of having pyloric stenosis. However, additional prospective studies are needed to refine the criteria for successful differentiation of the two groups of patients.

If it is impossible to fit the patient into either category, it is reasonable to start with sonography, as this is the least invasive examination and has been shown to have no false-positive results. No imaging is needed in patients who have unequivocal clinical signs and symptoms of pyloric stenosis

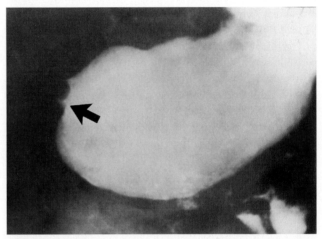

Figure 13–32
Pyloric stenosis: UGI series demonstrating the beak sign. The beak configuration results from contrast filling the proximal portion of the pyloric canal (*arrow*). Note the muscle mass in the distal antrum.

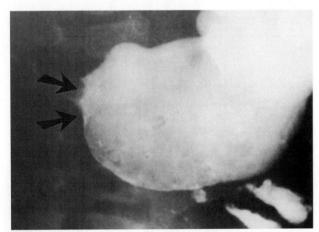

Figure 13–31
Pyloric stenosis: UGI series demonstrating the shoulder sign. Note the incursion of the hypertrophied muscle mass into the distal antrum. The up "shoulder" is more prominent than the lower shoulder because of the cephalic orientation of the pyloric channel.

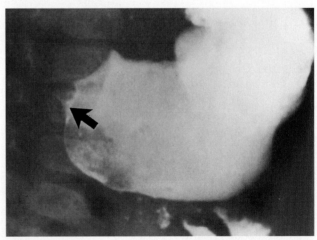

Figure 13–33
Pyloric stenosis: the beak sign. A peristaltic wave of the distal antrum has made the shoulder and beak appear more prominent. This radiograph is diagnostic for pyloric stenosis because it clearly demonstrates the presence of a large pyloric muscle mass.

as determined by experienced examiners. Clinical diagnostic accuracy can be as high as 85% under optimal circumstances.

Technique for Sonographic Examination[1,2,5,8,10,11,12,19,21,22,47,48] The infant is placed in the right lateral decubitus position, and transverse scanning is begun over the body of the stomach, slightly to the right of midline. By following the hypoechoic muscle layers of the distal antrum, the pyloric muscle mass can usually be identified. Most of the time the distal antrum is distended with gastric residual and easily visible (Fig. 13–34). If the stomach is empty because of vomiting or attempts to determine gastric residual volume, a small quantity of fluid can be administered. Oral intake is preferable, as the act of swallowing stimulates gastric peristalsis and antral emptying. Severe gastric distention may make it difficult to image a posteriorly displaced pyloric muscle mass (Fig. 13–35). A more lateral or upward angulation of the transducer is often helpful in locating the pylorus in this situation. Optimally the transducer should be perpendicular to the pyloric muscle and aligned with the center of the pyloric channel. Nonuniformity of the hypertrophied muscle mass is a characteristic sonographic finding caused by the orientation of the ultrasound beam with respect to the circular fibers of the pyloric muscle.[47]

Criteria for a positive diagnosis vary among institutions, as different measurements are obtained. The following are generally accepted criteria that should lead to no false-positive results:

1. Minimal pyloric muscle thickness 3.5 to 4.0 mm
2. Channel length equal to or greater than 17 mm
3. Muscle length equal to or greater than 19 mm
4. Gastric peristalsis that terminates abruptly at the pyloric muscle

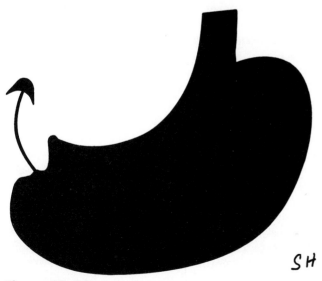

Figure 13–34
Pyloric stenosis: diagrammatic representation. The drawing depicts the shoulder sign, the teat sign, and the indentation of the duodenal bulb.

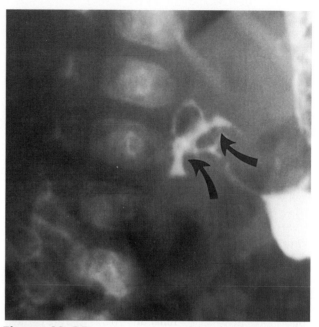

Figure 13–35
Pyloric stenosis: indentation of the duodenal bulb by the pyloric muscle mass (*arrows*). Mild compression of the distal antrum often facilitates filling of the pyloric canal and duodenal bulb. A string sign is also apparent

5. Minimal, if any, gastric emptying
6. An image that looks like pyloric stenosis

It should be mentioned that we and others[3] have seen infants who presented with moderate to severe failure to thrive and vomiting. The measurements obtained on these infants with pyloric stenosis were misleading because the pylorus itself was proportionately smaller. However, criterion 6 was diagnostic. This pitfall is a good example of the philosophical point that "a radiologist with a ruler is a radiologist in trouble."

It is important to retain credibility, and during the initial learning curve, it is probably wise to obtain a confirmatory UGI series in all questionable patients.

Technique for Upper Gastrointestinal Series The UGI series is a simple, quick, and efficient method for diagnosing or excluding pyloric stenosis.[45]

A soft polyethylene feeding tube is passed into the distal antrum at the beginning of the examination. This maneuver simplifies the examination by (1) making it possible to empty gastric secretions that tend to prolong the examination if left in the stomach (it takes longer for the contrast to mix with these thick secretions, and the mucosal coating is much decreased); (2) allowing the radiologist to introduce a small and controlled amount of contrast into the infant's stomach, which prevents gastric distention with contrast that can conceal the pylorus; and (3) facilitating removal of barium at the termination of the examination, which decreases the likelihood of aspiration (Fig. 13–36).

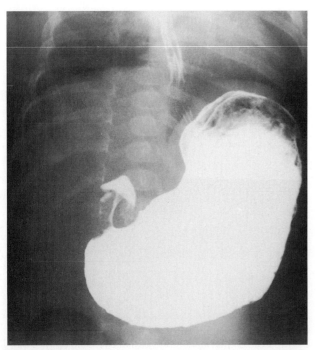

Figure 13–36

Pyloric stenosis: excessive residual barium following examination. This is the final film that accompanied a transferred infant. The stomach is distended with barium, and gastroesophageal reflux has occurred. Performing the UGI examination with a feeding tube offers numerous advantages. It permits emptying the stomach of secretions at the start of the study; it allows introducing graded amounts of contrast material; and it permits removing excessive contrast material after the examination is complete. The last maneuver is important to minimize the possibility of aspiration in these infants with obstructions.

After a small amount of contrast has been introduced into the distal antrum and it becomes obvious that transit from the stomach is going to be prolonged by either pyloric stenosis or pylorospasm, the infant is placed on the right side, and the examiner leaves the fluoroscopic suite for 5 minutes. This prevents repeated and nondiagnostic fluoroscopy of an empty pylorus. Almost always, after a 5-minute interval, diagnostic spot films showing either pyloric stenosis or a normal pylorus can be obtained.

Mild pressure placed on the distal antrum with a translucent palpation device often accelerates the passage of barium through the pyloric canal. Palpation with such a device can also define the muscle mass indenting the distal antrum. Demonstration of this muscle mass is sufficient confirmation of the diagnosis of pyloric stenosis.

If pyloric stenosis is absent, it is important to carefully check the position of the ligament of Treitz. The feeding tube is then withdrawn, and the infant is permitted to drink as much contrast as desired. When the stomach is full and the patient is satisfied, maneuvers are begun to demonstrate or exclude gastroesophageal reflux as the cause of vomiting.

The diagnosis of pyloric stenosis should never be made on the basis of plain films. Plain film findings, although suggestive of pyloric stenosis, cannot effectively exclude pylorospasm, which is a nonsurgical problem. The major plain film findings in pyloric stenosis include gastric dilatation, paucity of small bowel and colonic air, frothy gastric contents, absence of an air-filled duodenal bulb, gastric pneumatosis (rare), and normal appearance.

Diagnostic findings may be seen with the UGI series, the most important of which are given as follows, in order of their diagnostic value.

1. *Shoulder sign.* This sign is caused by the pyloric muscle mass indenting the distal antrum. Because of the upward angle of the muscle mass, the upper part of the distal antrum is more indented than is the lower part.

2. *Indentation of the duodenal bulb.* The base of the duodenal bulb may be indented convexly by the pyloric muscle; this sign, of course, depends on passing enough contrast material through the pylorus to fill the duodenal bulb.

3. *Beak sign.* As the barium column approaches the narrowed pyloric canal, it often concentrically narrows, forming a conical "beak."

4. *String sign.* This is a constantly narrowed, aperistaltic pyloric channel that curves slightly cephalad. This finding represents the elongated pyloric channel, which is no longer distensible because of the hypertrophied muscle bundle.

5. *Double track sign.* Compression of the mucosa in the elongated pylorus may cause the barium to be caught in the folded mucosa and to appear as two or more "tracks" rather than as a single lumen (Fig. 13–37).

6. *Teat sign.* This is a mammiform angle, formed by the distal lesser curvature and the pyloric pseudotumor as it indents the antrum.

7. *Gastroesophageal reflux.* This is a frequent but unimportant associated finding (Fig. 13–38).

All of these radiographic signs are merely a reflection of the pyloric muscle mass and the effects of this mass on the contrast column and the surrounding structures. Usually, only a few of these signs are seen in a given patient (Fig. 13–39).

Fluoroscopy must show that there is no significant change in the diameter of the pyloric canal and that this region is incapable of peristalsis. Isolated spot films of many normal UGI series may simulate pyloric stenosis, because this region is frequently contracted. The constancy of the elongation of the canal, the persistent aperistalsis of this region, and, most importantly, the demonstration of the muscle mass ensures the correct diagnosis.

The most common entity that may be confused with pyloric stenosis is pylorospasm. The following are basic differences between the two conditions:

1. In pylorospasm, a pyloric muscle mass is not suggested by the various signs previously mentioned.

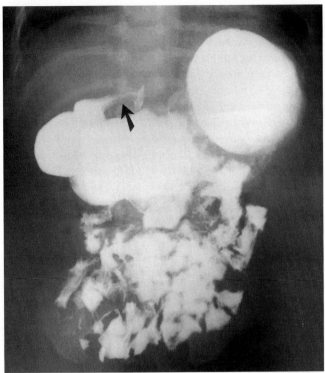

Figure 13–37
Pyloric stenosis: the double-track sign. The musculature of the elongated and narrowed pylorus may compress the mucosal folds so that barium enters two or more "tracks" *(arrow)* rather than a single apparent lumen.

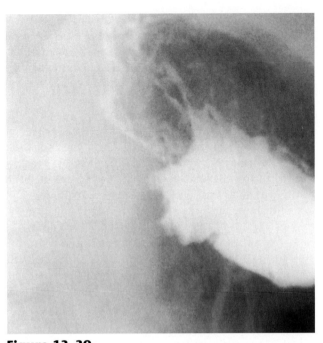

Figure 13–39
Pyloric stenosis: complete gastric outlet obstruction. This lateral view spot film demonstrates clear-cut shoulder and beak signs, without filling of the pyloric canal. Filling of the pyloric canal and duodenal bulb can sometimes be accomplished with compression of the distal antrum, but the findings shown here permit confident diagnosis, even in the absence of distal filling.

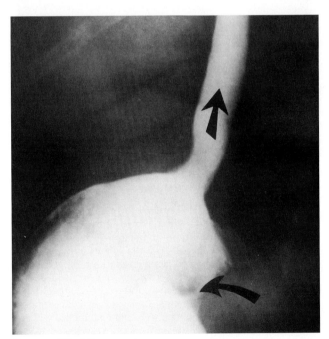

Figure 13–38
Pyloric stenosis: associated gastroesophageal reflux. Such reflux often accompanies gastric outlet obstruction. When marked reflux is observed in a patient with the symptom of vomiting, a midgut volvulus and (more commonly) pyloric stenosis must be excluded. This patient shows gastroesophageal reflux and a beak sign *(lower arrow)* reflecting pyloric stenosis.

2. Intermittent peristalsis through the involved segment occurs in pylorospasm.
3. Variability in the size of the narrowed lumen suggests pylorospasm.
4. Lack of a response to glucagon occurs in true pyloric stenosis.

Delayed gastric emptying is seen in both conditions and should not be the sole criterion for making either diagnosis. If questions remain, the examination can easily be repeated after a few days of medical management.

GASTROESOPHAGEAL REFLUX (CHALASIA)

Anatomy and Pathophysiology

The lower esophageal sphincter, a zone of high manometric pressure, is the junction between the esophagus and the stomach. It is under neural (vagus nerve) control and relaxes when swallowing occurs. Increases in serum gastrin levels result in lower esophageal sphincter tone. The precise physiologic mechanisms controlling the sphincter have not been completely defined, and at present, this subject is controversial.

Several important anatomic differences between infants and adults are evident. In the adult, about 3 cm of subdiaphragmatic intra-abdominal esophagus lie proximal to the stomach. In infants, this section is either nonexistent or very short. In addition, the adult esophagus joins the stomach at the cardia, where it forms an acute angle with the stomach. This angle is either absent or much less acute in infants; thus, in infants the esophagus and stomach tend to form a continuous straight tube. Many people think that these mechanical differences are important contributing factors in the high incidence of reflux in normal neonates.

For these reasons, some degree of gastroesophageal reflux is a normal phenomenon in many infants. The child with such reflux remains clinically unaffected, although the parents may be distressed because the child regurgitates or even vomits part of his food. This symptom tends to improve and is almost always totally resolved by the time the infant starts to walk (Fig. 13–40).

A few infants develop peptic complications of the esophagus. The esophageal mucosa tolerates the refluxed gastric acid secretions poorly and therefore may become inflamed, ulcerate, bleed, or even form a stricture. Anemia, melena, and dysphagia, all of which are secondary to esophageal mucosal damage, may be the presenting symptoms in such patients.

Occasionally, failure to thrive may result from excessive vomiting. This simply reflects inadequate nutrition due to caloric loss in the vomitus.

A large number of pulmonary disorders, such as asthma, recurrent pneumonia, bronchitis, bronchiolitis, and pulmonary fibrosis, have been linked to gastroesophageal reflux.[4] A causal relationship between recurrent respiratory problems and gastroesophageal reflux has been assumed to exist in such patients when other causes for the respiratory symptoms cannot be found. It is probably unjustified to assume a cause-and-effect relationship unless actual aspiration of refluxed material can be demonstrated. Reflux and regurgitation certainly can occur in infants without respiratory symptoms. The actual documentation of aspiration of gastric contents by radiography or by the more sensitive method of radionuclide esophagography and lung scanning remains rare (Figs. 13–41 and 13–42).

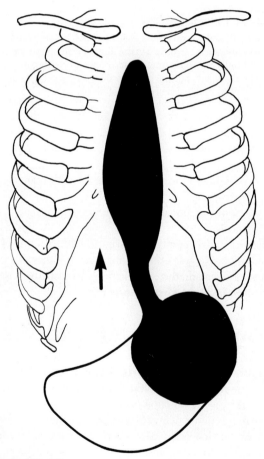

Figure 13–40
Gastroesophageal reflux: diagrammatic representation. In evaluating patients with reflux, it is important to document the level to which reflux ascends, to examine esophageal motility (e.g., did the refluxed contrast material clear quickly?), and to search for complications of reflux, such as esophagitis.

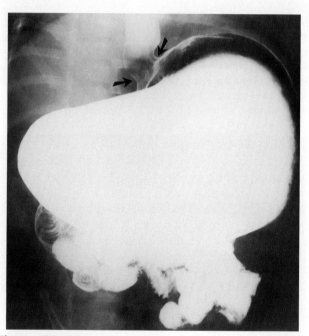

Figure 13–41
The gastroesophageal junction in infancy. A factor that may contribute to gastroesophageal reflux in infants is the anatomic configuration of the gastroesophageal junction, which, as shown in this patient *(arrows)*, can be widely patent. When the junction is open, the stomach and esophagus form an essentially straight tube. As the child matures, the junction forms an increasingly acute angle, and the length of the subdiaphragmatic intra-abdominal esophagus increases. The 2-month-old infant depicted was believed to have pyloric stenosis, but the pylorus was normal, and the vomiting reflected gastroesophageal reflux. Note the large volume of barium consumed by this patient. The volume administered should equal that routinely taken at feedings. Administering a smaller volume than that normally consumed often results in a false-negative examination for reflux.

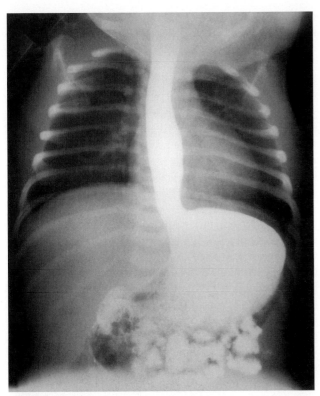

Figure 13–42
Severe gastroesophageal reflux. Note the patulous gastroesophageal junction.

Other entities that have been associated with gastroesophageal reflux include sudden infant death syndrome and neurologic symptoms such as irritability, apparent seizures, torticollis, and dystonia. The diagnostic modalities available for assessing gastroesophageal reflux include UGI series, radionuclide gastroesophagography, endoscopy, continuous pH monitoring of the distal esophagus, and measurement of lower esophageal pressures. Research indicates that there may not be uniform agreement by all modalities. Measurements of pH and prolonged monitoring by radionuclide methods are both more sensitive than is the intermittent fluoroscopic observation used during UGI examinations.

If a patient is suspected of having gastroesophageal reflux, the standard initial therapy is medical management consisting of smaller, thicker, and more numerous feedings along with a semi-upright posture after feeding or medication. Infants who are unresponsive to this regimen generally are referred for radiographic evaluation of gastroesophageal anatomy, severity of reflux, and associated peptic complications.

The surgical technique most frequently used to cure reflux is the Nissen fundoplication, in which the cardia is wrapped around the distal esophagus, creating a high-pressure zone. This technique cures reflux in 96% of patients. Indications for surgical intervention include persistent failure to thrive despite medical management, esophageal stricture with severe

reflux, and episodes of "near miss" sudden infant death syndrome.

Selecting patients for surgical cure of gastroesophageal reflux can be a difficult task, particularly in children with pulmonary problems. Even though the presence of reflux can be established with certainty by using several of the previously mentioned diagnostic modalities, the causal relationship between reflux and pulmonary disease remains largely circumstantial (Fig. 13–43). For this reason, nutritional failure to thrive and damage caused by reflux esophagitis have a much higher surgical cure rate than does pulmonary disease. In children with gastroesophageal reflux, the following major clinical questions must be answered:

1. In the child whose primary symptom is regurgitation or vomiting, is there simple reflux or a gastric outlet obstruction?
2. In the child shown to have gastroesophageal reflux, is the reflux uncomplicated or complicated by peptic acid damage such as esophageal edema, ulceration, or stricture?

Clinical Presentation

Excessive regurgitation or vomiting after feedings, beginning shortly after birth, is a common occurrence in normal infants. This is by far the most frequent and benign presentation of gastroesophageal reflux. Sometimes the vomiting can be so severe that reflux may be confused with gastric outlet obstruction. Other findings include anemia, melena, hematemesis, and dysphagia, all of which are related to

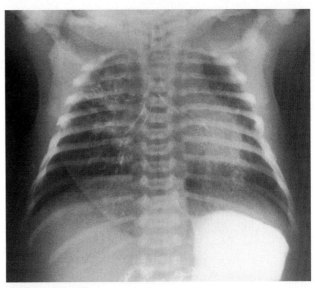

Figure 13–43
Gastroesophageal reflux with aspiration-delayed chest radiograph. The chest radiograph exposed following the UGI series documents the presence and extent of aspiration. In this patient, although all lobes of the lung contain contrast material, the right upper lobe is most markedly affected. Aspiration should be suspected in nonambulating infants who have recurrent right upper lobe infiltrates.

esophageal damage. Failure to thrive is secondary to retaining inadequate nutrition.

As previously mentioned, a variety of common pulmonary disorders, including asthma, recurrent pneumonia, bronchitis or bronchiolitis, pulmonary fibrosis, and bronchopulmonary dysplasia, are thought to be caused or exacerbated by gastroesophageal reflux. At times, neurologic or psychiatric disorders, such as irritability, apparent seizures, dystonia, and delayed motor development, may be the presenting symptoms of gastroesophageal reflux. Sandifer's syndrome, which is clearly related to reflux, presents with posturing of the head and neck in a torticollis-like configuration and with abnormalities of muscle tone.

In summary, clinical presentations in patients with gastroesophageal reflux may be extremely varied and are often confusing. The most common presentation in children is vomiting.

Radiographic Evaluation

UGI Series   Although esophagoscopy is a better method for evaluating the esophageal mucosa, the UGI series is needed for distal gastric and duodenal evaluation. For this reason, the UGI series remains the first examination to be performed, despite its overall lower sensitivity for reflux (38%, compared with 88% with radionuclide study). In all children who present with symptoms of reflux or with esophageal complications of reflux, the UGI series permits detailed examination of the esophagus, stomach, duodenum, and proximal small bowel. Pyloric stenosis is excluded, as are other obstructing duodenal lesions, and the normal position of the ligament of Treitz is verified. In those children who present with pulmonary symptoms, other causes of recurrent aspiration, such as vascular rings and an H-type tracheoesophageal fistula, are excluded. In every child, therefore, the esophagus should be examined in at least two projections.

The distal esophagus is studied for the presence of hiatus hernia, esophageal stricture, and the more subtle signs of esophagitis. The peristaltic activity, caliber, and tortuosity of the esophagus are evaluated. Only at the conclusion of the examination can the presence or absence of gastroesophageal reflux be assessed.

The most common error made by the examiner is inadequate filling of the stomach. This may produce a spuriously negative examination when gastroesophageal reflux is indeed the patient's problem. To avoid underfilling, the child's parents are asked how much the child drinks at each feeding; then, at least this amount of contrast is given. Frequently, the patient's own bottle is used, after a slightly larger hole has been made in the nipple. In assessing possible reflux, the swallowing mechanism is evaluated, with attention to normal tongue motion, lack of nasopharyngeal reflux, and normal upper and lower esophageal motility. After this evaluation has been completed, there is no further need for fluoroscopy during swallowing. We permit the infant to drink as much as is desired, encouraging consumption to be at least equal to the amount taken at home. The child is then held upright and burped. This maneuver usually clears contrast material from the esophagus. If it does not, a small sip of water generally will cleanse the esophagus. The child is then intermittently observed with brief bursts of fluoroscopy for 5 minutes, and the number of episodes of reflux is documented. No additional maneuvers, such as pressing on the abdomen or placing the child in the Trendelenburg position, are used. Because crying generally decreases reflux, every effort is made to keep the child calm.

If reflux occurs, the level to which the contrast rises in the esophagus is precisely noted.[7] The ability of the esophagus to effectively strip itself of the regurgitated contrast is also evaluated. Additional information (reflux or aspiration) may be obtained by including the chest on the gastrointestinal (UGI) overhead films. If the child is small, the radiograph is exposed to include the chest; if the child is older, a separate chest film is obtained. Occasionally, a child who has not shown reflux under fluoroscopic observation will show significant reflux on the overhead films.

Water Siphon Test   The lower esophageal sphincter relaxes during normal swallowing and, to a lesser degree, during sucking (Fig. 13–44). Significant reflux of contrast material may occur during swallowing. Because the radiologist cannot separate the contrast material that is being swallowed from the contrast material that is simultaneously being refluxed, another maneuver is used. This maneuver is the water siphon test, in which swallowing is initiated by water (nonopaque) and the refluxed gastric contrast material is readily identified.[6]

The water siphon test is performed at the conclusion of the UGI examination, when the infant's stomach is filled with contrast. The child is burped and then given a bottle of water to drink. The level and severity of the reflux contrast are documented. A small wisp of contrast that is rapidly cleared by normal esophageal peristalsis is considered a negative result; however, a persistent, wide column of contrast extending above the carina signifies a positive study.

The water siphon test has a high (30%) false-positive rate—that is, a positive test does not reliably indicate significant gastroesophageal reflux. However, a negative water siphon examination is a good indication that significant reflux is not the cause of the patient's symptoms. Because of the high false-positive rate, this examination has not gained wide acceptance.

Radionuclide Gastroesophagography   Radionuclide gastroesophagography is performed by feeding the patient a radionuclide-labeled drink. The child is burped and then monitored by the gamma camera, with multiple images taken during a 1-hour period. This examination has

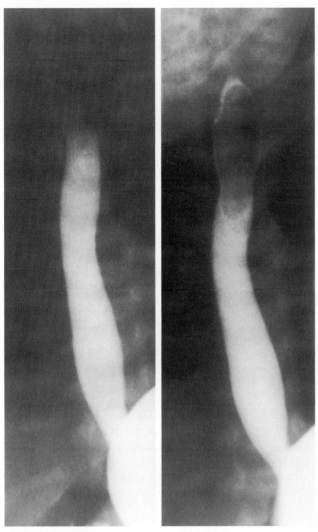

Figure 13–44
Water siphon test: fluoroscopic observation demonstrated a persistent column of barium when water was fed to this infant with gastroesophageal reflux.

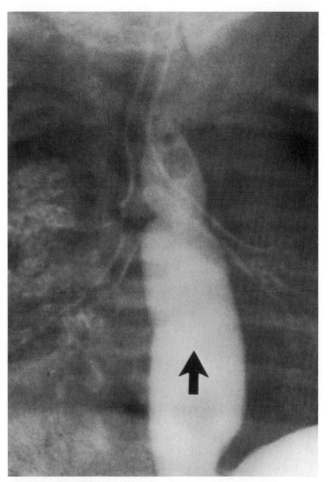

Figure 13–45
Gastroesophageal reflux with aspiration. This infant, who presented with recurrent pneumonias, demonstrates substantial gastroesophageal reflux and significant pulmonary aspiration. Note that the majority of aspiration was into the right upper lobe.

the advantage of providing monitoring that is both continuous and prolonged. The radiation dose is significantly lower than that received during routine UGI examination. Continuous imaging of the thorax permits identification of tracer aspiration. At present, there are difficulties in interpreting the significance of findings and in establishing controls. A strongly positive result is accepted as significant, and further examination by other modalities is indicated. However, a single negative radionuclide gastroesophagogram does not exclude pathologic symptomatic reflux.[9]

Radiographic Findings

There are no important plain film findings in gastroesophageal reflux, although some radiologists believe that the appearance of an air esophagram on chest radiography should raise the question of reflux, especially if this finding is seen repeatedly. Recurrent or chronic pneumonitis is also a somewhat indirect clue and is, of course, nonspecific; still, gastroesophageal reflux is one of the entities to consider when recurrent pneumonitis occurs (see Chapter 9).

The major radiographic features of gastroesophageal reflux to be assessed by the UGI series are as follows (Figs. 13–45 through 13–49):

1. Exclusion of gastric outlet obstruction
2. Evidence of disordered swallowing or nasopharyngeal reflux
3. Abnormal esophageal motility
4. Esophageal mucosal edema, ulceration, or stricture
5. Hiatus hernia
6. Gastroesophageal reflux

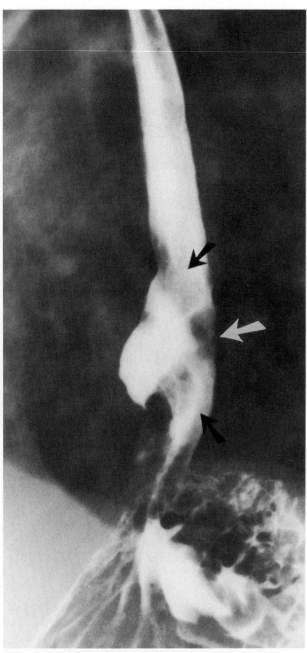

Figure 13–46
Gastroesophageal reflux with esophageal ulceration in a 5-year-old boy whose reflux was severe. Note the marked edema surrounding the ulcer crater *(arrows)*.

7. Documentation of the level of reflux, if reflux occurs
8. Aspiration of contrast

It is desirable to indicate on the spot films which films represent contrast being swallowed and which depict reflux. Several grading systems have been devised, but it is less complex and just as meaningful to simply state in anatomic terms the level of reflux demonstrated (e.g., carina or

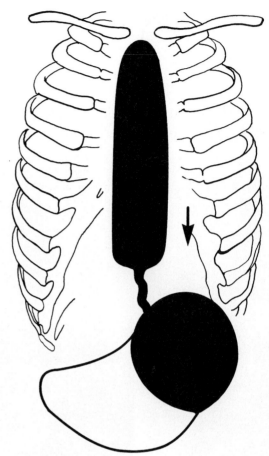

Figure 13–47
Gastroesophageal reflux with secondary stricture: diagrammatic representation. After an esophageal stricture has developed, gastroesophageal reflux may be difficult to document because the narrowing prevents swallowed barium from flowing back into the esophagus. Current modes of therapy in this situation are prevention of reflux (surgical fundoplication) with esophageal dilatation.

oropharynx) and the number of times it occurred during the 5-minute interval.[39]

SUMMARY

Vomiting is a common occurrence in childhood. It is most frequently a result of a pathologic process in an organ system other than the gastrointestinal tract. Infections of the middle ear and respiratory tract often result in temperature elevations that incite vomiting. The most common gastrointestinal cause of vomiting is viral gastroenteritis, a clinical diagnosis that seldom requires radiographic evaluation. Bowel atresias and pyloric stenoses are mechanical obstructing lesions that are readily diagnosed with the imaging procedures outlined in this chapter. Midgut volvulus is a medical emergency that

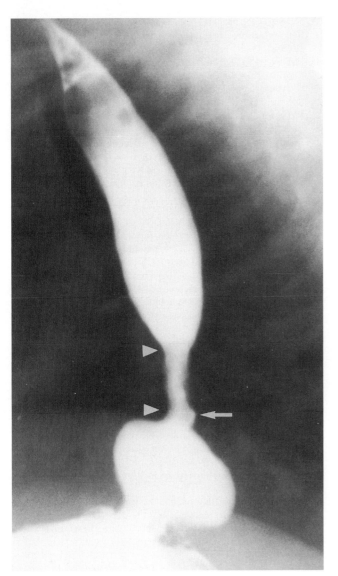

Figure 13–48
Gastroesophageal reflux with esophageal stricture, ulcer, and hiatal hernia. This 8-week-old premature infant was examined because of pulmonary problems. The lateral view of the esophagus, which was filled and distended with refluxed contrast material reveals a stricture *(arrowheads)* and a mucosal ulcer *(arrow)*. A hiatal hernia is seen beneath the ulceration. No aspiration of contrast material was documented.

requires prompt diagnosis and surgical intervention. The UGI series is the procedure that most reliably reveals a midgut volvulus. Gastroesophageal reflux is a common cause of vomiting in children younger than 1 year of age. Although there are many modalities that can be used to evaluate the presence of gastroesophageal reflux, pulmonary aspiration remains difficult to document in most children. The radiologist plays an important role in diagnosing the etiology of vomiting caused by mechanical obstructive lesions. In this

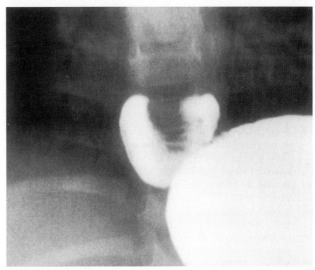

Figure 13–49
Nissen fundoplication. Contrast material administered through a gastrostomy tube reveals the normal postoperative appearance of this procedure.

chapter, the most common causes and their radiographic evaluations have been discussed.

REFERENCES

1. Atwell JD, Levick P. Congenital hypertrophic pyloric stenosis and associated anomalies in the genitourinary tract. J Pediatr Surg 16:1029–1035, 1981.
2. Ball TI, Atkinson GO Jr, Gay BB Jr. Ultrasound diagnosis of hypertrophic pyloric stenosis: Real-time application and the demonstration of a new sonographic sign. Radiology 147:499–502, 1983.
3. Bissett RAL, Gupta SC. Hypertrophic pyloric stenosis ultrasonic appearances in a small baby. Pediatr Radiol 18:405, 1988.
4. Bisset RA, Gupta SC, Zammit-Maempel I. Radiographic and ultrasound appearances of an intra-mural haematoma of the pylorus. Clin Radiol 39:316–318, 1988.
5. Blumhagen JD. The role of ultrasonography in the evaluation of vomiting in infants. Pediatr Radiol 16:267–270, 1986.
6. Blumhagen JD, Christie DL. Gastroesophageal reflux in children: Evaluation of the water siphon test. Pediatr Radiol 131:345–349, 1979.
7. Blumhagen JD, Maclin L, Krauter D, Rosenbaum DM, Weinberger E. Sonographic diagnosis of hypertrophic pyloric stenosis. AJR Am J Roentgenol 150:1367–1370, 1988.
8. Blumhagen JD, Noble H, George S. Muscle thickness in hypertrophic pyloric stenosis: Sonographic determination. AJR Am J Roentgenol 140:221–223, 1983.
9. Blumhagen JD, Rudd TG, Christie DL. Gastroesophageal reflux in children: Radionuclide gastroesophagography. AJR Am J Roentgenol 135:1001–1004, 1980.
10. Blumhagen JD, Weinberger E. Pediatric gastrointestinal ultrasonography. In Sanders RC, Hill MC, eds. Ultrasound Annual. New York: Raven Press, 1986, pp 99–140.
11. Bowen A. The vomiting infant: Recent advances and unsettled issues in imaging. Radiol Clin North Am 26:377–392, 1988.

12. Breaux CW Jr, Georgeson KE, Royal SA, Curnow AJ. Changing patterns in the diagnosis of hypertrophic pyloric stenosis. Pediatrics 81:213–217, 1988.

13. Carroll BA. US of the gastrointestinal tract. Radiology 172:605–608, 1989.

14. Carter CO, Evans KA. Inheritance of congenital pyloric stenosis. J Med Genet 6:233–254, 1969.

15. Carver RA, Okorie M, Steiner GM, Dickson JA. Infantile hypertrophic pyloric stenosis—Diagnosis from the pyloric muscle index. Clin Radiol 38:625–627, 1987.

16. Christie DL, O'Grady LR, Mack DV. Incompetent lower esophageal sphincter and gastroesophageal reflux in recurrent acute pulmonary disease of infancy and childhood. J Pediatr 93:23–27, 1978.

17. Cohen HL, Haller JO, Mestel AL, Coren C, Schechter S, Eaton DH. Neonatal duodenum: Fluid-aided US examination. Radiology 164:805–809, 1987.

18. Cremin BJ, Solomon DJ. Ultrasonic diagnosis of duodenal diaphragm. Pediatr Radiol 17:489–490, 1987.

19. Dawson KP. The use of ultrasound in the diagnosis of congenital pyloric stenosis. NZ Med J 101:1–2, 1988.

20. Finkelstein MS, Mandell GA, Tarbell KV. Hypertrophic pyloric stenosis: Volumetric measurement of nasogastric aspirate to determine the imaging modality. Radiology 177:759–761, 1990.

21. Foley LC, Slovis TL, Campbell JB, Strain JD, Harvey LA, Luckey DW. Evaluation of the vomiting infant. Am J Dis Child 143:660–661, 1989.

22. Forman GP, Leonidas JC, Kronfeld GD. A rational approach to the diagnosis of hypertrophic pyloric stenosis: Do the results match the claims? J Pediatr Surg 25:262–266, 1990.

23. Franken EA Jr, Smith WL. Gastrointestinal Imaging in Pediatrics. 2nd ed. Philadelphia: Harper & Row, 1982.

24. Gaines PA, Saunders AJS, Drake D. Midgut malrotation diagnosed by ultrasound. Clin Radiol 38:51–53, 1987.

25. Haller JO, Cohen HL. Hypertrophic pyloric stenosis: Diagnosis using US. Radiology 161:335–339, 1986.

26. Hayden CK Jr, Boulden TF, Swischuk LE, Lobe TE. Sonographic demonstration of duodenal obstruction with midgut volvulus. AJR Am J Roentgenol 143:9–10, 1984.

27. Hayden CK Jr, Swischuk LE, Rytting JE. Gastric ulcer disease in infants: US findings. Radiology 164:131–134, 1987.

28. Hicks LM, Morgan A, Anderson MR. Pyloric stenosis—A report of triplet females and notes on its inheritance. J Pediatr Surg 16:739–743, 1981.

29. Houston CS, Wittenborg MH. Roentgen evaluation of anomalies of rotation and fixation of the bowel in children. Radiology 84:1–17, 1965.

30. Is ultrasound really necessary for the diagnosis of hypertrophic pyloric stenosis? [Editorial]. Lancet 1:1146, 1988.

31. Jamroz GA, Blocker SH, McAlister WH. Radiographic findings after incomplete pyloromyotomy. Gastrointest Radiol 11:139–141, 1986.

32. Katz ME, Siegel MJ, Shackelford GD. The position and mobility of the duodenum in children. AJR Am J Roentgenol 148:947–951, 1987.

33. Keller H, Waldmann D, Greiner P. Comparison of preoperative sonography with intraoperative findings in congenital hypertrophic pyloric stenosis. J Pediatr Surg 22:950–952, 1987.

34. Lambrecht L, Robberecht E, Deschynkel K, Afschrift M. Ultrasonic evaluation of gastric clearing in young infants. Pediatr Radiol 18:314–318, 1988.

35. Lee DH, Lim JH, Ko YT, et al. Sonographic detection of pneumoperitoneum in patients with acute abdomen. AJR Am J Roentgenol 154:107–109, 1990.

36. Loyer E, Eggle KD. Sonographic evaluation of superior mesenteric vascular relationship in malrotation. Pediatr Radiol 19:173–175, 1989.

37. Lund Kofoed PE, Hest A, Elle B, Larsen C. Hypertrophic pyloric stenosis: Determination of muscle dimensions by ultrasound. Br J Radiol 61:19–20, 1988.

38. McAlister WH, Katz ME, Perlman JM, Tack ED. Sonography of focal foveolar hyperplasia causing obstruction in an infant. Pediatr Radiol 18:79–81, 1988.

39. McCauley RGK, Darling DB, Leonidas JC, Schwartz AM. Gastroesophageal reflux in infants and children: A useful classification and reliable physiologic technique for its demonstration. AJR Am J Roentgenol 130:47–50, 1978.

40. McKeown T, MacMahon B. Infantile hypertrophic pyloric stenosis in parent and child. Arch Dis Child 30:497–500, 1955.

41. Okorie NM, Dickson JA, Carver RA, Steiner AM. What happens to the pylorus after pyloromyotomy? Arch Dis Child 63:1339–1341, 1988.

42. Sauerbrei EE, Paloschi GGB. The ultrasonic features of hypertrophic pyloric stenosis, with emphasis on the postoperative appearance. Radiology 147:499–502, 1983.

43. Shaw D. Value of ultrasound in differentiating causes of persistent vomiting in infants [Letter]. Arch Dis Child 64:889, 1989.

44. Shuman FI, Darling DB, Fisher JH. The radiographic diagnosis of congenital hypertrophic pyloric stenosis. J Pediatr 71:70–74, 1967.

45. Simpson AJ, Leonidas JC, Krasna IH, Becker JM, Schneider KM. Roentgen diagnosis of midgut rotation: Value of upper gastrointestinal radiographic study. J Pediatr Surg 7:243–252, 1972.

46. Singleton EB, Wagner ML, Dutton RV. In Potchen EJ, ed. Radiology of the Alimentary Tract in Infants and Children. 3rd ed. Philadelphia: WB Saunders, 1977.

47. Spevak MR, Ahmadjian JM, Kleinman PK, Henriquez G, Hirsh MP, Cohen IT. Sonography of hypertrophic pyloric stenosis: Frequency and cause of nonuniform echogenicity of the thickened pyloric muscle. AJR Am J Roentgenol 158:129–132, 1992.

48. Stunden RJ, LeQuesne GW, Little KET. The improved ultrasound diagnosis of hypertrophic pyloric stenosis. Pediatr Radiol 16:200–205, 1986.

49. Swischuk LE, Fawcett HD, Hayden CK Jr, et al. Gastroesophageal reflux: How much imaging is required? Radiographics 8:1137–1145, 1988.

50. Swischuk LE, Hayden CK Jr, Stansberry SD. Sonographic pitfalls in imaging of the antropyloric region in infants. Radiographics 9:437–447, 1989.

51. Teele RL, Smith EH. Ultrasound in the diagnosis of idiopathic hypertrophic pyloric stenosis. N Engl J Med 296:1149–1150, 1977.

52. Tunell WP, Wilson DA. Pyloric stenosis: Diagnosis by real time sonography, the pyloric muscle length method. J Pediatr Surg 19:795–799, 1984.

53. Weinberger E, Winters WD, Liddell RM, Rosenbaum DM, Krauter D. Sonographic diagnosis of intestinal malrotation in infants: Importance of the relative positions of the superior mesenteric vein and artery. AJR Am J Roentgenol 159:825–828, 1992.

54. Weiskittel DA, Leary DL, Blane CE. Ultrasound diagnosis of evolving pyloric stenosis. Gastrointest Radiol 14:22–24, 1989.

55. Westra SJ, deGroot CJ, Smits NJ, Staalman CR. Hypertrophic pyloric stenosis: Use of the pyloric volume measurement in early US diagnosis. Radiology 172:615–619, 1989.

56. Wright LL, Baker KR, Meny RG. Ultrasound demonstration of gastroesophageal reflux. J Ultrasound Med 7:471–475, 1988.

57. Yip WC, Tay JS, Wong HB. Sonographic diagnosis of infantile hypertrophic pyloric stenosis: Critical appraisal of reliability and diagnostic criteria. J Clin Ultrasound 13:329–332, 1985.

ADDITIONAL READING

Ali KI, Haddad MJ. Early infantile hypertrophic pyloric stenosis: Surgery at 26 hours of age. Eur J Pediatr Surg 1996: 6:233–234, 1996.

Applegate KE, Goske MJ, Pierce G, Murphy D. Situs revisited: Imaging of the heterotaxy syndrome. RadioGraphics 19:837–852, 1999.

Chao H-C, Kong M-S, Chen J-Y, Sin SJ, Lin JN. Sonographic features related to volvulus in neonatal intestinal malrotation. J Ultrasound Med 19:371–376, 2000.

Chen EA, Luks FI, Gilchrist BF, Wesselhoeft CS Jr, DeLuca FG. Pyloric stenosis in the age of ultrasonography: Fading skills, better patients? J Pediatr Surg 31:829–830, 1996.

Helton KJ, Strife JL, Warner BW, Byczkowski TL, Donovan EF. The impact of a clinical guideline on imaging children with hypertrophic pyloric stenosis. Pediatr Radiol 34:733–736, 2004.

Hernanz-Schulman M. Infantile hypertrophic pyloric stenosis. Radiology 227:319–331, 2003.

Jamieson D, Stringer DA. Small bowel. In Stringer DA, Babyn PS, eds. Pediatric Gastrointestinal Imaging and Intervention. 2nd ed. BC Decker, Hamilton, Ontario, Canada, 2000, pp 311–474.

Latchaw LA, Jacir NN, Harris BH. The development of pyloric stenosis during transpyloric feeding. J Pediatr Surg 24:823–824, 1989.

Michalsky MP, Pratt D, Caniano DA, Teich S. Streamlining the care of patients with hypertrophic pyloric stenosis: Application of a clinical pathway. J Pediatr 71:70–74, 2000.

Miyakoshi K, Ishimoto H, Tanigaki S, et al. Prenatal diagnosis of midgut volvulus by sonography and magnetic resonance imaging. Am J Perinatol 18:447–450, 2001.

Ozsvath RR, Poustchi-Amin M, Leonidas JC, Elkowitz SS. Pyloric volume: An important factor in the surgeon's ability to palpate the pyloric "olive" in hypertrophic pyloric stenosis. Pediatr Surg 27:175–177, 1997.

Prasil P, Flageole H, Shaw KS, Nguyen LT, Youssef S, Laberge JM. Should malrotation in children be treated differently according to age? J Pediatr Surg 35:756–758, 2000.

Rohrschneider WK, Mittnacht H, Darge K, Troger J. Pyloric muscle in asymptomatic infants: Sonographic evaluation and discrimination from idiopathic hypertrophic pyloric stenosis. Pediatr Radiol 28:429–434, 1998.

Schlessinger AE, Parker BR. Acquired gastric and duodenal disorders. In Kuhn JP, Slovis TL, Haller JO, eds. Caffey's Pediatric Diagnostic Imaging. Philadelphia: Mosby, 2204, pp 1593–1615.

Skandalakis JE, Gray SW, Ricketts R, et al. The small intestines. In Skandalakis JE, Gray SW, eds. Embryology for Surgeons. 2nd ed. Baltimore: Williams &Wilkins, 1994, pp 184–241.

Strouse PJ. Disorders of intestinal rotation and fixation ("malrotation"). Pediatr Radiol 34:837–851, 2004.

THE CHILD WITH ABDOMINAL PAIN

Outline

CHAPTER
14

Simon C. S. Kao, MD

THE CHILD WITH ABDOMINAL PAIN

Abdominal pain is common in children. All physicians caring for infants and young children are familiar with "bellyache" as a complaint in a wide variety of conditions.[16,18] Similarly, chronic and recurrent abdominal pain is a major complaint in older children. The main decisions in evaluating children with either acute or chronic abdominal pain are to determine (1) which children require radiologic imaging for diagnosis or therapy and (2) which imaging techniques are most likely to give the information needed for clinical care. Both issues are discussed in this chapter.

PATHOPHYSIOLOGY OF ABDOMINAL PAIN

In considering abdominal pain, awareness of certain neurologic mechanisms is helpful. Pain sensation from the gut and other intra-abdominal organs reaches the spinal cord via the autonomic nervous system. Visceral pain sensation follows sympathetic nerves to the thoracic ganglia and from there to the spinal cord. Because afferent impulses are spread along the length of the thoracic and lumbar cord, localization of visceral pain is poor. In contrast, the parietal peritoneum, diaphragm, and abdominal wall are innervated by somatic nerves. These nerves show a well-localized distribution to the level and side of the spinal cord that corresponds to the dermatomes. Within the spinal cord, pain fibers ascend in the lateral spinothalamic tract to terminate in the thalamus. From the thalamus, the pain sensation reaches the cerebral cortex, where pain is perceived consciously.

One stimulus for abdominal pain is stretching or tension of an organ. Whereas crushing, tearing, or cutting of the gut is not perceived as being painful, traction on the peritoneum or rapid distention of a viscus is painful. Distention must be relatively sudden to cause pain. For example, gradual distention of the common bile duct by a slow-growing tumor is painless, whereas abrupt occlusion of the duct by a stone is accompanied by moderate to severe pain. Forceful contraction of the gut, as may occur in acute obstruction, usually causes pain. Inflammation, either chemical or microbial, causes pain as a result of local effects on nerve endings. In a similar fashion, the pain of ischemia results from accumulation of tissue metabolites within the involved region.

There are three types of pain caused by abdominal disease: visceral, parietal, and referred. *Visceral* pain, arising from the internal organs, is poorly localized and is usually perceived as occurring in a midline position because of bilateral and diffuse representation of the affected organ in the spinal cord. Nausea, vomiting, and pallor are autonomic effects that frequently accompany visceral pain. *Parietal* pain originates in the parietal peritoneum and is sharply localized to the affected dermatome. *Referred* pain is also localized in a dermatome distribution but is perceived only when the visceral stimulation is intense. For example, mild distention of a balloon within the gut produces poorly localized visceral pain. Not until the distention is considerable is referred pain perceived by the subject as back pain.

Although localization of pain is imprecise, the perceived site of visceral pain generally follows the embryonic origin of the viscera (Table 14–1).[42] *Epigastric* pain is associated with disease of the foregut derivatives: the stomach, duodenum, liver, biliary system, and pancreas. *Periumbilical* pain is produced by lesions of the midgut derivatives: the small bowel and proximal colon. *Infraumbilical* or hypogastric pain is associated with diseases of the hindgut derivatives (the distal two thirds of the colon), uterus, urinary bladder, and kidney. Visceral pain from the kidney and renal pelvis has a lateral localization, reflecting unilateral spinal cord representation. Renal pain, like pain from any other organ, is caused by distention of the renal capsule or collecting system.

TABLE 14-1 GENERAL LOCALIZATION OF ORGANIC ABDOMINAL PAIN

Epigastric Pain (Foregut Derivatives)
Stomach
Duodenum
Liver
Bile ducts
Periumbilical Pain (Midgut Derivatives)
Small bowel
Cecum
Infraumbilical Pain (Hindgut Derivatives)
Colon
Uterus
Bladder
Kidney (lateral localization)

Stress from any stimulus, including pain and psychophysiologic phenomena, has effects on the gastrointestinal tract (Fig. 14–1). These effects vary, depending on the patient's genetic makeup and previous life experiences. In many stressed experimental subjects, the gastric folds become prominent, and secretions increase. Similar changes occur in the stomachs of children with functional (psychogenic) abdominal pain. Pylorospasm is common in acutely stressed children and sometimes occurs merely from the psychologic trauma of undergoing radiographic examination or as a result of acute pain. Therefore, little importance can be attached to this radiographic finding as a sign of organic disease.

When acutely stressed, children may swallow considerable air. This tendency, when combined with a paralytic ileus resulting from sympathetic stimulation, may produce remarkable distention of the gastrointestinal tract, particularly of the stomach and colon, in children with acute pain from other sites. The physician evaluating the child with acute abdominal pain and a distended gut should consider the possibility that the pain is secondary to disease elsewhere.

Intestinal tonus also changes with stress, and an individual's perception of this change in tonus may or may not produce pain. Adults with functional bowel disease are much more likely to perceive pain as a result of distention or contraction of the gut than are those without functional disease.

THE "ACUTE ABDOMEN" (SURGICAL VERSUS MEDICAL)

The term *acute abdomen* generally indicates an acute disease of such severity that immediate surgical intervention must be considered.[19] The causes of an acute abdomen are usually divided into those of a medical nature and those necessitating surgical intervention. The medical causes can be subdivided into intra-abdominal and extra-abdominal causes. As in all other areas of pediatrics, the differential diagnosis of acute abdomen in children varies with the patient's age.[15] In *premature neonates*, necrotizing enterocolitis is the most common surgical cause of an acute abdomen. In *term neonates*, congenital intestinal obstruction, most commonly atresia, is the usual condition requiring surgery, whereas sepsis is the most frequent medical cause of acute abdomen. Septicemia is the most frequent cause of negative results for a laparotomy performed for an acute abdomen in neonates.

In *infants*, intussusception, strangulated inguinal hernia, complicated Meckel's diverticulum, malrotation with volvulus, and appendicitis are the most common indications for surgery (Fig. 14–2). Medical causes include primary peritonitis associated with nephrotic syndrome, colic, and gastroenteritis.

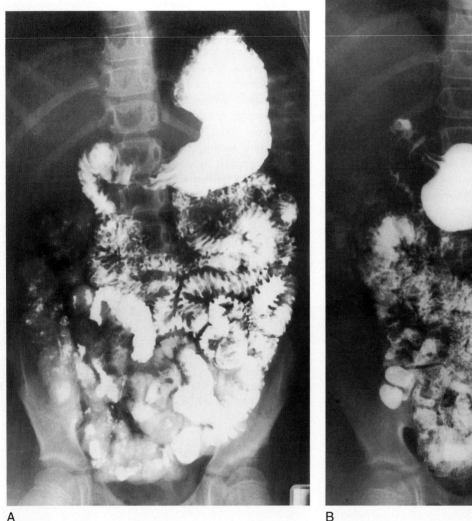

A   B

Figure 14–1
Small bowel changes presumed to be the effect of stress. *A,* An upper gastrointestinal examination, performed while the child was exceedingly apprehensive and frightened, is abnormal. Evident are a marked increase in intra-abdominal secretions, fragmentation of the barium column, and small bowel spasms. Fluoroscopic observation revealed marked and prolonged pylorospasm. *B,* A repeat examination with the child in a more tranquil state of mind was normal.

In *older children,* acute appendicitis is much more common than any other surgical ailment. Less frequent surgical conditions include acute cholecystitis, inflammatory bowel disease, and ruptured tumor (such as renal tumor). Principal medical intra-abdominal causes include nonspecific abdominal pain, gastroenteritis, primary peritonitis, bacterial enterocolitis, mesenteric adenitis, viral hepatitis, pancreatitis, urinary tract infection, sacroiliitis, pyomyositis, pelvic inflammatory disease, ectopic pregnancy or other gynecologic disorders, and perhaps constipation.

Lesions of the chest with involvement of the diaphragmatic pleura may cause *referred* pain to the abdomen. Pleural effusion and lower lobe pneumonitis are particularly apt to cause such pain. Pleural effusion not only may reflect thoracic disease but also may be associated with intra-abdominal

disease such as pancreatitis or renal abscess. Pneumonia of either lower lobe may simulate an acute "surgical abdomen" and may be missed without chest radiography. Spinal disorders of the bony spine or the spinal cord may be perceived as abdominal pain, particularly in younger children. Spinal cord tumors and, more commonly, inflammatory disk disease (diskitis) clinically mimic symptoms of abdominal pathologic conditions.

Acute abdominal pain may result from *systemic* diseases. Hematologic causes include sickle cell disease in crisis, Henoch-Schönlein purpura, hemolytic-uremic syndrome, and typhlitis in blood dyscrasia. The child with diabetic acidosis may present similarly. In adults with acute abdominal pain and diabetic acidosis, there is a possibility that a surgical abnormality is producing both the pain and diabetic acidosis,

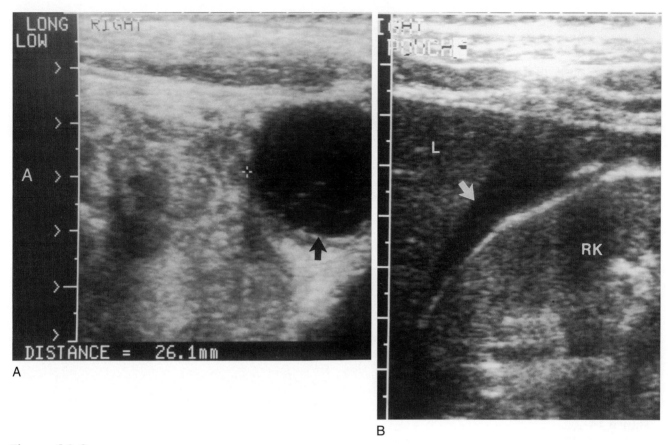

Figure 14–2
Perforative acute appendicitis with pelvic abscess and ascites. *A,* A longitudinal scan of the right lower quadrant shows a septated, cystic abscess *(arrow). B,* A longitudinal scan of the right upper quadrant reveals fluid *(arrow)* between the liver and right kidney. L, Liver; RK, right kidney.

but in children, the acute abdominal pain most often reflects the metabolic derangement of acidosis alone. Various types of poisoning, particularly from heavy metals such as lead, may manifest as acute abdominal pain along with neurologic signs and symptoms.

Few large series have been published on the relative incidence of diseases producing acute abdominal pain in the children. Jones[36] studied 363 consecutive children with acute abdominal pain who were admitted to the Royal Aberdeen Hospital for Children. Approximately one third of patients ultimately required surgery; acute appendicitis was the diagnosis in more than 90% of these. Nonsurgical diagnoses include upper respiratory infections, often in the form of lower lobe pneumonia, and constipation. In a series of 588 children from Dublin, O'Donnell[47] indicated a similar distribution of illnesses producing acute abdomen in children. In both series, acute nonspecific abdominal pain was a common symptom.

An *imaging workup* is often performed in children with suspected acute abdomen. Routine films include supine and horizontal-beam studies of the abdomen, as well as a chest radiograph. The horizontal-beam abdominal radiograph is frequently omitted on the attending physician's consultation request, but it is essential. The type may vary according to the preference of the radiologist and the condition of the patient; upright, left lateral decubitus, or lateral cross-table examinations are all satisfactory. In addition to demonstrating air-fluid levels within the gut, such a film is essential for detecting free intraperitoneal air (Figs. 14–3, 14–4, and 14–5).

Abdominal sonography is probably the next examination in evaluating a child with an acute abdomen, because it is noninvasive and sensitive for detecting common lesions causing acute abdomen in children (e.g., acute appendicitis, acute cholecystitis, obstructive uropathy, abdominal abscesses, and variable amounts of intraperitoneal fluid suggestive of peritonitis). Computed tomography (CT) is reserved for those patients in whom sonography yields normal results or is technically difficult because of gaseous distention or obesity.

Contrast studies of the gastrointestinal tract are seldom indicated in this setting, except in patients with suspected malrotation, congenital bowel obstruction, and intussusception and when a precise definition of an anatomic obstruction is needed. If arteriography, which is seldom indicated, is contemplated, it should be performed prior to any barium study.

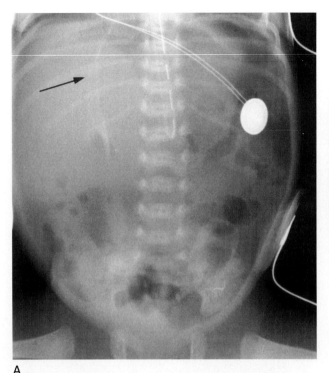

A

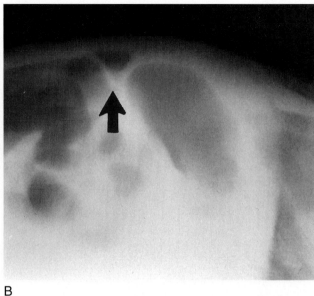

B

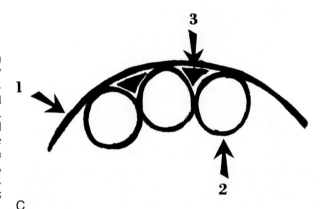

C

Figure 14–3

Free intraperitoneal air. *A,* A large pneumoperitoneum *(arrow)* clearly outlines the falciform ligament. *B,* the "triangle sign." A supine, cross-table lateral radiograph in an infant with pneumoperitoneum demonstrates a triangle of air *(arrow)* interposed between the stomach superiorly and a loop of bowel inferiorly. Such triangles have one side along the anterior abdominal wall when seen in this projection. Free air caught between multiple loops of bowel may produce several such triangles. This sign permits diagnosis of small amounts of free intraperitoneal air, which is an advantage of cross-table lateral, supine radiographs. *C,* Diagrammatic representation. 1, Abdominal wall; 2, bowel; 3, triangle sign.

Currently, the role of magnetic resonance imaging (MRI) in the investigation of the pediatric acute abdomen remains ill-defined.

CHRONIC, RECURRENT (FUNCTIONAL) ABDOMINAL PAIN

Chronic, recurrent abdominal pain is a common complaint of children and a frequent cause of referral for radiologic evaluation. Using Apley's criteria, the child who has had at least three episodes of pain, severe enough to interfere with activity, over a period longer than 3 months, is considered to have functional abdominal pain syndrome.[3] In almost all large series of patients with chronic abdominal pain, the incidence of organic disease is less than 10%. Functional abdominal pain is the most frequent cause of chronic abdominal pain. In the small percentage of children with an organic basis for chronic, recurrent abdominal pain, diseases of the gastrointestinal and genitourinary systems are seen with equal frequency. Thus, if it seems appropriate to evaluate a child with chronic pain using diagnostic procedures, radiologic evaluation of these two systems is most likely to be rewarding.

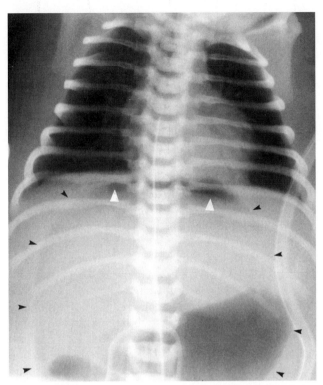

Figure 14–4
Free intraperitoneal gas: the "football sign." A large, oval lucency *(black arrowheads),* shaped roughly like a football, seen within the abdomen represents free intraperitoneal gas collecting anteriorly in a supine infant. White arrowheads indicate the top of the "football".

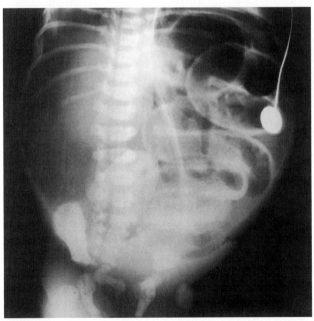

Figure 14–5
Free intraperitoneal gas. Term neonate with prolonged and severe peritonitis. There is severe swelling of the bowel wall, and air is clearly seen on both sides of the bowel wall. Also seen is a swollen and prominent falciform ligament.

DIFFERENTIAL DIAGNOSIS OF ABDOMINAL PAIN

GASTROINTESTINAL CAUSES

Esophagus

In diseases of the esophagus and gastroesophageal junction with pain as part of their clinical manifestations, the pain is usually substernal or thoracic rather than abdominal. Dysphagia, vomiting, and sometimes hematemesis are usually more prominent symptoms than pain.

Stomach

A relatively common cause of pain in patients older than 1 month of age is gastric outlet obstruction. Differential diagnosis includes pyloric stenosis, peptic ulcer disease, gastric volvulus, inflammatory disease of the stomach, bezoar, and, rarely, tumors. In most patients, symptoms of obstruction, nausea, and vomiting are predominant. Peptic gastric ulcer may present primarily as abdominal pain. Stress ulcer, usually seen in a child hospitalized for burns, trauma, sepsis, or other major illness, and the related entity, hemorrhagic gastritis, seldom produce abdominal pain; the usual clinical manifestations are hematemesis or peritonitis from perforation.

Small Bowel

Small bowel diseases are relatively frequent causes of organic abdominal pain in children. Crohn's disease is probably the most frequent organic cause of obscure abdominal pain in children. Other inflammatory small bowel diseases, with the exception of acute gastroenteritis, are rare in pediatric patients. In poverty-stricken areas, abdominal pain is one symptom of infestation by intestinal parasites such as *Ascaris lumbricoides.*

Incomplete obstruction of the small bowel often causes characteristic findings: abdominal distention, borborygmus, and vomiting. Occasionally, recurrent abdominal pain is the major clinical manifestation (Fig. 14–6). This is caused by distention of the intestine proximal to the obstruction. Causes of partial intestinal obstruction in children include duplication, polyps, tumor (especially lymphosarcoma), complications of cystic fibrosis, congenital or acquired stenosis of any cause, and Meckel's diverticulum.

Meckel's diverticulum is a vestige of the omphalomesenteric duct arising from the antimesenteric surface of the distal ileum. Only 25% to 40% become symptomatic, usually by one of the three following mechanisms:

1. If ectopic gastric mucosa is within the diverticulum (occurring in 56% of symptomatic patients), ulceration of adjacent small bowel with acute blood loss may occur; this usually occurs in the first 2 years of life.

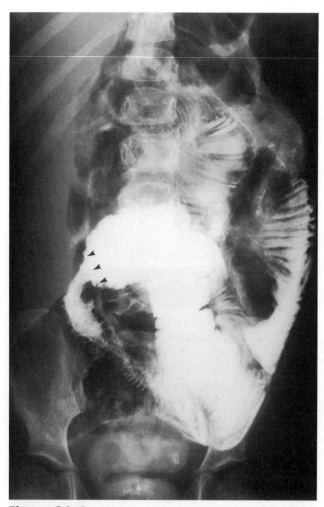

Figure 14–6
Adhesions causing partial bowel obstruction. An antegrade small bowel examination reveals a localized obstruction *(arrowheads)* with marked proximal bowel dilatation. An abrupt return to normal-caliber small bowel occurs beyond the point of obstruction. The patient, a 5-year-old boy, presented with recurrent abdominal pain and vomiting. Radiographic findings and a history of a previous laparotomy indicated adhesions as the cause of the obstruction. Laparotomy confirmed the diagnosis.

2. Intestinal obstruction can be caused by intussusception of the inverted diverticulum or by abnormal peritoneal bands around the diverticulum, producing kinking or volvulus.
3. If the orifice of the Meckel's diverticulum is partially obstructed, secretions may accumulate and become infected.

Symptoms of an inflamed Meckel's diverticulum resemble those of acute appendicitis but with a somewhat more subacute course. In addition, the inflammatory process is often medial to the usual site of appendicitis. If a barium enema reveals a normal cecum and appendix, barium refluxed into the terminal ileum may show extrinsic pressure from the inflamed Meckel's diverticulum.

If peptic disease causes lower gastrointestinal hemorrhage in a Meckel's diverticulum, detection by radionuclide scintigraphy (the Meckel's scan) is based on the affinity of sodium pertechnetate Tc 99m for ectopic gastric mucosa present in the diverticulum. This examination has an accuracy of about 95% in patients presenting with bleeding.[61] However, the role of scintigraphy in children presenting with abdominal pain alone has not been defined.

Henoch-Schönlein (anaphylactoid) purpura is a diffuse vasculitis. In most children, it appears as purpura with joint pain and sometimes nephritis. The gastrointestinal tract is often involved, and in about 10% of patients, primary manifestations occur there before the more diagnostic dermatologic findings appear. Intramural hemorrhage as a result of capillary damage and perivascular inflammation may involve both small and large bowel. Crampy abdominal pain and hematochezia result. Radiographic examination of the bowel reveals mucosal thickening, thumbprinting, and separation of bowel loops (Figs. 14–7 and 14–8). Occasionally, a hematoma may act as a lead point for intermittent intussusception. Sonography and CT may show bowel wall thickening and intussusception.

Intussusception occurs primarily in infants. Although colicky abdominal pain is associated with this disease, other manifestations, particularly abdominal mass and blood and mucus in the stool ("currant-jelly stools"), usually suggest the correct diagnosis.

Malrotation with intermittent or partial midgut volvulus may be associated with recurrent abdominal pain, intermittent intestinal obstruction, and chylous ascites in infants and older children.

Colon

Inflammatory disease of the colon may produce abdominal pain in children, usually accompanied by other indications of colonic disease, such as diarrhea, tenesmus, and, often, hematochezia. Acute gastroenteritis is the most common such condition and seldom needs radiographic investigation. Chronic symptoms suggest inflammatory bowel disease, particularly Crohn's colitis and ulcerative colitis. Other types of inflammatory colonic disease are rare in children.

Children with cystic fibrosis often present with symptoms and signs of distal intestinal obstruction. Differential diagnoses include meconium ileus equivalent, intussusception, volvulus, and fibrosing colonopathy. Characteristic radiographic findings in fibrosing colonopathy include colonic stricture, longitudinal shortening of the ascending colon, and an abnormal haustral pattern.[9]

For radiographic examination of the child with suspected inflammatory disease of the colon, we prefer the double-contrast barium enema. Its superiority over a single-contrast barium enema in detecting minimal colitis is well established.

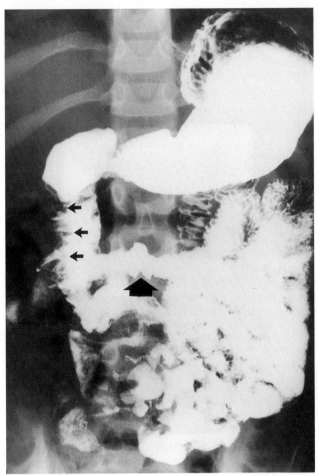

Figure 14–7

Abdominal pain and vomiting were the primary symptoms in this 8-year-old boy with diffuse vasculitis caused by Henoch-Schönlein purpura. The upper gastrointestinal examination demonstrates intramural masses *(small arrows)* and rigidity and deformity of the horizontal duodenum *(broad arrow)*. Intramural hematomas involving the small bowel and colon are frequently found in this disease.

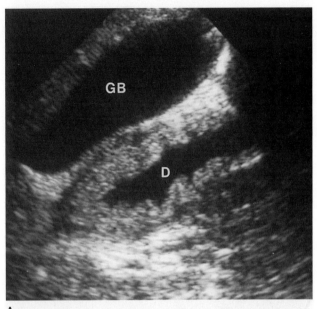

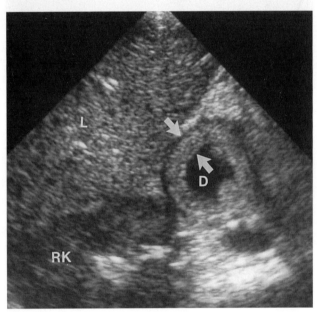

Figure 14–8

Duodenal hematoma in Henoch-Schönlein purpura. Longitudinal *(A)* and transverse *(B)* scans of the right upper abdomen show thickening of the duodenal wall *(arrows)*, which was confirmed by an upper gastrointestinal series. The patient developed skin manifestations of Henoch-Schönlein purpura 1 week later. D, Duodenum; GB, gallbladder; L, liver; RK, right kidney.

Acute appendicitis is the most frequent acute abdominal condition that requires laparotomy in children. Its manifestations are discussed in detail below.

Liver

Hepatic diseases causing distention of the hepatic capsule may elicit abdominal pain. As a result, acute hepatitis may occasionally simulate other causes of acute abdominal disease. Similarly, hepatic abscess and trauma may produce abdominal pain.

Gallbladder

Acute cholecystitis in children is usually of the acalculous variety. The typical occurrence follows bacterial inflammation elsewhere, particularly streptococcal pharyngitis, although

the exact relationship is unclear. Characteristically, there is acute right upper quadrant pain and tenderness, sometimes accompanied by jaundice. Abdominal sonography, the imaging procedure of choice, shows a distended gallbladder with thickening of its wall (3 mm), with or without gallstones. Single or multiple layers of sonolucency may be seen within

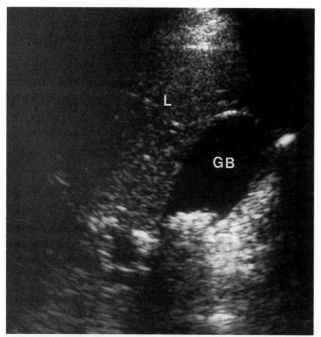

Figure 14–9
Gallstone sonography. A longitudinal scan of the gallbladder shows gallstones with distal acoustic shadowing. The patient was an asymptomatic 14-year-old girl with hereditary spherocytosis referred for evaluation of potential cholelithiasis. GB, Gallbladder; L, liver.

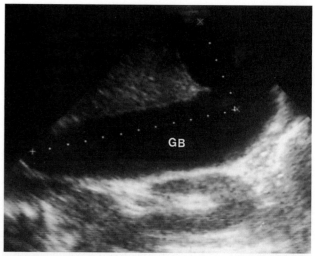

Figure 14–10
Hydrops of the gallbladder in a 15-year-old girl with fever of unknown origin, herpetic stomatitis, hepatitis, and right upper abdominal pain. A longitudinal scan of the right upper abdomen shows a markedly dilated gallbladder (17 cm in length) without wall thickening or gallstone. GB, Gallbladder.

the thickened hyperechoic wall, reflecting subserosal edema, inflammation, or hemorrhage.

Although calculous cholecystitis is rare in children, gallstone detection has increased in recent years as a result of therapeutic regimens predisposing to stone formation, heightened clinical suspicion, and the use of high-resolution sonography.[42] Gallstones in most children are nonhemolytic in origin, and about one third of cases in older children are idiopathic. Although gallstones are frequent in children with hemolytic anemia, they seldom cause symptoms in pediatric patients (Figs. 14–9). When gallstones do become symptomatic, intermittent, colicky, right upper quadrant pain is the usual complaint.

Hydrops, or acute distention of the gallbladder without cholecystitis or cholelithiasis, has been reported in children with systemic infectious disease, Kawasaki syndrome, and burns and in those who have undergone prolonged fasting accompanied by total parenteral nutrition. The mechanism involved is unknown. The patient usually presents with right upper quadrant or epigastric pain and a palpable mass. Sonography shows only a dilated gallbladder without wall thickening, a stone, or bile duct abnormalities (Fig. 14–10).

Choledochal cyst is the congenital dilation of a portion of the extrahepatic bile duct with or without dilation of the intrahepatic ducts. The etiology of choledochal cyst in children older than 1 month is thought to be an anomalous

relationship of the pancreatic and common bile ducts, causing reflux of pancreatic secretions into the bile duct, with secondary inflammation and subsequent dilatation of the bile duct. The triad of intermittent jaundice, recurrent right upper quadrant abdominal pain, and mass occurs in only about 25% of patients. A choledochal cyst may be identified by sonography, CT, MRI (including magnetic resonance cholangiopancreatography,), cholangiography, cholescintigraphy, or angiography; however, sonography remains the study of choice (Fig. 14–11).

Pancreas

Pancreatitis in children is more often acute than chronic, in contrast to that in adults, and the etiologic agents in children are different from those in adults; 25% to 50% of cases of acute pancreatitis are idiopathic.[42,83] Known causes of pancreatitis in children include accidental and nonaccidental trauma, mumps, steroid therapy, cystic fibrosis, and antimetabolic drugs. Familial hereditary pancreatitis with recurrent, mild attacks is rare during childhood and early adulthood and eventually results in pancreatic calcification in about half of patients.

Radiographic manifestations of pancreatitis in children are identical to those in adults. Secondary effects may be apparent in the duodenum, with persistent duodenal gas, dilatation, and stasis evident on contrast studies. More direct evidence of pancreatitis can be obtained by sonography or CT (Fig. 14–12).

Pancreatic pseudocyst in children is most often the result of pancreatitis from blunt abdominal trauma, and, in the

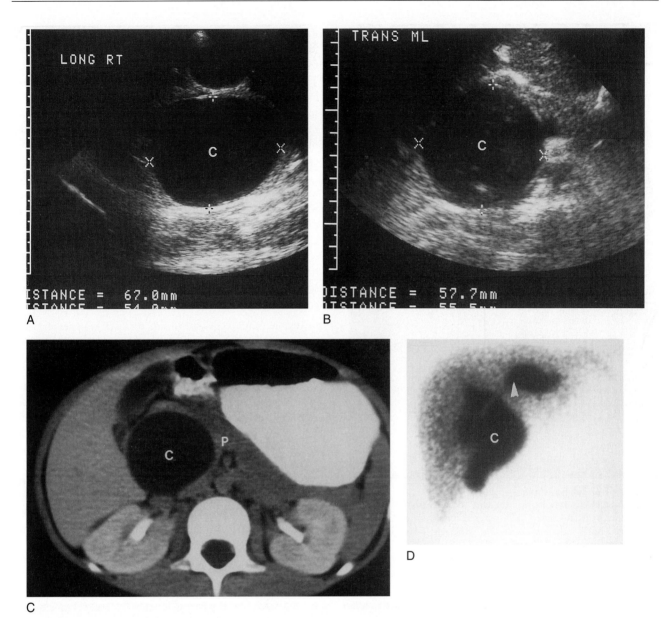

Figure 14–11
Choledochal cyst in a 6-year-old boy presenting with abdominal pain and jaundice. Longitudinal *(A)* and transverse *(B)* sonograms show dilatation of the extrahepatic duct. *C,* An axial computed tomography (CT) scan shows the lower end of the cystic mass in relation to the pancreatic head. *D,* A cholescintigram shows dilatation of the extrahepatic ductal system. C, Choledochal cyst; P, pancreas. Arrowhead points to delayed emptying of radionuclide from biliary system.

absence of a history of trauma, child abuse should be the primary diagnostic consideration. Pleural effusion, which is common in adults, is rare in children. The pseudocyst originates in the retrogastric region and commonly extends into the lesser sac but may dissect anywhere within the abdomen or even into the mediastinum. The usual clinical manifestations are vague, recurrent pain and abdominal mass. Sonography or CT invariably provides diagnostic images (Fig. 14–13).

GENITOURINARY DISEASE

Visceral abdominal pain of renal origin results from sudden dilatation of the renal pelvis and calyces. In the younger child, this may be manifested by midline pain in the periumbilical or suprapubic area. In older children, the pain is more suggestive of ureteral colic seen in adults. Dilatation of the ureter alone does not produce pain.

Ureteropelvic junction obstruction, either unilateral or bilateral, occasionally causes abdominal pain in children; in this setting the urinalysis is usually normal. Ureteral reflux may be associated with visceral renal pain because of distention of the collecting system. Obstructive renal stones produce pain in children by the same mechanism as in adults, although localization of the pain may be imprecise. Renal parenchymal disease produces pain by distention of the renal capsule. This usually has a somatic component so that the pain is localized to the flank; renal abscess is particularly likely to manifest in this way. Plain radiography, sonography, CT, nuclear medicine, and intravenous urograms are techniques often used to exclude stone diseases and associated complications, such as obstruction.

Gynecologic disorders that cause abdominal pain in girls include torsion of a normal ovary, an ovarian cyst, or a tumor, which may occur at any age (Fig. 14–14). Pelvic inflammatory disease and ectopic pregnancy seen in sexually active children and adolescents have findings similar to those in their adult counterparts; however, the diagnosis is frequently missed because it is not considered in the differential diagnosis. Pelvic sonography is the imaging modality of choice for these conditions.

MISCELLANEOUS

Mesenteric adenitis is often confused clinically with acute appendicitis. Although inflamed mesenteric lymph nodes may be detected by high-resolution sonography (Fig. 14–15), the significance of detection and the relationship to pain are uncertain. Infarction of an intra-abdominal organ, such as superior mesenteric artery occlusion with necrosis of the bowel, is a rare cause of abdominal pain in children. Occasionally, necrotic tumors, particularly Wilms' tumor, may cause pain. The child with lead intoxication can present with abdominal pain, constipation, and increased intracranial pressure (Fig. 14–16).

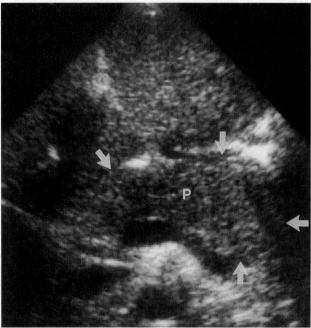

Figure 14–12
Acute pancreatitis (etiology unknown) in a 6-year-old girl with abdominal pain and sepsis. A transverse sonogram of the upper abdomen shows enlargement of the pancreas (arrows) without pseudocyst formation. P, Pancreas.

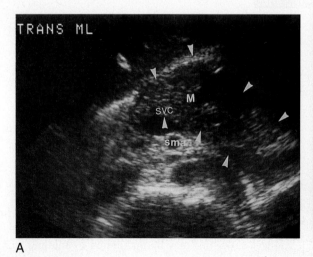
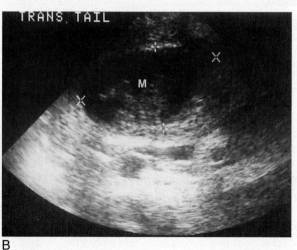

A   B

Figure 14–13
Hemorrhagic pancreatic pseudocyst in a 12-year-old boy after blunt abdominal trauma. Transverse sonograms of the upper abdomen show a complex cystic mass anterior to the body (A, arrows) and tail (B, cursors) of the pancreas.

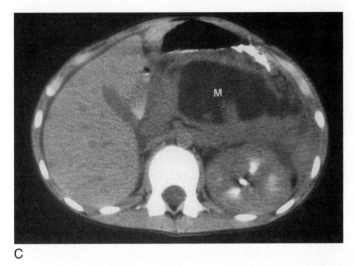

C

Figure 14–13—cont'd

C, A transverse CT scan shows a hypodense mass in the same region with an irregular soft tissue component arising from the posterior wall. Laparotomy revealed rupture of the pancreatic body with an infected hemorrhagic pseudocyst in the lesser sac. M, Pseudocyst; sma, superior mesenteric artery; svc, superior vena cava.

Figure 14–14

CT scan of ovarian torsion. A 6-year-old girl presented with a 2-day history of right lower quadrant pain, nausea, and vomiting. The pain gradually became periumbilical. Physical examination revealed abdominal tenderness without localizing signs or rebound tenderness. CT findings were similar to sonographic findings: a markedly enlarged ovary, which may be midline in position, with peripheral cysts, which are dilated follicles. Dynamic scanning after contrast administration revealed congested vessels at the periphery of the mass and heterogeneity in attenuation as a result of torsion. f, Peripheral foci of low attenuation; v, congested peripheral vessel. (From Bellah RD, Griscom NT. Torsion of normal uterine adnexa before menarche: CT appearance. AJR Am J Roentgenol 152:123–124, 1989.)

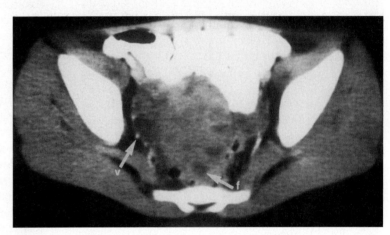

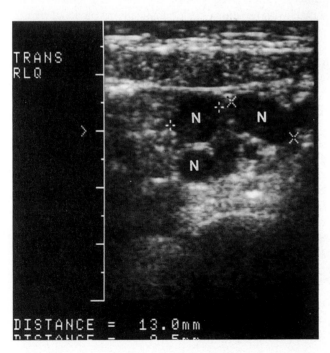

Figure 14–15

Mesenteric lymph node enlargement in an 8-year-old girl presenting with abdominal pain thought to be acute appendicitis. High-resolution sonography of the right lower quadrant shows several lymph nodes at the site of tenderness. Pain subsided with conservative management. N, Lymph node.

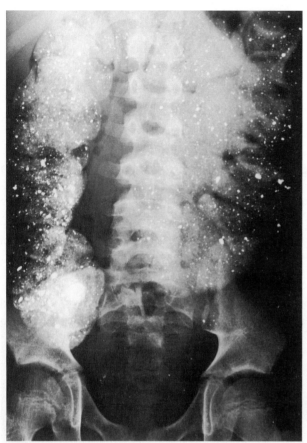

Figure 14–16
Lead intoxication, plain film. Patients with lead intoxication can present with abdominal pain, constipation, and increased intracranial pressure. The most common cause is lead-based paint, which is removed from a wall and ingested by the child. This patient, an 8-year-old boy, had ingested medication containing high quantities of lead; this medication is available in Mexico under the trade name of Azercon.

EVALUATION OF THE MOST IMPORTANT CONDITIONS CAUSING ABDOMINAL PAIN

RECURRENT FUNCTIONAL ABDOMINAL PAIN

Clinical Presentation

Recurrent functional abdominal pain is an extremely common ailment of children. In a study of 1000 unselected school children, Apley[3] noted that about 11% had some complaints of recurrent abdominal pain. In most studies of large groups of children with abdominal pain, functional abdominal pain constitutes 90% to 95% of all cases. Although this entity is well known to most pediatricians, radiologists are often less familiar with it. Functional abdominal pain is most common in children between the ages of 4 and 13 years and is slightly more frequent in girls than in boys. The characteristic feature of the syndrome is recurrent episodes of pain lasting from minutes to hours. A midline periumbilical or epigastric location is usual. A typical scenario is a child in apparently good health who has an acute onset of pain while playing; the pain is so severe that the child goes home to rest. Similarly, pain often occurs immediately before leaving for school, sometimes resulting in multiple absences from school. In contrast to other functional diseases, the pain may occur at night, awakening the child. When the painful episode ends, the child may become sleepy. Normal appetite and normal weight and growth are characteristic, in contrast to organic disease.

Other functional complaints, particularly headache, often accompany functional abdominal pain, and the family history often indicates other similarly affected family members. Results of physical examination and laboratory tests are invariably normal. Occasionally, minimal abdominal tenderness may be elicited.

There have been reports of various abnormalities producing functional abdominal pain; these include Meckel's diverticulum, superior mesenteric artery compression, and parasites. However, most authorities feel that the syndrome reflects a response to stress, with a resultant effect on the gastrointestinal tract. Studies of patients with functional pain have shown increased intestinal tonus and exaggerated response to intestinal dilatation. Other suggestions of autonomic dysfunction in these children include abnormal pupillary response to the cold pressor test and an exaggerated gastrointestinal response to neostigmine (Prostigmin). Apley's studies indicated that a child with functional abdominal pain has an equal chance of (1) becoming symptom free with time, (2) developing functional ailments of other types (such as headache), or (3) continuing into adult life with chronic gastrointestinal complaints.

Differentiation From Organic Disease

The task of the referring physician is to identify the child with functional abdominal pain, because radiologic investigation is not indicated for such pain. Findings in the child's history suggesting true organic disease include onset of pain before age 4 years or after age 13 years, pain located away from midline, genitourinary symptoms, and a family history of gastrointestinal disease (Tables 14–2 and 14–3). If there is evidence of growth failure, weight loss, fever, or abnormalities on the physical examination, radiologic investigation is indicated. Similarly, anemia, abnormal urinalysis results, or abnormal blood chemistry test results demand radiologic investigation. If the history suggests functional abdominal pain and no indicators of organic disease are present, radiologic investigation is not indicated, because the probability

TABLE 14-2 HISTORICAL FEATURES SUGGESTIVE OF ORGANIC DISEASE
Onset of pain before age 4 years or after age 13 years
Positive family history of gastrointestinal disease
Weight loss
Growth failure
Fever
Anemia
Genitourinary symptoms

TABLE 14-4 FEATURES SUGGESTIVE OF FUNCTIONAL ABDOMINAL PAIN
Age span 4 to 13 years
Normal appetite
Maintenance of normal weight and growth
Periumbilical or epigastric location of pain
Pain awakening child at night
Normal urinalysis and blood chemistries

of organic disease is extremely low (Table 14–4). In two series of children with recurrent abdominal pain evaluated by ultrasound, even the incidentally detected abnormalities present in 19% and 3.2% of patients, respectively did not account for the pain.[62,81] Abdominal sonography has evolved as the least invasive imaging modality used when there is parental pressure to "do everything." Fortunately, in this setting, the main advantage of sonography is that it is harmless. Yip et al.,[86] in their series of 644 children with recurrent abdominal pain, found abdominal abnormalities in 2% by sonography. They recommended that children with recurrent abdominal pain and atypical clinical features should have sonographic screening. If no abnormalities are found, the normal sonograms may be reassuring to parents.

MECHANICAL BOWEL OBSTRUCTION

Bowel obstruction occurs as a result of either a mechanical factor (mechanical obstruction) or lack of peristalsis (paralytic or adynamic ileus). However, in a child presenting with abdominal pain, both factors may contribute to the obstructive state. The following discussion mainly emphasizes acquired bowel obstruction beyond the neonatal period.

Common causes of mechanical bowel obstruction in childhood include intussusception (with or without lead point), incarcerated hernia, complicated acute appendicitis, and postoperative adhesions. Less common causes include

TABLE 14-3 CLINICAL FEATURES SUGGESTIVE OF ORGANIC DISEASE
Weight loss
Fever
Anemia
Abnormal urinalysis
Abnormal blood chemistries
Growth failure
Pain localization off the midline

superior mesenteric artery (cast) syndrome, volvulus around a Meckel's diverticulum, parasitic infestation, ingested foreign body, meconium ileus equivalent and fibrosing colonopathy in children with cystic fibrosis,[9] inflammatory bowel disease, and neoplasm.

Paralytic (adynamic) ileus is common after abdominal (including retroperitoneal) and spinal operation; it is often seen in response to inflammatory conditions (such as pneumonia, appendicitis, and enteritis) and after blunt trauma to the abdomen. Other causes include sepsis, metabolic (hypoglycemia and diabetic ketoacidosis) and electrolyte (potassium depletion) disturbances, medications affecting bowel motility (such as opiate narcotics), Henoch-Schönlein purpura, hemolytic-uremic syndrome, mucocutaneous lymph node syndrome, and primary intestinal pseudo-obstruction.

Clinical Presentation

Presenting clinical symptoms in children with an acute bowel obstruction vary with the etiology and the level of obstruction. In acute intestinal obstruction, abdominal distention and vomiting occur early, followed later by failure to pass flatus and stool. Pain of the spasmodic (colicky) type is usually present to a variable degree in mechanical obstruction; it is usually referred to the umbilical and epigastric regions. Severe pain often indicates a high-grade obstruction. A sudden decrease in abdominal pain accompanied by increasing systemic symptoms may indicate bowel gangrene with or without perforation. By contrast to mechanical obstruction, pain in adynamic ileus is much less prominent a symptom for the degree of distention. A high intestinal obstruction due to a mechanical cause is associated with profuse vomiting, which can result in electrolyte disturbance, ileus, and further distention.

Imaging Evaluation and Findings

Plain abdominal radiography is the imaging technique of choice in the initial evaluation of a child with a suspected bowel obstruction.[77] Supine and horizontal beam (upright or lateral decubitus) films of the abdomen are used. Apart from the bowel pattern, evidence for hernias and basal pneumonia should be looked for. Mechanical small bowel obstruction is characterized by disproportionate dilatation of the bowel proximal to the level of obstruction and paucity of air and fluid distal to the obstruction. A distal obstruction is associated with a larger number of dilated bowel loops than a proximal obstruction. Air-fluid levels are usually present with differential heights in the same bowel loop, and an orderly "step-ladder" appearance is produced on horizontal beam films when multiple loops are involved. A "string of beads" appearance may be seen when the dilated small bowel fills almost completely with fluid and traps small air bubbles along the nondependent portions of the bowel. An obstructive bowel with closed-loop strangulation may present with a pseudotumor of water density from trapped bowel contents. By contrast, paralytic ileus related to a recent abdominal operation and peritonitis is characterized by proportionate dilatation of both the small and large bowel with air-fluid levels at equal levels within the same bowel loop. A sentinel loop (localized ileus) may be seen associated with inflammation, such as acute pancreatitis and appendicitis. It is important to remember that in both mechanical or adynamic bowel obstruction, nasogastric or small bowel suctioning and repeated vomiting can reduce the amount of gas in dilated bowel loops, and when only fluid is present in these loops, confusing or subtle sausage-shaped mass shadows may be produced.

Contrast examination is only used when clinical symptoms and signs suggesting bowel obstruction are not supported by plain radiography. A contrast enema is obtained when the level of obstruction is in the colon or distal ileum and when there is no evidence of intestinal perforation (in which case water-soluble contrast material is used). A small bowel series or enteroclysis is performed when the suspected level of obstruction is higher. Attention is directed to observation of peristaltic activity (increased in mechanical obstruction until the late stages and decreased in late mechanical obstruction and adynamic ileus) and identification of a transition point between distended and normal or collapsed bowel lumen in mechanical obstruction.

Sonography can be used safely in critically ill patients with suspected small bowel obstruction when findings on plain radiography are equivocal.[59,77] Intestinal peristalsis can be observed and differentiation between mechanical and adynamic ileus may be possible, particularly when the abdomen is gasless.[60] The cause of obstruction may be determined with identification and characterization of the level of transition between dilated and collapsed bowel loops.

Although pediatric data are limited, *computed tomography* using oral and intravenous contrast material has been found to be a useful adjunct for evaluating the presence or etiology of small bowel obstruction in children.[32,77] The diagnosis of small bowel obstruction is based on the presence of a transition in the small bowel caliber or the presence of small bowel dilatation (greater than 2 to 2.5 cm) and a collapsed colon. This technique was reported to be able to identify specific causes for obstruction in 45% of patients, such as intussusception, Crohn's disease, and hernia. A proportional dilatation of the colon is consistent with an adynamic ileus. When no obvious cause for the obstruction is found, and particularly when a history of prior abdominal operation is present, adhesion is most likely the cause.

ACUTE APPENDICITIS

Epidemiology

Acute appendicitis is the most frequent indication for emergency abdominal surgery in children. The estimated incidence of appendicitis in the United States is 60,000 to 80,000 cases per year in the pediatric population.[69] Although the disease is rare in infancy, it becomes progressively more common with each year of childhood. Most cases occur in the first three decades, and the male-to-female ratio is approximately 2:1.

Acute appendicitis is produced by obstruction of the appendiceal lumen. Although many agents can be responsible, such as foreign body, lymphoid hyperplasia, and worms, the most common cause is a fecalith (appendicolith).[14] A fecalith is an inspissated fecal nidus covered with precipitates of mucus rich in calcium phosphate and produced by irritation of the mucous glands in the crypts of Lieberkühn. Intraluminal appendiceal obstruction, together with the local irritative effect of the fecalith, leads to secondary bacterial inflammation, edema, and vascular engorgement of the appendix. Compromised blood supply may produce necrosis, gangrene, and perforation with peritonitis. In milder cases, mucosal ulceration without obstruction may be evident. Bacteria can escape through an intact wall to produce peritonitis or an abscess that is locally confined by the omentum and adjacent intestine.

This sequence of events occurs more rapidly in infants and young children than in adults. Perforation may occur as rapidly as 2 hours after the onset of symptoms. The younger the child is, the greater the likelihood of perforation and diffuse peritonitis. In infants, peritonitis may be the initial clinical and radiographic sign of acute appendicitis.

Clinical Presentation

Appendicitis is more often diagnosed by the clinician than by the radiologist. The typical symptoms are abdominal pain, low-grade fever, anorexia, and vomiting. Usually the pain is initially periumbilical and fairly diffuse, reflecting visceral pain from stretching sensory receptors in the appendix (tenth thoracic dermatomes). With progression, the pain migrates to the right lower quadrant and is caused by irritation of the parietal peritoneum by the developing exudates. This is associated with focal and rebound tenderness. Concurrently, distention of the appendix initiates a vomiting reflex. Diarrhea is unusual except in patients with perforation and a pelvic abscess. Usually there is leukocytosis with a mean leukocyte count of 15,000/mm³. A clinical scoring system (MANTRELS) has been used, incorporating eight clinical and laboratory factors that have been found to be useful in making the diagnosis of appendicitis. These factors include *m*igration of pain to the right lower quadrant, *a*norexia, *n*ausea and vomiting, *t*enderness in the right lower quadrant, *r*ebound pain, *e*levated temperature, *l*eucocytosis, and a *s*hift of the white blood cell count to the left.[2]

In infants with appendicitis, the clinical manifestations are much less specific. The mother may describe only fretfulness in an infant, with a suggestion of a tender abdomen. Neonatal appendicitis has very nonspecific clinical findings. The diagnosis of neonatal appendicitis is rarely suspected until an exploratory laparotomy is done for an acute surgical abdomen.

Diagnostic delay increases morbidity and mortality. Although infertility caused by scarring of the fallopian tubes has been considered an important potential complication in girls, one study does not support this.[50]

Imaging Evaluation and Findings

Although acute appendicitis is usually diagnosed clinically, plain abdominal radiographs and contrast enema[21,58] may improve diagnostic accuracy. Sonography, CT, scintigraphy,[7,28] and MRI have increased the sensitivity and specificity of diagnosing acute appendicitis. These modalities are particularly helpful in atypical or equivocal cases. The ultimate choice of technique depends on clinical findings, local expertise, and availability of equipment.

Plain Radiographic Evaluation and Findings

Plain radiographs in appendicitis may be useful (1) to verify the diagnosis in children in whom clinical suspicion is present and the radiographs are highly diagnostic such as when an appendicolith is visible, (2) to exclude the presence of nonsurgical conditions simulating appendicitis (e.g., lower lobe pneumonitis), and (3) to exclude other surgical conditions of the abdomen masquerading as appendicitis (e.g., perforation, intussusception, and mechanical obstruction).

Most abdominal plain radiographs are normal in acute appendicitis; thus, normal radiographs do not exclude the condition. However, there are several plain film findings that, in the appropriate clinical setting, are diagnostic.[29,35,43,63,72,79,84] The younger the child is, the higher the incidence of radiographic abnormalities; this is a result of diagnostic delays in young children. Radiographic signs include the following:

1. Fecalith (Figs. 14–17 and 14–18). A calcified fecalith, varying from 5 to 20 mm in size, can be seen in 8% to 12% of patients. Detailed examination of the fecalith usually reveals a laminated calcified structure that is generally mobile when the supine and upright views are compared but may be positionally fixed in an abscess. Fecaliths can be multiple (in 30% of patients with this finding), and their alignment reflects that of the appendix. In patients with retrocecal appendices or malrotation, fecaliths lie in unusual locations. Identification of a calcified appendicolith in a child with an acute abdomen is virtually diagnostic, with a greater than 90% chance of appendicitis. The presence of an appendicolith in the setting of appendicitis increases the likelihood

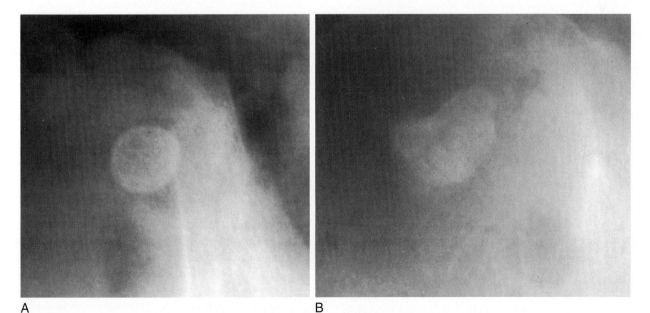

A   B

Figure 14–17
Appendicolith. Close-up views of appendicoliths in children.

Continued

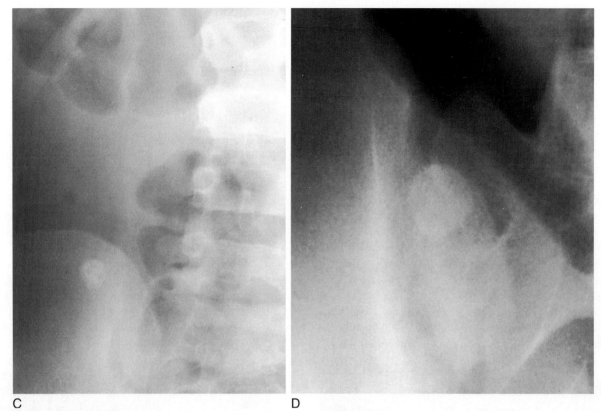

C   D

Figure 14–17—cont'd

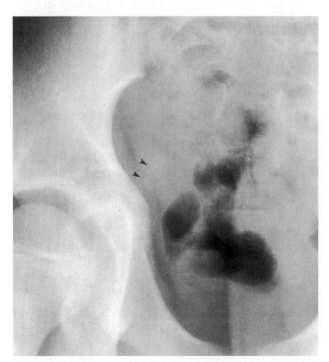

Figure 14–18
Multiple appendicoliths. Fecaliths can be multiple; this 5-year-old boy with appendicitis has two *(arrows)*. Appendicoliths are generally easily identified, but confusion may arise when they are unusually situated, as they may be in patients with malrotation or retrocecal appendices.

of complication by more than threefold, and in at least 50% of such patients, there is gangrene and perforation of the appendix. Prophylactic elective appendectomy is recommended in an asymptomatic child in whom a fecalith is identified on abdominal radiographs performed for other reasons.

2. An indistinct soft tissue mass in the right lower quadrant. With perforation and abscess formation, extraluminal air bubbles may appear within the mass. Appendiceal abscesses may also localize elsewhere in the abdomen; the cul-de-sac and subhepatic space are common sites.

3. Localized air-fluid levels in the cecum or terminal ileum on horizontal-beam views.

4. Thickening of the wall or mucosal folds of the cecum. The inflamed appendix may produce a mass indenting the cecal wall, often on the medial aspect. Inflammation of a retrocecal appendix may affect the ascending colon.

5. Mechanical small bowel obstruction. Acute small bowel obstruction sometimes accompanies acute appendicitis, especially after perforation (Fig. 14–19).

6. Paralytic ileus owing to reflex dilatation of the bowel. Marked reflex dilatation of the transverse colon and spasm of the ascending colon may result in the "colon cutoff" sign at the hepatic flexure, seen in at least 20% of children with appendiceal perforation.[78]

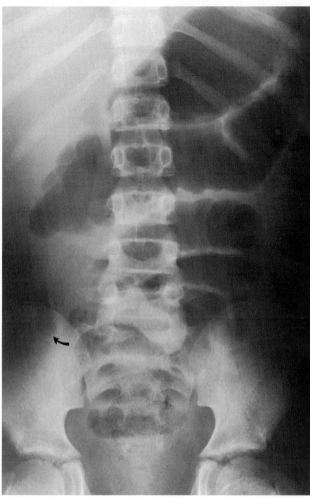

Figure 14–19
Appendicitis with mechanical small bowel obstruction. This supine radiograph of a 9-year-old boy demonstrates a mechanical bowel obstruction. Dilatation of the proximal bowel is pronounced, whereas the right lower quadrant is devoid of gas except for a small amount in a contracted cecum *(arrow)*. Colonic gas is absent.

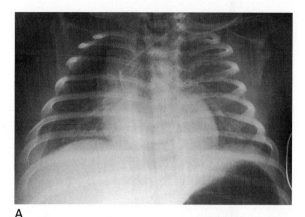

A

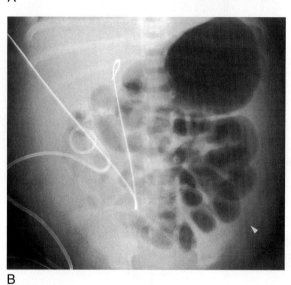

B

Figure 14–20
Neonatal appendicitis. A supine abdominal film demonstrates many of the radiographic findings common in neonates: obscuration of the right properitoneal fat line while the left one remains clearly evident *(arrowhead)*, focal abdominal wall edema, mass effect in the right lower quadrant, and ascites. Appendicitis with severe secondary peritonitis was found at autopsy.

7. Focal obliteration of the psoas margin.
8. Obliteration, complete or focal, of the properitoneal fat stripe in the right lower abdomen. In advanced cases, abdominal wall edema may be seen in the same area.
9. Right lumbar scoliosis.
10. Obliteration of pelvic fat planes around the urinary bladder and/or of the fat between the right obturator internus muscle and the intrapelvic contents; this is usually indicative of perforation.
11. Gas in the appendiceal lumen. However, this finding may also be seen in normal individuals (Figs. 14–20 and 14–21).

Sonography of the Appendix   The use of high-resolution transducers and the graded compression technique of Puylaert make it possible to directly visualize an acutely inflamed appendix in patients of any age.[1,27,37,51,66,68,82] These are currently used to increase preoperative diagnostic accuracy in atypical or equivocal presentations, thereby reducing the incidence of both negative laparotomy results (5% to 25%) and appendiceal perforation (23% to 73%) resulting from delayed diagnosis.[69]

Technique   The child's abdomen is examined with a 5- or 7.5-MHz phased linear array transducer without bowel preparation or sedation. Scanning is first performed in the transverse plane from the right upper quadrant to the right

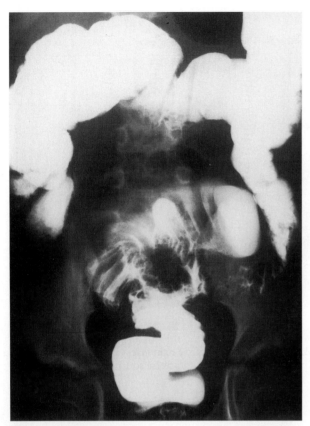

Figure 14–21
Perforative appendicitis. A 12-year-old boy with dehydration, abdominal pain, and heme-positive stools. Severe, persistent, inflammatory changes limited to the rectosigmoid region were caused by a large abscess due to appendiceal perforation.

lower quadrant of the abdomen. Graded compression is gently applied to achieve the following:

1. Displacement of most of the shadow-producing gas in the bowel
2. A decrease in distance between the transducer and intra-abdominal structures
3. Differentiation of normal compressible structures (i.e., cecum or terminal ileum) from a rigid, noncompressible, inflamed appendix

Demonstration of retroperitoneal structures such as the iliopsoas muscle and external iliac vessels indicates that compression is adequate. Care is taken not to elicit excessive tenderness or rebound tenderness with the compression maneuver. Subsequent longitudinal and oblique scans are obtained, starting laterally and progressing to the midline. The inflamed appendix is usually located medial and inferior to the tip of the cecum and anterolateral to the iliac vessels. When the appendix is retrocecal, examining the patient in the right anterior oblique position with the transducer on right flank without compression may facilitate identification.[4] A deep pelvic appendix can be examined using the suprapubic approach with the urinary bladder acting as an acoustic window.[4]

When no abnormal appendix is seen or complicated appendicitis is present, a survey of the rest of the abdomen and pelvis is performed with a 3- or 5-MHz sector transducer. Particular attention is paid to the subphrenic space, right kidney, gallbladder, portal vein, and pelvic cul-de-sac, along with the uterus, fallopian tubes, and ovaries in girls. An average examination takes 15 to 30 minutes.

An inflamed appendix is seen as a noncompressible, peristaltic, blind-ending, tubular structure when visualized along its longitudinal axis and as a "target" lesion on transverse section (Fig. 14–22).[37] The outer appendiceal diameter is usually greater than 6 mm, the maximum diameter of a normal appendix. In acute appendicitis, the appendiceal lumen is usually filled with anechoic or hypoechoic material (inflammatory exudates or pus). Hyperechoic structures with acoustic shadowing from appendicoliths may be seen in 15% to 50% of patients and are often associated with perforation (Fig. 14–23). Only one half to two thirds of appendicoliths identified by sonography can be seen on plain radiographs of the abdomen. The mucosa may be relatively intact, shaggy, or poorly defined, and the hypoechoic peripheral zone of the wall appears thickened. Echogenic foci of gas may be seen in the wall. Findings of perforation include the absence of the echogenic submucosal layer and the presence of loculated periappendiceal fluid or a mass of inhomogeneous echogenicities, interloop collections, or free peritoneal fluid or pus (Fig. 14–24).[53]

The use of color Doppler sonography has been shown to make interpretation of gray-scale sonographic findings easier and with increased confidence.[49,52] Appendiceal wall hyperemia is seen in approximately four fifths of those with nonperforated appendicitis and in 40% of those with perforated appendicitis.[52] In those with perforated appendicitis, a hyperemic, loculated periappendiceal or pelvic fluid collection appears specific for the diagnosis of an abscess.

In those with experience, the graded compression technique has sensitivity, specificity, and accuracy of more than 90% for diagnosing acute appendicitis in children. Limitations of the technique are excessive bowel gas or stool, obesity, or intolerable pain on compression. In a patient with intense pain, noncompressive sonography with the transducer placed in various positions can sometimes be useful.[4]

Conventional abdominal sonography is used to diagnose complications of acute appendicitis (including rare complications such as liver abscess and pyelophlebitis with portal vein thrombosis and portal hypertension)[70] and to exclude conditions that may clinically mimic the disease, such as ovarian torsion, ureteric calculus with obstructive hydroureteronephrosis, and adolescent pelvic inflammatory disease. Alternative diagnoses, usually gastrointestinal and gynecologic in nature, can be established in up to 25% to 30% of those referred for suspected appendicitis who do not have appendicitis.[64] Sonography is important in image-guided interventional drainage of appendiceal abscesses in children.[34]

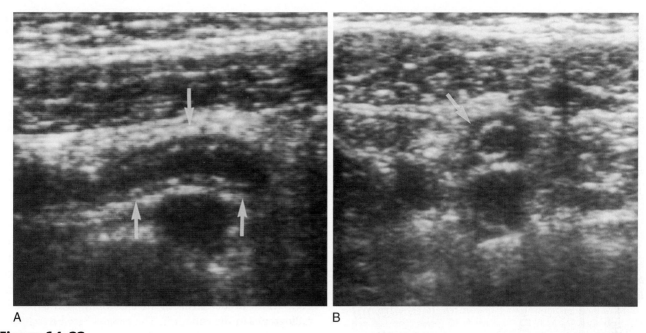

A   B

Figure 14–22

Acute appendicitis in an 18-year-old boy with right lower quadrant pain. *A,* A longitudinal scan of the right iliac fossa shows a blind-ending tubular structure *(arrows).* No peristalsis or compressibility was present during examination. *B,* A transverse scan of the appendicitis shows its "target" appearance *(arrow)* with a fluid-filled lumen.

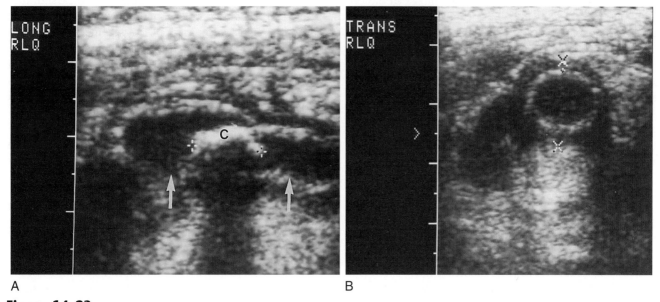

A   B

Figure 14–23

Appendicolith in acute appendicitis with perforation: sonography. *A,* A longitudinal view of the appendix *(arrows)* shows a large hyperechoic structure *(cursors)* in the lumen with distal acoustic shadowing caused by an appendicolith. *B,* A transverse section of the appendix shows a fluid-distended lumen *(cursors)* with a periappendiceal collection as a result of a local perforation. C, Calcification.

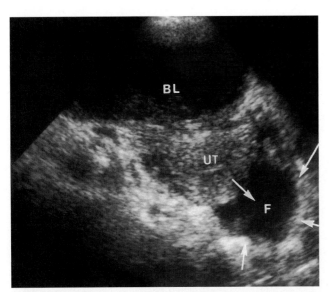

Figure 14–24
Perforative acute appendicitis in a 14-year-old girl: sonography. This transverse scan shows free peritoneal fluid *(arrows)* in the pelvis behind and to the left of the uterus. BL, Bladder; F, fluid; UT, uterus.

Computed Tomography   CT has been shown to be useful in the detection and diagnosis of acute appendicitis and its complications in adults. Experience in children has been limited owing to the wide use of sonography in the last decade.[5,33] However, the utility of CT has increased rapidly in the past few years with studies comparing its accuracy to that of sonography.[22,41,44,67] In a pediatric study, helical CT was found to have a significantly higher sensitivity and accuracy than sonography in the diagnosis of appendicitis, particularly in children older than 10 years of age.[67] In another study comparing unenhanced limited abdominal CT to sonography, the sensitivity, specificity, and accuracy were almost equal.[41] In a prospective study, radiologists were found to be more confident in their interpretation of CT than of sonography.[23]

CT preparation and scanning techniques have not been standardized. Variations include whether or not to use oral, rectal, or intravenous contrast media, the area of the abdomen scanned, and the thickness of collimation in the acquisition of images.[54] Scanning without contrast medium has the advantages of speed and simplicity at the expense of slightly decreased accuracy and negative predictive rate.[41,54] The use of oral contrast medium eliminates the diagnostic problem of confusing small bowel loops with the appendix, a phlegmon, or an abscess. Intravenous contrast medium helps in the identification of an enhancing appendiceal wall owing to inflammation and hyperemia and detection of the presence and extent of an abscess or an inflammatory mass. The use of rectal contrast medium assists in the visualization of a normal appendix (normal appendix visualized in 73% to 82%) and in the detection of cecal apical changes that are specific

for appendicitis.[44] Scanning a limited area reduces the radiation dose to the patient but has the disadvantage of possibly missing an alternative diagnosis. Thin-section collimation (5 mm) enhances the ability to trace a normal appendix in its entirety from the base to its blind-ending tip (Figs. 14–25, 14–26, and 14–27).

On CT, the normal appendix, varying in size between 3 and 8 mm (mean 6 mm), is tubular or ring-like and may be collapsed, air-filled, or fluid-filled.[54] Abnormal CT findings in appendicitis vary with the type and severity of the pathologic process. In milder appendicitis, the appendix, if visualized, may be only slightly distended (8 to 12 mm diameter) with wall thickening present. Periappendiceal inflammation is evidenced by linear fat stranding, local fascial thickening, and clouding of the adjacent mesentery. In more advanced appendicitis, the appendix may be fragmented, destroyed, and replaced by a phlegmon or an abscess with associated mesenteric inflammation. Abscesses distant from the cecal region may be detected. An appendicolith, seen by CT in 25% to 65% of patients with acute appendicitis, has a positive predictive value of 74% and a negative predictive value of 26%.[40] Finding an appendicolith on CT is not sufficiently specific to be the sole basis for the diagnosis of acute appendicitis. In perforative appendicitis, extraluminal gas may be seen in the retroperitoneal space or, rarely, free in the intraperitoneal cavity (Figs. 14–28 through 14–31).

Despite the high sensitivity, specificity, and accuracy of helical CT in the diagnosis of acute appendicitis, routine use is not recommended owing to concerns of higher cost, radiation exposure, and risk of contrast medium administration.[67] At the present time, its use should be limited to patients in whom sonography is inconclusive and to those with perforative appendicitis, for which sonography has lower sensitivity (38% to 55%).[8,53] CT can also be used to guide percutaneous abscess drainage as an alternative to immediate operative intervention.

Magnetic Resonance Imaging of Appendicitis
Experience using MRI in the diagnosis of acute appendicitis in children is limited. In one study of unenhanced MRI performed after sonography, nonperforated acute appendicitis appeared as a markedly hyperintense center, a slightly hyperintense thickened wall, and markedly hyperintense periappendiceal tissue on a T2-weighted ultra turbo spin-echo sequence.[30] Unenhanced axial T2-weighted spin-echo imaging was found to be the most sensitive sequence. Currently, cost and availability limit routine use of MRI.

CROHN'S DISEASE

Epidemiology and Pathology

In approximately 15% to 20% of patients with Crohn's disease (regional enteritis), the onset of symptoms occurs

Text continued on page 488

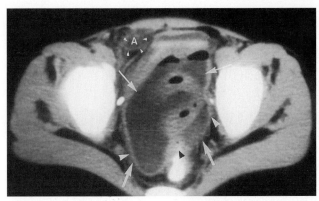

Figure 14–25
Perforative acute appendicitis with pelvic abscess in an 8-year-old boy. This CT scan of the pelvis shows a large pelvic abscess *(arrows* and *arrowheads)* and an inflamed appendix located to the right of the bladder and posterior to the right rectus abdominis muscle. A, Appendix.

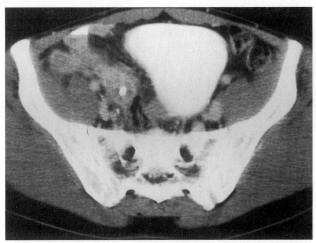

Figure 14–26
Appendicolith is seen within dilated appendix. The mass effect of appendiceal inflammation indents the bladder in this 13-year-old boy.

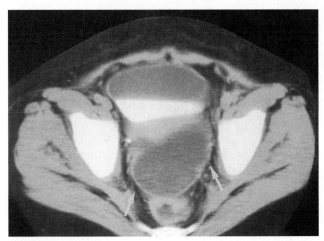

Figure 14–27
Large fluid collection *(arrows)* posterior to the bladder caused by an appendiceal perforation. CT is the modality of choice in appendicitis when percutaneous abscess drainage is being considered.

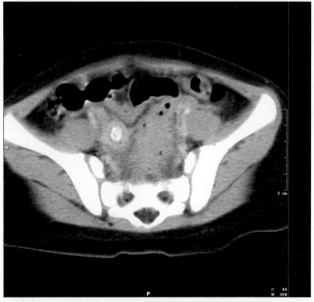

A

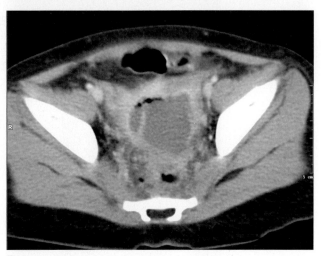

B

Figure 14–28
Appendicitis. *A,* Axial image with intravenous but no oral or rectal contrast medium. There is a large appendicolith and edema of the wall of the appendix. *B,* Axial image lower in the pelvis. A large fluid collection with rim enhancement and a small amount of air are seen. The diagnosis is ruptured appendix with a pelvic abscess.

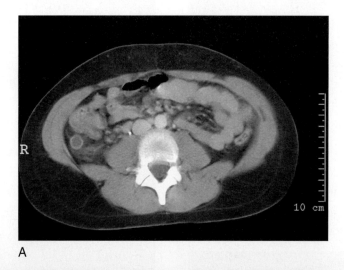

A

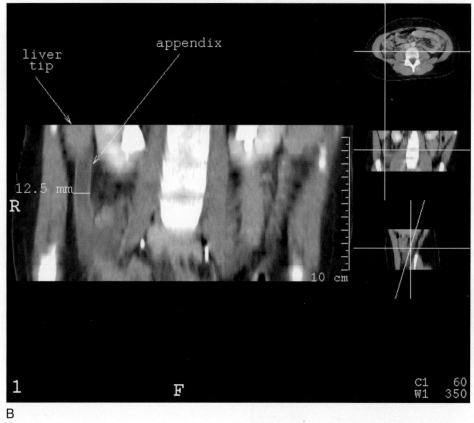

B

Figure 14–29

Appendicitis. *A*, Enlarged appendix (12.5 mm) posterior to the cecum with rim enhancement and edema in the adjacent fat. *B*, Oblique coronal reformation reveals an enlarged appendix that extends to the inferior margin of the liver.

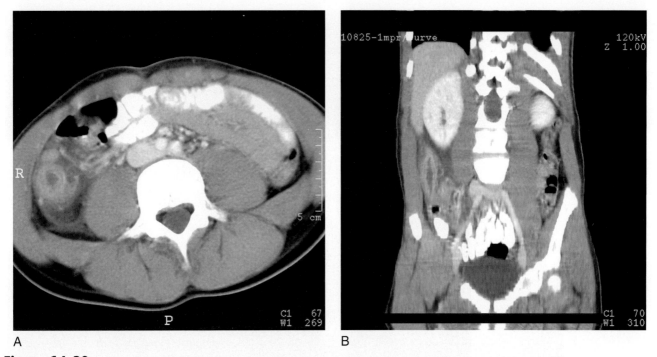

A

B

Figure 14–30
Appendicitis. Marked thickening of the wall of the appendix and edema of the adjacent fat in axial (A) and coronal refornet (B) images.

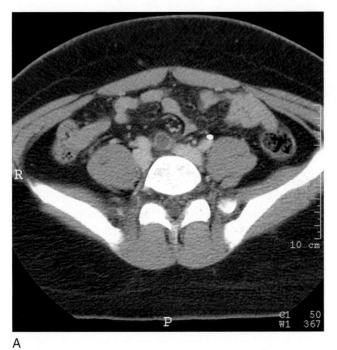

A

Figure 14–31
Appendicitis. *A*, Enlarged appendix (12.9 mm) near the midline with the mild periappendiceal edema.

Continued

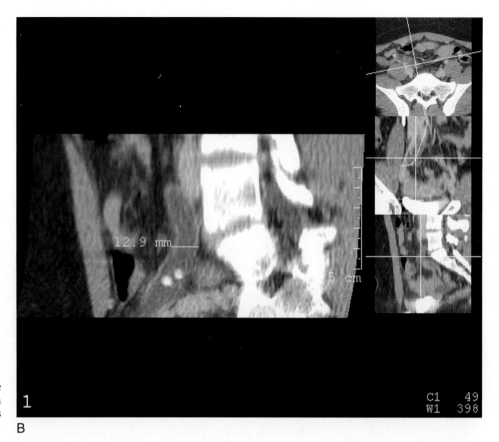

Figure 14–31—cont'd
B, Parasagittal reformation. The enlarged curvilinear appendix with two appendicoliths in the lumen is seen.

B

in childhood. The disease has been reported in children of all ages, but most cases are in children 10 years of age or older. The disease affects both sexes equally but is more common in whites, particularly Jews, and in families with known inflammatory bowel disease.[38]

The etiology of regional enteritis is unknown. There is some evidence of a transmissible agent, but no specific infectious organism has yet been found. Immune factors in affected individuals are probably relevant. It is uncertain whether the clustering of the disease in families indicates genetic factors or familial exposure to an unknown organism or agent. Emotional factors are important in exacerbation of symptoms in some cases but are not thought to be etiologic.

The pathologic characteristics of regional enteritis vary according to the stage of the disease in the area examined. Characteristic findings include focal, transmural, noncaseating granulomas. As the disease progresses, there may be luminal narrowing, with fibrosis of the involved bowel and deep ulcers extending into adjacent organs. The mucosa may be normal or may show minimal changes with ulcers and surrounding edema. Eventually, a "cobblestone" mucosa develops, formed by crisscrossing linear ulcers. The involvement may be asymmetric in a given loop of bowel, and "skip" areas of interposed normal bowel are frequent. Fistula formation occurs in 30% of patients.

The anatomic location of Crohn's disease in children is different from that in adults. In one series, 20% of patients had diffuse small bowel disease, 50% had both small and large bowel involvement, 20% had isolated terminal ileum involvement, and only 10% had isolated colonic disease.[25] In contrast to adults, involvement of the terminal ileum in children is not universal. Other sites of Crohn's disease in children are rare, but gastric, duodenal, and esophageal sites may be seen.

Clinical Presentation

The presenting clinical features of Crohn's disease in children also differ somewhat from those in adults. About one third of patients present with systemic symptoms, including arthritis, growth failure, delayed sexual maturation, fever of unknown origin, and anorexia nervosa. Less frequent systemic presentations include unexplained anemia, recurrent urinary tract infection, and dermatologic disorders.

In most children, the initial symptoms of Crohn's disease are related to the gastrointestinal tract. Abdominal pain is often the first or only symptom, occurring in about 80% of patients. The characteristics of the pain are nonspecific, with no typical diagnostic locations or types. Diarrhea, although present in about three fourths of the affected children, is usually mild. Anorexia may be a predominant feature, particularly in adolescents. In some instances, perianal disease without other gastrointestinal symptoms may be the presenting complaint. Blood in the stool can be detected in 40% of affected children.

This discussion does not include acute regional enteritis (acute Crohn's disease), which, as its name implies, is an acute syndrome resembling appendicitis. Laparotomy on these patients shows acute inflammation and edema of the ileum, sometimes with mesenteric adenopathy. This syndrome is currently thought to be different from Crohn's disease and often may be bacterial in origin; it resolves spontaneously. Occasionally it is difficult to distinguish this condition from exacerbations of Crohn's disease.

Possible complications of Crohn's disease are myriad, but in most series they are infrequent. In general, those complications associated with long duration of disease (i.e., obstruction, liver disease, and carcinoma) are uncommon in pediatric patients. As mentioned earlier, perianal fistulae are relatively common. Fistulae occurring in other areas of the gastrointestinal tract are found most often in the ileocolic region, usually following long-standing disease or surgery. Extraintestinal complications include growth failure, arthritis, gallstones, renal calculi, and hydronephrosis (Figs. 14–32, 14–33, and 14–34).

Radiographic Evaluation and Findings

Despite the increasing use of endoscopy in gastrointestinal diagnosis, radiographic examination remains important in managing Crohn's disease in children.[17,74] Plain abdominal radiographs may show mucosal abnormality in the colon and small bowel, an abnormal soft tissue mass in the right iliac region, or evidence of small bowel obstruction. Because feces do not accumulate adjacent to inflamed bowel, affected areas are typically devoid of stool. The increased peristalsis propels the stool distal to the site of involvement.

Technique   Further radiographic evaluation of a child with suspected Crohn's disease requires examination of the part of the bowel in which disease is clinically suspected.

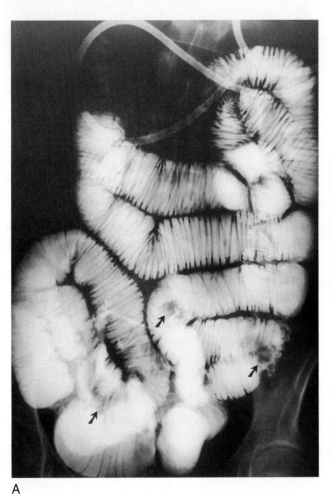
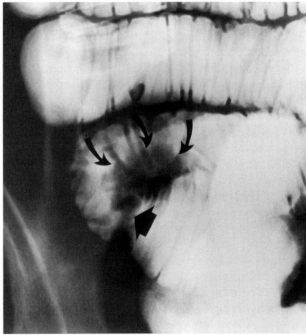

A

B

Figure 14–32
Crohn's disease demonstrated by enteroclysis. Results of a standard antegrade barium study had been normal in this 15-year-old patient. *A,* Focal, distal jejunal, and ileal disease is evident on this overhead radiograph *(arrows). B,* This ileal spot film demonstrates probable aphthous ulcers, eccentric nodular mucosa *(small arrows),* and luminal narrowing *(broad arrow).* The findings are characteristic of regional enteritis.

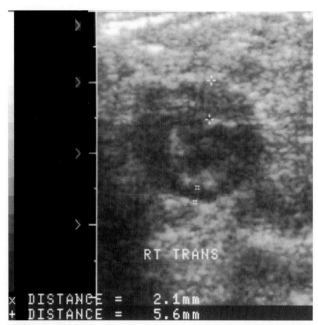

Figure 14–33
Crohn's disease: sonography. This patient, a 13-year-old boy, presented with abdominal pain and diarrhea. The right lower quadrant sonogram shows asymmetric thickening of the bowel wall *(cursors)* with a "target" appearance on transverse section.

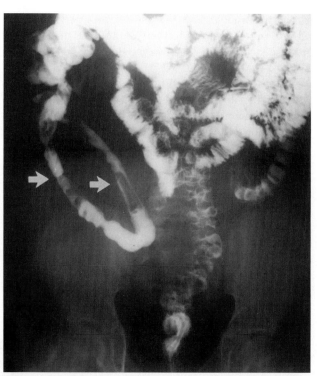

Figure 14–34
Crohn's disease: antegrade small bowel examination. This patient, a 15-year-old boy, presented with abdominal pain, anorexia, and weight loss. There is marked separation of the terminal ileal loops *(arrows)* with luminal narrowing owing to thickening of the bowel wall and adjacent mesentery.

If esophageal, gastric, or duodenal involvement is suspected, a double-contrast barium study or endoscopy is the examination of choice.

The small bowel is usually studied by an antegrade examination following barium study of the upper gastrointestinal tract (small bowel follow-through). It is important to use large amounts of barium; we customarily use 16 oz in teenagers. Serial films of the abdomen are taken after ingestion of barium. It is important that each film be examined by the radiologist as the study progresses so that fluoroscopy and spot filming may be performed if suspicious areas are identified. Because Crohn's disease is the cause of organic abdominal pain in children more frequently than is peptic ulcer disease, it is essential to examine the small bowel distal to the duodenum in patients being examined for peptic ulcer disease.

A standard examination for Crohn's disease includes serial radiographs of the abdomen with spot filming of the terminal ileum and ileocecal valve after the upper gastrointestinal series. Insufflation of air through the rectum in conjunction with the small bowel examination (peroral pneumocolon) has been advocated when the terminal ileum is poorly visualized or when an equivocal fistula from the terminal ileum is seen.[76]

If there is a high index of suspicion of small bowel disease, *enteroclysis* is a more valuable procedure. In enteroclysis, a tube is placed at the approximate level of the ligament of Treitz, and dilute barium is infused under fluoroscopic control.

This produces rapid but controlled filling and distention of small bowel and offers greater accuracy in detection of anatomic abnormality. It is important to place the tube distal in the duodenum, particularly in younger children. Otherwise, there is considerable reflux of barium into the stomach, with the attendant hazards of reflux and aspiration. We avoid this procedure in small infants because of the risk of water intoxication. Enteroclysis is used in the following three situations:

1. As the initial investigation in a child with strong clinical evidence of Crohn's disease
2. In a patient in whom the standard antegrade examination is equivocal
3. As a staging procedure for a child with demonstrated Crohn's disease

Because the ileocecal region is affected most often in pediatric Crohn's disease, contrast examinations of both small and large bowel are often required. The colon is best evaluated by double-contrast barium enema or colonoscopy.

Radiographic findings of regional enteritis are the same in adults and in children (see Fig. 14–34). Minimal changes are loss of definition of mucosal folds, perhaps with aphthous ulcers, and thickening of the bowel wall. Moderate disease is characterized by a cobblestone mucosa, rigidity of the bowel wall, and considerable thickening of the adjacent mesentery.

In advanced Crohn's disease, stenosis with loss of mucosal folds may be present. Because regional enteritis can affect more than one segment of bowel, the entire small and large bowel must be evaluated. Skip areas and eccentric involvement of diseased regions are common.

The differential diagnosis of Crohn's disease affecting the small bowel includes all entities that produce focal involvement of the jejunum and ileum. Other types of inflammation can be secondary to pancreatitis, appendicitis, intestinal tuberculosis, or other infection. Tumor, particularly lymphosarcoma, must also be considered. Traumatic disorders with focal disease of the small bowel include hematoma, ischemic stricture, and Henoch-Schönlein purpura. Occasionally, collagen disease in children can manifest as focal involvement of the small bowel. In the colon, the disease must be differentiated from ulcerative colitis.

Other Imaging Techniques

The use of high-resolution compression sonography has made it possible to directly visualize thickening of bowel (i.e., the target appearance on transverse section) in Crohn's disease (see Fig. 14–33).[39] The affected bowel also shows decreased peristalsis and loss of normal compressibility on real-time examination. The demonstration of abscess or fistula in association with bowel wall thickening and conglomeration strongly suggests the diagnosis of Crohn's disease. Some studies have shown that the extent of involvement is often underestimated, especially in early disease. In addition, the correlation between sonographic patterns and clinical activity is controversial. Although the role of sonography in screening and follow-up remains to be defined,[26,48,71] recent preliminary studies using color Doppler sonography have shown that vessel density in the diseased bowel, in addition to wall thickening (more than 3 to 5 mm), reflects the activity of the disease.[57,73]

CT, despite its ability to show thickened bowel loops and abscesses, is best reserved for patients in whom sonography results are equivocal and when CT-guided drainage of an abscess is contemplated.[31] Although MRI has been used in pediatric inflammatory bowel diseases (including use for identification of perianal involvement), colonoscopy with biopsy remains the most accurate tool for determination of the type and severity of inflammation.[12]

Although indium In 111–labeled and technetium Tc 99m hexamethylpropylene amine oxime (HMPAO)–labeled leukocyte scans have been used in the evaluation of Crohn's disease, their exact role has yet to be determined.[6,20,56]

PEPTIC ULCER DISEASE

Although peptic ulcer disease has become more widely recognized as a diagnostic consideration in the pediatric age group, it remains an uncommon entity in children. Few pediatric centers have more than five new cases per year, with an approximate incidence of 1 per 2500 hospital admissions.[11,65]

Peptic ulcer disease has generally been subdivided into primary and secondary types.[46] Primary ulcer occurs without an underlying systemic disease. Secondary, or stress, ulcer occurs in the presence of chronic systemic disease (e.g., renal failure, chronic pulmonary disease, cirrhosis, collagen vascular disease, chronic pancreatitis, cystic fibrosis, hyperparathyroidism, mastocytosis, multiple endocrine adenoma syndrome, and Zollinger-Ellison syndrome) or stress or in association with the use of ulcerogenic medications.

Primary Peptic Ulcer Disease

Although stress ulcers may occur in older children and adolescents, the majority of peptic ulcers in patients in these age groups (especially those older than 10 years of age) are primary, with a predominance of duodenal ulcers in most series. Peptic ulcer has been recognized with increasing frequency after the increased use of flexible endoscopy as a diagnostic and therapeutic procedure in children with upper gastrointestinal problems. Primary peptic ulcers are found more frequently in Anglo-Saxon, Scandinavian, and Eastern European children. Also of note are a male predominance and an increased incidence in those with type O blood or a positive family history for peptic ulcer disease in first-degree relatives.

The etiology of primary ulcer disease in children is thought to be the same as that in adults. Important factors include the effects of the aggressive forces of luminal acid and pepsin against the inherent gastric and duodenal mucosal defense, a genetic predisposition, psychologic factors, and the presence of *Helicobacter pylori* (also known as *Campylobacter pylori*), spiral gram-negative bacteria that colonize in the gastric surface mucous cells.[13,24,55,80,85] In addition to causing about one third of gastroduodenal ulcers, this bacteria has been found to be associated with various forms of gastritis (acute purulent, chronic, and nodular with lymphoid hyperplasia), duodenitis, duodenal gastric surface metaplasia, and disorders of the D cell–G cell axis, resulting in hypergastrinemia.[55]

Secondary Peptic Ulcer Disease

In neonates, the majority of ulcers of the upper gastrointestinal tract are stress ulcers, which occur in a clinical setting of prematurity and hypoxia. Gastric ulcers (stress ulcers) are more common than duodenal ulcers.

During infancy and early childhood, stress ulcers again account for more than 80% of peptic ulcer disease and are associated with shock, respiratory failure, sepsis, severe burns (Curling's ulcer), intracranial lesions (Cushing's ulcer), and the use of aspirin or other nonsteroidal anti-inflammatory medications. Gastric and duodenal ulcers are in this category.

Clinical Presentation

The clinical features of peptic ulcer disease in children are unlike those in adults. In neonates, who predominantly have secondary stress ulcers, hemorrhage and perforation are the main presentations. In infants, vomiting, sometimes associated with hematemesis, is the usual feature. In older children with primary disease, pain is more prominent, although it is still frequently accompanied by vomiting. The pain is chronic and recurrent and may be poorly localized or localized either to the epigastrium or to atypical sites such as the right lower quadrant. In contrast to adults, children with ulcer pain frequently have difficulty describing their pain, and the pain may be unaffected by or increased or decreased with food. The pain syndrome has a periodicity similar to that in adults, with symptoms lasting for 2 to 7 days, followed by several days of relief. Additional symptoms include heartburn and flatulence. In children with secondary gastric ulcers, vomiting and hematemesis are more common than recurrent abdominal pain. Physical examination is usually unrewarding. Melena may be found in some instances.

Radiographic Evaluation

Radiographic evaluation of peptic ulcer disease in children is similar to that in adults. The primary problem is selecting those patients who require thorough radiographic investigation—that is, differentiating the child with suspected ulcer from children with the much more common functional abdominal pain. With the advent of flexible endoscopy, the role of radiography has decreased. Single-contrast examinations are less accurate than endoscopy and may have a high incidence of false-positive results. There are few data comparing double-contrast radiography with endoscopy in children. Nevertheless, radiographic evaluation is more easily performed, as it does not require sedation, anesthesia, or intubation and may provide ancillary information about the upper gastrointestinal tract that may account for the pain.

Technique   When performing a single-contrast barium examination, we customarily expose spot films of the filled gastric antrum and both curvatures in prone and upright positions, along with mucosal relief spot films of the same areas. In adults, double-contrast examination of the stomach is usually performed to diagnose shallow gastric ulcers. This examination may be of similar value in appropriate pediatric patients, but its utility in such children has not been studied extensively.

In a child in whom a duodenal ulcer is a serious consideration, we expose eight spot films of the duodenum. The first two are taken with the child prone, one with and one without compression of the duodenal bulb. Four upright spot films of the filled duodenal bulb are then exposed: two in the right anterior oblique position (with and without compression), one in the left anterior oblique position, and one in the right anterior oblique position with maximal filling of the entire duodenum. We than expose at least two air-contrast spot films of the duodenal bulb with the patient in a supine left posterior oblique position. Equivocal studies may be repeated using a double-contrast technique and paralysis of the proximal bowel with glucagon.

Radiographic Findings

In a sick child with a perforated peptic ulcer, plain radiographs of the abdomen may demonstrate free intraperitoneal gas. The site of leakage may be confirmed using iso-osmolar, water-soluble contrast media.

The radiographic findings in peptic ulcer in children are identical to those in adults (Figs. 14–35 and 14–36). The ulcer crater, seen as an outpouching from the gastric or duodenal wall on single-contrast studies, varies from 1 mm to 1 cm in size; larger ulcers are rare. Convergence of mucosal folds toward the ulcer site may be seen. Deformity of the duodenal bulb, which is characteristic of peptic disease, is presumptive evidence of an ulcer, either past or present, but the crater itself should be identified for definitive diagnosis.

Endoscopic studies have indicated that duodenitis is often associated with peptic ulcer. Duodenitis is characterized endoscopically by mucosal edema and inflammation, but the relationship of these findings to the radiographic findings of prominent duodenal mucosa is undetermined.

Differential diagnosis of peptic ulcer disease in children includes findings that are also seen in normal children. A child's duodenal bulb seldom fills to the same extent as that of an adult, and rapid emptying is the rule. This does not suggest peptic disease. Similarly, pylorospasm is a frequent phenomenon in children undergoing barium examination and is usually not related to ulcer disease. In some patients, the common bile duct indents the duodenal bulb, particularly on its greater curvature aspect and thereby resembles the deformity of peptic ulcer.

Radiographic evaluation of a child who has undergone previous surgery for peptic ulcer disease is similar to that of an adult, with special attention given to areas of surgical deformity and anastomosis.

Other Imaging Techniques

High-resolution sonography can detect gastric or duodenal wall thickening and ulcer; however, it has not been reliable enough to be used routinely.[10,75] The role of technetium Tc 99m sucralfate scanning in the localization of gastric ulcers has not been defined.

▌SUMMARY

In children, abdominal pain is a common symptom that may reflect disease unrelated to the gastrointestinal tract. In older children, functional abdominal pain is much more common than organic disease. The clinical history, physical examination, and clinical laboratory findings can usually distinguish between functional and organic disease, thus suggesting which patients require radiologic evaluation.

When radiographic examination of the upper gastrointestinal tract is warranted, small bowel examination should be included to evaluate the possibility of Crohn's disease.

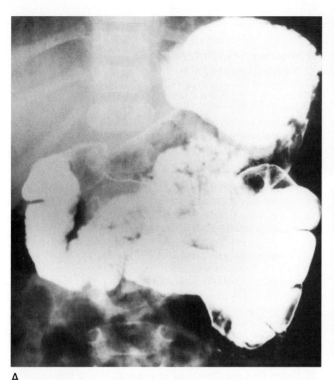
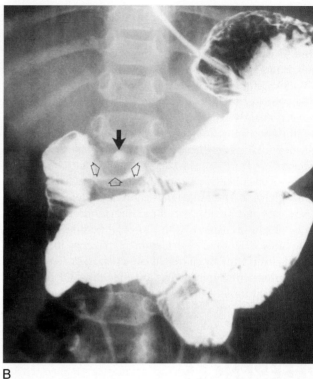

A   B

Figure 14–35
Duodenal ulcer masked by positioning in a 3-year-old boy with recurrent midepigastric pain and vomiting. *A,* An air-contrast study of the distal antrum and duodenal bulb appears normal while the patient is supine. *B,* A prone radiograph of the barium-filled distal antrum and duodenal bulb reveals a typical duodenal ulcer crater *(solid arrow)* with extensive surrounding edema *(open arrows)*. The crater was hidden on the supine view because it was located on the anterior duodenal wall.

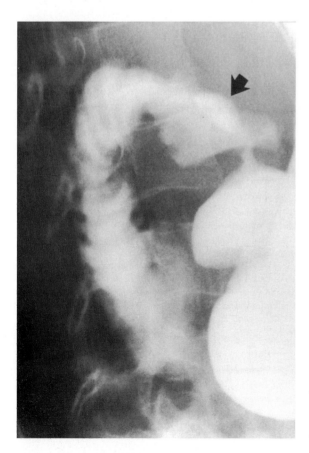

Figure 14–36
Duodenal ulcer in an 8-year-old boy who presented with recurrent bouts of abdominal pain accentuated by eating and accompanied by nausea and vomiting. Features suggestive of organic disease were a positive family history of peptic ulcer disease and failure to maintain normal growth. This upright spot film of the duodenal bulb demonstrates an ulcer crater *(arrow)* that extends beyond the confines of the duodenal lumen.

Peptic ulcer disease, although a common cause of pain in the adult, is rare in children.

With careful attention to the plain radiographic pattern of the bowel gas, differentiation between mechanical bowel obstruction and adynamic ileus is possible. Contrast examination, sonography, and CT may be used in patients with equivocal findings or when a specific cause for an obstruction is sought.

Acute appendicitis is a common disease in children and young adults. Its clinical manifestations are often confusing in neonates and infants. Barium examination of the colon can be helpful in patients with equivocal findings but very rarely adds diagnostic information in patients in whom appendicitis is strongly suggested clinically. High-resolution compression sonography and helical abdominal CT provide direct visualization of the inflamed appendix and are most useful in children with atypical presentations of appendicitis.

REFERENCES

1. Abu-Yousef MM, Franken EA Jr. An overview of graded compression sonography in the diagnosis of acute appendicitis. Semin Ultrasound CT MR 10:352–363, 1989.
2. Alvarado A. A practical score for the early diagnosis of acute appendicitis. Ann Emerg Med 15:557–564, 1986.
3. Apley J. The Child with Abdominal Pains. 2nd ed. Oxford, England: Blackwell Scientific Publications, 1975.
4. Baldisserotto M, Marchiori E. Accuracy of noncompressive sonography of children with appendicitis according to the potential positions of the appendix. AJR Am J Roentgenol 175:1387–1892, 2000.
5. Balthazar EJ, Gordon RB. CT of appendicitis. Semin Ultrasound CT MR 10:326–340, 1989.
6. Barabino A, Gattorno M, Cabria M, et al. 99mTc-white cell scanning to detect gut inflammation in children with inflammatory bowel diseases or spondyloarthropathies. Clin Exp Rheumatol 16:327–334, 1998.
7. Barron B, Hanna C, Passalaqua AM, Lamki L, Wegener WA, Goldenberg DM. Rapid diagnostic imaging of acute, nonclassic appendicitis by leukoscintigraphy with sulesomab, a technetium 99m-labeled antigraulocyte antibody Fab' fragment. Surgery 125:288–296, 1999.
8. Birnbaum BA, Wilson SR. Appendicitis at the millennium. Radiology 215:337–348, 2000.
9. Crisci KL, Greenberg SB, Wolfson BJ, Geller E, Vinocur CD. Contrast enema findings of fibrosing colonopathy. Pediatr Radiol 27:315–316, 1997.
10. Derchi LE, Ierace T, DePra L, Solbiati L, Rizzatto G, Musante F. The sonographic appearance of duodenal lesions. J Ultrasound Med 5:269–293, 1986.
11. Drumm B, Rhoads JM, Stringer DA, Sherman PM, Ellis LE, Durie PR. Peptic ulcer disease in children: Etiology, clinical findings, and clinical course. Pediatrics 82:410–414, 1988.
12. Durno CA, Sherman P, Williams T, Shuckett B, Dupuis A, Griffiths AM. Magnetic resonance imaging to distinguish the type and severity of pediatric inflammatory bowel diseases. J Pediatr Gastroenterol Nutr 30:170–174, 2000.
13. Ernst PB, Gold BD. *Helicobacter pylori* in childhood: New insights into the immunopathogenesis of gastric disease and implications for managing infection in children. J Pediatr Gastroenterol Nutr 28:462–473, 1999.
14. Faegenburg D. Fecaliths of the appendix: Incidence and significance. AJR Am J Roentgenol 89:752–759, 1963.
15. Franken EA Jr, Kao SCS, Smith WL, Sato Y. Imaging of the acute abdomen in infants and children. AJR Am J Roentgenol 153:921–928, 1989.
16. Franken EA Jr, Smith WL. Gastrointestinal Imaging in Pediatrics. New York: Harper & Row, 1982.
17. Franken EA Jr, Smith JA, Fitzgerald J. Regional enteritis in children: Clinical and roentgen features. CRC Crit Rev Diagn Imaging 10:163–185, 1977.
18. Franken EA Jr, Smith JA, Smith WL. Radiology of abdominal pain in children. Appl Radiol 8:29–36, 1979.
19. Frimann-Dahl J. Roentgen Examination in Acute Abdominal Diseases. 3rd ed. Springfield, IL: Charles C Thomas, 1974.
20. Froelich JW, Field SA. The role of indium-111 white blood cells in inflammatory bowel disease. Semin Nucl Med 18:300–307, 1988.
21. Garcia C, Rosenfield NS. The barium enema in the diagnosis of acute appendicitis. Semin Ultrasound CT MR 10:314–320, 1989.
22. Garcia Peña BM, Mandl KD, Kraus SJ, et al. Ultrasonography and limited computed tomography in the diagnosis and management of appendicitis in children. JAMA 282:1041–1046, 1999.
23. Garcia Peña BM, Taylor GA. Radiologists' confidence in interpretation of sonography and CT in suspected pediatric appendicitis. AJR Am J Roentgenol 175:71–74, 2000.
24. Grahm DY. Campylobacter pylori and peptic ulcer disease. Gastroenterology 96:615–625, 1989.
25. Gryboski JD, Spiro HM. Prognosis in children with Crohn's disease. Gastroenterology 74:807–817, 1978.
26. Haber HP, Busch A, Ziebach R, Stern M. Bowel wall thickness measured by ultrasound as a marker of Crohn's disease activity in children. Lancet 355:1239–1240, 2000.
27. Hahn HB, Hoepner FU, Kalle T, et al. Sonography of acute appendicitis in children: 7 years experience. Pediatr Radiol 28:147–151, 1998.
28. Henneman PL, Marcus CS, Inkelis SH, Butler JA, Baumgartner FJ. Evaluation of children with possible appendicitis using technetium 99m leukocyte scan. Pediatrics 85:838–843, 1990.
29. Hilton SvW, Edwards DK. Plain film findings of appendicitis in the neonate and premature infant. Presented at the 24th Annual Meeting of the Society for Pediatric Radiology, San Francisco, March 1981.
30. Hormann M, Paya K, Eibenberger K, et al. MR imaging in children with nonperforated acute appendicitis: Value of unenhanced MR imaging in sonographically selected cases. AJR Am J Roentgenol 171:467–470, 1998.
31. Hyer W, Beattie RM, Walker-Smith JA, NcLean A. Computed tomography in chronic inflammatory bowel disease. Arch Dis Child 76:428–431, 1997.
32. Jabra AA, Fishman EK. Small bowel obstruction in the pediatric patient: CT evaluation. Abdom Imaging 22:466–470, 1997.
33. Jabra AA, Shalaby-Rana EI, Fishman EK. CT of appendicitis in children. J Comput Assist Tomogr 21:661–666, 1997.
34. Jamieson DH, Chait PG, Filler R. Interventional drainage of appendiceal abscesses in children. AJR Am J Roentgenol 169:1619–1622, 1997.
35. Johnson JF, Coughlin WF. Plain film diagnosis of appendiceal perforation in children. Semin Ultrasound CT MR 10:306–313, 1989.
36. Jones PF. The acute abdomen in infancy and childhood. Practitioner 222:373–378, 1979.
37. Kao SCS, Smith WL, Abu-Yousef MM, et al. Acute appendicitis in children: Sonographic findings. AJR Am J Roentgenol 153:375–379, 1989.
38. Kelts DG, Grand RJ. Inflammatory bowel disease in children and adolescents. Curr Probl Pediatr 10:5–40, 1980.
39. Limberg B. Sonographic features of colonic Crohn's disease: Comparison of in vivo and in vitro studies. J Clin Ultrasound 18:161–166, 1990.

40. Lowe LH, Penney MW, Scheker LE, et al. Appendicolith revealed on CT in children with suspected appendicitis: How specific is it in the diagnosis of appendicitis? AJR Am J Roentgenol 175:981–984, 2000.

41. Lowe LH, Penney MW, Stein SM, et al. Unenhanced limited CT of the abdomen in the diagnosis of appendicitis in children: Comparison with sonography. AJR Am J Roentgenol 176:31–35, 2001.

42. Merten DF. The acute abdomen in childhood. Curr Probl Diagn Radiol 15:340–395, 1986.

43. Meyers MA, Oliphant M. Ascending retrocecal appendicitis. Radiology 110:295–299, 1974.

44. Mullins ME, Kircher MF, Ryan DP, et al. Evaluation of suspected appendicitis in children using limited helical CT and colonic contrast material. AJR Am J Roentgenol 176:37–41, 2001.

45. Navarro DA, Weber PM. Indium 111 imaging in appendicitis. Semin Ultrasound CT MR 10:321–325, 1989.

46. Nord KS. Peptic ulcer disease in the pediatric population. Pediatr Clin North Am 35:117–140, 1988.

47. O'Donnell B. Abdominal Pain in Children. Oxford, England: Blackwell Scientific Publications, 1985.

48. Papi C, Iscaro D, Salvatori V, et al. Sonographic evaluation of Crohn's disease. Ital J Gastroenterol 21:257–262, 1989.

49. Patriquin HB, Garcier JM, Lafortune M, et al. Appendicitis in children and young adults: Doppler sonographic-pathologic correlation. AJR Am J Roentgenol 166:629–633, 1996.

50. Puri P, McGuinness EPJ, Guiney EJ. Fertility following perforated appendicitis in girls. J Pediatr Surg 24:547–549, 1989.

51. Puylaert JBCM. Acute appendicitis: US evaluation using graded compression. Radiology 158:355–360, 1986.

52. Quillin SP, Siegel MJ. Diagnosis of appendiceal abscess in children with acute appendicitis: Value of color Doppler sonography. AJR Am J Roentgenol 164:1251–1254, 1995.

53. Quillin SP, Siegel MJ, Coffin CM. Acute appendicitis in children: Value of sonography in detecting perforation. AJR Am J Roentgenol 159:1265–1268, 1992.

54. Rhea JT. CT evaluation of appendicitis and diverticulitis. Part 1: Appendicitis. Emerg Radiol 7:160–172, 2000.

55. Riddell RH. Pathobiology of *Helicobacter pylori* infection in children. Can J Gastroenterol 13:599–603, 1999.

56. Roddie ME, Peters AM, Danpure HJ, et al. Inflammation: Imaging with Tc-99m HMPAO-labeled leukocytes. Radiology 166:767–772, 1988.

57. Ruess L, Nussbaum Blask AR, Bulas DI, et al. Inflammatory bowel disease in children and young adults: Correlation of sonographic and clinical parameters during treatment. AJR Am J Roentgenol 175:79–84, 2000.

58. Schey WL. Use of barium in the diagnosis of appendicitis in children. AJR Am J Roentgenol 118:95–103, 1973.

59. Schmutz GR, Benko A, Fournier L, Peron JM, Morel E, Chiche L. Small bowel obstruction: Role and contribution of sonography. Eur Radiol 7:1054–1058, 1997.

60. Seibert JJ, Williamson SL, Golladay ES, Mollitt DL, Siebert RW, Sutterfield SL. Distended gasless abdomen: Fertile field for ultrasound. J Ultrasound Med 5:301–308, 1986.

61. Sfakianakis GN, Conway JJ. Detection of ectopic gastric mucosa in Meckel's diverticulum and in other aberrations by scintigraphy: 1. Pathophysiology and 10-year clinical experience. J Nucl Med 22:647–654, 1981.

62. Shanon A, Martin DJ, Feldman W. Ultrasonographic studies in the management of recurrent abdominal pain. Pediatrics 86:35–38, 1990.

63. Shaul WL. Clues to the early diagnosis of neonatal appendicitis. J Pediatr 98:473–476, 1981.

64. Siegel MJ, Carel C, Surratt S. Ultrasonography of acute abdominal pain in children. JAMA 266:1987–1989, 1991.

65. Singleton EB. Incidence of peptic ulcer as determined by radiologic examinations in the pediatric age group. J Pediatr 65:858–862, 1964.

66. Sivit CJ. Diagnosis of acute appendicitis in children: Spectrum of sonographic findings. AJR Am J Roentgenol 161:147–152, 1993.

67. Sivit CJ, Applegate KE, Stallion A, et al. Imaging evaluation of suspected appendicitis in a pediatric population: Effectiveness of sonography versus CT. AJR Am J Roentgenol 175:977–980, 2000.

68. Sivit CJ, Newman KD, Boenning DA, et al. Appendicitis: Usefulness of US in a pediatric population. Radiology 185:549–552, 1992.

69. Sivit CJ, Siegel MJ, Applegate KE, Newman KD. When appendicitis is suspected in children. RadioGraphics 21:247–262, 2001.

70. Slovis TL, Haller JO, Cohen HL, Berdon WE, Watts FB Jr. Complicated appendiceal inflammatory disease in children: Pylephlebitis and liver abscess. Radiology 171:823–825, 1989.

71. Sonnenberg A, Erckenbrecht J, Peter P, Niederau C. Detection of Crohn's disease by ultrasound. Gastroenterology 83:430–434, 1982.

72. Soter CS. The contribution of the radiologist to the diagnosis of acute appendicitis. Semin Roentgenol 8:375–388, 1973.

73. Spalinger J, Patriquin H, Miron M-C, et al. Doppler US in patients with Crohn's disease: Vessel density in the diseased bowel reflects disease activity. Radiology 217:787–791, 2000.

74. Stringer DA. Imaging inflammatory bowel disease in the pediatric patient. Radiol Clin North Am 25:93–113, 1987.

75. Stringer DA, Daneman A, Brunelle F, Ward K, Martin DJ. Sonography of the normal and abnormal stomach (excluding hypertrophic pyloric stenosis) in children. J Ultrasound Med 5:183–188, 1986.

76. Stringer DA, Sherman P, Liu P, Daneman A. Value of the peroral pneumocolon in children. AJR Am J Roentgenol 146:763–766, 1986.

77. Suri S, Gupta S, Sudhakar PJ, Venkataramu NK, Sood B, Wig JD. Comparative evaluation of plain films, ultrasound and CT in the diagnosis of intestinal obstruction. Acta Radiol 40:422–428, 1999.

78. Swischuk LE, Hayden CK. Appendicitis with perforation: The dilated transverse colon sign. AJR Am J Roentgenol 135:687–689, 1980.

79. Tegtmeyer CJ, Thistlethwaite JR, Sneed TF. Roentgen findings in acute appendicitis. Med Ann 38:127–130, 1969.

80. Thomson M, Walker-Smith J. Dyspepsia in infants and children. Baillieres Clin Gastroenterol 12:601–624, 1998.

81. Van der Meer SB, Forget PP, Arends JW, Kuijten RH, van Engelshoven JM. Diagnostic value of ultrasound in children with recurrent abdominal pain. Pediatr Radiol 20:501–503, 1990.

82. Vignault F, Filiatrault D, Brandt ML, Garel L, Grignon A, Ouimet A. Acute appendicitis in children: Evaluation with US. Radiology 176:501–504, 1990.

83. Weizman Z, Durie PR. Acute pancreatitis in childhood. J Pediatr 113:24–29, 1988.

84. Wilkinson RH, Bartlett RH, Eraklis AJ. Diagnosis of appendicitis in infancy: Value of abdominal radiograph. Am J Dis Child 118:687–690, 1969.

85. Yeomans ND. Bacteria in ulcer pathogenesis. Baillieres Clin Gastroenterol 2:573–591, 1988.

86. Yip WCL, Ho TF, Yip YY. Chan KY. Value of abdominal sonography in the assessment of children with abdominal pain. J Clin Ultrasound 26:397–400, 1998.

ADDITIONAL READING

Alberini JL, Badran A, Freneaux E, et al. Technetium-99m HMPAO-labeled leukocyte imaging compared with endoscopy, ultrasonography, and contrast radiology in children with inflammatory bowel disease. J Pediatr Gastroenterol Nutr 32:278–286, 2001.

Andronikous S, Welman CJ, Kader E. The CT features of abdominal tuberculosis in children. Pediatr Radiol 32:75–81, 2002.

Applegate KE, Sivit CJ, Salvator AE, et al. Effect of cross-sectional imaging on negative appendectomy and perforation rates in children. Radiology 220:103–107, 2001

Bremner AR, Pridgeon J, Fairhurst J, Beattie RM. Ultrasound scanning may reduce the need for barium radiology in the assessment of small bowel Crohn's disease. Acta Paediatr 93:479–481, 2004.

Bruno I, Martelossi S, Geatti O, et al. Antigranulocyte monoclonal antibody immunoscintigraphy in inflammatory bowel disease in children and young adolescents. Acta Pediatr 91:1050–1055, 2002.

Callahan MJ, Rodriguez DP, Taylor GA. CT of appendicitis in children. Radiology 224:325–332, 2002.

Carty HM. Paediatric emergencies: Non-traumatic abdominal emergencies. Eur Radiol 12:2835–2848, 2002.

Charron M. Pediatric inflammatory bowel disease imaged with Tc-99m white blood cells. Clin Nucl Med 25:708–715, 2000.

Cohen HL, Smith WL, Kushner DC, et al. Imaging evaluation of acute right lower quadrant and pelvic pain in adolescent girls. American College of Radiology. ACR Appropriateness Criteria. Radiology 215(Suppl):833–840, 2000.

Garcia Peña BM, Cook EF, Mandl KD. Selective imaging strategies for the diagnosis of appendicitis in children. Pediatrics 113:24–28, 2004.

Hagendorf BA, Clarke JR, Burd RS. The optimal initial management of children with suspected appendicitis: A decision analysis. J Pediatr Surg 39:880–885, 2004.

Hogan MJ. Appendiceal abscess drainage. Tech Vasc Interv Radiol 6:205–214, 2003.

Karakas SP, Guelfguat M, Leonidas JC, Springer S, Singh SP. Acute appendicitis in children: Comparison of clinical diagnosis with ultrasound and CT imaging. Pediatr Radiol 30:94–98, 2000.

Klein MD, Rabbani AB, Rood KD, et al. Three quantitative approaches to the diagnosis of abdominal pain in children: Practical applications of decision theory. J Pediatr Surg 36:1375–1380, 2001.

Kosloske AM, Love CL, Rohrer JE, Goldthorn JF, Lacey SR. The diagnosis of appendicitis in children: Outcomes of a strategy based on pediatric surgical evaluation. Pediatrics 113:29–34, 2004.

Pena BM, Taylor GA, Fishman SJ, Mandl KD. Effect of an imaging protocol on clinical outcome among pediatric patients with appendicitis. Pediatrics 110:1088–1093, 2002.

Sandrasegaran K, Maglinte DD, Howard TJ, Kelvin FM, Lappas JC. The multifaceted role of radiology in small bowel obstruction. Semin Ulrasound CT MR 24:319–335, 2003.

Sivit CJ. Imaging the child with right lower quadrant pain and suspected appendicitis: Current concepts. Pediatr Radiol 34:447–453, 2004.

Stephen AE, Segev DL, Ryan DP, et al. The diagnosis of acute appendicitis in a pediatric population: To CT or not to CT. J Pediatr Surg 38:367–371, 2003.

Strouse PJ. Imaging and the child with abdominal pain. Singapore Med J 44:312–322, 2003.

Strouse PJ, Bates DG, Bloom DA, Goodsitt MM. Non-contrast thin-section helical CT of urinary tract calculi in children. Pediatr Radiol 32:326–332, 2002.

Vayner N, Coret A, Polliack G, Weiss B, Hertz M. Mesenteric lymphadenopathy in children examined by US for chronic and/or current abdominal pain. Pediatr Radiol 33:864–867, 2003.

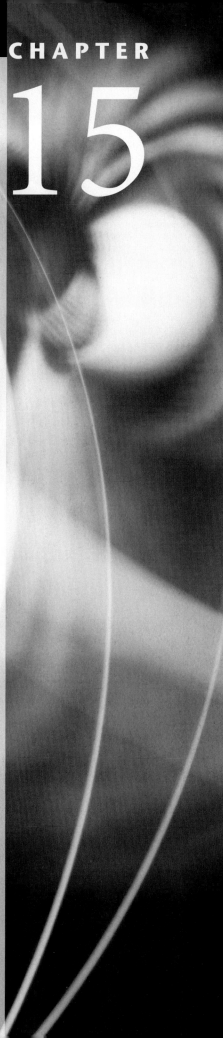

CHAPTER 15

THE CHILD WITH DIARRHEA

Outline

Alan David Hoffman, MD

THE CHILD WITH DIARRHEA

Diarrhea has been defined as "an increase in frequency, fluidity, or volume of bowel movements relative to the usual habit of the individual."[70] The consequences of acute diarrheal illness range from the mild irritation of a diaper rash in the infant with irritable colon syndrome to the life-threatening complications of severe colitis (sepsis, toxic megacolon, and perforation). The etiology of acute diarrhea in the majority of children is enteric infection. Dehydration is the most common serious complication of acute diarrheal diseases, particularly in very young or debilitated patients. Worldwide, especially in developing nations, diarrheal disease is a problem of enormous proportions. Chronic diarrheal illness is important because of the potential for malnutrition and growth failure. In general, because most entities causing childhood diarrhea are due to a physiologic disturbance rather than to a gross anatomic abnormality, roentgen evaluation is rarely done. Radiographic evaluation is indicated only in a limited number of well-defined clinical situations.

DIFFERENTIAL DIAGNOSIS OF DIARRHEA

The following factors are important in the formulation of a differential diagnosis of childhood diarrhea: patient's age, duration of illness (acute or chronic), general state of health (well or sick), severity of diarrhea, types of stool (e.g., watery, bloody, or fatty), associated symptoms (e.g., symptoms of parenteral infection or fever), associated signs (e.g., dehydration or malnutrition), and clinical history (e.g., dietary changes, siblings or schoolmates being ill, use of antibiotics, weight loss, or constipation). The patient's age is a convenient, initial branching point in the decision tree analysis of pediatric diarrheal disease.

Neonates (Birth to 1 Month)

The important causes of diarrhea in the newborn are listed in Table 15–1. The consequences of diarrhea are likely to be of greater importance in neonates than in patients of any other age. This is particularly true for diarrheal illness due to enteric infections, the most common cause of diarrhea in the neonate. The alimentary tract of the newborn, although initially sterile, is rapidly colonized by bacterial organisms. If pathogens are present in the environment when colonization occurs, intestinal infection can readily result. Enteropathogenic *Escherichia coli* (EPEC) may cause acute severe enteritis in the newborn. Newborn nursery epidemics caused by this organism are often quite serious and difficult to eradicate. Nursery-acquired EPEC infection may present at home soon after the newborn has been discharged from the hospital. Other bacteria (e.g., *Salmonella*) and viruses may also be responsible for enteritis in the newborn.

Postenteritis carbohydrate intolerance, usually a secondary lactase deficiency, may develop after any intestinal disease that damages the mucosa of the small bowel; it is a more common cause of milk intolerance than is milk protein allergy. Neonatal gastroenteritis is often responsible for secondary lactase deficiency, which occurs when the return of normal lactase activity lags behind epithelial repair and regeneration.

TABLE 15-1 Causes of Diarrhea in Neonates (Birth to 1 Month)

Common
Enteric infection
Parenteral infection (respiratory tract, urinary tract, otitis media)
*Iatrogenic (associated with antibiotic therapy)
*Postenteritis carbohydrate intolerance
Necrotizing enterocolitis
Uncommon
*Cow's milk protein and soy protein allergy
*Cystic fibrosis
*Hirschsprung's disease with enterocolitis
*Endocrine abnormalities
*Metabolic defects (commonly primary enzyme deficiency)
*Neural tumor
*Cholestasis (hepatitis, intrahepatic or extrahepatic biliary atresia, choledochal cyst)
*Hemolytic-uremic syndrome
*Congenital partial small bowel obstruction (malrotation, bands, stenosis, duplication)

*Chronic or recurring conditions.

In the neonate and infant, symptoms of cow's milk protein sensitivity may mimic bacterial gastroenteritis, with fever, vomiting, and watery diarrhea of short duration. There may be blood in the stool. Often, eosinophilia is present in the peripheral blood and in the stool. Colitis with gross bleeding, suggesting ulcerative or bacterial colitis, may also result from milk protein sensitivity.

The stressed premature infant may develop necrotizing enterocolitis, an idiopathic intestinal disease characterized by varying degrees of mucosal or transmural necrosis, most commonly involving the ileum or right colon. Occasionally, necrotizing colitis develops in term babies, but it most commonly presents in premature infants with respiratory distress syndrome. Abdominal distention, systemic toxicity, and bloody diarrhea are common symptoms. Perforation and peritonitis often forewarn a fatal outcome, which occurs in one fourth to one half of affected patients. Radiographic recognition depends on detection of ectopic intra-abdominal gas, usually associated with bowel dilatation.

An uncommon but serious and potentially fatal enterocolitis can develop in children with Hirschsprung's disease. Enterocolitis may be the initial manifestation of Hirschsprung's disease in the neonate or infant. In such presentations, the child may be severely ill; prompt diagnosis and treatment are essential to avoid a fatal outcome.

Cystic fibrosis is the most common cause of chronic malabsorption in children. The clinical manifestations of this pancreatic exocrine insufficiency typically become apparent in the neonate or infant. Liver disease (cholestasis or cirrhosis) may also impair absorptive function in these children and may be clinically significant in neonates.

Infancy (1 Month to 2 Years)

The important causes of diarrhea in infancy are listed in Table 15–2. There is considerable overlap in the conditions that cause diarrhea in neonates and in infants.

Enteric infection is the most common cause of diarrhea in infants as well as in all pediatric age groups. Infections of organ systems other than the gastrointestinal tract and treatment of such conditions with antibiotics (e.g., ampicillin) may be associated with diarrhea.

Pseudomembranous enterocolitis, a very uncommon and frequently fatal condition in infants and children, has been related to the use of antibiotics, severe systemic illness, or postoperative states. The pathogenesis of pseudomembranous enterocolitis is unknown. Pathologically, the disease is similar to necrotizing enterocolitis, Hirschsprung's enterocolitis, and the colitis of hemolytic-uremic syndrome. Variable amounts of transmural edema, mucosal ulceration, and plaques of white-yellow exudate (pseudomembranes) are present. Onset of symptoms is usually within 1 week following surgery or initiation of antibiotic therapy. A related condition,

TABLE 15-2 CAUSES OF DIARRHEA IN INFANTS
(1 MONTH TO 2 YEARS)

Common
Enteric infection
Parenteral infections (respiratory tract, urinary tract,
  otitis media)
*Iatrogenic (associated with antibiotic therapy)
*Postenteritis carbohydrate intolerance
*Irritable colon syndrome
*Cow's milk protein and soy protein allergy
Uncommon
*Cystic fibrosis
*Celiac disease
*Hirschsprung's disease with enterocolitis
Necrotizing enterocolitis
Small intestinal stasis
    *Congenital partial small bowel obstruction
      (malrotation, bands, stenosis, duplication)
    *Postsurgical (blind loop, short bowel, partial
      obstruction)
Pseudomembranous enterocolitis
*Neutropenic colitis
*Endocrine abnormalities
*Metabolic defects (commonly primary enzyme
  deficiency)
*Neural tumor
*Specific food allergy
*Malnutrition
*Immunodeficiency
*Cholestasis (hepatitis, intrahepatic or extrahepatic
  biliary atresia, choledochal cyst)
*Intractable diarrhea of infancy
*Hemolytic-uremic syndrome

*Chronic or recurring conditions.

neutropenic colitis, is particularly evident in debilitated or immunocompromised patients. A high mortality rate is characteristic of severe disease, which typically has a sudden onset and a fulminant course.

Irritable colon syndrome, a common functional disorder, typically presents in healthy infants. Increased stool frequency and fluid content possibly are related to rapid intestinal transit, but malabsorption is absent. Physical examination is normal, and spontaneous resolution before 4 years of age is usual.

Celiac disease typically becomes manifest in infancy, with onset of symptoms following the introduction of cereals in the diet. In some children, the disease presents after 2 years of age, and almost all occurrences of childhood celiac disease

are manifest by 10 years of age. Celiac disease is the most common etiology of diffuse mucosal disease causing malabsorption.

Rarely, milk protein allergy may cause a syndrome of diarrhea and protein-losing enteropathy that presents in early infancy.

YOUNG CHILDREN (2 TO 5 YEARS)

The important causes of diarrhea in young children are listed in Table 15–3. As in the neonate and infant, enteric infection, postenteritis carbohydrate intolerance, parenteral infection, and antibiotic therapy are common etiologies of diarrhea. After the age of toilet training, functional megacolon with encopresis can cause intermittent paradoxical diarrhea. Inflammatory bowel disease may occur in children younger than 5 years of age but is uncommon. Diarrhea can also be the initial manifestation of acute appendicitis in young children. Occasionally, neuroblastoma is

TABLE 15-3 CAUSES OF DIARRHEA IN YOUNG
CHILDREN (2 TO 5 YEARS)

Common
Enteric infection
Parenteral infections (respiratory tract, urinary tract,
  otitis media)
Postenteritis carbohydrate intolerance
*Functional megacolon (fecal impaction or paradoxical
  diarrhea)
*Iatrogenic (associated with antibiotic therapy)
*Irritable colon syndrome
Uncommon
*Appendicitis
*Cow's milk protein and soy protein allergy
*Cystic fibrosis
*Celiac disease
*Hirschsprung's disease with enterocolitis
*Food allergy
*Inflammatory bowel disease
    *Ulcerative colitis
    *Crohn's disease
*Neural tumors
*Cholestasis (hepatitis, cirrhosis, choledochal cyst)
*Hemolytic-uremic syndrome
*Pseudomembranous enterocolitis
*Neutropenic colitis
*Postsurgical small intestinal stasis (blind loop, short
  bowel, partial obstruction)

*Chronic or recurring conditions.

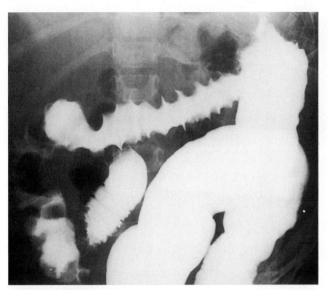

Figure 15–1
Colitis of hemolytic-uremic syndrome. This 3-year-old girl presented with mild diarrhea, fever, and heme-positive stools. A clinical diagnosis of infectious enterocolitis was made but could not be confirmed by appropriate cultures. This anteroposterior (AP) supine view of a barium enema shows spasm and thickening of the colon wall in the ascending and transverse colon. These changes are due to hemorrhage, edema, and inflammation. Rapidly progressive azotemia began 2 days after the barium enema. Usually in patients with hemolytic-uremic syndrome, azotemia is present when intestinal symptoms begin, and a barium enema is not necessary.

associated with chronic diarrhea, which results from poorly defined neurohumoral effects on bowel secretions and motility.

Hemolytic-uremic syndrome is a rare disorder in which renal failure, hemolytic anemia, and coagulopathy develop after a prodrome that suggests localized or systemic infection. Infants and young children are those usually affected. Renal, central nervous system, and gastrointestinal symptoms predominate. Bloody diarrhea, simulating acute colitis, often occurs. Barium enema may show nonspecific evidence of acute colitis (Fig. 15–1) but has no role in the diagnosis or management of patients with this disorder.

OLDER CHILDREN (5 YEARS AND OLDER)

The important causes of diarrhea in older children are listed in Table 15–4. Infectious enteritis, inflammatory bowel disease, and appendicitis are the common causes of diarrhea in children 5 years of age and older. The list of uncommon causes includes lymphoma and diarrhea of psychogenic origin.

TABLE 15-4 CAUSES OF DIARRHEA IN OLDER CHILDREN (5 YEARS AND OLDER)
Common
Enteric infections
*Inflammatory bowel disease
*Ulcerative colitis
*Crohn's disease
*Functional megacolon (fecal impaction or paradoxical diarrhea)
Appendicitis
Uncommon
*Psychogenic
*Neural tumors or lymphoma
*Cholestasis (hepatitis, cirrhosis, choledochal cyst)
*Pseudomembranous enterocolitis
*Neutropenic colitis

*Chronic or recurring conditions.

IMPORTANT CONDITIONS CAUSING DIARRHEA

ACUTE ENTERIC INFECTIONS

Susceptibility to acute enteric infection, one of the most prevalent infections of humans, is greater in the first 2 years of life than at any other age. Compared with adults, infants have a higher risk of exposure to enteric pathogens, a greater likelihood of acquiring enteric infection, relatively fewer immunologic defenses, and fewer physiologic reserves against dehydration, the major cause of morbidity and mortality in patients with enteric infection.

Acute enteric infections associated with diarrhea are conventionally termed *acute gastroenteritis*, although gastric infection is unusual. *Acute infectious enteritis* is a more accurate descriptive term, because the majority of cases involve the small intestine. Occasionally, invasive bacterial infection of the small bowel and colon develops, a condition properly termed *infectious enterocolitis*. *Dysentery* is enterocolitis with severe and predominantly colonic disease, typically manifested by grossly bloody stools of small volume accompanied by systemic symptoms.

Almost all acute enteritides are self-limited. Supportive treatment consisting primarily of rehydration, followed by maintenance of hydration, is generally the only therapy required. Oral rehydration with glucose electrolyte solutions (50 or 90 mmol of sodium per liter and 111 mmol of glucose per liter) has been shown to be a safe and effective substitute for intravenous therapy in most well-nourished children

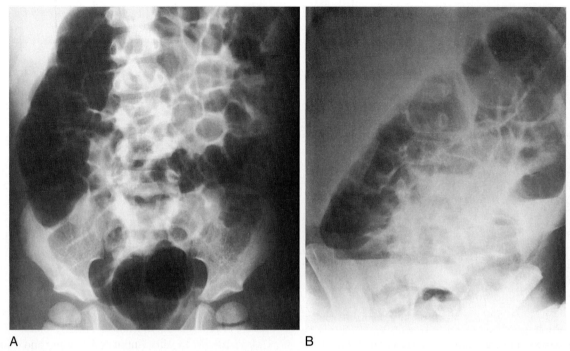

A   B

Figure 15–2
Acute gastroenteritis in a 2-year-old child. *A,* A supine abdominal radiograph demonstrates mild small bowel and colon dilatation. Gas fills the entire colon, including the rectum. *B,* An upright abdominal radiograph reveals air-fluid levels in both the small bowel and the colon. This intestinal gas pattern is indicative of acute enteritis or acute enterocolitis.

hospitalized with acute diarrhea.[75] Antibiotic therapy is not indicated for most cases of bacterial enteritis; however, documentation of bacterial disease by culture assists in identification and treatment of the occasional patient who require such therapy. When acute bacterial enterocolitis or dysentery mimics acute idiopathic inflammatory bowel disease, stool culture is the most reliable method of differentiation. In such clinical situations, barium enema is reserved for those patients in whom infectious causes have been excluded by multiple stool cultures and microscopic examinations.

Epidemiology and Pathophysiology

Acute enteric infection may be the most prevalent infectious disease of humans and is probably the leading cause of death in the world (Fig. 15–2). Microorganisms responsible for acute diarrheal illnesses include viral, bacterial, and parasitic agents (Table 15–5). Viral pathogens are by far the most common cause of infectious enteritis; bacterial enteritis is documented in only 10% to 15% of patients investigated by stool culture. Parasitic organisms are relatively uncommon etiologic agents in patients with acute enteritis.

Humans and animals serve as reservoirs for enteric pathogens. Occasionally, pets have been implicated in household outbreaks of bacterial enteritis. Transmission is fecal-oral and usually indirect, through food, drink, clothing, or various other contaminated objects. Direct person-to-person transmission occurs but is less common.

TABLE 15-5 MICROBES COMMONLY RESPONSIBLE FOR DIARRHEAL ILLNESS
Viral
Rotavirus
Parvovirus
Other (coxsackievirus, echovirus, etc.)
Bacterial
Campylobacter jejuni
Salmonella spp.
Shigella spp.
Escherichia coli
Enterotoxigenic (ETEC)
Enteropathogenic (EPEC)
Enteroinvasive (EIEC)
Yersinia enterocolitica
Staphylococcus aureus
Clostridium perfringens
Parasitic
Giardia lamblia
Entamoeba histolytica

In underdeveloped countries, breast-fed infants experience less morbidity and mortality from acute diarrheal illness than bottle-fed infants. Similarly, in societies with modern medical care, there is less morbidity and there are fewer infants requiring hospitalization for acute enteritis among those who are breast-fed than among those who are bottle-fed.

Most cases of acute enteritis are sporadic or associated with a household outbreak, but some result from epidemics in nurseries, schools, and camps and common-source exposures (e.g., food or water). Illness from "food poisoning" results when the common source is contaminated by preformed bacterial enterotoxins (e.g., *Staphylococcus*) or by many organisms (e.g., *Salmonella*).

Of viral agents, human rotaviruses are the agents most commonly responsible for acute gastroenteritis in infants and children younger than 9 years. Biopsy of the proximal small bowel infected with rotavirus shows changes in the epithelium and lamina propria inflammation. This mild invasion of the intestine is not significantly destructive; the associated diarrhea is watery and devoid of leukocytes and erythrocytes and simulates the secretory diarrhea induced by bacterial enterotoxins. Transient malabsorption of xylose, lactose, and fat also occurs with rotavirus and other enteric viruses. Other important viral causes of childhood gastroenteritis include parvo-like viruses and, less likely, adenoviruses, astroviruses, and caliciviruses.[35]

Bacterial infection begins when ingested pathogens attach to specific intestinal mucosal binding sites. In healthy individuals, large numbers of indigenous bacterial flora compete for and occupy these sites. However, when the number of indigenous flora is reduced by broad-spectrum antibiotics or by malnutrition, the probability that ingested pathogens will successfully bind to the mucosa is increased. Conversely, colostrum and breast milk immunoglobulin (Ig) A prevent bacterial adhesion to the intestinal mucosa, which explains the high degree of immunity of breast-fed babies to EPEC gastroenteritis.

After adhesion of pathogenic bacteria, diarrhea may be induced by two mechanisms: (1) enterotoxin stimulation of fluid and electrolyte secretion (secretory diarrhea), and (2) enteroinvasion, with varying degrees of mucosal destruction and inflammation.[56]

Enterotoxin production by various bacterial pathogens (e.g., enterotoxigenic *E. coli, Vibrio cholerae, Salmonella* species, *Staphylococcus aureus,* and *Clostridium perfringens*) activates adenylate cyclase in intestinal epithelial cells, stimulating intracellular accumulation of cyclic adenosine monophosphate (cAMP) that causes massive Na^+ and Cl^- secretion into the gastrointestinal lumen. The prototype organism for enterotoxin-induced (secretory) diarrhea is *V. cholerae,* a microbe associated with the production of voluminous, watery diarrhea. Tissue biopsy of intestines affected by enterotoxin diarrhea shows no histologic alteration. Other than the effects of dehydration, systemic symptoms are absent or minimal when diarrhea is provoked solely by enterotoxins.

Enteroinvasive bacterial organisms (e.g., *Shigella* species, *Salmonella* species, *Campylobacter jejuni, Yersinia enterocolitica, S. aureus,* and enteroinvasive *E. coli*) penetrate the intestinal mucosa and cause variable degrees of inflammation and ulceration. Leukocytes are often present in the diarrheal stool, reflecting significant small bowel or colon mucosal inflammation or both. The presence of microscopic or macroscopic blood in the stool indicates that infection and ulceration involve the colon. Systemic symptoms are more common with enteroinvasive bacterial infections, in which enteritis is usually self-limited but which occasionally can produce severe enterocolitis or a dysenteric syndrome. In addition, most enteroinvasive bacteria produce enterotoxin or have an enterotoxin-like effect (e.g., *Salmonella* species, *Shigella* species, and *S. aureus*). Biopsy of an intestine infected with enteroinvasive organisms often shows mucosal inflammation. Colon biopsy may reveal moderate to severe mucosal and submucosal inflammation and variable degrees of mucosal ulceration.

The major parasites capable of causing diarrheal illness are the protozoans *Giardia lamblia* and *Entamoeba histolytica. Giardia* invades the duodenum and jejunum and causes mild mucosal inflammation, histologically similar in degree to the inflammation caused by rotaviruses. An acute or subacute malabsorption accompanies infection caused by *Giardia. E. histolytica* invades and ulcerates the colonic mucosa.

Clinical Presentation

In viral gastroenteritis, an abrupt onset of illness is typical. Vomiting is often the only symptom during the first few hours of illness. Rotavirus enteritis is almost always accompanied by vomiting in the first 24 to 48 hours of illness. Diarrhea soon ensues and lasts from 3 to 10 days. Fever is usually absent or, if present, of low grade. Associated parenteral infection, particularly of the upper respiratory tract, is common. Occurrences may be sporadic or associated with outbreaks within the family, neighborhood, or school. Affected children are not systemically ill or "toxic." Viral enteritis is self-limited; replacement of gastrointestinal fluid and electrolyte losses is the only therapy required.

Rotaviruses are responsible for sporadic and epidemic outbreaks of gastroenteritis in infants and young children, most frequently occurring in the fall or winter. In communities in which it has been studied, rotavirus infection has been found in 40% to 80% of children who are hospitalized for acute diarrheal illness. Between 50% and 90% of 2-year-old children have rotavirus antibodies. Infection can be verified by electron microscopy, immunoabsorbent assay of stool specimens, or a rise in complement-fixing antibody titers.

Parvovirus infection is not as common as is rotavirus infection in children, and it usually affects older children. Parvovirus causes a mild enteritis that usually lasts a maximum of 2 to 3 days. Viral particles can be identified in stool specimens by electron microscopy.

Usually, bacterial enteritis is clinically indistinguishable from viral enteritis. The diagnosis of bacterial enteritis is strengthened by (1) the presence of high fever and toxicity; (2) a history of exposure to people with documented bacterial enteritis; (3) the absence of a family, school, or community outbreak of disease; (4) the presence of persistent or relapsing diarrhea; and (5) illness severe enough to require hospitalization. A septic clinical picture obviously signifies a serious bacterial enteritis. Fecal leukocytes are sometimes present with mild invasive bacterial enteritis but are commonly present with severe invasive bacterial enteritis; they are absent in viral or noninvasive bacterial infection. Fecal erythrocytes or gross blood are present with invasive bacterial colitis but are absent in viral or noninvasive bacterial infection.

EPEC is the most common bacterial cause of acute gastroenteritis in infants, particularly in those younger than 6 months of age. Infants with EPEC enteritis may be severely ill with vomiting, dehydration, electrolyte imbalance, and fever. Mild cases of EPEC enteritis are characterized by mild fever, absence of systemic symptoms, and no significant dehydration. Stools are watery but without pus or blood, and the illness is self-limited, typically resolving in a week or less. Unfortunately, outbreaks of EPEC enteritis in hospital nurseries are not rare and are often difficult to control. Infants whose diet consists solely of breast milk almost never acquire EPEC infection. EPEC infection does occur in children older than 2 years of age but is typically mild.

Enterotoxigenic *E. coli* (ETEC) infections are responsible for a self-limited type of enteritis that is rarely associated with significant vomiting or fever. Diarrhea varies from mild to severe and is caused solely by enterotoxin. ETEC is the leading cause of traveler's diarrhea[88] and is occasionally identified in sporadic cases of enteritis and in outbreaks of enteritis in hospital nurseries.

Other *E. coli* gastroenteritides that are seen, particularly in adults, are enteroinvasive *E. coli* (EIEC) infection, epidemics that resemble shigellosis, and enterohemorrhagic *E. coli* infection, a condition that has been seen sporadically in epidemics caused by contaminated beef distributed through fast-food chains.[67,72]

C. jejuni, possibly the most common cause of bacterial enteritis in the pediatric age group, produces diarrheal illness ranging in severity from a mild enteritis of short duration to a severe, persistent, relapsing enterocolitis simulating acute idiopathic inflammatory bowel disease. *C. jejuni* infection may mimic appendicitis when pain and fever are the dominant symptoms; these often occur early in the illness, prior to the onset of diarrhea. Grossly bloody stools and high fever are common symptoms, but significant vomiting and dehydration are unusual. The illness is often self-limited, typically resolving within 7 to 10 days. Persistent or relapsing disease occurs in a minority of patients and responds promptly to erythromycin.

Domestic animals (both farm and household) are important reservoirs for *C. jejuni*. Documentation of *C. jejuni*

infection can be accomplished by direct-phase contrast microscopy of stools or by stool culture, utilizing special bacteriologic methods (i.e., either differential filtration or selective antibiotic media with microaerophilic conditions).

Diarrheal illness caused by nontyphoid *Salmonella* species may be quite mild, as in the secretory diarrhea that occurs in infants, or quite severe, as in the rare cases of severe enterocolitis or *Salmonella* dysentery. The most common manifestation of *Salmonella* intestinal infection is a self-limited gastroenteritis characterized by a gradual onset of symptoms with high fever. Fecal leukocytes are often present in the diarrheal stool. In most patients, spontaneous resolution occurs in 2 to 5 days, but symptoms may persist for up to 2 weeks. Antibiotic therapy is not given routinely for *Salmonella* gastroenteritis because, according to Nelson, "…antibiotic therapy does not abbreviate the symptomatic period or prolong the carrier state."[63] Antibiotic therapy, however, is necessary for patients with severe *Salmonella* enterocolitis or dysentery. In such patients, colon biopsy and barium enema, if done, reveal nonspecific acute ulcerating colitis. Routine culture techniques for enteric pathogens will document *Salmonella* infection.

Shigella enteritis causes an acute diarrheal illness of short duration (2 to 3 days), typically accompanied by high fever, which occasionally results in febrile convulsions. *Shigella* dysentery (bacillary dysentery) is manifested by bloody diarrhea of 1 to 2 weeks' duration, accompanied by cramping abdominal pain, tenesmus, and fever. *Shigella* dysentery is often clinically indistinguishable from acute idiopathic inflammatory bowel disease. *Shigella* can be isolated with routine culture techniques for Enterobacteriaceae organisms.

Invasion of the distal small bowel or colon by *Y. enterocolitica* may result in a variety of clinical presentations, including acute, subacute, and chronic diarrheal illness. Mesenteric adenitis caused by *Yersinia* infection may mimic appendicitis. Many cases of acute regional enteritis are caused by *Yersinia* infection and may be mistaken for chronic regional enteritis (Crohn's disease) because of a similar appearance on small bowel barium examination.[16,76]

Outbreaks of *Yersinia* infection have been reported in families, schools, and hospitals, but sporadic cases are most common. Usually, fever, diarrhea, and vomiting are present. The diarrhea lasts between 1 and 2 weeks, and fecal leukocytes may be present. Occasionally, acute, severe enterocolitis that is clinically similar to acute idiopathic inflammatory bowel disease develops from *Yersinia* infection. The diagnosis may be established by stool culture, but special bacteriologic methods are required. Serologic testing can also be used. Cases of moderate or severe yersiniosis usually require antibiotic therapy.

Parasitic intestinal disease, although uncommon when compared with viral and bacterial enteritis, is important, because drug therapy is routinely necessary. *G. lamblia*, the most common intestinal parasite in the United States, causes acute, subacute, and chronic diarrheal illness.[19] Children are infected by *Giardia* considerably more often than are adults.

Prevalence rates of giardiasis are highest in children between 5 and 10 years of age; in some communities, more than 10% of children are infected. Patients with immunoglobulin deficiency apparently have increased susceptibility to giardiasis.

Transmission is commonly by contaminated food or water. The protozoan invades the duodenum and jejunum, inducing a mild to moderate mucosal inflammation, occasionally with associated villous atrophy. Clinically, a mild, subacute diarrheal illness is typical. Patients with chronic infection may develop significant malabsorption. *Giardia* is a cause of traveler's diarrhea, which usually develops toward the end of the trip, presumably because of the long incubation period (10 to 20 days). Diagnosis is established by examination of stools or aspirated duodenal contents. In chronic cases, excretion of the organism may be intermittent, making detection by stool examination more difficult. Rarely, a small intestine biopsy is necessary to establish the diagnosis. Contrast radiographs show edema and spasm of the duodenum and proximal jejunum with sparing of the more distal bowel. These radiographic findings of giardiasis are, strictly speaking, nonspecific. However, in practice, this appearance is highly suggestive of giardiasis in the clinical setting of a diarrheal illness (Figs. 15–3 and 15–4). This is probably a result of the greater frequency of giardiasis compared with other causes of mucosal fold thickening involving both the duodenum and jejunum. Therapy with quinacrine or furazolidone is usually successful.

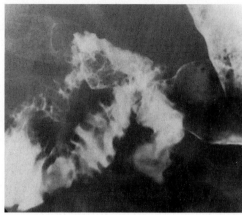

Figure 15–4
Giardiasis: spot film of the duodenum in a 2½-year-old girl with diarrhea. The second part of the duodenum was persistently narrowed by spasm and inflammation. *Giardia lamblia* was recovered from duodenal aspirates.

Tissue invasion by the protozoan *E. histolytica* in the colon and occasionally in the terminal ileum results in diarrheal illness, ranging from a mild, chronic form to an acute fulminant amebic dysentery. However, the asymptomatic cyst carrier state is the most common form of amebiasis, in which *E. histolytica* lives as a commensal in the gastrointestinal tract, and tissue invasion occurs only rarely. Humans are the principal hosts and reservoirs of these protozoa.

Amebic ulcerations are most common in the cecal and rectosigmoid regions; however, any pattern of disease may occur, including pancolitis. With sigmoidoscopy, rectal ulcerations are visible in most patients; the mucosa between ulcerations is relatively normal. Simple amebic ulcerations of the colon are not associated with suppuration, and there are no fecal neutrophils. Secondary bacterial infection, however, may result in the appearance of fecal leukocytes. Fecal erythrocytes are often present.

Symptoms of amebic colitis are generally nonspecific and compatible with most forms of infectious colitis or idiopathic inflammatory bowel disease. With most cases of amebic colitis, onset of disease is gradual, and fever and leukocytosis are either absent or mild. The onset of fulminant amebic dysentery is often abrupt, and high fever is common.

The diagnosis of amebic colitis depends on identification of cysts or motile trophozoites in the stool. Colon cleansing or contrast enema prior to stool collection will greatly reduce the probability of finding amebae. Contrast examination reveals nonspecific evidence of an ulcerating colitis and, if performed, should be the last diagnostic procedure done. A number of serologic tests are available and are particularly sensitive in the diagnosis of invasive amebic dysentery. Treatment with appropriate amebicides is indicated for all symptomatic patients and in asymptomatic cyst carriers.

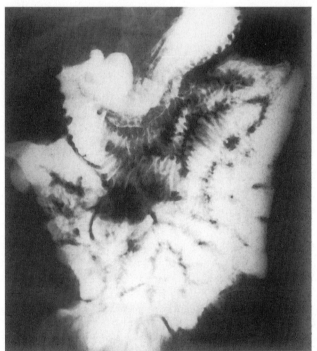

Figure 15–3
Giardiasis. Moderate thickening of the duodenal and proximal jejunal folds is shown on this film from a small bowel series in an 8-year-old girl with a subacute diarrheal illness and weight loss. *Giardia* organisms were recovered from a stool specimen.

Radiographic Evaluation

Radiographic evaluation is not used for most children with acute enteritis or acute enterocolitis because confident diagnosis is almost always possible with clinical and laboratory assessments. Radiographic examination is of limited use as a confirmatory test because of the nonspecific nature of the roentgenographic findings in acute enteritis.

Radiographic evaluation may be useful in atypical cases when bowel obstruction or appendicitis is a differential diagnostic consideration. Ileus, abdominal distention, and vomiting may be the initial manifestations of acute enteric infection, preceding the onset of diarrhea and simulating obstruction. Plain films of the abdomen can assist in excluding obstruction, particularly an established high-grade obstruction. Early small bowel obstructions, however, may not be distinguishable from nonobstructive ileus and gastroenteritis on plain film examination. Prompt exclusion of obstruction may be accomplished with a small bowel barium series, but this is very rarely necessary.

In children, acute bacterial enterocolitis or dysentery typically has a clinical course and contrast enema findings that are indistinguishable from those of acute idiopathic inflammatory bowel disease. Exclusion or diagnosis of bacterial causes of enterocolitis or colitis relies mainly on stool culture. Contrast examination, if done, should be the last diagnostic procedure performed in such situations and should be undertaken only after multiple adequate stool specimens have been obtained for microscopic and bacteriologic evaluation. Some laboratories do not routinely culture for *Y. enterocolitica* or *C. jejuni* because special methods are required. If these organisms have not been sought, barium enema is delayed until results of specific cultures for them are available.

Cleansing of the colon or contrast enemas greatly reduce the chances of finding amebae on wet mounts. The protozoans are found in debris adjacent to ulcers, and any kind of enema will remove both the debris and the organisms.

Radiographic Findings

Plain film examination may show a variety of patterns in patients with acute enteritis (see Fig. 15–2). The most characteristic pattern consists of air-fluid levels in nondilated small bowel and colon. However, the intestinal gas pattern may mimic partial small bowel obstruction, distal colonic obstruction, or nonobstructive ileus.

Contrast examination of the acutely infected small bowel primarily reveals motility disturbances. Because of altered peristalsis, intestinal motility may be found to be increased. Conversely, if ileus is prominent, transit of barium in the small intestine may be slow. Small intestinal edema and inflammation may cause thickening of mucosal folds, generally with preservation of basic fold architecture.

G. lamblia and *Y. enterocolitica* each cause fairly specific radiologic changes in the small bowel (Figs. 15–5 through 15–8) that should suggest their diagnosis in the clinical setting

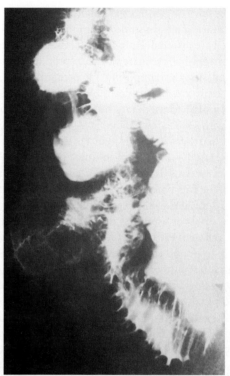

Figure 15–5
Yersiniosis. Moderate to marked mucosal edema and inflammation are present in the terminal ileum of an adolescent with a presumptive diagnosis of Crohn's disease. Stool cultures were positive for *Yersinia enterocolitica*. The condition responded promptly to antibiotic therapy.

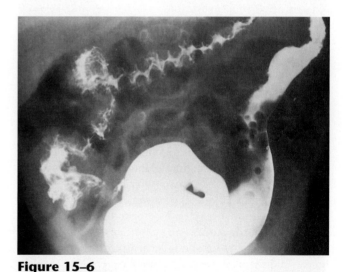

Figure 15–6
Bacterial enterocolitis. A barium enema was difficult to perform in this 15-month-old infant with bloody diarrhea because of spasm, particularly of the right colon. Spasm and edema are present in the ascending and transverse segments of the colon. Ulcerations are visible in the hepatic flexure and proximal descending colon. Idiopathic inflammatory bowel disease is highly unlikely because of the patient's age. A diagnosis of *Shigella* enterocolitis was made on the basis of a positive stool culture.

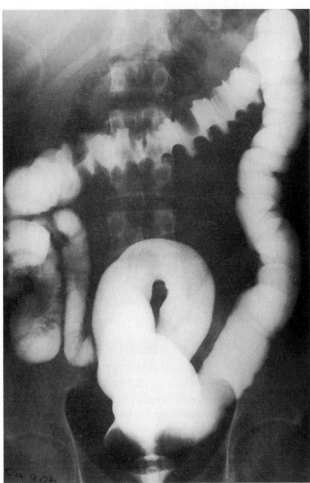

Figure 15–7
Salmonella colitis. A nonspecific pattern of segmental colitis is noted, characterized by spasm of the cecum and transverse colon and moderate edema of the transverse colon. *Salmonella* organisms were recovered from the stool of this 16-year-old boy with bloody diarrhea.

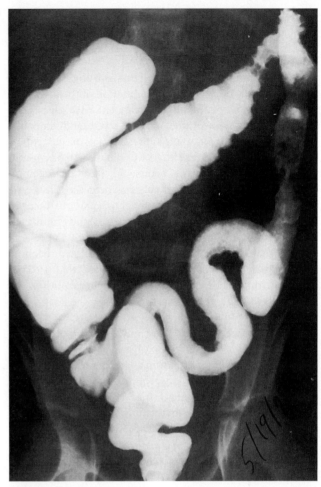

Figure 15–8
Amebic colitis. Spasm, edema, and ulceration involve the rectum, the sigmoid colon, and the descending and distal transverse segments of the colon in a continuous and symmetric circumferential distribution; this pattern is typical of idiopathic ulcerative colitis. Amebic trophozoites were recovered from the stool of this 7-year-old child with bloody diarrhea.

of acute or subacute enteritis. Inflammation of the small intestine, manifested by flexible thickening of the mucosal folds of the duodenum and proximal jejunum, is highly suggestive of giardiasis. Delayed filming of the small bowel may be necessary to demonstrate findings consistent with inflammation.[6] In areas of endemic giardiasis, recognition of this pattern will often persuade the referring physician to treat the infection empirically and forgo duodenal aspiration or duodenal biopsy. In general, however, diagnosis depends on recovery of the organism from duodenal aspirate or stool.

Acute regional enteritis caused by *Yersinia* may cause edema or nodularity of the terminal ileum or both. These changes are indistinguishable from those in nonstenotic Crohn's disease. Such terminal ileal findings are, strictly speaking, nonspecific but limit the diagnostic possibilities to Crohn's disease and yersiniosis in the majority of patients.

In yersiniosis, complete resolution of these ileal changes occurs by the time of repeat examination 6 to 8 weeks later, thereby distinguishing it from Crohn's disease.[16] Results of culture and serologic studies should also be positive with *Yersinia* infection.

Invasive colon infection may cause motility disorder, inflammation, edema, superficial ulceration, deep ulceration, and, in chronic infections, stricture. In cases of infectious enterocolitis or infectious colitis, barium enema findings range from normal or suggestive of a mild segmental or nonsegmental colitis to suggestive of moderate or severe segmental or nonsegmental colitis (see Figs. 15–6 and 15–8). The radiographic appearance is not distinguishable from that of acute idiopathic inflammatory bowel disease. Radiologic evidence of ulcerating colitis has been reported for all enteroinvasive pathogens, most recently *Campylobacter* colitis.

ENTEROCOLITIS OF HIRSCHSPRUNG'S DISEASE

Enterocolitis may complicate Hirschsprung's disease at any time; it may be the initial manifestation of the disease or may occur after successful surgical treatment.[92] Hirschsprung's enterocolitis may present with an acute, severe, and fulminant clinical course that is often fatal, or it may cause malabsorption syndrome due to recurrent bouts of mild disease or chronic low-grade enterocolitis. The incidence of Hirschsprung's enterocolitis in patients of all ages has decreased in recent years, probably because of earlier diagnosis and treatment as well as refinement of surgical techniques. In a study from 1945 to 1961, Bill and Chapman[4] reported that 24 of 47 patients with Hirschsprung's disease (51%) developed enterocolitis. In a more recent large series, it was noted that 15% of patients with Hirschsprung's disease had enterocolitis at the time of diagnosis, and with this complication the fatality rate was 30%.[23]

The incidence, severity, morbidity, and mortality of Hirschsprung's enterocolitis are greatest in neonates and young infants, in whom the mortality rate can be as high as 50%. Enterocolitis is particularly common when Hirschsprung's disease is neither diagnosed nor treated in the first month of life. A survey of American pediatric surgeons shows that the diagnosis of Hirschsprung's disease is still delayed beyond the first year of life in 20% of patients.[49] It has been suggested that a delay in the diagnosis of Hirschsprung's disease beyond 1 week of age is a risk factor in the development of enterocolitis. Furthermore, in patients with Down syndrome, who have an increased incidence of Hirschsprung's disease, there is a significantly increased chance of development of enterocolitis compared with patients with Hirschsprung's disease but without Down syndrome.[90] The association of Down syndrome has been reported in as many as 9% of patients with Hirschsprung's disease.[24]

The diagnosis of Hirschsprung's enterocolitis is straightforward when the diagnosis of Hirschsprung's disease has been previously established. However, a diagnostic challenge exists in the patient who is not known to have Hirschsprung's disease and presents with enterocolitis of uncertain etiology. Particularly in the neonate or young infant, enterocolitis can be the initial recognized manifestation of Hirschsprung's disease. Rapid emergency diagnosis, usually with radiologic assistance, is essential to allow immediate colon decompression, generally with a diverting colostomy. The precarious situation of patients with Hirschsprung's enterocolitis and undiagnosed Hirschsprung's disease is emphasized in an older series in which a 4% mortality rate was found when enterocolitis developed after colostomy, compared with a 33% mortality rate when enterocolitis developed before colostomy.

Pathophysiology

Inflammation, ulceration, and ischemic necrosis of a variable length of the ganglionic bowel characterize Hirschsprung's enterocolitis; these abnormalities may extend into the small bowel.

Obstruction and ischemia have been thought to be important in the pathogenesis of this disease. However, obstruction cannot by itself be responsible for Hirschsprung's enterocolitis because of the recurrence of enterocolitis after decompression and because the frequency of enterocolitis does not correlate with the severity of obstruction. For the same reasons, ischemia due to extreme bowel dilatation cannot by itself explain the development of enterocolitis.

New observations have been made that can help explain the pathophysiology of the enterocolitis of Hirschsprung's disease. Studies have begun to show how patients with Hirschsprung's disease who develop enterocolitis are different from those who do not develop this complication. Wilson-Storey and Scobie[92] have shown significantly reduced levels of IgA in the serum and saliva of patients with Hirschsprung's disease who have developed enterocolitis compared with those who do not have this complication. Some of these patients were infants, but others were older, and screening might be done to determine which patients are at risk. This lack of mucosal defense may render these patients more prone to mucosal invasion by pathogenic and commensal organisms. Definition of a subgroup of patients with Hirschsprung's disease with diminished immune defenses could explain the recurrent and late development of enterocolitis. A percentage of patients with Hirschsprung's disease with associated enterocolitis have enterocyte-adherent organisms (*E. coli*, *Clostridium difficile*, and *Cryptosporidia*), and 35% of those with Hirschsprung's disease with colitis in one series[7] had histologic findings of pseudomembranous colitis. In these patients, appropriate antibiotic therapy (vancomycin) is used. In addition, there is evidence of a subset of patients with Hirschsprung's disease with enterocolitis who have alterations of intestinal mucins. It is hypothesized that these patients have greater susceptibility to enterocyte-adherent organisms, which release toxins causing local mucosal destruction (crypt abscess, ulceration, and perforation) or systemic disease (sepsis and coagulopathy). A grading system has been developed that can be applied to tissue specimens of patients with Hirschsprung's disease to establish a prognostic basis for follow-up.[89]

Clinical Presentation

A newborn who develops enterocolitis associated with Hirschsprung's disease generally appears well initially, without associated abnormalities. Although delayed passage of meconium and subsequent obstruction are the usual symptoms of Hirschsprung's disease, profound diarrhea with foul, liquid, and often bloody stools may be the first and only signs of neonatal Hirschsprung's disease in some infants. In others, initial mild constipation, which is often overlooked, may suddenly evolve into explosive, foul diarrhea. Abdominal distention with signs of obstruction, including bilious vomiting, may occur. In infants with severe disease, listlessness may progress to systemic symptoms of sepsis, with high fever, prostration, dehydration, and bowel perforation.[35] Shock and death may occur within 24 hours. In infants with such fulminant disease, resuscitative measures, even if undertaken immediately, may not be successful.

After the patient's condition has been stabilized and a diagnosis has been established with contrast enema and suction biopsy, immediate colon decompression with colostomy is the method of treatment preferred by most pediatric surgeons. A rectal tube may be inserted as a temporary measure. The often dramatic decompressing effect of rectal tubes and colostomy indicates that obstruction has some role in the pathogenesis of this disorder. If the patient is too ill for general anesthesia, a right transverse colostomy can be done under local anesthesia.

Episodes of enterocolitis may develop after colostomy or definitive surgery, but these are usually mild and diminish in frequency, enabling normal bowel habits after 12 to 18 months. When the recurrent enterocolitis is mild, such infants are often treated with a rectal tube and rectal irrigation at home.

When a term neonate or young infant presents with symptoms and signs of colitis or enterocolitis of uncertain etiology, the main diagnostic considerations include Hirschsprung's enterocolitis, infectious enterocolitis, milk protein allergy, and the rare occurrence of necrotizing enterocolitis in the term baby. Idiopathic inflammatory bowel disease is extremely rare in patients in this age group. When bilious vomiting, distention, and bloody diarrhea are present, a midgut volvulus must also be considered.

Radiographic Evaluation

The radiographic evaluation of Hirschsprung's enterocolitis will be discussed with regard to two distinct presentations: (1) neonatal or infantile enterocolitis of uncertain etiology, and (2) enterocolitis in patients with proven Hirschsprung's disease.

Neonatal or Infantile Enterocolitis of Uncertain Etiology
Plain film examination (supine and horizontal-beam films) is done in these patients primarily to detect findings that contraindicate performance of a barium enema (free intraperitoneal air, toxic megacolon, intestinal pneumatosis, or portal venous gas). The presence of any of these findings in this clinical setting indicates a very sick child with a high risk of contrast extravasation or sepsis if a contrast enema is performed. Supine and horizontal-beam plain films in these patients usually show several dilated bowel loops with air-fluid levels, an appearance that neither distinguishes colon obstruction from nonobstructive ileus nor suggests a specific cause for the enterocolitis.

Plain films may also reveal nonspecific evidence of colitis, such as toxic megacolon, haustral blunting, thumbprinting (reflecting moderate to severe edema and inflammation), pseudopolyps, and membranes outlined by luminal gas. If the child is severely ill or if a significant risk of enema-induced perforation or sepsis is thought to exist, contrast enema is not done.

Contrast enema is performed primarily to demonstrate the aganglionic segment or, if an aganglionic segment cannot be demonstrated, to confirm the presence of enterocolitis. Confirmation of enterocolitis will exclude the possibility of midgut volvulus in the infant with bilious vomiting and bloody diarrhea. Radiologic diagnosis of Hirschsprung's enterocolitis depends on demonstration of the narrowed aganglionic segment, because the appearance of the inflamed colon is nonspecific and compatible with enterocolitis from any cause. As an aid to surgical planning, the proximal extent of colitis may be delineated; however, a complete colon examination is done only when considered safe. The decision of whether to perform a limited examination (the aganglionic segment and distal colitic segment only) or a complete examination is a clinical determination based on the patient's general condition and the severity and duration of the illness.

As a general rule, demonstration of the aganglionic segment of Hirschsprung's disease by contrast enema is more difficult in neonates than in older pediatric patients. Enterocolitis exacerbates the problem, because diarrheal stool may dilate or distend the aganglionic segment. Because demonstration of the aganglionic segment may be difficult and because of the risk of sepsis, the technique by which contrast enema examination is done is very important. The patient is hydrated and stabilized before the examination is begun. Optimal results are obtained with these patients using the following techniques:

1. Powdered barium is mixed with isotonic saline to avoid the risk of water intoxication associated with tap water.
2. A soft red catheter is used for the enema tip; balloon catheters are avoided.
3. The total volume of contrast is limited, using only enough to fill the aganglionic segment and the distal portion of the ganglionic colon; if a complete colon examination is done, the entire colon is filled carefully.
4. Contrast must be introduced slowly, in small volumes and at low pressures, to avoid distention of the aganglionic segment; this is best accomplished by multiple 5-mL hand injections with a 50-mL syringe.
5. Fluoroscopy is performed in the lateral projection, and overhead films always include a lateral view, as anteroposterior (AP) views may not show the narrowed segment.
6. Hypertonic water-soluble contrast agents are not used because of the risk of patient dehydration. Newer nonionic, water-soluble contrast materials have lower osmolality and are optimal in this setting.

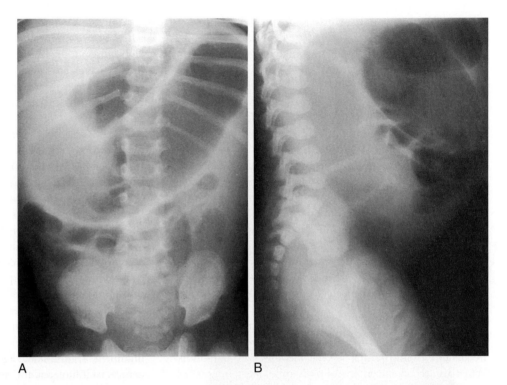

Figure 15–9
Hirschsprung's disease: entero-colitis and toxic megacolon. *A,* This supine anteroposterior abdominal film shows marked dilatation of the transverse colon. Rectal gas is absent. *B,* The left lateral abdominal film also shows marked colon distention. Again, no rectal gas is seen. This 7-week-old boy presented with sepsis and died soon after admission. Rectosigmoid aganglionosis and thick pseudomembranes were discovered in the colon at autopsy.

Enterocolitis in Patients With Proven Hirschsprung's Disease Radiographic evaluation of patients with proven Hirschsprung's disease is generally not required, except in rare situations. Plain films are indicated if there is clinical suspicion of perforation. In a patient in whom Hirschsprung's disease was diagnosed by rectal suction biopsy but who has not had a barium enema, barium examination may be useful if the surgeon, in preparing for colostomy, would like an estimate of aganglionic segment length. In most other situations, radiographic investigation will not add any new knowledge to the clinical findings.

Radiographic Findings

Plain radiographs usually show bowel dilatation suggestive of, but not specific for, low mechanical obstruction. The extreme colon dilatation of toxic megacolon can be easily demonstrated with plain films (Figs. 15–9 through 15–12). Intestinal gas may outline the colonic lumen on plain films and show irregularity of the luminal surface, reflecting edema, ulceration, spasm, and even pseudopolyps and pseudomembranes. Horizontal-beam films will show free air if bowel perforation has occurred.

Contrast enema often, but not invariably, demonstrates the narrowed or spastic aganglionic segment and the transition zone (see Fig. 15–10). The colitic segment shows variable degrees of bowel wall thickening due to inflammation and irregularity of the luminal bowel surface from ulceration, edema, debris, and pseudomembranes. The ganglionic segment may or may not be dilated in neonates; dilatation is

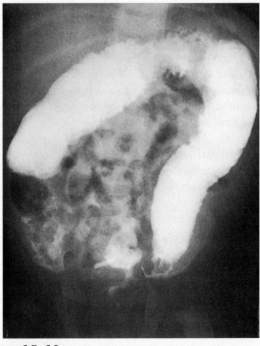

Figure 15–10
Hirschsprung's disease and enterocolitis. This 4-month-old infant presented with signs of intestinal obstruction. A prolonged diarrheal illness of uncertain origin had been extensively evaluated and symptomatically treated in the second and third months of life. A contrast enema was performed to exclude intussusception. The characteristic findings of Hirschsprung's disease, including rectosigmoid spasm and mucosal irregularity in the distal descending colon, were demonstrated by the barium enema.

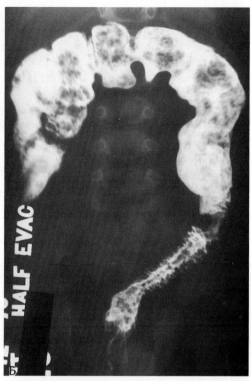

Figure 15–11
Hirschsprung's disease and enterocolitis: postoperative study. Enterocolitis after a Soave pull-through operation for Hirschsprung's disease. Postevacuation film demonstrates a shortened colon with moderate edema and inflammation of the distal segment of colon.

a more common feature in patients with long-standing obstruction. Opacification of only the distal part of the inflamed ganglionic colon is necessary. Although the colitic segment extends proximal from the transition zone for a variable distance, definition of the proximal extent of colitis with barium is not essential, particularly in children whose enterocolitis is severe and in whom the risk of perforation is high.

IDIOPATHIC INFLAMMATORY BOWEL DISEASE

Idiopathic inflammatory bowel diseases (i.e., ulcerative colitis and Crohn's disease) are not common childhood disorders but are important causes of growth failure, chronic illness, and recurrent temporary disability in children. Mortality from these disorders remains significant despite advances in diagnosis and treatment. The incidence of both diseases, particularly Crohn's disease, appears to be increasing in the pediatric age group.

Most children with inflammatory bowel disease who present with gastrointestinal symptoms have diarrhea; however, rectal bleeding (particularly with ulcerative colitis) and

abdominal pain (particularly with Crohn's disease) are often the primary symptoms. A significant percentage of children with inflammatory bowel disease present solely with extraintestinal symptoms (growth failure, delayed sexual maturation, arthritis, fever, anemia, or weight loss). Diagnostic delays of several months and, occasionally, years are common with such presentations.

Radiographic investigation is an important part of the diagnosis and surveillance of inflammatory bowel disease. Confident radiographic distinction between ulcerative colitis and Crohn's colitis can usually, but not invariably, be made.[9] Cross-sectional imaging has an important role in the follow-up of patients in whom inflammatory bowel disease has been diagnosed. This is particularly true in the evaluation of extraintestinal complications, which includes cross-sectional imaging, particularly computed tomography (CT) and ultrasonography. Radionuclide imaging and magnetic resonance imaging have less defined roles.

Pathophysiology

The causes of ulcerative colitis and Crohn's disease are unknown. Transmissible agents, immunologic mechanisms, emotional influences, and hereditary factors have been investigated, but no satisfactory etiologic mechanisms have been identified. Certain groups of people—those with a family history of inflammatory bowel disease and whites, particularly Jews—develop these diseases more commonly than the general population.

Pathologically, ulcerative colitis may be defined as an idiopathic inflammation of the mucosa and submucosa of the colon. Crohn's disease is characterized pathologically by an idiopathic, noncaseating, granulomatous inflammation of the mucosa, submucosa, tunica muscularis, serosa, lymph nodes, and mesentery of any portion of the gut from the esophagus to the anus, but most commonly involving the small bowel, colon, or both. The transmural inflammation of Crohn's disease accounts for the much greater occurrence of severe ulceration, acute inflammatory stenosis, chronic fibrotic stenosis, fistulas, abscess, and perianal disease than in ulcerative colitis. Involvement of the regional lymph nodes and mesentery in Crohn's disease may cause inflammatory enlargement and thickening of these structures, features not usually present in ulcerative colitis. Encroachment of mesenteric fat onto the intestinal serosal surface ("creeping fat") is characteristic of Crohn's disease.

Ulcerative colitis causes symmetric, circumferential involvement of the colon, whereas Crohn's disease causes noncircumferential or asymmetric circumferential involvement of the intestine. With ulcerative colitis, the longitudinal distribution of disease characteristically is continuous, beginning in the rectum and involving contiguous proximal colon for a variable distance. Crohn's disease is usually discontinuous in longitudinal distribution, with normal areas of bowel between abnormal areas (i.e., skip lesions). Continuous or discontinuous right colon disease, extending distally from the cecum, is typical of Crohn's colitis. Rectal involvement occurs in approximately one third of patients with Crohn's disease and in 95% of patients with ulcerative colitis.

Mucosal damage and secondary functional impairment are responsible for diarrhea in both disorders. Lymphatic obstruction may also contribute to diarrhea in Crohn's disease. Bleeding is due to ulceration of inflamed mucosa and fragile granulation tissue. Pain is caused by abnormal motility and bowel edema. Obstructive pain is relatively common with Crohn's disease. Chronic undernutrition and anorexia are more important causes of growth failure than are malabsorption, enteric protein loss, or hormonal influences. Reduced caloric intake has been found to be a major factor in growth retardation in children with Crohn's disease.

Clinical Presentation

Approximately one fifth of all patients with inflammatory bowel disease experience onset of the disease in childhood, commonly in the second decade of life. A significant number of children develop disease in the first decade of life, almost always in the latter half of this decade. Presentation before

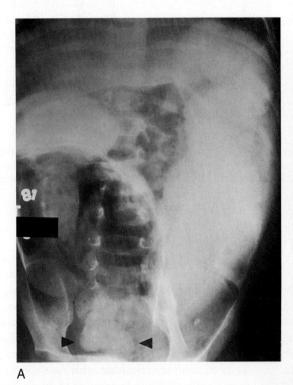

A

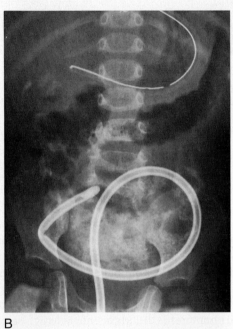

B

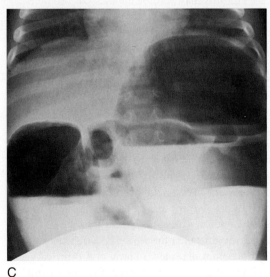

C

Figure 15–12
Hirschsprung's disease and enterocolitis in a 12-month-old infant with a history of constipation and abdominal distention. Diarrhea then developed, and 2 days before referral, a barium enema was performed. The patient was severely ill with a shock-like syndrome. *A,* The supine abdominal radiograph reveals marked dilatation of the colon and a normal caliber rectum *(arrowheads).* The small bowel gas pattern is unremarkable. *B,* The upright film demonstrates several moderately long air-fluid levels. All of these findings are typical of colon obstruction at the level of the rectum. *C,* Supine abdominal radiograph done 2 days after the radiograph shown in *B.* Treatment with a rectosigmoid tube resulted in colon decompression and marked clinical improvement.

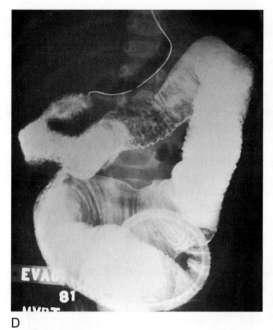 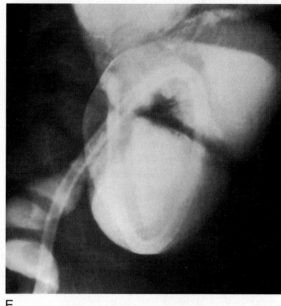

D   E

Figure 15–12—cont'd
D, Postevacuation film of a barium enema performed through the rectal tube. Dilatation, jejunization, and mucosal irregularity are present, indicative of Hirschsprung's disease and enterocolitis. *E,* The transition zone could be identified only on the lateral view, because it was obscured by the sigmoid colon on the AP view. The rectum was filled with contrast, which was administered through a second tube (not visible) in the distal rectum.

the age of 5 years is uncommon, particularly for Crohn's disease, and presentation before the age of 1 year is rare, reported only for ulcerative colitis.

Gastrointestinal symptoms are the dominant initial signs of inflammatory bowel disease in most patients. However, a smaller but significant number of patients have mainly extraintestinal symptoms as the first manifestation of disease. Extraintestinal symptoms may precede the onset of intestinal symptoms by months or years. Common extraintestinal symptoms include growth failure, arthritis, weight loss, fever of unknown origin, and anemia. All of these symptoms and signs are more frequent principal manifestations of Crohn's disease than of ulcerative colitis.

Ulcerative Colitis

Clinical Features Ulcerative colitis typically occurs in children who were previously healthy. The most characteristic initial symptoms of ulcerative colitis are diarrhea and rectal bleeding. Often there are frequent stools that are loose or watery, with variable amounts of mucus, pus, and blood. Early morning stooling is typical; nighttime bowel movements suggest more severe disease. Painless passage of red blood may initially be mistaken for a benign anal process.

Lower abdominal pain is usually present and is probably related to nonpropagation of peristaltic contractions in the diseased colon. A sensation of urgency to defecate is common and may approach constant tenesmus. Anorexia is common during acute exacerbations of ulcerative colitis and may persist because of abdominal pain associated with eating. Nausea and vomiting are signs of severe ulcerative colitis.

Patients may appear relatively healthy or chronically ill. Toxicity is present in those with severe disease. Physical examination reveals minimal or no abdominal tenderness in patients with mild disease. Moderate and severe colitis causes localized (usually left lower quadrant) or diffuse abdominal tenderness, depending on the proximal extent of colon involvement. Bowel sounds are typically increased, and rectal examination is often painful. Skin lesions are not commonly present, but erythema nodosum and erythema multiforme may be present in acute stages of the disease. A small minority of children with ulcerative colitis have arthritis, typically a peripheral polyarthritis involving the large joints. Growth failure may be the most important extracolonic manifestation of ulcerative colitis in children, occurring in approximately 15% of patients.

In the acute stages of ulcerative colitis, proctoscopy reveals a diffusely inflamed and hyperemic rectal mucosa with obscuration of the normal vascular pattern and increased mucosal friability. Ulcers, pseudopolyps, and mucosal granularity are rarely identified. Fecal leukocytes and erythrocytes are typically present. Histologically, acute and chronic inflammatory cell infiltrates of the lamina propria, distortion of the rectal glands, disruption of the surface epithelium, and crypt abscesses are evident. Appropriate antibiotic therapy will result in rapid improvement in the histologic findings of infectious colitis; idiopathic ulcerative colitis will not show such a response. However, the histologic features of ulcerative colitis and infectious colitis on rectal biopsy are not distinct enough from one another to allow reliable diagnosis based on a single biopsy. Thus, serial rectal biopsies are considerably more useful than is a single biopsy for distinguishing ulcerative colitis from infectious colitis. Confident histologic differentiation between ulcerative colitis and Crohn's disease on rectal biopsy primarily depends on the demonstration of granulomas in the latter.

The most common abnormal findings on laboratory evaluation are anemia due to chronic intestinal blood loss and the marrow depression of chronic disease. The sedimentation rate is usually elevated in active disease. Leukocytosis may be present, and platelet counts may be depressed. Indicators of protein metabolism are usually normal, but hypoalbuminemia may accompany severe or chronic disease. Abnormal liver function studies are seen in 25% of patients with ulcerative colitis, but clinical liver disease is rare.

The onset and progression of the disease may take several forms in childhood. The most common presentation is an insidious onset, with bloody diarrhea. Systemic symptoms of fever and weight loss are typically often absent. There is intermittent, low-grade disease activity, generally limited to the rectum. Patients with such symptoms usually do not have extraintestinal symptoms of ulcerative colitis. Another group of patients, constituting about one third of the children with this condition, present with more acute, overt evidence of the disease, including bloody diarrhea, cramps, urgency, and systemic symptoms (weight loss, malaise, low-grade fever, and mild anemia). About 10% of children with ulcerative colitis present with serious systemic involvement in the form of severe anemia, hypoalbuminemia, fever, tachycardia, significant weight loss, and several bloody diarrheal stools daily.

The outcome of ulcerative colitis in pediatric patients varies, as it does in adult patients. About 10% of children have a single episode, without recurrence. Even if a complete evaluation is done during the acute episode, the diagnosis may subsequently be questioned. Approximately one third of patients have only occasional exacerbations, often preceded by stress or illness. In the remaining majority, the disease continues in a chronic, unremitting course.

Treatment goals are control of symptoms, preservation of adequate nutrition, maintenance of growth, and return to a normal life. Specific therapy includes consideration of medical and surgical alternatives. Sulfasalazine, steroids, and a low-residue diet are the major medical means of dealing with ulcerative colitis. Hyperalimentation and appropriate antibiotics may be useful in selected patients.

Acute complications of childhood ulcerative colitis are rare and include fulminant or unremitting colitis, toxic megacolon (with or without perforation), and colonic hemorrhage. Toxic megacolon occurs in approximately 1% of patients with ulcerative colitis at any stage or age. Its etiology is unknown, but pathologically there is marked dilatation of the colon with thinning of its wall. Transmural inflammation and necrosis of a variable extent are present. Perforation leading to peritonitis is not uncommon. Clinically, generalized sepsis is often present, even before perforation. On physical examination, the child's condition appears to be toxic, with a distended abdomen and diminished or absent bowel sounds.

Chronic complications of ulcerative colitis include growth failure, undernutrition, chronic debility from intestinal or extraintestinal disease, and colon malignancy. The risk of developing colon carcinoma is 3% in the first decade of disease and 20% in the second, with increasingly higher percentages in succeeding decades. Children with pancolitis and continuous disease activity have an additional risk of colon malignancy. The tumors are adenocarcinomas, and they may be multicentric. Colon lymphoma has also been reported as a complication of chronic ulcerative colitis. Dysplastic alteration of colon mucosa is thought to predict malignant conversion.

Children with these acute or chronic complications are treated surgically with proctocolectomy, which is curative for ulcerative colitis. Eventually, most patients with early onset of ulcerative colitis undergo colectomy for cancer prophylaxis. The mortality rate for emergency colectomy is about 10 times higher than that for elective colectomy. Advances in surgical procedures, including total colectomy, mucosal proctectomy, and ileoanal anastomosis, hold the promise of earlier elective surgery, with less disruption of normal functioning. These procedures remove all colonic mucosa that might be affected by primary disease and prone to developing carcinoma, while avoiding long-term ostomies and allowing patients to have a relatively normal stooling pattern. The ileoanal anastomosis is the procedure of choice in the surgical treatment of ulcerative colitis in children.[66]

Radiographic Evaluation Plain film evaluation of the abdomen in children with ulcerative colitis is useful primarily for detection of free air when perforation is suspected clinically, usually in a clinical setting of an ill child with possible toxic megacolon. Plain films are also useful for confirmation of toxic megacolon by showing colon dilatation.

Contrast enema (single- or double-contrast), performed at the time of presentation and initial evaluation, is useful (1) to define the extent and severity of colitis proximal to the rectum, (2) to support a clinical diagnosis of idiopathic ulcerative colitis by excluding colitis with radiographic features typical of Crohn's colitis, and (3) to exclude terminal ileal disease compatible with Crohn's disease, assuming ileal reflux is sufficient for confident evaluation of the terminal ileum. The clinical diagnosis of idiopathic ulcerative colitis is one of exclusion. The main differential diagnostic considerations, apart from Crohn's disease, include infectious colitis, pseudomembranous colitis, and hemolytic-uremic syndrome; these are most reliably excluded by history, proctoscopic examination, stool culture, and laboratory evaluation.

Contrast evaluation plays a secondary but important role in the diagnosis of idiopathic ulcerative colitis and is most valuable when the differential diagnosis has been narrowed to ulcerative colitis and Crohn's disease. Both single- and double-contrast barium enema examinations are highly accurate in the diagnosis of advanced ulcerative colitis. However, double-contrast examinations are more sensitive in the detection of early disease.[93] With the availability of smaller, more technically advanced equipment and better techniques, colonoscopy performed by experienced endoscopists has become the primary modality in many centers in the initial diagnosis of inflammatory bowel disease of the colon. The ready availability of biopsy allows diagnosis in early stages of the disease when direct visualization of the mucosa appears normal. Although sedation is necessary, current protocols for sedation of children allow safe and successful endoscopy in the majority of patients.[84,91]

Upper gastrointestinal (UGI) and small bowel series are performed in all patients at the time of initial presentation to exclude the possibility of Crohn's disease.

Contrast enema is useful at the time of follow-up for assessment of the extent and severity of disease when required clinically and for surveillance for carcinoma proximal to the rectum. However, annual colonoscopy with biopsy and biannual proctoscopy with biopsy are the primary methods of surveillance for malignancy when colitis has been evident for 5 to 10 years.

Contraindications to contrast enema include free air evident on the plain film, toxic megacolon or suspected toxic megacolon, and recent rectal or colon biopsy. It is prudent to wait at least 48 hours before proceeding with the contrast enema in patients who have had a rectal or colon biopsy.

The preparation of patients is important in obtaining maximal diagnostic information. High-quality contrast enemas (i.e., capable of detecting the early and subtle changes of ulcerative colitis) require excellent colon preparation. However, the patient with colitis who is acutely ill colitis has excessive colon fluid and mucus, which preclude confident detection of the ulceration and mucosal granularity that are otherwise apparent on air-contrast examination. Accurate determination of the extent of disease in such patients is not possible. Colon preparation in patients with ulcerative colitis is often deliberately limited because of concern about (1) increasing fluid and electrolyte losses by thorough purgation of a child who may already be electrolyte- and volume-depleted, (2) the discomfort associated with purgation, and (3) the potential for exacerbation of colitis. The concerns about fluid and electrolyte depletion and patient discomfort are valid. However, a cause-and-effect relationship between colon preparation and

clinical deterioration has not been shown. We do not recommend barium enema in children with acute colitis until the disease has been controlled to the point that the child can tolerate adequate colon preparation. This approach is justified for two reasons: (1) barium examination is generally not needed in the initial stages of diagnosis and treatment of colitis in children, and (2) the patient's and physician's interests are best served by an examination that is as accurate as possible in defining the extent and pattern of colitis. This method of treatment also avoids the additional radiation that the child would receive from a second examination, necessitated by the uncertainty of the results of the first examination.

Rarely, an unusual clinical situation requires barium enema in an acutely ill child with significant diarrhea. In such patients, thorough purgation is neither necessary nor appropriate, and a single-contrast contrast enema is done. Preparation of these patients consists of consumption of a clear liquid diet and gentle saline enemas given the morning of the study. When the patient's colitis has been controlled to the point that the child can tolerate more complete colon cleansing, we use the following: (1) cleansing saline enemas or Fleet Phospho-soda the evening before the study and again in the early morning or oral colon preparation products such as Golytely; and (2) a low-residue or clear liquid diet for 24 hours prior to the examination. This preparation is usually adequate for an air-contrast examination.

Enema tips equipped with inflatable balloons are not used to avoid damage to friable rectal mucosa. High-density nonflocculating barium is instilled by gravity to the distal or midtransverse colon. Air is introduced after gravity drainage of as much rectosigmoid barium as possible. Subsequently, the patient is asked to roll over several times, and filming is done in multiple positions, which always include left and right lateral decubitus views. Double-contrast examinations, although often uncomfortable for patients with considerable colon distention, are better tolerated by children than by adults. Currently, many radiologists use air-contrast contrast enemas for suspected inflammatory bowel disease, because this method is capable of showing early changes substantially better than does the single-contrast examination.

Radiographic Findings In patients with ulcerative colitis, plain films are most often normal, regardless of the level of disease activity. Occasionally, gross features of ulcerative colitis (e.g., spasm, haustral loss or thickening, colon shortening, edema or inflammation, large ulcers, and pseudopolyps) may be detected if sufficient intraluminal gas is present to outline these features (Fig. 15–13). Toxic megacolon is often evident on plain films as marked colon distention, which on supine films is most obvious in the transverse colon because of the anterior location of this segment (Fig. 15–14). Horizontal-beam abdominal radiographs (decubitus or upright) reveal air-fluid levels that are generally quite long. Free air from perforation (with or without toxic megacolon) is best shown with horizontal-beam films.

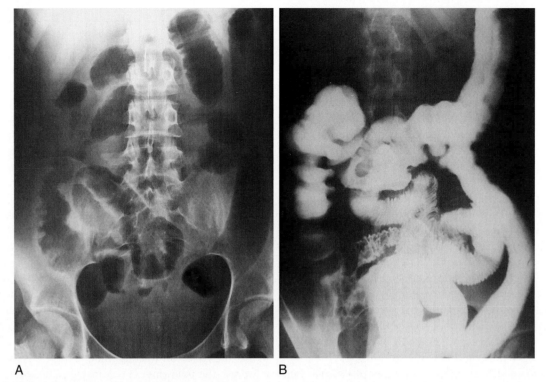

A   B

Figure 15–13
Images of a 15-year-old patient with bloody diarrhea. *A,* This plain abdominal film demonstrates air distending the descending colon, with some scattered dilated loops of small intestine. The wall of the descending colon appears irregular, suggesting the possibility of inflammatory bowel disease in this region. *B,* After administration of a single-contrast contrast enema, the left colon has a fine, spiculated appearance, consistent with the diagnosis of ulcerative colitis.

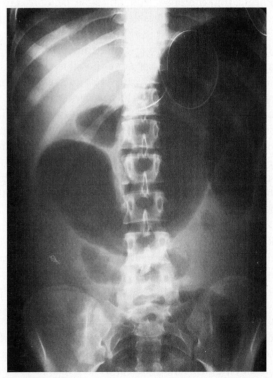

Figure 15–14
Toxic megacolon in ulcerative colitis: supine abdominal radiograph of a 16-year-old adolescent with clinical features of toxic megacolon. Marked distention of the transverse colon and moderate distention of the sigmoid and proximal descending colon are apparent. The patient was treated with proctocolectomy.

The distribution of colon involvement is continuous along the bowel axis. Disease begins in the rectum in 95% of patients and involves contiguous proximal colon for a variable length. Pancolitis may be associated with dilatation of the ileocecal valve and the terminal ileum, a finding termed *backwash ileitis,* despite the fact that actual inflammation of the terminal ileum in such patients is uncommon. However, some patients with backwash ileitis show evidence of mucosal disease (Fig. 15–15).

The radiographic findings of active ulcerative colitis reflect the presence of disordered motility, edema, inflammation, ulceration, and pseudopolyps. These findings are discussed in the following subsections.

Active Ulcerative Colitis[57]

Disordered Motility Disordered motility in the acute phase of ulcerative colitis is obvious by focal, multifocal, or diffuse spasm (contraction of the circular muscularis), haustral effacement (Fig. 15–16) or blunting (contraction of the muscularis mucosa and longitudinal muscularis), and reversible colon shortening (generalized longitudinal muscularis contraction). Severe spasm can completely obstruct retrograde barium flow. These abnormalities of motility are nonspecific and may be seen in acute colitis from any cause. Reduced haustration in the left colon can be a normal variant.

Edema and Inflammation Mild edema and inflammation of the mucosa and submucosa result in indistinctness, "fuzziness," or fine granularity (see Fig. 15–16) of the mucosal surface (best seen on air-contrast studies). This appearance

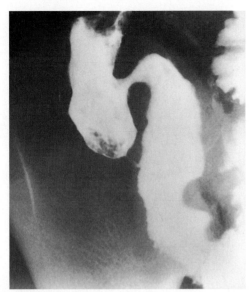

Figure 15–15
Ulcerative colitis: backwash ileitis. In this film of a 14-year-old girl with chronic ulcerative colitis, note the reduced cecal caliber, absence of haustration, and mild dilatation of the terminal ileum, which also demonstrates mild mucosal irregularity. Mucosal disease is an uncommon manifestation of the backwash ileitis of ulcerative colitis.

may also be caused by retained colonic fluid and mucus, with resultant poor coating of the colon surface (Fig. 15–17). The only evidence of edema and inflammation may be found on postevacuation films, which show thickening of the mucosal folds or a longitudinal orientation of mucosal folds

that are normally haphazardly oriented (Fig. 15–18). Haustral thickening and blunting may also result from more advanced degrees of edema and inflammation. These indications of edema and inflammation are nonspecific findings seen with acute colitis of any kind.

Ulceration Small ulcers are identified most confidently on air-contrast examination, which reveals a fine serration or spiculation of the colon surface in tangent and a fine stippling en face (Fig. 15–19). The fine spiculation seen in tangent must be differentiated from normal innominate grooves and from the poor coating caused by retained fluid or a fine fecal residue. The stippled appearance en face must be differentiated from poor coating due to excess mucus, excess fluid, or a fine fecal residue. As the ulcers enlarge or become confluent, coarse spiculation in tangent and coarse granularity en face are evident. Granulation tissue also contributes to the coarsely granular appearance. Larger ulcers are often irregular in shape and typically vary in size to a moderate degree. Enlargement of the base of ulcers may undermine the mucosa and create "collar button" ulcerations. These patterns of ulceration are not specific for idiopathic ulcerative colitis and may be identified in any ulcerating type of colitis (e.g., infectious colitis or Crohn's disease).

Pseudopolyps A polypoid or "cobblestone" pattern may be produced when "islands" of inflamed and hyperplastic mucosa develop in a "sea" of extensive ulceration. The morphologic appearance and size of these inflammatory pseudopolyps vary from patient to patient, but the size in any given patient is usually fairly uniform. Occasionally, these inflammatory

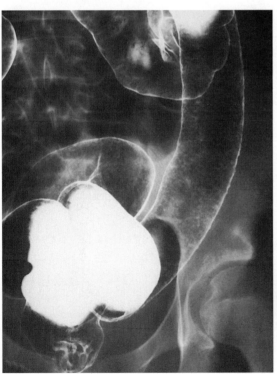

A

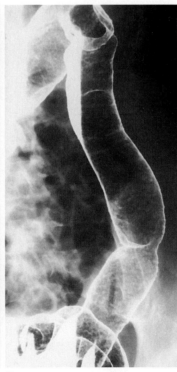

B

Figure 15–16
Ulcerative colitis, mild changes: double-contrast contrast enema in a 13-year-old girl with ulcerative colitis and moderate symptoms. *A,* This radiograph demonstrates the granular pattern of early ulcerative colitis in the sigmoid segment. This appearance reflects the presence of mild edema and inflammation. Haustrations are absent. *B,* This right decubitus view of the descending colon shows fine spiculation of the lateral aspect of the distal descending colon, representing small ulcerations.

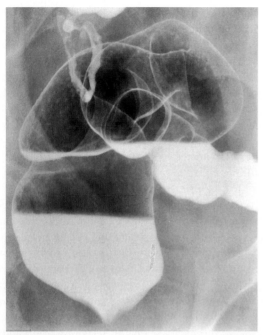

Figure 15–17
Poor coating simulating the granular pattern of early ulcerative colitis: double-contrast view of the rectosigmoid region in an adolescent. The granular appearance is compatible with either mild edema/inflammation or poor coating from excess fluid and mucus. The latter cause was confirmed by endoscopic examination, results of which were normal.

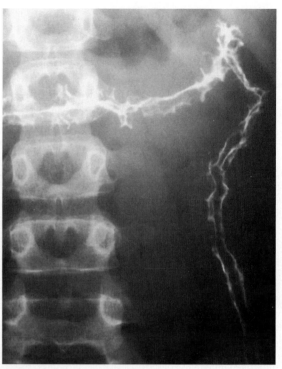

Figure 15–18
Ulcerative colitis: postevacuation film of a 10-year-old child. The longitudinal orientation of mucosal folds in the descending colon indicates edema and inflammation. Edematous and inflamed mucosal folds are also present in the transverse colon.

Figure 15–19 Ulcerative colitis: double-contrast contrast enema in a 5-year-old boy who had had both intestinal and extraintestinal symptoms intermittently since the age of 3 years. *A,* Small ulcerations are distributed uniformly about the colonic circumference and continuously from the rectum to the proximal transverse colon. This pattern of involvement is typical of ulcerative colitis. *B,* In this coned view of the sigmoid colon in the same patient, small ulcerations are represented by fine spiculation of the colonic contour in tangent and by fine stippling of the colon surface en face.

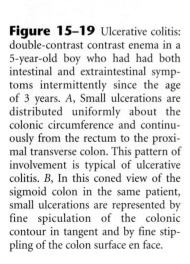

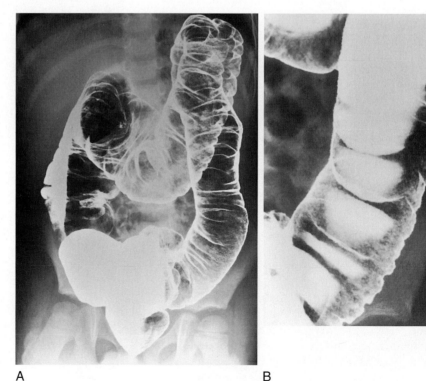

A   B

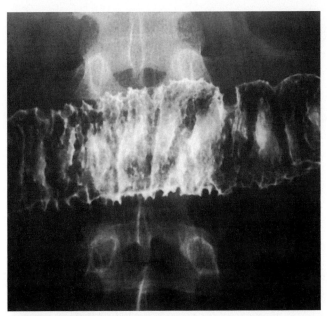

Figure 15–20
Innominate grooves. These grooves, noted in the transverse colon, simulated early ulcerative colitis in this 12-year-old boy with abdominal pain. The colon was endoscopically normal.

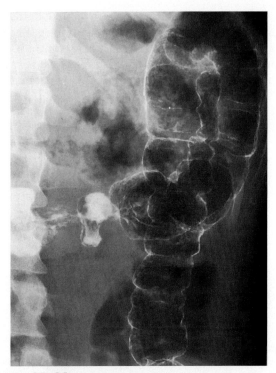

Figure 15–21
Ulcerative colitis: double-contrast barium enema in a 16-year-old boy with a long history of ulcerative colitis. A coarsely granular mucosal pattern is visible in the splenic flexure, secondary to confluent ulceration and granulation tissue.

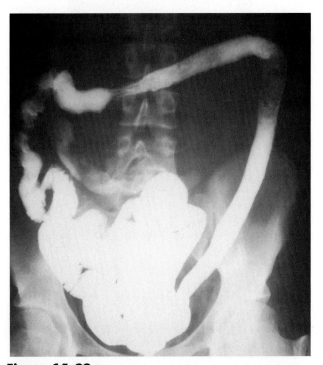

Figure 15–22
Ulcerative colitis: late changes. This double-contrast contrast enema shows the late changes of ulcerative colitis in a 15-year-old girl. The colon is featureless, reduced in caliber, and shortened. Dilatation of the terminal ileum (backwash ileitis) is present.

polyps simulate a luminal mass. Typically, the polyps mimic true sessile polyps, suggesting familial polyposis. Sometimes, tubular bands of mucosa (mucosal bridges or filiform polyps) result when these inflamed islands of mucosa are extensively but incompletely undermined (tunneled) (Figs. 15–20, 15–21 and 15–22).

Inactive Ulcerative Colitis After an episode of active colitis has subsided, the radiographic appearance of the colon often returns to normal or may show abnormalities reflecting irreversible chronic changes. "Inactive" may not be an accurate term, because abnormal histologic findings are frequently seen in biopsy specimens from asymptomatic patients. Radiographic findings of inactive disease reflect the presence of mucosal atrophy, healed pseudopolyps, hypertrophy and contracture of muscular layers, and, rarely, mild submucosal fibrosis. These findings are discussed in the following subsections (Figs. 15–23 and 15–24).

Mucosal Atrophy With healing, mucosal atrophy may occur, and the mucosa may lose its mobility over the underlying muscularis mucosa, causing a featureless mucosal surface. The colon may then have a smooth, tubular appearance involving a segment of the colon or the entire colon (see Fig. 15–22).

Hypertrophy and Contracture of the Muscular Layers Irreversible segmental or generalized shortening of the colon is the result of permanent muscular hypertrophy and contracture (longitudinal muscularis).[61] An irreversible segmental or generalized reduction in colon caliber is also due to permanent muscular changes. In advanced stages, haustrations are absent, and a short, narrow, featureless colon results, with loss of normal redundant areas such as flexures and sigmoid regions (see Fig. 15–22).

Benign strictures are usually the result of focal hypertrophy of the muscularis mucosa and focal separation of the inner

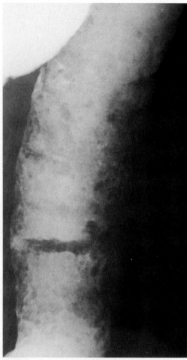

Figure 15–23
Ulcerative colitis: pseudopolyps. Multiple small nodules of varying size are present in the descending colon of this adolescent with ulcerative colitis; the disease was not active at the time of the examination.

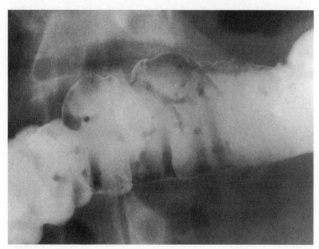

Figure 15–24
Ulcerative colitis: filiform polyposis. Multiple thin, tubular filling defects are present in the transverse colon of this adolescent girl with inactive ulcerative colitis.

(circular) layer of the muscularis mucosa from the outer (longitudinal) layer. Because these strictures are related to hypertrophy, some of them may resolve if the hypertrophy regresses. Benign strictures are typically mild, symmetric stenoses that taper gradually and are pliable.

Pseudopolyps The deformity of the colon surface created by pseudopolyps may persist, even though healing and epithelial regeneration take place. These "chronic" pseudopolyps will persist unless recurrent active disease destroys their architecture. They may have nodular or filiform shapes.

Submucosal Fibrosis Mild degrees of shortening and narrowing of the colon may occasionally occur due to submucosal fibrosis. In general, however, fibrosis is not present to a degree that would account for the changes in colon caliber and length.[61]

Colonic Malignancy Colonic malignancy from chronic ulcerative colitis generally appears similar to carcinoma unrelated to inflammatory bowel disease. Carcinoma may present as an annular, constricting ring; as a sessile polypoid mass; or as a stricture. In patients with chronic ulcerative colitis, polypoid lesions of any size must be regarded as carcinoma until proved otherwise. Malignant strictures are usually asymmetric but may mimic symmetric, gradually tapered, benign strictures.

Cross-Sectional Imaging Ulcerative colitis generally involves only the mucosa, and thus cross-sectional imaging adds little information to barium enemas and endoscopy (Figs. 15–25 and 15–26). However, wall thickness may be increased (see Fig. 15–25) or, with toxic megacolon, decreased. For further discussion of cross-sectional imaging findings, see "Crohn's Disease."

Crohn's Disease

Clinical Features A diagnostic delay of several months is common with Crohn's disease, probably because of the high frequency of initial symptoms at extraintestinal sites and

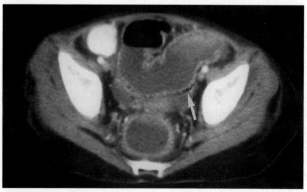

Figure 15–25
Computed tomography (CT) image: chronic ulcerative colitis. In this 6-year-old girl with chronic ulcerative colitis, an irregular, thickened wall *(arrow)* can be seen in the dilated rectosigmoid colon.

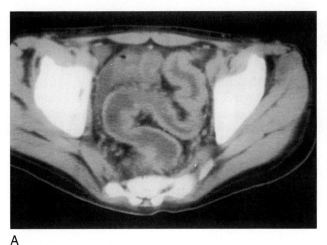 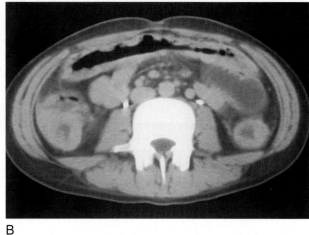

A   B

Figure 15–26
CT without oral contrast material of an older patient with ulcerative colitis. *A,* Thickening of the upper ascending and descending colon. Across the middle of the upper portion of the CT slice, the transverse colon is seen with air in it, but the wall is also thickened. *B,* Scan through the pelvis shows the considerable thickening of the entire sigmoid colon.

the typically insidious nature of gastrointestinal symptoms. Occasionally, however, disease onset is abrupt, with acute abdominal symptoms suggesting acute infectious enteritis, obstruction, intestinal perforation, or acute appendicitis.

Idiopathic growth failure is the sole presenting symptom in 5% of the children with Crohn's disease, and approximately 30% to 40% of patients with Crohn's disease are below normal in stature at the time of diagnosis. Early abdominal symptoms are often nonspecific and include vague and poorly localized pain, anorexia, and bloating. Three fourths of children have diarrhea and abdominal pain at the time of diagnosis. Initially, pain is often periumbilical but eventually may localize to the right lower quadrant. Gross rectal bleeding is uncommon except when isolated Crohn's colitis is present. Fever may occur, and weight loss is almost always reported at the time of diagnosis.

On physical examination, many patients appear chronically ill, although some are relatively healthy. Chronic disease can be manifest by pallor, digital clubbing, retarded growth, and delayed development of secondary sexual characteristics. Tenderness and mass may be detectable in the right lower quadrant. Anal disease in the form of fissure, fistula, or infection is often present. Arthritis, cutaneous lesions (erythema nodosum or pyoderma gangrenosum), and stomatitis occur but are infrequent at the time of diagnosis.[62,68] One study suggested a higher incidence of UGI involvement in children with Crohn's disease than previously believed.[5] When rectal disease is present, proctoscopy reveals patchy involvement and anal disease. Biopsy of the rectal mucosa may reveal a variety of findings, including normal appearance, appearances identical to that of "classic" ulcerative colitis, and submucosal inflammation with relatively normal mucosa.

Granulomas are seen about 50% of the time, permitting confident diagnosis of Crohn's disease.

Laboratory data reveal evidence of both acute and chronic disease. The sedimentation rate is elevated initially in almost all patients. Anemia from blood loss, chronic disease, or both is common. Hypoproteinemia is present in about one third of patients with Crohn's disease, and abnormal liver function is present in about one fourth of patients. As with ulcerative colitis, clinical liver disease is rare. Malabsorption of carbohydrate, fat, or both can be shown in about one third of the patients, presumably those with severe proximal small bowel disease. About one third of the patients have abnormal vitamin B_{12} absorption, but B_{12} deficiency is commonly prevented by the large amount of stored B_{12}. Low or absent serum IgA is noted in approximately 20% of patients.

Undernutrition can be the most debilitating of all intestinal complications. A few patients have urinary tract problems, primarily oxalate stones resulting from increased oxalate absorption in the colon. Urinary tract obstruction and enterovesical fistulas rarely develop.

In general, the course of childhood Crohn's disease is slowly progressive and relentless. Disease control, rather than cure, is the object of treatment.

In a report of 86 children with Crohn's disease seen in a referral center during a 10-year period, Gryboski and Spiro[31] concluded that

(1) ileocolitis is now the most common type of disease in children referred to this center, (2) the long-term prognosis depends in part upon the segment of bowel most involved at the time of diagnosis, (3) disease of the small bowel alone, no matter how extensive, is associated with a more benign

course than in cases with coexistent colonic disease, and (4) ileocolitis is the most difficult form of the disease to treat satisfactorily by either medical or surgical methods.

In addition, children with isolated colonic disease had fewer operations and complications than children with ileocolitis. Gryboski and Spiro[31] also found that the small group of children with duodenal disease usually did not respond well to medical therapy. Treatment goals include minimization of disability and preservation of normal growth or reversal of growth failure. Sulfasalazine, steroids, and dietary therapy are commonly used for medical management; hyperalimentation is useful for severe disease. Surgical treatment is reserved for intestinal complications of the disease and sometimes for reversal of growth failure. In general, the objective of surgical intervention is palliation rather than cure because of the high rate of recurrence of Crohn's disease after resection. However, proctocolectomy and ileostomy for isolated Crohn's colitis may yield results comparable to those of proctocolectomy for ulcerative colitis. This is probably due to the fact that isolated Crohn's colitis rarely progresses to ileocolitis.

The intestinal complications most frequently encountered are obstruction and fistula formation (bowel, bladder, and skin). Intestinal hemorrhage, perforation, and abscess, including psoas abscess, are relatively less common. Toxic megacolon is unusual and is less common than in ulcerative colitis. Carcinoma of the colon and small bowel may also complicate Crohn's disease[79]; the risk of colon carcinoma is considerably less than that in chronic ulcerative colitis. The presence of surgically bypassed bowel loops adds to the risk of malignant complications, which increases with time in all patients with Crohn's disease.

Gryboski and Spiro[31] recommended that a child with ileocolitis should not have surgery for growth failure unless the patient is showing early signs of puberty. They believed that

…children with early pubertal changes, operated on between 12 and 16 years of age while their bone age is still retarded, show the best response in growth and in sexual development. Those operated on before puberty often fail to develop secondary sexual characteristics because of recurrent disease. Those who are sexually mature and small at the time of surgery usually grow poorly. The greatest dilemma occurs in that group of children who are at adolescent age but whose pubarche is yet retarded

Long-term studies show that a large number of children with Crohn's disease require surgery. After 15 years, 87% of 67 children needed surgery. Those with ileocecal disease were more likely to require surgical intervention. The most common indications were obstructive symptoms, fistula formation with possible perforation, and significant growth failure. These patients did not respond adequately to conventional, medical, and nutritional therapy. The ability to better diagnose extraintestinal disease such as fistula and abscess

formation and to treat selectively with nonoperative techniques such as CT-guided drainage may reduce the need for surgical intervention.[18,71]

Radiographic Evaluation Plain films are useful primarily for estimation of the presence or absence of small bowel or colon obstruction and for detection of extraintestinal gas (abscess or free air). Other associated abnormalities may also be seen, such as urinary stones, enteroliths, sacroiliitis, or large mesenteric masses.

Because Crohn's disease may affect any segment of the gastrointestinal tract, an esophagram, UGI series, small bowel series, and contrast enema are done at the time of initial diagnosis. However, in many centers, upper and lower gastrointestinal endoscopy has supplanted the initial evaluation with barium studies. Biopsies of involved or suspected areas are routinely done at the time of endoscopy.

Esophageal, gastric, and duodenal disease are less common in children than in adults. Small bowel examination is usually an initial part of the evaluation because the endoscopic visualization does not include the majority of the small intestine. Routine surveillance with repeated endoscopy or contrast studies is not recommended because the results of such examinations rarely reveal anything significantly inconsistent with the clinical evaluation. When complications (e.g., fistula, obstruction, hemorrhage, or abscess) are suspected clinically, plain films, barium evaluations, and CT (discussed later) may be indicated for diagnosis, surgical planning, or drainage procedures.

When a small bowel examination is performed it may either be with routine techniques or enteroclysis. The latter method is more sensitive for detection of mild, early disease. When routine small bowel examination is done, frequent fluoroscopic observations (usually at 10- to 15-minute intervals) are often needed to delineate potential complications such as fistulas. If contrast enema is performed, it is best to use a double-contrast technique; however, a solid-column study is appropriate for demonstration of fistulas. If the patient is acutely ill with significant diarrhea, it is recommended that the barium enema be postponed until a good colon preparation and a high-quality air-contrast contrast enema can be performed. This approach is recommended both at the initial presentation and at follow-up examinations. Obstruction and stenosis often limit the use of purgatives, and good preparation of the colon may necessitate consumption of a clear liquid or low-residue diet for 2 or 3 days. CT is often used in follow-up, particularly when complications outside the lumen of the bowel are suspected.

Radiographic Findings Intestinal barium studies usually show abnormal results at the time of initial evaluation. In children, longitudinal (axial) progression of initially defined small bowel and colon disease occurs with or without surgery but is more common after surgery.[30] With progression of Crohn's disease, affected segments of the intestine develop stenosis or, if they are already stenotic, become more stenotic. Ulceration may extend to sinus formation, from which a fistula or abscess may result. An "improvement" in the radiographic appearance of Crohn's disease is uncommon, and when it does occur, it is probably due to reversal of motility disturbances (spasm and irritability) in normal or diseased intestine.

The distribution of Crohn's disease is typically discontinuous (segmental) along the gastrointestinal axis and is asymmetric or discontinuous around the circumference of the gut. The term *skip lesion* refers to the discontinuous pattern of involvement in which the disease skips the normal intestine that is between two foci of disease.

Gross patterns of intestinal involvement and their approximate frequency in childhood Crohn's disease are as follows[21,46]: ileocolitis, 40% to 55%; isolated small bowel, 35% to 50%; and isolated colon, 10%.

Small Intestine Crohn's enteritis exhibits three basic patterns of disease distribution: isolated terminal ileum disease; diffuse small bowel disease, including the terminal ileum; and small bowel disease with sparing of the terminal ileum (Fig. 15–27). In one series, 20% of the children who presented with small bowel Crohn's disease exhibited terminal ileal sparing.[46] Duodenal Crohn's disease is uncommon, occurring less frequently in childhood Crohn's disease than in adult Crohn's disease (Figs. 15–28 and 15–29). Nevertheless, because of the rarity of peptic disease in children, Crohn's disease is a differential diagnostic consideration any time an abnormal duodenum is demonstrated on barium radiographs.

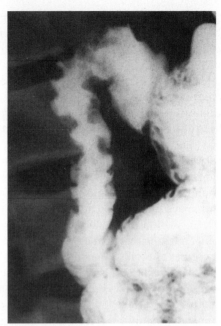

Figure 15–28
Crohn's duodenitis in a 15-year-old adolescent who presented with abdominal pain. There is mucosal fold thickening in the duodenal bulb and the second portion of the duodenum, representing the moderate inflammatory changes of Crohn's disease. Peptic duodenitis can cause an identical radiographic appearance.

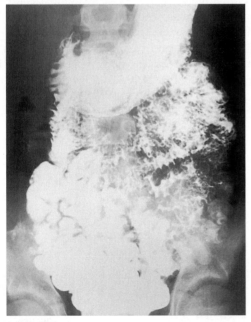

Figure 15–27
Crohn's enteritis: ileal sparing. This radiograph shows mild to moderate inflammatory changes involving the jejunum. There is sparing of the ileum, including the terminal ileum.

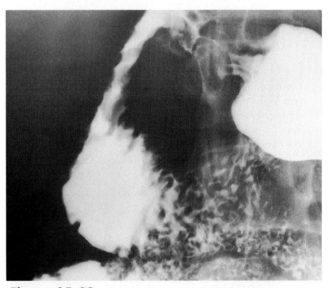

Figure 15–29
Crohn's duodenitis. Moderate to severe inflammatory stenosis of the second portion of the duodenum is present in this 16-year-old boy. Ulceration and mucosal fluid effacement are evident in the involved segment.

The radiographic appearance of small bowel Crohn's disease reflects the presence of varying degrees of edema, inflammation, ulceration, and fibrosis involving the bowel wall, lymphatic system, and mesentery. Spasm and irritability of normal and diseased segments may also contribute to the radiographic findings (see Figs. 15–27, 15–28, and 15–29).

Mild changes of Crohn's disease in the small bowel are due to slight degrees of edema and inflammation without stenosis or visible ulceration. These changes are manifested by mild enlargement of the mucosal folds. Basic fold architecture and bowel pliability are preserved. With moderate edema and inflammation, the mucosal folds become larger, vary somewhat in size, become mildly distorted (Figs. 15–30 and 15–31), and demonstrate reduced pliability during fluoroscopic observation with palpation. Moderate edema and inflammation may also cause a nodular pattern of mucosal fold enlargement (Figs. 15–32 and 15–33). Some separation of these loops may be observed secondary to inflammatory thickening of the bowel wall. With marked degrees of edema and inflammation, the mucosal folds become so distorted that the regular fold pattern is lost (Figs. 15–29 and 15–34). Complete effacement of the mucosal folds may occur. Stenosis of the lumen is common with this marked degree of edema and inflammation (see Figs. 15–29 and 15–34). Severe transmural and mesenteric edema and inflammation cause the affected segment to become relatively inflexible, straightened, and separated from adjacent bowel loops. A thickened

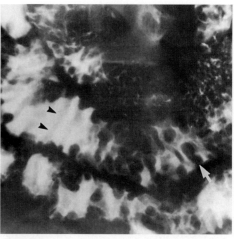

Figure 15–31
Crohn's enteritis. Moderate inflammation and edema have caused moderate mucosal fold enlargement with straightening of some folds *(black arrowheads)* and distortion of others *(white arrow)*. Ulceration is not present.

terminal ileum often causes a mass impression on the medial cecum (see Figs. 15–30 through 15–35).

Ulceration may be present with any degree of inflammation but is more common and extensive with moderate and severe degrees of inflammatory change. Small ulcerations are represented by punctate or short, linear accumulations of barium projecting from the lumen margin. Aphthous lesions are occasionally identified in the small bowel and are caused by a small central ulceration in an enlarged lymph follicle or in a small inflammatory focus. Medium-size ulcerations appear as linear or spike-like projections from the lumen boundary. With more extensive and confluent ulceration, deep linear, longitudinal, and circumferential ulcerations form.

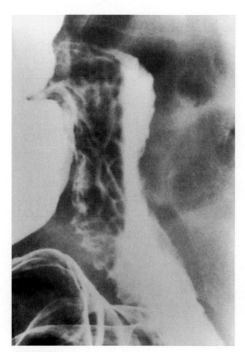

Figure 15–30
Crohn's ileitis. Mild to moderate mucosal fold thickening and mild distortion of fold architecture are present in the nonstenotic terminal ileum of this 14-year-old girl.

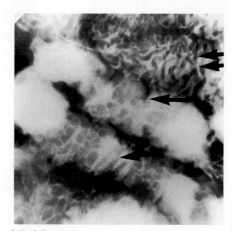

Figure 15–32
Crohn's jejunitis: nodular mucosal fold thickening in an 11-year-old boy. Moderate inflammation of the jejunal loops has caused nodular fold thickening *(single arrows)*. Normal jejunum *(double arrows)* is present proximal to the affected loops.

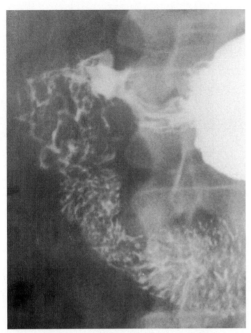

Figure 15–33
Crohn's duodenitis. This adolescent had Crohn's disease and duodenal involvement. Nodular thickening of the folds is present in the proximal second portion of the duodenum.

These deep fissures may isolate multiple focal areas of thickened and inflamed bowel wall, resulting in a multinodular (cobblestone) appearance (Fig. 15–36).

Ulceration may extend through the serosa to form sinuses, contained perforations, abscesses, and fistulas. Free perforation is the exception. Sinuses and fistulas are visible as irregular, linear, extraintestinal tracts and communications that

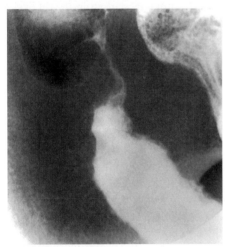

Figure 15–34
Stenotic Crohn's disease. Severe stenosis of the terminal ileum is present in this 16-year-old boy. Inflammatory effacement of the mucosal folds and small ulcerations characterize the proximal nonstenotic segment.

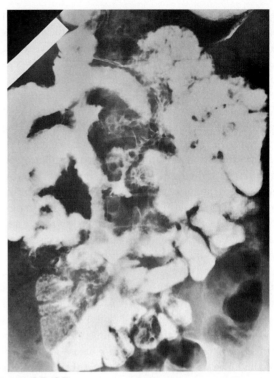

Figure 15–35
Crohn's disease. Inflammatory thickening of the bowel wall and mesentery has separated multiple loops of ileum in this 16-year-old girl. Moderate to severe ulceration is present in the affected segments.

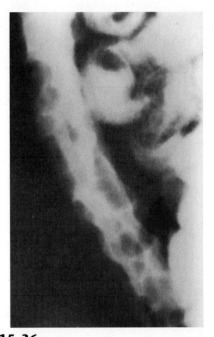

Figure 15–36
Crohn's disease: cobblestone pattern in a 9-year-old girl. Multiple deep linear ulcers (fissures) are separated by hyperplastic and markedly inflamed tissue. This pattern of severe disease is known as *cobblestone*. The nodular inflamed mucosal lesions are inflammatory pseudopolyps.

may be quite numerous in a given segment of affected intestine (see Fig. 15–32). Fistulas may form with any adjacent organ (e.g., small bowel, colon, bladder, psoas, and skin). Enteroenteric and enterocolic are the most common types of fistulas. Fistulization between the terminal ileum and cecum is very common (Figs. 15–37 and 15–38).

As a rule, early Crohn's disease is nonstenotic. With progression of the disease, however, intestinal stenosis of variable degrees develops in most patients. Stenoses of the small intestine from Crohn's disease can be due to spasm, inflammation and edema, or fibrosis. In the early stages of stenotic disease, stenosis is more likely to be due to a combination of spasm, inflammation, and edema. With progression of the disease, areas of inflammation and edema are gradually replaced by fibrotic tissue. With advanced disease, stenoses may predominantly be due to transmural fibrosis. Stenoses in Crohn's disease have a great variety of appearances; they may be short or quite long. The proximal and distal margins of stenoses are usually sharply defined, with an abrupt transition from normal to abnormal bowel. However, stenoses may also be tapered, with a broad transition zone reflecting a gradual decrease in severity of the disease at the stenosis boundary. The "string sign" is a relatively long stenosis with a narrow lumen diameter. Such stenoses may be caused

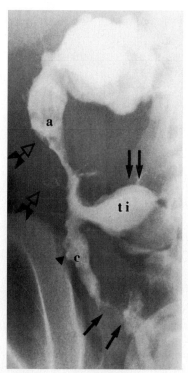

Figure 15–38
Crohn's disease: sinuses and fistula. Severe ileocolitis has resulted in an ileocecal fistula *(single arrows, lower)* and sinus formation in the ascending colon (a) *(arrows on platform)*. c, Cecum *(arrowhead);* ti, terminal ileum *(paired arrows)*.

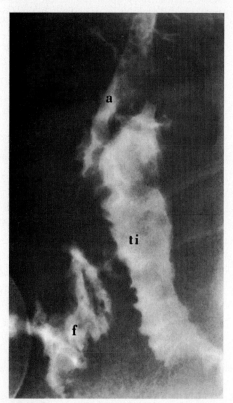

Figure 15–37
Crohn's disease: sinuses and fistula. The terminal ileum (ti) is severely diseased and is the origin of an enterocutaneous fistula (f). The ascending colon (a) is also severely diseased and stenotic and gives rise to two sinus tracts.

by spasm, inflammation, edema, or fibrosis. Irregularity of these stenoses may be present and is due to ulceration, causing a frayed string appearance. Resolution or significant improvement in some stenoses suggests that spasm contributes significantly to them. Marked intestinal dilatation proximal to the stenoses implies chronicity and an increased likelihood that fibrosis is the cause (Fig. 15–39).

Pseudodiverticuli may develop when a short, eccentrically diseased segment of bowel is isolated between two obstructing stenoses. "Ballooning" of the normal portion of the isolated segment produces an eccentric dilatation, simulating a diverticulum.

Edema and inflammation of the mesentery contribute to the appearance of straightened and separated loops of intestine. Focal mesenteric inflammation or abscess can cause kinking or separation of bowel loops or a focal extraintestinal mass (Fig. 15–40). These masses are recognized by noting a roughly circular area devoid of bowel loops that impresses filled bowel loops adjacent to the mass's margin.

The radiographic differential diagnosis of small bowel Crohn's disease is quite limited. Yersiniosis may cause nodular inflammation of the terminal ileum, a condition that commonly resolves in 6 to 8 weeks, thereby allowing differentiation from Crohn's disease. The gross pathologic and radiographic features of tuberculosis may appear identical to

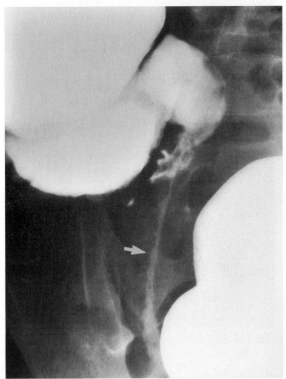

Figure 15–39
Crohn's disease: string sign *(arrow)*. Ulcerations are present in this severely stenotic terminal ileum, giving a "frayed string" appearance. The cecal wall is thickened and irregular. The patient is a 13-year-old boy with long-standing disease.

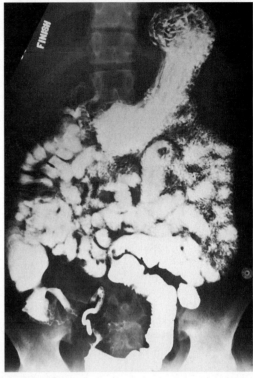

Figure 15–40
Crohn's disease: mesenteric mass in a 16-year-old boy. An inflammatory mesenteric mass can be inferred from the relative paucity of bowel loops in the right lower quadrant medial and inferior to the cecum. Severe stenosis of the terminal ileum and moderate cecal deformity are also demonstrated. The cecal deformity could be the result of primary cecal disease or a secondary effect of adjacent terminal ileal disease.

those of Crohn's disease; however, intestinal tuberculosis is quite rare in the United States. Lymphoma must also be included in the differential diagnosis, particularly when localized nonstenotic disease is present, with or without an associated mass.

Colon Typically, Crohn's colitis is initially concentrated in the right colon. Continuous or discontinuous disease of the right colon from the cecum distally is common. Rectal disease is present in approximately one third of patients. Anal disease is common, with or without colon disease.

Isolated Crohn's colitis progresses longitudinally in a significant number of cases; however, progression to ileocolitis is rare. Pancolitis from Crohn's disease is uncommon but does occur.

The basic pathologic processes of Crohn's colitis (Figs. 15–41 through 15–44) are identical to those of Crohn's enteritis. Mild edema and inflammation are somewhat more difficult to detect in the colon than in the small bowel but are identifiable when haustral thickening, mild mucosal fold thickening (on postevacuation films), and a hazy or slightly irregular bowel margin (on air-contrast studies) are observed. Moderate or severe edema and inflammation are easily perceived when a markedly thickened and irregular colon wall (thumbprinting) is present. As in ulcerative colitis, pseudopolyps may be seen in the acute or chronic phases of the disease.

Aphthous lesions, thought by many to be the earliest sign of Crohn's disease, are identified more commonly in the colon than elsewhere in the gut. Aphthous lesions are focal, raised lesions (similar to papules) of varying size (1 to 15 mm), with central ulceration that is often irregular in shape and size. The nodular component of the lesion is caused by either focal inflammation (mucosal and submucosal) or an inflamed lymph follicle. Aphthous lesions are specific for Crohn's disease and may also be seen in Behçet's disease, amebiasis, and yersiniosis.[72] Aphthous lesions are easily distinguished from normal lymphoid follicles. The normal lymphoid follicular pattern of the pediatric colon and terminal ileum also has been termed *lymphoid hyperplasia* (Fig. 15–46), reflecting the original concept that these follicles were apparent because of

Text continued on page 530

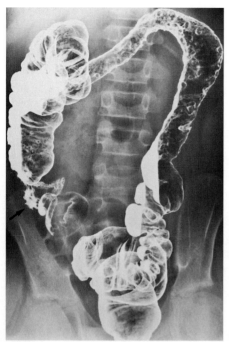

Figure 15–41

Crohn's colitis in a 14-year-old boy. Segmental involvement of the cecum *(arrow)* and the transverse and descending colon is present. Note the cecal stenosis. The rectosigmoid and ascending segments are free of disease.

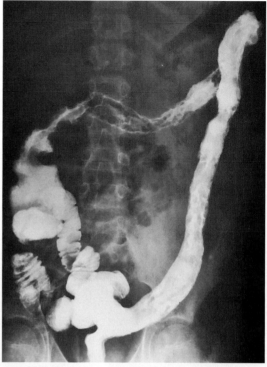

Figure 15–42

Crohn's colitis in a 13-year-old boy. Colon disease extends from the hepatic flexure to the rectum, sparing a segment of distal sigmoid colon. Affected segments are moderately narrowed. Stenosis involving the hepatic flexure was constant.

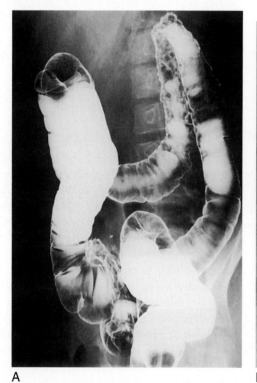

A

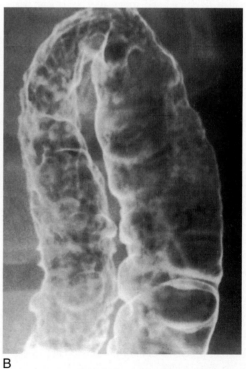

B

Figure 15–43

Crohn's colitis in an 8-year-old girl with severe growth retardation. Her upper gastrointestinal tract and small bowel were radiographically normal. *A,* Segmental colitis involves the distal transverse colon, splenic flexure, and proximal descending colon. Note the haustral blunting; ulcerations; moderate, irregular inflammatory changes; and mild luminal narrowing in the involved segment. *B,* The splenic flexure spot film demonstrates these features with greater clarity. Aphthous lesions are an early manifestation of Crohn's disease and are seen in the distal transition zone from abnormal to normal colon, near the junction of the splenic flexure and descending colon.

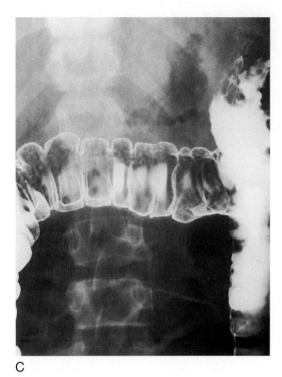

C

Figure 15–43—cont'd
C, Aphthous lesions are also present in the proximal portion of the midtransverse colon.

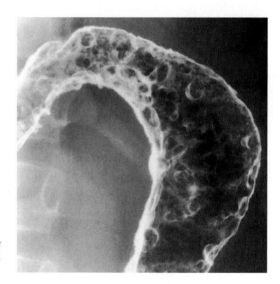

Figure 15–44
Crohn's colitis: pseudopolyps. Multiple mucosal "nodules" are present in the splenic flexure in this 14-year-old boy with Crohn's colitis. The appearance is typical of pseudopolyps associated with quiescent disease.

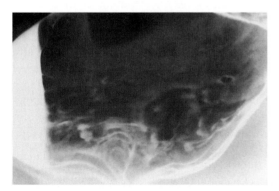

Figure 15–45
Aphthous lesion: distal rectum. Aphthous ulcers signify early rectal disease in this 16-year-old boy with Crohn's colitis.

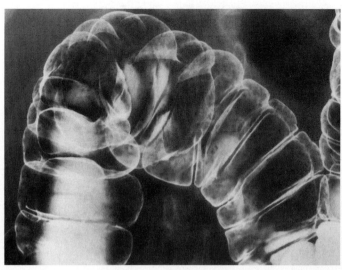

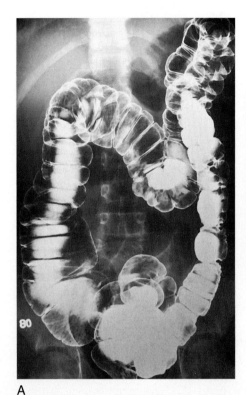

A

B

Figure 15–46

Normal lymphoid follicles. Lymphoid follicles are prominent on this contrast enema, the results of which were normal. *A,* Supine double-contrast examination reveals lymphoid follicles in the right and proximal transverse segments of the colon. *B,* Hepatic flexure spot film demonstrates multiple small, rounded filling defects of uniform size and distributed in a regular pattern. The colonic wall is visible in profile in several areas and has good coating, revealing no evidence of ulceration.

viral disease or other stimuli that provoke hyperplasia. Normal lymphoid follicles in the pediatric intestine differ from aphthoid lesions in the following ways:

1. Normal lymphoid follicles are 4 mm or less in diameter and vary little in size.
2. Central umbilications may or may not be present but, when present, are fairly uniform in size and shape.
3. Most importantly, there is no evidence of associated colon or ileal abnormality.

Aphthous lesions (Fig. 15–45), although considered an early manifestation of disease when they occur, are almost always accompanied by evidence of more advanced disease in adjacent or distant portions of the colon or small bowel. Large lymphoid follicles (greater than 4 mm but less than 8 mm in diameter) have been described as a rare, early manifestation of inflammatory bowel disease.[45] Large lymphoid follicles are differentiated from normal lymphoid follicles primarily on the basis of size and from aphthous lesions by the relatively greater uniformity of nodule size and size and shape of the central umbilication (Figs. 15–47, 15–48, and 15–49). In Table 15–6 the characteristics of these various nodular umbilicated entities are summarized. The progression or regression of aphthous ulcers may be related to disease

activity or treatment, but in some patients they may act independently of these factors.[3] The radiographic differential of Crohn's colitis from ulcerative colitis is shown in Table 15–7.

Cross-Sectional Imaging   Since the 1980s, the widespread availability of CT has had a major impact on the evaluation of patients with inflammatory bowel disease. Whereas endoscopy and barium studies only directly visualize the intraluminal surfaces of the bowel, these studies cannot directly determine extraluminal manifestations of Crohn's disease. The use of cross-sectional imaging, particularly CT, allows radiologists to define mural and extraluminal involvement. Attention to technique requires that excellent bowel opacification be achieved. Unopacified loops may simulate a mass, lymph nodes, or abscess. Luminal opacification is also necessary to define wall thickness. CT in Crohn's disease shows wall thickness increasing from the normal 2 to 3 mm to a measurement of 1 cm or more. Areas of luminal narrowing may not be demonstrated as well with CT as on barium studies. The demonstration of mesenteric disease including abscess, phlegmon, and fibrofatty proliferation and large mesenteric lymph nodes can be particularly well accomplished on high-grade CT examinations.[28,37] Because endoscopy and

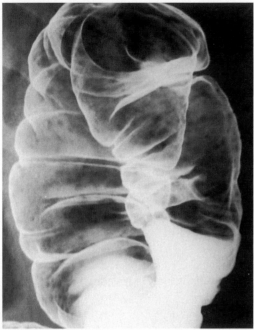

Figure 15–47

Normal lymphoid hyperplasia. Multiple small nodules of uniform size are visible in the splenic flexure of a 13-year-old boy with *Shigella* enteritis. The entire colon distal to the hepatic flexure was similarly involved but otherwise is normal.

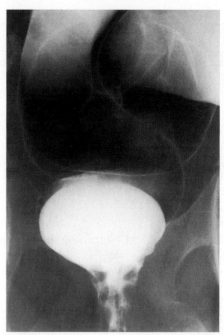

Figure 15–49

Lymphoid nodules. Multiple small nodules are present in the distal rectum. Benign lymphoid aggregates were identified on biopsy from the rectum of this 8-year-old girl with rectal bleeding. The remainder of the colon was normal. Proctoscopic examination revealed a normal rectum proximal to the lymphoid nodules, which were not ulcerated. Idiopathic proctitis was the final diagnosis.

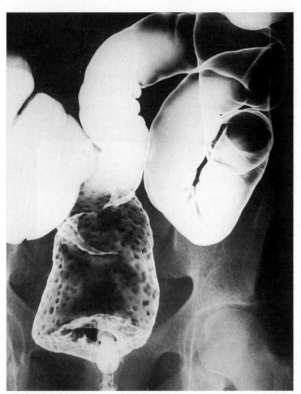

Figure 15–48

Large lymphoid follicles. Lymphoid follicles, confirmed by rectal biopsy, ranged in size up to 6 mm and were confined to the rectosigmoid region. This 12-year-old girl had rectal bleeding caused by nonspecific proctitis. (From Kenney PK, Koehler RE, Shackelford GD. The clinical significance of large lymphoid follicles of the colon. Radiology 142:41–46, 1982.)

contrast studies are superior in defining mucosal lesions, including aphthous ulcers, pseudopolyps, and ulcerations, they remain the primary methods of initial evaluation of patients with inflammatory bowel disease. However, CT is a powerful adjunct.[25] Additional information was obtained in 28% of symptomatic patients with CT.[20] Fistula and abscess formation was the most frequent and important finding.

As with contrast examinations and endoscopy, CT can distinguish well-established ulcerative colitis from Crohn's disease. However, it does not differentiate disease that is indeterminate by clinical and barium studies (Figs. 15–50 through 15–54).[2] In patients with Crohn's disease, contrast studies remain the primary method for detecting and determining the extent of enteroenteric fistulas, sinus tracts, and strictures, as well as for evaluating postoperative anastomoses. CT, however, is better for mesenteric inflammation, abscess, and enterovesical and enterocutaneous fistulas.[6] Another role for CT in the management of patients with idiopathic bowel disease is in the percutaneous drainage of abscesses. Some authors have found that the likelihood of curing an abscess with an enteric communication is minimal with percutaneous drainage alone.[15,53] However, even incomplete treatment of such abscesses minimizes the amount of surgery and frequently obviates the need for surgical intervention.[7,10] Abdominal sonography has also been found to be useful in determining wall thickness in both ulcerative colitis and Crohn's disease. In the latter, wall thickening is more pronounced and more

Text continued on page 535

TABLE 15-6 CHARACTERISTICS OF LYMPHOID FOLLICLES AND APHTHOUS LESIONS

SIZE	NORMAL LYMPHOID FOLLICLES (LYMPHOID HYPERPLASIA, SMALL LYMPHOID FOLLICLES)	APHTHOUS LESIONS	LARGE LYMPHOID FOLLICLES
Variation in size in individual case	Small (1–4 mm)	Large (1–15 mm)	Moderate (4–8 mm)
Central defect (ulceration or umbilication)	+ or – (umbilication)	+ (ulceration)	+ or – (umbilication)
Shape and size of central defects	Uniform size and regular shapes	Often nonuniform sizes and irregular shapes	Uniform size and regular shapes
Pathology of nodule	"Normal" submucosal lymph follicle	Inflamed lymph follicle or focus of mucosal and submucosal	Hyperplastic submucosal lymph follicle
Location	Anywhere, but most common in right colon	Any location in colon: occasionally identified in stomach or small bowel	Anywhere, but most common in rectosigmoid region
Significance	Normal variation (very common under 5 years; common up to 15 years; found in 15% to 25% of adults)	Abnormal; Crohn's disease is usual etiology; other evidence of Crohn's colitis is present	Abnormal; very uncommon manifestation of inflammatory colon
Differential diagnosis	Nonspecific immune response of intestinal lymphoid system (?)	Crohn's colitis Ulcerative colitis Herpes colitis Monilial colitis	Idiopathic inflammatory bowel disease is usual etiology Ulcerative colitis Ulcerative proctitis Crohn's disease Lymphoma Dysgammaglobulinemia

TABLE 15-7 INFLAMMATORY BOWEL DISEASE—RADIOLOGIC DIFFERENTIAL

FEATURE	ULCERATIVE COLITIS	CROHN'S DISEASE
Involvement (portion of intestine)	Colon + backwash ileitis	Esophagus through colon
Distribution	Continuous	Continuous or skip
Involvement (portion of bowel wall)	Mucosa, initially	Lesions
Fistula/sinus tracts	Rare	All layers
Deep ulcers	Symmetrical	Common
Strictures	Frequently seen	Asymmetrical
Toxic megacolon		Uncommon

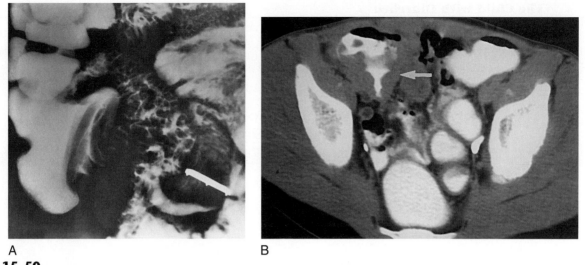

A

B

Figure 15–50
Crohn's disease of the distal ileum in a 12-year-old girl. *A*, A spot film from a small bowel examination shows large, nodular changes of the distal ileum. *B*, The CT scan correlates well, showing large nodules and considerable wall thickening *(arrow)*.

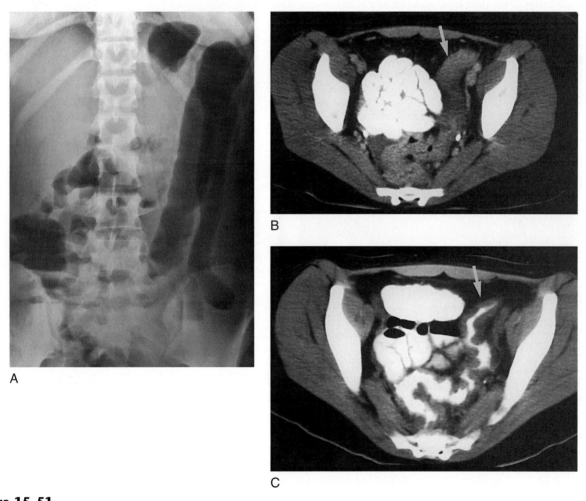

A

B

C

Figure 15–51
Crohn's colitis in a 16-year-old adolescent. *A*, A plain film showing air distending left colon; the descending colon is somewhat featureless. *B*, A CT scan through the upper pelvis shows contrast material in normal small bowel loops in the right and midportion of the pelvis. There is a thickened tubular structure coursing from anterior to posterior in the left pelvis and presacral region. *C*, Only with delayed filming has contrast material filled the lumen of the structure seen in *B*; the extent of infection and wall thickening is clearly demonstrated.

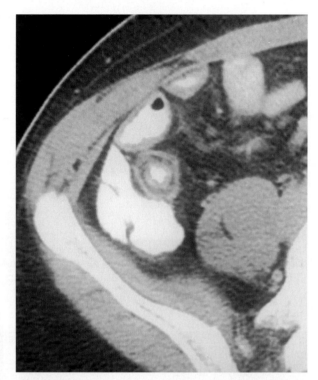

Figure 15–52
Localized CT image of the right lower quadrant of an older patient with Crohn's disease, a "target" sign can be seen in the terminal ileum with contrast material and then alternating layers of thickened mucosa, submucosa, and muscle/serosa. At this time, the patient did not have any other involvement of his Crohn's disease.

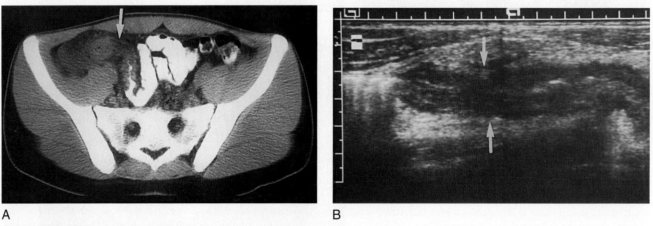

A   B

Figure 15–53
Crohn's disease involving the distal ileum in a 17-year-old adolescent. *A*, A CT scan with contrast material in a narrowed loop shows fibrofatty proliferation *(arrow)*. *B*, This sonographic depiction of very thickened bowel *(arrows)* was the first indication of inflammatory bowel disease in this patient, who presented with abdominal pain.

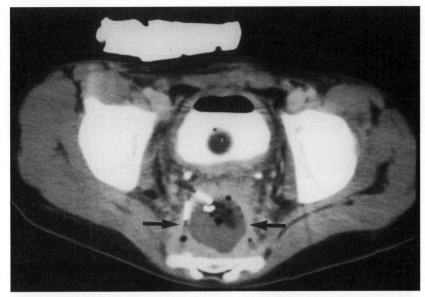

A

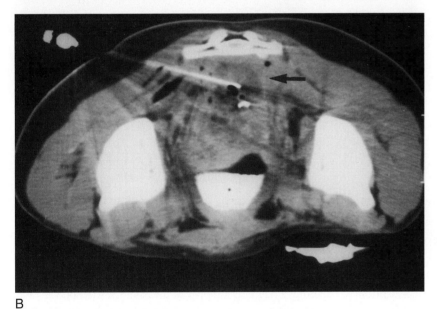

B

Figure 15–54
Images of a 14-year-old boy who had previously had a proctocolectomy for treatment of ulcerative colitis. *A*, This CT scan demonstrates a low-density collection with air bubbles in the presacral space. *B*, With the patient in a prone position, CT was used to guide abscess drainage.

often detected (see Fig. 15–54*B*).[95] Extraluminal involvement, particularly in Crohn's disease, can also be detected with sonography. The most frequent finding is conglomeration: an irregular mass with a mixed echo pattern reflecting matted, inflamed bowel loops and mesentery. Target or "bull's-eye" lesions were seen with abscesses,[40] and fluid in the cul-de-sac was easily identified with sonography. Definition of the colon wall can be enhanced with the addition of a water enema in the detection of Crohn's colitis.[5] Recently, magnetic resonance (MR) has been shown to be of use in the evaluation of perirectal fistulas in sinus tracts in patients with Crohn's disease. Although fistulograms using contrast material and aided by CT and ultrasound may be of use, MR, with its

excellent tissue resolution and planes of view may be helpful in the diagnosis of this complication.[50] Scintigraphy using technetium Tc 99m white blood cell scans has been found to be a sensitive, noninvasive test to determine the extent and distribution of inflammation in children with inflammatory bowel disease.[11]

CELIAC DISEASE

Celiac disease is the most common diffuse mucosal disease responsible for malabsorption. It was among the first diseases to be associated with malabsorption and is a prototype of

---

TABLE 15-8 Classification of Malabsorption

Luminal Phase Deficiency
Pancreatic insufficiency
  Cystic fibrosis
  Chronic pancreatitis
  Pancreatic insufficiency and bone marrow failure
    (Shwachman-Diamond syndrome)
Zollinger-Ellison syndrome
Enterokinase deficiency
Insufficient conjugated bile acids
Hepatic disease
Biliary atresia
Acute hepatic disease
Chronic hepatic disease
Biliary obstruction
Intestinal disease
  Bacterial overgrowth
    Chronic partial obstruction
    Blind loop
  Short bowel syndrome
Intestinal Phase Deficiency
Mucosal disease
  Celiac disease
  Regional enteritis
  Milk protein allergy
  Enteric infection
  Enteric parasites (*Giardia lamblia*, etc.)
  Secondary disaccharidase deficiency
  Drug-induced (antibiotics, methotrexate)
  Radiation enteritis
  Ulcerative colitis
  Eosinophilic enteritis
  Other

Metabolic deficiencies
  Primary disaccharidase deficiency
  Glucose-galactose malabsorption
  Fructose intolerance
  Abetalipoproteinemia
  Others
Endocrine abnormality
  Hyperthyroidism
  Neuroblastoma
  Diabetes
  Addison's disease
  Other
Transport Phase Deficiency
Regional enteritis
Congestive heart failure
Intestinal lymphangiectasia
Lymphoma
Whipple's disease
Other
Intractable diarrhea of infancy
Primary immune defects
Collagen diseases
Wolman's disease
Mastocytosis

---

such conditions. In Table 15–8, a list of these malabsorption syndromes is given.

There is some confusion related to the variety of names applied to celiac disease. It was initially described in 1888 by Samuel Gee as *coeliac affliction*. Its relationship to wheat was discovered by Dicke et al.,[14] who noted clinical improvement in those with the disease in Holland during World War II, when wheat was unavailable. At that time, it was referred to as *coeliac disease*. Other terms that have been used include *idiopathic steatorrhea, nontropical sprue*, and *gluten-sensitive enteropathy*, the last reflecting the pathogenesis of the disorder.

The disease results from ingestion of certain gluten-containing grains that produce a variety of symptoms in individuals with gluten-sensitive small bowel mucosa. Characteristic radiographic changes are present in many patients; however, laboratory tests and radiographic studies are not specific enough to permit accurate diagnosis.

Peroral small bowel biopsy is the essential method for both diagnosis and therapeutic assessment in children with celiac disease. Treatment includes a diet that restricts the offending foods, to which there is lifelong sensitivity.

Pathophysiology

Celiac disease is a disorder in which the small bowel mucosa is damaged by ingested gluten. Gliadin, the alcohol-soluble fraction of gluten, is the toxic component of wheat gluten. Other grains related to wheat, including oats, rye, and barley, may cause symptoms and contain alcohol-soluble proteins termed prolamins.[42] The affected mucosa shows atrophy with villous flattening, cuboidal epithelial cells, and infiltration of the lamina propria by lymphocytes and plasma cells. This lesion leads to malabsorption of one or more food components, which include carbohydrates, fats, proteins, minerals, and vitamins. Absorptive functions most affected are those located at or near the tips of villi. Disaccharidases, which normally reside in the brush border, are severely disturbed early in the development of this disorder. Restriction of gluten-containing foods from the diet of children generally results in recovery of the intestinal mucosa and regression of clinical symptoms related to malabsorption.

Celiac disease is a familial condition, with 10% of an affected person's immediate family having typical mucosal changes. This percentage increases to 44% if only individuals with clinical disease are considered. Further, celiac disease is closely associated with the presence of certain human leukocyte antigens (i.e., HLA-B8, HLA-DR3, and HLA-DQw2 tissue antigens), which occur three or four times more often in people with celiac disease than in the normal population. Also, an antigen on the B lymphocyte has been found in 5 to 10 times as many affected people as in the normal population.

Although early researchers clearly established the link between gluten ingestion and the clinical and pathologic changes of celiac disease, the precise mechanism by which the mucosal lesion is produced remains unknown. Currently there is considerable interest in invoking immunologic mechanisms that involve both humoral and cellular cytotoxicity in the intestinal mucosa of patients with celiac disease. There has been a great deal of interest in the use of IgA and IgG antigliaden antibodies,[77] IgA antireticulin antibodies,[13] and IgA anti-endomysium antibodies[73] to define and monitor disease activity. Whereas these laboratory measurements are not specific enough to replace a small bowel biopsy, they may be used for monitoring compliance to diet in patients with established celiac disease and for determining the optimal timing for biopsy in patients undergoing evaluation for celiac disease.[44] There may be cross-reactivity of a gliadin fraction with adenovirus serotype 12, which is often isolated from human intestines. Both share a region of amino acid sequence homology.[41] Thus, cell-mediated immunity may play a role in the pathogenesis of celiac disease, as the gliadin fraction of gluten causes sensitization of lymphocytes. Studies using an in vitro model based on organ culture techniques support such a hypothesis. Steroids have been used with success as alternative therapy in patients with severe, life-threatening symptoms from celiac disease when the response to a gluten-free diet is too slow. These factors suggest that genetically predisposed patients have an immunologic derangement permitting gluten-induced mucosal damage.

Clinical Presentation

Generally, celiac disease is limited to people in Europe, North America, and Australia; however, it has been reported in geographic areas as diverse as India, West Pakistan, and the Middle East but appears to be rare in Africa and Japan. The rate of occurrence is similar for males and females.

Celiac disease usually presents in infancy following weaning and shortly after the introduction of grain cereals. In the past, this occurred in children between 9 months and 3 years

of age, but when these gluten-containing foods are introduced earlier, symptoms may appear earlier. Most cases are manifest by the age of 10 years; another peak in incidence occurs in the third decade of life in previously asymptomatic people. Gluten sensitivity is lifelong, but clinical remissions occur in some patients, particularly during adolescence.

The most common presentation includes diarrhea with bulky, foul-smelling stools or, in some cases, watery, diarrheal stools. Initially, the diarrhea may be intermittent and associated with episodes of gastroenteritis or upper respiratory infection. Loss of appetite, with consequent decreased caloric intake, results in weight loss, failure to thrive, and wasting. Patients fall progressively behind their expected weight percentiles and show little growth in height. Affected children are noticeably irritable, a symptom that resolves with surprising rapidity after initiation of a gluten-free diet. Vomiting, abdominal distention, and pain are sometimes the most notable features at the time of presentation.

There is a variable inability to absorb all food components, leading to specific clinical manifestations. Disaccharidase deficiency may cause accentuation of the diarrhea by osmotic mechanisms. Fats are incompletely absorbed, leading to steatorrhea and fat-soluble vitamin deficiencies. Rickets or osteomalacia may result from a deficiency of vitamin D, night blindness from a deficiency of vitamin A, and bleeding difficulties from a deficiency of vitamin K. Peripheral edema due to hypoproteinemia may be seen in children with celiac disease. Anemia can occur, most often from iron deficiency or occasionally as a result of folate malabsorption. Clubbing of the fingers is seen in severely afflicted individuals.

Generally, the clinical picture of most patients with celiac disease is dominated by diarrhea, failure to thrive, and malabsorption. However, occasionally a patient presents with constipation or alternating diarrhea and constipation.

After the appropriate diagnostic evaluation has been completed and has resulted in a diagnosis of celiac disease, treatment is begun with a gluten-free diet. Although the term *gluten-free* is commonly used, the diet is actually gluten restricted, because gluten from wheat, rye, barley, and oats is excluded, but gluten from rice and corn is not. In children, unlike in adults, there is an almost universal clinical response to such a diet, with rapid and dramatic improvement or cessation of symptoms. A definite subjective sensation of well-being may be evident as soon as 24 hours after restriction of gluten has begun. Within days, there is a decrease in diarrhea and fecal fat excretion, with significant weight gain. Complete clinical recovery usually is achieved within a few months.

A poor response may be the result of continuous ingestion of a significant amount of gluten. However, diagnostic error must also be considered.

Small bowel biopsy is a widely available technique and remains the cornerstone of diagnosis in celiac disease. Traditionally, the standard has been peroral small bowel biopsy for the diagnosis of celiac disease. Increasingly, gastroenterologists are using endoscopically derived biopsies; fewer diagnostic failures, the ability to obtain multiple biopsies, and direct observation of intestinal mucosa are cited as advantages of this technique.[47] Biopsies are usually performed at the ligament of Treitz to ensure a consistent biopsy site. This is an important factor when changes in mucosal morphology on rebiopsy following therapy are considered. If celiac disease is seriously considered to be the diagnosis, many believe that it is appropriate to proceed immediately to biopsy, bypassing the multitude of laboratory tests that have been advocated in the past. In the affected patient, a well-oriented set of histologic sections from the duodenum or jejunum shows characteristic flattened mucosa with absent or short villi, hypertrophied crypts, and intense infiltration of the lamina propria with lymphocytes and plasma cells. The surface epithelium is cuboidal rather than columnar. This striking pattern, although characteristic of celiac disease and necessary for its diagnosis, is nonspecific. In children, a variety of conditions exist that cause flat small bowel mucosa, including malnutrition, severe iron-deficiency anemia, bacterial gastroenteritis, giardiasis, milk protein allergy, and immune disorders. However, in pediatric patients who have celiac disease, adherence to a gluten-free diet will result in the return of the small bowel mucosa to normal or near normal. In adults, the jejunal biopsy will frequently not return to normal. It is believed that in children, the degree of initial mucosal abnormality is proportional to the amount of gluten ingested.

Because of the nonspecificity of the mucosal biopsy, it has generally been considered appropriate to perform a second biopsy after a patient has adhered to a gluten-free diet for several months. At that time, the small bowel mucosa should be normal or near normal if the diagnosis was correct and the patient has maintained the appropriate diet. To avoid overdiagnosis if the original cause of the abnormal biopsy was transient and unrelated to celiac disease, a third biopsy is recommended 2 weeks after gluten has been reintroduced into the diet. However, the Working Group of the European Society of Pediatric Gastroenterology and Nutrition has offered a simpler protocol for patients with uncomplicated disease.[94] First, a biopsy is needed to document the characteristic histologic abnormalities of the small bowel mucosa. Second, a gluten-free diet should produce a clear-cut clinical remission with relief of all symptoms. The response should be rapid, occurring within a matter of weeks rather than many months. If these two conditions are met, the diagnosis is certain, and a gluten challenge is not mandatory. In asymptomatic patients, however, as in first-degree relatives with celiac disease, baseline biopsies are needed to define mucosal recovery with a gluten-free diet.[3] If these patients do not have a clear-cut remission on biopsy, a repeat biopsy and perhaps a gluten challenge may be necessary.[7,60] The intolerance to gluten is believed to be lifelong, although gluten is reintroduced into the diet of some patients without resulting in the

onset of clinical deterioration. However, long-term analysis of patients shows that histologic relapse is likely to occur in the vast majority of patients.[78] Furthermore, in children the risk exists for growth retardation during periods of gluten ingestion. In adult patients, there is an increased incidence of malignancy, particularly gastrointestinal lymphoma; this has not been shown in children. Long-term follow-up of adults has shown that a restrictive diet prevents the added risk of malignancy.[36]

Radiographic Evaluation

As previously stated, contrast radiographic examination is not the definitive means of investigation in patients suspected of having celiac disease. This statement has been particularly true since the widespread availability of safe, peroral small bowel biopsy.

In patients with celiac disease, an abnormal small bowel appearance on contrast radiograph examination is characteristically present, although false-negative results occasionally occur. Radiographic findings are neither sufficiently specific nor consistent enough to obviate small bowel biopsy. Radiographic evaluation in patients with suspected malabsorption is useful for (1) confirmation of the presence of proximal jejunal abnormality, suggesting a positive peroral biopsy result (Table 15–9); (2) exclusion of distal small bowel

TABLE 15-9 BIOPSY RESULTS AT THE LIGAMENT OF TREITZ

Diagnostic Biopsy
Celiac disease
Whipple's disease
Abetalipoproteinemia
Thymic alymphoplasia
Acquired agammaglobulinemia
Diagnostic or Nondiagnostic Biopsy
Intestinal lymphangiectasia
Eosinophilic gastroenteritis
Giardiasis
Crohn's disease of the proximal jejunum
Isolated IgA deficiency
Dysgammaglobulinemia
Mastocytosis
Lymphoma
Nonspecific Changes
Malnutrition
Intractable diarrhea of early infancy
Antibiotic- or methotrexate-induced malabsorption
Contained small bowel syndrome
Radiation enteritis

From Roy CC, Silverman A, Cozetto FJ. Pediatric Clinical Gastroenterology. St. Louis: CV Mosby, 1975, p 225. Published by permission of the publisher and authors.

disease (e.g., Crohn's disease), which generally cannot be diagnosed by peroral biopsy (Table 15–9); and (3) delineation of congenital and postsurgical causes of partial small bowel obstruction (duodenal and jejunal stenosis or diaphragm, malrotation with obstructing bands, blind loops, or anastomotic stenosis). Malabsorption in these partial obstructions results from stasis and secondary bacterial overgrowth (Fig. 15–55).

Radiographic examination may also be performed in patients in whom celiac disease is not a primary diagnostic consideration but whose symptoms, such as abdominal pain, anemia, diarrhea, or vomiting, suggest Crohn's disease or an anatomic abnormality. When a small bowel examination is done in such patients, the radiographic features of celiac disease should also be sought. Small bowel biopsy is encouraged in such patients if an atrophic, dilated jejunum or transient intussusception is discovered.

Although a one- or two-film study has been advocated to exclude celiac disease, we prefer to do our routine small bowel examination when this diagnosis is suggested. Using nonflocculating barium, routine fluoroscopic examination of the esophagus, stomach, and duodenum, with only a few spot films, precedes the small bowel study. Emphasis, as in all pediatric UGI examinations, is placed on the position of the ligament of Treitz. Generally, right anterior oblique and AP radiographs are obtained with an overhead tube. Subsequently,

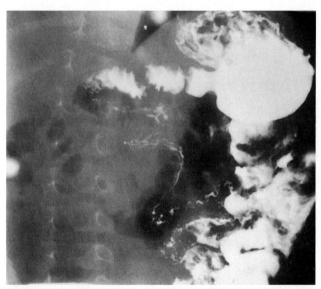

Figure 15–55
Image of a 3-year-old girl who presented with chronic diarrhea and failure to thrive. After 48 hours of continuous gastric aspiration via a nasogastric tube, a small bowel series was performed. The right anterior oblique abdominal film from the small bowel series displays a spiral configuration of the duodenum and proximal jejunum, the classic appearance of a midgut volvulus. This rare presentation of midgut volvulus (i.e., chronic partial obstruction and malabsorption) contrasts with the far more common presentation of midgut volvulus (i.e., an acute, high-grade obstruction, which commonly causes intestinal vascular compromise) (see Chapter 13).

intermittent fluoroscopic examination of the small bowel is done. The intervals vary from 10 or 15 minutes, when Crohn's disease and fistulas are a possibility, to about 30 minutes in more routine examinations. Overhead films, usually posteroanterior views, are made after some fluoroscopic views have been obtained. Attempts are made to obtain a film of the jejunum and ileum. A spot film of the distended terminal ileum completes the examination.

In most patients with celiac disease, the radiographic appearance of the small bowel will generally parallel the clinical diagnosis, and a return to a normal radiographic pattern is expected after adequate diet therapy for 6 months. If the radiographic appearance remains abnormal after a 6-month period, then adherence to the diet may be inadequate or the diagnosis may be incorrect.

Radiology plays an adjunctive role during small bowel biopsy when fluoroscopy is used to help with the passage of the Crosby capsule into the proximal jejunum.

Evaluation of patients with active celiac disease is aided by skeletal radiographs, which in patients with severe disease may show osteoporosis or osteomalacia (rickets). Bone age may show significant delay of maturation. After successful treatment, bone age and height may not reach the normal range for 1 to 2 years or perhaps longer.

Radiographic Findings

Dilatation The most prevalent and characteristic finding on small bowel radiographic examinations in patients with active celiac disease is dilatation, which is most pronounced in the jejunum but usually extends to some degree throughout the small bowel, including the duodenum (Figs. 15–56 and 15–57). In rare instances, megacolon has been reported in celiac disease. The dilated intestinal loops are long and tortuous and pliable on palpation during fluoroscopy. There are no areas of fixed narrowing causing proximal dilatation, as is seen with congenital bands or the inflammatory strictures of Crohn's disease. The cause of small bowel dilatation in celiac disease is unknown, but it is a more prominent feature of celiac disease than of any other cause of malabsorption with abnormal small bowel radiographs.

Mucosal Changes After dilatation, abnormal mucosal folds are the most reliable radiographic finding in celiac disease (Figs. 15–58 and 15–59). An abnormal fold pattern is typically present in the jejunum; however, the duodenum may also be involved. A normal transverse mucosal fold pattern may not be present until the third or fourth month of life. Abnormal thinning of the mucosal folds is characteristic of celiac disease and occurs in many patients, correlating with atrophy present on biopsy; however, a normal fold thickness is often present. Abnormal thickness of the mucosal folds is seen in some patients with celiac disease. It is likely that in some patients, the apparent thickening results from the adherence of secretions to mucosal folds and consequent poor coating of the bowel surface with barium.

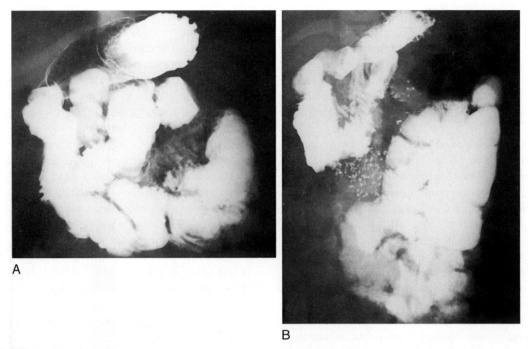

Figure 15–56
Celiac disease. Typical radiographic findings of celiac disease are demonstrated on these films from a small bowel series of a 3-year-old girl with failure to thrive, osteoporosis, delayed bone age, anemia, and steatorrhea. *A*, The 30-minute film shows dilatation and an atrophic fold pattern in the duodenum and jejunum. *B*, The 2-hour film shows some precipitation of barium, dilatation, and atrophic mucosa. Note the slow transit of contrast.

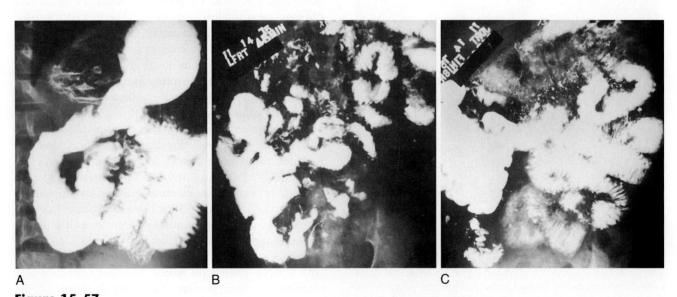

Figure 15–57
Celiac disease: small bowel examination in an 11-year-old child. *A*, This radiograph shows dilatation of duodenum and jejunum with normal mucosal folds. *B*, Segmentation of the contrast column by the relatively large amount of intestinal fluid can be seen. *C*, There is precipitation of barium caused by excessive intestinal fluid.

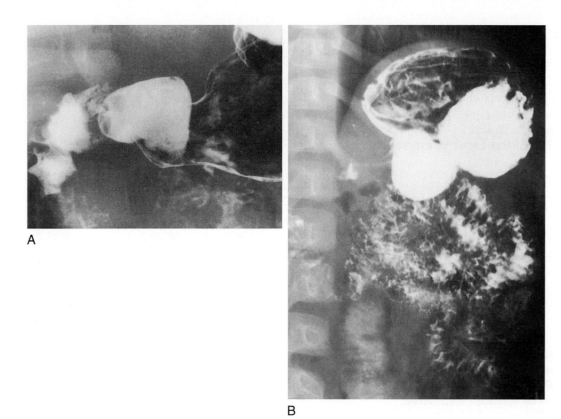

A

B

Figure 15–58
Duodenal and jejunal celiac disease in a 3-year-old boy. Note the thickened and distorted duodenal folds *(A)* and thickened but regular jejunal folds *(B)*. Dilatation is absent.

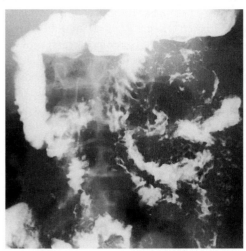

Figure 15–59
Celiac disease. Precipitation, segmentation, and flocculation of barium are shown on this small bowel radiograph of a 4-year-old boy with celiac disease. Dilatation is not present.

In other patients, thickened folds may reflect relatively severe acute celiac disease with hypoproteinemia. The combination of moderate or marked proximal small bowel dilatation and normal or atrophic folds is characteristic of gluten-sensitive enteropathy. Other possible causes of this pattern are either rare (e.g., idiopathic pseudo-obstruction or collagen disease) or easily excluded (e.g., obstruction or ileus) (Table 15–10).

Hypersecretion The phenomenon conventionally termed *hypersecretion* may actually be secondary to diminished absorption of fluids or stasis. This phenomenon results in poor mucosal coating, precipitation, flocculation, segmentation, and moulage formation—all signs formerly thought to have relative specificity for celiac disease. However, these findings are the result of an excessive volume of fluid in the gut relative to the volume of administered barium and are thus nonspecific evidence of stasis and increased intestinal fluid. These signs are less frequently observed with colloidal barium, which is currently in common use, than they were with noncolloidal barium, which was used in the past.

Motility Transient intussusception is very rare in normal children and reflects the presence of abnormal bowel motility. If transient intussusception, a feature of the abnormal motility of gluten enteropathy, is observed in a child with a suggestive clinical history, small bowel biopsy is encouraged (Fig. 15–60).

TABLE 15-10 RADIOGRAPHIC CLASSIFICATION
OF MALABSORPTIVE CONDITIONS

Pattern I. Normal small intestine
Pancreatic insufficiency other than cystic fibrosis
Drug-induced malabsorption: antibiotics, methotrexate,
  para-aminosalicylic acid
Pattern II. Dilated small intestine with normal folds
Obstruction and ileus
Celiac disease
Collagen diseases: systemic lupus erythematosus,
  dermatomyositis, scleroderma
Chronic idiopathic pseudo-obstruction
Pattern III. Thickened regular folds with or without dilatation
Celiac disease
Hypoproteinemia
Edema
Lymphangiectasia
Amyloidosis
Lymphoma
Pattern IV. Thickened irregular or nodular folds with or without dilatation
Cystic fibrosis
Crohn's disease
Lymphoid nodular hyperplasia
Whipple's disease
Mastocytosis
Eosinophilic gastroenteritis
Abetalipoproteinemia
Zollinger-Ellison syndrome
Lymphoma

From Roy CC, Silverman A, Cozetto FJ. Pediatric Clinical
Gastroenterology. St. Louis: CV Mosby, 1975, p 224. Published
by permission of the publisher and authors.

Abnormal small bowel transit time is difficult to diagnose because of the wide normal variability; however, a prolonged transit time is characteristic of celiac disease.

SUMMARY

Conservative use of radiographic studies in children with diarrheal illness is warranted because of the absence of specific radiographic findings in most childhood diarrheal diseases. However, in well-defined situations, children with diarrhea will benefit from radiographic investigation. Plain film evaluation may be used as a diagnostic indicator when diarrhea is due to necrotizing enterocolitis. Plain films are essential

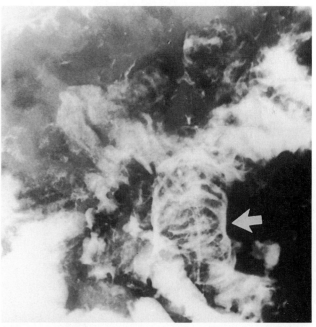

Figure 15–60
Celiac disease: transient intussusception. These images are from a small bowel series performed in a 3-year-old child with celiac disease. *A*, Precipitation and fragmentation of barium in the proximal jejunum reflect the small amount of contrast relative to intestinal fluid. A transient intussusception is present in the midjejunum *(arrow)*. The lumen of the intussusceptum is visible as a linear collection of barium oriented along the central longitudinal axis of the intussuscipiens.

if perforation or toxic megacolon from severe colitis is considered clinically. Children with known Crohn's disease usually need only plain films for evaluation of acute obstructive episodes that respond to medical therapy.

For patients with suspected acute inflammatory bowel disease, infectious colitis must be excluded by stool cultures and microscopy before barium enema is performed. In such situations, barium enema is delayed until the colitis is controlled and the patient can tolerate good colon preparation. The absence of obscuring fluid and fecal residue permits the radiologist to perform a high-quality barium enema, which will optimize the radiographic assessment of disease distribution and severity. When clinically indicated, follow-up barium studies aid in the care of children with inflammatory bowel disease. Fistula, obstruction, abscess, and stenosis caused by Crohn's disease are often well defined by barium studies, and additional information may be obtained by cross-sectional imaging, which may be useful in the guidance of nonsurgical treatment.

When enterocolitis is the initial recognized manifestation of Hirschsprung's disease, a carefully performed contrast examination of the colon will facilitate an immediate diagnosis of Hirschsprung's disease as the cause for the enterocolitis.

A small bowel series in children with malabsorption is useful for the following:

1. Confirmation of proximal small bowel mucosal disease. This predicts a successful peroral jejunal biopsy.
2. Demonstration of mucosal disease primarily in the distal small bowel. This implies that peroral biopsy may not be diagnostic and a negative biopsy finding is of limited value.
3. Exclusion of congenital or postsurgical partial small bowel obstruction, which can cause malabsorption due to stasis with bacterial overgrowth.

Results of a small bowel contrast examination are abnormal in most children with celiac disease, and the characteristic radiographic appearance of the disorder is evident in many patients.

REFERENCES

1. Agha FP, Ghahremani GG, Panella JS, Kaufman MW. Appendicitis as the initial manifestation of Crohn's disease: Radiologic features and prognosis. AJR Am J Roentgenol 149:515–518, 1987.
2. Anderson CM, Burke V. Coeliac disease. In Anderson CM, Burke V, eds. Paediatric Gastroenterology. Oxford, England: Blackwell Scientific Publications, 1975, pp 175–197.
3. Auricchio S, Mazzacca G, Tosi R, et al. Coeliac disease as a familial condition: Identification of asymptomatic coeliac patients within family groups. Gastroenterol Int 1:25–31, 1988.
4. Bill AH Jr, Chapman ND. The enterocolitis of Hirschsprung's disease: Its natural history and treatment. Am J Surg 103:70–74, 1962.
5. Blaser MJ, Reller LB. Campylobacter enteritis. N Engl J Med 305:1444–1452, 1981.
6. Brandon J, Glick S, Teplick SK. Intestinal giardiasis: The importance of serial filming. AJR Am J Roentgenol 144:581–584, 1985.
7. Brearly S, Armstrong GR, Nairn R, et al. Pseudomembranous colitis: A lethal complication of Hirschsprung's disease unrelated to antibiotic usage. J Pediatr Surg 22:257–259, 1987.
8. Capitanio MA, Kirkpatrick JA. Lymphoid hyperplasia of the colon in children. Radiology 94:323–327, 1970.
9. Caroline DF, Evers K. Colitis: Radiographic features and differentiation of idiopathic inflammatory bowel disease. Radiol Clin North Am 25:47–66, 1987.
10. Casola G, vanSonnenberg E, Neff CC, Saba RM, Withers C, Emarine CW. Abscesses in Crohn's disease: Percutaneous drainage. Radiology 163:19–22, 1987.
11. Charron M, del Rosario FJ, Kocoshis SA. Pediatric inflammatory bowel disease: Assessment with scintigraphy with ^{99m}Tc white blood cells. Radiology 212:507–513, 1999.
12. Desai AG. Diarrheal disorders in childhood. Q Med Rev 30:1–33, 1979.
13. Dias J, Unsworth DJ, Walker-Smith JA. Antigliadin and antireticulin antibodies in screening for coeliac disease [Letter]. Lancet 2:157–158, 1987.
14. Dicke WK, Weijers HA, van de Damer JH. Coeliac disease: II. The presence in wheat of a factor having a deleterious effect in cases of coeliac disease. Acta Paediatr 42:34, 1953.
15. Domemeny JM, Burke DR, Meranze SG. Percutaneous drainage of abscesses in patients with Crohn's disease. Gastrointest Radiol 13:237–241, 1988.
16. Eckberg O, Sjostrum B, Brahme F. Radiological findings in *Yersinia* ileitis. Radiology 123:15–19, 1977.
17. Falchuck ZM. Update on gluten-sensitive enteropathy. Am J Med 67:1085–1096, 1979.
18. Farmer RG, Whelan G, Fozzio VW. Long-term follow-up of patients with Crohn's disease. Relationship between clinical patterns and prognosis. Gastroenterology 88:1818, 1985.
19. Fisher CH, Oh KS, Bayless TM, Siegelman SS. Current perspectives in giardiasis. AJR Am J Roentgenol 125:207–217, 1975.
20. Fishman EK, Wolf EJ, Jones B, Bayless TM. Siegelman SS. CT evaluation of Crohn's disease: Effect on patient management. AJR Am J Roentgenol 148:537–540, 1987.
21. Franken EA Jr. Gastrointestinal Radiology in Pediatrics. New York: Harper & Row, 1975, pp 172–190.
22. Franken EA, Smith JA, Fitzgerald JR. Regional enteritis in children: Clinical and roentgen features. CRC Crit Rev Diagn Imaging 10:163–185, 1977.
23. Franks JD, Nixon HH. Cause of death in Hirschsprung's disease. Analysis and conclusion for therapy. Prog Pediatr Surg 13:199–205, 1979.
24. Goldberg E. An epidemiological study of Hirschsprung's disease. Int J Epidemiol 13:479–485, 1984.
25. Goldberg HI, Gore RM, Margulis AR, et al. Computed tomography in the evaluation of Crohn disease. AJR Am J Roentgenol 140:277–282, 1983.
26. Goldberg HI, Jeffrey RB. Recent advances in the radiographic evaluation of inflammatory bowel disease. Med Clin North Am 64:1059–1081, 1980.
27. Goldberg HI, Reeder MM. Infections and infestations of the gastrointestinal tract. In Margulis AR, Burhenne HJ, eds. Alimentary Tract Roentgenology. 2nd ed. St. Louis: Mosby, 1973, pp 1575–1591.
28. Gore RM, Balthazar EJ, Ghahremani GG, Miller FH. CT features of ulcerative colitis and Crohn's disease. AJR Am J Roentgenol 167:3–15, 1996.
29. Gore RM, Marn CS, Kirby DF, Vogelzang RL, Neimann HL. CT findings in ulcerative granulomatous and indeterminate colitis. AJR Am J Roentgenol 143:279–284, 1984.
30. Gryboski J, Hillemeier C. Inflammatory bowel disease in children. Med Clin North Am 64:1185–1202, 1980.
31. Gryboski JD, Spiro HM. Prognosis in children with Crohn's disease. Gastroenterology 74:807–817, 1978.
32. Hamilton JR. Diarrhea and malabsorption in children. In Sleisinger MH, Fordtran JS, eds. Gastrointestinal Disease. 2nd ed. Philadelphia: WB Saunders, 1978, pp 336–353.
33. Haworth EM, Hodson CJ, Pringle EM, Young WF. The value of radiological investigation of the alimentary tract in children with coeliac syndrome. Clin Radiol 19:65–76, 1968.
34. Hizawa K, Iida M, Aoyagi K, Fujishima M. The significance of colonic mucosal lymphoid hyperplasia and aphthoid ulcers in Crohn's disease. Clin Radiol 51:706–708, 1996.
35. Hodes HL. Gastroenteritis with special reference to rotavirus. Adv Pediatr 27:195–245, 1980.
36. Holmes GKT, Prior P, Lane MR, Pope D, Allan RN. Malignancy in coeliac disease—Effect of a gluten-free diet. Gut 30:333–338, 1989.
37. Jabra AA, Fishman EK, Taylor GA. CT findings in inflammatory bowel disease in children. AJR Am J Roentgenol 162:975–979, 1994.
38. Jaffe N. Radiographic appearances and course of discrete mucosal ulcers in Crohn's disease of the colon. Gastrointest Radiol 5:371–378, 1980.
39. Joseph VT, Sim CK. Problems and pitfalls in the management of Hirschsprung's disease. J Pediatr Surg 23:398–402, 1988.
40. Kaftori JK, Pery M, Kleinhaus U. Ultrasonography in Crohn's disease. Gastrointest Radiol 9:137–142, 1984.
41. Kagnoff MF. Celiac disease: Adenovirus and alpha gliadin. Curr Top Microbiol Immunol 145:67–78, 1989.
42. Kagnoff MF. Celiac disease. In Yamada T, ed. Textbook of Gastroenterology. Vol 2. Philadelphia: JB Lippincott, 1991, pp 1503–1520.

43. Kalser MH. Celiac sprue (gluten-induced enteropathy, nontropical sprue, idiopathic steatorrhea). In Bockus HL, ed. Gastroenterology. Vol 2. 3rd ed. Philadelphia: WB Saunders, 1976, pp 244–284.

44. Kapuscinska A, Zalewski T, Chorzelski TP, et al. Disease specificity and dynamics of changes in IgA class anti-endomysial antibodies in celiac disease. J Pediatr Gastroenterol Nutr 6:529–534, 1987.

45. Kelts DG, Grand RJ. Inflammatory bowel disease in children and adolescents. Curr Probl Pediatr 10:1–40, 1980.

46. Kemey PJ, Koehler RE, Shackelford GD. The clinical significance of large lymphoid follicles of the colon. Radiology 142:41–46, 1982.

47. Kirberg A, Latorre JJ, Hartard ME. Endoscopic small intestinal biopsy in infants and children: Its usefulness in the diagnosis of celiac disease and other enteropathies. J Pediatr Gastroenterol Nutr 9:178–181, 1989.

48. Kirks DR, Currarino G. Regional enteritis in children: Small bowel disease with normal terminal ileum. Pediatr Radiol 7:10–14, 1987.

49. Kleinhaus S, Bokey SJ, Sheran M, Sieber WK. Hirschsprung's disease—A survey of the members of the surgical section of the American Academy of Pediatrics. J Pediatr Surg 14:588–597, 1979.

50. Koelbel G, Schmiedl U, Majer MC, et al. Diagnosis of fistulae and sinus tracks in patients with Crohn's disease: Value of MR imaging. AJR Am J Roentgenol 152:999–1003, 1989.

51. Kollitz JPM, Davis GB, Berk RN. Campylobacter colitis: A common infectious form of colitis. Gastrointest Radiol 6:227, 1981.

52. Krugman S, Ward R, Katzl SL. Infectious Diseases of Children. 6th ed. St. Louis: CV Mosby, 1977, pp 69–82.

53. Lambiase RE, Cronan JJ, Dorfman GS, et al. Percutaneous drainage of abscesses in patients with Crohn's disease. AJR Am J Roentgenol 150:1043–1045, 1988.

54. Lenaerts C, Roy CC, Vaillancourt M, et al. High incidence of upper gastrointestinal tract involvement in children with Crohn's disease. Pediatrics 83:777–781, 1989.

55. Leonidas JC, Krasna IH, Strauss L, et al. Roentgen appearance of the excluded colon after colostomy for infantile Hirschsprung's disease. Am J Roentgenol Nuclear Med Radiol Ther 112:116–122, 1971.

56. Levine M. Escherichia coli infections. N Engl J Med 313:445–447, 1985.

57. Lichtenstein JE. Radiologic-pathologic correlation of inflammatory bowel disease. Radiol Clin North Am 25:3–24, 1987.

58. Limberg B. Sonographic features of colonic Crohn's disease: Comparison of in vivo and in vitro studies. J Clin Ultrasound 18:161–166, 1990.

59. McNeish AS, Harms HK, Rey J, Shmerling DH, Visakorpi JK, Walker-Smith JA. The diagnosis of coeliac disease: A commentary on the current practices of members of the European Society for Paediatric Gastroenterology and Nutrition (ESPGAN). Arch Dis Child 54:783–786, 1979.

60. McNicholl B, Egan-Mitchell B, Fottrell PF. Variability of gluten intolerance in treated childhood coeliac disease. Gut 20:126–132, 1979.

61. Morson BC. Pathology of ulcerative colitis. In Kirsner JB, Shorter RB, eds. Inflammatory Bowel Disease. Philadelphia: Lea & Febiger, 1980, pp 281–310.

62. Navab F, Boyd CM, Diner WC, Subramani R, Chan C. Early and delayed indium 111 leukocyte imaging in Crohn's disease. Gastroenterology 93:829–834, 1987.

63. Nelson JD. Antibiotic therapy for Salmonella syndromes. Am J Dis Child 135:1093–1094, 1981.

64. O'Donovan AN, Somers S, Farrow R, Mernagh JR, Sridhar S. MR imaging of anorectal Crohn disease: A pictorial essay. RadioGraphics 17:101–107, 1997.

65. Orel SG, Rubesin SE, Jones B, Fishman EK, Bayless TM, Siegelman SS. Computed tomography vs. barium studies in the acutely symptomatic patient with Crohn's disease. J Comput Assist Tomogr 11:1009–1016, 1987.

66. Orkin BA, Telander RL, Wolff BG. The surgical management of children with ulcerative colitis. The old vs. the new. Dis Colon Rectum 33:947–955, 1990.

67. Pai CH, Gordon R, Sims HV, Bryan LE. Sporadic cases of hemorrhagic colitis associated with Escherichia coli O157:H7. Clinical, epidemiologic, and bacteriologic features. Ann Intern Med 101:783–742, 1984.

68. Palder SB, Shandling B, Bilik R, Griffiths AM, Sherman P. Perianal complications of pediatric Crohn's disease. J Pediatr Surg 26:513–515, 1991.

69. Park RH, McKillop JH, Duncan A, Mackenzie JF, Russell RI. Can 111 indium autologous mixed leucocyte scanning accurately assess disease extent and activity in Crohn's disease? Gut 29:821–825, 1988.

70. Philips SF. Diarrhea: Pathogenesis and diagnostic techniques. Postgrad Med 57:65, 1975.

71. Puntis J, McNeish AS, Alan RN. Long-term prognosis of Crohn's disease with onset in childhood and adolescence. Gut 25:329, 1984.

72. Remis RS, MacDonald KR, Riley LW, et al. Sporadic cases of hemorrhagic colitis associated with Escherichia coli O157:H7. Ann Intern Med 101:624–626, 1984.

73. Rossi TM, Kumar V, Lerner A, Heitlinger LA, Tucker N, Fisher J. Relationship of endomysial antibodies to jejunal mucosal pathology: Specificity towards both symptomatic and asymptomatic celiacs. J Pediatr Gastroenterol Nutr 7:858–863, 1988.

74. Safrit HD, Mauro MA, Jaques PF. Percutaneous abscess drainage in Crohn's disease. AJR Am J Roentgenol 150:1043–1045, 1987.

75. Santosham M, Daum RS, Dillman L, et al. Oral rehydration therapy of infantile diarrhea. N Engl J Med 306:1070–1076, 1982.

76. Schrago G. Yersinia enterocolitica ileocolitis findings observed on barium enema. Br J Radiol 49:181–183, 1976.

77. Scott H, Ek J, Havnen J, et al. Serum antibodies to dietary antigens: A prospective study of the diagnostic usefulness in celiac disease. J Pediatr Gastroenterol Nutr 11:215–220, 1990.

78. Shmerling DH, Francx J. Childhood coeliac disease: A long term analysis of relapses in 91 patients. J Paediatr Gastroenterol Nutr 5:565–569, 1986.

79. Shorter RG. Risks of intestinal cancer in Crohn's disease. Dis Colon Rectum 7:35–41, 1985.

80. Sieber WK. Hirschsprung's disease. In Ravitch MM, et al, eds. Pediatric Surgery. 3rd ed. Chicago: Year Book Medical, 1979, pp 1035–1054.

81. Silverman A, Roy CC, Cozzetto FJ. Pediatric Clinical Gastroenterology. St. Louis: CV Mosby, 1971, pp 132–148, 199–210.

82. Simpkins KC. Aphthoid ulcers in Crohn's colitis. Clin Radiol 28:601–608, 1977.

83. Singleton EB, Wagner ML, Dutton RV. Radiology of the Alimentary Tract in Infants and Children. 2nd ed. Philadelphia: WB Saunders, 1977, pp 225–237, 316–333.

84. Squires RH Jr. Assessment of inflammatory bowel disease [Editorial]. J Pediatr 130:10–12, 1997.

85. Stringer DA, Sherman PM, Jakowenko N. Correlation of double-contrast high-density barium enema, colonoscopy, and histology in children with special attention to disparities. Pediatr Radiol 16:298–301, 1986.

86. Swenson O. Hirschsprung's disease. In Raffensperger JG, ed. Swenson's Pediatric Surgery. 4th ed. New York: Appleton-Century-Crofts, 1980, pp 507–531.

87. Swenson O, Davidson FZ. Similarities of mechanical intestinal obstruction and aganglionic megacolon in the newborn infant. A review of 64 cases. N Engl J Med 262:64–67, 1960.

88. Taylor DN, Echeverria P, Blaser MJ, et al. Polymicrobial aetiology of traveler's diarrhea. Lancet 1:381, 1985.

89. Teitelbaum DH, Caniano DA, Qualman SJ. The pathophysiology of Hirschsprung's-associated enterocolitis: Importance of histologic correlates. J Pediatr Surg 24:1271–1277, 1989.

90. Teitelbaum DH, Qualman SJ, Caniano DA. Hirschsprung's disease. Identification of risk factors for enterocolitis. Ann Surg 207:240–244, 1988.

91. Williams CB, Nicholls S. Endoscopic features of chronic inflammatory bowel disease in childhood. Bailliere's Clin Gastroenterol 8:121–131, 1994.

92. Wilson-Storey D, Scobie WG. Impaired gastrointestinal mucosal defense in Hirschsprung's disease: A clue to the pathogenesis of enterocolitis? J Pediatr Surg 24:462–464, 1989.

93. Winthrop JD, Balfe DM, Schackelford GD, McAlister WH, Rosenblum JL, Siegel MJ. Ulcerative and granulomatous colitis in children. Comparison of double and single contrast studies. Radiology 154:657–660, 1985.

94. Working Group of European Society of Paediatric Gastroenterology and Nutrition: Revised criteria for diagnosis of coeliac disease. Arch Dis Child 65:909–911, 1990.

95. Worlicek H, Lutz H, Heyder N, Matek W. Ultrasound findings in Crohn's disease and ulcerative colitis: A prospective study. J Clin Ultrasound 15:153–163, 1987.

ADDITIONAL READING

Bartlett JG: Antimicrobial agents implicated in *Clostridium difficile* toxin-associated diarrhea or colitis. Johns Hopkins Med J 149:6–9, 1981.

Brazowski E, Rozen P, Misonzhnick-Bedny F, Gitstein G. Characteristics of familial juvenile polyps expressing cyclooxygenase-2. Am J Gastroenterol 100:130–138, 2005.

Bridger S, Evans N, Parker A, Cairns SR. Multiple cerebral venous thromboses in a child with inflammatory bowel disease. J Pediatr Gastroenterol Nutr 25:533–536, 1997.

Dundas SA, Dutton J, Skipworth P: Reliability of rectal biopsy in distinguishing between chronic inflammatory bowel disease and acute self-limiting colitis. Histopathology 31:60–66, 1997.

Laghi A, Paolantonio P, Catalano C, et al. MR imaging of the small bowel using polyethylene glycol solution as an oral contrast agent in adults and children with celiac disease: Preliminary observations. AJR Am J Roentgenol 180:191–194, 2003.

Navarro OM, Daneman A, Chae A: Intussusception: The use of delayed, repeated reduction attempts and the management of intussusceptions due to pathologic lead points in pediatric patients. AJR Am J Roentgenol 182:1169–1176, 2004.

Ojha S, Menon P, Rao KL. Meckel's diverticulum with segmental dilatation of the ileum: Radiographic diagnosis in a neonate. Pediatr Radiol. 34:649–651, 2004.

Oktar SO, Yucel C, Ozdemir H, Uluturk A, Isik S. Comparison of conventional sonography, real-time compound sonography, tissue harmonic sonography, and tissue harmonic compound sonography of abdominal and pelvic lesions. AJR Am J Roentgenol 181:1341–1347, 2004.

Proujansky R, Fawcett PT, Gibney KM, Treem WR, Hyams JS. Examination of anti-neutrophil cytoplasmic antibodies in childhood inflammatory bowel disease. J Pediatr Gastroenterol Nutr 17:193, 1993.

Shmuely H, Samra Z, Ashkenazi S, Dinari G, Chodick G, Yahav J. Association of *Heliobacter pylori* infection with *Shigella* gastroenteritis in young children. Am J Gastroenterol 99:2041–2045, 2004.

Sugita A, Sachar DB, Bodian C, Ribeiro MB, Aufses AH Jr, Greenstein AJ. Colorectal cancer in ulcerative colitis: Influence of anatomical extent and age at onset of colitis-cancer interval. Gut 32:167–169, 1991.

Xin W, Brown PI, Greenson JK. The clinical significance of focal active colitis in pediatric patients. Am J Surg Pathol 27:1134–1138, 2003.

Zerin J, Kuhn-Fulton J, White S, et al: Colonic strictures in children with cystic fibrosis. Radiology 194:223–226, 1995.

THE CHILD WITH CONSTIPATION

Outline

CHAPTER
16

Saskia von Waldenburg Hilton, MD

THE CHILD WITH CONSTIPATION

Constipation, or difficulty in passing stool, is an important problem not only because it is very common, but also because it may be the first symptom of a potentially life-threatening illness. When constipation results from psychogenic factors, the accompanying fecal soiling often may affect peer relationships and thereby seriously retard the child's social development. Most commonly, constipation is due to environmental factors that are often temporary and of no medical significance. The challenge confronting the clinician is in deciding when this symptom warrants additional investigation and when it represents an insignificant, temporary derangement of bowel function.

Constipation is defined as infrequent stooling, although some authorities stress that the character of the stool and associated symptoms are more important than the frequency of defecation. "Normal" frequency varies widely among people of various ages and cultures and even in the same individual at different times. Factors most commonly responsible for constipation include anorectal disease (especially fissures); decreased fluid intake; dietary changes; some drugs; and altered routines, such as bedrest, travel, or environmental change. When so many different factors are involved and such a wide range of normal stooling exists, how does one decide when to further investigate or treat constipation? In general, further evaluation is required in the following circumstances:

1. When there is failure to pass meconium within the first 24 hours after birth, followed by obstructive symptoms or an abnormal stooling pattern
2. When constipation is associated with failure to thrive
3. When a fever of unknown etiology or diarrhea is seen in a child who was previously constipated
4. When neurologic symptoms are present
5. When a presumed psychogenic megacolon is unresponsive to adequate treatment

Treatment is generally indicated in the following circumstances:

1. When bloody stools or painful defecation indicate the presence of anorectal disease
2. When encopresis is present
3. When rectal examination reveals that true constipation exists in a normal child whose history suggests no other disease
4. When recurrent abdominal pain is present

Insignificant constipation usually presents as an isolated symptom in an otherwise healthy child. If additional signs or symptoms are present or if the patient is a neonate, the failure to stool should not be ignored (Diagram 16–1; Figs. 16–1 through 16–5).

DIFFERENTIAL DIAGNOSIS OF CONSTIPATION

NEONATES (BIRTH TO 1 MONTH)

Failure to stool in the neonatal period should always be considered abnormal until proved otherwise. This is not true

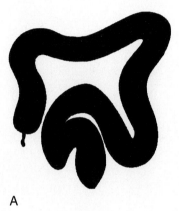

A

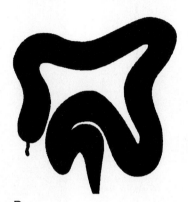

B

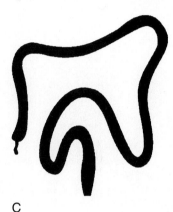

C

A, Normal neonatal colon. The normal neonatal colon is markedly redundant, and at all ages, the rectum is wider in caliber than the sigmoid. Cecal location is occasionally slightly higher than above the right lower quadrant, where it is normally seen in older children or adults. Reflux of barium into the terminal ileum during barium enema is difficult to achieve in normal neonates.

B, Colon in a patient with Hirschsprung's disease. In neonates, a true transition zone is usually not present. A difference in colonic caliber is usually evident, with the aganglionic segment narrower than the normal proximal distal colon. Spasm of the aganglionic portion is usually visible fluoroscopically. This diagram demonstrates the relatively narrowed distal aganglionic segment and the normal proximal colon.

C, Microcolon. A microcolon is a normal but unused colon that appears markedly diminished in width but otherwise is of normal proportions. It is not normally distended with meconium because of a proximal mechanical obstruction (e.g., meconium ileus or ileal atresia). Once the obstruction is relieved, the colon begins to function and then radiographically appears normal.

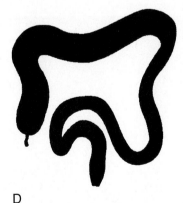

D

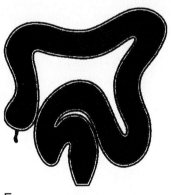

E

D, Neonatal small left colon syndrome. This entity, which some authorities believe to be a variant of meconium plug syndrome, is characteristically seen in infants of diabetic mothers. Obstructive signs of abdominal distention and vomiting are seen shortly after birth. Once the meconium plug is evacuated, the colon demonstrates a relative transition zone, typically at the splenic flexure. The colon distal to the splenic flexure is narrowed without evidence of spasm or the abnormal rectosigmoid ratio that characterizes Hirschsprung's disease.

E, Meconium plug syndrome. In this entity, meconium is not evacuated and obstruction results. Most commonly, these infants respond to rectal stimulation, but sometimes a contrast enema is needed to initiate evacuation. The contrast material surrounds the cast of meconium as schematically illustrated here. Meconium plug syndrome may be the initial presentation of Hirschsprung's disease.

Diagram 16–1
Schematic representation of mechanical and functional obstruction in the neonatal period.

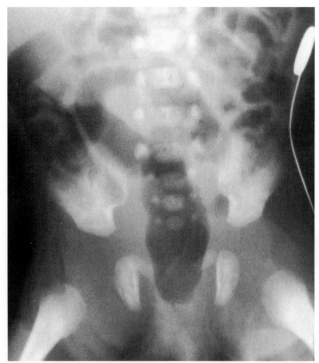

Figure 16–1
Normal neonatal colon. Note the generous amount of air in the rectum. The sigmoid colon is seen in the left mid abdomen and is smaller in diameter than the rectum. Note also that the colon is circuitous.

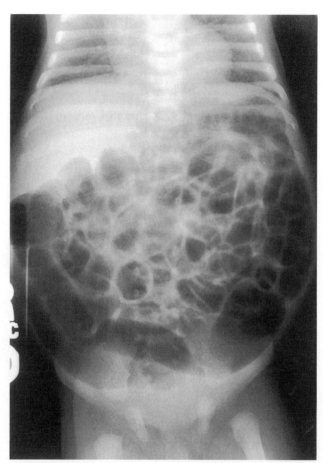

Figure 16–2
Hirschsprung's disease. Classic findings are present. Abdominal distention is seen and is more pronounced distally. Note the absence of rectal gas.

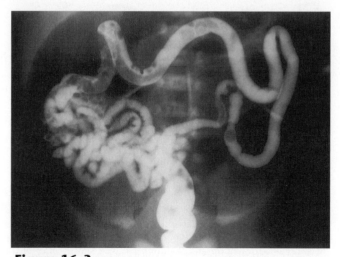

Figure 16–3
Microcolon. A microcolon is a normal, unused colon. An obstruction prevents the passage of meconium into the colon. Once the obstruction is removed, the colon appears and functions normally.

for children in other age groups. Ninety-four percent of normal, term newborn infants spontaneously pass meconium within 24 hours after birth, and 99.8% stool within the first 48 hours. Exceptions to this rule include premature infants whose bowels may be immature or who are severely ill from respiratory disease and term infants who were severely asphyxiated or subjected to large quantities of maternal analgesics.[15,39] These infants may fail to stool but do not have abdominal distention that would suggest bowel obstruction.

Infants whose failure to stool represents a mechanical or functional obstruction usually develop clinical as well as radiographic evidence of obstruction. Clinical evidence consists of abdominal distention and vomiting. Radiographs show dilation of the small bowel that initially may be uniform but with time becomes more pronounced in the loops just proximal to the obstruction. The major diagnostic possibilities, in decreasing order of frequency, are meconium plug syndrome,[21,28,33] Hirschsprung's disease, ileal atresia, meconium ileus, neonatal small left colon syndrome,[7,8,27,34] and colonic atresia.

Contrast enema examination is often used to distinguish these entities from one another. A microcolon will be present in infants with ileal atresia, colonic atresia, and meconium

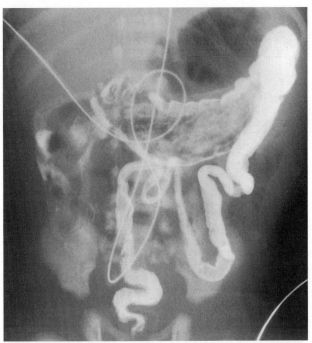

Figure 16–4

Neonatal small left colon syndrome in an infant of a diabetic mother who presented with abdominal distention and vomiting. Narrowing of the colon, starting at the splenic flexure, is evident. Spasticity of the distal segment was absent, and the colon, apart from being narrowed, was normal. A suction biopsy confirmed the absence of Hirschsprung's disease. An umbilical arterial line is present.

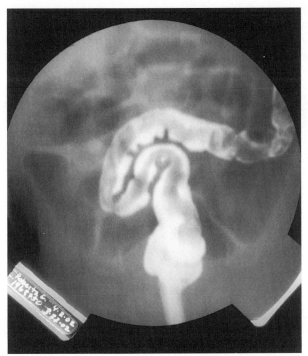

Figure 16–5

Meconium plug. A neonate with a meconium plug has a colon of normal size and length. The plug causes a temporary obstruction.

ileus. In meconium ileus, plain films often show bubbly meconium in the right lower quadrant. Because of the tenacious nature of meconium, air-fluid levels are uncommon in meconium ileus. Thus, absence of air-fluid levels is a suggestive sign, although their presence does not exclude a positive diagnosis. Reflux of a water-soluble hyperosmotic contrast agent into the terminal ileum (as in a diatrizoate meglumine [Gastrografin] enema) shows pellets of meconium. This is a diagnostic and often therapeutic procedure for relieving the obstruction.

Colonic atresia will be evident as the flow of contrast material halts at the atretic segment (often in the transverse colon); ileal atresia precludes reflux of contrast material into the terminal ileum. Despite multiple attempts, the radiologist may be unable to reflux contrast material into the terminal ileum in meconium ileus, rendering the findings indistinguishable from those for ileal atresia. This problem is unimportant clinically, however, because an inability to reflux and thereby relieve the obstruction converts meconium ileus from a medical to a surgical condition (Fig. 16–6).

In meconium plug syndrome, Hirschsprung's disease, and neonatal small left colon syndrome, the colon is of normal size. In meconium plug syndrome, the contrast material outlines a large cast of meconium within the colon. A similar finding may be present in neonatal small left colon syndrome, but once the plug is evacuated, the entire distal left colon is seen to be smaller in diameter than the proximal, normal colon. The transition from normal to small colon characteristically occurs near the splenic flexure. Often, the patient's history reveals maternal diabetes. Aganglionosis is seldom confused with neonatal small left colon syndrome because of the typical site of transition of the latter and because the narrowed segment does not demonstrate shortening or spasm. The radiographic diagnosis of Hirschsprung's disease in neonates is described in detail in the next section.

In older neonates, dietary problems may cause infrequent stooling but do not produce bowel obstruction. Low breast milk production, improperly diluted formula, and inadequate feedings are the conditions most commonly responsible for constipation (Table 16–1).

INFANTS (1 MONTH TO 2 YEARS)

Dietary factors and anorectal disease are the two major causes of benign constipation in infants. The most common dietary reason for constipation is decreased fluid intake and early introduction of solid foods, particularly cereals and vegetables. Excessive intake of cow's milk with its associated casein or whey may also produce hard or infrequent stools. Painful stooling from anal fissures can cause withholding of stool even at this early age, before toilet training has been initiated. Anal fissures are readily diagnosed by direct

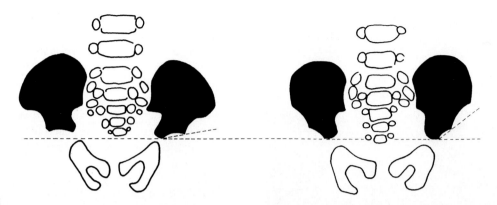

Figure 16–6
This diagram shows the characteristic appearance of the pelvis in trisomy 12 (Down syndrome) *(A)* compared with that in a normal infant *(B)*. Note the eversion of the ilia in trisomy 21, producing flared and apparently large ilia suggestive of "Mickey Mouse ears." The other difference is a shallow acetabular angle (i.e., the angle formed by a line drawn through the medial- and lateral-most aspect of the acetabulum and intersecting a line drawn through both triradiate cartilages) in the patient with trisomy 21 compared with the normal patient. Because the acetabular angle normally decreases with age, this assessment is most valid in the neonate.

inspection of the anal ring; they usually heal with the aid of stool softeners and increased fluids.

When evaluating an infant with constipation, the clinician must keep the following question in mind: Is the constipation an isolated symptom in an otherwise healthy, thriving child, or is it one part of a larger complex of symptoms? If the latter is true, additional investigation, which may reveal significant and often treatable conditions, is indicated.[5,14] These conditions include aganglionosis undiagnosed in the neonatal period, hypothyroidism, renal tubular acidosis, and neurologic disease (Table 16–2; Figs. 16–7, 16–8, and 16–9).

Young Children (2 to 5 Years)

The most common causes of constipation that appears in the second and third years of life are related to toilet training and diet. This is the age at which functional constipation starts in most children. Toilet training that is punitive, unrealistically early, or tension filled is the major cause of constipation in children in this age group. Conscious withholding of stool may cause anorectal fissures, which make defecation painful and augment stool withholding. Hirschsprung's disease and constipation due to neurogenic problems are uncommon

TABLE 16-1 CAUSES OF CONSTIPATION IN
NEONATES (BIRTH TO 1 MONTH)

Common
Maternal medication or anesthesia
Neonatal asphyxia
Bowel immaturity (premature infants)
Breastfeeding
Meconium plug syndrome
Uncommon
Hirschsprung's disease
Ileal atresia
Colon atresia
Meconium ileus
Small left colon syndrome
Imperforate anus
Duplication cyst

TABLE 16-2 CAUSES OF CONSTIPATION IN
INFANTS (1 MONTH TO 2 YEARS)

Common
Dietary factors
Anorectal disease
Early toilet training
Uncommon
Hirschsprung's disease
Hypothyroidism
Tethered cord
Sacral agenesis
Cerebral palsy
Cerebral atrophy (neonatal hemorrhage; cerebral
   ischemia, post-traumatic; post-nonaccidental trauma)
Meningomyelocele
Pseudo-obstruction
Segmental dilatation of the colon
Spinal tumors

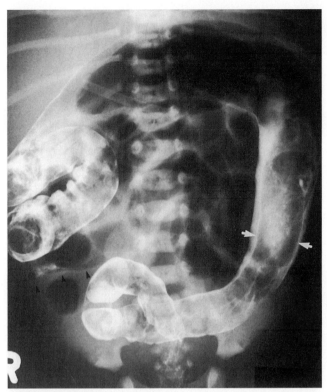

Figure 16–7

Hirschsprung's disease with appendiceal dilatation. This neonate presented with trisomy 21 (Down syndrome) and abdominal distention. A meconium plug *(white arrows)* is seen as a defect in the contrast-filled colon. Once the plug was evacuated, the transition zone was evident at the junction of the sigmoid and descending colon. Appendiceal dilatation, seldom seen in normal neonates, is evident *(black arrowheads)*. Appendiceal or transverse colonic rupture may occur in infants with Hirschsprung's disease, presumably because of ischemia resulting from chronic dilatation. Idiopathic perforation at either of these sites mandates exclusion of aganglionosis. The diagnosis of trisomy 21 is easily made by the characteristic appearance of the pelvis. The probability of dealing with Hirschsprung's disease is increased when a neonate with an obstruction also has trisomy 21.

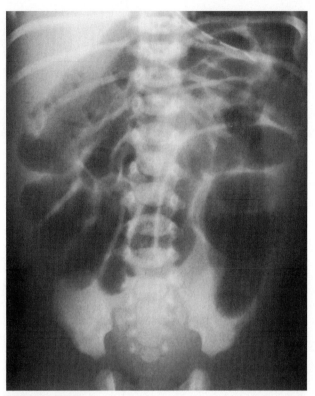

Figure 16–8

Neonatal Hirschsprung's disease. Note the complete absence of gas overlying the pelvis, with moderate dilatation of the entire small bowel despite nasogastric tube decompression.

of Hirschsprung's disease, a suction biopsy of the rectum to detect ganglion cells is an effective and easy method for distinguishing psychogenic constipation from the rare case of low-segment aganglionosis (Table 16–3; Figs. 16–14, 16–15, and 16–16).

EVALUATION OF MAJOR CONDITIONS CAUSING CONSTIPATION

HIRSCHSPRUNG'S DISEASE

Hirschsprung's disease is the most common and most important disease to be excluded in neonates with mechanical bowel obstruction and in older children with constipation. Its recognition requires familiarity with its typical clinical and radiographic findings.[37] Failure to suspect or confirm the diagnosis may have serious consequences for the child. Colitis is not an uncommon complication of untreated Hirschsprung's disease and has a high mortality rate.

diagnostic possibilities. An older child with Hirschsprung's disease is not a healthy child clinically; a neurologic examination is usually abnormal in a child whose constipation is neurogenic in origin (Figs. 16–10 through 16–13).

OLDER CHILDREN (5 TO 18 YEARS)

The older the child, the more likely it is that any stooling difficulties are functional in origin. Although aganglionosis has been found in children of all ages, it is rarely undiagnosed in older children. If a patient has a history of normal stooling between birth and 1 year of age, Hirschsprung's disease is unlikely; however, if there is even the slightest clinical suspicion

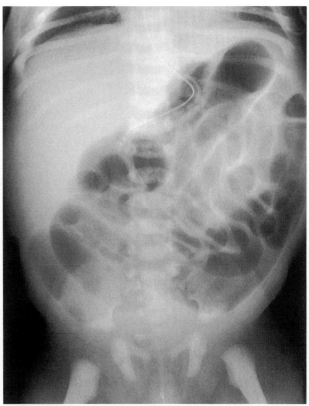

Figure 16–9
Hirschsprung' disease. Note mild increasing bowel dilatation distally. Normal rectal gas. The normal appearance of the rectum in neonates is shown in this supine frontal view. Notice the normal caliber of the small bowel. Although rectal gas is not always present in normal infants, its continued absence in a child with obstructive signs or symptoms should strongly suggest the possibility of aganglionosis. In neonates, plain film differentiation of the small bowel from the large bowel is not possible. The only exception to this rule is bowel lying within the confines of the pelvis, which represents the rectosigmoid region.

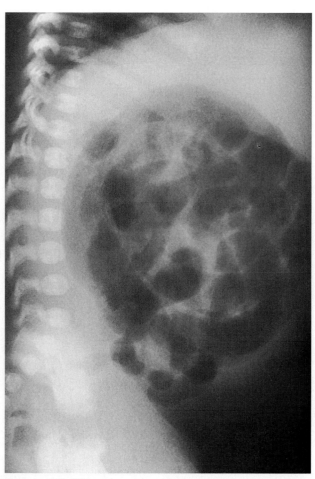

Figure 16–10
Neonatal Hirschsprung's disease. This overhead lateral view demonstrates small bowel dilatation and abnormally attenuated rectal gas. The disadvantage of this view is that it cannot be used to either evaluate the possibilities of free intraperitoneal air nor assess the presence and extent of air-fluid levels. If this view is used, the patient should be positioned with the right side down so that the rectum is higher than the sigmoid colon.

Of the available methods of diagnosing Hirschsprung's disease, radiographic evaluation is used to suggest or verify the diagnosis, to determine the proximal extent of aganglionosis, to exclude other diseases, and to alert the surgeon if the patient has developed enterocolitis. The second method, rectal suction biopsy, has markedly simplified management by permitting pathologic confirmation of the lesion; such proof is a necessity prior to surgical intervention. A suction biopsy can be performed at the bedside without general anesthesia. The specimen obtained may confirm the radiographic diagnosis; more importantly, it may exclude the disease with confidence when the radiographic findings are equivocal (Figs. 16–17, 16–18, and 16–19).

Rectal manometric examination has also been shown to be helpful when performed by experienced personnel. It has been most useful in differentiating low-segment Hirschsprung's

disease (a controversial condition) from psychogenic constipation. None of these methods have supplanted the enema examination, as all three procedures tend to be complementary rather than competitive (Fig. 16–20).

Anatomy and Pathophysiology

The pathologic abnormality in Hirschsprung's disease is absence of myenteric and submucosal ganglion cells in a variably long segment of distal bowel. Embryologically, primitive neuroblasts migrate caudally, appearing at the gastroesophageal junction at 6 weeks' gestation and at the rectum, completing innervation of the colon by 12 weeks. Presumably, and for uncertain reasons, migration of the neuroblasts is arrested, resulting in a distal segment that is not innervated, lacking both Auerbach's plexus (located between longitudinal

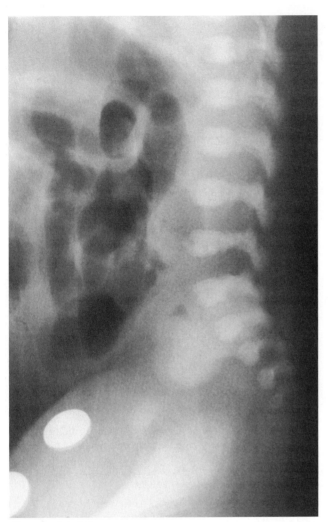

Figure 16–11
Neonatal Hirschsprung's disease. The prone cross-table lateral view most reliably demonstrates the rectum to best advantage. Because the rectum is superior in this position, air tends to rise and fill it. The infant is placed prone, and the beam is directed as for a cross-table lateral view. Note the almost complete absence of rectal gas in this patient, along with multiple air-fluid levels and small bowel distention.

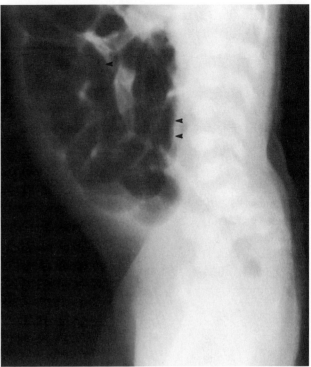

Figure 16–12
Neonatal Hirschsprung's disease. This supine cross-table lateral view demonstrates suspiciously attenuated rectal gas and small bowel dilatation. Air does not reliably outline the rectum to best advantage in this view because the rectum is dependent. Small bowel air-fluid levels (*arrowheads*) and dilatation indicate a functional mechanical obstruction in this neonate with Hirschsprung's disease.

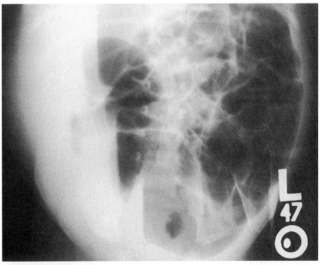

Figure 16–13
Bowel obstruction in Hirschsprung's disease. Another example demonstrating the severity of the mechanical obstruction that can result in this condition. Multiple air-fluid levels, dilated bowel, and a lack of rectal gas are clearly evident on this film. The most common plain film finding in neonatal Hirschsprung's disease is an obstruction.

and circular muscle) and Meissner's plexus (located in the submucosa).[24] The most significant radiographic finding of this disease, the transition zone, is the boundary between the aganglionic and ganglionic segments. The aganglionic colon is spastic, narrowed, and empty of stool, whereas the ganglionic, or normal, colon is dilated, has muscular hypertrophy, and is filled with feces. In 80% of patients, the transition zone is located in the rectosigmoid region. Rarely, the entire colon and small bowel may be involved (3% of patients) (Figs. 16–21 through 16–24).

Disordered motility in the form of denervation hyperspasticity is seen in the distal segment. The inability of the colon to move feces effectively to the rectum results in a

TABLE 16-3 CAUSES OF CONSTIPATION IN
YOUNG AND OLDER CHILDREN

Common
Functional
Anorectal disease
Dietary factors
Uncommon
Hirschsprung's disease
Tethered cord
Sacral agenesis
Cerebral atrophy
Meningomyelocele
Pseudo-obstruction
Spinal tumors
Hypothyroidism
Pelvic masses

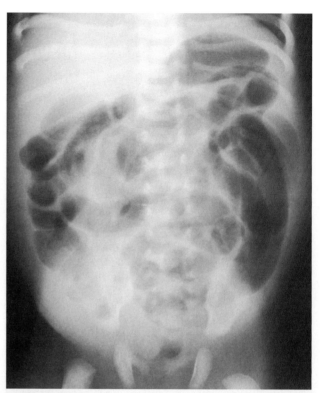

Figure 16–15
Neonatal Hirschsprung's disease. A lack of normal rectal gas and
mild dilatation of small bowel loops are evident. Clinically, this
premature male infant was initially suspected of having necrotizing
enterocolitis. Although Hirschsprung's disease is distinctly unusual
in preterm infants, the diagnosis of aganglionosis should not be
dismissed solely because of prematurity.

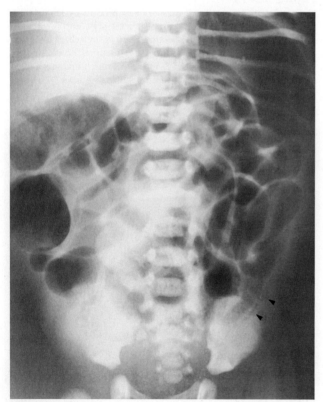

Figure 16–14
Neonatal Hirschsprung's disease. Markedly distended loops of
small bowel and a lack of rectosigmoid gas are evident. Also present
in this neonate with an obstruction is pneumatosis cystoides intestinalis *(arrowheads)*. Note the typical pelvic appearance in this trisomy
21 patient compared with the normal pelvis in Figure 16–6.

mechanical obstruction of varying severity. In normal patients,
the internal anal sphincter relaxes when the rectum distends.
This reflex relaxation of the internal sphincter does not occur
in Hirschsprung's disease and forms the basis for the diagnosis of aganglionosis by rectal manometry. Some authorities
believe that this failure of the internal sphincter to relax
causes the major obstructive component in Hirschsprung's
disease. It has clearly been shown that the length of the aganglionic segment does not correlate with either the severity of
obstructive symptoms or the age of the patient on presentation
(Figs. 16–25 through 16–28).

Pathologic diagnosis of the presence and extent of
Hirschsprung's disease requires confirmation of the absence
of ganglion cells. A submucosal suction biopsy is customarily done prior to a diverting colostomy, with a full-thickness
biopsy performed at the time of definitive surgical repair.

Failure to thrive in this disease results from chronic obstruction. Of patients with Hirschsprung's disease, 18% develop
enterocolitis, and in these infants, the mortality rate is 30%.
Enterocolitis is most frequently seen during the first 3 months
of life. Colonic distention results in ischemia, bacterial inva-
sions, and stercoraceous ulcers. Overgrowth with *Clostridium*

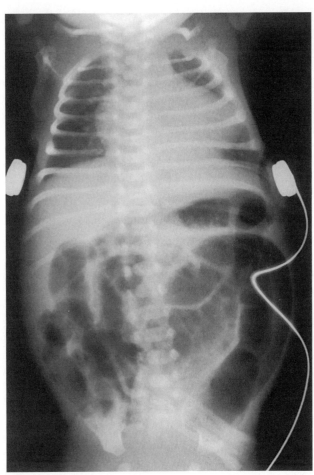

Figure 16–16
Hirschsprung's disease. Neonate with trisomy 21. Note cardiomegaly, increased pulmonary vascularity, and abdominal distention. A moderate ventricular septal defect was present.

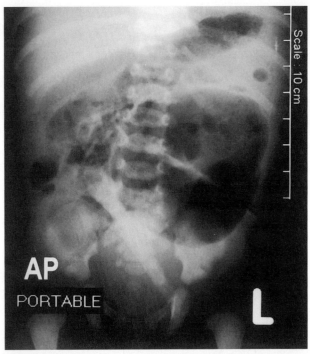

Figure 16–17
Hirschsprung's disease. Neonate with severe abdominal distention and a large loop of bowel in the left abdomen. No gas is present in the rectum.

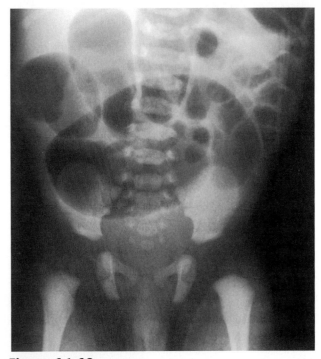

Figure 16–18
Hirschsprung's disease. In a 24-hour delayed view a bizarre gas pattern persists.

difficile occurs with associated toxin production. If the obstruction and fecal stasis become prolonged and severe, the incidence of enterocolitis may be as high as 50%. Perforation of the appendix or proximal colon (presumably a result of ischemia from chronic dilatation) is a less frequent complication and most commonly occurs in infants.[20]

Clinical Presentation

The incidence of Hirschsprung's disease is 1 per 5000 live births (0.02%). This incidence increases to 3.6% in families in which Hirschsprung's disease has already affected one male member and to 8% when a female member has been affected. Of the patients with Hirschsprung's disease 80% are male, and 3% have trisomy 21 (Down syndrome).[18] Because the clinical presentation in the neonatal period is distinctly different from presentation later in life, each is discussed separately (Figs. 16–29 and 16–30).

Neonates Of patients with Hirschsprung's disease, 70% to 80% become symptomatic within the first week

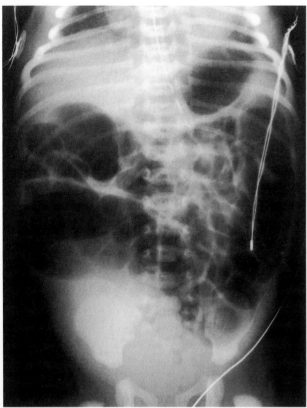

Figure 16–19
Hirschsprung's disease. In a 24-hour delayed view, the largest loops of bowel are distal. A suction biopsy was positive for Hirschsprung's disease. The most consistent indicator of Hirschsprung's disease is the lack of air over the rectum.

of life. Most affected children are term neonates, although this disease occasionally occurs in premature infants. Affected infants show delayed passage of the first stool. As previously mentioned, 99% of normal children pass meconium within the first 48 hours of life, whereas 90% of children with Hirschsprung's disease do not. Abdominal distention with vomiting begins at 2 to 7 days of life. The vomiting may initially be mild but eventually becomes severe, with bilious staining.[2] The obstructive symptoms may abate when feedings are stopped, only to resume when oral intake is again attempted. Failure to thrive becomes a pronounced symptom in infancy if the diagnosis is delayed. The triad of failure to thrive, abdominal distention, and intermittent vomiting strongly suggests aganglionosis (Figs. 16–31 and 16–32).

Enterocolitis is seen in one fifth of neonates. Symptoms of enterocolitis include explosive diarrhea, fever, severe prostration, sepsis, and eventual circulatory collapse. For a more extensive discussion of this problem, see Chapter 15.

Occasionally, Hirschsprung's disease masquerades as meconium plug syndrome.[11] A false sense of security may be obtained when an obstruction is relieved by the removal of a plug, either by rectal stimulation or by contrast enema. A few of these patients return, however, with either symptoms of Hirschsprung's disease or full-blown enterocolitis. Thus, any infant with meconium plug syndrome should be suspected of having aganglionosis, and any symptoms such as recurrent obstruction, fever, diarrhea, or constipation warrant full investigation by enema or suction biopsy (Figs. 16–33, 16–34, and 16–35).

Figure 16–20
Distal segment aganglionosis (Hirschsprung's disease): anteroposterior *(A)* and lateral *(B)* views of a barium enema in a 3-day-old neonate with severe abdominal distention and vomiting. The spastic distal segment is best seen on the lateral view *(arrow)* but is also evident on the frontal view *(arrow)*. The aganglionic segment was not in spasm at the time the frontal view was obtained, so the transition zone is not as clearly defined as on the lateral view. Note that even on the frontal view the distal segment is smaller than the more proximal normal colon. Contrast examination to exclude Hirschsprung's disease is always commenced with the patient in the lateral position, because this view demonstrates the rectum to best advantage.

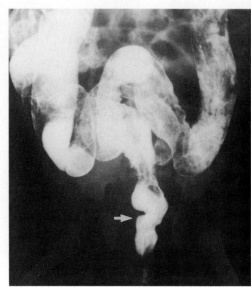

A

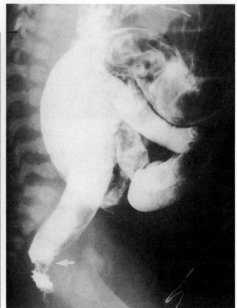

B

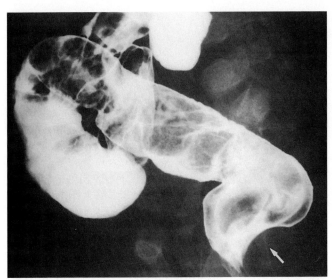

Figure 16–21
Normal colon This lateral view of a normal colon demonstrates a normal posterior indentation *(arrow)* caused by the puborectal sling. The puborectal muscle, which is attached to the posterior pubis, is important in maintaining fecal continence. Note that the diameter of the rectum is normally wider than that of the sigmoid colon. Abundant stool is almost always present in patients being examined for Hirschsprung's disease, because cleansing of the colon is purposefully omitted. Cleansing of the colon makes identification of the transition zone more difficult.

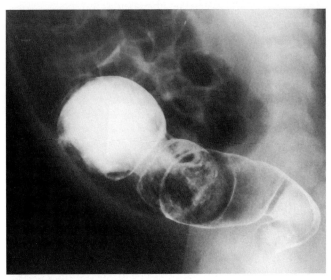

Figure 16–22
Hirschsprung's disease: lateral view of a 2-month-old boy with Hirschsprung's disease. Note the relative narrowing of the distal colonic segment when compared with the normal sigmoid colon. This reversal of relative width of the rectum and sigmoid is diagnostic of Hirschsprung's disease. In very distal segment disease, this sign may be overlooked unless lateral views are obtained and the finding is specifically sought. In patients with aganglionosis proximal to the sigmoid colon, both the rectum and the sigmoid are narrowed. This infant demonstrates significant proximal obstruction as evidenced by small bowel dilatation.

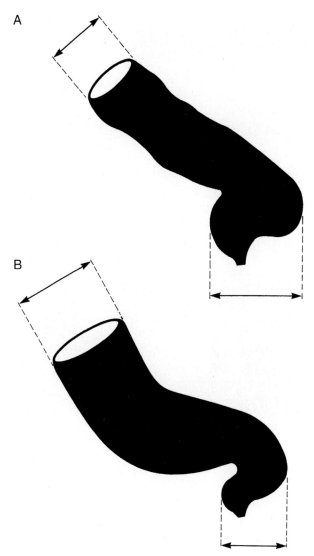

Figure 16–23
Rectosigmoid ratio: diagrammatic representation. *A,* The normal rectum is wider in caliber than the normal sigmoid colon. *B,* In aganglionosis distal to a normal sigmoid colon, the rectum is smaller in diameter than the sigmoid. This finding, which is occasionally overlooked, is important, because it may be the only clue to the diagnosis of Hirschsprung's disease in patients in whom the rectum has been distended and no spasm is evident. A clearly abnormal rectosigmoid ratio is virtually pathognomonic for distal aganglionosis.

Another complication (4%) of Hirschsprung's disease is perforation of the large bowel, most commonly the proximal colon (68%) or the appendix (17%). This complication is most commonly associated (62%) with total aganglionosis and generally occurs by 4 months of age.[22] At the time of perforation, the neonate may have no other findings of aganglionosis, and thus the true diagnosis may not be considered. Unexplained perforation of the colon or appendix is another indication for biopsy to exclude Hirschsprung's disease.[23]

Children Children with aganglionosis usually present by 2 or 3 years of age. Occasionally, however, the diagnosis

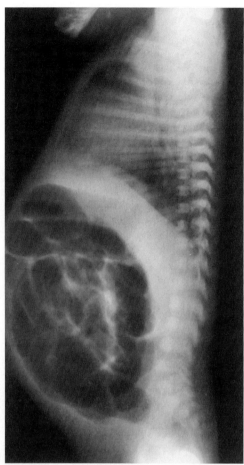

Figure 16–24
Hirschsprung's disease. A clear demonstration of the rectosigmoid ratio in Hirschsprung's disease is seen in this lateral view.

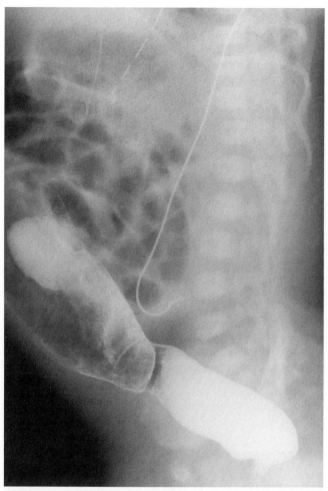

Figure 16–25
Hirschsprung's disease. A lateral view demonstrates the transition zone and the rectosigmoid ratio. The rectum is smaller than the sigmoid colon.

is not made until the late teenage years or even adulthood. Lethal complications of perforation and enterocolitis are rare in young children. Symptoms are chronic (lifelong) constipation, abdominal enlargement with prominent veins and visible peristalsis, intermittent bouts of intestinal obstruction due to fecal impaction, ribbon-like stools, failure to thrive, anemia, and sometimes hypoproteinemia. Rarely, a patient may present with a fecaloma. Fecal soiling is conspicuously but not invariably absent. Rectal examination usually reveals an anal canal and rectum devoid of stool. Spasm of the rectum may be felt compressing the examining finger, or the rectum may be perceived as narrow and tight (Fig. 16–36).

In summary, the majority (80%) of children with Hirschsprung's disease initially present as neonates, with signs of a distal bowel obstruction. A high incidence of complications, especially lethal enterocolitis and perforation, makes prompt diagnosis in this age group mandatory. Beyond infancy, the presenting symptoms predominantly relate to constipation and malnutrition.

Radiographic Evaluation

In Hirschsprung's disease, the role of the radiologist is to confirm the diagnosis, determine the length of the aganglionic segment for subsequent surgical treatment, and exclude other causes of obstruction.[16,38] Because aganglionosis accounts for one third of all neonatal bowel obstructions, the exclusion of Hirschsprung's disease is a relatively common procedure. Contrast enema examination for this disease is one of the few pediatric radiology emergencies, because affected infants may develop the potentially lethal complication of fulminant enterocolitis within 24 hours. Once aganglionosis is suspected, no delay in diagnosis or treatment (usually diverting colostomy) is safe (Fig. 16–37).

Radiographic evaluation consists of plain films, which are necessary to exclude perforation and other diagnoses such as necrotizing enterocolitis stenoses and atresias, and a contrast

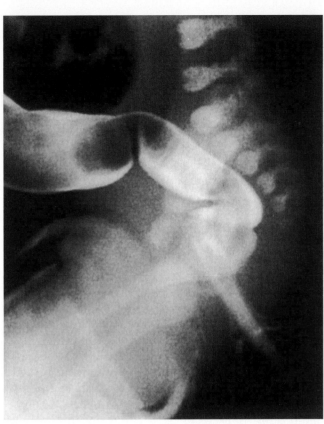

Figure 16–26
Hirschsprung's disease. Another example of a transition zone. The rectum is narrower than the sigmoid colon. Most transition zones are located in the rectosigmoid region.

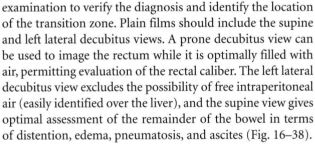

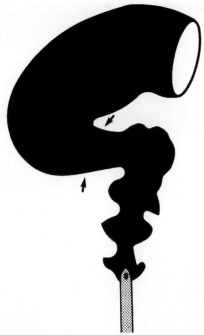

Figure 16–27
Transition zone and aganglionic spastic segment: diagrammatic representation. The transition zone is between the normal (proximal) and abnormal (distal) segments *(arrows)*. Spasm of the distal aganglionic portion accentuates visibility of the transition zone. The aganglionic segment is usually empty, whereas the ganglionic portion is filled with stool. Cleansing of the colon, thereby diminishing the width of the proximal dilated segment, decreases the visibility of the transition zone. The catheter is carefully placed distally in the colon so that the aganglionic segment is filled with contrast material.

examination to verify the diagnosis and identify the location of the transition zone. Plain films should include the supine and left lateral decubitus views. A prone decubitus view can be used to image the rectum while it is optimally filled with air, permitting evaluation of the rectal caliber. The left lateral decubitus view excludes the possibility of free intraperitoneal air (easily identified over the liver), and the supine view gives optimal assessment of the remainder of the bowel in terms of distention, edema, pneumatosis, and ascites (Fig. 16–38).

Contrast enema examination is contraindicated if plain films reveal pneumoperitoneum, pneumatosis, or the clearly abnormal mucosal pattern of enterocolitis. Administering an enema to a patient with active colitis may precipitate sepsis and secondary circulatory collapse. Known enterocolitis due to Hirschsprung's disease, with grossly evident abnormal mucosa (on plain films), is a relative contraindication to contrast examination of the colon; in such patients, an immediate suction biopsy is a safer method of establishing the diagnosis. Supportive medical management along with diverting colostomy (usually done at the splenic flexure) probably offers the best chance for survival in severely ill neonates.

Bowel cleansing prior to contrast enema is contraindicated because it makes the transition zone less obvious and, more importantly, bowel evacuants may precipitate a fulminant colitis. The tendency of affected children to retain cleansing enemas may also cause serious electrolyte imbalance. Inadvertent lowering of body temperature is also a danger to the neonate, and to prevent loss of body heat, the mixture is heated to about 85°F by placing it in a water bath or sink. Heat lamps, radiant warmers, or other adequate methods are used to ensure that the infant's body temperature does not drop during the procedure. Plastic-tipped catheters and retention balloons are not used in infants because of the likelihood of rectal trauma in a spastic and narrowed rectum. Instead, a soft, red rubber catheter (No. 16 to 30 French) is used. To ensure that the tip is not placed proximal to the aganglionic segment, we tape an adhesive marker around the tubing approximately 2 cm from its tip. This marker also helps to create a seal when the buttocks are taped together with paper tape.

The examination is begun in the lateral projection to detect a distal transition zone. Contrast material is introduced slowly,

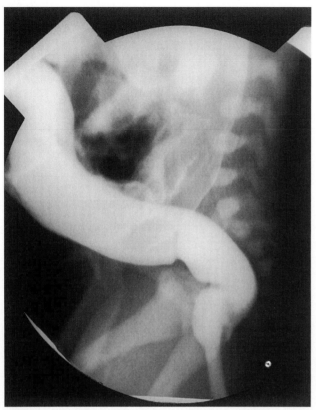

Figure 16–28

Hirschsprung's disease. In this infant the findings are less pronounced than in the previous examples. The diagnosis of Hirschsprung's disease can be confirmed and the transition zone identified.

either by gravity or by using a large syringe, to best demonstrate denervation hyperspasticity. The rate of filling is carefully controlled; no more than 5 mL of contrast are introduced incrementally. Then time is allowed for equilibration of intracolonic pressure. Multiple initial spot films are done in the lateral position, which delineates the distal rectum to best advantage. It is possible to dilate the aganglionic distal segment to a normal caliber, and if films are taken while the bowel is distended, the diagnosis may be missed. Typically, radiologists are trained to obtain spot films of the bowel during maximum distention to avoid false-positive diagnoses of bowel strictures or cancer. Hirschsprung's disease is a notable exception to this rule, because documentation of spasm during the unfilled state confirms the diagnosis. This denervation hyperspasticity is often an intermittent occurrence and may be accentuated with inflammation resulting from colitis (Fig. 16–39).

The colon is slowly filled until the transition between the aganglionic and normal colon is encountered, most commonly in the rectosigmoid region. In neonates, hypertrophy and dilatation of the proximal segment have not developed as yet, but a transition zone is still visible most of the time as a change in caliber between the spastic and normal bowel. When the transition zone has been identified, the proximal colon does not need to be examined because no additional information is likely to be obtained and because the predictably poor emptying will leave a colon needlessly filled

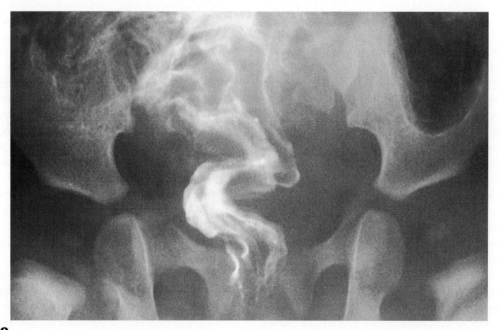

Figure 16–29

Hirschsprung's disease: delayed frontal view. A 24-hour delayed view in a 4-month-old male infant with aganglionosis demonstrates a spastic rectal segment that was not recognized previously on the barium enema examination. It is helpful to obtain delayed films in patients with negative or equivocal barium enema findings and in whom the clinical suspicion is low. In patients with a high index of clinical suspicion, we do not delay suction biopsy while waiting for 24- or 48-hour delayed films. If the barium enema is inconclusive, a suction biopsy is done immediately, as life-threatening colitis may supervene before 24 hours have passed. Delayed films are especially helpful in patients whose aganglionosis was not appreciated fluoroscopically and who did not evacuate. In this group, delayed films often demonstrate the empty, narrowed aganglionic segment.

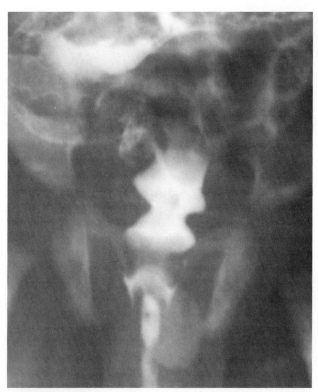

Figure 16–30
Denervation spasticity in Hirschsprung's disease. Note the typical sawtooth appearance of the aganglionic segment as the bowel displays spasticity. This finding is demonstrated to best advantage by introducing the contrast material as distally and as slowly as possible. Maximal control is obtained by using a syringe to inject the contrast material very gradually. Rapid distention of the colon may dilate the spastic segment and make it appear deceptively normal.

with contrast, which may complicate the procedure for the surgeon performing a diverting colostomy.

If initial films of the colon show no spastic segments or transition zone, delayed lateral and frontal views at 24 or 48 hours may reveal the transition zone. Delayed films in Hirschsprung's disease often show the barium to be mixed with feces and sometimes even to be refluxed into the small bowel. Little, if any, contrast is effectively propelled distally in a bolus. If the infant is ill, however, waiting for delayed films may be hazardous; we usually perform a suction biopsy as soon as an enema is judged to provide inconclusive results.

In summary, the contrast enema examination is diagnostic if a spastic distal segment is revealed or if a transition zone is identified. Rapid overdistention of the colon with barium is the most common reason for missing both the spasm and the transition zone. Delayed films may be diagnostic if results of the initial examination are normal or inconclusive by demonstrating a transition zone and barium mixed with stool.

Radiographic Findings

Plain films are helpful in neonatal Hirschsprung's disease because they frequently suggest the diagnosis by revealing a distal small bowel obstruction.[6] Furthermore, plain film evidence of colitis indicates that biopsy may be a safer diagnostic tool than a barium enema. Finally, in older children, plain films often suggest the diagnosis by showing a large amount of colonic stool when there is an empty rectal vault.

The important plain film findings in Hirschsprung's disease are the following:

Obstructive findings:
1. Dilatation of the entire small bowel.
2. Air-fluid levels on decubitus examination.
3. No evidence of air in the rectum.

Signs of enterocolitis:
1. Pneumatosis cystoides intestinalis.
2. Edematous or irregular mucosa in dilated bowel. Thick, edematous mucosa outlined by air is most often seen in the transverse colon because this structure is usually filled with air when the patient is in the supine position. A very similar pattern of mucosal edema and dilatation of the bowel is present in adults with acute megacolon caused by ulcerative colitis.

Findings in older children with constipation:
1. Dilatation of feces-filled colon distal to the rectum.
2. Empty rectal vault.

The important findings of barium enema examination with Hirschsprung's disease are as follows:

1. Denervation hyperspasticity (narrowing) of the distal segment, a highly specific fluoroscopic finding. Spot films show a spastic or "sawtooth" configuration.
2. A transition zone, or an abrupt change in bowel width between the spastic segment and the innervated portion that has dilated from obstruction.
3. Decreased rectosigmoid ratio.[29] In aganglionosis, the rectum is smaller than the dilated sigmoid, whereas normally the reverse is true. This sign is valid when aganglionosis does not involve the sigmoid colon. We have found this to be an exceedingly reliable sign, especially in infants, in whom a definite transition zone may be absent.
4. Work hypertrophy ("jejunization"). In a child older than 3 months, the proximal colon develops hypertrophy of the circular and longitudinal muscle fibers in response to the obstruction of the aganglionic segment. This causes a prominence of the muscle fibers that radiographically resembles the plicae circulares of the jejunum. This jejunization is a useful supportive sign of aganglionosis.
5. Delayed and disordered evacuation. The normal colon propels the barium distally in a single, continuous bolus. In aganglionosis, the barium is interspersed with feces and, instead of being propelled distally, often appears proximal to its location of 24 or 48 hours previously.

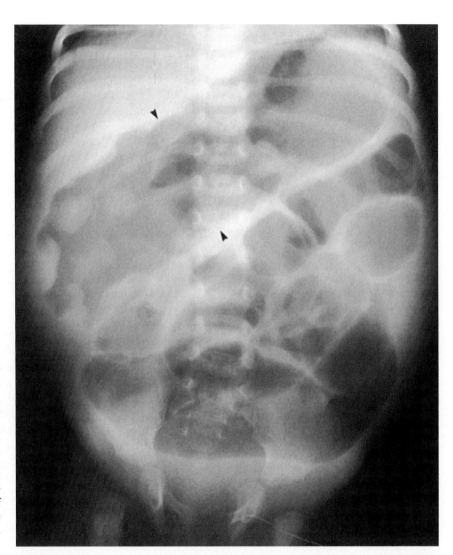

Figure 16–31

Enterocolitis secondary to Hirschsprung's disease. This 3-week-old boy had severe diarrhea, sepsis, and an abnormal stooling history suggestive of Hirschsprung's disease. The supine plain film shows clear evidence of colitis. The transverse colon *(arrowheads)* is markedly dilated and has multiple nodules seen in tangent and en face. Small bowel dilatation is evident, as is the absence of rectal gas. If Hirschsprung's disease is likely, as judged by historical factors, then suction biopsy and immediate decompression offer these critically ill children the best chance of survival. A contrast enema may precipitate sepsis or circulatory collapse. This infant did not survive.

This reverse propulsion is especially pronounced in total colonic aganglionosis, in which retrograde filling of the small bowel is common.

6. Bowel shortening. One manifestation of aganglionosis is loss of the redundancy of the sigmoid colon that is seen in normal infants. This shortening becomes more pronounced in total aganglionosis.[3] The colon has been described as resembling a question mark.

7. Meconium plug. Meconium plug and Hirschsprung's disease coexist in 10% to 30% of patients. Frequently, a meconium plug is assumed to be the sole cause of a neonatal obstruction, and the diagnosis of Hirschsprung's disease is missed. In this setting, it is important that the clinician not overlook the radiographic and clinical findings of aganglionosis.

The advent of suction biopsy of the rectum has simplified the diagnosis of Hirschsprung's disease and has shifted the main role of the contrast enema to defining the transition zone when surgical intervention is planned. Suction biopsy is an easily performed bedside procedure that does not require general anesthesia, and the results are highly reliable. It is most useful for excluding the diagnosis in patients whose radiographic findings are questionable and for diagnostic verification prior to surgical intervention. Contrast enema examination should precede suction biopsy. Because the depth of tissue is removed during biopsy is variable, it cannot be predicted whether the potentially high pressures generated during an enema might produce perforation at the biopsy site. In patients in whom suction biopsy was the initial mode of diagnosis and a contrast enema examination is needed to evaluate the length of the aganglionic segment, it is safest to wait 1 week to ensure healing of the biopsy site, if possible.

With experienced personnel, rectal manometry has also proved helpful in the diagnosis of Hirschsprung's disease. Reflex relaxation of the internal rectal sphincter follows distention of the rectum by a balloon in normal individuals

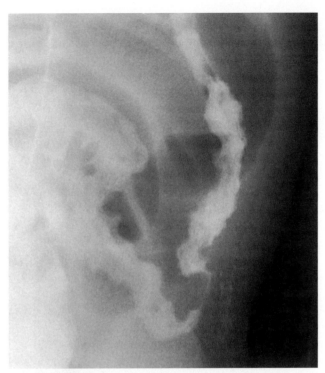

Figure 16–32

Hirschsprung's disease with superimposed colitis. Residual colonic contrast material is present in this male infant with proven distal segment Hirschsprung's disease. The proximal left colon demonstrates marked mucosal irregularities indicative of colitis. Proximal small bowel dilatation due to functional obstruction is also evident.

but does not occur in individuals who have aganglionosis. Rectal manometry may be superior to contrast examination in patients in whom the aganglionic segment is very short, although the existence of true short-segment Hirschsprung's disease remains controversial. The use of rectal manometry is limited to term infants because normal, reflex relaxation of the internal sphincter does not occur in premature infants whose maturational age is less than 39 weeks or who weigh less than 6 lb (2.7 kg).

When a contrast study cannot be done and immediate colostomy is required because of the patient's poor clinical condition, splenic flexure colostomy is adequate for 85% of patients. Rectal tube decompression is useful as a temporizing measure until colostomy is performed. At the time of operation, frozen section will verify the presence or absence of ganglion cells.

Summary

Occasionally Hirschsprung's disease remains undiagnosed. Failure to consider the diagnosis is probably the most frequent error. This is especially true when the presenting symptoms are atypical (e.g., fever of unknown origin, diarrhea, failure to thrive, or fecal soiling). Fecal soiling, although very unusual in aganglionosis, does not exclude the presence of

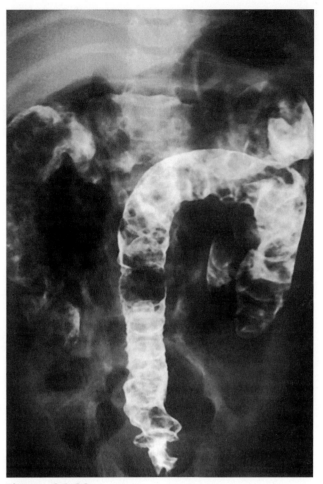

Figure 16–33

Colonic shortening. Another child with total colonic aganglionosis whose contrast enema demonstrates more pronounced colonic shortening than the patient in Figure 16–38. Note that the normal redundancy of the sigmoid colon is absent. The overall shape of the colon has been likened to that of a question mark.

Hirschsprung's disease with certainty. The same is true with prematurity, a setting that is also distinctly unusual but should not lead the clinician away from the diagnosis if there are suggestive clinical signs. In premature infants with Hirschsprung's disease, symptoms abate with cessation of oral feedings, only to return with resumption of oral intake. An awareness of the association of Hirschsprung's disease with Down syndrome and its familial tendency is also helpful.

Common pitfalls in radiologic diagnosis of Hirschsprung's disease include (1) too-rapid distention of the aganglionic segment with contrast material, (2) failure to recognize spasm in the aganglionic segment when the spasm subsides after slow filling of the colon, (3) failure to examine the rectum in the lateral position during fluoroscopy or with overhead films, and (4) a lack of awareness that Hirschsprung's disease and meconium plug syndrome often coexist. Recognition of a meconium plug should lead the clinician to carefully

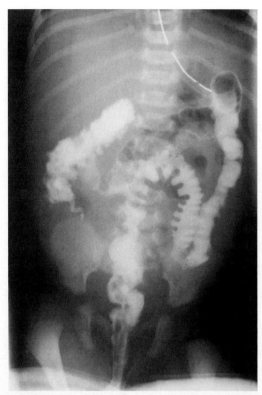

Figure 16–34
Total aganglionosis. Note the shortening of the entire colon and diffuse spasm. The rectum and sigmoid colon follow a straight, vertical line. Spasms are best seen in the appendix.

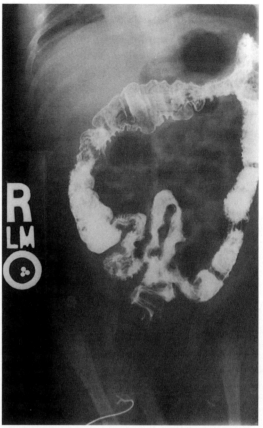

Figure 16–35
Acute enteric infection in the neonate. Bacterial colitis is manifested with spasm and mucosal edema. The infant had minimal bloody stools. Note that the colon was normal in length.

examine the colon for concomitant signs of Hirschsprung's disease.

Hirschsprung's disease is a common cause of bowel obstruction in the neonate and causes constipation when it remains unrecognized. Prompt, accurate diagnosis is important, as it will alleviate symptoms and may be lifesaving when the disease is recognized and treated before enterocolitis supervenes.

PSYCHOGENIC MEGACOLON

Psychogenic megacolon (also known as *idiopathic megacolon* and *psychogenic constipation*) is the most common cause of severe constipation in childhood. Most cases are easily diagnosed by obtaining a patient history and performing a physical examination. Diagnostic maneuvers are usually not required in straightforward cases. Prompt and adequate response to treatment serves as convincing proof that the diagnosis of psychogenic megacolon was correct.

Generally speaking, radiographic evaluation is sought when failure of therapy or atypical features suggest another diagnosis. The differential diagnostic possibilities are few, with the most prominent being Hirschsprung's disease in older children. In the following section, the problem of establishing

the diagnosis of psychogenic megacolon, which is essentially a process of exclusion, is discussed (Figs. 16–40 through 16–44).

Anatomy and Pathophysiology

The development of psychogenic megacolon may be initiated by several predisposing factors, including a low-roughage diet, familial tendency, gastroenteritis causing dehydration, fear of the toilet, anorectal disease, and unrealistically early or punitive toilet training. There are many variations in abnormal parent-child interactions. A common parent-child history, however, is that stress between the young child and a coercive parent results in "holding back" stool to gain parental approval. Withholding stool may also be a learned response associated with previous painful stooling from a rectal tear or fissure. This often initiates a vicious cycle that compounds the problem of painful stooling and consciously withholding stool. Whatever the primary cause of withholding stool, the normal afferent sensations that signal the urge to defecate diminish with progression of the disease until the child no longer perceives the need to stool. The colon propels fecal material normally and effectively to the rectum, where it

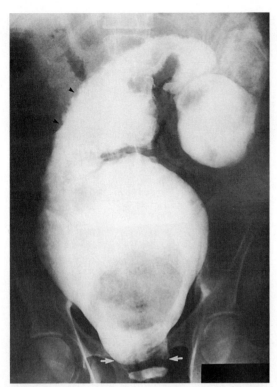

Figure 16–36

Hirschsprung's disease. This 23-year-old man had been constipated since birth and had been erroneously diagnosed as having functional constipation. A contrast enema revealed a dilated proximal segment and a narrowed distal (aganglionic) colon. *White arrows* indicate the approximate transition zone. Note that the proximal colon demonstrates irregular mucosal markings *(black arrows)* consistent with superimposed colitis, which was verified endoscopically at the time of suction biopsy. In the majority of patients, Hirschsprung's disease is diagnosed in the neonatal period, but occasionally the diagnosis is delayed until several years of age or even adulthood.

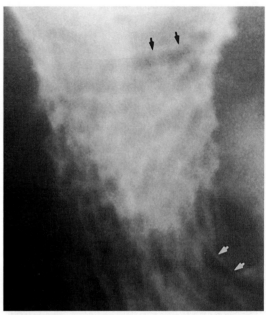

Figure 16–37

Work hypertrophy: close-up view of the proximal sigmoid in a 6-month-old boy with constipation. Note the prominent circular ridges *(black arrows)* and longitudinal ridges *(white arrows)*. Longitudinal and circular muscle hypertrophy produces prominence of these muscles, which is a useful supportive sign of aganglionosis. Work hypertrophy is usually not present until several months of age and represents a physiologic adaptation of the proximal normal colon to overcome the obstruction resulting from Hirschsprung's disease. The orderly and symmetric pattern of muscle hypertrophy should be distinguished from the irregular pattern of mucosal edema due to superimposed colitis.

collects and causes distention. The puborectal sling becomes relaxed, and the normal length of the anal canal is reduced to the skin-lined anus. The external sphincter alone cannot retain all the feces; thus, it permits intermittent or constant leakage of liquid stool around the large fecal mass (encopresis). Fecal soiling may cause the child to be ostracized by friends and playmates and thus may retard normal social development.

Clinical Presentation

The typical age of onset of psychogenic constipation coincides with or slightly precedes the time of toilet training. The two most common presenting symptoms are constipation and fecal incontinence, which is sometimes perceived as diarrhea. This "diarrhea" is actually liquid stool that leaks around the fecal impaction, unretained by an incompetent anal sphincter.

A thorough history of normal stooling habits during the neonatal period and early infancy is important in making

the diagnosis of psychogenic constipation. Boys are more commonly affected (80% of cases) than girls.

Physical examination reveals a normally developed child without abdominal distention. Fecal material can be palpated through the abdominal wall, and rectal examination reveals a rectal ampulla filled with hard stool. The anal canal is markedly shortened, and there is minimal sphincter tone. When children with psychogenic megacolon do evacuate, they may have antecedent colicky abdominal pain. In contradistinction to the thin, ribbonlike stools of Hirschsprung's disease, stools in this condition are huge and voluminous. Failure to thrive is so uncommon in this disease that its presence should encourage the clinician to exclude psychogenic megacolon as a diagnostic possibility.

Parental concern is often more vocal and intense than that of the patient, who commonly is withdrawn and tries to hide the fecal soiling. Patient prognosis is uniformly good, and symptoms rarely persist beyond the second decade of life.

Radiographic Evaluation

As previously mentioned, the confirmation of psychogenic constipation is centered on excluding the presence of

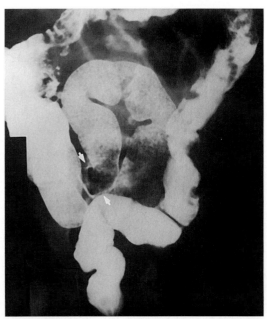

Figure 16–38
Abnormal evacuation: a 24-hour delayed film in a 2-month-old girl who presented with a history of abnormal stooling since birth. Results of the contrast enema were judged to be normal, but this 24-hour postevacuation film demonstrates reflux into the small bowel that was not present during the initial examination. The barium is well mixed with stool in the distal terminal ileum (*arrows*) and dilated small bowel. Reverse propulsion is a common finding, but one that is quite pronounced in total aganglionosis. In retrospect, the colon, although not demonstrating spasm, is abnormally short in this patient with total colonic aganglionosis.

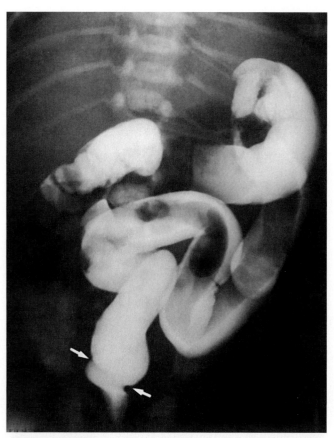

Figure 16–39
Meconium plug with Hirschsprung's disease. This term male infant presented with abdominal distention and failure to pass meconium at 24 hours of life. Note the cast of meconium within the contrast column. Distal colonic narrowing exists, representing distal segment aganglionosis (*arrows*). All patients with meconium plug syndrome deserve a careful and critical examination of the distal colon to exclude the possibility of Hirschsprung's disease.

aganglionosis, postsurgical rectal stenosis, obstructing pelvic masses, neurogenic causes, and rare cases of hypothyroidism.

Three clinical parameters that are very important in confirming the diagnosis include a history of normal stooling early in life, evidence of a dilated, feces-filled rectum, and response to treatment. The radiologist becomes involved only if the history, physical examination, or both are suggestive of aganglionosis or if therapy is not effective in relieving the constipation.

If the patient has a great deal of fecal material in the rectal vault on plain films, contrast enema examination will rarely give additional information that is helpful in distinguishing Hirschsprung's disease from psychogenic megacolon. A suction biopsy of the rectum is the diagnostic modality of choice in this situation.

Radiographic Findings

The important radiographic findings in psychogenic megacolon are as follows:

1. Absence of previously described radiographic findings of Hirschsprung's disease.
2. Normal lumbosacral spine.
3. Absence of an extrinsic mass pressing on the rectum.
4. Dilatation of the rectum and sigmoid colon to form a pear-shaped chamber that extends from the anal canal vertically out of the pelvis. The proximal colon is normal.
5. Mild dilatation of the entire colon, with feces from the anal canal to the level of the ascending colon

In summary, the patient history and physical examination are usually typical and permit ready diagnosis of psychogenic megacolon. Plain films show variable fecal distention of the rectum, with stool extending to the anal canal. Usually, additional investigation is carried out only when the condition is atypical or unresponsive to conventional medical management.

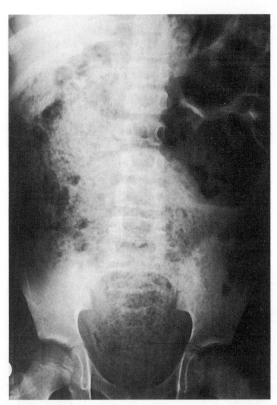

Figure 16–40
Psychogenic constipation: plain film of a 7-year-old boy with severe constipation. Note the massively distended rectosigmoid colon and rectum. On plain films, a contrast enema will yield no additional information. This patient responded to conservative medical management.

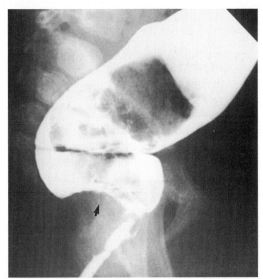

Figure 16–41
Psychogenic constipation: lateral rectum. This radiograph of a 4-year-old boy with encopresis demonstrates a normal rectal caliber with a posterior indentation secondary to the puborectal sling *(arrow)*. The puborectal sling in this patient is normal and does not demonstrate relaxation, as is often seen in patients with severe psychogenic constipation.

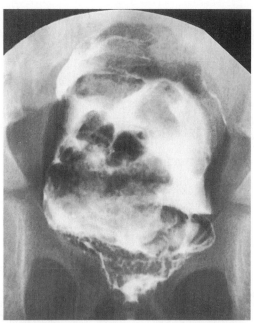

Figure 16–42
Psychogenic constipation: frontal view of a 6-year-old boy, demonstrating the typical radiographic findings of psychogenic constipation. Dilatation of the colon and fecal residue extend all the way to the anus. Physical examination revealed a rectal ampulla full of stool.

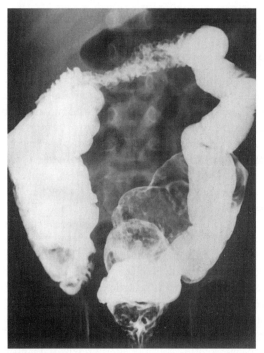

Figure 16–43
Psychogenic constipation: frontal view. In this 5-year-old boy, a feces-filled colon is seen extending out of the pelvis to involve the entire rectosigmoid colon. The contrast enema revealed no evidence of Hirschsprung's disease.

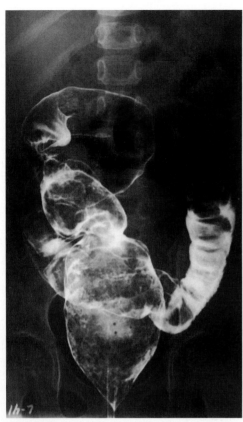

Figure 16–44
Psychogenic constipation: Contrast enema reveals stool only in the rectal vault.

Other Causes of Constipation

The conditions that follow are rare causes of constipation. Fortunately, all are treatable and readily diagnosed if they are considered.

Segmental Dilatation of the Colon

Segmental dilatation of the colon is a rare entity of unknown etiology in which a portion of the colon is markedly dilated and aperistaltic.[9,30] The site and extent of involvement are variable. The proximal and distal bowel segments are normal, without the spasticity and narrowing that accompanies Hirschsprung's disease. The muscular layers of the dilated segment are markedly hypertrophied, although normal ganglion cells are seen in the entire colon.

Symptoms of this disorder mainly include failure to thrive, abdominal distention, and severe constipation commencing at birth. Infants with this disease are almost always brought to medical attention because they present with profound symptoms early in life.

The diagnosis is made by barium enema examination, which reveals persistent dilatation of a segment of the colon (Fig. 16–45). A suction biopsy, if performed, reveals normal

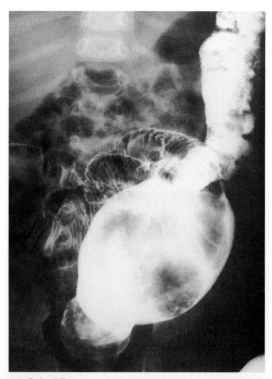

Figure 16–45
Segmental dilatation of the colon in a 2-month-old girl with severe constipation. A contrast enema demonstrates a well-defined portion of the colon, which is filled with feces and dilated. The remainder of the colon, both distally and proximally, was normal. Pathologically, the muscular layers of the dilated segment are markedly hypertrophied. Ganglion cells were identified in the dilated portion as well as distally. This disease entity is a rare cause of unremitting constipation commencing at the time of birth.

ganglion cells. The proximal and distal colon segments function normally after the dilated obstructive portion has been removed. With relief of chronic constipation, the child begins to thrive normally.

Occult Spinal Dysraphism

Occult spinal dysraphism is a general term for unrecognized spinal defects that insidiously cause progressive neurologic defects that variably affect the bladder and lower extremities. Although signs of neurogenic bladder and lower extremity muscle atrophy are the most common presenting features, some children may present with constipation as a primary symptom.

Local intraspinal masses may gradually compress the cord or cauda equina as they grow within the rigid confines of the bony spinal canal. Intraspinal masses may also cause traction on nerve roots or create local nerve ischemia. Less commonly, the normal cephalic migration of the spinal cord is restricted by an underlying malformation (tethered cord[12] and diastematomyelia[15]). This failure of migration leads to progressive deficits as traction on the cord and nerve roots

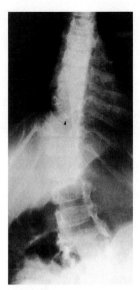

Figure 16–46

Occult spinal dysraphism. This 8-year-old patient was known to have congenital scoliosis caused by multiple congenital vertebral abnormalities involving the lower thoracic spine. Constipation and recurrent urinary tract infection were prominent symptoms. The plain film demonstrates a bony spur overlying the body of the tenth thoracic vertebra. The spur of diastematomyelia is sometimes cartilaginous instead of ossified, as in this patient. Insidious, progressive neurologic symptoms are clinical hallmarks of diastematomyelia.

becomes increasingly pronounced. Loss of normal innervation to the colon results in decreased peristalsis and loss of the incompletely understood "urge to defecate" (Fig. 16–46).

A complete physical examination will often reveal neurologic abnormalities. Additional findings include muscle wasting of the lower extremity; pes cavus; talipes equinovarus; and

signs of neurogenic bladder, such as incontinence or recurrent urinary tract infections. Half of the patients who have occult spinal dysraphism also have spinal cutaneous abnormalities such as lipomas, hypertrichosis, dimples, nevi, hemangiomas, hypopigmented patches, asymmetric gluteal folds, or a rudimentary tail.

Radiographic evaluation is important in children with these abnormalities, because many of the plain film findings reveal spinal dysraphism on the abdominal film. If feces obscure the sacrum, lateral plain films are required. Barium enema examination, if performed, usually reveals normal findings except for increased fecal residue.

Plain film findings include failure of fusion of the posterior neural arches above L5 in an older child, widened interpedicular distance, erosion of the medial margins of the pedicles, a midline bony spur, absence of one or all sacral segments, or a scalloped lateral defect in the lower sacral segments ("scimitar sign"). In children younger than 5 years of age, the neural arches of the sacrum of L5 are so commonly unfused that no significance can be attached to this observation when it is the sole plain film abnormality. Precise preoperative evaluation of the type and extent of the spinal lesion is best performed using magnetic resonance imaging (MRI). Ultrasound is the examination of choice in the neonate.

Pelvic Masses

Constipation in children is sometimes caused by a pelvic mass that compresses the distal colon or rectum. If a pelvic mass is suspected, abdominal sonography is the study of choice followed by computed tomography or MRI (Figs. 16–47, 16–48, and 16–49).

The following mass lesions may cause rectal compression and resultant constipation: cul-de-sac abscess due to perforative appendicitis, sacrococcygeal teratoma hydrometrocolpos,

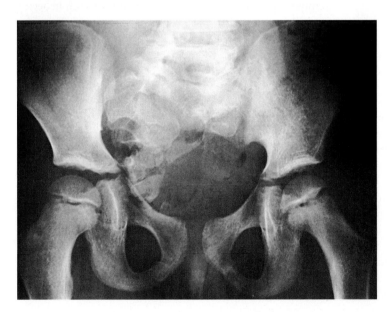

Figure 16–47

Anterior sacral meningocele. This 6-year-old boy presented with constipation and a pelvic mass. Note the abnormal, bowed sacrum. This characteristic anomaly has been termed the *scimitar sign* and is most often associated with an anterior meningocele.

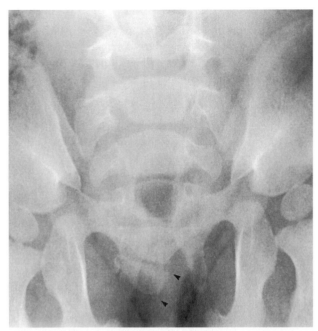

Figure 16–48
Sacrococcygeal teratoma: plain film of a 3-year-old girl with a pelvic mass and constipation. The lower sacrum is abnormally deviated *(arrowheads)*.

partial duplication of the distal colon, sarcomas of the pelvis, or anterior meningocele.[1,25]

Hypothyroidism

Hypothyroidism is a rare cause of stooling difficulties in infants and young children. The diagnosis is an important one to exclude, because adequate levels of thyroid hormone are necessary for normal cerebral development in the first year of life. Thus, the diagnosis must be made early so that treatment can be instituted to minimize the accompanying irreversible brain damage. Screening for neonatal hypothyroidism is routinely performed in many nurseries, but this practice is not universal.

The clinical findings in congenital hypothyroidism usually include high birth weight; feeding difficulties; noisy respiration; nasal obstruction; a large tongue; somnolence; sluggishness while awake; a large abdomen, frequently with umbilical hernia; heart murmurs with cardiomegaly; constipation; and anemia. Both constipation and anemia are refractory to symptomatic treatment and transfusion. The barium enema examination reveals a normal colon in these patients; however, the following radiographic findings should alert the radiologist to the true diagnosis:

1. Delayed bone age. The capital femoral epiphysis normally ossifies between 3 and 6 months of age. Its absence in a constipated child who is older than

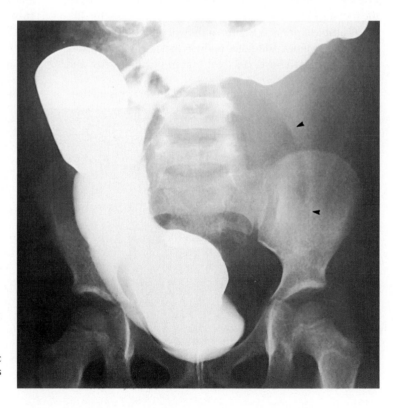

Figure 16–49
Lipomeningocele. This 4-year-old girl presented with a pelvic mass and mild constipation. Note the large, lucent mass *(arrowheads)* displacing the entire colon.

6 months is significant. Additional bone age markers in the neonate are distal femoral epiphysis at 36 to 38 weeks' gestational age and proximal tibial epiphysis at 38 to 40 weeks' gestational age.

2. Rounded vertebral bodies. Vertebral bodies appear rounded instead of rectangular, especially in the thoracolumbar region. This finding is present in newborns and becomes more pronounced with advancing age.

3. Cardiomegaly. Occasionally, this is erroneously thought to reflect congenital heart disease.

4. Large fontanelles, prominent, wide sutures, and a rounded, enlarged sella turcica revealed on skull films. Wormian bones are commonly but not invariably present.

In summary, hypothyroidism is an exceedingly rare cause of constipation. It is essential to diagnose the condition in infancy, because prompt therapy with thyroid hormone can prevent mental retardation and relieve all symptoms that develop in untreated conditions.

SUMMARY

Constipation is a common complaint that only rarely is symptomatic of significant disease. The aim of diagnosis is to excluding a few treatable causes, the most important of which is Hirschsprung's disease. Aganglionosis, if unrecognized, can cause severe growth retardation, chronic constipation, and death from superimposed enterocolitis. Because of the unpredictable and lethal complication of enterocolitis, we have tried to emphasize the urgency of correctly identifying Hirschsprung's disease.

Psychogenic constipation, a far more common cause of stooling difficulties, rarely requires radiologic investigation because the diagnosis is established clinically. Additional diagnostic maneuvers are indicated only if therapy is ineffective or if the patient's history, physical examination, or both suggest Hirschsprung's disease.

Neurogenic causes, pelvic masses, hypothyroidism, and the rare entity of segmental dilatation of the colon have been included in our discussion because the radiographs may contain the first clue that these diseases are the cause of constipation.

REFERENCES

1. Anderson FM, Burke BL. Anterior sacral meningocele. JAMA 237:39–42, 1977.
2. Berdon WE, Baker DH. Roentgenographic diagnosis of Hirschsprung's disease in infancy. AJR Am J Roentgenol Am J Roentgenol 93:432–446, 1965.
3. Berdon WE, Koontz P, Baker DH. Diagnosis of colonic and terminal ileal aganglionosis. AJR Am J Roentgenol 91:680–689, 1964.
4. Bradley MJ, Pilling D. The empty rectum on plain x-ray. Does it have any significance in the neonate? Clin Radiol 43:265–267, 1991.
5. Clayden GS, Lawson J. Investigation and management of long standing chronic constipation in childhood. Arch Dis Child 51:918–923, 1976.
6. Davis WS, Allen RP. Conditioning value of plain film examination in the diagnosis of neonatal Hirschsprung's disease. Radiology 93:129–133, 1969.
7. Davis WS, Allen RP, Favera BE, Slovis TL. Neonatal small left colon syndrome. AJR Am J Roentgenol 120:322–329, 1974.
8. Davis WS, Campbell JB. Neonatal small left colon syndrome. AJR Am J Roentgenol 129:1024–1027, 1975.
9. DeLorimer AA, Benzian SR, Gooding CA. Segmental dilatation of the colon. AJR Am J Roentgenol 112:100–104, 1971.
10. Ehrenpreis T. Hirschsprung's Disease. Chicago: Year Book Medical, 1970.
11. Ellis DG, Clatworthy HW. The meconium plug revisited. J Pediatr Surg 1:54–61, 1966.
12. Fitz CR, Harwood-Nash DC. The tethered conus. AJR Am J Roentgenol 125:515–523, 1975.
13. Fleisher DR. Diagnosis and treatment of disorders of defecation in children. Pediatr Ann 5:700–722, 1976.
14. Foster P, Cowan G, Wrenn EL Jr. Twenty-five years' experience with Hirschsprung's disease. J Pediatr Surg 25:531–534, 1990.
15. Guthkelch AN. Diastematomyelia with median septum. Brain 97:729–742, 1974.
16. Hope JW, Borns PF, Berg PK. Roentgenologic manifestations of Hirschsprung's disease in infancy. AJR Am J Roentgenol 95:217–229, 1965.
17. James HE, Walsh JW. Spinal dysraphism. Curr Probl Pediatr 11:1–25, 1981.
18. Kilcoyne RF, Taybe H. Conditions associated with congenital megacolon. AJR Am J Roentgenol 108:615–620, 1970.
19. LeQuesne GW, Reilly BJ. Functional immaturity of the large bowel in the newborn infant. Radiol Clin North Am 13:331–342, 1975.
20. Martin LW, Perrin EV. Neonatal perforation of the appendix in association with Hirschsprung's disease. Ann Surg 166:799–802, 1967.
21. Mikity VG, Hodgman JE. Meconium blockage syndrome. Radiology 88:740–744, 1967.
22. Newman B, Nussbaum A, Kirkpatrick JA Jr. Bowel perforation in Hirschsprung's disease. AJR Am J Roentgenol 148:1195–1197, 1987.
23. Newman B, Nussbaum A, Kirkpatrick JA Jr, Coody A. Appendiceal perforation, pneumoperitoneum and Hirschsprung's disease. J Pediatr Surg 23:854–856, 1988.
24. Okamoto E, Takasi U. Embryogenesis of intramural ganglia of the gut and its relation to Hirschsprung's disease. J Pediatr Surg 2:437–443, 1967.
25. Oren M, Lorber B, Lee SH, Truex RC Jr, Gennaro AR. Anterior sacral meningocele. Dis Colon Rectum 20:492–505, 1977.
26. Peters ME, Li BU, Kalayoglu M. Giant colonic ulcers associated with Hirschsprung's. J Pediatr Gastroenterol Nutr 7:466–468, 1988.
27. Philippart AI, Reed JO, Georgeson KE. Neonatal small left colon syndrome: Intramural not intraluminal obstruction. J Pediatr Surg 10:733–740, 1975.
28. Pochaczevsky R, Leonidas JC. Meconium plug syndrome—Roentgenographic evaluation and differentiation from Hirschsprung's disease and other pathologic states. AJR Am J Roentgenol 120:342–352, 1974.
29. Pochaczevsky R, Leonidas JC. "The recto-sigmoid index"—A measurement for the early diagnosis of Hirschsprung's disease. AJR Am J Roentgenol 123:770–777, 1975.
30. Ratcliffe J, Tait J, Lisle D, Leditschke JF, Bell J. Segmental dilatation of the small bowel: Report of three cases and literature review. Radiology 171:827–830, 1989.
31. Rosenfield NS, Ablow RC, Markowitz RI, et al. Hirschsprung disease: Accuracy of the barium enema examination. Radiology 150:393–400, 1984.

32. Roshkow JE, Haller JO, Berdon WE, Sane SM. Hirschsprung's disease, Ondine's curse, and neuroblastoma-manifestations of neurocristopathy. Pediatr Radiol 19:45–49, 1988.

33. Siegel M, Shackelford GD, McAlister WH. Neonatal blockage in the ileum and proximal colon. Radiology 132:79–82, 1979.

34. Stewart DR. Neonatal small left colon syndrome. Ann Surg 186:741–745, 1977.

35. Suberman RI. Constipation in children. Pediatr Ann 5:32–48, 1976.

36. Swenson D, Rathauser F. Segmental dilatation of the colon: New entity. Am J Surg 97:734–738, 1959.

37. Swenson O, Sherman JO, Fisher JH. Diagnosis of congenital megacolon an analysis of 501 patients. J Pediatr Surg 8:587–593, 1973.

38. Taxman TL, Ylish BS, Rothstein FC. How useful is the barium enema in the diagnosis of infantile Hirschsprung's disease? Am J Dis Child 140:881–884, 1986.

39. Van Houtte JR, Katzman DO. Roentgenographic manifestations of immaturity of the intestinal neural plexus in premature infants. Radiology 106:363–367, 1973.

ADDITIONAL READING

Catto-Smith AG, Coffey CM, Nolan TM, Hutson JM. Fecal incontinence after the surgical treatment of Hirschsprung's disease. J Pediatr 127:954–957, 1995.

Coran A, Teitelbaum D. Recent advances in the management of Hirschsprung's disease. Am J Surg 180:382–387, 2000.

Cremin BJ. The early diagnosis of Hirschsprung's disease. Pediatr Radiol 2:23–28, 1974.

Diseth TH, Bjornland K, Novik TS, Emblem R. Bowel function, mental health, and psychosocial function in adolescents with Hirschsprung disease. Arch Dis Child 76:100–106, 1997

Fonkalsrud EW. Long-term results after colectomy and ileoanal pull-through procedure in children. Arch Surg 131:881–885; discussion 885–886, 1996.

Fotter R. Imaging of constipation in infants and children. Eur Radiol 8:248, 1982.

Haney PJ, Hill JL, Sun C-C. Zonal colonic aganglionosis. Pediatr Radiol 12:258–261, 1982.

O'Donovan AN, Habra G, Somers S, Malone DE, Rees A, Winthrop AL. Diagnosis of Hirschsprung's disease. AJR Am J Roentgenol Am J Roentgenol 167:517–520, 1996.

Roshkow JE, Haller JO, Berdon WE, Sane SM. Hirschsprung's disease, Ondine's curse, and neuroblastoma-manifestations of neurocrisopathy. Pediatr Radiol 19:45–49, 1988.

Skinner MA. Hirschsprung disease. Curr Probl Surg 33:389–460, 1996.

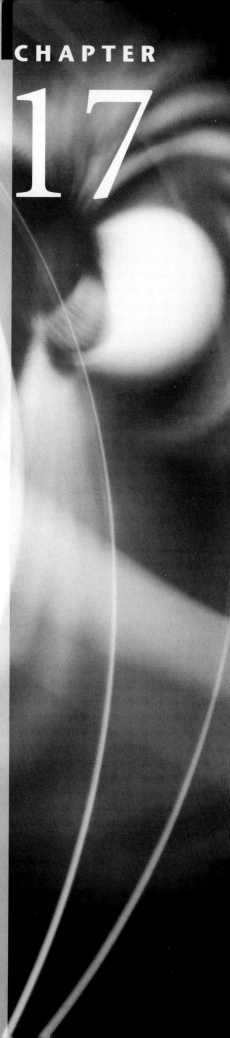

DIFFERENTIATING THE ACCIDENTALLY INJURED FROM THE PHYSICALLY ABUSED CHILD

Outline

Saskia von Waldenburg Hilton, MD

CHAPTER 17

DIFFERENTIATING THE ACCIDENTALLY INJURED FROM THE PHYSICALLY ABUSED CHILD

Although significant increases in survival rates have been achieved in premature infants, children with neoplasms, and those with congenital malformations, the incidence of accidental death in childhood remains essentially unchanged from year to year. Approximately one tenth of all emergency department admissions for children younger than 5 years are related to nonaccidental trauma. Conservative calculations indicated that approximately 250,000 children are physically abused each year and at least 2000 to 5000 of these die as a result of their injuries. Among survivors, irreversible brain damage of variable degree is common.

Distinguishing abuse from accidental trauma is possible most of the time with a relatively high degree of certainty. The distinction can be made by careful analysis of the imaging findings, the clinical picture, and a detailed history of the traumatic event. The intent of this chapter is to facilitate this task for physicians who care for infants and children. Accidental trauma is discussed only when it is likely to be mistaken for abuse. Selected medicolegal aspects of abuse, including physician testimony, are discussed in greater detail in Chapter 18. The imaging of accidental injuries, such as those sustained in motor vehicle accidents or other major nonintentional trauma, is described in Chapter 10.

Establishing and documenting the diagnosis of child abuse is important for both medical and legal reasons. Confirmation of the medical diagnosis establishes a cause for the illness and directs appropriate treatment for the child's presenting symptoms, as well as for occult injuries. In addition, the diagnosis of child abuse sometimes dramatically clarifies a constellation of puzzling symptoms, including partial blindness, seizures, hydrocephalus, unusual abdominal injuries, burns, and failure to thrive. Confirmation of abuse also initiates legal proceedings to remove the child and any siblings from a volatile and dangerous home environment until the abuser can be identified and the safety of the child's home guaranteed.

The radiologist often plays a major role in diagnosing child abuse. Radiographs with positive findings are legal documents that often reveal uncontestable evidence of battering. Although skeletal radiographs are used most commonly, any imaging modality that reveals lesions typical of abuse can be employed as legal evidence, including varied studies such as computed tomography (CT) or magnetic resonance (MR) images of typical brain injury, sonography of pancreatic pseudocyst, contrast examination of duodenal hematoma, and bone scans of multiple fractures.

Although the exact mechanism of many abuse injuries remains uncertain, a general understanding of the typical forces and methods of injury is helpful to diagnose abuse confidently. The most important factors are the patient's developmental stage and age. Thus, the significance of a spiral tibial fracture is quite different in a 2-month-old, nonambulating infant than in a 2-year-old toddler; in the absence of a convincing history, the infant is probably abused, whereas the 2-year-old has probably suffered an accidental toddler's fracture.

Familiarity with common and typical accidental injuries of childhood is also important to permit distinguishing accidental from nonaccidental trauma.[59] The dictum that high-quality pediatric radiology requires both close cooperation and communication with the pediatrician and detailed clinical information is doubly true when possible child abuse is encountered. Correlating the history of the accident with the severity and type of injury forms the basis for confident diagnosis of nonaccidental trauma.

This chapter is divided into three sections. In the first section, common accidental, iatrogenic, and nonaccidental injuries are discussed as they occur in patients of different ages up to 5 years. The second section outlines injuries that are common in childhood and should not suggest abuse; included are brief descriptions of birth injury and automobile trauma. The last section describes the diagnosis of nonaccidental trauma in detail. Although skeletal injury is emphasized, the cranial, abdominal, and cutaneous stigmata of abuse are also included. Neglect, emotional abuse, and sexual abuse, although ultimately much more damaging to the child than physical trauma, are beyond the scope of this textbook. An outstanding textbook by Kleinman is highly recommended for readers interested in the subject of physical abuse in greater detail.[41]

DIFFERENTIAL DIAGNOSIS OF TRAUMA ACCORDING TO AGE

The types of injuries that children incur are closely related to their developmental milestones, which depend on age. For simplicity, the relevant ages are divided into three groups: nonambulating children (birth to 10 months), toddlers (10 months to 3 years), and young children (3 to 5 years).

NONAMBULATING CHILDREN (BIRTH TO 10 MONTHS)

Statistics from the National Safety Council show that although accidents account for only 2% of all deaths during the first year of life, the total number of accidental deaths during this time is greater than that at any other age from 2 through 14 years. Included in this figure and decreasing in frequency are deaths from mechanical suffocation, motor vehicle accidents, fires, drowning, falls, and poisonings.[19] Whether some of these accidental deaths represent unrecognized child abuse or the first 12 months are simply a perilous time is uncertain.

The common causes of trauma during the first year of life can be grouped into birth trauma, accidental injury in the home, motor vehicle injury, and child abuse.

Birth trauma is usually a result of a difficult delivery and is more common in large or neurologically impaired infants. Skull injuries that result from birth trauma include fractures, cephalhematomas, and subdural hematomas from suction extractions. The three bones, other than the skull, that are most commonly fractured as a result of birth trauma are the clavicle, humerus, and femur. Callus formation at these fracture sites is usually visible by 5 to 11 days of age; this feature can be used to date the injury if abuse is questioned.[4]

Accidentally dropping an infant is the most common cause of trauma during infancy. Evaluation of emergency department visits revealed that falls were the leading cause of unintentional injury for children during the first year of life.[15] The falls commonly occur when an adult stumbles while carrying the child or when an infant seat falls from a countertop, table, or couch. Sometimes the infant is dropped when an unsupervised sibling attempts to play with or care for an infant. The resulting injuries consist mainly of soft tissue bruises, but occasionally the skull is fractured. In these accidents, there is almost always a plausible clinical history, as well as parental grief, concern, and guilt that are appropriate to the injury. Such injuries are rarely serious.

By contrast, motor vehicle trauma involving unrestrained infants is frequently fatal.[19] The infant's body tends to accelerate head first, with the brain incurring severe damage on impact. An infant held by a nonrestrained adult in an automobile passenger seat may be crushed between the dashboard and the adult's body. An infant seated on an adult's lap and included in the adult's seat belt may also be crushed by the adult's body. Such accidents are rarely diagnostically difficult, because documentation is readily available.[78]

An abused infant is often severely injured because of the small size of the body and the strength and violence of the adult abuser. Multiple metaphyseal fractures are common in this age group, because the abused infant is often severely shaken, and its extremities may be used as "handles" by which to grab the infant prior to throwing the child across a bed or room. Fractures of the femur and humerus also occur in child abuse at this age, often reflecting rotatory (twisting) forces applied to the extremities. Thoracic trauma is evident from multiple rib fractures and costochondral separations or costovertebral fracture, which usually result from compression of the thorax during shaking or from direct impact. Often multiple stages of healing are present, confirming the fact that multiple assaults occurred. Intracranial injury (hemorrhage, edema, and infarction) may be manifested by signs of increased intracranial pressure or seizures and is the most common cause of death in this age group.

TODDLERS (10 MONTHS TO 3 YEARS)

As infants learn to ambulate, they may injure themselves by bumping into household furniture such as coffee tables, television sets, and chairs. Soft tissue bruises and facial lacerations constitute most resulting injuries. Climbing becomes another favorite pastime as toddlers explore and expand their domain. Falls from couches, tables, and ladders ensue but rarely cause severe injuries. Some accidents are caused by toddlers ambulating with a walker. If fractures do occur, the midclavicle, distal radius, and skull are the most common sites. It has been my experience that cranial trauma accidentally incurred in a typical household bump or fall is usually clinically benign, even when a skull fracture is present.

If a toddler exerts a rotatory force on the tibia when jumping or falling with a foot caught between the bars of a playpen or crib, the resulting spiral fracture of the tibia may be confused with abuse. This typical "toddler's fracture" is described in greater detail in Chapter 20. The leading causes of accidental deaths that occur during the second year of life include motor vehicle accidents (33%), drowning (24%), fires (22%), falls (3%), and airway obstruction (1%).[19] An appropriate history is invariably available.

Abuse in toddlers occurs through several mechanisms, some of the more common of which are twisting of the extremities, slaps or punches to the head, and direct blows to the midabdomen. The head is often the focal point of parental blows, producing facial bruises and intracranial or ocular damage in the form of retinal hemorrhage and detachment. Superficial lacerations such as those that often result from accidental bumps and falls are uncommon in battered children. Cutaneous burn injuries of the extremities or the buttocks resulting from forceful immersion in hot water become more frequent.

YOUNG CHILDREN (3 TO 5 YEARS)

Normal 3- to 5-year-old children become increasingly adept at climbing and thus more apt to fall. They learn to run faster and begin to ride Big Wheels and tricycles. The ability to ride a bicycle, however, is not usually mastered by a 5-year-old child; bicycle riding becomes a major source of morbidity and, occasionally, mortality at 6 to 7 years of age. The enforcement of the use of helmets has decreased the number of injuries. Common accidental fractures in young children include distal radial torus fractures that result from the child attempting to break a fall with an outstretched hand. Clavicular and occasional skull fractures are seen from ordinary accidental falls.

The types of fractures produced by abuse are not markedly different in this age group from those in the toddler age group, but their incidence plummets as the child increases in age. In my experience, asymptomatic, unrecognized fractures are rare in patients older than 3 years of age. In a review of our patient population, skeletal surveys performed on children older than 3 years or on asymptomatic older siblings of abused children have yielded no useful clinical or legal information.[5]

ACCIDENTAL TRAUMA

This section discusses the mechanisms of injury and the radiographic findings in birth trauma and common accidental trauma, showing the consistent relationship between the mechanism of injury and the ensuing injury. The contrast between the radiographic findings of accidental and nonaccidental trauma is emphasized when it exists.

BIRTH TRAUMA

Birth trauma can mimic child abuse and may even be seen with cesarean sections.[16,38] Whenever abuse involves a neonate, the question of obstetric trauma arises, both in daily practice and in court. Skeletal trauma caused by birth injury and that caused by abuse are usually distinguishable by history alone and sometimes by the radiographic age of the injury. Other than the skull, the bones involved in birth injury, in decreasing order of frequency, are the clavicle, humerus, and femur (Fig. 17–1). Rib fractures are rare.[23]

An isolated midshaft fracture of the clavicle is the most common skeletal birth injury. Affected infants are usually large, and their delivery is often difficult. Usually, the fracture is recognized at or soon after delivery. The parents may seek medical advice when callus formation causes a palpable mass at about 1 month of age. In cases of abuse, the distal portion of the clavicle is fractured more commonly, as opposed to the midshaft fractures seen in obstetric trauma (Fig. 17–2). In birth fractures, callus formation is visible, depending on the quality of the radiograph, within 5 to 14 days of delivery and may be quite exuberant. Thus, in an infant older than 2 weeks of age whose fracture has no radiographically visible callus, the injury is clearly not a result of obstetric trauma.

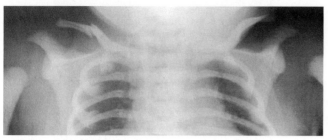

Figure 17–1
Acute clavicular fracture. This 3-kg infant of a diabetic mother whose delivery was difficult had a suspected right clavicular fracture. The radiograph confirms a right midshaft fracture. Such birth injuries are easily differentiated from abuse because they almost invariably constitute an isolated injury.

Additionally, an isolated clavicular fracture is rarely the sole fracture in abused infants.

Birth injury of the humerus may involve the diaphysis (midshaft) or may cause a fracture-separation of the distal or proximal epiphysis. Although the epiphyseal injury may be undetected, diaphyseal fractures usually are obvious clinically. A history of a difficult delivery and the presence of periosteal new bone is helpful in differentiating birth trauma from abuse.

Femoral fractures may occur during difficult breech extraction and may consist of a diaphyseal fracture or a fracture-separation of the distal epiphysis (Figs. 17–3 through 17–6). Proximal epiphyseal separations (i.e., of the unossified capital femoral epiphysis) are uncommon in both birth trauma and child abuse.

There is no question that femoral injuries from abuse can mimic those resulting from birth trauma. Furthermore, isolated long-bone fractures may be the sole presenting sign of abuse during this time. A typical history in cases of abuse is "The baby's thigh suddenly became swollen." It is the infant's incessant crying and irritability from the pain of the nonimmobilized fracture that usually brings the family to medical attention (Fig. 17–7).

In summary, to distinguish etiologies of femoral fracture, the most helpful factors are a history of a difficult delivery and the presence of periosteal new bone within 5 to 14 days of

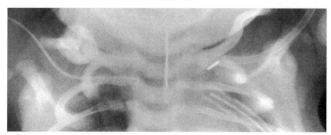

Figure 17–2
A 28-day-old clavicular fracture in a large infant with cyanotic congenital heart disease whose right clavicle was fractured at delivery. A large amount of callus is evident at this time.

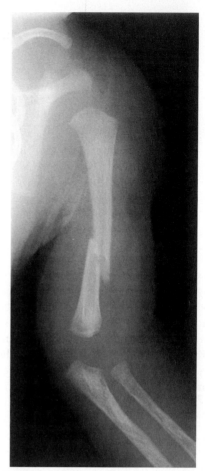

Figure 17–3
Birth trauma: oblique diaphyseal fracture. This was a difficult delivery for a large newborn. The injury was obvious at birth. Periosteal new bone may be evident as early as 5 days and should be visible by 12 days.

age, which indicate birth trauma. The presence of additional fractures indicates abuse (Fig. 17–8).

COMMON ACCIDENTAL TRAUMA

Statistics reveal that accidental trauma is the most significant threat to the lives and welfare of children and adolescents.[61,62,66–69,100] As noted earlier, motor vehicle accidents, burns, poisonings, and drownings are the most common causes of fatal accidents. Falls, minor burns, nonlethal poisonings, and aspiration or ingestion of foreign bodies cause most nonlethal accidents. In healthy children, such accidents result in isolated injuries. There is always an appropriate history of the accident, and appropriate parental concern and grief.

Young children sustain injuries that are common and typical for a particular mechanism of trauma. Familiarity with these injuries helps prevent the false diagnosis of abuse.

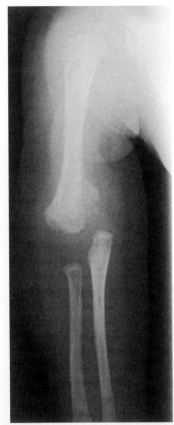

Figure 17–4
Birth trauma: fracture–dislocation of the distal humeral epiphysis. Two weeks after delivery there is marked periosteal new bone at the medial aspect of the distal humerus.

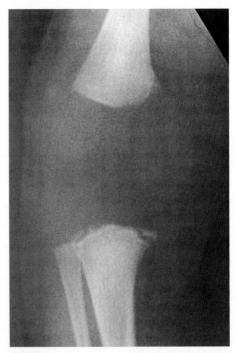

Figure 17–5
Metaphyseal avulsion secondary to birth trauma. This frontal view of the right knee at 17 days of age demonstrates metaphyseal avulsions of the lateral and medial proximal tibia. This male infant of 34 weeks' gestation had required a difficult breech extraction. Radiographically, birth injury can mimic child abuse, but the two can almost always be reliably differentiated by combining clinical information with radiographic findings. Incidentally, note the absence of the distal femoral epiphysis and the distal tibial epiphysis, which normally appear at 36 and 38 weeks gestational age, respectively.

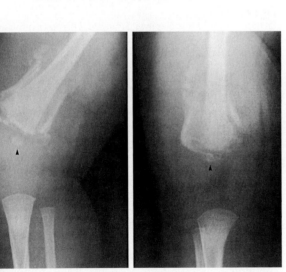

Figure 17–6
Distal femoral epiphyseal fracture-separation. Frontal and lateral radiographs of the right knee exposed at 28 days of age. This premature infant required a difficult breech extraction, but the distal femoral epiphyseal separation was not clinically suspected at the time of delivery. Mature periosteal new bone is evident, and the capital femoral epiphysis *(arrowhead)* is posterolaterally displaced from the femoral shaft. An absent proximal tibial epiphysis is consistent with the patient's prematurity of 35 weeks gestational age.

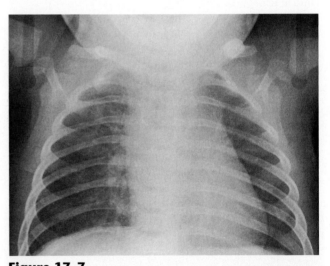

Figure 17–7
Accidental clavicular fracture. A 4-week-old clavicular fracture was incidentally noted on this chest film done to exclude pneumonia. The infant had rolled off a changing table while the mother had momentarily left the room to attend to a sibling who was having a temper tantrum. Irritability and supraclavicular swelling prompted the mother to seek medical help at that time. The history and parental reaction were appropriate for the injury. Note the mature callus formation at the midshaft of the left clavicle. The lungs are normal.

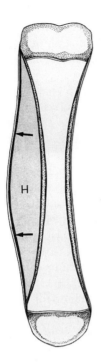

Figure 17–8
Schematic representation of a subperiosteal hematoma (H), which lies between the cortex and the periosteum. The earliest new bone formation *(arrows)* occurs beneath the osteogenic layer of the periosteum. (From Kleinman PK: Diagnostic Imaging of Child Abuse. 2nd Edition. Philadelphia, Mosby Year Book, Inc. May 1998.)

TABLE 17-1 DEVELOPMENT IN INFANTS, TODDLERS, AND YOUNG CHILDREN
4 months: Raise head
5–6 months: Roll over
7 months: Pivot prone in pursuit of object
8–9 months: Maintain sitting position
8 months: Stand with support
9 months: Take steps with support
15 months: Walk alone
18 months: Climb stairs, run stiffly
24 months: Run well, without frequent falls
3 years: Ascend stairs, using alternate feet
4 years: Descend stairs, using alternate feet
3–4 years: Ride tricycle
4–5 years: Begin riding bicycle

Table 17–1 indicates the developmental capabilities of children at various ages.

Falls are the most common cause of injury in infants and young children (Fig. 17–9). Children who have experienced accidental falls usually tumble from identifiable heights, such as cribs, kitchen counters, and stairs. Tripping and falling to the ground rarely cause severe injuries in young children because the distance to the ground is short. Falls are usually broken by outstretched hands, preventing or diminishing the impact of the face and skull on the ground. However, when a child falls backward from a significant height, moderate or severe cranial injury may occur. The type of surface covering is relevant in these cases. Skull fractures rarely occur when a child falls onto a carpeted surface, but such fractures can result from falling on a concrete or tile floor.

In a study of 250 documented falls (severe enough to warrant medical attention) from sofas, beds, and examining tables, superficial bruises and scratches were the only injuries evident in 70% of children.[29] In 3% of children, skull or clavicular fractures were present, and one infant had an isolated humeral fracture.[18] In such accidents, there is almost always an appropriate, plausible history of the incident, unlike in cases of abuse, in which the history is often absent or bizarre. Parents of infants who are accidentally injured generally exhibit grief and guilt, blaming themselves for inadequately

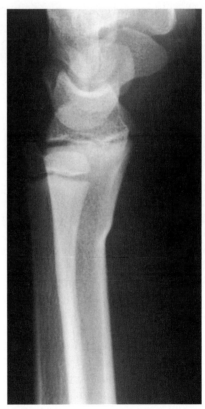

Figure 17–9
Distal radial torus fracture. This 5-year-old boy fell on his outstretched right hand while jumping from a 4-foot fence. The lateral radiograph demonstrates the typical appearance of an incomplete (torus) fracture of the distal radius. These fractures are invariably more easily identified on the lateral than on the frontal view. Healing without sequelae is the rule; the forearm is placed in a cast primarily to diminish pain. This is an injury commonly seen in accidental falls.

protecting their offspring. Physical and radiographic examinations of genuine accidents reveal the common fractures of the clavicle, distal radius and ulna, skull, tibia, and distal phalanges; these are isolated or all of the same age.

The clavicle is the most commonly fractured bone in children. The cause of injury is usually a fall on the shoulder, with the direct impact causing a midshaft fracture with variable displacement. The fall may be from surprisingly low heights, such as from a sofa to the floor. Pain is the most common reason for seeking medical help. An isolated fracture of the midshaft of the clavicle should not arouse suspicion of abuse.

Distal radial or ulnar fractures are caused by falling on an outstretched hand. Such fractures present no diagnostic problems, and although they are more common in older age groups, they can occur in any ambulating child.

Isolated skull fractures, although rare, occur in young children who have fallen from moderate heights onto their heads. The radiographic appearance of a calvarial injury caused by abuse may be the same as that of such an injury incurred accidentally. However, accidental skull fractures tend to be linear, narrow, and uncomplicated, whereas a larger percentage of fractures caused by abuse are complex, depressed, and diastatic. In accidental skull fractures, the severe intracranial damage seen in battered children is distinctly unusual. Again, accidental cranial injuries are accompanied by an appropriate history, whereas those from abuse are not.

An important accidental injury that may erroneously raise suspicion of abuse is the toddler's fracture (Fig. 17–10). This characteristic spiral or oblique fracture of the distal tibia is considered to be a result of normal trauma and is almost always self-inflicted in young children. The fracture can occur when the foot is immobilized (as between the bars of a playpen or crib) and a rotational force is exerted on the tibia as the child's body falls. Another mechanism for this fracture in young children is a direct lengthwise tibial impact when the child jumps from a considerable height (e.g., dresser, bunk bed, or piano). The mode of injury is seldom perceived as an accident by either the parents or the child. The usual presenting complaints are refusal to bear weight or walk or a limp. The onset of symptoms may be delayed, which adds further confusion and accounts for the absence of a history of trauma.

Persisting limp is sometimes the reason for radiographic evaluation of a toddler's fracture. In these instances, periosteal new bone is present if the fracture occurred more than 12 days previously. The lack of an appropriate history and the presence of periosteal new bone may erroneously raise suspicion of abuse, tumor, or infection. The toddler's fracture is a notable exception to the rule that long-bone fractures are highly suggestive of abuse (Fig. 17–11).

Distal phalangeal soft tissue injuries, with or without fractures and soft tissue amputation, constitute most hand injuries in children. The most common mechanism of injury is the fingers being closed in a door. These accidental injuries result in distal phalangeal trauma, as opposed to the metacarpal fractures seen more commonly in abuse. Metacarpal injuries may occur when the hand is accidentally crushed, but in these rare instances, there is usually an appropriate history.

In children older than 5 years, significant skeletal trauma is incurred during sports and vehicular accidents. These events are almost always witnessed and clearly defined; confusion with abuse is unlikely (Fig. 17–12). Bicycle accidents, contact sports, and motor vehicle and pedestrian accidents can cause abdominal trauma in older children; however, visceral injuries in children younger than 5 years of age are very rare. Young children who step on each other, who are stepped on by a dog, or who punch each other rarely have visceral injuries; thus, visceral injury is not included in expected "traumas" of children in this age group. Finally, it should be emphasized that *any* fracture in a nonambulating child should be viewed with great suspicion (Fig. 17–13).

To summarize, the important nonintentional injuries of children younger than 5 years are as follows:

1. Clavicular fractures (usually midshaft), with variable degrees of displacement.
2. Skull fractures that are usually narrow, linear, uncomplicated, and seldom associated with neurologic sequelae.
3. Toddler's fracture, an oblique, hairline fracture of the tibia, usually best seen on the external oblique view and sometimes invisible on frontal or lateral views. Soft tissue edema may be absent, reflecting a lack of soft tissue injury with only minimal subperiosteal bleeding.
4. Torus fractures, or incomplete distal radial and ulnar fractures.
5. Complete fractures of both the radius and the ulna or variations thereof.
6. Distal phalanx injury, a soft tissue injury, with or without a fracture of the distal phalanx.

NONACCIDENTAL TRAUMA

The concept of physical abuse of children is best understood in the context of family violence.[9,26,31] Society has become aware of the plight of battered wives, physical abuse of the elderly, and even physical abuse of parents by teenagers. In many dysfunctional families, verbal and physical abuse toward family members who are unable or unwilling to defend themselves is common. Low self-esteem is frequent among battered wives, and beatings may continue for years. Similarly, abused children erroneously assume responsibility for their plight. Children of abusive parents often believe that they "deserved" the beatings because they were "naughty" or "bad." The child's ready acceptance of guilt makes it more comprehensible that abused children continue to love their dangerous parents and often wish to return to them.

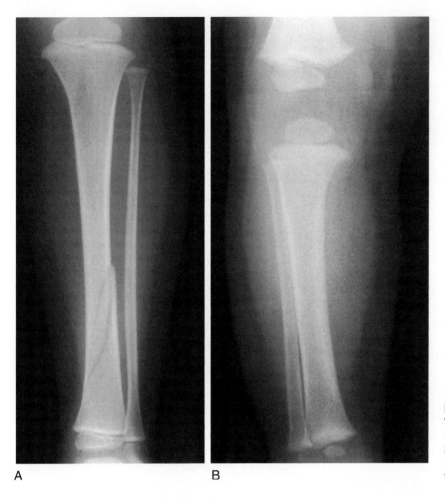

A   B

Figure 17–10
Toddler's fracture. *A,* Radiograph of an 18-month-old infant with moderate displacement of a spiral fracture. *B,* Radiograph of a 1-year-old boy with acute refusal to walk. No trauma was witnessed by the parents.

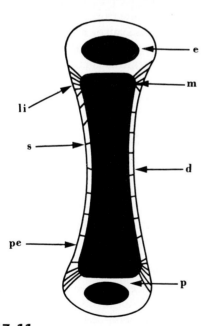

Figure 17–11
Growing bone: diagrammatic representation. d, Diaphysis; e, epiphysis; li, ligamentous insertion; m, metaphysis; p, physis (growth plate); pe, periosteum; s, Sharpey's fiber.

Few problems in pediatrics evoke more emotional response than that of parents who mutilate or kill their children. Disbelief, disgust, anger, and an intense desire for punitive action are common responses of health professionals who encounter child abuse. Unfortunately, excessively emotional responses are seldom appropriate or effective.

It is important to remember that the radiologist's sole function is to establish or refute the diagnosis of abuse. Two issues that the radiologist and pediatrician should consciously avoid are establishing the identity of the perpetrator (the function of the police) and ensuring that justice is carried out (the function of the courts).[20,47] Competent, unbiased diagnosis is more effective when the radiologist allows other professionals to deal with interrogation, confrontation, and prosecution.

In this setting, most experienced pediatric radiologists deliberately avoid any interaction with the parents, because such interaction serves little purpose and may complicate an already difficult situation. The approach to giving accurate and effective testimony in court is discussed in Chapter 18, which addresses selected legal aspects of child abuse.

Some physicians are reluctant to diagnose abuse because of potential legal involvement. In addition, these cases tend

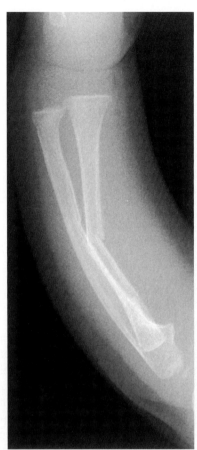

Figure 17–12
Accidental injury. The infant was lying on the floor while an adult accidentally stepped on the child's arm. Multiple witnesses were present and appropriate medical care was sought immediately.

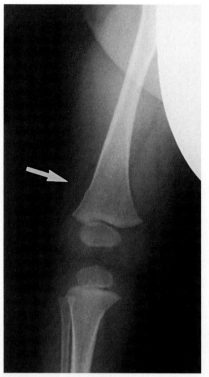

Figure 17–13
Accidental femoral fracture in a 7–month–old boy who accidentally rolled off a changing table and fell to the ground. Note the torus fracture of the distal radius. Although femoral fractures should certainly raise intense suspicion of abuse, not all femoral fractures during infancy are caused by nonaccidental trauma.

to be very time consuming and are seldom rewarded by either positive interactions or financial compensation. To ensure the reporting of cases of potential abuse, all states have passed laws that hold the physician liable for overlooking or not reporting abuse, and most states have adopted laws that protect physicians in cases of false-positive abuse diagnosis. As early as 1976, the State Supreme Court of California ruled that a physician who fails to identify or report a case in which there is physical, historical, or radiographic evidence of abuse is guilty of professional negligence. Thus, knowledge of the radiographic findings of child abuse, much like malpractice insurance, cannot be considered optional for radiologists.

"Reporting" means notifying the social services department responsible for child protection.[3] The referring physician is usually the one to send the official notice of potential abuse; however, if nonaccidental trauma is a rare diagnosis, it is advisable for the radiologist to verify that such a report has been sent. California laws have expanded the obligation to report abuse to include all professionals who work with children, such as nurses, school teachers, and guidance counselors.

The official radiology report should be thoughtfully and carefully dictated without errors and equivocation. Although an unequivocal diagnosis can be made from the radiographs alone, it is important to fully understand the proposed mechanism of injury and to include in the report the fact that the findings seen on imaging could not have resulted from the described mechanism of injury.

DIAGNOSIS BY SKELETAL RADIOGRAPHS

Skeletal radiographs can provide irrefutable evidence that abuse has occurred; therefore, the films should be considered a legal document.[9,11,19,37,45,58,60,65,80,91,98,99] In Table 17–2, the standard radiographic views obtained for child abuse are listed. Close monitoring of the examination is helpful, including looking briefly at the patient as well as at the films, because in court, the radiologist is often asked to verify that the films presented as evidence were actually taken of the child in question and not of some other child. The radiographs should be of good quality and correctly labeled. Additional views should be obtained of any areas with questionable findings so that equivocation on the final radiographic report is minimized or eliminated.

TABLE 17-2 COMPLETE SKELETAL SURVEY

Thorax (AP), lateral and both obliques to include
   thoracic spine and ribs
Abdomen (AP), lumbarsacral spine, and bony pelvis
Lumbar spine, lateral
Skull, frontal and lateral
Arms (AP)
Forearms (AP)
Hands (PA)
Thighs (AP)
Feet (PA or AP)

AP, Anteroposterior; PA, posteroanterior.
Adapted from ACR Practice Guidelines.

TABLE 17-3 ESTIMATING THE AGE OF BRUISES
IN CHILDREN

APPROXIMATE AGE	SKIN APPEARANCE
0–2 days	Tender and swollen
2–5 days	Blue, purple, red
5–7 days	Green
7–10 days	Yellow
10 or more days	Brown
2–4 weeks	Cleared

The rate of resolution of bruises can be affected by the depth of
   the bruise and by the amount of bruises.
Reprinted from Reece RM. Cutaneous Manifestation of Abuse,
   Child Abuse Medical Diagnosis and Management. Lea &
   Febiger, 1994, p. 169.

Occasionally, the fractures seen on trauma surveys are virtually pathognomonic for abuse (e.g., metaphyseal corner fractures, acromial fractures, and multiple rib fractures). More commonly, it is the type of fracture, together with the clinical history and the age of the patient, that permits diagnosis of abuse (e.g., femoral or humeral fractures, fracture-separation of the distal humeral epiphysis, and tibial fractures in a nonambulating child). Evidence of multiple fractures in different stages of healing helps verify the diagnosis and documents the fact that multiple episodes of abuse have occurred. However, a child does not need to be abused on multiple occasions before a competent radiologist can make a firm diagnosis of such abuse (Table 17–3).

The bones of children younger than 5 years differ from the bones of adults in several respects. These differences warrant brief emphasis, because they improve understanding of skeletal injuries in children. In young children, the strongest parts of the skeleton are the ligaments, and the weakest parts are the cartilaginous growth plates (epiphyses); the bones are of intermediate strength. Thus, sprains or ligamentous tears, which are common in adults and adolescents, are rare in young children. Instead of ligamentous tears, young children suffer disruption of the epiphyses (Salter type I injuries) and fractures of the underlying bones, especially the most immature portions of the metaphyseal primary spongiosa.

Another notable skeletal difference in young children is the presence of considerable woven bone. Woven bone is weaker in structure than the haversian bone that eventually replaces it, and it tends to wrinkle or bend rather than shatter when subjected to stress. As a result, torus and bowing fractures are common in young children.

During childhood, the periosteal membrane is loosely attached to most of the underlying cortex except at the cartilaginous physis and epiphyses. This contrasts with the uniform, tight, periosteal adherence present in adults. Thus, subperiosteal elevation from bleeding occurs readily in children and is manifested radiographically by calcification of the subperiosteal hematoma in 5 to 15 days. The volume of subperiosteal bleeding is greatest at the diaphysis and least at the physis, producing a gently, outward, diaphyseal ballooning.

Although loosely adherent, the periosteum is much stronger and thicker in children than in adults, functioning as a strong envelope to protect the growth plate and bone. This membrane is rarely torn in children, although it is easily and frequently displaced. Thus, it functions as a splint by protecting the delicate growth plate and minimizing the displacement of fracture fragments. In young children, the healing of fractures occurs rapidly and completely; anatomic remodeling is the rule. The rate of remodeling depends on the rate of bone growth; thus, complete remodeling of a fracture takes less time in a 2-month-old infant than in a 5-year-old child. Healing is facilitated by proper immobilization and optimal nutrition, both of which may be lacking in an abused child.

In the following section, the mechanisms and typical appearances of skeletal trauma resulting from nonaccidental injury are discussed; such trauma includes metaphyseal corner fractures, long-bone fractures, thoracic injuries, fracture-separation of the distal humeral epiphysis, vertebral fractures, and other miscellaneous fractures. The validity of this discussion assumes the presence of normal underlying bone. If the skeleton is globally or focally abnormal (e.g., as a result of metabolic bone disease, infection, genetic abnormalities, or tumor), the radiographic features of abuse as presented here may be unreliable indicators.

Extremity Trauma

Metaphyseal Injuries or Classic Metaphyseal Lesions Metaphyseal injuries are seen commonly in physically abused infants and are virtually pathognomonic of nonaccidental trauma. The most common names for these are *corner fracture* and *bucket-handle fractures,* although the terms *avulsion fracture* or *metaphyseal infraction* are sometimes used. Periosteal new bone is usually not seen with small corner fractures because subperiosteal bleeding rarely occurs;

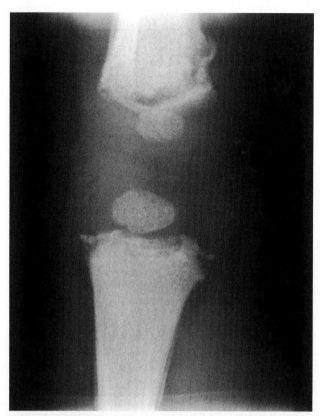

Figure 17–14

Metaphyseal injury. The distal femur is a common site for metaphyseal injuries. Periosteal new bone is visible along the more proximal aspect of the femoral shaft. Bucket–handle fracture. A bucket–handle fracture is a more extensive metaphyseal avulsion. In this case, the entire superior cortical margin of the tibia has been torn off. Note the extensive periosteal new bone along the distal medial tibial shaft. This patient had additional rib fractures, a left acromial avulsion, and bilateral distal humeral metaphyseal avulsions.

bleeding and elevation of the periosteum are requisites for the formation of periosteal new bone (Fig. 17–14).

Histopathologic analysis of the anatomy of metaphyseal injuries, performed by Kleinman et al.[13] in the mid-1980s, revealed that this lesion is not an isolated fragment of bone, but instead a complete or partial disc of metaphyseal bone that has fractured and separated from the primary spongiosa of the metaphysis. The periphery of this disc is thicker than the thin center and therefore appears as two isolated triangles of bone when radiographed in tangent. The thickness of the changes in orientation of the bony disc may result in different radiographic appearances, varying from the usual corner fracture to a bucket-handle appearance as the crescentic portion of the disc is imaged. Variations in appearance are influenced by the configuration of the metaphysis and the x-ray beam angulation. Other factors that may give an atypical appearance to metaphyseal injuries are incomplete circumferential fractures and superimposed healing. Repeated trauma at the same site can also produce an atypical appearance.

Additional studies by Kleinman et al.[14] indicated that metaphyseal trauma frequently causes vascular injury and disruption. Vascular insufficiency results in an abnormal persistence of epiphyseal cartilage instead of the orderly transformation of such cartilage to bone. Persistent vertical cartilaginous columns extend into the metaphysis and become visible radiographically as zones of lucency that are contiguous with the growth plate (Fig. 17–15).[51]

The precise etiology of metaphyseal fractures remains uncertain. It is theorized that the extremities of small infants may be used by the abuser as "handles" to grab the child's body prior to throwing or violently moving it. Shaking the infant's body violently while holding the thorax produces deceleration and acceleration forces that can cause metaphyseal injuries of the extremities. It appears reasonable that symmetric metaphyseal injuries result from shaking, whereas focal or unilateral metaphyseal damage is probably related to

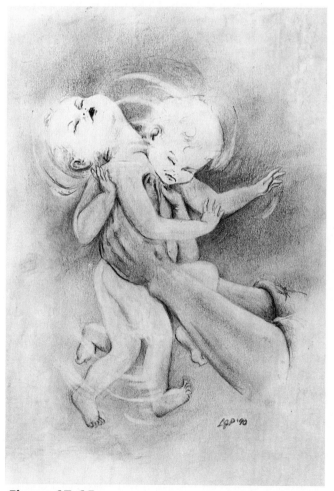

Figure 17–15

The shaken infant. (Illustrated by Laura Perry, M.D., based on descriptions by assailants. Reproduced with permission from Kleinman PK: Diagnostic imaging in infant abuse. Review article, AJR 155:703-712, 1990.)

using the extremities as handles. A second study, which has verified the predominance (60%) of left-sided fractures,[5] makes a plausible case for the scenario in which a right-handed abuser faces the child and uses the left extremity to hold the infant during episodes of abuse (Fig. 17–16).

Metaphyseal lesions are most commonly seen in nonambulatory abused infants, and in this age group they are highly specific for abuse. These metaphyseal lesions are not the result of the child's own actions nor are they seen in accidental trauma.

The most common locations for metaphyseal fractures of abuse are the knee, ankle, and distal humerus (Table 17–4). Although these injuries are most often seen in association with other fractures, they can occur in isolation. It is important to understand that normal handling of an infant (such as bathing and diapering), rough play with siblings or parent, and accidental falls from any height may produce other injuries, but not the metaphyseal lesions of abuse (Fig. 17–17).

In the presence of normal bones, even a single metaphyseal lesion in an infant is virtually pathognomonic of abuse. Unfortunately, it is sometimes difficult to convince the referring clinician that this benign-appearing lesion signifies such an ominous etiology. I once encountered a solitary corner fracture that was the sole skeletal abnormality in a child who subsequently died of visceral injuries; it was also the sole fracture in another 18-month-old girl who returned to the

TABLE 17-4 PHYSICAL SIGNS OF ABUSE
Refuse to move an extremity
Hard, irregular masses on the extremities caused by callus
Bead like masses palpable over the rib cage caused by healing rib fractures
A grating sound over the rib cage caused by the movement of multiple acute broken ribs
Twitching motions of fingers or extremeties caused by cerebral trauma
Bruises in nonambulating infants
Imprints of the human hand anywhere on the body
Human bite marks
Belt marks
Cigarette marks
Immersion burns

hospital 2 weeks later with a femoral fracture, a depressed skull fracture, and severe neurologic damage.

Spiral Long-Bone Fracture In my experience, an isolated, usually oblique, long-bone fracture has been the initial presentation in 15% of children radiographed for suspected abuse. In the absence of trauma, an oblique fracture of the femur or humerus is highly suggestive, but not

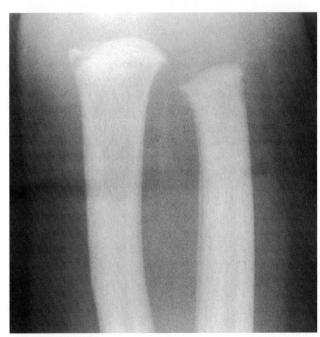

Figure 17–16
Metaphyseal injury: anteroposterior view of the distal radius and ulna demonstrating a metaphyseal avulsion. Also seen is minimal periosteal new bone along the ulnar shaft. This 4-month-old girl had multiple other fractures.

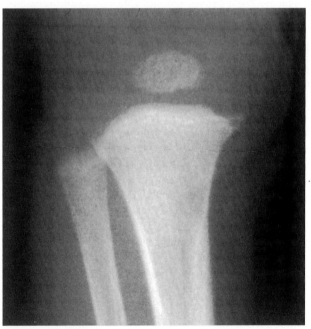

Figure 17–17
Classic metaphyseal lesion. This lateral view of the ankle demonstrates a metaphyseal injury of the distal tibia and the fibula. Note the normal skeleton and the absence of periosteal new bone. In small infants, a hospital identification band placed around the ankle may occasionally obscure enough detail that the subtle findings of a small metaphyseal injury may be overlooked.

invariably diagnostic,[24] of abuse. Certainly, there should be no doubt about the cause of this injury in a nonambulating infant. The most common history given in these infants is "sudden swelling of the thigh or arm."[4,92] Medical help is usually sought because the child cries incessantly, as a nonimmobilized fracture of this magnitude is very painful. These infants and children will also refuse to bear weight on the affected side. Extensive periosteal new bone is sometimes seen in children in whom medical help is delayed and the extremity is not immobilized. Although femoral fractures in ambulating children are highly suggestive of abuse, they can be incurred accidentally. An appropriate, plausible history must be obtained and carefully analyzed in these unusual cases. We once encountered a 2-year-old boy who fell from the top of a bunk bed and broke his femur (Figs. 17–18, 17–19, and 17–20).

A possible mechanism of femoral injury in abuse is a rotatory force applied to the leg. The resulting fracture is often spiral, and most such fractures are diaphyseal. If the extremity is grasped above the knee, a more proximal spiral femoral fracture results. External signs of bruising are often absent, as is disruption of the fat muscle interface, because the fracture results from a rotational stress on the femoral diaphysis instead of a blow that injures the soft tissues. Many femoral fractures are incurred while diapers are being changed, and they most often happen when no other person is in the room. The perpetrators describe not only an audible "pop" when the bone breaks, but some also describe feeling the bone break (Figs. 17–21 through 17–29).

A similar mechanism may cause spiral fractures of the humerus. Again noteworthy is the increased frequency of left-sided diaphyseal fractures, reflecting the preponderance of right-handedness (87%) in the general population. The majority of abuse is apparently carried out with the abuser facing the child. Although the mechanism just described is probably the most common way by which a humerus or femur is fractured, there are many ways a bone can be broken during abuse. For example, I have encountered a transverse femoral fracture in which the abuser subsequently admitted to stepping on the child's thigh.

Falls from a bed, couch, or highchair seldom fracture long bones. In considering the clinical history of the accident, the physician must remember that children younger than 3 years of age rarely climb trees or roof tops. When such injuries occur accidentally, there is almost always a caregiver to witness the event and give an appropriate history. By contrast, an abuser often initially denies any trauma, specifying that swelling of the extremity and evidence of pain were the first untoward events noted. Conspicuously absent is a plausible explanation of how the injury occurred.

Epiphyseal Displacement It is fortunate that irreversible disruption of the growth plate as seen in a Salter type V injury is rare in child abuse, as such lesions create considerable growth disturbances.[17] Epiphyseal displacement,

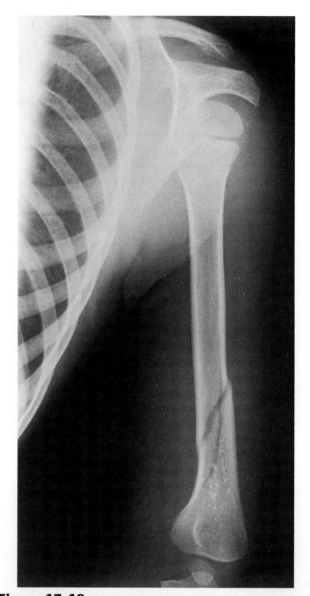

Figure 17–18
Spiral humeral fracture in a 3 1/2-year-old boy with pain and swelling of the left arm. The mother stated that the child had fallen off his tricycle, thus incurring the injury. This anteroposterior view of the left arm reveals a distal spiral fracture. An important finding is mild periosteal new bone along the medial aspect of the distal humeral shaft. This indicates that the injury occurred at least 7 to 10 days earlier. Abuse was subsequently proved.

or a Salter type I injury of the distal humeral epiphysis, has become increasingly recognized as an injury suggestive of abuse. The entire epiphysis is likely to slip when subjected to a rotatory shearing force.[63] Such forces most frequently result from abuse but are also seen in accidental injury or birth trauma (Fig. 17–30).

The mechanism of injury is external rotation, usually of the left forearm. This rotatory force causes posteromedial

Text continued on page 595

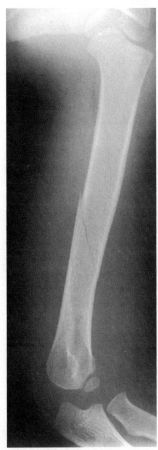

Figure 17–19
Spiral humeral fracture: lateral *(right)* views of the left humerus of a child with clinical suspicion of abuse. Multiple other fractures were identified on the trauma survey. The spiral fracture in this child is located more proximally than in the patient shown in Figure 17–21.

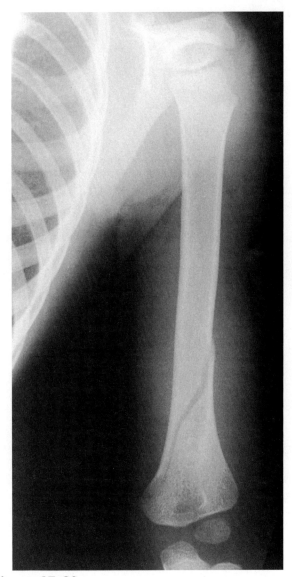

Figure 17–20
Acute distal humeral fracture. Note the sharp edges of this 2-day-old fracture.

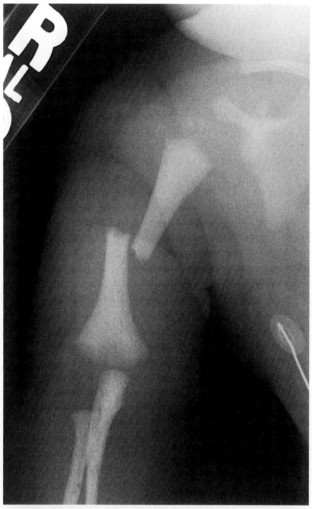

Figure 17–21
Femoral fracture. The 2-month-old infant presented with a swollen
thigh and no history of trauma. This was the only abnormality seen
in this infant. This is a common presentation.

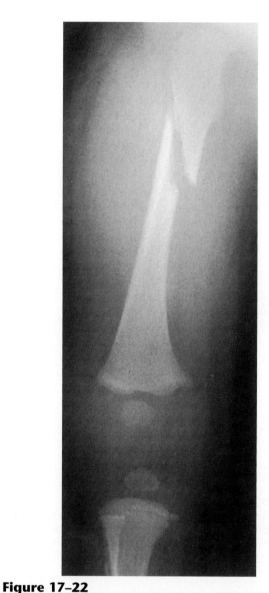

Figure 17–22
Acute femoral fracture. This 4-month-old infant presented with
swelling of his left thigh. There was no history of trauma. Note that
there is a lot of soft tissue swelling and also there is a classic metaphyseal lesion at the lateral aspect of the femur. No other injuries
were identified. This obviously reveals that this child had previously been abused.

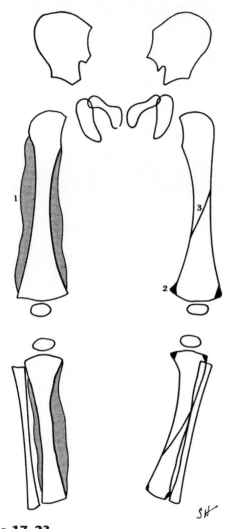

Figure 17–23
Characteristic lower extremity injuries of child abuse: diagrammatic representation. 1, Periosteal new bone; 2, metaphyseal injuries; 3, diaphyseal spiral fractures.

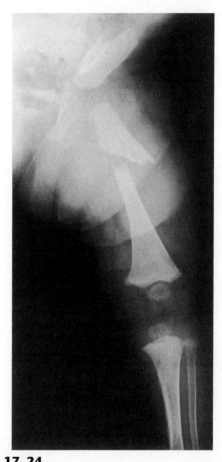

Figure 17–24
Acute femoral fracture. This infant presented without a history of trauma. Note an acute fracture of the left femur. The fracture is more distal than the other patient's. Also seen are multiple classic metaphyseal lesions, most notably on the medial aspect of the left femur and the tibia as well.

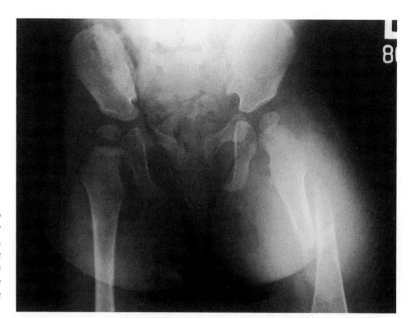

Figure 17–25
Femoral fracture. Six month old infant was brought to the hospital for inability to bear weight. The father relayed that while changing diapers the father heard a pop. Note that there is extensive soft tissue swelling. The history of hearing a distinct pop is highly suggestive that that was the time that the bone was broken. The break can also be felt if the fracture is close to where the perpetrator was grasping the child.

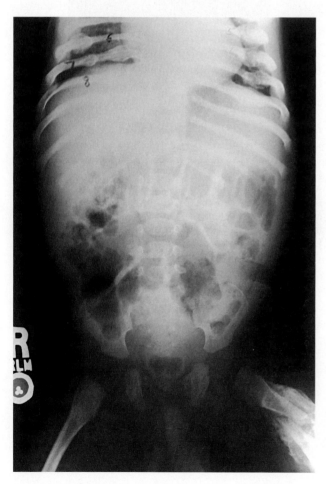

Figure 17–26
Untreated femoral fracture. This fracture was incidentally identified during a nonaccidental trauma survey. Note the exhuberant preiosteal new bone and multiple bilateral rib fractures.

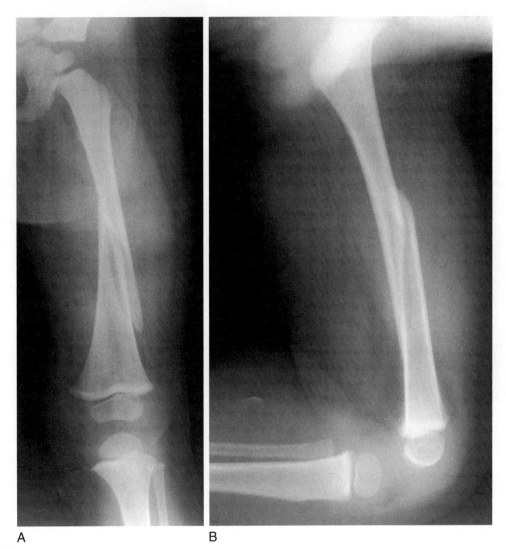

A   B

Figure 17–27
Spiral long–bone fracture. Frontal *(A)* and lateral *(B)* views show a 10-month-old boy who was brought to the emergency department with a history of sudden swelling of the left thigh.

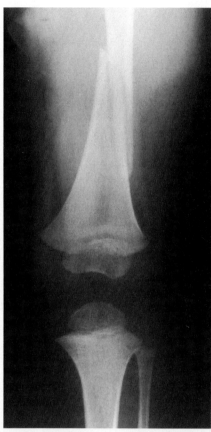

Figure 17–28
Spiral long–bone fracture: frontal view of a 12-month-old ambulating girl who was noted to be irritable and refused to bear weight on the left leg. The mother stated that the child "fell off the couch." A frontal view of the left femur reveals a spiral distal metaphyseal fracture. The remainder of the trauma survey was normal. The child may well have fallen off the couch, but that event did not result in a femoral fracture. Abuse was eventually verified.

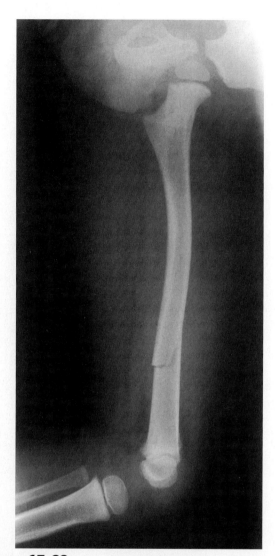

Figure 17–29
Transverse long–bone fracture: lateral view of the femur of a 4-year-old boy who was brought to the emergency department because of pain and swelling of the left thigh. The mother and her boyfriend had been camping with the child and stated that the injury occurred when the boy tripped and fell. Abuse was suspected, and the boyfriend eventually admitted to having stepped on the child's leg "because the boy had wet his sleeping bag." Although most of the injuries of child abuse have a well–defined pattern, any fracture can be the result of nonaccidental trauma.

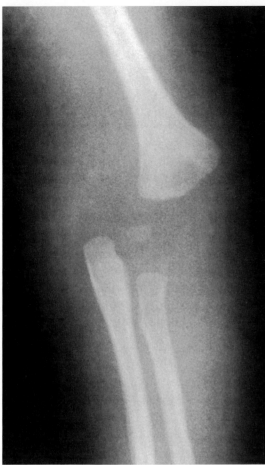

Figure 17–30
Fracture–separation of the distal humeral epiphysis. This 9-month-old boy presented with swelling of the left arm. This frontal radiograph of the left arm revealed an acute fracture–separation of the distal humeral epiphysis. Note that the capitellum has maintained its normal relationship with the long axis of the radius.

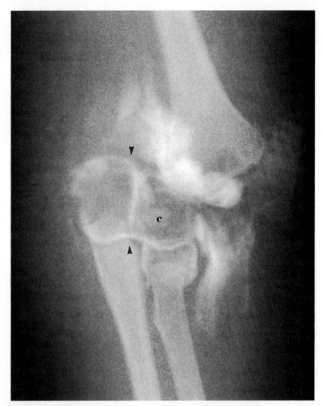

Figure 17–31
Fracture–separation of the distal humeral epiphysis. An arthrogram clearly defines the anatomic abnormality. Note that the distal (cartilaginous) humeral epiphysis (*arrowheads*) has been separated from the ossified portion of the distal humerus. The normal anatomic relationship of the elbow has been maintained. This is a Salter type I injury very suggestive of abuse. C, Capitellum.

displacement of the entire distal humeral epiphysis. The ossification centers of the elbow remain intact and maintain their normal relationship to each other. Thus, the capitellum, if visibly ossified, retains its normal anatomic alignment with the long axis of the radial shaft. In injuries that result from such abuse, the forearm is displaced medially, whereas in accidental elbow dislocations, displacement is lateral (Fig. 17–31).

The most significant physical finding acutely is a markedly swollen, painful elbow. Clinically, children with such injuries usually are suspected of having a dislocated elbow, and the true diagnosis of fracture-separation often is made solely by the characteristic radiographic appearance. The possibility of nonaccidental trauma should be entertained if a fracture-dislocation of the distal humeral epiphysis is noted and a plausible history is lacking. In such instances, a trauma survey is indicated and can be conclusive if it reveals occult fractures (Figs. 17–32, 17–33, and 17–34).

During the healing of this injury, the medial periosteum of the humerus is more markedly elevated. The extensive periosteal ossification may produce a hard mass that is palpable around the elbow. This late-onset physical finding may be the first abnormality that prompts the parents to seek medical attention. Typically, referral is made to "rule out bone tumor." Prognosis for normal elbow function is excellent, and no treatment is indicated in injuries that are not acute. In most children, the distal radius remodels without residual deformities. The same type of epiphyseal dislocation can occur at the proximal femoral head, but this is far less common in cases of abuse.

Injuries of Hands and Feet   Accidental injuries to the hands usually involve the phalanges. These injuries often result from fingers getting slammed in doors. Almost all accidental hand injuries are accompanied by an appropriate trauma history from the parent and, often, the patient. Child abuse more commonly results in fractures of the metacarpals or metatarsals but may include injury to the digits as well.

Many of these injuries are clinically unsuspected. The significance of documenting these lesions lies not in their

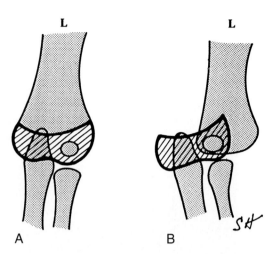

Figure 17–32
Fracture–dislocation of the distal humeral epiphysis: diagrammatic representation. *A,* Normal. *B,* Shearing of the left distal humeral epiphysis.

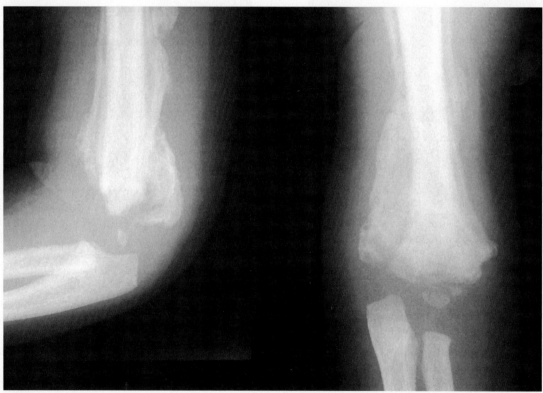

Figure 17–33
Fracture–separation of the distal left humeral epiphysis. This 3-year-old boy was brought to his pediatrician because of a palpable left elbow mass. No history of trauma was elicited. Extensive periosteal new bone secondary to a healing fracture–separation of the distal left humeral epiphysis is evident. The capitellum is medially displaced. Note that the periosteal new bone is more extensive medially because of more marked elevation of the medial periosteum of the humerus when the epiphysis is separated. This injury is more common on the left because it occurs while the abuser is facing the child, using the right hand to externally rotate the child's left arm.

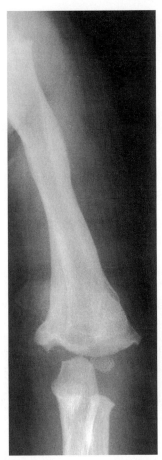

Figure 17–34
Healing fracture–separation in the same child shown in Figure 17–29, 9 months later. This frontal view demonstrates incorporation of periosteal new bone into the remodeling shaft.

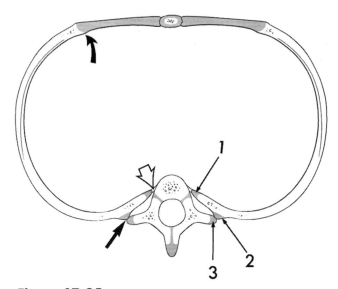

Figure 17–35
Diagram of normal anatomy. The rib head articulates with the costal facet of the vertebra anteriorly *(open arrow);* posteriorly the rib tubercle articulates with the transverse process facet *(solid straight arrow).* Generous cartilaginous apophyses are noted at the rib head 1) tubercle 2) and transverse processes 3). There is slight expansion of the costochondral junctions *(curved arrow).* (From Kleinman PK: Diagnostic Imaging of Child Abuse. 2nd Edition. Philadelphia, Mosby Year Book, Inc. May 1998.)

specificity for abuse, but in their ability to serve as additional evidence of child abuse in children with suspicious skeletal trauma. A single anteroposterior view of both hands and feet is a routine part of my radiographic skeletal survey, and these regions are also included in skeletal scintigraphy for abuse.

Central Skeletal Trauma

Thoracic Injuries The bony thorax as seen on routine chest radiography is a high-yield examination for documenting, and often for first suspecting, the presence of child abuse (Fig. 17–35). The chest film includes the ribs, proximal humeri, acromion, scapula, sternum, and upper spine.[49,50,52,90] Fractures of any of these structures are highly suggestive of abuse; rib fractures are especially common in nonaccidental trauma. Thus, a "routine" chest radiograph in a subgroup of children at risk for abuse should be carefully scrutinized for these fractures. A high index of suspicion is indicated under the following circumstances: shunt tube placement for idiopathic hydrocephalus (Fig. 17–36).

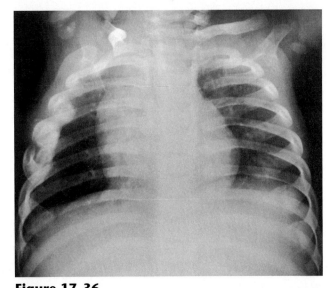

Figure 17–36
Rib fractures. Multiple and obvious healed rib fractures and anterior costochondral fractures are evident on this frontal chest film. This 4-year-old boy and his brother were severely and repeatedly beaten by their father. Fortunately, neither one sustained cerebral injuries.

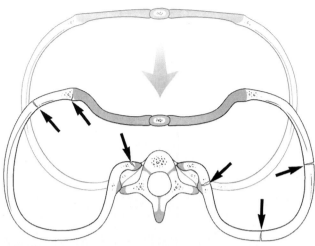

Figure 17–37

Mechanisms of injury. With anteroposterior compression of the chest there is excessive leverage of the posterior ribs over the fulcrum of the transverse process. This places tension along the inner aspect of the rib heads and necks, resulting in fractures at these sites *(arrows)*. This mechanism is also consistent with morphologic patterns of injury at other sites along the rib arc at the costochondral junctions *(arrows)*. (From Kleinman PK: Diagnostic Imaging of Child Abuse. 2nd Edition. Philadelphia, Mosby Year Book, Inc. May 1998.)

While giving careful scrutiny to the bony thorax, the clinician must recognize the limitations of conventional frontal chest radiography. This examination rarely demonstrates acute, nondisplaced fractures in the medial half of the posterior rib arc. The fractures that do occur here cause subsequent callus formation along the inner aspect of the rib, with the outer cortex often remaining intact.[13] Such fractures become easily visible when periosteal new bone has formed. Equally difficult to visualize are injuries close to the costochondral junction and fractures of the lower ribs, if the lower portion of the thorax is underexposed. Coned and oblique views can be used in infants in whom there is a high degree of suspicion for abuse. The presence of focal pleural thickening should alert the radiologist to the high likelihood of a recent rib fracture in a child suspected of being abused. Meticulously performed scintigraphy reveals more fractures of the thorax than conventional radiography and is often helpful in selected children (Figs. 17–37, 17–38, and 17–39).

Fractured ribs are highly suggestive of abuse because they are rare in normal children subjected to the daily trauma of childhood and most minor accidents. The normal pediatric thorax is highly resilient, and minor trauma almost never results in fractures. In addition, although rib fractures from birth trauma can simulate child abuse in the axial skeleton, rib fractures are only very rarely incurred during delivery. By contrast, premature infants with bronchopulmonary dysplasia and diffuse osteopenia may develop multiple rib fractures during pulmonary toilet (Figs. 17–40, 17–41, and 17–42).

Sometimes the legal question arises as to whether closed chest massage during cardiopulmonary resuscitation (CPR) was the cause of rib fractures. Studies by Kleinman and Feldman and Brewer[6] revealed that despite prolonged resuscitation performed by people with variable degrees of skill,

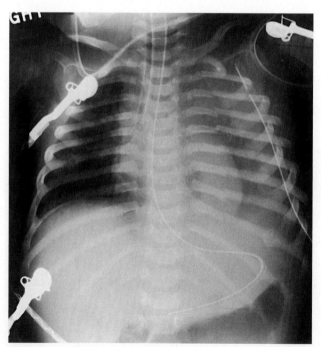

Figure 17–38

Flail chest. A 4-month-old infant was hospitalized for severe respiratory distress. He had multiple acute rib fractures on the left side. Also note multiple healing rib fractures in different stages of healing on the right side. The endotracheal tube is in the right mainstem bronchus.

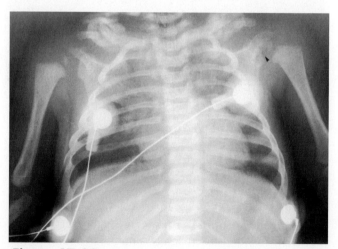

Figure 17–39

Acromial fracture. This frontal chest film of a moribund 4-month-old girl demonstrates a left acromial fracture *(arrow)*. Also present are bilateral clavicular fractures and periosteal new bone along the medial aspect of the right humeral shaft. This child died because of severe intracranial hemorrhage.

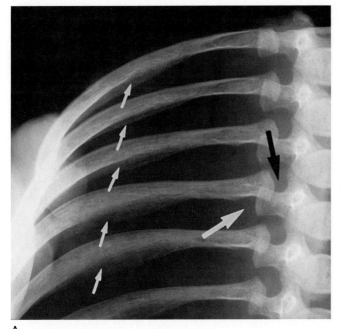

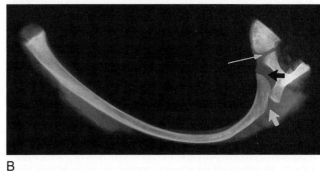

A

B

Figure 17–40

Normal anatomy: radiologic and histologic correlates. Right ribs with vertebral articulations in a normal 2-month-old infant. *A,* Frontal projection. The rib heads are partially superimposed over the transverse processes. The rib head *(black arrow)* and transverse process *(large white arrow)* apophyses are radiolucent. Note the normal, inferiorly flanged appearance of the posterolateral ribs *(small white arrows)*. *B,* Axial specimen radiograph. The rib head articulates with the vertebral body *(black arrow)* near the neurocentral synchondrosis *(thick white arrow)*. The rib tubercle articulates with the transverse process posteriorly *(short white arrow)*. Substantial radiolucency is evident at both articulations. (From Kleinman PK: Diagnostic Imaging of Child Abuse. 2nd Edition. Philadelphia, Mosby Year Book, Inc. May 1998.)

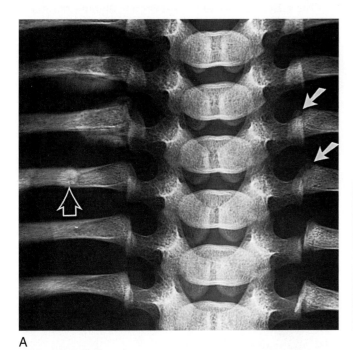

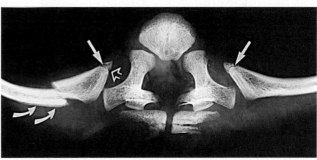

A

B

Figure 17–41

Posterior rib fractures in a 2 1/2-month-old abused infant. *A,* A specimen radiograph of the sixth to tenth posterior ribs demonstrates vague radiolucencies involving the heads of the left seventh and eighth ribs *(solid arrows)*. Also evident are healing fractures at the costotransverse process articulations of the right sixth and seventh ribs. There is a more recent fracture of the neck off the right eighth rib *(open arrow)*. *B,* Axial specimen radiograph of the eighth ribs and their vertebral articulations. There are bilateral rib head fractures *(solid arrows)*. Note the extension of radiolucency from the rib head apophysis into the fracture site *(open arrow)*. The fracture of the lateral aspect of the rib neck shows posterior displacement with subtle subperiosteal new bone formation (SPNBF) *(curved arrows)*. (From Kleinman PK: Diagnostic Imaging of Child Abuse. 2nd Edition. Philadelphia, Mosby Year Book, Inc. May 1998.)

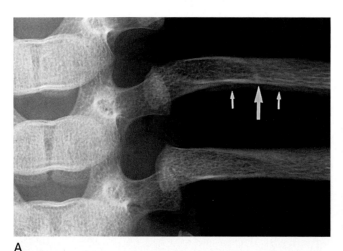

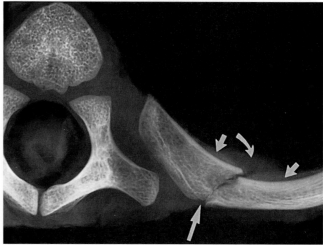

A   B

Figure 17–42

Rib neck fracture with early healing in a 2-month-old abused infant. *A,* Specimen radiograph of the left sixth and seventh ribs with vertebral articulations. A faint area of radiodensity crosses the left sixth rib *(large white arrow).* The fracture site appears to lie well lateral to the level of the transverse process. Note also the fine recent SPNBF *(small white arrows).* *B,* An axial specimen radiograph of the left seventh rib shows an oblique fracture through the rib neck *(long arrow).* Early SPNBF, approximately 7 to 10 days old, is noted only ventrally *(short arrows).* Note that the fracture appears to lie well lateral to the costotransverse process articulation. Radiolucent callus *(curved arrow)* is visible along the ventral (inner) aspect of the rib. (From Kleinman PK: Diagnostic Imaging of Child Abuse. 2nd Edition. Philadelphia, Mosby Year Book, Inc. May 1998.)

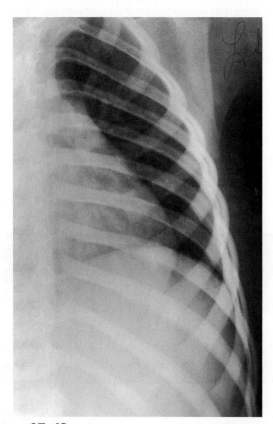

no fractures could be attributed to CPR in children with normal bones (Figs. 17–43 and 17–44).[22,86]

The major postulated mechanism for thoracic trauma is anteroposterior compression of the chest caused by shaking an infant. The typical posterior rib fracture, located on the inner surface of the rib opposite the costotransverse articulation, is most likely caused by anteroposterior compression.

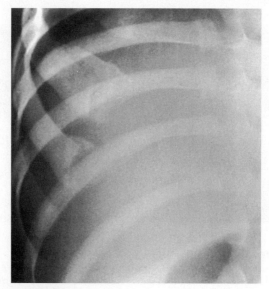

Figure 17–43

Healing rib fractures. Healed rib fractures in older children can be very subtle. Note the residual periosteal new bone which appears as a ridge. Abnormal contour and increased density are other findings that may be subtle. Bone scanning is an excellent method for further evaluation of questionable rib fractures when these represent the sole radiographic finding.

Figure 17–44

Costochondral fracture separations. This close-up view of anterior costochondral fractures shows splaying of the anterior aspect of ribs. Purely cartilaginous injuries will not be visible radiographically unless they have caused subperiosteal hemorrhage.

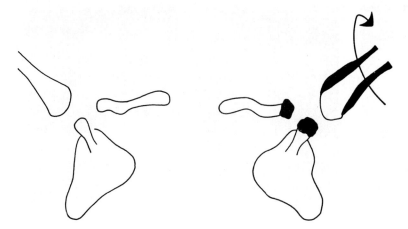

Figure 17–45
Chest injuries caused by arm twisting: diagrammatic representation. Rotatory forces exerted on the upper extremity may cause distal clavicular and acromial fractures.

Suffice it to say that to date much remains to be learned about the precise mechanisms of injury.

Clavicular Injuries The clavicle is the bone most commonly fractured during delivery, and clavicular fractures are quite common in accidental childhood injuries. By contrast, the clavicle is relatively rarely injured in child abuse (2% to 6%).[9] Although medial and lateral clavicular injuries are more likely to be seen with abuse than are midshaft fractures, the specificity of an isolated occult clavicular fracture for abuse is so low as to be almost useless in an ambulating child. Falling on the shoulder or breaking a fall with an outstretched hand may not be perceived by the child or parent as forceful enough to cause a fracture. Thus, these fractures may be truly accidental but unsuspected. When these patients are radiographed for persistent pain or a clavicular mass, the radiologist's discovery of a healing clavicular fracture should

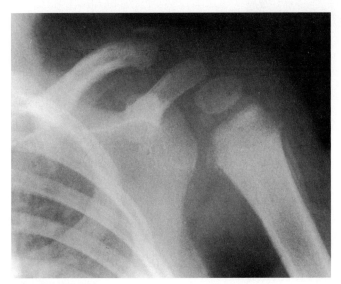

Figure 17–46
Classic findings of clavicular injuries in abuse. Note that the distal portion of the clavicle is avulsed. There is also periosteal new bone around the acromion and the distal left humerus.

not cause concern for abuse unless there is clinical suspicion (Figs. 17–45 and 17–46).

Distinguishing abuse from birth trauma is seldom a problem with a fractured clavicle. A clavicular fracture incurred during delivery invariably constitutes an isolated injury; documentation is usually available, and periosteal new bone is seen as early as 11 days.[4] By 1 month of age, mature callus is evident around the fracture site. Conversely, any clavicular fracture without periosteal new bone in an infant older than 2 weeks of age did not result from birth trauma. It must be noted that an acute, isolated clavicular fracture in an infant is very worrisome.

Acromial Injuries An important injury of the scapula in child abuse involves the acromion, a curved protrusion of bone arising from the scapular spine that serves as the tendinous insertion for several shoulder girdle muscles. This lesion is easily identified when specifically sought and is virtually pathognomonic for abuse.[54] As mentioned previously, the shoulder girdle is often injured when an upper extremity is used as a lever or handle to manipulate the child's body (Figs. 17–47 and 17–48).

Partial avulsion of bony fragments or complete fracture of the acromial process may occur. Although an acute injury may be invisible, periosteal new bone soon renders this lesion obvious on the frontal chest film or shoulder view (Table 17–5). An easy method of identification is to compare both acromial processes. In my experience, the lesion is usually unilateral and more often left sided. The asymmetry caused by periosteal new bone or residual deformity is easily discernible. Confident diagnosis requires careful scrutiny of and familiarity with this highly specific lesion. Normal variants may cause confusion and must be differentiated from true fractures.[16]

Other Scapular Injuries Less common but equally specific for abuse are other fractures to the scapula. A sudden force exerted on a ligamentous insertion may avulse portions of the coracoid, the inferior angle of the scapula, or portions of the glenoid.

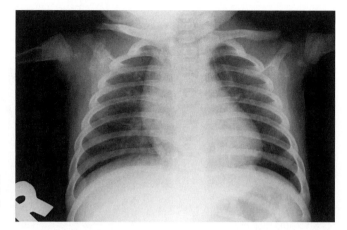

Figure 17–47
Acromial injury. This radiograph of the chest reveals a healing acromium on the left. No other injuries are present. This injury is highly specific for abuse. Side-to-side comparison makes the diagnosis with a certainty.

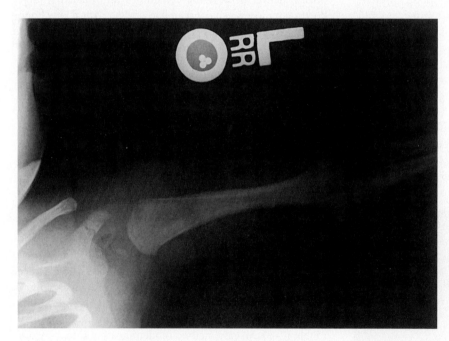

Figure 17–48
Acromial fracture. This infant has an acute acromial fracture. No periosteal new bone is evident. Multiple fractures were seen elsewhere.

TABLE 17-5 LIKELIHOOD TO BE THE ABUSER
1. New boyfriend
2. Father
3. Mother
4. Baby-sitter

Sternal Injuries Sternal fractures or sternomanubrial dislocations are rarely documented lesions that are nonetheless highly specific for abuse. These lesions are easily seen on scintigraphy but are invisible on a frontal view of the chest. Identification is often possible when the sternum is included on the lateral view of the thoracic spine, and this projection should be carefully scrutinized.

Injuries to the Spine Vertebral trauma is thought to be relatively rare in child abuse, although it is also possible that subtle abnormalities remain undetected.[57,89] The lateral view of the spine is optimal for detecting such abnormalities and is therefore included in a routine trauma survey. Injuries to the thoracic spine fall into three categories (Figs. 17–49 and 17–50).

1. *Compression fractures of the vertebral body.* Findings can range from severe compression of the anterior portion of the vertebral body to a subtle decrease in height that may be difficult to recognize. Sometimes the compression extends uniformly across the vertebral body, producing variable degrees of platyspondyly. Variations include a burst fracture of the thoracolumbar spine and a "hangman's fracture" in the cervical region. The relative instability of the thoracolumbar junction makes this location a common site for vertebral body abnormalities caused by forceful flexion of an abused infant.

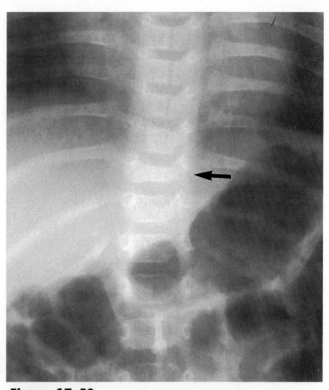

Figure 17–50
Vertebral fracture: compression fracture of T10 vertebra. Note asymmetric platyspondyly *(arrow)*. Without high–resolution spine films, this fracture might have been missed. Multiple rib fractures were also present.

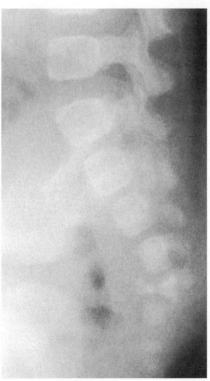

Figure 17–49
Vertebral fracture. A sacral fracture is evident in this abused child with multiple additional fractures.

2. *Disk herniation.* Herniation of the nucleus pulposus usually occurs into the anterosuperior portion of the vertebral body with concomitant loss of intervertebral disk height. The resulting abnormality has a characteristic appearance, with variable degrees of notching of the anterosuperior part of the vertebral body. This may be due to a growth disturbance due to involvement of the growth plate of the ring apophysis.

3. *Avulsion of the posterior elements.* Avulsion of cartilaginous and bony fragments of the spinous process can be identified on the lateral view of the spine. However, cartilaginous avulsions and paraspinal hematomas are not seen unless periostitis has formed.

Vertebral compression fractures and disk herniation are caused by an axial force exerted through the length of the spine (Fig. 17–51). Most children in the 18- to 24-month age range who have spinal injuries are ambulatory. The resulting radiographic changes, when not recognized as indications of abuse, are sometimes mistaken for infection, leukemic infiltration, or eosinophilic granuloma. No neurologic symptoms occur unless there is dislocation or the spinal cord or nerve roots have been injured by transection, contusion, or hemorrhage. MR imaging is the modality of choice for these children. The most common physical finding in vertebral

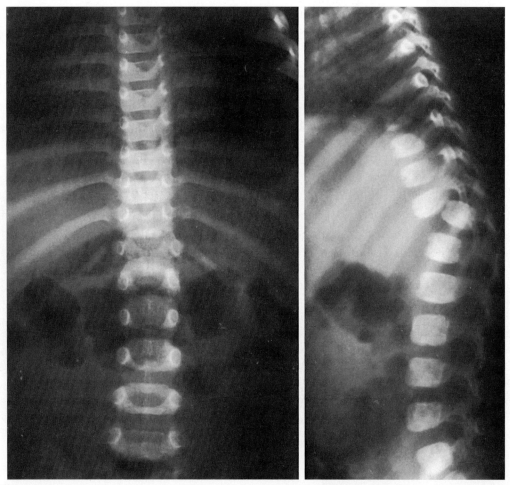

Figure 17–51
Vertebral fracture–dislocation: Fracture–dislocation of T11 on T12. This patient presented with a progressive inability to walk. Note the dislocation in the vicinity of the thoracolumbar junction.

trauma is unexplained kyphosis at or near the thoracolumbar junction. Rarely are these injuries seen in isolation, and a trauma survey usually documents additional fractures, thereby establishing the true diagnosis (Fig. 17–52).

SKELETAL SCINTIGRAPHY IN CHILD ABUSE

Some authorities have advocated skeletal scintigraphy as the primary method of investigation in questionable cases of abuse. They recommend that only scintigraphically questionable or abnormal areas be further evaluated radiographically. When supervised and interpreted by personnel who have a high level of experience and expertise, there is no doubt that the bone scan is more sensitive than the radiographic trauma survey.[40,84,88]

A drawback to the use of skeletal scintigraphy in young children is that adequate studies are technically very demanding.

High-quality images are obtained consistently only under the following conditions:

1. Adequate patient immobilization, sedation, or both are needed. (Heavy sedation is usually required in young children.)
2. Positioning is done without patient rotation.
3. Homologous joints that cannot be positioned neutrally must be imaged with the same degree of joint rotation, flexion-extension, and abduction-adduction.
4. A high-resolution technique must be used (i.e., 3-mm pinhole collimator views).
5. Adequate densities (i.e., counts per square centimeter) are obtained.
6. Separate images of the diaphysis and the metaphysis are obtained to exclude the presence of metaphyseal corner fractures.

The primary theoretical problem with scintigraphic examination is that metaphyseal fractures located at the ends of actively growing bone lie in regions of maximal normal radionuclide uptake. Despite these problems, if high-quality

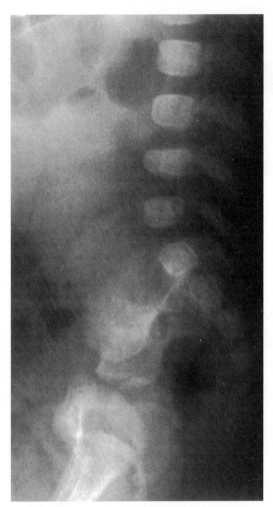

Figure 17–52
Vertebral injuries. Note platyspondyly.

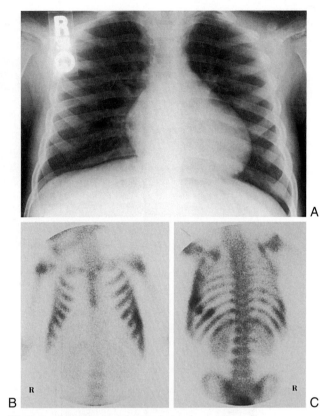

Figure 17–53
Skeletal scintigraphy in abuse. *A,* Frontal chest film showing bilateral small, focal pleural effusions. Scintigraphy performed in the anterior *(B)* and posterior *(C)* projection reveals multiple bilateral rib fractures.

images can be obtained consistently, the accuracy of bone scans should supersede or at least equal that of radiographs in the diagnosis of child abuse[22] (Fig. 17–53).

The bone scan often detects many more fractures in the central skeleton, as acute rib fractures and chondral injuries may be invisible on plain films. A negative result on a technically poor bone scan is not acceptable, because on such a scan, pathognomonic metaphyseal injuries may be missed.

Radiography is used as a primary imaging modality. Scintigraphic examination is used as a supplemental procedure (1) if the sole radiographic finding is focal pleural thickening, suggesting that acute but occult rib fractures (scintigraphically demonstrable) have caused pleural bleeding, (2) if only a single fracture, which is very suggestive of abuse, is present and if the presence of additional unrecognized skeletal trauma would simplify testimony, and (3) on very rare occasions when clinical suspicion is exceedingly high but all test results, including those on radiographs, are negative, and a positive bone scan would permit the child to be removed from a presumptively dangerous home (Fig. 17–54).

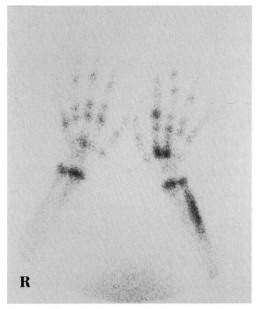

Figure 17–54
Metacarpal fractures; scintigraphy. Increased radioisotope uptake is present in the distal left ulna, the proximal second and third metacarpals, and the proximal phalanx of the index finger of the left hand.

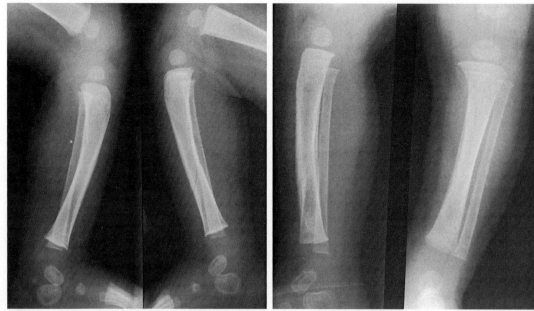

Figure 17–55

Acute distal tibial fracture. *A,* The lateral view demonstrates a sharp, oblique fracture line in a 2-month-old infant. The injury was 48 hours old. The normal leg is shown for comparison. *B,* 28-day-old tibial fracture. The frontal and lateral views *(right)* demonstrating moderate periosteal new bone best seen posteromedially. The fracture edge has become markedly unclear.

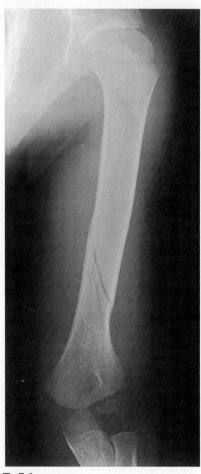

Figure 17–56

Spiral humeral fracture in an abused infant. The injury was acute and clearly reveals a sharp fracture line. Acute fractures have very sharp edges and appear as does broken glass.

The choice of plain films or skeletal scintigraphy as the primary method of examination is a matter of personal preference, expertise, and technical capability.

INJURY DATING BY SKELETAL RADIOGRAPHY

Precise dating of bony injury based on radiographic appearance can be important for establishing evidence that multiple episodes of skeletal trauma have occurred and for temporally defining a single assault or multiple assaults. Multiple fractures that occurred at different times have long been considered the most significant indication of child abuse. In the absence of some of the more pathognomonic injuries, the identification of multiple episodes of trauma is indeed very helpful in verifying the diagnosis of abuse. Such identification requires determination of the ages of the fractures.

Dating the injury is sometimes crucial in eliminating the possibility of abuse or identifying potential abusers. For instance, it is necessary if the child was temporarily in the care of someone other than the parents or, more commonly, if a man has joined the household of a previously single or divorced mother (Figs. 17–55 through 17–63).

Accurate radiographic dating is possible in acute or relatively new fractures, but such dating is less specific with old injuries. It is important that the radiologist date the injuries as accurately as possible, but it is equally important for all involved to understand the limitations of this procedure.

Text continued on page 610

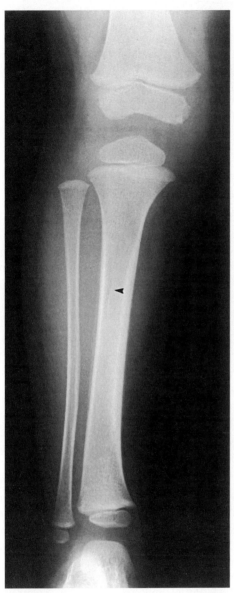

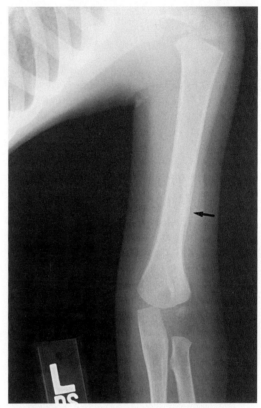

Figure 17–58
Periosteal new bone: relatively mature periosteal new bone 24 days after acute injury. Note the delicate stripe of periosteal new bone at the medial aspect of the humerus.

Figure 17–57
Toddler's fracture. This 3-year-old boy presented with a limp of several days' duration. This frontal film of the right tibia shows minimal periosteal new bone along the lateral tibial shaft. The spiral tibial fracture is not visible on this radiograph. Lucency just proximal to the mid–diaphysis *(arrowhead)* represents the normal nutrient canal. Because the possibility of osteomyelitis could not be excluded with confidence, a bone scan was performed (not shown), demonstrating the oblique fracture and excluding the possibility that the periostitis was due to hematogenous infection typically seen in the metaphysis.

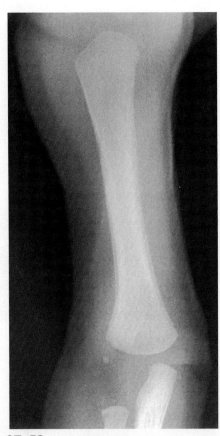

Figure 17–59
Periosteal new bone in a 20-day-old injury. Definite and relatively thick periosteal new bone is apparent.

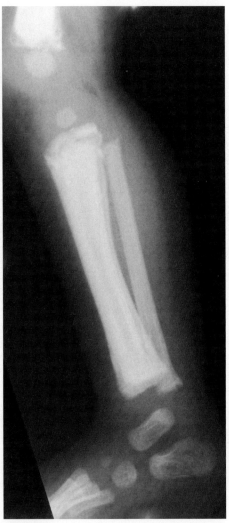

Figure 17–60
Periosteal new bone in an 8-week-old injury. The amount of elevated periosteum is extensive. The entire tibia is denser than normal because there was repetitive injury.

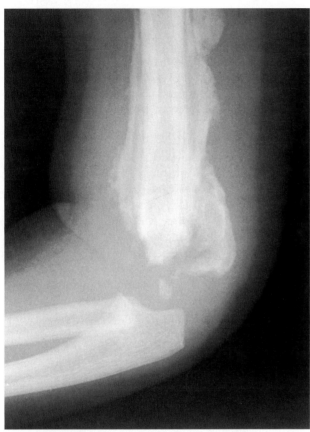

Figure 17–61
Periosteal new bone. This injury incurred a large amount of bleeding and therefore there is exuberant callus. The injury was 3 months old.

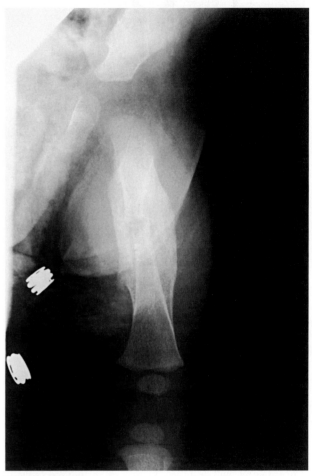

Figure 17–62
Fracture healing. Note that there is a large amount of periosteal new bone. However, it is well contained. The injury was 3-1/2 months old.

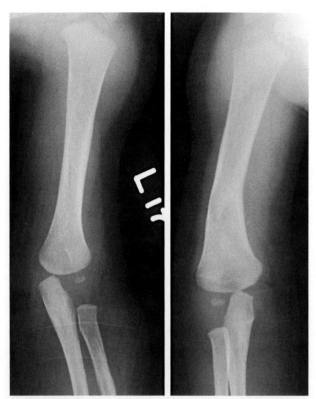

Figure 17–63
Healed humeral fracture: anteroposterior view of the left and right forearms in a girl suspected to have been abused. The obvious healed right humeral fracture shows significant diaphyseal and distal metaphyseal deformity. The oblique fracture line is still minimally visible. The injury was 4 months old.

The following discussion is a general guide to the sequence of radiographic findings in skeletal healing.

1 to 3 Days

With the initial injury, there is disruption of the normal sharp interface of muscle and subcutaneous fat planes, caused by diffuse edema of soft tissues. Frequently, the soft tissue abnormalities will not be obvious or even detectable by physical examination. If subperiosteal bleeding has occurred without distinct fracture, the soft tissue abnormalities will be the sole radiographic finding of abuse. If a fracture has occurred, its edges will be sharp. In fact, the sharpness of the fracture line is similar to that of the edge of a piece of shattered glass.

5 to 15 Days

Resorption around fracture lines makes the edge of the fracture less crisp and more indistinct. Hyperemia and associated osteoclastic activity will sometimes resorb enough bone to enable the radiologist to conclude with moderate certainty that the fracture is not acute but several days old. The indistinctness of a fracture line, however, is a subjective assessment that usually cannot be made with great confidence.

An unequivocal sign during this time period is calcification of subperiosteal hemorrhage, which appears as periosteal new bone. Subtle but definite periosteal new bone may be seen as early as 5 days in young infants. Generally, in older children, periosteal new bone is commonly seen by 1 week and should be present by 15 days after the injury. Rib fractures usually take slightly longer (15 to 20 days) to clearly show callus formation.

The definite presence of slight callus formation accurately indicates that the fracture is not acute and is probably between 1 and 2 weeks old.

15 Days to 6 Weeks

During this period, the callus formation becomes more mature and the fracture begins to remodel. Usually, it is impossible to date the fracture precisely during this period.

6 Weeks to 8 Months

During this period, remodeling of bone and incorporation of periosteal new bone into the growing skeleton takes place. A slightly asymmetric bone contour persists for several months, but this may not be obvious unless side-to-side comparisons are made. The rapidity with which bone remodeling occurs depends on the following factors:

1. *Age of the patient.* The younger the child, the more rapid are healing and remodeling.
2. *Nutritional status of the patient.* Suboptimal nutrition, which may be a factor in some abused infants and children, retards bone healing and remodeling.
3. *Lack of proper immobilization.* Most central and some extremity fractures that are incurred in child abuse are diagnosed retrospectively and therefore have not been treated with immobilization.[18]

Thus, residual deformity and exuberant callus formation are more common in untreated fractures than in properly casted injuries.

Skull fractures are notoriously difficult to date accurately because there is no periosteal new bone. The only criteria that are used are sharpness of the fracture edge and visibility of the fracture. Most fractures will be visible for a minimum of 6 weeks, and many can still be seen at 12 to 16 weeks, after which they may be invisible or persist for a variable time. Precise determination of the age of skull fractures is seldom possible.

The following rules are helpful in determining the age of fractures (Fig. 17–64):

1. A fracture without periosteal new bone is less than 7 to 12 days old depending on the quality of the film.
2. A fracture with definite but slight periosteal new bone is more than 10 days old.
3. A fracture with a large amount of periosteal new bone is more than 2 weeks old.

In conclusion, the dating of fractures is not a science and as such cannot be used to pinpoint the precise date of injury.

POSTMORTEM RADIOGRAPHY

It has been our practice to obtain postmortem radiographs on any child whose cause of death is unknown or uncertain. Cases from the coroner's office are transported to the radiology department, where postmortem radiographs are obtained under the direct supervision of a pediatric radiologist. High-detail technique and multiple views are used to obtain maximal information. Any abnormalities found on this examination are further evaluated by the pathologist during the autopsy. High-yield areas in infants under 1 year of age include the metaphyses around the shoulder, knee, and ankle. On several occasions, exhumation of a child's body has revealed unequivocal evidence of child abuse. If the diagnosis of abuse remains in question a forensic pathologist well versed in child abuse can confirm the diagnosis (Figs. 17–65 and 17–66).[97]

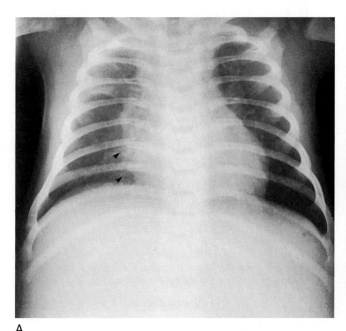

A

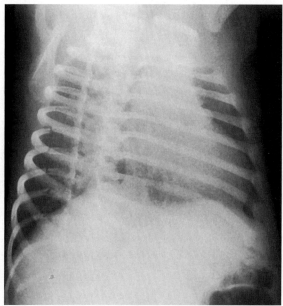

B

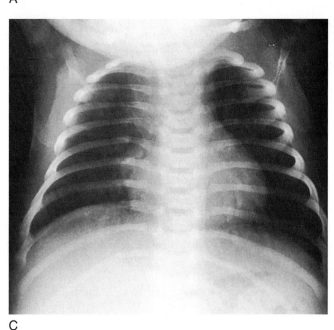

C

Figure 17–64

Rib fractures: sequence of healing. *A,* This appears to be a normal frontal chest radiograph of a 4-week-old infant until one appreciates the overlap of the right posterior seventh and eighth rib *(arrow). B,* An oblique view, done on the same day, demonstrates that the fifth through ninth ribs have been broken. The distance from the fifth to the ninth rib approximates the size of an adult fist. *C,* A radiograph taken 7 days later; the fractures are again difficult to appreciate. Periosteal new bone is not yet apparent.

Continued

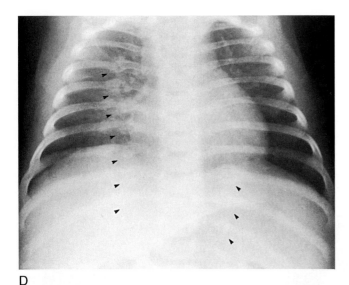

D

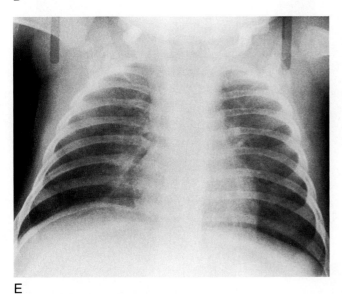

E

Figure 17–64—cont'd

D, A radiograph taken 10 days later; all the rib fractures are optimally visible because of moderate periosteal new bone. Also seen for the first time are healing posterior rib fractures of the ninth, tenth, and eleventh ribs on the left side *(arrows)* and fourth and tenth ribs on the right. *E,* A radiograph taken 56 days after *A* and *B;* the rib fractures are again difficult to see because of resorption of callus and bone remodeling. However, side–to–side comparison of the ribs clearly demonstrates asymmetry. Note that the lower rib fractures are the most difficult to appreciate on a light chest film. They are visualized optimally on a frontal view of the abdomen. Because the rate of healing is dependent on the rate of growth, the older the child, the longer the fractures remain visible.

DIFFERENTIAL DIAGNOSIS OF SKELETAL LESIONS

In the medical practice of pediatric radiology, the most common differential diagnosis for skeletal abuse is accidental

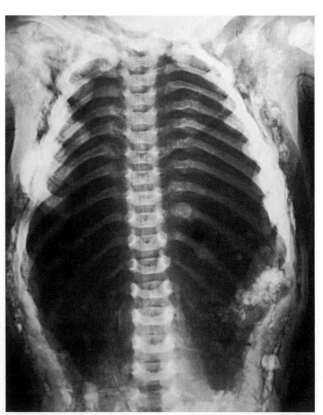

Figure 17–65
Postmortem radiography. This 2-year-old girl had supposedly died of sudden infant death syndrome; however, the grandparents demanded a criminal investigation with exhumation of the body for full evaluation. The right humerus had an acute fracture (not shown). Note the healing fractures of most thoracic ribs close to the costovertebral junction. These findings made conviction of the abuser possible.

injury. In related legal proceedings, however, the question of abnormal bones is an issue that is often raised. If the skeleton is radiographically abnormal (i.e., severe osteoporosis, rachitic changes, superimposed infection or tumor, skeletal dysplasia, or osteopetrosis), child abuse cannot be diagnosed radiographically with certainty. In those rare cases of possible abuse in children who have skeletal abnormalities that produce fragile bones, the diagnosis of abuse is preferably established clinically.

Conditions that can cause confusion with abuse include normal variants, metabolic abnormalities, infections, neoplasms, and miscellaneous entities; these are discussed in this section. Knowledge of these diseases is essential in the legal arena and occasionally useful in daily practice.

Normal Variants

Normal variants are described by Kleinman et al.[46] (based on postmortem high-detail radiography) and fall into four categories: spurring, beaking, metaphyseal step-off, and proximal tibial cortical irregularity.

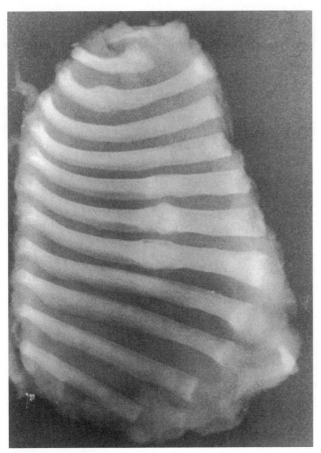

Figure 17–66
Postmortem radiography: dissection of the thorax. Note multiple rib fractures. High-quality, high-detail radiography should be performed by a radiologist, as coroner's offices rarely have the expertise and equipment to obtain optimal films. This is not an optimal film.

A normal spur is a continuous metaphyseal projection of bone that may be seen in the lateral aspect of the distal femur or in the radius, ulna, or metacarpals. This contour variation is not a separated fractured fragment as is seen in child abuse.

A beak is a well-defined, dense projection from the medial aspects of the humerus. Beaking of the proximal tibia is less well defined. The typical location, appearance, lack of cortical separation, and bilaterality (77%) differentiate beaking from corner fractures.

A metaphyseal step-off is an almost horizontal extension of cortical bone. The margins may be indistinct; involvement can be seen in the distal portion of the femur, radius, and ulna or proximal tibia. Bilaterality was seen in 44% of patients in Kleinman et al.'s study.

The tibia may demonstrate a focal, cortical irregularity medially and proximally.

Metabolic Abnormalities

Of all the metabolic diseases, rickets is the most frequently encountered, usually due to renal or, occasionally, biliary disease.

Rickets causes extensive osteoporosis, splaying of the metaphyses, and widening of the growth plate or physis. Invariably the renal or biliary disease is evident clinically (Fig. 17–67).

Osteogenesis Imperfecta

Osteogenesis imperfecta is an inherited disorder of connective tissue characterized by abnormal bone fragility with osteoporosis, defective dentition, presenile hearing impairment, and blue sclera.[1,43] Less common clinical features include easy bruising, fragile skin, hyperplastic healing, ligamentous laxity, short stature, wormian bones, progressive scoliosis, and premature vascular calcification[1] (Figs. 17–68, 17–69, and 17–70).

Osteogenesis imperfecta types I and II should be clinically apparent by the presence of blue sclera. Although the sclera are normal in type III osteogenesis imperfecta, there is severe osteoporosis and progressive deformity of long bones and spine. Wormian bones and typical clinical features help differentiate the milder forms of type III from injuries caused by abuse.

Type IV osteogenesis imperfecta, an autosomal dominant subtype, is very rare, and radiologic evaluation of the disease is limited.[1] Most patients demonstrate radiographic abnormalities, and those with mild disease in whom radiographs are normal can usually be identified by clinical findings (dentinogenesis imperfecta and hearing loss) or a positive family history. Problems can arise if the patient has a new dominant mutation of type IV osteogenesis imperfecta without clinical findings and with normal radiographs. This combination is highly unlikely, because the incidence of new mutations in type IV is between 1 and 3 per 1 million births. These statistics translate into a single child with the

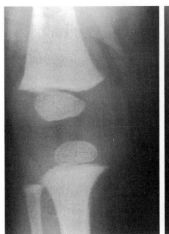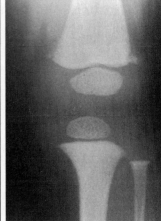

Figure 17–67
Renal osteodystrophy in a patient with renal failure caused by complications of prune-belly syndrome. Note the lateral ulnar metaphyseal avulsion. Severe osteoporosis indicates abnormal bones, precluding the confident diagnosis of abuse.

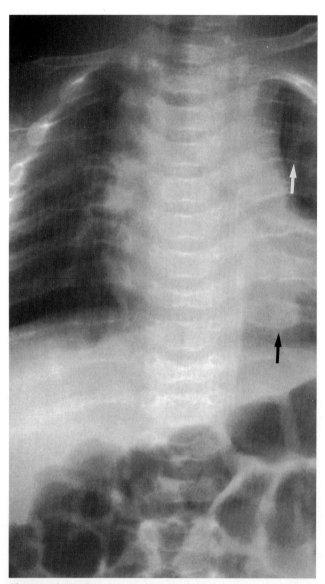

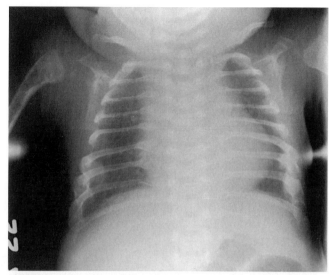

Figure 17–69
Osteogenesis imperfecta. The patient was a term newborn. Note multiple healing fractures of the ribs and distal humeri. Also seen is a healing acromial fracture on the left. The ribs are very thin and gracile and the bone density is diminished.

parents. Clinical symptoms include anorexia, pruritus, soft tissue swelling, coarse and sparse hair, hepatosplenomegaly, and digital clubbing. Periosteal new bone is present in a unique, characteristic, and symmetric distribution: the medial aspect of the ulnar diaphysis, the metatarsal diaphysis, and, less commonly, the clavicles, tibia, and fibula. An acute and chronic

Figure 17–68
Osteogenesis imperfecta in a 2-day-old boy with significant growth retardation. Note that the ribs are thin *(white arrow)* except where fractures have occurred *(black arrow)*. Note that most of the rib fractures exhibit significant healing. The thoracolumbar spine has extensive platyspondyly caused by compression fractures. Severe osteoporosis is present. This patient has osteogenesis imperfecta type II.

autosomal dominant mutation being born in a city with a population of 500,000 every 100 to 300 years.[10] Although these rare sporadic patients with normal bone density may be relatively susceptible to fracture, it is uncertain whether any resulting injuries mimic the typical fractures of child abuse and even whether fractures in osteogenesis imperfecta type IV occur in the absence of recognizable trauma.

Hypervitaminosis A

Toxic doses of vitamin A in childhood are usually administered orally as dietary supplements by well-meaning, misguided

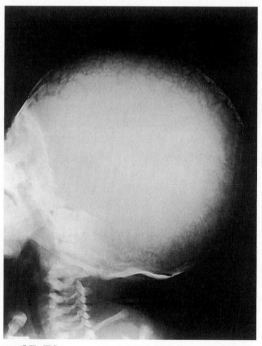

Figure 17–70
Osteogenesis imperfecta. Newborn infant with osteogenesis imperfecta. Note the multiple Wormian bones.

increase in cerebrospinal fluid results in splitting of cranial sutures. The split sutures and periosteal new bone may be mistaken either for cranial and osseous trauma in abuse or for systemic disease such as metastatic neuroblastoma or leukemia. Symmetric involvement, characteristic predilection for the ulna, and verification of excess vitamin intake differentiate hypervitaminosis A from other diseases.

Metastatic Malignancies

Metastatic neuroblastoma or leukemia can cause painful focal or diffuse destructive skeletal changes. There may be associated reactive new bone with a mixed lytic and blastic appearance. These changes result in abnormal bones whose etiology is easily distinguished from abuse. Isolated periosteal

new bone may be seen in such malignancies, and, when present, the major differential diagnostic considerations are osteomyelitis and trauma. Rarely, pancreatitis from pancreatic trauma in abuse may produce mixed lytic and blastic bony lesions that mimic neuroblastoma or leukemia.

Physiologic Periosteal New Bone

Physiologic periosteal new bone is a normal phenomenon seen in approximately one third of neonates younger than 3 months. The tibia, femur, and humerus are most commonly involved (Fig. 17–71). Spevak and Kleinman[21] performed a postmortem comparison between a group of 79 infants who died from sudden infant death syndrome and 20 infants who suffered fatal abuse. In the normal infants, the thickness of

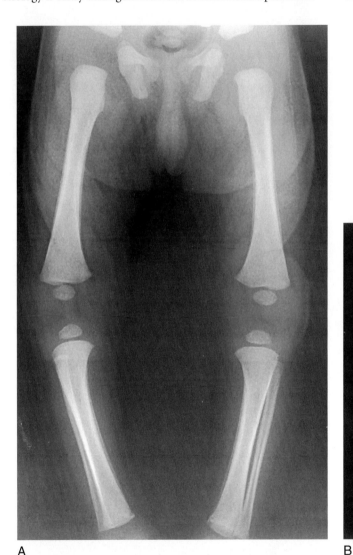

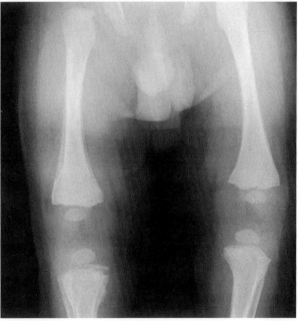

A   B

Figure 17–71

A, Differentiating physiologic periosteal new bone from other causes of periosteal new bone, namely child abuse. 1) Note that in physiologic periosteal new bone there is perfect asymmetry from side-to-side in terms of the thickness and the distribution of the periosteal new bone. 2) Physiologic periosteal new bone is seen up to 3 months of age. 3) Physiologic periosteal new bone should not exceed 1 mm of thickness. *B,* Periosteal new bone secondary to abuse in a 5-month-old girl. Note several diagnostic features: periosteal new bone varies in thickness when comparing the medial and lateral aspects of both femurs. Periosteal new bone along the lateral aspect of the right femur is greater than 1.8 mm. This infant is more than 3 months old. Note that metaphyseal injuries of both tibias are also diagnostic of abuse.

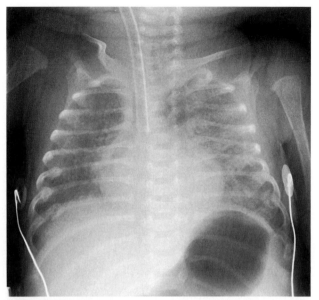

Figure 17–72
Bone disease of prematurity in an 8-week-old infant who initially had respiratory distress syndrome. Minimal changes of bronchopulmonary dysplasia are evident in the lungs. Furosemide (Lasix) was administered to treat a patent ductus arteriosum, and the infant was given chest physiotherapy for recurrent atelectasis. Note multiple healing rib fractures bilaterally; most easily seen are those in the right hemithorax on ribs 6, 7, and 8.

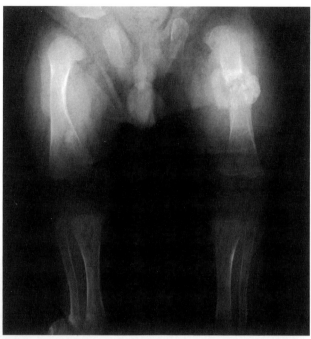

Figure 17–74
Bone disease of prematurity. The frontal view of both femora reveal a healing left femur with moderate-to-severe periosteal new bone. This finding was seen incidentally on an abdominal radiograph. At the time of its discovery it had become stable. It must be remembered that premature infants may have fractures which were incurred in the hospital rather than due to child abuse.

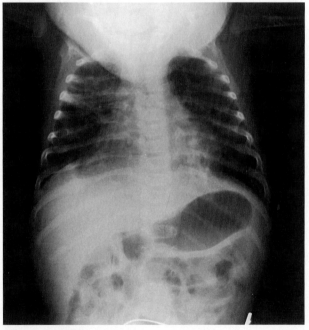

Figure 17–73
Bone disease of prematurity. Note multiple rib fractures and slightly decreased bone density. This premature infant underwent extensive hyperalimentation due to complications of necrotizing enterocolitis. Note that the rib fractures incurred in the hospital appear identical to those of physical abuse. Also noted is chronic pulmonary disease.

the periosteal reaction was usually 1 mm; a thickness of 1.8 mm was never seen. They concluded that normal infants older than 3 months did not demonstrate physiologic periosteal new bone and that a periosteal reaction greater than 1 mm in thickness was unlikely to represent a physiologic phenomenon.[87] In addition, it is important to note that normal periosteal new bone is bilaterally perfectly symmetric, whereas traumatic injuries almost never have this characteristic.

Bone Disease of Prematurity

Metabolic bone disease in premature infants results in moderate to severe demineralization and mild rachitic changes. Affected premature infants often require intubation because of respiratory distress syndrome or prolonged apnea. Segmental atelectasis is a common problem when these infants are weaned from the respirator or after extubation. Chest physiotherapy to relieve the atelectasis may cause multiple rib fractures that simulate those caused by abuse (Figs. 17–72, 17–73, and 17–74).

Complete healing of rib fractures usually occurs within 2 to 4 months after cessation of physical therapy. A history of prematurity, pulmonary disease, and chest physical therapy distinguish iatrogenic rib fractures from those of abuse.

Congenital Syphilis

Congenital syphilis may produce trophic changes of the entire skeleton, most commonly involving the metaphyseal regions. Symmetric involvement of the proximal humeri and distal femurs is common. The changes seen are metaphyseal irregularities, fragmentation, and periosteal new bone. Clinical signs include splenomegaly, rhinorrhea, rash, and anemia. Radiographic abnormalities can be present at birth but may not develop until 2 months after delivery, depending on the time of intrauterine infection. The symmetric skeletal involvement of congenital syphilis usually is not confused with abuse.

Neonatal Osteomyelitis

Neonatal osteomyelitis produces moderate to severe destructive changes with exuberant callus formation. Usually there is a single focus, but hematogenous infection may result in multiple lesions. The "moth-eaten" lytic lesions of osteomyelitis are almost always metaphyseal and can be distinguished from fractures by their lytic component. Abundant periosteal new bone may cause some confusion, but clinical differentiation between abuse and osteomyelitis is usually not a problem.

Prostaglandin Inhibitor Therapy

Prostaglandin inhibitors may be used in neonates with congenital heart disease that requires a patent ductus arteriosus for survival; prostaglandin E_1 prevents closure of the ductus arteriosus until palliative shunting or surgical correction is possible. The use of this drug frequently causes diffuse periosteal new bone formation along the ribs and long bones. The uniform, symmetric involvement of the skeleton and the clinical history make confusion with child abuse unlikely.

Schmid-like Metaphyseal Chondrodysplasia

Schmid-like metaphyseal chondrodysplasia is a hereditary disorder that frequently produces short stature, metaphyseal flaring, and irregularity.[11] The metaphyseal abnormalities are most marked in the femur and tibia. The spine in these patients is normal. To the unwary, the metaphyseal irregularity and spurring may be confused with child abuse, especially when one is viewing isolated films of the knee. The diagnosis is not clinically obvious during infancy. A family history of this disorder is helpful diagnostically, as is a complete trauma survey demonstrating the typical findings and their symmetry (Fig. 17-75).

Menkes' Kinky-Hair Syndrome

Menkes' kinky-hair syndrome is a rare disease of copper metabolism deficiency that results in severe retardation, seizures, hypotonia, failure to survive, and coarse hair (e.g., affected sheep produce an unacceptably poor grade of wool). Radiographic findings include metaphyseal spurring and wormian bones. The spurring may be confused with

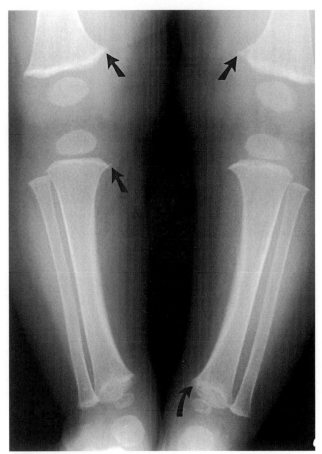

Figure 17–75

Schmid–like metaphyseal chondrodysplasia. Note marked metaphyseal irregularity *(arrow)*, which may be confused with a child abuse injury. A complete trauma survey will show symmetric metaphyseal flaring and irregularity that is most pronounced in the femur and tibia. A family history of short stature is helpful. (From Kleinman PK. Schmid–like metaphyseal chondrodysplasia simulating child abuse. AJR 156:576–578, 1991.)

a corner fracture, but the spur is not separated from the metaphysis. The presence of wormian bones and the clinical features of Menkes' kinky-hair syndrome make the distinction from child abuse apparent (Fig. 17-76).

OROPHARYNGEAL INJURIES

Oropharyngeal injuries are common in abused children, although they rarely come to the attention of the radiologist. Feeding a child is sometimes a volatile event as is dealing with the child's stools. The soft tissues of this region are bruised or torn by forceful insertion of foreign bodies, and occasionally, pharyngeal or esophageal perforations occur. Although spoons are commonly used during "forced feedings," I have seen a child whose esophagus was injured by a coat hanger and a 4-week-old girl who had the base of her

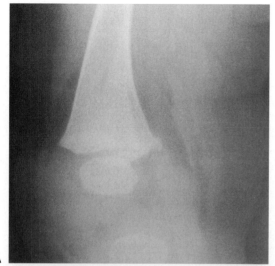

A

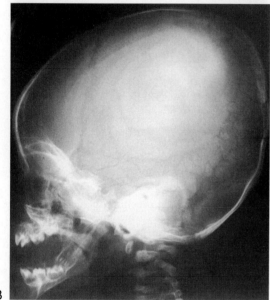

B

Figure 17–76
Menkes' kinky–hair syndrome. *A,* Metaphyseal spurring is seen in this rare disorder of copper metabolism. Particularly marked spurring of the medial aspect of the distal femur exists. However, the spur is not separated from the rest of the metaphysis. Distinguishing this from a healing reunited corner fracture caused by abuse may be difficult. *B,* Lateral view of the skull in the same patient showing extensive wormian bones (intrasutural bones).

tongue torn during a sexual assault by her father. Kleinman and Spevak[56] reported a 5-week-old boy with an esophageal perforation who initially presented with stridor resulting from airway obstruction.

VISCERAL INJURIES

Most children with visceral injuries present with strange symptoms, and frequently the diagnosis of abuse is made only with great difficulty.[44,67,71,74]

Although precise data are lacking, visceral injury is a common cause of death in child abuse. In children younger than 5 years, significant abdominal trauma related to accidents is extremely rare, except when children are struck by motor vehicles (a setting in which documentation is virtually always available). Thus, in the absence of such an accident, the finding of visceral trauma in a child younger than 5 years is highly suggestive of abuse. The average age of fatal visceral injury is 2 years, but children older than 5 years can be affected.

The precise mechanism of abdominal injury is often unknown, but it appears that most cases of visceral trauma result from a direct blow to the abdomen. This blow is most commonly delivered to the center of the abdomen, compressing the viscera against the spine. At greatest risk are the underlying duodenum, pancreas, mesentery, and left lobe of the liver.

The most significant problem in visceral injuries caused by abuse is that their magnitude is seldom appreciated. The absence of any external signs of abuse and the lack of a history of trauma can mislead the physician into believing that the child's vomiting, abdominal distention, and pain result from gastroenteritis, a urinary tract infection, or other medical disorder. The extent and often the presence of severe visceral damage are frequently appreciated only after hypotension, caused by blood loss or septic shock due to peritonitis, supervenes. Commonly a child with vague abdominal symptoms and no history of trauma presents at the emergency department. Abdominal disease requiring surgery may be unsuspected, because a variable period of well-being may precede the onset of circulatory collapse. Thus, the child may be sent home, only to return later in a moribund state.

A revealing accidental model for abdominal injury is the child with seat belt ecchymosis sustained during vehicular accidents.[81] The single lap belt is intended to immobilize the iliac crest of adult passengers. On a child, this belt usually crosses the midabdomen. A sudden blow to the abdomen is delivered as the child is catapulted forward against the fixed belt.

The most common injuries in a group of 59 children with seat belt ecchymoses resulting from immobilization with an adult lap belt involved the jejunum and duodenum. Some patients had partial or total small bowel transection and intramural hematoma formation. Mesenteric injury, when present, consisted of contusions and lacerations. Solid organ injury was most common in the liver, spleen, and pancreas. Bowel strictures, presumably owing to mesenteric injury, were noted 2 to 3 weeks following the accident.[20]

A series of 21 intestinal perforations in abused children demonstrated the following distribution: duodenum 30% and jejunum 60% just distal to the ligament of Treitz and 10% in the ilium. The average age of these children was 2 years.

Stomach

Perforation of the stomach is the most serious complication of gastric trauma in abuse.[10,24,77,94] When the injury occurs after a meal, gastric distention makes the organ more vulnerable to rupture. The most common site of perforation is the anterior gastric wall. Radiographic recognition is rarely a problem, as there is usually a massive pneumoperitoneum. Contrast studies to define the site of perforation are not indicated, because immediate surgery is required to prevent hypovolemic or septic shock (Figs. 17–77 and 17–78).

Another important entity, which is seen in child neglect rather than physical abuse, is acute gastric dilatation. This complication follows ingestion of a large meal in children who are chronically starved. If abundant food is made available, the child eats voraciously and then becomes severely ill, with abdominal distention, pain, and vomiting.[23,79] Early recognition of this complication and exclusion of gastric outlet obstruction ensure the institution of correct therapy: suction to decompress the atonic stomach and gradual resumption of small quantities of food thereafter; intravenous fluids may be needed to counteract systemic circulatory collapse. In many of these children, neglect may already be known to be an underlying problem, but sometimes acute gastric dilatation may be the first indication of chronic abuse by starvation.

Duodenum

An intramural hematoma is the most frequently documented small bowel injury in nonlethal cases of child abuse with abdominal trauma. Most commonly involved is the duodenum or proximal jejunum. Maximal damage occurs at the sites of small bowel fixation, the retroperitoneal duodenum, and the jejunum proximal to the ligament of Treitz.

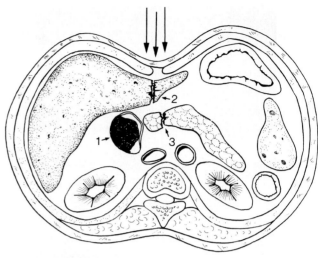

Figure 17–78
Distribution of visceral injuries from blunt abdominal trauma. A midline abdominal blow will compress the abdominal viscera against the spine, resulting in injury to the duodenum (1), left lobe of the liver (2), and pancreas (3). More laterally positioned blows may cause injury to the right lobe of the liver, the kidneys, the adrenal, and occasionally the spleen. Shearing forces generated by a direct blow or sudden deceleration will result in intestinal-mesenteric injuries. (From Kleinman PK: Diagnostic Imaging of Child Abuse. 2nd Edition. Philadelphia, Mosby Year Book, Inc. May 1998.)

The immobilized bowel is compressed between the anterior abdominal wall and the spine, typically resulting in a hematoma at the junction of the first and second portions of the duodenum.[23] The usual clinical symptoms are abdominal pain and vomiting; variable degrees of mechanical obstruction also occur (Figs. 17–79 and 17–80). Upper intestinal examination is helpful to diagnose and document this injury.[48,101] In the absence of accidental trauma, this finding is highly suggestive of abuse, and the injury should be documented for legal purposes. Occasionally, the importance of legal evidence is overlooked when the patient is improving, and clinical management would not be altered by imaging the gastrointestinal findings.

Plain films of the abdomen may be normal and show varying degrees of obstruction. Contrast examination of the duodenum reveals an intramural mass of variable size and extent that is typically located in the outer aspects of the curvature of the duodenum. Conservative treatment and exclusion of pancreatic injury constitute the current management of choice.

Mesentery

Mesenteric tears are a frequent postmortem finding in fatal cases of abuse. Avulsion of arteries and veins causes severe and usually fatal hemorrhage. Mesenteric contusion and thrombosis may result in bowel ischemia with pneumatosis intestinalis or portal venous gas. Stricture formation is another complication of bowel ischemia, which in the

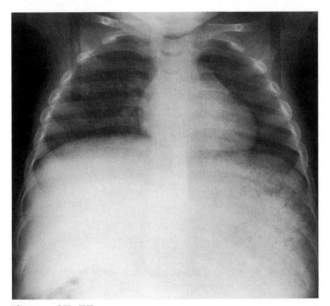

Figure 17–77
Overeating in a chronically starved child. Note the severe gastric dilatation in this 2-year-old child. After overeating, the child experienced abdominal pain and distention.

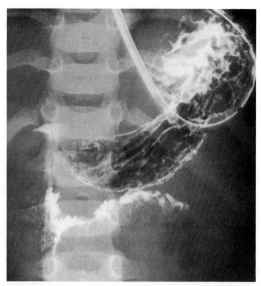

Figure 17–79
Duodenal hematoma in a 7-year-old abused child who presented with vomiting. This frontal view of the barium–filled stomach and duodenum demonstrates an extensive hematoma of the duodenum. The fixed retroperitoneal structures are those most frequently injured (duodenum and small bowel near the ligament of Treitz).

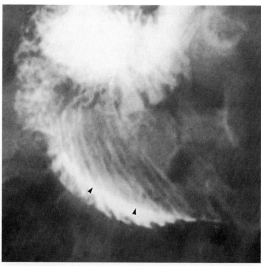

Figure 17–80
Proximal ileal hematoma. This small bowel spot film demonstrates the valvulae conniventes stretched over a large intramural hematoma (*arrowheads*) of the proximal ileum. The child had been kicked in the abdomen by the father.

accidental model occurs within 2 to 3 weeks of the traumatic event[19] (Figs. 17–81 and 17–82).

Liver

The liver is frequently injured, because it is susceptible to traumatic lacerations. The left lobe of the liver is especially vulnerable because it is pushed against the spine. In lethal cases of abuse, liver lacerations are common, resulting in substantial bile and blood spillage into the peritoneum. In milder injuries, hematomas remain subcapsular, and contusions often are undetected. Although CT is the imaging modality of choice, abdominal sonography affords adequate diagnosis and documentation of most complications, including free intraperitoneal fluid. It is interesting to note that rib fractures are rarely associated with hepatic injury,[8,34] presumably because the periumbilical blows avoid the bony thorax (Figs. 17–83 and 17–84).

Spleen

Although the spleen is frequently injured in accidental trauma, splenic injuries are rare in abuse. The reason for this is unclear.

Pancreas

Acute hemorrhagic pancreatitis with or without subsequent development of a pancreatic pseudocyst is a highly suggestive indicator of abuse if accidental injury and hereditary pancreatitis are excluded.[7,8,39,83,93] Imaging of pancreatitis and its complications is best accomplished with

sonography or CT. Percutaneous drainage of pancreatic pseudocysts has proven useful in children and is a good alternative to surgical intervention in selected patients.

Pancreatitis may cause periostitis with mixed lytic and blastic lesions in tubular bones of the lower extremities, particularly the feet. These changes, caused by osseous fat necrosis, may be associated with soft tissue swelling over the dorsum of the foot. Bony abnormalities have been identified from 2 to 10 weeks after the onset of abdominal symptoms.[9,13,35,70,76,82,85,102] Because the clinical symptoms of pancreatitis (abdominal pain, fever, and an abdominal mass) may lead to an erroneous search for leukemia, neuroblastoma, or infection, it is important to be aware of the similarities of osseous changes caused by this group of diseases and child abuse.

Adrenal Glands

Adrenal injury is seen in child abuse. For unknown reasons the right adrenal gland only is almost always involved. The presence these findings can indicate trauma.

Summary

Visceral trauma is frequently fatal in child abuse because the injuries are severe and often belatedly recognized. As soon as child abuse is suspected as a cause of abdominal signs and symptoms, pneumoperitoneum, hemoperitoneum, and peritonitis must be excluded, as the mortality rate is very high with these complications. Pancreatitis, pancreatic pseudocyst,

Text continued on page 623

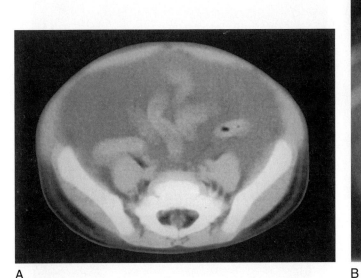

A

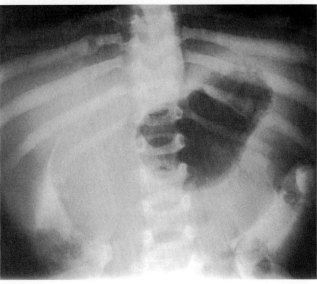

B

Figure 17–81

Bladder rupture. This 3-year-old male presented with abdominal distention and renal failure. *A,* A lengthy evaluation ensued and a CT was performed which revealed a large amount of fluid in the peritoneum. It is common for child abuse to present in strange ways because the true diagnosis of trauma is never revealed. *B,* A plain film of the abdomen revealed multiple rib fractures in different stages of healing. The father finally confessed and admitted that he kicked his son in the abdomen. The stomach and the bladder are more prone to rupture if they are distended at the time that the trauma occurs.

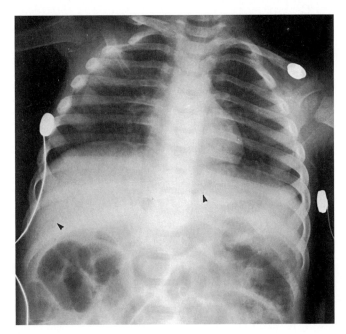

Figure 17–82

Mesenteric tears. This 3-year-old boy who presented to the emergency department with vague abdominal pain was diagnosed as having gastroenteritis. He returned 6 hours later with severe hypotension and abdominal distention. This radiograph shows dilated bowel, portal venous gas *(arrowheads),* and fractures of the seventh and eighth right posterior ribs at the costovertebral junction. Despite all efforts, circulatory collapse was irreversible, and the patient died.

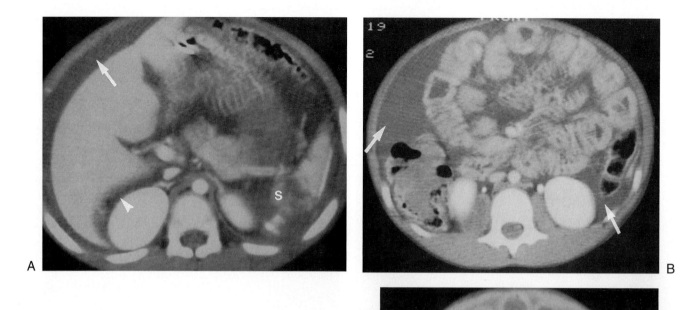

Figure 17–83
Hypovolemic shock and hemoperitoneum. *A,* A computed tomographic (CT) scan through the upper abdomen shows a fragmented spleen (S) and blood in the subphrenic *(arrow)* and subhepatic *(arrow)* spaces. *B,* A more caudal CT scan reveals a large volume of blood in the right and left paracolic gutters *(arrows)*. *C,* A scan through the lower abdomen demonstrates dilated small bowel with intensely enhancing walls and a large amount of blood.

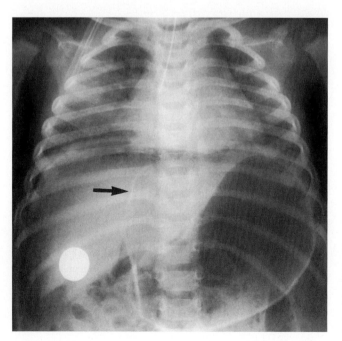

Figure 17–84
Gastric rupture. This 18-month-old abused girl was brought to the hospital moribund and could not be resuscitated. Autopsy revealed gastric rupture and severe peritonitis. Note extensive intraperitoneal air outlining the falciform ligament *(arrow)*.

and duodenal or hepatic hematomas should always suggest abuse unless a well-documented traumatic episode explains the findings. CT is the preferred imaging modality.

It is pointless and potentially hazardous to subject a critically ill child to a radiographic trauma survey. However, unless the diagnosis of abuse can be excluded on clinical grounds, skeletal examination should be performed when the child's condition is stable. Documentation of abdominal trauma by any imaging modality is also important. The need for legal proof may be overlooked by the physician caring for the moribund child whose course and treatment will remain unaltered by documentation. It is the policy at my institution to obtain postmortem trauma surveys of any child whose cause of death is uncertain. There have been several instances in which exhumation of the body and radiographic examination of the skeleton of abused children have provided sufficient legal evidence to obtain a criminal conviction.

INTRACRANIAL INJURY

The brain is the organ of greatest concern in nonaccidental trauma. Although skeletal injuries are important in diagnosing child abuse, they seldom result in permanent damage or functional impairment. By contrast, intracranial injuries are the major cause of death and significant permanent, neurologic, visual, and mental deficits. In one study, cerebral atrophy developed in all abused children who had abnormal CT findings at the time of initial diagnosis.[15,25,27,28,30,33,64]

CT and MR imaging have made it possible to assess acute and chronic brain injury accurately and noninvasively. CT is capable of detecting small amounts of fresh blood and therefore is the imaging modality of choice in children with acute head trauma. Although CT is capable of defining acute or subacute hemorrhage, MR imaging is superior for detecting very small amounts of subacute blood and hematoma residuals. In the subacute phase of injury, MR imaging can clarify questionable areas of hemorrhage identified on an initial CT scan (Fig. 17–85). MR imaging is also more sensitive for the detection of subtle focal and diffuse cerebral edema.

The sensitivity of MR imaging for detection of small quantities of breakdown products of blood makes it a useful tool in child abuse.[2,5,6,36,75,96,103,104] The content of methemoglobin in an intracerebral hemorrhage increases with time and produces a strong signal on T1-weighted images. This phenomenon is similar to callus formation in skeletal fractures. The amount of callus and the degree of remodeling clearly indicate multiple fractures in different stages of healing, just as the documentation of separate episodes of intracranial hemorrhage clearly points toward abuse as the cause of the abnormality (Figs. 17–86 through 17–89).

A conservative estimate of the incidence of symptomatic head trauma in cases of child abuse is 25%. Approximately one tenth of all neurologic disease in children is caused by abuse,[55] but this figure rises to 64% in infants younger than 11 months of age in whom acute head trauma is identified on CT or clinical examination.[22] Approximately 40% of battered children have ocular involvement, most commonly retinal hemorrhage, periorbital edema, retinal detachment, and lens subluxation. Permanent visual defects are frequent in such children.

Many authorities believe that retinal hemorrhages in children who are older than neonates but younger than 3 years of age are pathognomonic for abuse. Other forms of head trauma, including automobile accidents, show a conspicuous absence of this lesion. Unfortunately, 15% to 30% of retinal hemorrhages occur at the time of delivery, making this finding less useful in the neonatal period (Fig. 17–90).

Although much remains to be learned about the precise mechanisms of neurologic injury, shaking of the crying child "until it stops" is a mechanism described by abusers in numerous testimonies. The cause of calvarial fractures is less certain, but they obviously reflect a direct impact to the skull.

Plain skull radiography is an important part of imaging in child abuse, because it can document that trauma occurred. Skull fractures are often missed with CT, MR imaging, and skeletal scintigraphy. Thus, plain films of the calvarium are needed to supplement all of these imaging modalities. CT bone windows are a helpful addition to document fractures or split sutures, but a skull fracture parallel with the plane of section may be missed.

Kleinman[8] divided skull fractures into simple and complex. A simple fracture is a single line, no more than 2 mm wide, that is straight, curved, or jagged and is confined to one bone in the calvarium. Thus, simple fractures do not cross sutures or synchondroses and are not diastatic or depressed. Complex fractures are composed of more than one fracture line that may branch or radiate from a single point. Isolation of a fracture fragment in a complex injury is termed a *comminuted fracture* and carries with it the potential complication of a displacement of the fragment into the brain (*depressed fracture*). A *compound fracture* is a fracture associated with a laceration of the scalp. Subgaleal hematomas may be produced when the abuser pulls the child's hair or delivers a blow to the head (Figs. 17–91, 17–92, and 17–93). Both accidental injuries and child abuse can result in simple skull fractures, which are most commonly seen in the parietal bone. One important difference is that skull fractures are very rare (2%) in accidental injury[8] and common (10% to 38%) in abuse. Second, 95% of accidentally incurred fractures are simple, whereas 79% of fractures caused by abuse are complex. Finally, accidentally incurred skull fractures are almost never associated with intracranial injury, whereas those caused by child abuse have a high (65%)[8] correlation.

Although skull fractures are important, their absence does not exclude serious neurologic injury. Retrospective analyses of abused children show that intracranial injury is more

Text continued on page 627

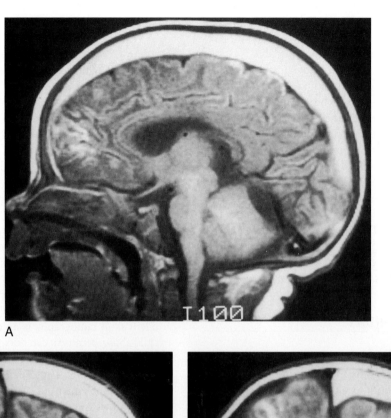

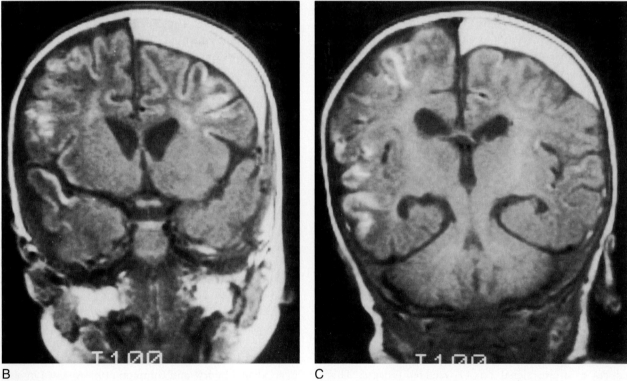

Figure 17–85

Child abuse: subdural hematoma. These magnetic resonance (MR) images are from a 15-month-old abused girl with a large, left-sided subdural hematoma. *A*, A parasagittal image to the left reveals a subdural hematoma and petechial hemorrhage anteriorly and in the parieto-occipital region. *B*, The coronal image shows cortical hemorrhage over both convexities as well as in the right temporal lobe. *C*, Minimal mass effect is seen on the left.

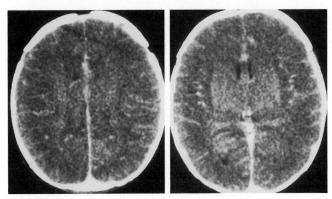

Figure 17–86
Child abuse: interhemispheric subdural hematoma. These nonenhanced, computerized axial tomographic scans through the supratentorial region demonstrate the typical appearance of interhemispheric blood. Note the dense stripe of blood, which is thicker than the normal falx and has more irregular edges. Ventricular compression and effacement of the gyri indicate diffuse edema.

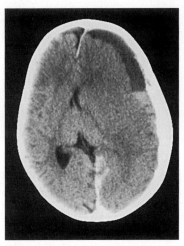

Figure 17–88
Child abuse: interhemispheric subdural hematoma and mass effect. Note the gyral effacement and the horizontal fluid interface, the latter caused by breakdown of blood products, a recurrent hemorrhage, or, less likely, a low hematocrit level.

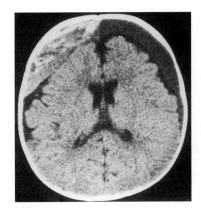

Figure 17–87
Child abuse: chronic and acute or subacute subdural hematoma. This MR image shows a chronic subdural hematoma on the left and a more recent episode of hemorrhage on the right, thus documenting two separate episodes of cranial trauma.

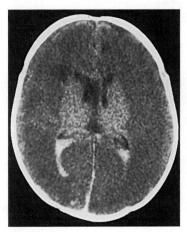

Figure 17–89
Child abuse: reversal sign. Acute injury has caused diminished density of the cortical gray and white matter, which contrasts with unaffected structures such as the thalamus, brain stem, and cerebellum. Note interhemispheric, subdural blood and blood in the dependent portion of the ventricles.

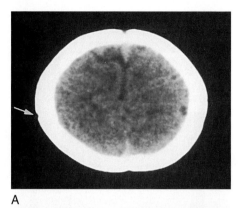

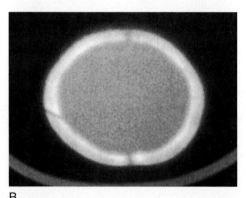

Figure 17–90

Child abuse: skull fracture computerized tomography scan. A, Note the small notch *(arrow)*. Normal sutures cannot account for this subtle finding. B, This bone window scan clearly shows a skull fracture. The brain of this abused child was otherwise normal.

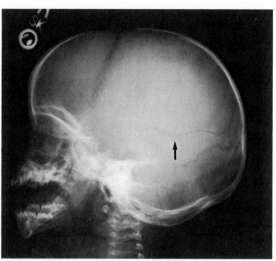

Figure 17–92

Child abuse: complex skull fracture with increased intracranial pressure. This 2-year-old boy had skeletal evidence of abuse. A linear fracture is seen in the parieto–occipital region. The anterior portion of the fracture crosses the squamosal suture, and posteriorly the fracture branches. The coronal and lambdoid sutures are split, indicating increased intracranial pressure.

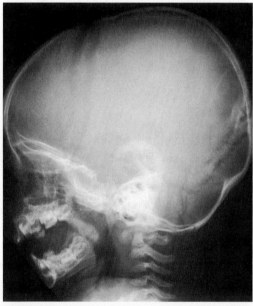

Figure 17–91

Child abuse: split sutures. In this lateral view of the skull of a 5-month-old infant with severe seizures, the coronal sutures are markedly separated. It should be noted that unless bone window scans are done with computerized tomography, split sutures and skull fractures may be missed. Plain skull films therefore play a significant role in defining cerebral abnormalities that are of uncertain origin noted on computerized tomography.

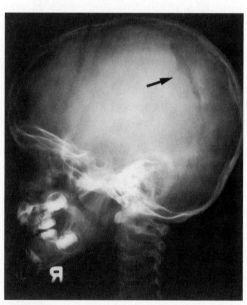

Figure 17–93

Child abuse: leptomeningeal cyst as a delayed sequela of an occipital skull fracture secondary to abuse. Note the scalloped, widened fracture margins *(arrow)*. A dural defect caused herniation of arachnoid and cerebrospinal fluid through the bony defect. Surgical repair was necessary.

commonly seen with an intact calvarium than with an associated fracture (78% versus 65%).[3] This is especially true for subarachnoid hemorrhage.

Subdural hematomas result from the tearing of veins that run from the brain surface to large superficial venous structures such as the superior sagittal sinus. Movement of the brain substance within the confines of the calvarium, as produced by shaking or deceleration in blunt trauma, ruptures these bridging veins, resulting in hemorrhage into the interhemispheric subdural space. Blood may then dissect the subdural space over the cerebral convexities. An interhemispheric subdural hematoma is often unilateral and is most commonly identified on CT in the posterior interhemispheric space as an increased density that is broader, slightly more irregular, and more ill defined laterally than the pristine, sharply marginated falx. One study demonstrated this finding in 65% of abused infants with acute head injury.[25] Epidural hemorrhage is unusual in abuse.

Contusion is the most common brain injury in child abuse. On CT, parenchymal injuries may appear isodense or of high or low density, depending on the relative extent of hemorrhage and edema. Parenchymal lesions of low density may represent ischemic infarcts.

Cerebral edema may be generalized or focal; when diffuse, it may be recognized by compression or obliteration of the ventricles and cisternal spaces.[12,14,25] Early, diffuse edema may cause indistinctness of the gray-white matter interface. Severe, diffuse edema produces diminished density of the gray and white matter, which contrasts with the high density of the unaffected cerebellum, brainstem, and thalamus. This phenomenon has been called the *reversal sign*.[8]

Focal edema is more readily visible than mild diffuse edema and may cause a mass effect. Ipsilateral ventricular compression, obliteration of the cortical sulci and cisterns, and a midline shift may result. It is important to understand that a normal CT scan may be seen soon after injury in children with neurologic damage of sufficient magnitude to cause death. The patient may expire before abnormalities become visible or a repeat scan is performed.

REFERENCES

1. Ablin DS, Greenspan A, Reinhart M, et al. Differentiation of child abuse from osteogenesis imperfecta. AJR 154:1035–1046, 1990.
2. Alexander RC, Schor DP, Smith WL Jr. Magnetic resonance imaging of intracranial injuries from child abuse. J Pediatr 109:975–979, 1986.
3. American Association for Protecting Children, Inc. Highlights of official child neglect and abuse reporting 1983. Denver: The American Humane Association, 1985, pp 1–36.
4. Anderson WA. The significance of femoral fractures in children. Ann Emerg Med 11:174–177, 1982.
5. Ball WS Jr. Nonaccidental craniocerebral trauma (child ab use): MR imaging. Radiology 173:609–610, 1989.
6. Billmire ME, Meyers PA. Serious head injury in infants: Accident or abuse? Pediatrics 75:340–342, 1985.
7. Blauvelt H. A case of acute pancreatitis with subcutaneous fat necrosis. Br J Surg 34:207–208, 1946.
8. Boswell SH, Baylin GJ. Metastatic fat necrosis and lytic bone lesions in a patient with painless acute pancreatitis. Radiology 106:85–86, 1973.
9. Caffey J. Multiple fractures in the long bones of infants suffering from chronic subdural hematoma. AJR 56:163–173, 1946.
10. Case MES, Nanduri R. Laceration of the stomach by blunt trauma in a child: A case of child abuse. J Forensic Sci 28:496–501, 1983.
11. Chadwick DL. Child abuse. JAMA 235:2017–2018, 1976.
12. Chakeres DW, Bryan RN. Acute subarachnoid hemorrhage in vitro comparison of magnetic resonance and computed tomography. AJNR 7:223–228, 1986.
13. Cohen H, Haller JO, Friedman AP. Pancreatitis, child abuse, and skeletal lesions. Pediatr Radiol 10:175–177, 1981.
14. Cohen RA, Kaufman RA, Myers PA, et al. Cranial computed tomography in the abused child with head injury. AJR 146:97–102, 1986.
15. Craft AW, Shaw DA, Cartlidge NEF. Head injuries in children. Br Med J 4:200–203, 1972.
16. Cumming WA. Neonatal skeletal fractures. Birth trauma or child abuse? J Can Assoc Radiol 30:30–33, 1979.
17. DeLee JC, Wilkins KE, Rogers LF, et al. Fracture–separation of the distal humeral epiphysis. J Bone Joint Surg 62A:46–51, 1980.
18. DeSmet AA, Kuhns LR, Kaufman RA, et al. Bony sclerosis and the battered child. Skeletal Radiol 2:39–41, 1977.
19. Dunbar JS, Owen HF, Nogrady MB, et al. Obscure tibial fracture of infants the toddler's fracture. J Can Assoc Radiol 15:136–144, 1964.
20. Edwards DK. The battered child: Your day in court. In Gosink BB, ed. Syllabus of 12th Annual San Diego Postgraduate Radiology Course. San Diego: University of California, San Diego, 1987, pp 47–59.
21. Ellerstein NS. The cutaneous manifestations of child abuse and neglect. Am J Dis Child 133:906–909, 1979.
22. Feldman KW, Brewer DK. Child abuse, cardiopulmonary resuscitation, and rib fractures. Pediatrics 73(3):339–342, 1984.
23. Franken EA, Fox M, Smith JA, et al. Acute gastric dilatation in neglected children. AJR 130:297–299, 1978.
24. Fulcher AS, Das Narla L, Brewer WH. Gastric hematoma and pneumatosis in child abuse. AJR 155:1283–1284, 1990.
25. Gentry LR, Godersky JC, Thompson B, et al. Prospective comparative study of intermediate–field MR and CT in the evaluation of closed head trauma. AJR 150:673–682, 1988.
26. Hamlin H. Subgaleal hematoma caused by hair–pull. JAMA 205:314, 1968.
27. Harley RD. Ocular manifestations of child abuse. J Pediatr Ophthalmol Strabismus 17:5–13, 1980.
28. Harwood–Nash DC. Craniocerebral trauma in children. Curr Probl Radiol 3(3):3–42, 1973.
29. Helfer RE, Slovis TL, Black M. Injuries resulting when small children fall out of bed. Pediatrics 60:533–535, 1977.
30. Hesselink JR, Dowd CF, Healy ME, et al. MR imaging of brain contusions: A comparative study with CT. AJNR 9:269–278, 1988.
31. Hight DW, Bakalar HR, Lloyd JR. Inflicted burns in children: Recognition and treatment. JAMA 242:517–520, 1979.
32. Jaffe AC, Lasser DH. Multiple metatarsal fractures in child abuse. Pediatrics 60:642–643, 1977.
33. James HE. The neurosurgeon and the battered child. Surg Neurol 2:415–418, 1974.
34. Kaufman RA, Babcock DS. An approach to imaging the upper abdomen in the injured child. Semin Roentgenol 19:308–320, 1984.
35. Keating JP, Shackelford GD, Shackelford PG, et al. Pancreatitis and osteolytic lesions. J Pediatr 81:350–353, 1972.
36. Kelly AB, Zimmerman RD, Snow RB, et al. Head trauma: Comparison of MR and CT experience in 100 patients. AJNR 9:699–708, 1988.

37. Kempe CH, Silverman FN, Steele BF, et al. The battered–child syndrome. JAMA 181:105–112, 1962.
38. Kennedy PC. Traumatic separation of the upper femoral epiphysis: A birth injury. Am J Roentgenol Rad Ther Nucl Med 51:707–719, 1944.
39. Kilman JW, Kaiser GC, King RD, et al. Pancreatic pseudocysts in infancy and childhood. Surgery 55:455–461, 1964.
40. Kimmel RL, Sty JR. 99mTc–methylene diphosphonate renal images in a battered child. Clin Nucl Med 4:166–167, 1979.
41. Kleinman PK. Diagnostic Imaging of Child Abuse. Philadelphia: Williams & Wilkins, 1987.
42. Kleinman PK. Diagnostic imaging in infant abuse. AJR 155:703–712, 1990.
43. Kleinman PK. Differentiation of child abuse and osteogenesis imperfecta: Medical and legal implications. AJR 154:1047, 1990.
44. Kleinman PK. Schmid–like metaphyseal chondrodysplasia simulating abuse. AJR 156:576–578, 1991.
45. Kleinman PK, Akins CM. The "vanishing" epiphysis: Sign of Salter type I fracture of the proximal humerus in infancy. Br J Radiol 55:865–867, 1982.
46. Kleinman PK, Belanger PL, Karellas A, et al. Normal metaphyseal radiologic variants not to be confused with findings of infant abuse. AJR 156:781–783, 1991.
47. Kleinman PK, Blackbourne BD, Marks SC, et al. Radiologic contributions to the investigation and prosecution of cases of fatal infant abuse. N Engl J Med 320:507–711, 1989.
48. Kleinman PK, Brill PW, Winchester P. The resolving duodenal–jejunal hematoma in abused children. Radiology 160:747–750, 1986.
49. Kleinman PK, Marks SC, Adams VI, et al. Factors affecting visualization of posterior rib fractures in abused infants. AJR 150:635, 1988.
50. Kleinman PK, Marks SC, Blackbourne B. The metaphyseal lesion in abused infants: A radiologic–histopathologic study. AJR 146:895–905, 1986.
51. Kleinman PK, Marks SC, Spevak MR, et al. Extension of growth–plate cartilage into the metaphysis: A sign of healing fracture in abused infants. AJR 156:775–779, 1991.
52. Kleinman PK, Marks SC Jr, Spevak MR, et al. Fractures of the rib head in infant abuse. Radiology 185:119–123, 1992.
53. Kleinman PK, Raptopoulos VD, Brill PW. Occult nonskeletal trauma in the battered–child syndrome. Radiology 141:393–396, 1981.
54. Kleinman PK, Spevak MR. Variations in acromial ossification simulating infant abuse in victims of sudden infant death syndrome. Radiology 180:185–187, 1991.
55. Kleinman PK, Spevak MR. Soft tissue swelling and acute skull fracture. J Pediatr, 121:737–739, 1992.
56. Kleinman PK, Spevak MR, Hansen M. Mediastinal pseudocyst caused by pharyngeal perforation during child abuse. AJR 158:1111–1113, 1992.
57. Kleinman PK, Zito JL. Avulsion of the spinous processes caused by infant abuse. Radiology 15:389–391, 1984.
58. Kogutt MS, Swischuk LE, Fagan CJ. Patterns of injury and sig–nificance of uncommon fractures in the battered child syndrome. AJR 121:143–149, 1974.
59. Kravitz H, Driessen G, Gomberg R, et al. Accidental falls from elevated surfaces in infants from birth to one year of age. Pediatrics 44(suppl):869–876, 1969.
60. Lauer B, Broeck ET, Grossman M. Battered child syndrome: Review of 130 patients with controls. Pediatrics 54:67–70, 1974.
61. Mayer T, Walker ML, Johnson DG, et al. Causes of morbidity and mortality in severe pediatric trauma. JAMA 245:719–721, 1981.
62. McCort J, Vaudagna J. Visceral injuries in battered children. Radiology 82:424–428, 1964.
63. Merten DF, Kirks DR, Ruderman RJ. Occult humeral epiphyseal fracture in battered infants. Pediatr Radiol 10:151–154, 1981.
64. Merten DF, Osborne DRS. Craniocerebral trauma in the child abuse syndrome: Radiological observations. Pediatr Radiol 14:272–277, 1984.
65. Merten DF, Radkowski MA, Leonidas JC. The abused child. A radiological reappraisal. Radiology 146:377–381, 1983.
66. Meyer RJ, Roelofs HA, Bluestone J, et al. Accidental injury to the preschool child. J Pediatr 63:95–105, 1963.
67. Mukherji SK, Siegel MJ. Rhabdomyolysis and renal failure in child abuse. AJR 148:1203–1204, 1987.
68. National Safety Council. Accident Facts, 1989.
69. Oliver JE, Cox J, Buchanan A. The extent of child abuse. In Smith SM, ed. The Maltreatment of Children. Baltimore: University Park Press, 1979, p 121.
70. Pena SDJ, Medovy H. Child abuse and traumatic pseudocyst of the pancreas. J Pediatr 83:1026–1028, 1973.
71. Rimer RL, Roy S III. Child abuse and hemoglobinuria. JAMA 238:2034–2035, 1977.
72. Rivara FP. Epidemiology of childhood injuries. Am J Dis Child 136:399–405, 1982.
73. Rivara FP, Kamitsuka MD, Quan L. Injuries to children younger than one year of age. Pediatrics 81:93–97, 1988.
74. Rosenberg HK, Gefter WB, Lebowitz RL, et al. Prolonged dense nephrograms in battered children. Urology 21:325–330, 1983.
75. Sato Y, Yuh WTC, Smith WL, et al. Head injury in child abuse: Evaluation with MR imaging. Radiology 173:653–657, 1989.
76. Scarpelli DG. Fat necrosis of bone marrow in acute pancreatitis. Am J Pathol 32:1077–1087, 1956.
77. Schechner SA, Ehrlich FE. Gastric perforation and child abuse. J Trauma 14:723–725, 1974.
78. Scherz RG. Fatal motor vehicle accidents of child passengers from birth through four years of age in Washington state. Pediatrics 68:572–575, 1981.
79. Shulman BH, Evans HE, Manvar D, et al. Acute gastric dilatation following feeding of nutritionally abused children. Clin Pediatr 23:108, 1984.
80. Silverman FN. The roentgen manifestations of unrecognized skeletal trauma in infants. AJR 69:413–427, 1953.
81. Sivit CJ, Taylor GA, Newman KD, et al. Safety belt injuries in children with lap belt ecchymosis. AJR 157:111–114, 1991.
82. Slovis TL, Berdon WE, Haller JO, et al. Pancreatitis and the battered child syndrome. AJR 456–461, 1975.
83. Slovis TL, VonBerg VJ, Mikelic V. Sonography in the diagnosis and management of pancreatic pseudocysts and effusions in childhood. Radiology 135:153–155, 1980.
84. Smith FW, Gilday DL, Ash JM, et al. Unsuspected costovertebral fractures demonstrated by bone scanning in the child abuse syndrome. Pediatr Radiol 10:103–106, 1980.
85. Sperling MA. Bone lesions in pancreatitis. Aust Ann Med 17:334–340, 1968.
86. Spevak MR, Kleinman PK. Does cardiopulmonary resuscitation cause rib fractures in infants? A post–mortem radiologic–pathologic study. Present at the Seventy–sixth Assembly and Annual Meeting of the Radiological Society of North America, Chicago, IL, November 25–30, 1990.
87. Spevak MR, Kleinman PK. Differences between physiologic and post–traumatic periosteal reaction in infants. Presented at the Annual Meeting of the Society for Pediatric Radiology, Orlando, FL, May 1992.
88. Sty JR, Starshak RJ. The role of bone scintigraphy in the evaluation of the suspected abused child. Radiology 146:369–375, 1983.
89. Swischuk LE. Spine and spinal cord trauma in the battered child syndrome. Radiology 92:733–738, 1969.
90. Thomas PS. Rib fractures in infancy. Ann Radiol 20(1):115–122, 1977.
91. Thomas M, Cameron A. Rarity of non–accidental penetrating injury in child abuse. Br Med J 1:375–376, 1977.

92. Thomas SA, Rosenfield NS, Leventhal JM, et al. Long–bone fractures in young children: Distinguishing accidental injuries from child abuse. Pediatrics 88(3):471–476, 1991.

93. Thomford NR, Jesseph JE. Pseudocyst of the pancreas. A review of fifty cases. Am J Surg 118:86–94, 1969.

94. Tollner J, Henrichs I, Bittner R, et al. Rupture of the stomach caused by child–battering. Monatsschr Kinderheilkd 132:801–802, 1984.

95. Touloukian RJ. Abdominal visceral injuries in battered children. Pediatrics 42:642–646, 1968.

96. Tsai FY, Zee C–S, Apthorp JS, et al. Computed tomography in child abuse head trauma. CT: J Comput Tomogr 4:277–286, 1980.

97. Wecht CH, Larkin GM. The battered child syndrome: A forensic pathologist's viewpoint. Leg Med 1–23, 1989.

98. Wilkinson RH. Imaging of the abused child. In Newberger E, ed. Child Abuse. Boston: Little, Brown, 1982, p 159–175.

99. Wilkinson RH, Kirkpatric JA Jr. Pediatric skeletal trauma. Curr Probl Diagn Radiol 6:3–38, 1976.

100. Williams AF. Children killed in falls from motor vehicles. Pediatrics 68:576–578, 1981.

101. Woolley MM, Mahour GH, Sloan T. Duodenal hematoma in infancy and childhood: Changing etiology and changing treatment. Am J Surg 136:8–14, 1978.

102. Young LW, Adams JT. Roentgenographic findings in localized trauma to the pancreas in children. AJR 101(3):639–648, 1967.

103. Zimmerman RA, Bilaniuk LT, Bruce D, et al. Computed tomography of pediatric head trauma: Acute general cerebral swelling. Radiology 126:403–408, 1978.

104. Zimmerman RA, Bilaniuk LT, Bruce D, et al. Computed tomography of craniocerebral injury in the abused child. Radiology 130:687–690, 1979.

ADDITIONAL READING

Kleinman PK, Kleinman PL. Suspected infant abuse: Radiographic skeletal survey practices in pediatric healthcare facilities. Radiology 233:477-485, 2004.

Kleinman PK, Marks SC Jr, Nimkin K, Rayder SM, Kessler SC: Rib fractures in 31 abused infants: postmortem radiologic-histopathologic study. Radiology 200:807-810, 1996.

Kleinman PK, Marks SC Jr, Richmond JM, Blackbourne BD: Inflicted skeletal injury: A postmortem radiologic-histopathologic study in 31 infants. AJR 165:647-650, 1995.

Kleinman PK, Marks SC Jr: A regional approach to the classic metaphyseal lesion in abused infants: the proximal tibia. AJR 166:421-426, 1996.

Kleinman PK, Marks SC Jr: A regional approach to the classic metaphyseal lesion in abused infants: the distal tibia. AJR 166:1207-1212, 1996.

Kleinman PK, Marks SC Jr: A regional approach to the classic metaphyseal lesion in abused infants: the proximal humerus. AJR 167:1399-1403, 1996.

Kleinman PK, Marks SC Jr: A regional approach to the classic metaphyseal lesion in abused infants: the distal femur. AJR 170:43-47, 1998.

Kleinman PK, Marks SC Jr: Relationship of the subperiosteal bone collar to metaphyseal lesions in abused infants. J Bone Joint Surg 77A(10):1471-1476, 1995.

Kleinman PK, Nimkin K, Spevak MR, Rayder SM, Madansky DL, Shelton YA, Patterson MI: follow-up skeletal surveys in suspected child abuse. AJR 167:893-896, 1996.

Kleinman PK, O'Connor B, Nimkin K, Rayder SM, Spevak MR, Belanger PL, Getty DJ,

Karellas A. Detection of rib fractures in an abused infant using digital radiography: a laboratory study. Pediatr Radiol 32(12):896-901, 2002. Epub 2002 Aug 08.

Kleinman PK, Schlesinger AR: Mechanical factors associated with posterior rib fractures: laboratory and case studies. Pediatr Radiol 27:87-91, 1997.

Kwon DS, Spevak MR, Fletcher KE, Kleinman PK. Physiologic subperiosteal new bone formation: prevalence, distribution and thickness in infancy. AJR Am J Roentgenol 179(4):985-8, 2002.

Nimkin K, Kleinman PK, Teeger S, Spevak MR: Distal humeral physeal injuries in child abuse: MR imaging and ultrasonography findings. Pediatr Radiol 25:562-565, 1995.

Nimkin K, Kleinman PK: Imaging of child abuse. Radiol Clin North Am 39:843-864, 2001.

Nimkin K, Spevak MR, Kleinman PK: Fractures of the hands and feet in child abuse: imaging and pathologic features. Radiology 203:233-236, 1997.

Spevak MR, Kleinman PK, Belanger PL, Primack C, Richmond JM: Cardiopulmonary resuscitation and rib fractures in infants. A postmortem radiologic-pathologic study. JAMA 272(8):617-618, 1994.

COURT TESTIMONY IN CASES OF NONACCIDENTAL TRAUMA

Outline

David K. Edwards, III, MD

COURT TESTIMONY IN CASES OF NONACCIDENTAL TRAUMA

T he pediatric radiologist is often called to testify in court in cases concerned with nonaccidental trauma, primarily child abuse. The testimony of the physician may often be the pivotal factor in determining the outcome of the case—whether a child is removed from the home or a child abuser is punished.

Although the child in question generally benefits considerably from the court suit, the physician's appearance is usually a nerve-wracking, time-consuming, and scientifically uninteresting experience. It is important, therefore, that the radiologist be aware of general courtroom procedures and how to prepare for them. The intent of this chapter is to describe these procedures in hopes of making the court appearance a little easier for those who have little experience in this arena.

Although the material in this chapter is based on courtroom experience in the state of California, with some variation, the process and procedures are similar in most other areas. The need for solid preparation and a calm, confident attitude remains the same in any courtroom.

The courtroom environment is an arena in which science, the rigors of diagnosis, and even common sense often seem to be absent. When faced with this situation, it is important to remember the potential benefit to the child that may result from your testimony and the physician's testimony.

THE SUBPOENA

The subpoena is a notice in which one is instructed to appear in court, threatening arrest to anyone who does not comply. In our community, subpoenas are "served" by uniformed, armed police officers whose appearance in the quiet radiology suite causes invariable alarm. On the subpoena itself are written the names of the defendant, the plaintiff, and, often, the attorneys involved. These names and parties may be unrelated to the child whose films were reviewed; thus, one may have to search for the required information. The time and place for the court appearance should also be indicated on the subpoena.

The various attorneys and court officials involved are generally quite sympathetic to the needs of physicians and are usually (but not invariably) willing to make whatever changes are needed in the court calendar to permit testimony at an acceptable time. Often the court permits testimony to be given out of the usual sequence if this is helpful to the physician. Furthermore, because the timing of court cases on a given day is approximate at best, standby call can usually be arranged, thereby minimizing wasted time. It is important, however, to be on time. To make arrangements, one usually needs only to telephone the attorney whose name is on the subpoena.

In any event, one must contact the attorney to learn what is involved in the legal action, the name of the patient, other physicians who have been subpoenaed, and whether one is subpoenaed as an expert witness or as a witness of fact. A second call or visit with this attorney should be scheduled after the relevant films have been located and reviewed.

In cases that are not of a criminal nature or on the rare occasion when the attorney is defending rather than prosecuting the case, an expert witness is generally sought in a manner less abrasive than a subpoena. The attorney in question arranges to meet the physician to discuss the case, to schedule the physician's appearance at any pretrial procedures, and to agree on a fee.

PREPARATION FOR TESTIFYING

In any endeavor, adequate preparation is often responsible for attaining the best results (by contrast, there is no substitute for a total lack of preparation); this is especially true in preparing to testify in court. Careful attention to details well in advance of the actual court appearance significantly helps to minimize wasted time and to maximize the effectiveness of the testimony. In Table 18-1, a checklist for advanced preparation for testifying as an expert witness in a child abuse case is given.

ESTABLISH GROUND RULES

CAN THE TRIAL APPEARANCE BE AVOIDED?

The first order of business is to talk with the attorney responsible for the subpoena and find out whether a court appearance is in fact necessary. In some instances, a formal

TABLE 18-1 PREPARATION FOR TESTIFYING AS AN EXPERT WITNESS IN A CHILD ABUSE CASE

Initial Contact with Sponsoring Attorney
Determine whether court appearance can be avoided with a pretrial procedure, such as a deposition
Determine witness status (expert witness or witness of fact)
Establish expert witness fee
Obtain schedule for appearing in court
Arrange for subsequent meeting
Homework
Do background reading about child abuse, especially features pertinent to the case in question
Review witness's personal professional history
Review of Relevant Films and Radiographic Reports
Discussion of Case with Attorney
Establish general strategy of case
Prepare for specific questions
Determine probable thrusts of the cross-examination
Film Preparation
Label films with date and identifying letters or numbers
Highlight specific abnormalities
Make explanatory drawings
Place films in order for viewing
Assemble Items Helpful in Testifying
Films of the case
Copies of radiographic reports
Subpoena
Viewbox and pointer
Normal films for comparison, if indicated

deposition may be taken at a time and place that are suitable for the radiologist to present the findings and to be questioned by attorneys from both sides. For the radiologist, a deposition is definitely preferable to a court appearance. However, there are difficulties associated with depositions. Depositions are taken in a less formal atmosphere than the courtroom, and it should be kept in mind that one's testimony is sworn testimony that is likely to be read into a transcript at the subsequent trial. Preparation for a deposition should be as extensive as that for a court appearance, with an equal amount of care taken concerning the presentation of the material.[2]

A court appearance can sometimes be avoided by offering to review the films and findings with the attorney to provide the substance of the radiographic examinations. Unfortunately, in most cases of child abuse, the radiographs are an essential part of the evidence, and the radiologist's direct testimony is mandatory. Because criminal actions are often involved in child abuse cases, it is uncommon that a deposition alone will be sufficient. Only rarely are cases handled outside the courtroom.

Expert Witness Versus Witness of Fact

At the beginning of a court case, shortly after the subpoena has been served, it is necessary to determine whether one has been subpoenaed to testify as an expert witness or as a witness of fact. The difference between the two types of witnesses is substantial. As a witness of fact, one is obliged to testify only about the facts of a particular case: names, dates of examination, and interpretation of films from the patient's file. If necessary, one may be asked to identify the films, point out any abnormalities, and so on, but one does not provide an opinion or make a judgment. As a witness of fact, the radiologist's role is to establish "the chain of evidence" tying a crime to its perpetrators; the radiologist's testimony is supposedly given no more intrinsic weight than, for example, the testimony of the technologist who exposed the films.

An expert witness, on the other hand, is expected to provide the court with opinions and judgments based on real or court-assumed expertise. An expert witness is expected to indicate, for example, the most likely mechanism of injury, whether a hypothesized mechanism is or is not plausible in the particular case, or the probable age of a particular fracture. Evidence of opinion is ordinarily inadmissible. The expert witness is thus permitted reasoned and experienced conjecture, not merely the recitation of facts. In addition, an expert witness is expected to translate medical facts, techniques, and observations into understandable, everyday parlance for the benefit of the court and the jury.

It is obvious that such "expert" testimony bears with it a tremendous responsibility. On the basis of such testimony, abused children may be taken from their homes, and abusive parents may be sent to jail. In addition to this responsibility, expert witnesses may be publicly challenged and attacked in a variety of distasteful ways, and their professional competence may be questioned.

Expert witnesses are paid a much higher rate for their testimony than are other witnesses. However, most expert witnesses agree that this recompense is small indeed, considering the effort involved in preparing for a court case. However, the fee is a part of the contemporary legal system and should be demanded, even if one subsequently donates the monies to a child welfare agency. The fee should be agreed upon prior to the court appearance and should represent a reasonable compensation for the radiologist's time away from work.

For the remainder of this chapter, it will be assumed that the radiologist is serving as an expert witness. If the radiologist is called as a witness of fact, there is relatively little preparation required, other than to be well-versed in the facts regarding the case. A witness of fact should not also testify as an expert witness in the same case (thus exposing oneself to cross-examination). However, even a witness of fact may find aspects

of this chapter helpful in gaining an understanding of the courtroom situation.

HOMEWORK

In some ways, it is relatively easy to become an expert witness.[3] The only requirement is that one must be accepted as such by the judge. It is important to remember that what constitutes expertise according to the law is not necessarily considered expertise in the medical community.

Nonetheless, if expert testimony is demanded, it is in one's best interest to become as much of an expert as possible within the constraints of one's time and interest. It is helpful to read selected papers or texts on the subject of child abuse and to research specific technicalities that are relevant to the case. Although it is acceptable to say "I don't know"—and this is the recommended response if one does not know the answer to a question—it is better to have some knowledge of possible questions that may arise concerning the types and frequencies of injuries that occur in child abuse and to prepare answers to these questions. It is appropriate to spend at least as much time in this sort of "homework" as one would in preparing a seminar for colleagues. It is advisable to be a scholar and a teacher in court; pretrial preparations allow these roles to become a reality.

It is also useful to review one's own professional history. The radiologist may be asked to recount aspects of training, background, and professional experience in specific detail. Reviewing personal facts such as one's date of graduation from medical school, dates of postgraduate training, approximate number of child abuse cases encountered, and any relevant research or presentations, honors, and awards may be helpful. If such reviewing is done ahead of time, one is able to present this information more coherently in the courtroom.

REVIEW OF FILMS AND RADIOGRAPHIC REPORTS

The most "radiologic" portion of the preparation involves critically examining all imaging studies performed of the patient. Fractures are noted, and their approximate age is estimated. If there are numerous fractures, it is a good idea to list the specific fractures on paper and have this information with you in the courtroom. Equivocal findings, as well as any technical limitations that hamper particular views, should also be noted.

The radiologist must be absolutely sure that the films being reviewed are indeed those of the child involved in the legal action.

The radiologist must also be certain that the diagnosis made is correct. The defense attorney will surely inquire about possible diagnoses other than nonaccidental trauma, particularly diagnoses associated with fragile bones that might break in the course of ordinary handling of the child or diseases whose manifestations simulate child abuse. Thus, particular care must be taken to assess bone mineralization, to seek wormian bones, to examine the character of the fractures, and to exclude the possibility of fragile bones due to severe prematurity and malnutrition (see Chapter 17).[6] In theory, this effort will have already been made and the diagnosis established, but in light of the scrutiny to which the films and the findings will be subjected, reacquainting oneself with the case and critically reassessing the films and findings may be extremely valuable.

At this time, one should strongly consider peer review (advice from colleagues or experts in the field), an action that is too often ignored in preparing a case for court.[1] One should encourage one's peers to review the films critically and to make suggestions. It is better that ideas and findings that you may have overlooked emerge at this time rather than in court. It is likely that the opposing attorney will also seek such advice and will arrive in court prepared to divulge whatever weaknesses the radiographic examination may contain; peer review reduces the probability of a distressing surprise.

The radiologist should also review the radiographic report of the study. Because it is a part of the child's medical record, this dictated report will almost certainly be reviewed with great care by all attorneys involved. Thus, one may expect comprehensive and explicit questioning concerning this document. If the report does not accurately describe the findings of the films, the reason for the disparity should be sought and recognized.

DISCUSSION OF THE CASE WITH THE ATTORNEY

The only attorney with whom it is proper to discuss the case is the one who arranged for your appearance as a witness (i.e., the sponsoring attorney). It is improper to discuss the case with attorneys from the opposing side unless this is done openly in the consenting presence of all attorneys concerned. It is also improper and unwise to discuss the case with the child's family or local news media. One should inquire as to the identity of anyone who telephones and wishes to discuss the case.

Sometime prior to the court appearance, it is important to review the case in detail with the sponsoring attorney. It is a legal adage that, on direct examination, a question should not be asked unless the answer is known in advance; therefore, the attorney will probably insist on such a discussion. At this time, the format of the questions to be asked, as well as the strong and weak points of the testimony, should be established. Another useful result of this discussion should be to uncover

the "methods of attack" that will probably emerge during cross-examination. Such methods tend to be similar in most child abuse cases, but the eccentricities of each case may result in unexpected variations of the usual.

If the sponsoring attorney does not suggest a pretrial conference, the radiologist should suggest it. Such a conference can be quite helpful, particularly if the physician is a neophyte in the courtroom.

FILM PREPARATION

Frequently in cases of child abuse, the radiographs are taken as evidence of the actual physical abuse. Each film should be marked by affixing a gummed paper label to it on which an identifying letter or number is written. This enables the radiologist to refer to the findings on "film G," rather than having to say "this film here."

I also mark on the films, with film-marking crayon, the date of the examination, making the numbers large enough so that they are easily apparent from a distance, and drawing arrows pointing to the various abnormalities. The latter is done so that, in the heat of the moment, I do not forget important information; additionally, it makes my testimony more clear and easier to understand to any individual who demands to examine the film personally.

If the films are overexposed or the findings are particularly subtle, it may be useful to make a drawing showing the findings on a piece of clear film. This may be particularly helpful in revealing small corner fractures in infants. A normal bone can be drawn for comparison. The sketch should be made much larger than the original film so that it can be seen from a distance.

The films should be arranged in a reasonable order and should be placed in an envelope so that when they are removed they will be in the correct order. Shuffling through a disorganized pile of films, turning them this way and that and finally climaxing the performance by showing the film upside down is embarrassing and conveys an impression of incompetence. In general, the radiographic findings are better understood if the patient's left is also the film's left, but to avoid personal confusion, I do not display films this way.

ITEMS TO BRING TO COURT

The radiologist should bring the following items to court (or have them available): all relevant films, a copy of the radiographic reports, the subpoena, a pointer, a viewbox, and normal films for comparison. In most courts, the original films, not copies, are desired; the radiologist may consult the attorney about this. The radiographic reports are useful in cases in which parts of them are read aloud. One can then follow the reading, being wary of omissions or misinterpretations.

The subpoena contains information that will enable the clerks at the court building to show one the way to the correct room.

The importance of having a pointer and a viewbox cannot be overemphasized. They enable one to display the radiographic findings easily. Many courts furnish a pointer and a viewbox if notified in advance; if this is not the case, it is worthwhile to bring a viewbox, preferably the slim, single-panel variety.

Normal films for comparison are seldom necessary in cases of child abuse, because fractures are generally blatantly apparent and the contralateral extremity or rib can serve as the norm. However, with subtle fractures, such as small and symmetric "corner" fractures, normal films from a child of the same approximate age as the child in question may be useful in confirming the abnormality to nonradiologists.

Finally, it is important to be dressed professionally in the courtroom. Perhaps this should go without saying, but I have been involved in cases in which it had obviously not been made clear. Courts are conservative places, and cavalier clothing is often thought to be disrespectful.

IN COURT

This section provides an overview of what can generally be expected in the courtroom, particularly the different phases of the testimony in which the physician will be involved. Specific details about testifying are presented in the subsequent section.

PHILOSOPHICAL DIFFERENCES BETWEEN LAW AND MEDICINE

It is important, if difficult, to keep in mind the fact that legal ethics and legal truth are different from medical ethics and medical truth in several important ways. I will attempt to state these differences in a way that may risk excessive simplicity. To attorneys, truth is whatever can be established in the adversarial context of the courtroom by employing the legally legitimate tools of evidence, examination, and cross-examination. To physicians, truth is whatever actually occurred or whatever most likely occurred, as established by observation or science. There is an enormous difference between the two, and unawareness of this difference can result in the physician and the attorney inadvertently being at cross-purposes.

It is well to remember that to attorneys the business of courtroom law is very much a "game." This is the way the law works, this is the way attorneys are trained, and this is entirely legally ethical. The strategy and tactics of the game, not the actual truth or falsity of the legal question at issue, dominate the courtroom situation. If the testifying physician

becomes flustered and momentarily incoherent or if he loses his temper in an unseemly way or accidentally misspeaks himself, the damage that is done to the case is quite real, despite the fact that the factual testimony was crucial to the case. The witness has then lost credibility.

The differences between medical and legal truths should always be kept in mind in the courtroom. Recalling the game that is taking place, which will continue regardless of whether one approves of it, is invaluable in maintaining one's equanimity. Recognizing and admitting the limitations of medical truth in establishing legal truths helps to prevent one from falling into uncomfortable legal traps in which the probabilistic assessments of medicine conflict with the arbitrarily defined absolutes of the law.

THE COURTROOM

On arriving at the courtroom, one should notify the bailiff or appropriate court officer of one's presence. A period of waiting then ensues. During this time one may be outside the courtroom and out of earshot of the proceedings within or inside the courtroom. In either case, it is best not to converse with anyone, because the people who are milling about may be witnesses, and conversation with them may result in a mistrial. Eventually, one is summoned inside the courtroom.

Even people who have not been in many courtrooms will be familiar with the general layout, personnel, and procedures from watching movies or television. A testifying physician is "on stage" from the moment he is called by the attorney to the time he is excused by the judge. The procedure begins with the physician's recitation of his name and the oath to be truthful, after which he is seated in the witness stand and examination begins. The witness stand is usually close to the court reporter, who will be typing a shorthand transcript of the proceedings.

QUALIFYING AS AN EXPERT WITNESS

If one is to testify as an expert witness, it is at this time that the sponsoring attorney will attempt to convince the judge that the physician he has brought is indeed an expert in the matter at hand—in this case, child abuse and, more generally, the radiography of children. The attorney may ask only for a statement of qualifications, or, instead, he may pose questions concerning the physician's training or status. At any time during this procedure, the opposing attorney can short-circuit the proceedings by stipulating that the physician is acceptable to him as an expert witness. He may do this because he is sure that the judge is going to accept the witness in any case, and he either wants to save time or prevent the recitation of qualifications that might be harmfully impressive.

The opposing attorney may choose to dispute the witness's expertise. If this is the case, the situation may become unpleasant for the physician. The opposing attorney, despite knowing that a challenged witness will ultimately be accepted, may take the opportunity to belittle the physician's expertise as much as possible, to blunt the effects of the subsequent testimony. Browbeating and the use of personal invectives are not allowed, but the challenging attorney may make vigorous efforts to demean, denigrate, and otherwise impugn the physician's skill, competence, experience, and even personal traits. Here, as in cross-examination, equanimity, if preserved, can be very gratifying. Indeed, the more bombastic the attack, the better the physician may appear if he plays the game properly.

DIRECT EXAMINATION

Once it has been determined that the testifying physician is an expert witness, the sponsoring attorney proceeds to elicit testimony from him. The manner in which this is done is determined by the way in which the attorney views the witness. If the attorney is willing to risk some loss of control and if the witness is a good speaker, the attorney may permit the witness to develop the case with a minimum of questions and a maximum of narrative from the witness. In other instances, the attorney may develop the case question by question, with only brief responses demanded by each. With either technique, the expectation or at least the hope is that there will be no surprises, because the material should have been covered during the pretrial conference between the attorney and the physician.

During direct examination, the overall strategy is to present the case in the strongest and most convincing manner possible. Although the strong points of the testimony should be emphasized, the weak aspects may also be brought to light to explain them and minimize their impact during cross-examination.

In direct examination the radiographs and other imaging studies will usually be introduced. Here, preparation, if it has been done carefully, will be beneficial. If a jury is present, the radiographs should be directed to the jury members. If the procedure is a hearing without a jury, one should try to angle the viewbox so that everyone in the room, including the judge, can see.

CROSS-EXAMINATION

The cross-examination is the second part of the proceedings. Here the situation may get rough for the testifying physician. The opposing attorney will attempt to minimize or negate the testimony. The range of possible questions and attacks is considerably broader than it is in direct examination. If the sponsoring attorney has done his job well, the witness will be prepared for the most likely forms of attack.

There are two major forms of attack that the opposing attorney is apt to take during cross-examination.[5] The first of these, the "nice guy" attack, involves disputing the evidence

that has been presented. The thrust of this challenge is based on the possibility that there might be other interpretations of the radiographs or that entities other than child abuse may have produced the abnormalities. In this type of cross-examination questions of osteogenesis imperfecta and Menkes' syndrome arise. Some opposing attorneys will have done their homework well, and the questions may be somewhat scholarly. This type of cross-examination can be very seductive, and the physician must be wary.

The second form of refutation, the "bad guy" attack, involves attempting to impeach the witness. Usually this type of cross-examination is limited to procedures with juries; judges by themselves have little tolerance for it. This variety of attack is considerably livelier. The attorney may attack the witness's observations, judgments both medical and otherwise, and even honesty. Insinuation often plays a major role in this form of attack; the physician may be asked if he discussed the case in advance with the sponsoring attorney, suggesting by intonation that this is somehow illicit (of course, it is not). Questions may involve the witness's fee, suggesting that accepting money is improper or that the sum is contingent on a favorable outcome.

If the witness has made inconsistent statements or statements that may seem to be inconsistent, such testimony is resurrected and emphasized. Typographic and grammatical errors in the radiographic reports are mentioned to reveal the witness's illiteracy, carelessness, or uncertainty about the findings. A favorite question in child abuse cases is a variation of "You mean you did not take these films yourself? Someone else took them?" The implication of such a question is professional dereliction coupled with uncertainty that the radiographs actually depict the child in question.

It is often demanded that questions be answered with either "yes" or "no." The favorite of such questions is one that requires both a "yes" and a "no" answer: "Are you quite certain—could this be anything except child abuse?" The answer might be "yes" to the first part, and "no" to the second part. It is legitimate for the witness to emit the prized "yes" or "no," followed by an explanatory remark, if needed. It is also legitimate to protest that the question cannot be answered correctly with either "yes" or "no," when this is in fact the case. Sometimes one is required to answer thus anyway; it is hoped that the sponsoring attorney will seek clarification during redirect testimony.

REDIRECT TESTIMONY

Redirect testimony gives each attorney another chance to question the physician. The sponsoring attorney generally attempts to clear up any misconceptions that may have arisen in cross-examination and to strengthen, if possible, any weaknesses that have appeared in his case. The opposing attorney does likewise from his point of view. It is relatively uncommon for anything new to be uncovered during this portion of the testimony, and usually it does not last very long. However, it can be continued until both attorneys are satisfied that all possible progress has been made. When completed, the physician is free to leave the courtroom.

TESTIFYING: DETAILS

In this section, details of the moment-to-moment process of testifying are discussed. Some of these details seem obvious; nevertheless, all are based on blunders that have been made. The most important details in testifying are one's attitude and demeanor.

ATTITUDE AND DEMEANOR

The attitude and courtroom demeanor adopted by the testifying physician are of crucial importance in any case. They are important not only in making the evidence presented more compelling but also in keeping the witness personally calm, unrattled, and coherent. The best attitude to adopt is that of scholar and teacher.[1] That is, questions should be answered and remarks should be presented in a solemn and formal manner, as though one were a scholar teaching a group of intelligent, interested laymen. This technique cannot be recommended too strongly. If pretrial preparation has been adequate, so that one is familiar with the general subject matter as well as details of the case at hand, then one is fully qualified for such a role. As much as possible, one should respond to both attorneys in the same manner, as though everyone involved is seeking together to discover the truth. It is proper and helpful to understand that the trial is essentially a game, but one's demeanor should remain that of a teacher. Inasmuch as one is a partisan, one should be a partisan for the child.

It is astonishing how profoundly one's attitude can affect the courtroom atmosphere. The preservation of a calm, reasoning equanimity may greatly upset a hostile attorney. Of course, sensitive attorneys notice this before the situation gets out of hand and change their tactics.

A calm, reasoning attitude can markedly truncate cross-examination and may even obviate it. It has been observed that "…the cross-examination of a truthful, honest, efficient, and capable medical expert witness who is not given to exaggeration is not only dangerous but usually harmful to the trial lawyer."[4]

GENERAL FEATURES OF ANSWERING QUESTIONS

At the outset, it is a good idea to identify the audience to whom one's remarks and responses will be directed. In the case of a jury trial, the audience is the jury, which means that one should address remarks toward the jury, even though the question was asked by one of the attorneys. Looking frequently at the jury is desirable. If there is no jury, the audience can be defined as the attorney who is asking the questions.

One should not begin to answer a question until it has been asked in its entirety. Even then, one should think first and formulate the best answer that is possible. This tactic not only reduces the number of regrettable answers but also conveys an impression of thoughtfulness. Furthermore, if the question is a hostile or emotionally laden one, pausing before answering helps one to maintain one's composure.

The physician must never enter into an argument with an attorney. One should try to maintain a calm, clear, even voice throughout the questioning, with a tone that is authoritative without being argumentative.

As an expert witness, one should explain medical terms and avoid jargon. In the context of explaining films, it is useful to use proper medical terms followed immediately by the common name (e.g., the left tibia, or shinbone, is fractured). The court reporter may request that you spell medical and anatomic words.

If a question is confusing or if you do not understand a question, ask for clarification.

Do not disparage or criticize any other physician or any other findings, treatment, or testimony; respectfully disagree, if necessary. Confine your answer to the question asked; do not needlessly volunteer information that is not directly related to the question. The best answer is a "yes" or "no," followed by any necessary explanations, exceptions, or qualifications. Keep these succinct. Do not be sarcastic or ironic; this not only creates a bad impression, but also risks misinterpretation. Intonations of voice are not preserved in the court record, and a sarcastic answer may be interpreted as a lie. Similarly, do not be jocular; the demeanor of responses should reflect the fact that the business at hand is of a serious nature.

TYPES OF QUESTIONS

Certain specific questions and types of questions are almost invariably encountered in child abuse cases. Familiarity with these can expedite testifying considerably.

Hypothetical Questions

Attorneys acquire a vast amount of information from medical expert witnesses by asking hypothetical questions. Such questions involve recitation of a series of facts and events, all of which are presumably evidence in the case at hand, followed by asking the witness to assume the truth of these and, on that basis, to render an opinion about a particular question. Frequently, these questions originate from the sponsoring attorney, in which case the witness should have already formulated an answer. However, the opposing attorney may also employ these tactics, in which case the facts and events to be assumed commonly represent the defendant's explanation of the injuries. One must simply answer hypothetical questions as well as possible.

Questions to Which the Answer Is Unknown

There are two types of questions for which the answer is unknown: those for which the answer is not known to medical science, and those for which the answer, whether known to medical science or not, is certainly unknown to the witness at that particular moment. To either of these questions, the correct answer is "I don't know." If the witness is quite certain that the answer is medically unknown, it is appropriate to add this fact.

"I don't know" is a very legitimate answer and the only answer that should be given if one does not know. Bluffing or guessing may result in distress and embarrassment, because a medical textbook with the correct answer can be brought forth as factual information.

Rhetorical questions do not require an answer.

Percentage Questions

Witnesses are frequently asked to quantify something that cannot be quantified, such as one's degree of certainty. My response to this type of question is usually 1% or 99.9%.

Questions About Force

A common question is how much force was required to break a particular bone. For some time, I answered in terms of bundles of so many pencils; now I estimate by the size of a comparable bone in a chicken or turkey, specifying that the estimate is very rough at best, which is generally considered to be a satisfactory answer.

Objections

At any time during the testimony, the opposing attorney may object; this objection may be to a question or to the witness's response. Objections should not be regarded as personal attacks, although they may be disruptive and irritating. The proper response to an objection is to stop talking at once and wait until the judge rules on the matter and gives instructions about the question.

The Big Question

Sooner or later, usually in direct examination, the big question arrives: "In your expert opinion, doctor, how do you believe these injuries were sustained?" It should be answered in a direct, forthright manner: "I believe the injuries were sustained as a result of deliberate child abuse." Unless there is some other plausible cause, hemming and hawing or equivocating at this point may be harmful to the case.

SUMMARY

The courtroom is an alien environment to many physicians, an arena that sometimes seems entirely divorced from medical verities, scientific thought, reason, and even elemental common sense. The physician called to testify as an expert witness is encouraged to remember that medical ethics and truths differ markedly from legal ethics and truths. The legal system is not intended to seek absolute truths; instead, it functions on the model of a "game," with the truth defined by the winning side in a rigorous but essentially arbitrary contest of strategies, tactics, and showmanship.

The physician witness is encouraged to prepare extensively for the courtroom endeavor, because the effort thus spent will make testifying much easier. Preparation includes film review, arranging the films for smooth presentation, studying the case in question and child abuse in general, and conferring with peers and the sponsoring attorney. The latter consultation should include seeking to avoid the courtroom appearance by pretrial deposition, as well as settling fees, discussing the case's overall strategy, and establishing specific questions that will be addressed.

In the courtroom, the physician witness is urged to assume the role of scholar and teacher, rather than the role of a partisan. It is hoped, indeed, that after the pretrial preparations the physician will be capable of assuming this role legitimately, at least regarding the matter at hand. As a scholar and a teacher, the witness's testimony should be medically sound as well as convincingly presented. By observing a few rather minor rules and protocols and being prepared for certain unpleasant events, a physician has an excellent chance of being a capable and effective witness. It is hoped that the beneficiary of such preparation and presence will be the child.

REFERENCES

1. Brent RL. The irresponsible expert witness: A failure of biomedical graduate education and professional accountability. Pediatrics 70:754—762, 1982.
2. James AE Jr, ed. Legal Medicine With Special Reference to Diagnostic Imaging. Baltimore: Urban and Schwarzenberg, 1980.
3. Miller M. The radiologist as expert witness. Diagn Imag 4:51, 1982.
4. Neal JF, Doramus JV. Cross-examination. In James AE Jr, ed. Legal Medicine With Special Reference to Diagnostic Imaging. Baltimore: Urban and Schwarzenberg, 1980, p 91.
5. Renner RR. The radiologist as expert witness. In James AE Jr, ed. Legal Medicine With Special Reference to Diagnostic Imaging. Baltimore: Urban and Schwarzenberg, 1980, pp 103–116.
6. Stinson R, Stinson P. On the death of a baby. Atlantic Monthly 244:64, 1979.

ADDITIONAL READING

Barnes PD. Ethical issues in imaging nonaccidental injury: Child abuse. Top Magn Reson Imaging. 13:85–93, 2002.

PSYCHOLOGIC APPROACH TO THE PEDIATRIC PATIENT

Outline

Calvin A. Colarusso, MD

PSYCHOLOGIC APPROACH TO THE PEDIATRIC PATIENT

Approaching and interacting with a sick child is difficult under the best of circumstances, but is particularly so for the radiologist who needs to perform a complicated procedure that requires the child's participation and cooperation. An understanding of child development, especially the pertinent psychologic variables when the child is ill, can be of great practical utility. Knowing patients' limitations, needs, and desires at various ages increases the physician's sensitivity and empathy. This understanding, coupled with minor age-specific procedural modifications, contributes significantly to obtaining the child's cooperation. The following gains may be anticipated:

1. A higher quality examination
2. Timely completion of the procedure
3. Reduced stress on the radiologist and staff
4. A relieved patient and grateful parents
5. A sense of mastery and accomplishment for the child

THE NATURE OF THE CHILD

Prior to the twentieth century, children were misleadingly considered to be miniature adults, smaller physically but similar mentally. Failure to recognize important mental and emotional differences between children and adults significantly hinders successful interaction between a child and an adult, particularly when the child is ill and the interaction is strange or painful. An understanding of such differences, which are relatively few and simple, can benefit the radiologist and enhance the child's cooperation in any setting.

The major differences between adults and children fall into four categories: cognitive capacities, sense of time, egocentricity, and regression.

Because the young child's ability to think in logical, rational terms is limited,[8] such a patient may misinterpret the intentions and actions of the radiologist, even when detailed explanations are provided, because the meaning of these explanations cannot be comprehended or integrated. This limited cognitive capacity may result in incorrect and strange perceptions. Thus, being placed alone in a dark room or a confined space may lead to tears or a refusal to remain immobile because of fear of harm or punishment. For example, after radiographs were obtained for his broken arm, one 4-year-old boy complained for several days that "everybody ran away from me because I was bad," referring to being left alone during the radiographic exposure. He also perceived that he was abandoned for hours, which illustrates the young child's inability to use measures of time such as minutes or hours the way older children and adults do.[1,2] Even children who have recently learned to tell time (usually at age 6 or 7) may regress in the presence of illness or stressful procedures resulting in a distortion of the sense of time. Ongoing involvement with parents assists the child's ability to remain temporally oriented despite unfamiliar surroundings, strange adults, and pain.

Young children's cognitive immaturity and temporal disorientation augment a tendency to view events solely from the limited vantage point of their own understanding and needs. This egocentricity results in misinterpretation of events. In the earlier example, the boy perceived that he was left alone with the physician or technician because he was naughty, not because his injury required diagnosis. This reaction is common. Similarly, painful procedures may be perceived as punishment rather than as necessary steps in a medical process.

Regression, or temporary abandonment of mental and physical functions acquired at earlier phases in life, is a common, normal phenomenon in childhood, even in the best of circumstances. Furthermore, the tendency to regress is greatly accentuated by illness, fear, or pain, and so the radiologist must often interact with a child who is not functioning in an age-appropriate manner. An appreciation of regression encourages tolerance, empathy, and the adoption of measures to minimize the young patient's regression. Encouraging parental presence and participation and ensuring that the child does not needlessly wait for extended periods are particularly helpful with children ages 3 months to 6 years. It is also helpful at the time an appointment is made to encourage the parent to bring the child's favorite toy and to permit the child to retain as many personal items of clothing as possible during the procedure.

DEVELOPMENTAL STAGES

Children are different at different ages. This deceptively simple statement has profound implications for understanding and treating children, because it recognizes that not only are children qualitatively different from adults but they are also qualitatively different from each other. Thus, to work effectively with children, the radiologist must have some knowledge of age-related developmental differences.

A detailed discussion of developmental theory is beyond the scope of this chapter, which focuses solely on the interaction between the radiologist, the family and the child. For a more detailed presentation of clinically relevant developmental theory, the reader is referred to *Encounters With Children: Pediatric Behavior and Development*, by Dixon and Stein.[8]

Childhood is most conveniently subdivided into developmental phases, or intervals of time characterized by particular and fairly stereotyped modes of thinking and behavior. In the context of diagnostic imaging, childhood may be divided into the following phases: infancy, birth to 2 years; early childhood, ages 2 to 6 years; middle childhood, ages 6 to 12 years; early adolescence, ages 12 to 15 years; and late adolescence, ages 15 to 19 years (Table 19–1).

The following sections describe the major aspects of each of these phases and present techniques for interacting with children of these ages as suggested by developmental theory.

INFANCY (BIRTH TO 2 YEARS)

Infants are extremely sensitive to the treatment they receive from their caretakers. By a few weeks of age they begin to distinguish one familiar person from another, and by 6 to 8 months of age they are normally anxious in the presence of strangers. *Dependence on parental presence for a sense of well-being, particularly during stress, continues through the early years of life.* When left alone with a stranger, many infants react as if they were abandoned by the loving parent. In addition, the ability to understand language develops rapidly between the ages of 6 and 12 months, preceding the appearance of speech, which begins at about 1 year of age.

Techniques for Interaction

1. During the first 3 months of life, no special precautions are needed to prepare the patient.
2. Allow older infants time to become familiar with the surroundings and the individuals involved in the procedure.
3. If the infant is older than about 3 months, allow the mother or primary caretaker to remain with the infant throughout the procedure, if possible. If this is impossible, designate a caring substitute to perform this function.
4. Allow the infant to keep a special blanket, stuffed animal, or toy during the procedure. Such familiar objects help the infant tolerate stress and separation from parents.[10]
5. With patients older than 3 months, be circumspect with speech during the procedure. Receptive language begins to develop during the first year, and infants understand more than is generally recognized and may become needlessly anxious or upset.

TABLE 19-1 THE PEDIATRIC EXAMINATION: A DEVELOPMENTAL APPROACH

AGE (APPROXIMATE)	DEVELOPMENTAL STAGE	APPROACH TO THE PHYSICAL EXAMINATION
Birth to 6 months	**Symbiotic** (not fearful of strangers)	It is usually easy to examine the infant on the table; start with the least invasive parts of the examination (abdominal, cardiac, pulmonary, lymphatic, etc.).
6 months to 3 years	**Separation-individuation** (fear of strangers initially, followed by the toddler clinging to the parent)	Perform the examination while a standing parent holds the child or while the infant is in the parent's lap; approach the child gently; the use of toys, peekaboo games, keys, flashing otoscope may be helpful.
3 to 6 years	**Preschool age:** age of initiative (a period of fantasy play and increasing verbal ability)	Communicate with the child in simple language; explain the procedures and ask the child to participate in the examination; make use of the child's interest in fantasy.
6 to 12 years	**School age:** age of industry (a period of cognitive growth; growing interest in and ability to understand cause and effect)	Recognition of the child's ability to understand the procedures leads to cooperation; an explanation of bodily functions and the results of assessment is helpful.
12 to 19 years	**Adolescence:** age of identity (heightened awareness of the body and its perceived effect on others)	Respect the patient's privacy during the examination; careful explanations help.

Adapted from Dixon S, Stein M. Encounters With Children: Pediatric Behavior and Development. 2nd ed. St. Louis: Mosby-Year Book, 1992.

EARLY CHILDHOOD (AGES 2 TO 6 YEARS)

Although toddlers and young children are in the process of psychologically separating from their parents and acquiring their own individuality, they are still deeply attached to their parents for a sense of well-being. These children are normally quite active physically and release their emotions physically as well as vocally; for these reasons children of this age respond poorly to parental absence and forced immobilization. By age 3, young children are intrigued by their bodies, particularly the genital area. They are often apprehensive about strangers touching them, especially if the examination involves undressing and inspection of the genitals. Because they have become aware of their small size and lack of power in a world controlled by adults, many of their fantasies about adults are competitive, filled with aggressive wishes to replace them. Consequently they interpret painful interactions with adults as punishment administered in retaliation for their own hostile wishes.

Techniques for Interaction
1. Be honest: tell the child in precise detail what will happen. Describe various steps in the procedure, using language the child can understand. Answer questions directly and simply.

2. Allow the parents to be involved in the procedure as much as possible. This will improve the child's cooperation and minimize regression.
3. Respect the child's newly emerging need for privacy and modesty. If possible, allow children to retain their own clothing, removing only those garments that impede the examination.
4. Encourage the child to ask questions during and after the procedure. Encourage the parents to let the child express feelings about the experience through play.

MIDDLE CHILDHOOD (AGES 6 TO 12 YEARS)

Children of this age admire and respect adults; this improves cooperation during the medical procedure if they are approached sensitively. Their intellectual and cognitive capacities are sufficiently developed that they can understand explanations of what is being done (and why) at a more sophisticated level than preschool children. Furthermore, particularly toward the end of the elementary school years, they can function in most situations without significant parental support and involvement. Prepuberty begins as early as ages 8 or 9 in some children, and the number of children in puberty increases steadily through the fifth, sixth, and seventh grades. The physical changes of prepuberty and the psychological responses to them produce an increasing preoccupation with, and sensitivity to, the body and all its functions.

Techniques for Interaction

1. Because of the development of an integrated sense of right and wrong and increased intellectual abilities, children in this age group pay close attention to what adults tell them and expect to be treated accordingly. Because of their own preoccupation with right and wrong, they deeply resent dishonesty. Thus, the radiologist should explain what will happen in a detailed, straightforward manner and should not deviate from the outline presented to the child.
2. Although most children in this age group can cooperate in the examination without direct parental involvement, certain younger children may require their parent's presence.
3. Look for signs of prepuberty (e.g., growth spurt, gangliness, pubic hair, or breast buds). If these signs are present, be extremely sensitive to the need for modesty. Do not make unnecessary comments or jokes about body parts, functions, or appearance or the child's style of dress and grooming.

ADOLESCENCE (AGES 12 TO 19 YEARS)

Adolescents are in the process of psychologically separating from their parents and establishing their independence. They prefer to be treated as individuals and with dignity and respect. Cognitively, they are capable of abstract thought[8] and, for the most part, think and understand like adults. Once puberty has occurred, they have sexually mature bodies that are a source of pleasure and pride, as well as exquisite sensitivity and embarrassment. Comfortable acceptance of the sexually mature body and its functions occurs gradually as adolescence progresses.

Techniques for Interaction

1. Do not invite the parents of an adolescent to participate in the examination unless the adolescent requests their involvement.
2. At all times, treat the adolescent with the same dignity and respect accorded to adult patients. Explain the procedure fully in a noncondescending manner and request the adolescent's cooperation.
3. As with the preadolescent, be extremely sensitive to issues of modesty and privacy. During adolescence, procedures involving the sexual parts of the body should be performed, if possible, by a member of the same sex.
4. Once the procedure has been completed, speak directly to the adolescent about the results.

THE SICK CHILD

When a child is ill, particularly a young child, certain normal developmental processes are temporarily compromised while others are accentuated. Withdrawal into the self and a diminished interest in people, play, and surroundings replace the usual curiosity, exuberance, and physical activity. Although the psychologic symptoms that may occur with illness vary with the individual child and the age and level of development, the most common are emotional withdrawal, loss of confidence and self-esteem, and all forms of regressive behavior (e.g., wetting, soiling, temper tantrums, and eating and sleep disturbances).[5]

Illness confronts the child with feelings and experiences that, depending on previous experience and level of cognitive development, are difficult or impossible to comprehend and integrate. For instance, the young child may be unable to distinguish between suffering caused by the disease inside the body and suffering imposed from the outside in an attempt to cure the illness. The child must submit passively and uncomprehendingly to both types of feelings. A kind, sensitive adherence to the principles of interaction presented earlier helps minimize the patient's emotional confusion and turmoil (Table 19–2).

In addition, children (and patients of any age) must renounce ownership and control of their own bodies and permit them to be handled passively, producing a regressed state similar to that of infancy, when care of the body was performed by others. This regressive period, which is necessarily present during diagnostic imaging, should be kept as brief as possible, while allowing the child to participate actively in the process to the greatest possible extent; for example, "Are you ready for your examination" or "Let's you and I go and look at the x-ray machine."[3]

INTERACTING WITH PARENTS

Parents play an important role in their child's illness. It is only with parental permission that examinations are performed or treatments initiated.

The presence and support of parents can diminish the emotionally traumatic effects of procedures and increase cooperation of the child. Therefore, every effort should be made to facilitate their presence during imaging procedures.

Parental cooperation will be maximized if the following concepts and techniques are taken into consideration:

1. Because of the depth of parental emotional investment in their children, the parents are usually more anxious than if the procedures were being performed on themselves.

TABLE 19-2 Communicating With Hospitalized Children

Ages Birth to 3 Years

Allow the child prior, nonstressful exposure to new perceptual experiences: lights, masks, uniforms, smells, restraints.

Allow the child to establish a sense of control by handling the equipment or performing the procedures on dolls.

Provide information to the parents and allow expression of concerns.

Assure the child that the parents will return.

Ages 3 to 6 Years

Provide the child with models of coping responses.

Allow the child to rehearse coping responses to a painful/stressful procedure.

Help the child distinguish attainable goals: blood tests cannot be avoided but can be shortened by the child's action.

Explore concepts of illness, hospitalization, and procedures.

    Misconceptions include the following:

        Illness and procedures are punishment.

        Do not believe what can't be seen (e.g., spots are only caused externally).

        Organ systems are often "lumped": e.g., the heart pumps when you breathe.

        Blood is a fixed quantity that can be permanently depleted.

        All diseases are contagious.

        Procedures that hurt are not therapeutic.

Explore concerns about separation, mutilation, physical pain, guilt.

Ages 6 to 12 Years

Explore concerns about the impact on peer relations, especially a sense of inferiority.

Explore illness concepts.

    Misconceptions include the following:

        Inability to consider simultaneously numerous causes or factors in disease.

        Failure to recognize changes in mood, motivation, state, and role accompanying the illness.

        Failure to understand the interdependency among organ systems.

        No awareness of preventive action.

Ages 12 to 19 Years

Explore concerns about body image, independence, and sexual identity; interference with the ability to establish an identity is especially likely.

Recognize the tendency to deny or minimize severity of illness.

The patient may desire more information about etiology and prognosis than the physician provides.

Adapted from Dixon S, Stein M. Encounters With Children: Pediatric Behavior and Development. 2nd ed. St. Louis: Mosby-Year Book, 1992.

2. Parental anxiety and concern can be minimized by a brief meeting with the radiologist and parents alone to express concerns or fears without affecting the child.

3. The parents need to understand that their sole function throughout the imaging procedure is to comfort their child and increase the level of cooperation.

PREPARATION FOR IMAGING PROCEDURES

The setting in which the child is examined and the personal interactions with all staff members should be as predictable, comfortable, and nonthreatening as possible. It is valuable for the parent and child to have a general understanding of the examination so that they can prepare themselves both mentally and physically (e.g., fasting, hydration, colonic cleansing, or prolonged waiting for delayed images). The necessary transfer of information often requires more than one explanation. Usually, the referring physician informs the parent of the procedure's general nature and its clinical goals. At the time the appointment is made, it is desirable to provide a written description of the examination so that the parent can understand the procedure and prepare the child.

There is an optimal time interval between informing the child and performing the procedure. The patient must be given sufficient time to comprehend and integrate the diagnostic procedure. The amount of time required depends on the patient's age. Children under 5 are told 2 to 3 days in advance, children ages 6 to 12 are given about 5 days, and adolescents can optimally process the information in 1 week. During this time the parents must be available to discuss the procedure and address any questions or fears that their child may have (Table 19–3).

Children are very sensitive to their surroundings and to the adults who interact with them, particularly in unfamiliar settings and under stressful circumstances. Thus, considerable thought should be given to the appearance of waiting areas and examination rooms and to the manner in which children are greeted and accompanied through diagnostic procedures.

Waiting areas should be friendly, calm places equipped with comfortable, home-like furnishings and pictures and toys that have universal appeal to children. Diagnostic imaging rooms tend to be sterile and barren, often containing anatomic diagrams that may be frightening to children and generally serve no useful function. Recognizing that space is usually limited, a small number of well-chosen, comfortable, and familiar items can greatly enhance the child's sense of comfort and security.

TABLE 19-3 REACTIONS TO HOSPITALIZATION AND PROCEDURES

Regression
Immature behavior: thumb sucking, enuresis, encopresis, baby talk, clinging, crying
Feeding dysfunction
Increased dependency
Decreased attention span
Refusal to attend school
Sleep Disturbance
Anxiety
Refusal to leave home (separation anxiety)
Fear of physicians/nurses
Aggressive Behavior
Increased temper tantrums
Hitting and biting
Self-mutilation
Progression
Increased self-esteem
Accelerated development

Adapted from Dixon S, Stein M. Encounters With Children: Pediatric Behavior and Development. 2nd ed. St. Louis: Mosby-Year Book, 1992.

Another source of anxiety for children is fear of the dark; the darkness needed to view the fluoroscopic or sonographic image may be perceived by the child as fearful and ominous. This problem can often be solved by a 15- to 25-watt light surrounded by a small, warm-colored shade that suffuses the room with sufficient illumination to assuage the child's anxiety. Syringes, vials, and similar equipment are best kept out of the child's view, and when these are used, the clinician should be careful to explain each step of the process.

Several items in the examination room warrant an explanation to the child. These include the imaging device, the monitor, and the child's location during the procedure. An acceptable explanation is that the patient is being photographed by a large television camera. The radiologist may invite the patient to "watch yourself on TV," which provides an opportunity to clarify and explain the need to remain still or assume specific positions.

The young child should be encouraged to bring a "companion," such as a stuffed animal or doll, who can also undergo the examination, or a favorite blanket that can cover the child or remain within reach. The most important sources of comfort and security for the child from birth to 6 years of age are the parents, whose presence in the examination room often has a desirable, calming effect.

The child should not be exposed to the hectic and impersonal parts of a busy radiology department such as the main processor area, special procedure rooms, and radiologist's interpretation and consultation areas. These locations are typically filled with people who are concentrating on their work and who cannot be expected to acknowledge or interact with the child. Exposure to this impersonal and foreign environment may cause needless anxiety in a child who is expecting to be the center of attention and who may misinterpret what is seen.

The most important individual in the procedure is the technologist. This individual should greet the child in the waiting area and spend sufficient time to develop a rapport with the child and familiarize the child (and parent) with the planned procedure. The technologist is then in a position to be a source of comfort, continuity, and information to the child by remaining by the child's side throughout the procedure, thus increasing the likelihood of cooperation and diminishing emotional trauma.

TECHNIQUES

1. Carefully choose a technologist who is interested in children and has the ability to make them feel comfortable and secure. If circumstances require a technologist who dislikes children or exhibits anxiety in their presence, contact between this individual and the patient should be minimized.
2. If possible, designate a corner of the adult waiting room for children. An inexpensive, comfortable decor can be achieved using
   a. A box filled with commonly used toys
   b. A lamp to supplement overhead lighting
   c. Several posters or pictures suited for children (e.g., Disney characters)
   Both parents and children will welcome this oasis of familiarity in a stressful, high-technology environment. The distractions provided can help decrease the anxiety that occurs while waiting for a procedure to begin. "Play is the work of childhood,"[8] and playing permits the child to express concerns while providing a sense of mastery and control.
3. Designate a route for children through the department that bypasses the sight of seriously ill patients, other examinations in progress, and high-activity work areas.
4. Choose one examination room to be used routinely for pediatric procedures. Special pediatric equipment can be stored here; the following may be helpful:
   a. A few posters or pictures suited for children
   b. A small lamp with a shade that can be placed in the line of vision of the patient
   With appropriate explanation, this room can be used for all patients, including adolescents.
5. Whenever possible, permit children to wear their own clothing (especially undergarments) instead of a hospital gown. The child thereby retains an increased sense of

security, comfort, and identity. If disrobing is necessary, care should be taken to preserve patients' sense of modesty and control over their own bodies.

6. Be scrupulously truthful about procedures. If aspects of a procedure are painful or uncomfortable, prepare any child older than age 2 in advance, using words that can be understood.

7. Encourage the child to participate in producing the best possible examination. Give the patient a sense of importance that can be translated into playing a vital role. Permit the child to make individual choices whenever possible (e.g., placement of a toy or blanket, the position of a parent, the flavor of oral contrast material, or the selection of a bandage).

The following sections focus on psychologic considerations for imaging procedures that demand more cooperation or are more invasive. Each situation is discussed from the standpoint of infants and young children (birth to 6 years), those in middle childhood (ages 6 to 12 years), and adolescents (ages 12 to 20 years).

Fasting and Drinking Contrast Material

Ages Birth to 6 Years Because of the need to abstain from eating before drinking contrast material, young children should be scheduled as early in the morning as possible. When hungry, infants and toddlers tend to regress and become irritable and uncooperative. Their ability to follow simple commands and remain still decreases as their hunger increases. Although "nothing after midnight" may be an appropriate instruction for adults, it is unreasonable for an infant who gets fed every 3 to 4 hours. Ideal scheduling should permit the time of fasting to be reduced to an absolute minimum.

The unfamiliar taste and the strange situation may make children unwilling to drink contrast medium. It is useful to have the mother or another primary caretaker encourage the child to drink.

Ages 6 to 12 Years Children in this age group can tolerate hunger better than younger children but still should be scheduled early in the morning. A detailed explanation of the reason for drinking the contrast medium usually increases cooperation.

Contrast Enema of the Colon

Because plain film radiography is painless and noninvasive, it is not traumatic for most children. Procedures that include injection or ingestion of contrast medium are more traumatic but still relatively benign experiences. Unfortunately this is not true for contrast enemas, which are difficult for children of all ages because they expose parts of the body that are associated with private, complex feelings and powerful physical sensations. For these reasons they have the potential to produce severe emotional trauma with far-reaching consequences.

Ages Birth to 6 Years Children in this age group are likely to be most affected by the intense physical sensations of enema tip placement and the flow of contrast material into the colon. For those children who are old enough to think and imagine, the experience may stimulate fantasies about being attacked. Children who are in the midst of toilet training or who have only recently gained control of bowel function are likely to perceive the procedure as an episode of soiling. The idea of soiling oneself in public is intensely embarrassing for both children and adults. Patients frequently express their worry about impending soiling by requesting that the procedure be terminated.

In girls between the ages of 4 and 6, the enema may stimulate fantasies of pregnancy or birth, as these girls tend to associate birth with the gastrointestinal tract.

Ages 6 to 12 Years Young children of school age will experience many of the feelings and fantasies of their younger counterparts. Because of their increased ability to understand the details of the procedure and a more developed sense of integrity and modesty, most will become frightened, anxious, and embarrassed.

Ages 12 to 20 Years Adolescents are fully capable of understanding the procedure and its purpose. In early and middle adolescence the central developmental task is the acceptance of a physically and sexually mature body. During this time adolescents are exceedingly sensitive about their bodies, particularly the genital area, and experience embarrassment and discomfort when these areas are exposed. Procedures involving the anus may stimulate sexual as well as aggressive fantasies, particularly regarding anal intercourse, in patients of both sexes. For these reasons it is best for the technologist to be the same sex as the patient. In addition, the emphasis should be on modesty and performing the examination in as expeditious a manner as possible.

Catheterization of the Bladder

Ages Birth to 6 Years Because bladder catheterization involves the genitals, this procedure is likely to be the most difficult for all children to experience. Once toilet training has begun and the child is aware of sexual sensations and masturbation (usually between the ages of 2 and 3), the genitals have emotionally charged meaning for the child. Because of the child's cognitive immaturity, touching or washing the perineum in preparation for sterile catheterization will be experienced as sexual stimulation and insertion of the catheter as an assault. Being asked to delay voiding until the bladder is full and to urinate in front of another person will be both stimulating and embarrassing for the child.

Ages 6 to 12 Years Children in this age group will experience the same feelings as those described previously. However, because of their greater intellectual understanding and their need to please adults, they may be more cooperative and appear to be less affected.

Ages 12 to 20 Years This procedure will be difficult for most adolescents because of the power of their nonintegrated sexuality. In addition to the embarrassment associated with exposure of the genitals, boys will fear an erection from the sexual stimulation of cleansing.

Catheterizing an adolescent requires the greatest degree of sensitivity and patience and should be performed only by those individuals who are comfortable with children. If possible, the person performing the catheterization should be the same sex as the patient.

Sonography

Sonography is a psychologically ideal imaging modality for children of all age groups because neither the transducer nor the warmed coupling gel is painful or invasive. The parent's ability to comfort the child while remaining physically close is also helpful. As previously mentioned, a small, low-wattage, shaded lamp will offset the fear of the dark in younger children.

Computed Tomography

Computed tomography is a relatively benign procedure from a psychologic viewpoint. Before the acquisition of speech, young children use physical motion as a means of expression and release of anxiety. It is unreasonable to expect young children to lie still for a long time, and thus heavy sedation or general anesthesia is usually required.

Older children may also find it difficult to lie still for extended periods of time and may react adversely to being confined to a small tubular space. A detailed explanation of the function of the apparatus and continuous verbal and visual contact during the procedure will enhance cooperation and may make sedation unnecessary.

Magnetic Resonance Imaging

Although painless, magnetic resonance imaging (MRI) places substantial demands on the child. The problem is sensory deprivation during the examination, and this relatively little sensory input is often unfamiliar and ominous. The important psychologic factors are related to mental responses to confinement in an extremely limited space, as well as immobility and isolation. A small number of children (and adults) experience a genuinely claustrophobic reaction, but many more react adversely to the absence of familiar stimuli and the inability to release anxiety through physical motion. When the mind is deprived of the constant input of familiar auditory, visual, and tactile stimuli, mental regression can occur within minutes, producing disorientation, frightening fantasies, and intense anxiety. Unless they are well prepared, many normal individuals will interrupt the examination at this point. Although children may dislike the machine's noise, the relative sensory deprivation is far more difficult to tolerate for prolonged periods of time.

This problem can be minimized by informing older children in advance about what they are likely to experience, maintaining verbal contact, keeping image acquisition time as short as possible, and removing patients from the machine between sequences and encouraging physical movement at that time.

Headphones with music can help retain mental organization and orientation, but a human voice has a more calming influence because of its connectedness to another person. Because of the lack of ionizing radiation with MRI, the parent can safely accompany the patient, and at some institutions the mother sits at the patient's head, providing reassurance or reading aloud; indeed, in some instances, the mother may recline partly within the scanner, again offering reassurance, consolation, and encouragement. It can be suggested to older children that mental disorganization can be inhibited by simple tasks such as reciting the multiplication tables, recalling events during the past few days, or concentrating on a close friend or family member.

▌SUMMARY

The performance of complicated diagnostic procedures is a difficult experience for children to understand, integrate, and master. It is important for each patient to receive sufficient emotional support during these stressful times. Emerging from the experience with a sense of mastery will help the child grow emotionally. A long-term benefit for the child who successfully mastered the stress and pain of being sick is the perception that illness can be overcome.

REFERENCES

1. Azarnoff P. Parents and siblings of pediatric patients. Curr Probl Pediatr 14:19–40, 1984.
2. Bibace R, Walsh M. Development of children's concept of illness. Pediatrics 66:912–917, 1980.
3. Coffey BJ. Pediatric psychopharmacology. In Sadock BJ, Sadock VA, eds. Comprehensive Textbook of Psychiatry 7th ed. Baltimore: Lippincott Williams & Wilkins, 2000, p 283.
4. Colarusso CA. The development of time sense. From birth to object constancy. Int J Psychoanal 60:243–251, 1979.
5. Colarusso CA. The development of time sense. From object constancy to adolescence. J Am Psychoanal Assoc 35:119–144, 1987.
6. Colarusso CA. Child and adult development. New York: Plenum Publishing, 1992.
7. Cotton NS. Normal adolescence. In Sadock BJ, Sadock VA, eds. Comprehensive Textbook of Psychiatry 7th ed. Baltimore: Lippincott Williams & Wilkins, 2000, pp 2550–2557.
8. Dixon S, Stein M. Encounters With Children: Pediatric Behavior and Development. 3rd ed. St. Louis: Mosby-Year Book, 2000.
9. Drell M, Hanson White, T. Children's reaction to illness and hospitalization. In Sadock BJ, Sadock VA, eds. Comprehensive Textbook of Psychiatry. 7th ed. Baltimore: Lippincott Williams & Wilkins, 2000, pp 2889–2995.

10. Freud A. The role of bodily illness in the mental life of children. Psychoanal Study Child 7:69–81, 1952.

11. Gordon M. Normal child development. In Sadock BJ, Sadock VA, eds. Comprehensive Textbook of Psychiatry. 7th ed. Baltimore: Lippincott Williams & Wilkins, 2000, pp 2534–2550.

12. Parmelee AH. Childhood Illness as a Source of Psychological Growth. Presidential address, Society for Research in Child Development, 1985.

13. Perrin EC, Gerrity PS. There's a demon in your belly: Children's understanding of concepts regarding illness. Pediatrics 12:19–14, 1981.

14. Peterson L, Shigetomi C. The use of coping techniques to minimize anxiety in hospitalized children. Behav Ther 12:19–14, 1981.

15. Piaget J. The Construction of Reality in the Child. New York: Basic Books, 1954.

16. Winnicott DW. Adolescent process and the need for personal confrontation. Pediatrics 44:752–756, 1969.

17. Zeltzer LK, Dolgin MJ, LeBaron S, Le Baron C. A randomized, controlled study of behavioral intervention for chemotherapy distress in children with cancer. Pediatrics 88:34–42, 1991.

18. Zeltzer LK, Jay SM, Fisher DM. The management of pain associated with pediatric procedures. Pediatr Clin North Am 36:19–24, 1989.

ADDITIONAL READING

Dixon S, Stein M. Encounters with Children: Pediatric Behavior and Development. St. Louis: Mosby, 2006.

McGee K. The role of a child life specialist in a pediatric radiology department. Pediatr Radiol 33:467–474, 2003.

Stokland E, Andreasson S, Jacobsson B, Jodal U, Ljung B. Sedation with midazolam for voiding cystourethrography in children: a randomized double-blind study. Pediatr Radiol 33:247–249, 2003.

Whitfield MF. Psychosocial effects of intensive care on infants and families after discharge. Semin Neonatal 8:185–193, 2003.

THE CHILD WITH A LIMP

Outline

Gerald A. Mandell, MD
H. Theodore Harcke, MD

THE CHILD WITH A LIMP

Children with acute or recent onset of limping or refusal to walk are frequently seen in emergency departments, outpatient clinics, and offices of family physicians and pediatricians. Most of these patients have minor soft tissue injuries that resolve within days without treatment. If the child or parent relates the onset of symptoms to an appropriate and significant episode of trauma, care of the patient is straightforward. Radiographic evaluation excludes fracture and provides therapeutic guidance when a fracture is present. Minor trauma is experienced daily by normal children, however, and a history of trauma can be misleading unless it unequivocally explains the symptom. Because young children may not accurately localize pain or effectively communicate symptoms to the physician, trauma cannot be assumed to be the etiology, and other conditions must be considered. In this chapter, the focus is on acute or newly discovered limping for which an acute traumatic cause is not clearly obvious (Figs. 20–1 and 20–2).

Almost all congenital causes of limping are manifest at birth or within the first months of life. Some congenital causes present late as a limp around 1 year of age, however, when the child begins to ambulate. Developmental dysplasia, one such condition, is included here because occasional cases are overlooked in neonates and only present when walking begins. Occult spinal dysraphism and tarsal coalition typically become manifest during early childhood and adolescence. Child abuse, always a consideration in a limping toddler, is discussed in detail in Chapter 17.

Symptomatic primary bone neoplasms are almost always visible on initial radiographs. Because of their relative rarity, such neoplasms are not discussed in detail here. Osteoid osteoma, Ewing's sarcoma, and osteogenic sarcoma are mentioned as differential diagnostic considerations where appropriate (Fig. 20–3). Secondary bone neoplasms, particularly leukemia and neuroblastoma, may present with musculoskeletal complaints and are included as differential diagnostic considerations in children with arthritis or bone pain. Normal radiographs do not rule out these conditions.

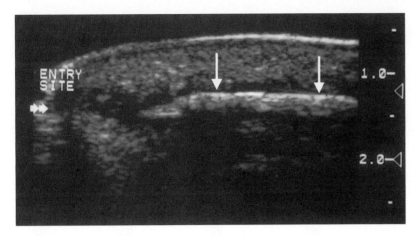

Figure 20–1
Nonopaque foreign body in the foot. Sonogram of the plantar soft tissues of the foot in a 9-year-old boy with a puncture wound and normal radiographs. A wooden toothpick fragment is easily visible with bright reflective echoes from the surface and acoustic shadowing.

DIFFERENTIAL DIAGNOSIS OF THE CHILD WITH AN ACUTE LIMP

When possible, it is important to obtain a detailed history of the limp, with particular emphasis on time of onset, persistence, and association with episodes of trauma and illness. Birth and developmental history may be useful.

Observe the gait of the child with the child unclothed, and examine the patient's shoes for proper fit and abnormal patterns of wear. If gait is normal and careful examination fails to reveal any limitation of joint motion or deep bone tenderness, it is usually safe to assume that the limp results from minor soft tissue injury and rapid resolution can be anticipated. The major forms of gait disturbances can be categorized by the examining physician.[128] This often considerably narrows the range of likely etiologies.

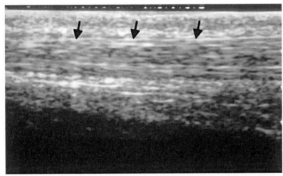

A

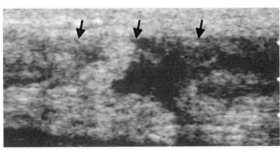

B

Figure 20–2
Achilles tendon rupture. An 18-year-old male adolescent with a complete tear of the Achilles tendon 8 cm above the calcaneal insertion. The sonograms of the normal (A) and affected (B) tendons (arrows) show fluid between retracted ends of the torn tendon with disruption of the normal fibrillar tendon architecture.

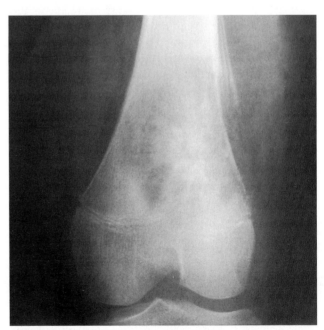

Figure 20–3
Osteogenic sarcoma. Initial radiograph of the distal right femur in a 10-year-old boy with right knee pain. Bone destruction, laminated periosteal reaction, and osteoid matrix characterize this osteosarcoma.

AGE

The age of the child with an acute limp limits diagnostic considerations and provides a useful framework for discussion of the differential diagnosis. The younger the child, the more difficult it is to localize the site of the pathologic condition. It may be impossible to distinguish a lower leg problem from a hip problem. Selected laboratory tests, particularly those reflecting the presence or absence of infection, should be ordered and considered in the decision to order further imaging studies when plain films are normal. In younger children, a more aggressive approach to the use of multiple studies is required to ensure that infection is not overlooked.

Trauma is, by far, the most common cause of limping in all age groups. The immaturity of the skeleton results in fractures unique to children. These fractures, classified by Salter and Harris[103] and expanded upon by others,[95] are found at all ages until skeletal maturity (Fig. 20–4). The classification is used because it has therapeutic and prognostic implications. The weakest plane of the physis is the zone of earliest calcification. The prepubertal growth spurt may further weaken the calcifying cartilage zone, increasing the likelihood of epiphyseal fractures. A fracture through the growth region may result in serious deformity because it can cause premature fusion of a portion of the growth center.

Preschool Children (1 to 4 Years Old)

The common causes of limping in toddlers are listed in Table 20–1. As noted earlier, trauma is the most common cause of limping in all age groups. Even if the toddler is able to give a history, it may not be reliable or accurate, making clinical assessment difficult.

Diagnosis of most fractures using routine radiographs is straightforward, although the relatively greater resilience of cortical bone and the looser attachment of the periosteum to the shaft of the bone result in different types of fractures in young children than in older patients. Specifically, torus fractures, incomplete fractures (greenstick and buckle), epiphyseal fractures, and metaphyseal corner fractures are seen commonly in young children. Metaphyseal corner fractures are almost always caused by child abuse. A spiral fracture of the tibia ("toddler's fracture") may be invisible on standard frontal and lateral radiographs and, occasionally, it is also difficult to discern on oblique views. Stress fractures generally occur in older children and adults.

Inflammatory conditions are also common causes of acute limping in toddlers and young children. Transient synovitis of the hip is by far the most common inflammatory condition (Fig. 20–5). Differentiation of transient synovitis from septic arthritis is made using clinical criteria and, if necessary, by analyzing aspirated joint fluid. Early diagnosis of septic arthritis is essential to avoid irreversible joint damage. Other arthritides, such as acute juvenile rheumatoid arthritis

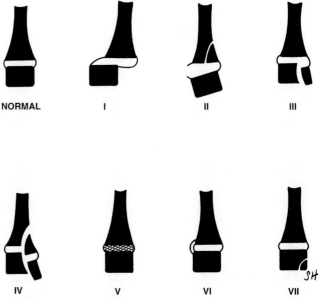

Figure 20–4

Salter-Harris classification of growth plate and epiphyseal injuries as modified by Ozonoff.[95]

I. Slippage of the epiphysis often causes widening or displacement of the growth plate. Because the periosteum usually remains intact, spontaneous reduction occurs frequently, resulting in apparently normal radiographs. Local soft tissue swelling and subtle growth plate widening are often evident when specifically sought. Apart from a slipped capital femoral epiphysis (SCFE), this injury is most commonly seen in children ages 1 through 5 years.

II. The shearing or avulsive force of this injury causes unilateral tearing of the periosteum, splitting of the growth plate, and fracture of a small portion of the metaphysis. Unilateral widening of the growth plate, epiphyseal displacement, and contralateral metaphyseal fracture make this injury readily apparent radiographically. These easily reducible fractures constitute approximately 50% to 75% of all growth plate injuries.

III. An intra-articular fracture causes vertical splitting of the epiphysis. The growth plate is variably widened, and the periosteum remains intact.

IV. This fracture, involving the metaphysis, growth plate, and epiphysis, results in offset of the growth plate and articular surface. Surgical reduction is necessary for satisfactory results. The epiphyseal periosteum remains intact bilaterally.

V. A compressive force injures the vascular supply and the germinal cells of a variable amount of the growth plate without resulting in definable epiphyseal widening or displacement. Therefore, radiographs are normal at the time of acute injury. Epiphyseal growth may be affected by this injury.

VI. Perichondrial injury may induce bone formation external to the growth plate. Focal perichondrial ossification may restrict normal epiphyseal growth and cause angulation of the epiphysis. Radiographs of the initial injury are normal.

VII. Only epiphyseal damage is present in this important and relatively common injury. Osteochondritis dissecans, a transchondral fracture, is included in this category, as is epiphyseal injury due to avascular necrosis, as in Köhler's disease (post-traumatic necrosis of the tarsal navicular).

TABLE 20-1 COMMON CAUSES OF LIMPING IN TODDLERS (2 TO 4 YEARS OLD)

Congenital
Spinal dysraphism
Club foot
Congenital dislocation of the hip
Coxa vara
Traumatic
Soft tissue injuries
Toddler's fracture
Other fractures
Nonaccidental trauma
Improperly fitting shoes and clothes
Foreign body
Inflammatory
Transient synovitis
Osteomyelitis
Septic arthritis
Cellulitis
Soft tissue abscess
Diskitis
Neuromuscular
Cerebral palsy
Spina bifida and/or meningomyelocele

(JRA), acute rheumatic fever, Lyme disease, rubella immunization arthritis, and tuberculous arthritis, are much less common in toddlers than are transient synovitis and pyogenic arthritis. Approximately 20% of patients with seronegative JRA present with monoarticular arthritis; the knee is the most frequent site of involvement. Symptoms resulting from bone involvement in patients with leukemia and neuroblastoma may mimic those of arthritis, and these conditions warrant consideration when pain is not responsive to standard therapy. Lyme disease is the most common tick-borne disease in the United States. The asymmetric involvement of one or more joints, especially the knees, is typical. Cases of Lyme arthritis usually begin appearing in the summer. Children usually have acute arthritis and not the chronic form that features joint destruction. The acute arthritis usually has joint swelling out of proportion to the pain and lasts approximately 8 days.

Osteomyelitis affects toddlers as well as children in all other pediatric age groups. Approximately 75% of cases in children involve the lower extremity. Cellulitis, or soft tissue abscess, occasionally develops spontaneously or after localized trauma. The toddler who limps for a period of time and then refuses to walk or even sit up should be suspected of having diskitis.

Unfortunately, developmental dysplasia of the hip (DDH) is occasionally overlooked during evaluation of the newborn infant. Congenital dislocation should be detected in infancy by appropriate repeated physical examinations (the Barlow and the Ortolani tests). After 3 months of age, the clinical

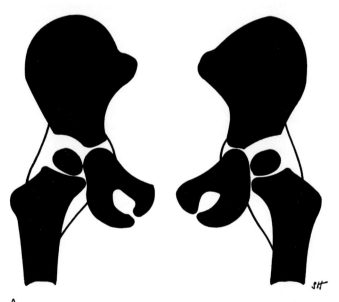 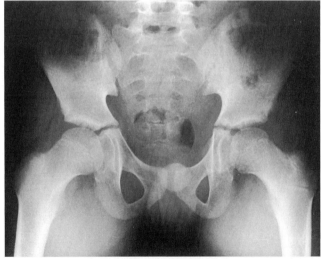

A   B

Figure 20–5
Fat planes of the hip. *A,* Diagrammatic representation. The three fat planes around the hip are the psoas, obturator, and gluteal planes. The psoas line parallels the medial femoral neck and represents fat between the iliopsoas muscle and the medial hip joint capsule. The obturator line represents fat medial to the obturator internus muscle and is visible medial to the acetabulum, roughly parallel to the pelvic wall. The gluteal line courses between the greater trochanter and the iliac bone and represents fat medial to the gluteus minimus muscle. *B,* Radiographic representation. Normal fat planes about the right hip are clearly demonstrated.

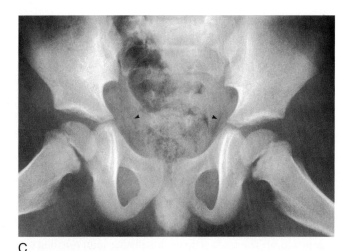

C

Figure 20–5—cont'd
C, Displacement of the obturator fat plane. Inflammatory disease of the left hip has displaced the obturator fat line medially. Of the three fat planes (radiolucent lines), only the obturator line can be evaluated accurately on frog-position pelvic films.

finding is limited abduction. The condition is difficult to assess on plain radiographs until ossification centers appear.[7]

Sonography is highly accurate in assessing infant development and stability of the hip joint.[9,62] The role of plain radiography for DDH in infants younger than 6 months of age is limited. In older infants, in whom the femoral head has begun to ossify, radiographs may provide useful information about development of the hip joint.

Toddlers with undiagnosed unilateral DDH present with limping characterized by features of both the short-leg and Trendelenburg gaits, with increased lumbar lordosis. Chung[18] discovered 6 children with congenital dislocation of the hip (now termed DDH) that were overlooked in a referral group of 148 children with an acute limp. Confident radiologic recognition of overlooked congenitally dislocated hip, whether unilateral or bilateral, is simple because acetabular dysplasia invariably is present, almost always with femoral head subluxation. In the young toddler, developmental coxa vara typically manifests as a painless limp and is readily revealed radiographically.

Occult spinal dysraphism, a congenital disorder, may not become apparent until the child is between the ages of 3 and 6 years and may first manifest as a painless limp. Intraspinal lesions (lipoma, dermoid, tethered cord, and diastematomyelia) typically are associated with cutaneous lesions (dermal sinus, hypopigmented areas, hairy tufts, pigmented nevi, hemangiomas, and subcutaneous lipoma). The symptomatic state results when growth of bony structures, dysplastic lesions, or both causes compression of or traction on the spinal cord or spinal nerves. Hip films of limping children usually include

the lower lumbar spine on the anteroposterior (AP) pelvic view; routine evaluation of this area is useful to detect dysraphic changes (e.g., arch defects or fusion anomalies, widened interpediculate distance, vertebral deformity, and sacral deformity). Radiographic abnormality of the lumbar spine (often subtle or minor) is present in 90% of patients who have occult spinal dysraphism. A definitive diagnosis is best achieved with magnetic resonance imaging (MRI), although there may be a role for computed tomography (CT) in patients in whom more information about osseous structures is desired (diastematomyelia). The average age at onset of symptoms (orthopedic, neurologic, or urologic disturbances) in occult dysraphism syndromes is 3 years; however, the average age at diagnosis is 7 years. Urologic complications are discussed in Chapter 4.

Elementary School Children (5 to 10 Years Old)

The common causes of limping in children between 5 and 10 years of age are listed in Table 20–2. As noted, trauma is the most common cause of newly acquired limping, with soft tissue injuries occurring more frequently than fractures. Ankle sprain is the most common injury. Assessment of joint stability is primarily clinical, but stress radiographs of a joint may be helpful. Generally, fractures in children in this age group are not difficult to detect on standard radiographs, although a Salter type I fracture through the cartilage plate may be subtle without a comparison view of the contralateral epiphysis. Characteristic fractures of toddlers, such as the spiral tibial fracture and the metaphyseal corner fracture of

TABLE 20-2 Common Causes of Limping in Children (5 to 10 Years Old)
Traumatic
Soft tissue injuries
Fractures
Improperly fitting shoes
Foreign body
Inflammatory
Transient synovitis
Septic arthritis
Juvenile rheumatoid arthritis
Osteomyelitis
Cellulitis
Abscess
Diskitis
Tendinitis
Other
Legg-Calvé-Perthes disease

child abuse, essentially are not seen in children of this age group. However, torus and greenstick fractures still occur. Osteochondral injuries and osteochondritis dissecans may occur (see "Preadolescents and Adolescents") but are less common in this age group than in adolescents. Normal developmental irregularities of the subchondral bone of the femoral condyles are very common and may mimic osteochondritis dissecans (Fig. 20–6). These irregularities of condylar ossification may be differentiated from osteochondritis dissecans by their tendency to involve the posterior (non–weight-bearing) surfaces of the condyles and by their propensity to develop in both condyles or in the lateral condyle alone.[68]

The pattern of long-bone fractures in older children and adolescents differs from that in younger children. With increasing age, cortical bone becomes less resilient and the periosteum more firmly attached, and torus and greenstick fractures become uncommon. Instead, there are relatively more fractures involving the epiphysis, metaphysis, and growth plate.

The same inflammatory conditions that occur in toddlers also affect children in this age group. Older children are able to describe and localize their pain more clearly than toddlers, but referred pain (often knee pain in hip disease) remains a common source of confusion. Occasionally, multiple radiographic examinations of the knee are performed before attention is finally (and correctly) directed to the hip. Transient synovitis is by far the most frequent inflammatory condition encountered in children of this age group. Differentiation of transient synovitis from other inflammatory arthritides such as septic arthritis, JRA, rheumatic fever, and tuberculous

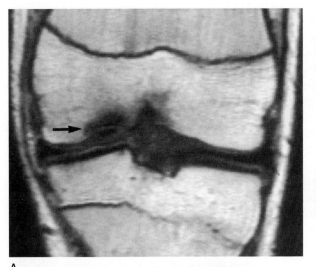

A

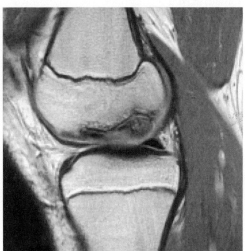

B

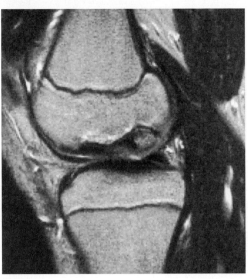

C

Figure 20–6

Magnetic resonance imaging (MRI) in osteochondritis dissecans. Knee imaging: *A,* Coronal T1-weighted image of the left knee shows loss of normal marrow signal in the osteochondritis fragment on the lateral aspect of the medical femoral condyle *(arrow).* A proton-density sagittal view *(B)* and a T2-weighted sagittal view *(C)* also reveal loss of signal in the bony fragment. No complications are evident.

arthritis must be made on clinical grounds and by aspiration of the joint.

In this age group, osteomyelitis can be revealed by scintigraphy and MRI with greater accuracy (i.e., fewer false-negative diagnoses) than in neonates and toddlers.

In its early phase, avascular necrosis of the femoral head, from Legg-Calvé-Perthes (LCP) disease or other causes, may result in symptoms that suggest inflammatory disease. Typically, LCP disease affects children between 5 and 10 years of age.

Preadolescents and Adolescents (11 to 18 Years Old)

Common causes of limping in older children and adolescents are listed in Table 20–3. Trauma continues to be the most common etiology, and ankle sprains are the most frequent injuries. Radiographic evaluation of traumatic injuries is similar to that used in younger children. Radiographs should supplement, not substitute for, a thorough physical examination. Findings on physical examination may indicate the need for specific stress views to reveal joint instability or suggest additional injuries. The presence of soft tissue abnormalities, including joint effusion, fat pad displacement, edema, and intra-articular fat-fluid level, is indicative of bone trauma and may prompt CT or MRI examination.

The number of children and adolescents involved in organized sports has increased dramatically over recent decades. Participation in organized sports is now regarded as a common rite of childhood for both boys and girls in the United States. Older children and adolescents participating in athletics are likely to suffer injuries characteristic of specific activities.

For example, gymnasts or cheerleaders tend to suffer avulsion fractures of the ischial tuberosities. In older adolescents, particularly those who participate in contact sports such as football, intra-articular cartilage injuries are frequently seen. It is appropriate to evaluate these with MRI or arthrography. Meniscal tears, discoid lateral meniscus, cruciate ligament disruption, and joint capsule disruption are familiar diagnoses that may be established using these techniques.

Osteochondritis dissecans results from avascular necrosis of a localized portion of articular cartilage and an underlying osseous fragment. It typically occurs in older children, adolescents, and young adults.[42] The majority of patients relate a history of trauma consistent with an acute chondral or osteochondral fracture, but other proposed etiologies include chronic mechanical stress, familial dysplasia, avascular necrosis, and fat emboli.[24] The usual sites of involvement in the lower extremity are the distal femur, talar dome, and posterior patella (Fig. 20–7). The classic femoral lesion occurs in the medial femoral condyle adjacent to and extending into the intercondylar notch. This location correlates with the nonmeniscal weight-bearing region of the articular surface when the knee is extended. After osteonecrosis has occurred and evolved, a linear semicircular or crescent-like

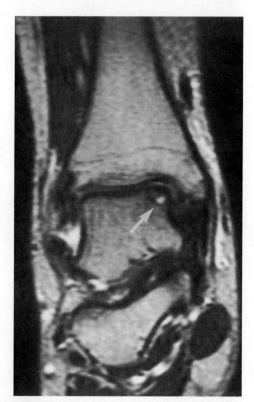

Figure 20–7
Ankle imaging: A T2-weighted coronal view of the right ankle shows an area of osteochondritis dissecans in the superior medial aspect of the dome of the talus. A small amount of high-signal fluid *(arrow)* can be seen between the fragment and the talus, indicating a fissure or a break in the overlying articular cartilage of the talus.

TABLE 20-3 COMMON CAUSES OF LIMPING IN OLDER CHILDREN AND ADOLESCENTS (11 TO 18 YEARS OLD)
Traumatic
Soft tissue injuries
Fractures
Stress fractures
Osteochondritis dissecans
Osgood-Schlatter disease
Inflammatory
Juvenile rheumatoid arthritis
Ankylosing spondylitis
Septic arthritis
Cellulitis
Abscess
Osteomyelitis
Tendinitis
Other
Slipped capital femoral epiphysis

subchondral radiolucent osseous defect demarcates the subchondral bone fragment on plain radiographs. Careful observation of the articular cartilage during arthrography may reveal a chondral fracture in which a fragment has been detached from the joint surface. MRI can demonstrate a chondral or osteochondral injury long before plain radiographs show any abnormality, and it can also usually demonstrate whether the fragment is attached or unstable.[23,24] Inadequate healing of this and other intra-articular lesions may result in long-term disability from degenerative joint disease.

When hip pain presents in the prepubertal adolescent, there is a strong possibility of a slipped capital femoral epiphysis (SCFE). This can present as an acute onset of limp or may manifest as chronic pain depending upon the nature of the slip.

Older children and adolescents are more likely to develop stress fractures than are younger children, probably as a result of more rigid cortical bone combined with a greater tendency to perform prolonged, repetitive physical activities such as running. Commonly occurring stress fractures in children are seen in the proximal and distal tibia (41%), fibula (27%), and proximal neck or shaft of the femur (12%) (Fig. 20–8).[112] Other areas of involvement include the distal metatarsals and calcaneus. After weeks of symptoms, a stress fracture usually manifests a transverse sclerotic line, a lucent line, or both, often with periosteal new bone. Later, as healing progresses, bony callus develops. Pain should subside promptly with immobilization.

Early in the course of a tibial stress fracture, it may be difficult to distinguish such a fracture from traumatic periosteal

reaction ("shin splints") on clinical grounds, and radiographs are typically normal in both conditions. Because the sensitivity of skeletal scintigraphy for stress fracture approaches 100%, it is generally considered the "gold standard." Bone scintigraphy will show obvious increased activity extending transversely through the cortex of the bone at a stress fracture site. In periostitis, increased radiotracer deposition is noted over a broad area of the posterior tibial cortex, often affecting both lower extremities.[54,85] Because the course of healing is much longer for a stress fracture than for periosteal reaction, differentiation soon after presentation may be desirable for the competitive athlete who is anxious to return to play.

It is not unusual for stress fractures or reactions of the pars interarticularis (spondylolysis) to become evident during participation in organized athletics. The reported incidence is 4.4% in children.[38] Spondylolysis is most often an overuse injury associated with repetitive hyperextension of the spine. Gymnastics, ballet, diving, and football line play are particularly common predisposing activities. These lesions may be unilateral or bilateral and occur predominantly at L4 or L5. Bone scintigraphy with single photon emission computed tomography (SPECT) can identify lesions not obvious on plain radiographs. CT confirmation is sometimes necessary if the diagnosis is equivocal or does not explain the patient's symptoms. Children and adolescents usually present with pain due to spasm of the lumbar-ischial and hamstring muscles.[104] Another characteristic post-traumatic lesion encountered in older children and adolescents is Osgood-Schlatter disease, or osteochondrosis of the tibial tuberosity. The pathologic fracture is a small avulsion of the tibial tubercle near the attachment of the patellar tendon. Physical examination is the appropriate method of diagnosis in Osgood-Schlatter disease, because affected patients have obvious soft tissue swelling and point tenderness over the tibial tuberosity. Radiographic assessment is warranted, but only to exclude other possible conditions (i.e., stress fracture, osteomyelitis, or neoplasm). The radiographic findings of Osgood-Schlatter disease are soft tissue swelling over the tuberosity and edema in the infrapatellar tendon.[108] A fragmented configuration to the ossified portion of the tibial tuberosity is nonspecific because it also may be seen in normal children.

The same inflammatory diseases described in younger patients also affect older children. Radiography and bone scintigraphy are more accurate methods of examination in older children and adolescents than in younger children. Immobility is more easily attained, soft tissue planes are more clearly outlined, and the metaphyseal growth zones are less intensely active on scintigraphy, making interpretation of findings in these regions easier.

Tarsal coalition is an important cause of foot or ankle pain in children and adolescents. Tarsal coalition is a failure of segmentation or an abnormal fusion between tarsal bones, most commonly the calcaneus with the talus (talocalcaneal coalition) or navicular (calcaneonavicular coalition).

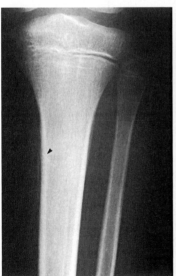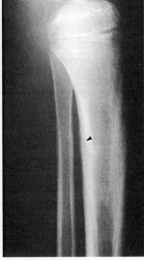

Figure 20–8

Stress fracture. Anteroposterior (AP) and lateral radiographs of the left tibia of an 11-year-old boy with pain in the region of the proximal tibia. Periosteal new bone is seen about the proximal shaft of the tibia, and a transverse lucency with sclerotic borders *(arrowhead)* is evident, representing the stress fracture. Symptoms had been present for 6 weeks.

Patients with congenital tarsal coalition typically present in the second decade of life with a painful and rigid foot. Coalition (i.e., fusion of tarsal ossification centers) is fibrous or cartilaginous during the first decade of life. With further maturation in the second decade, the coalition becomes less flexible and creates intertarsal rigidity with secondary symptoms. A rigid foot with peroneal muscle spasm is a characteristic symptom. Talocalcaneal coalition, the most common form of tarsal coalition, most often involves the middle facet (sustentaculum) of the subtalar joint. This site is best revealed on plain films with an axial calcaneal (Harris) view. Talocalcaneal coalition is manifested radiographically by secondary signs of dorsal talar beaking, broadening, and rounding of the lateral process surface of the ankle joint, and the "C sign," an abnormal outline formed on a lateral projection by the medial talar dome and inferior sustentaculum tali.[73] These radiographic changes are apparent in disease of long duration. The facet joints of the subtalar joint are best revealed on a 45-degree posterior axial oblique (Harris) projection. Calcaneonavicular coalition is easily revealed in an oblique view of the foot.

CT is useful for the diagnosis of coalitions when suspicion is high and plain radiographs are negative or inconclusive and for surgical planning when radiographs are positive. For CT of talocalcaneal coalition, the hip and knee should be flexed and the feet placed flat on the gantry. A bony bridge connecting the talus to the calcaneus is easy to recognize, whereas a fibrous or cartilaginous bridge is manifested by irregularity and sclerosis of the adjacent osseous surfaces. Subtalar joints are demonstrated best on coronal slices and calcaneonavicular joints on longitudinal slices. MRI is useful for demonstrating nonosseous coalitions, which (except for secondary joint sclerosis and irregularity) are difficult to detect with CT. Bone scintigraphy with pinhole collimation and SPECT can be used effectively if radiographic and CT changes are equivocal.[80] The earlier the coalition can be extirpated, the less likely degenerative changes are to develop in the foot. The coexistence of calcaneonavicular and talocalcaneal coalition occurs in 17% and 30% of patients.[26]

EVALUATION OF IMPORTANT CONDITIONS CAUSING ACUTE LIMP

DEVELOPMENTAL DYSPLASIA OF THE HIP

Hip dislocation and dysplasia are included in the discussion of childhood limping because recognition in infancy and appropriate early treatment may prevent changes that cause a limp after walking progresses.

Pathophysiology

The term *congenital dysplasia of the hip* was changed to *developmental dysplasia of the hip* (DDH) to better convey the scope of this condition, which has a range of abnormalities and changes over time. DDH is regarded as a spectrum of findings related to femoral head position, stability, and morphology of the acetabulum. The conditions of patients with bilateral DDH, who manifest variable severity from side to side, support the concept that this is a single but variable pathologic entity.

Laxity of the hip joint, often found at birth, is influenced by maternal hormones. The sex of the child plays a role in DDH and is thought to account for the 6:1 female-to-male incidence. Other genetic factors also appear important, because DDH is more likely to occur in infants with a sibling or parent with DDH.[78]

Near the time of birth, when the joint capsule is elastic and stretched, there is a tendency for the femoral head to dislocate. The shape of the joint and the soft tissues are nearly normal, however, so if the femoral head is kept in the acetabulum, the joint capsule will tighten and return to normal configuration in a few weeks. Although this can occur spontaneously without treatment, in some patients the hip remains unstable or frankly dislocates. When DDH is undetected and the hip is not successfully reduced, adaptive changes in the acetabulum (pseudoacetabulum formation and femoral head or small flattened delayed ossification), ligaments, and muscles (contractures) occur. With a greater deformity to reverse, obtaining a satisfactory reduction is difficult. Surgery is required in patients with severe DDH.[52]

Clinical Presentation

In the first 2 to 3 months of life, it is easy to overlook DDH, as it is not painful, and there is no apparent deformity. DDH is generally detected after that period by clinical examination. The American Academy of Pediatrics recommends that all infants be examined periodically for DDH.[3] Incorporated into the examination are the Ortolani and Barlow maneuvers, done to detect a dislocated hip reducing or an unstable hip dislocating. The abnormal hip produces a vibratory sensation felt by the examiner, described as a "clunk." After several months of being dislocated, the soft tissues around the hip tighten, the hip will not reduce, and an Ortolani sign will not be elicited. At this time, there is limited abduction of the hip, which becomes the key sign of DDH. As walking begins, the toddler with undiagnosed unilateral DDH presents with limping characterized by a short leg or Trendelenburg gait with increased lumbar lordosis.[7]

Diagnostic Imaging

The immature hip is composed of cartilage, which is not visible on radiographs. This has limited the accuracy of plain films prior to the appearance of the femoral head ossification center (between ages 4 and 8 months) (Fig. 20–9).

In assessing infant plain films for hip anatomy, several guidelines assist in radiographic diagnosis.[11] Use of these

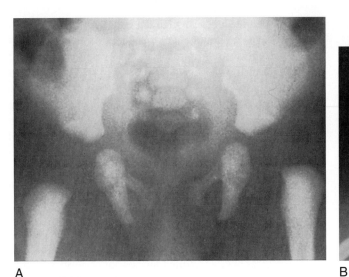
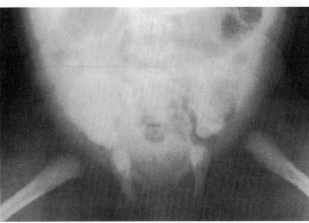

A   B

Figure 20–9
Congenital hip dislocation. *A,* AP view. The left femoral neck is slightly displaced laterally and superiorly, indicating a femoral head dislocation. There is no evidence of acetabular dysplasia. Clinical examination revealed a congenital dislocation of the hip in this neonate. *B,* von Rosen view. A maneuver to dislocate the hips is performed by internal rotation and abduction (45 degrees from midline) of the femurs. Care is taken not to rotate the pelvis. In this patient, the von Rosen view markedly accentuates the left hip dislocation; the right hip maintains a normal relationship to the acetabulum. The von Rosen view is especially helpful in dislocatable (rather than dislocated) hips that are normal on the frontal view.

parameters is highly dependent upon proper positioning. Rotation of the pelvis and asymmetric positioning of the femora can distort normal anatomic relationships, making them seem abnormal.

Over the years, real-time sonography has been found to reliably assess three key features of the infant hip joint[44,49]: (1) *position,* the relationship of the femoral head to the acetabulum; (2) *stability,* the change in position of the head in response to movement and stress—typically, this is modeled after the Barlow and Ortolani maneuvers and is referred to as dynamic examination, and (3) *morphology,* the development of the bony and cartilaginous components of the acetabulum. Acetabular angles and coverage measurements that reflect the severity of dysplasia have been used in quantification of development.

Most sonographers have adopted a technique that incorporates both morphologic and dynamic assessment. The relationships of the femoral head to the acetabulum at rest and with stress (position and stability) are examined along with the development of the acetabular roof components (morphology)[4] (Figs. 20–10 and 20–11).

Use of ultrasound to manage patients with DDH has focused on evaluation in the Pavlik harness, a dynamic splint

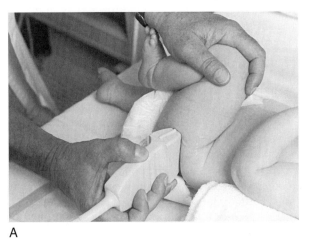
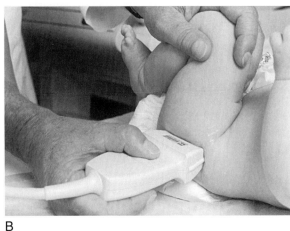

A   B

Figure 20–10
Flexion views of the hip. *A,* Positions of the hip and transducer for transverse-flexion view. *B,* Transducer is rotated 90° clockwise for the coronal-flexion view.

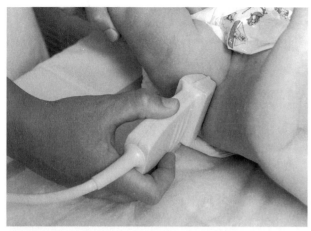

Figure 20–11
Transverse neutral view of the hip. Positions of the hip and transducer.

used for treating infants with uncomplicated DDH. Dynamic sonography detects instability and posterior displacement.[46] Discrepancies may exist in the sonographic appearance of the bony acetabulum and the appearance on pelvic radiographs. For this reason, an AP pelvic view is recommended when the harness is discontinued.[98]

CT is usually reserved for cases requiring surgical intervention. Axial sections through the hip show displacement of the femoral head from the acetabulum. Radiation exposure can be significantly reduced by using a scout radiograph to select planes of examination. Frequently, one may use only one or two slices when assessing a patient in a cast after closed or open reduction. By lowering the radiographic dosage level (milliamperes), exposure is further reduced. Although the images may be of lesser quality, they are adequate to make the diagnosis.[47]

The anatomy of the infant is well demonstrated by MRI. In single hips, detailed images obtained with small surface coils result in excellent visualization of all clinically important soft tissue and cartilaginous structures.[61] Three-dimensional MRI images of infant hips have been obtained. Because it is relatively small, the infant hip is greatly affected by partial volume averaging, low contrast, and other technical factors. MRI is principally used in preoperative planning for patients with DDH that did not respond to treatment, but it is also being used to assess operative reduction.[86] The development of avascular necrosis in the femoral head as a complication of DDH treatment is well recognized. MRI with contrast enhancement has the potential to detect early avascular changes in the developing epiphysis.

TODDLER'S FRACTURE

A toddler's fracture historically has been considered a nondisplaced oblique or spiral fracture of the tibia in a preschool child. It is seen characteristically in children 1 to 3 years of age.[30] Presentation of the toddler's fracture, however, can be extended to span the period of 9 months to 6 years.[87] Although healing occurs regardless of whether or not therapy is administered, recognition of the fracture at the time of presentation limits the symptomatic period and precludes the cost, concern, and wasted time of unnecessary diagnostic maneuvers. The sometimes confusing history and the frequent paucity of obvious signs of fracture on physical examination and standard radiographs render this entity a diagnostic challenge in many instances. Clinicians became more aware of the other fractures of the foot (calcaneus, cuboid, talus, and metatarsal) in toddlers because of the use of scintigraphy in the investigation of preschool children with lower extremity pain, gait disturbances, or both. These foot fractures have accounted for 50% of abnormal findings in bone scans.[6,33] Fractures of the metatarsal and tarsal bones were once considered rare in children. Another recently described toddler's fracture involves the upper tibial metaphysis.[116]

Pathophysiology

A nondisplaced spiral fracture of the tibia is the most common toddler's fracture. These fractures probably result during normal play activities. Jumping from heights and sliding, perhaps followed by a difficult landing, or catching a foot between bars of a playpen can create enough twisting or longitudinal driving force to cause either a spiral fracture of the tibia or a compression fracture of a foot bone. The torsion forces tend to be mild, so displacement of fracture fragments is usually minimal, and the fibula is rarely involved. The fibula is resilient enough to remain intact. The tibial periosteal sleeve remains intact. Jumping from a height with impaction and twisting usually results in a fracture of the base of the first metatarsal. Calcaneal fractures can be caused by impaction injuries.[114] Forced dorsiflexion usually causes a talar fracture, whereas forced plantar flexion results in a cuboidal fracture from compression between the calcaneus and the metatarsals.[13] Upper tibial fracture results from forces applied to the hyperextended knee bone. Most foot fractures are subtle. Certainly, the frequency of tarsal fractures should prompt the inclusion of radiographic images of the feet in the screening examination of the limping preschool child.[60]

Clinical Presentation

A history of appropriate trauma is elicited in about half of children, but often the episode is not witnessed, and the toddler cannot effectively relate the history or specific symptoms of the injury. Toddler's fracture produces an abrupt onset of pain. Often, the child suddenly refuses to walk or walks with an antalgic limp. Typically, the child is irritable and may cry frequently or continually. Fever, leukocytosis, and other systemic signs are absent. Accurate localization of deep tenderness on physical examination may be difficult unless the child can first be calmed and the normal side examined before one proceeds to performing gentle palpation of the symptomatic extremity. Pathologic abnormality in the knee or foot is often suspected. Skin temperature over the fracture area may be increased. Deformity and significant swelling are not discernible initially, because the fracture is not displaced and is stable with its intact periosteal sleeve. If the fracture is assumed to involve the tibia, and the child is immobilized with a long-leg cast, symptoms can persist if the fracture involves the foot. Symptoms persist for many days, and the parents must contend with an unhappy child. Nevertheless, healing proceeds satisfactorily. A tender swelling resulting from periosteal new bone may be palpated over the area of involvement about 1 week after the traumatic episode.

It is important to note that the vast majority of toddler's fractures result from accidental trauma.[87] Even if the trauma seems minor or was not observed, child abuse is not likely.

Diagnostic Imaging

Imaging of the limping toddler should include an AP pelvis view to compare the hip joint spaces, anterior images, and posterior images of the symptomatic lower extremity, including the foot. Tibial fracture may be invisible, owing to the lack of displacement and the curving oblique course of the hairline crack. Oblique views, particularly the internally rotated oblique view, may reveal the fracture line. Some examiners have used fluoroscopy to find the exact degree of rotation to show the fracture. If the clinical diagnosis is reasonably certain despite normal radiographs, follow-up films at 10 to 14 days are appropriate to confirm the fracture.

Because a significant minority of cases of osteomyelitis present without fever or an elevated white blood cell (WBC) count, bone infection may be considered in children with toddler's fracture. In such circumstances, a bone scan usually reliably distinguishes the two entities. Most fractures display increased radiotracer uptake on scintigrams within 48 hours of injury, and most patients with osteomyelitis have positive findings within 24 to 48 hours after the onset of symptoms.[103,107] If the scintigraphic findings are not classic for toddler's fracture, the entire skeleton should be imaged to search for an occult metastatic neoplasm.

The lower two thirds of the tibia is the usual site of fracture. Extension into the upper third may occur, however, particularly in children older than 3 years (Fig. 20–12). The fracture must be distinguished from the canal for the normal nutrient artery. After 10 to 14 days, healing processes make the fracture more evident, with resorption of the bone around the fracture line and formation of periosteal new bone (Figs. 20–13 and 20–14).

On skeletal scintigraphy, the cortical bone adjacent to the fracture line shows increased activity, usually within hours

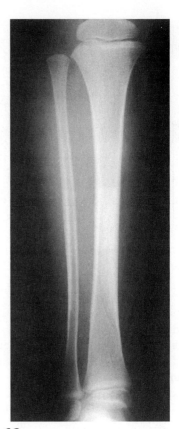

Figure 20–12
Toddler's fracture. An oblique lucency of the distal right tibia is clearly evident on this frontal radiograph. This 18-month-old boy presented with a limp of acute onset. A history of trauma could not be elicited. Few toddler's fractures are as clearly visible as this example, and many require oblique views to define the spiral fracture.

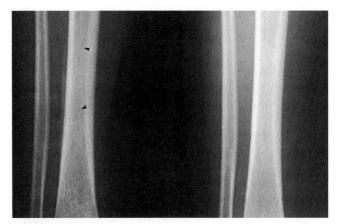

Figure 20–13
Toddler's fracture. Frontal and lateral views obtained at the time of initial injury were normal. Thirteen days later, the AP radiograph *(left)* demonstrates a faint oblique lucency *(arrowheads)* and definite periosteal new bone. Bone resorption associated with healing will often make fracture lines more visible.

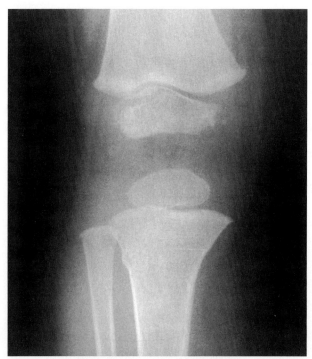

Figure 20–14
Toddler's fracture variant in a 23-month-old female. A buckle fracture of the proximal tibia shows localized cortical disruption at the lateral tibial metaphysis. This shows the importance of radiographing the entire extremity when examining the limping toddler.

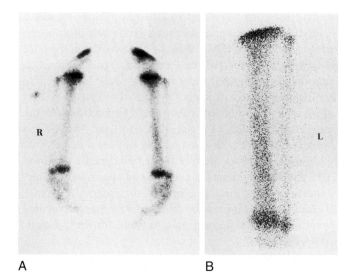

A   B

Figure 20–15
Toddler's fracture. *A*, A technetium 99m medronate disodium (Tc-MDP) high-resolution collimator scintigram was performed in this 20-month-old limping boy because frontal, lateral, and even oblique plain films did not confirm a fracture. Because there was no history of trauma, osteomyelitis was a diagnostic possibility that required exclusion. The left spiral tibial fracture is seen as an oblique area of increased activity. *B*, A pinhole collimator image again shows the spiral tibial fracture and, more importantly, excludes the possibility of hematogenous osteomyelitis with confidence.

after the injury. Pinhole collimator images often reveal the distinctive spiral configuration, notably different from the focal metaphyseal or occasional epiphyseal lesion seen in osteomyelitis (Fig. 20–15). In the small bones of the feet, osteomyelitis might be difficult to differentiate from a traumatic lesion without association of abnormalities in the sedimentation rate and blood count.

TRANSIENT SYNOVITIS

Transient synovitis of the hip (or sometimes of the knee or ankle[57]) is the most common nontraumatic cause of an acute limp in a child. This condition has a variety of names, including observation hip, transitory synovitis, toxic synovitis, and coxitis fugax. Throughout its history, its diagnosis has been one of exclusion. The fact that complete recovery tends to occur within 5 to 14 days excludes serious conditions such as LCP disease, tuberculosis, and childhood malignancy (particularly leukemia and neuroblastoma).

Pathophysiology

The etiology of transient synovitis is unknown. The most appealing proposed etiology is a nonspecific inflammatory response to antecedent viral or, perhaps, streptococcal infection. Activation of the interferon system in about 80% of patients with transient synovitis provides nonspecific laboratory evidence for active viral infection as a primary factor.[76] Trauma and allergy have been proposed as etiologies, but careful comparisons of affected and normal children have not supported such theories. Microscopic examination of the affected synovium shows only a nonspecific inflammatory reaction.

Clinical Presentation

The typical patient with transient synovitis is a Caucasian boy between 3 and 10 years of age who gradually, over 1 to 2 days, develops a limp associated with pain in the hip, thigh, or knee. Occasionally, the onset is sudden. Boys are affected more commonly than girls by a ratio of 2:1. Average age of onset is 6 years. Bone age can be delayed in either transient synovitis or LCP disease.[121] Sometimes there is a history of recent viral illness, usually an upper respiratory infection, in more than half of patients. A minority of patients have mild fever, and about half have modestly elevated erythrocyte sedimentation rates. Among children hospitalized with transient synovitis, more than 90% have normal leukocyte counts.

On physical examination, the patient usually does not appear systemically ill, although the affected joint may be very painful. Limited motion of the hip joint is evident, and usually there is pain with passive motion. Joint aspiration yields 1 to 3 mL of clear or slightly blood-tinged fluid containing only a few granulocytes in about 80% of patients.

Although transient synovitis and septic arthritis often can be distinguished without joint aspiration,[118] arthrocentesis is indicated with appropriate analysis of the fluid in patients with suspected septic arthritis. When septic arthritis is excluded, the major differential diagnoses besides transient synovitis are trauma, osteomyelitis, LCP disease, acute rheumatoid arthritis, acute rheumatic fever, and tuberculosis. Early in the course of these diseases, the distinction is made typically without radiography, but skeletal scintigraphy or MRI can be useful in identifying osteomyelitis and early LCP disease.

Periarticular bone lesions from leukemia and neuroblastoma can produce a clinical picture that closely resembles acute or subacute arthritis (Fig. 20–16). Intra-articular hemorrhage and cellular infiltration are additional mechanisms of joint involvement present in leukemia. When "synovitis" persists despite standard therapy, blood smear and bone marrow examinations should be considered to exclude such malignancies.

Complete bed rest, followed by limitation of weight bearing, relieves the pain of transient synovitis and allows recovery of full range of motion within an average of 13 days, often within 4 to 6 days. Although acute symptoms usually subside rapidly, a small number of patients (2.5%)[50] develop avascular necrosis of the femoral head within several months, usually with no cessation of symptoms during the interval.[92] The increased volume of sterile joint fluid creates an elevation of intra-articular pressure. Maintenance of elevated pressure for more than 12 to 24 hours has been shown experimentally to produce irreversible ischemia of the femoral head.[127] There is no convincing etiologic link between transient synovitis

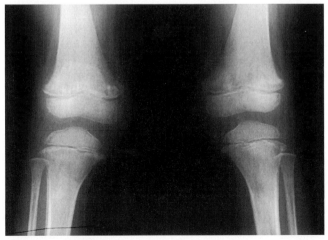

Figure 20–16
Leukemia in a 4-year-old boy presenting with lower extremity pain. Bilateral metaphyseal changes are present in the distal femur and proximal tibias. Lucency adjacent to the growth plates has a "band-like" appearance owing to loss of the trabecular architecture. Note the periosteal reaction along the proximal tibias.

and LCP disease, despite the relative ischemia of the femoral head observed in some patients with transient synovitis.[66] Recurrences of transient synovitis also occur, sometimes years later and usually without any more severe outcome than that for the original episode.[58] The frequency of long-term sequelae is low.[25,110] Coxa magna and widening of the femoral neck can occur. Arthrograms have shown hypertrophied cartilage in some patients with transient synovitis.[40] Joint space narrowing, osteoarthritis, and cystic changes of the femoral neck are rare but can occur.[110]

Diagnostic Imaging

Imaging of patients with suspected transient synovitis is done primarily to exclude other pathologic conditions. Radiographs are the first step to rule out trauma and specific radiographic lesions seen with primary neoplasm, LCP disease, and chronic osteomyelitis. Radiographs in transient synovitis usually appear normal; if abnormal, they demonstrate changes in the hip joint space that are nonspecific and reflect joint effusion. Ultrasound can be useful in documenting the presence of joint fluid. This is a nonspecific finding but lets the physician know that aspiration, if performed, will yield a specimen for laboratory analysis. Some physicians perform aspiration routinely because it relieves pain as well as provides fluid for analysis.

Most workups conclude following aspiration. Additional imaging with scintigraphy or MRI is necessary only when there is a high index of suspicion for infection or avascular necrosis. If pain persists after a trial of conservative treatment, these other modalities may reveal occult infection outside the joint, such as psoas abscess, iliac osteomyelitis, sacroiliitis, or disc space infection in the spine.

Radiographic signs of hip joint effusion are subtle and not always present. Displacement of fat planes around the hip have historically been described as signs of hip joint effusion, particularly in transient synovitis.[31] Anatomic studies have shown that fat plane changes are more related to variations in leg position (abduction) than to distension of the joint capsule.[5,14] A 2-mm variation in medial joint space dimension on a very straight radiograph suggests joint effusion (Fig. 20–17).

Sonography is performed from an anterior approach in the long axis of the femoral neck. A linear transducer is used, and both the affected and asymptomatic hips are scanned. Fluid collects preferentially in the inferior recess of the joint capsule. Echoes from the tissue planes are displaced, and convex bowing is noted (Fig. 20–18).

The distance from the anterior margin of the capsule to the bone can then be measured.[2] Fluid character is not helpful, and there are no constant distinguishing sonographic signs for hemorrhagic, purulent, or sterile effusions.[84,90]

The radiographic density of the periarticular bones is usually normal in transient synovitis. However, some patients

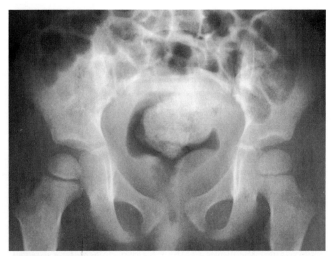

Figure 20–17
Hip effusion with femoral subluxation due to transient synovitis in a 2¹/₂-year-old girl. A right hip joint effusion displaces the right femur laterally and slightly inferiorly. Note that the pelvis is not rotated and the femurs are positioned neutrally.

who have symptoms for a week or longer develop regional osteoporosis, due presumably to hyperemia or disuse.

Scintigraphic findings in transient synovitis vary. The immediate soft tissue ("blood-pool") images may be normal or may exhibit slightly increased activity, reflecting the hyperemia associated with synovial inflammation. Delayed scans may be normal or may display slightly increased uptake

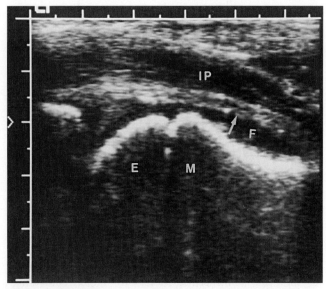

Figure 20–18
Joint effusion. This parasagittal image obtained from an anterior approach shows a collection of hypoechoic fluid (F) in the anterior part of the joint capsule displacing the joint capsule away from the femoral neck *(arrow)* in a convex arc. E, epiphysis; M, metaphysis; IP, iliopsoas.

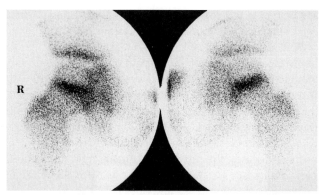

Figure 20–19
Transient synovitis. Pinhole collimator scintigrams of the hips in a 6-year-old boy with transient synovitis on the right (R). A generalized, symmetric increase in radiotracer deposition in and about the right hip is evident. Plain films of the pelvis (not shown) demonstrated the hip effusion by displacement of the obturator, iliopsoas, and gluteal fat lines. These findings are compatible with synovitis from any cause.

on both sides of the joint (Fig. 20–19). Characteristically in LCP disease, part or all of the proximal femoral epiphysis is "cold" or photopenic. This can be confusing in some instances of large joint effusions, when there is reduced activity or photopenia involving the entire hip. The increased intra-articular pressure exceeds the venous pressure, which results in compression of the venous circulation and, in turn, decreased arterial supply. The tamponade can be reversed either by aspiration or by physiologic resorption of the fluid. Reversible ischemia can also occur with effusions of septic arthritis, hemarthrosis, and sympathetic joint effusion related to osteomyelitis. The reversal of the photopenia of the femoral head can be demonstrated by a repeat bone scan[126] (Fig. 20–20).

If MRI is used to exclude LCP disease or septic arthritis, the key to diagnosis of transient synovitis is normal bone marrow signal intensity on T1-weighted and fat-suppressed T2-weighted fast spin-echo images. Joint fluid is seen, but without juxta-articular abnormality or diffuse marrow alteration.[75]

LEGG-CALVÉ-PERTHES DISEASE

Although there is debate about both the necessity for therapy and the efficacy of specific therapeutic maneuvers in LCP disease, early diagnosis is desirable if only to exclude other conditions.

Pathophysiology
By definition, LCP disease is idiopathic avascular necrosis (AVN) of the femoral head in childhood. Some of the numerous known causes of AVN of the femoral head are listed in Table 20–4. The etiology of idiopathic AVN is related to the

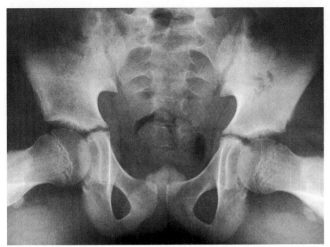

A

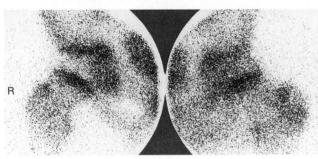

B

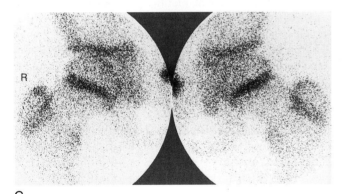

C

Figure 20–20

Femoral head ischemia in a 10-year-old boy with a 5-day history of right hip pain. *A,* AP frog-leg pelvis radiograph. Slight bulging of the right obturator fat plane is present. This is a reliable observation because the pelvis is not rotated. *B,* In a bone scintigram (made with pinhole collimation) of the hips obtained the next day, there is marked reduction in right femoral head uptake, consistent with significant ischemia. *C,* A bone scintigram (made with pinhole collimation) 3 months later shows a normal femoral head image. A program of non–weight-bearing and a nocturnal abduction splint had been enforced throughout this period. Radiographs taken 1 year later were normal, and the patient was asymptomatic.

TABLE 20-4 CONDITIONS ASSOCIATED WITH AVASCULAR NECROSIS OF THE FEMORAL HEAD

Legg-Calvé-Perthes disease
Femoral neck fracture
Steroid therapy
Slipped capital femoral epiphysis
Congenital dislocation of the hip
Sickle cell anemia
Cushing's disease
Diabetes mellitus
Sprue
Radiation
Familial dysautonomia
Gaucher's disease
Pancreatitis
Caisson disease
Trichorhinophalangeal syndrome
Multiple epiphyseal dysplasia

interruption of the blood supply to the proximal femoral epiphysis. Multiple or repetitive episodes of infarction have been implicated. The changing pattern of the vascular supply to the femoral head during growth may explain the vulnerability of the proximal epiphysis to AVN. The major blood supply to the infant femoral head and neck is derived from the multiple small branches of the medial and lateral femoral circumflex arteries, which either pass through or around the physis. By the time the child reaches 2 to 3 years of age, the femoral neck becomes elongated and the physis is intra-articular. If there is regression of the lateral circumflex system and poor development of the medial circumflex artery, the blood supply in the child 4 to 9 years of age preferentially perfuses the posterior half of the femoral head and predisposes the anterior lateral half to ischemia. Later, when the physis starts closing, the barrier to metaphyseal-epiphyseal anastomoses is removed, and idiopathic AVN does not occur. However, the exact etiology is not known.

Clinical Presentation

LCP disease affects boys four times more frequently than girls. The age range at onset of disease is 3 to 12 years, with the highest incidence occurring in children between the ages of 6 and 8 years. The incidence of LCP disease is greatest among Japanese, Mongolian, Eskimo, and Central European children and is low among African Americans and Native Americans.[119] Delayed osseous maturation of a mild degree is characteristic of LCP disease, especially in boys. LCP disease is bilateral in 10% to 13%[36] of patients, but the onset of infarction is seldom bilateral simultaneously. Therefore, the disease is rarely in the same stage of evolution on both sides.

When bilateral simultaneous infarction occurs, the primary causes of avascular necrosis (sickle cell anemia, Gaucher's disease, steroid therapy, and so on) should be sought.

The typical child with LCP disease has an insidious onset of mild hip or knee pain, provoking an antalgic limp. Many children are not brought to medical attention until symptoms have been present for months. There are no systemic symptoms or signs and, initially, the condition may be indistinguishable clinically from transient synovitis of the hip.

Treatment objectives include minimizing stress on the femoral head (particularly the anterolateral portion), limiting lateral subluxation of the femoral head, and optimizing congruity between the deformed femoral head and the acetabulum. Strategies may include bed rest, abduction bracing, innominate osteotomy, and varus derotational osteotomy. Prognosis depends primarily upon the age at diagnosis and the fraction of the femoral head that undergoes necrosis.[59] A poorer prognosis accompanies larger infarcts and disease that presents after 9 years of age.[37] The prognosis for female patients is generally worse than that for male patients.[36]

Diagnostic Imaging

Plain radiographic examination of the hip (neutral and frog-leg views) has been the only useful diagnostic imaging procedure available. Plain radiographs remain very important for excluding other conditions and for delineating osseous structure during the later course of the disease.

Early in the course of LCP disease, both MRI and scintigraphy are more accurate than radiography in assessing patient prognosis. Except for assessment of the length of the initial subcortical fracture, radiographic indicators of poor patient prognosis (i.e., persistent lateral subluxation, large metaphyseal lucencies, total head deformity, and ossification in laterally extruded cartilage) appear later.

The most significant radiographic findings are listed in Table 20–5. No pathognomonic radiographic changes are seen in the early stage of the disease, and for up to 4 weeks, the only abnormal findings may be lateral displacement of the femoral head and perhaps bulging of the so-called capsular shadows. Some patients show a slight widening of the joint space on early radiographs, a finding very similar to that seen in arthritis of the hip but due to thickening of acetabular and femoral head cartilage and cessation of growth of the ossific nucleus, rather than to joint effusion. The radiographic appearance is similar to that for toxic synovitis. A small joint effusion may also contribute to the widening. This is followed by the avascular state, with an increase in density in part or all of the femoral epiphysis. Within weeks, a small, crescent-like subcortical lucency, representing a subcortical fracture, becomes visible in many patients (Fig. 20–21). This fracture is often more easily seen on views of the hip in the frog-leg lateral position, because it predominantly involves the anterior articular surface. The extent of the subcortical

TABLE 20-5 Radiographic Findings in Legg-Calvé-Perthes Disease
Initial Phase
Epiphysis small compared with contralateral epiphysis
Normal epiphysis
Lateral subluxation of femoral head
Subcortical fracture
Degenerative Phase (18 months)
Impaction of femoral epiphysis
Sclerosis of femoral epiphysis
Fragmentation of femoral epiphysis
Metaphyseal lucencies
Widening of femoral neck and head
Regenerative Phase (3 years)
Further widening of femoral neck and head
Reossification
Inhibition of femoral neck growth

fracture corresponds to the amount of the head affected by AVN. The subcortical fracture disappears after several months, but the lateral displacement of the femur tends to progress and persist for years.

Sclerosis and impaction of the femoral head then progress over a period of several months until the femoral head becomes a flattened collection of sclerotic fragments (referred to as *coxa plana*). The entire degenerative phase of the disease takes an average of 18 months. Focal metaphyseal lucencies, usually contiguous to the most severely affected portion of the epiphysis, commonly appear during this phase. These metaphyseal defects are small masses of cartilage that may persist for many years (Fig. 20–22).

The apparent space left by the shrinking epiphyseal bone is taken up by thickened articular cartilage and subchondral fibrous tissue, which subsequently reossifies from several foci during the regenerative phase. The regenerative phase lasts an average of 3 years. The femoral neck and metaphysis gradually widen during both the degenerative and regenerative phases. Inhibition of femoral neck growth may falsely suggest overgrowth of the greater trochanter. The remodeled femoral head enlarges to match the widened metaphysis and epiphyseal plate, becoming considerably wider and flatter than normal (referred to as *coxa magna*). This mushroom-like proximal femur fits the acetabulum poorly, often causing secondary severe degenerative joint disease in early adulthood. Surgical widening of the acetabular roof to better cover the femoral head has been attempted to ameliorate the joint degeneration. Few patients recover from LCP disease without hip deformity, but most suffer no significant disability.

An irregular, fragmented appearance of the femoral capital epiphysis may be an incidental finding on radiographs of

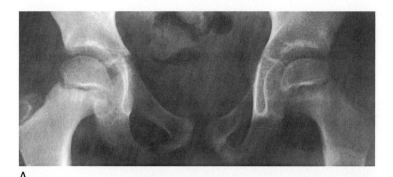

A

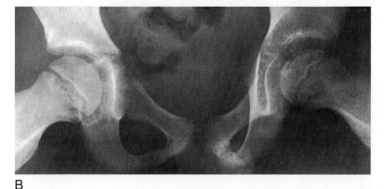

B

Figure 20–21

Legg-Calvé-Perthes (LCP) disease. *A*, Frontal radiograph of a 7-year-old boy with early LCP disease demonstrates widening of the apparent joint space of the left hip and the proximal femoral cartilage plate (physis) in comparison with the normal right side. A subcortical fracture is also present. *B*, Frog-leg view of the same patient shows the subcortical fracture of the left femoral head to better advantage. Medial joint space widening remains evident.

a young child (2 to 4 years) without hip symptoms. This uncommon condition, known as *Meyer's dysplasia*, is bilateral in approximately 50% of children and may be a limited form of multiple epiphyseal dysplasias. Bilateral irregularity of femoral head ossification is also seen in hypothyroidism. These conditions should not be mistaken for bilateral LCP disease, which is almost never symmetric. A patient with epiphyseal dysplasia can develop AVN superimposed on dysplasia.[82] Bone scintigraphy readily differentiates the complicated form (dysplasia with AVN) from the uncomplicated form (dysplasia alone). In multiple epiphyseal dysplasias without AVN, the distribution of the tracer activity matches the ossification pattern on the radiograph. A normal, nondysplastic epiphysis has uptake similar to that of the femoral neck (Fig. 20–23).

Both skeletal scintigraphy and MRI are highly accurate in the early diagnosis of LCP disease, beginning days or weeks before plain radiographs become abnormal (Fig. 20–24).[115] With 2-mm to 3-mm pinhole collimator magnification views, the anatomy of the infarct within the femoral head can be seen clearly as a region devoid of activity early in the process. Changes on bone scintigraphy predate radiographic changes by 4 to 6 weeks.[65] Scintigraphy can be helpful later in demonstrating the earliest evidence of revascularization. Revascularization of bone can occur by recanalization of existing vessels or by neovascularization through the development of new vessels. Recanalization is a rapidly occurring process (minutes to weeks), whereas neovascularization is a prolonged process (months to years). The recanalization process has a characteristic scintigraphic pattern beginning

with the visualization of a "lateral column" and is associated with a good prognosis for eventual outcome in LCP disease. Neovascularization also has a characteristic scintigraphic appearance ("base filling" and "mushrooming"), associated with a poorer prognosis. The extended interval required for healing places the femoral head at risk for complications such as fracture, collapse, and extrusion.[21] Sedation is usually required in young children because of the long imaging times (approximately 10 to 15 minutes per image).

MRI is clearly more accurate than scintigraphy in detecting osteonecrosis in adults, and in children it is reportedly more sensitive, although not invariably.[51] Comparison of the two modalities in children with LCP disease depends significantly on the technical aspects of the procedures (Fig. 20–25). Sometimes the positive scintigram predates the positive MRI findings.[32] MRI is not always the most sensitive way to diagnose or exclude LCP disease. On MRI, the earliest appearance of the avascular region is a well-demarcated area of low signal intensity on T1-weighted spin-echo images. The lesion is usually isointense on T2-weighted images early on. A decreased signal on T1-weighted images may persist for many years in patients with LCP disease despite complete healing demonstrated radiographically.[51] An increased signal supposedly develops on T2-weighted images with revascularization of the infarct, but this has not been a reliable finding. Although MRI does not accurately demonstrate revascularization, it shows the cartilaginous and synovial structures of the hip better than any other method.[102] Subtraction MRI depicts ischemia as a widespread absence of enhancement and is in good agreement with bone scintigraphy. The subtraction

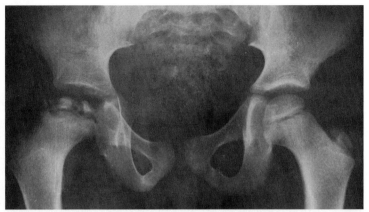

A

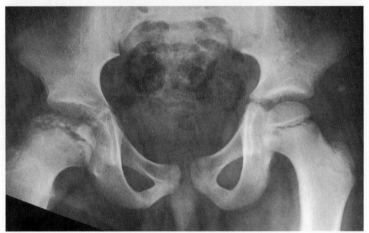

B

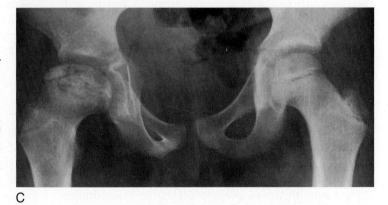

C

Figure 20–22

LCP disease. *A,* Coxa plana on the right at the conclusion of the degenerative phase of LCP disease. The femoral head has degenerated into a group of sclerotic fragments after 12 months of symptoms. *B,* Early in the regenerative phase, 2 years after the onset of the disease. The femoral neck displays widening and lucent metaphyseal regions caused by masses of cartilage. The flattened femoral head is beginning to reossify. *C,* Four years after onset, healing has progressed further. The reconstituted, enlarged femoral head fits poorly in the acetabulum.

technique improves the sensitivity and the specificity of MRI.[109] Although patients generally experience irreversible necrosis of a significant portion of the femoral head and then proceed through the usual sequence of degeneration and healing, in some, the ischemia is completely reversible.[41,89,97] A variety of insults may be associated with transient ischemia of the femoral head, including trauma, SCFE, hemarthrosis, and synovitis. Scintigraphy has been helpful in identifying the return to normal. Some relationship to reflex neurovascular dystrophy is possible in idiopathic occurrences of transient

ischemia and edema of the bone marrow, which may be analogous to an adult condition termed *transient osteoporosis.*[74,125]

SEPTIC ARTHRITIS

In children, septic arthritis affects the knee in 40% of patients, the hip in 23%, and the ankle in 13%.[35] As a result, 75% of patients with this infection present with limping

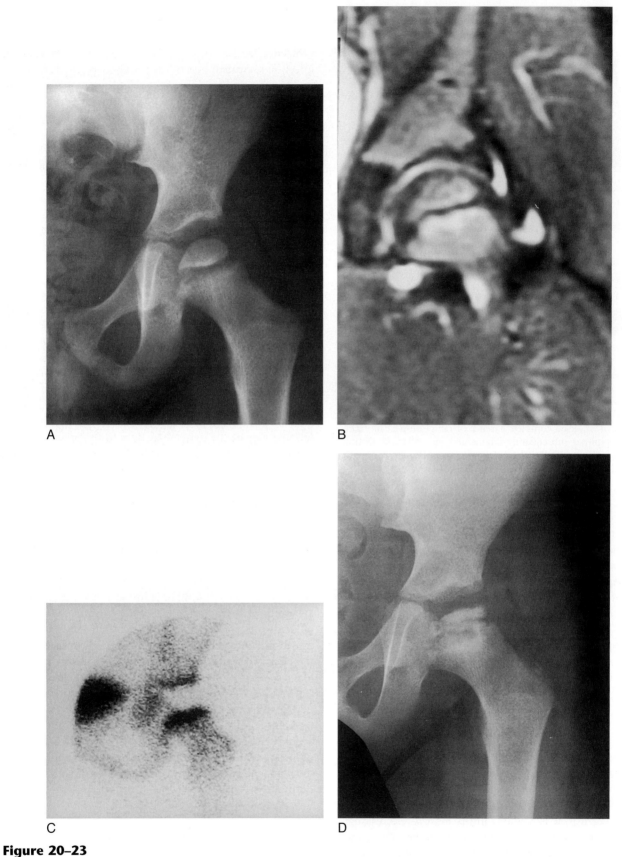

Figure 20–23
Avascular necrosis (AVN) in a 5-year-old male with multiple epiphyseal dysplasia and left hip pain. *A,* The plain film shows a normal appearance to the capital femoral epiphysis. MRI and scintigraphy were performed within 24 hours of presentation. *B,* The inversion recovery (T2-weighted) image reveals the presence of a mottled signal in the epiphysis and a joint effusion, whereas the scintigraphic study showed complete absence of the uptake in the epiphysis on *(C)* a pinhole delayed image of the hip. *D,* A follow-up radiograph 11 months later shows the flattened, sclerotic femoral head and cystic metaphyseal changes noted in the healing stage of AVN.

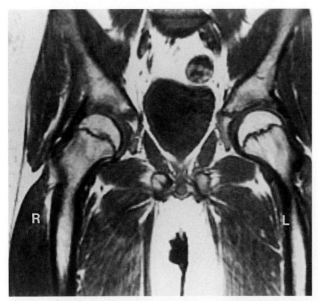

Figure 20–24

Early LCP disease: coronal T1-weighted scan of the hips. There is a subtle asymmetry of the marrow signal from both femoral epiphyses. The left side has a normal high and uniform signal, whereas the signal from the right side is slightly decreased and mottled. Plain films were normal, but pinhole collimator views of the right hip (not shown) revealed complete absence of radioisotope. The right femoral epiphysis subsequently fragmented and collapsed. (From Moore SG, Bisset GS, Siegel HJ, Donaldson JS. Pediatric musculoskeletal MR imaging. Radiology 179:345–360, 1991.)

or pseudoparalysis. Septic arthritis is a surgical emergency. The consequences of delayed diagnosis or unsuccessful treatment include bone growth disturbance, chronic degenerative arthritis, ankylosis, and osteonecrosis. Septic hips are the cause of most permanent joint damage and deformity, with or without disability, in children with septic arthritis.

Pathophysiology

The most common route of infection is hematogenous deposition of bacteria in the synovium. Approximately 75% of cases of septic arthritis involve the lower extremities.[55] The hip is the most common site. Seeding of the joint may come directly from the bloodstream or by extension from the pyogenic focus in an adjacent bone. Contiguous spread from metaphyseal osteomyelitis in the hip region can occur as a result of the intracapsular direct inoculation of organisms from the femoral metaphyses. This combination of septic arthritis and contiguous osteomyelitis often is complicated by osteonecrosis, which results in the most severe residual deformity and disability. In children younger than 1 year, the adjacent focus of osteomyelitis can be in the epiphysis because the transepiphyseal blood supply allows bacteria in the metaphysis to cross the growth plate into the epiphysis. These transepiphyseal vessels are obliterated after infancy, and a more

protective barrier to the invasion of the joint by metaphyseal infection is created.

The enzymatic products of pyogenic bacterial inflammation are potent chondrolytic agents. This chondrolysis accounts for the rapid development of permanent joint damage when appropriate therapy is delayed. Rapid accumulation of fluid in the hip joint can elevate intracapsular pressure sufficiently to cause vascular compression, producing ischemia of the femoral head.

Clinical Presentation

Pyarthrosis is frequently accompanied by bacteremia. The typical patient appears systemically ill and has rapidly progressive joint pain, limitation of motion, and fever. Joint pain and reduced mobility may sometimes precede signs of sepsis. The presenting symptom may be an antalgic gait or contracture limp, which results from spasm of the muscles irritated by the adjacent inflammation. In preambulatory infants, pseudoparalysis is typical. The age distribution for this disease is lower than that for transient synovitis: about half of the patients are younger than 2 years old. The frequency is nearly equal in boys and girls.

Although most patients have significant fever, leukocytosis, or an elevated erythrocyte sedimentation rate, pain and limping may be the only initial clues to the presence of the disease. Prompt arthrocentesis and blood culture are necessary for diagnosis and therapeutic guidance. The concentration of granulocytes in infected joint fluid varies and overlaps significantly with that seen in other forms of arthritis. Gram stain of the fluid reveals organisms in about one third of patients, and cultures are positive in 50% to 80% of patients, depending upon prior antibiotic therapy. Blood cultures are less frequently compromised by prior therapy and yield additional positive results. Organisms in the neonatal period are usually coliform or gram-positive cocci. In patients 6 months to 2 years of age, *Haemophilus influenzae* is the predominant organism. Meningitis accompanies *H. influenzae* pyarthrosis in about 25% of cases in younger children and infants.[35] Most cases in older infants and children are due to *Staphylococcus aureus*, but other frequent pathogens include streptococci, *Neisseria gonorrhoeae*, and *Neisseria meningitidis*.

The differential diagnoses of septic arthritis include transient synovitis, acute rheumatoid arthritis, osteomyelitis, acute rheumatic fever, and Lyme disease. Therapy consists of intravenous antibiotics, aspiration and immobilization of the joint, and (depending upon the clinical situation) surgical drainage. Open drainage is often indicated for hip joint infections.

Diagnostic Imaging

Clinical and laboratory diagnoses of septic arthritis are usually accurate, which is fortunate because imaging procedures typically yield nonspecific results. Initial radiographic assessment is warranted in all patients, however, because

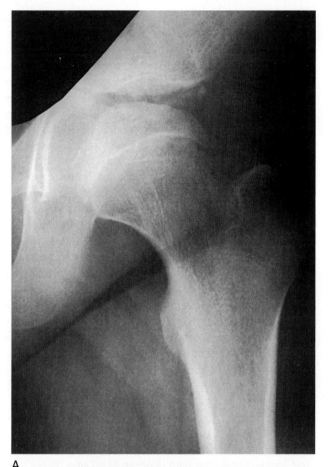

A

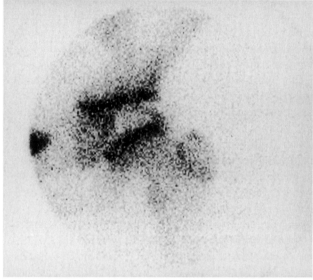

B

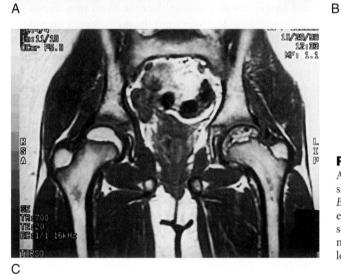

C

Figure 20–25
Avascular necrosis of the hip in an 8-year-old female. *A*, Plain films show some flattening and sclerosis in the capital femoral epiphysis. *B*, The bone scan (pinhole image) reveals patchy uptake in the epiphysis and ischemia due to synovitis was a differential diagnosis. *C*, The T1-weighted coronal image shows unequivocal involvement of the capital epiphysis with heterogenous intermediate and low signal intensity.

drainage of both the joint and the bone is usually performed when there is radiographic evidence of associated metaphyseal osteomyelitis. Sonography can reliably demonstrate the joint effusion, especially in the hip, but it cannot accurately indicate infection as the cause. Radiographic evaluation is also helpful in assessing delayed complications.

Initial radiographs of infected joints frequently reveal synovial fluid, easily recognized on the lateral view of the knee as distention of the suprapatellar bursa. Effusion is more difficult to recognize in the hip or ankle. In the hip, the most reliable sign is displacement of the femur away from the acetabulum, which results from large effusions or marked synovial swelling associated usually with septic arthritis.[122] Lateral displacement of the femur is very frequent in patients younger than 1 year of age but is far less common in older children.[67] Such displacement of the femur is rarely seen in transient synovitis. Displacement of the psoas line and obturator fat pad may also indicate hip joint effusion. In ankle joint effusion, the anterior fat plane is often recognizably displaced away from the joint on the lateral view. A lytic change in the metaphysis, with or without periosteal new bone, identifies osteomyelitis, which may be isolated or accompanied by a septic joint (Fig. 20–26).

If the disease process is not stopped, articular cartilage destruction rapidly ensues. After synovial fluid and swelling have subsided, significant cartilage destruction may be identified radiographically by narrowing of the joint space. Subchondral osseous erosions reflect destruction of subchondral bone by the thickened, inflamed synovium. Late radiographic changes of inadequately treated septic arthritis include bony ankylosis, growth disturbance, and osseous necrosis. Growth disturbances may produce leg shortening or leg lengthening, and abnormal angulation may develop at the end of the affected bone as a result of asymmetric growth. Osteonecrosis in the proximal femur may result in a flattened (coxa plana) or enlarged (coxa magna) femoral head.

Periarticular accumulation of technetium 99m phosphates in septic arthritis is usually detectable within 3 days of the onset of symptoms. Periarticular radiotracer deposition results from hyperemia and, thus, is a nonspecific finding that does not differentiate septic arthritis from other causes of acute arthritis. Focal radiotracer deposition in an adjacent

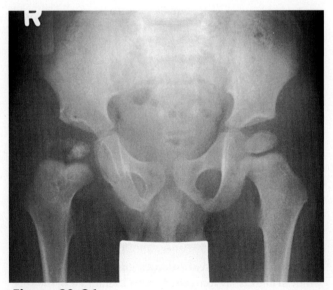

Figure 20–26
Septic arthritis due to osteomyelitis; late changes from osseous necrosis. This film, taken 1 year after diagnosis, demonstrates femoral head deformity, femoral neck widening, lateral subluxation, and poor congruity between the femoral head and acetabulum.

metaphysis implies associated osteomyelitis but may be difficult to visualize if there is significant regional uptake as a result of hyperemia. Ischemia of the femoral head, resulting from vascular compression, spasm, or thrombosis, is more easily recognized on scintigrams. The resultant photopenia of the femoral head can be relieved by aspiration if the increased intra-articular pressure has been present for less than 24 hours. If saline washing or arthrography was performed during arthrocentesis, it is advisable to wait at least 45 minutes before performing bone scintigraphy.[79] The volume of iatrogenic fluid placement can produce transient photopenia of the femoral head.[79]

Septic arthritis of the sacroiliac joint differs from that in most other joints, as bony involvement occurs early in the course of the disease, and most cases result from a primary osseous infection. This joint is usually affected in preadolescents and adolescents. Skeletal scintigraphic results are appropriately positive at an early stage of the disease. Acute pyogenic sacroiliitis is most often caused by *Staphylococcus* organisms, but other pathogens are possible, and aspiration of the joint is frequently desirable. CT may provide useful anatomic definition of the arthritic process and is preferred over plain radiographic tomography (Fig. 20–27).

ACUTE OSTEOMYELITIS

Acute osteomyelitis is an important cause of morbidity and temporary disability in children of all ages. When acute osteomyelitis is treated promptly, permanent crippling and clinically significant deformity are rare. Prompt diagnosis is desirable, because therapeutic delay increases the risk of bone necrosis and chronic osteomyelitis. False-positive diagnoses should be avoided, however, owing to prolonged antibiotic therapy, the possibility of drug toxicities, discomfort, and considerable expense. Fortunately, drug therapy can be administered on an outpatient basis with indwelling venous lines (peripherally inserted central catheters and Broviac catheters). The lower extremity is affected in about 65% of children with osteomyelitis. Boys outnumber girls by a ratio of 2:1. An acute limp is a common manifestation of lower extremity osteomyelitis and is often associated with lumbar vertebral and iliac osteomyelitis.

The diagnosis of acute osteomyelitis may be quite challenging when leukocytosis and fever are absent, as in about one third of children early in the course of the disease.

Pathophysiology

Hematogenous delivery of organisms to osseous tissue is the most common mechanism of bone infection in children. Although bone infection can occur by contiguous spread from adjacent soft tissue and by direct implantation of organisms as a result of penetrating trauma, these mechanisms are comparatively uncommon in children.

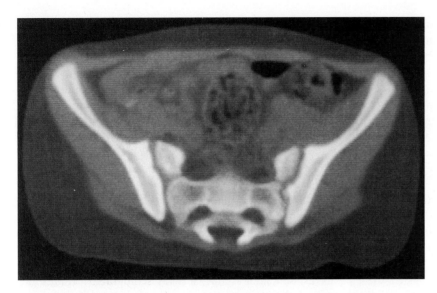

Figure 20–27
Septic arthritis of the sacroiliac joint in a young boy. Destruction and thinning of iliac subchondral bone of the left sacroiliac joint are present. Destruction of the sacral subchondral bone is also visible, particularly along the posterior portion of the joint. Note swelling of the left iliacus muscle and edema of fat adjacent to the posterior joint margin on the left.

The usual primary locus of infection lies in the metaphysis of a long bone, because of the vascular architecture in these regions. The blood supply arrives primarily from the medullary space in longitudinally oriented terminal arterioles, which turn abruptly as they near the epiphyseal cartilage plate to empty into wide venous sinusoids. The sudden decrease in flow velocity and deficient phagocytosis in this venous capillary network provide a favorable environment for deposition and proliferation of bacteria.[123] Certain other regions of the skeleton have an analogous vascular network and are typical, although less frequent, sites of hematogenous osteomyelitis; these other sites have been termed *metaphysis-equivalent sites* and are typically located immediately subjacent to the cartilage plates of apophyseal growth centers, articular cartilage, or fibrocartilage.[94] The pediatric skeleton between 6 and 16 years of age is susceptible to infection at these locations, which resemble the long-bone metaphyses. In preadolescents and adolescents, the causative organism is usually *S. aureus*. The most important of these metaphysis-equivalent sites are the vertebral end plate and the iliac bone adjacent to the sacroiliac joint.

The concept of a predisposing vascular architecture that changes with skeletal maturity fits well with the fact that more than 85% of cases of hematogenous osteomyelitis occur in children younger than 16 years of age. Cartilage impedes the spread of osteomyelitis much more effectively than does the periosteum, so it is very uncommon for infection to spread through articular cartilage to involve a joint. When a portion of the metaphysis is enclosed within the joint capsule, septic arthritis often complicates osteomyelitis. This occurs in the hip, ankle, shoulder, and elbow. The growth plate also impedes the spread of infection, but numerous vascular channels connect the epiphysis to the metaphysis at birth, allowing frequent concomitant osteomyelitis in both compartments

in the infant. This is found to occur in the distal femoral and proximal tibial epiphyses. In most children, these perforating channels usually regress by 18 months of age. Hematogenous infection may occur in the subarticular bone of the mature skeleton, although less predominantly. Isolated epiphyseal infection in children between 2 and 4 years of age is now recognized.[45,101] At times, the infection is subacute, and the aspirates may be sterile. Uncommonly, infection can arise in the subperiosteal cortex of a long bone[53,101] (Fig. 20–28).

Clinical Presentation

Acute osteomyelitis involving the lower extremity typically presents with fever, rapidly developing local pain, and an antalgic limp. Young children and infants may manifest a pseudoparalysis. Although an acute clinical presentation is typical, relatively mild symptoms may occur with minimal or no systemic manifestations. This is particularly true in older children and in patients who receive antibiotic therapy for systemic symptoms, which partially controls the localized infection before it becomes clinically apparent. Children with a chronic, localized osseous abscess (i.e., Brodie abscess) generally have regional pain without systemic symptoms.

The extremity with acute osteomyelitis is often swollen, and tenderness can be elicited over the metaphysis. Soft tissue swelling, when present, is centered over the metaphysis and typically is poorly marginated compared with cellulitis, which also typically displays erythema and induration of the skin and subcutaneous tissues, unlike the deeper swelling associated with osteomyelitis. In contrast to septic arthritis, which usually results in marked limitation of motion, mild limitation is variably present in the articulation adjacent to osteomyelitis. The joint may also contain a small sympathetic effusion. Approximately one third of children with iliac osteomyelitis or lumbar osteomyelitis present with an

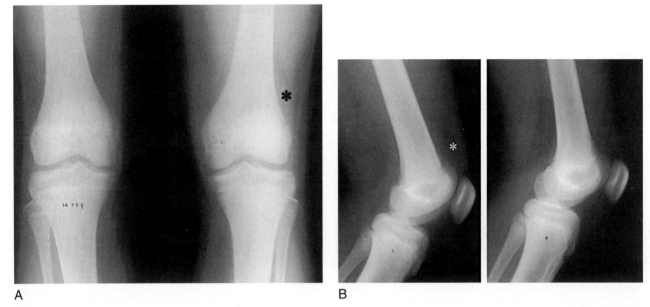

A   B

Figure 20–28
Acute osteomyelitis of the distal left femur in a 14-year-old female. Early radiographic changes are in the deep soft tissues adjacent to bone. The anterior *(A)* and lateral fat muscle planes *(B)* show convex bowing and displacement by soft tissue inflammation *(asterisks)*. A normal right femur is shown for comparison.

acute limp. The casual examiner may misdiagnose such conditions as primary lower extremity problems.[8] Careful examination, however, should reveal bone tenderness over the spine or pelvis.

Laboratory data suggest an infectious etiology in most patients, with an elevated WBC count and erythrocyte sedimentation rate, although the WBC count is normal in a significant minority of patients (40% in one series).[27] The best way to establish the causative organism is culture of material aspirated directly from the infected site in the bone. Blood and any joint fluid that can be aspirated should also be cultured. *S. aureus* accounts for slightly more than half of the cases, and various strains of *Streptococcus* account for about 10%.[35] In patients with sickle cell disease, *Salmonella* accounts for the majority of cases.[10,16] The role of surgical drainage is controversial, but drainage is usually performed when a significant amount of suppuration is suspected.

Differential diagnostic considerations in patients presenting with the typical symptoms of infection include septic arthritis, cellulitis, and acute rheumatic fever. When systemic manifestations are mild or absent and local symptoms are less specific, the differential diagnosis extends to a broader spectrum of possibilities, including childhood malignancies such as Ewing's sarcoma, leukemia, and neuroblastoma.

Diagnostic Imaging

The ability of imaging techniques to demonstrate osseous infection lags behind the pathologic processes in the acute and healing phases of osteomyelitis (Table 20–6). Early in the course of the disease, this delay is more significant for radiographically demonstrable osseous destruction than for deep soft tissue swelling, as shown with MRI, and for alterations in blood flow to the infected site and surrounding region, as seen with bone scintigraphy. In the healing phase, clinical parameters more accurately reflect the response to treatment than radiologic images.

When the child's clinical presentation suggests acute osteomyelitis and appropriate cultures have been obtained, treatment is often initiated without imaging confirmation of the diagnosis. Treatment with appropriate antibiotics within 4 days of onset may prevent bone lysis, preclude gross destruction of bone, and reduce the incidence of premature epiphyseal closure.

Often no deep soft tissues can be seen. There is a 7- to 14-day delay in the radiographic appearance of lytic bone changes, because more than 50% of the mineralized osseous matrix must be destroyed before lysis becomes visible on plain films. A similar delay in the appearance of reactive bone reflects the time required for adequate mineralization of the reactive bony matrix. Plain radiographs are an effective, practical method of demonstrating soft tissue gas collections and radiopaque foreign bodies. Skeletal scintigraphy, CT, and MRI typically show the changes of infection earlier than plain radiography.

Early imaging of osteomyelitis can be done with skeletal scintigraphy, and results become positive within 24 to 72 hours of the onset of symptoms. Phosphate radiotracers localize osteomyelitis by the associated focal increase in bone metabolism and blood flow. Occasional false-negative results occur due to vascular spasm or occlusion associated

TABLE 20-6 Classic Pattern* of Pathologic Correlation With Radiographic (R) and Scintigraphic (S)† Findings in Acute Hematogenous Osteomyelitis

Modality	Findings	Time of Observation After Onset of Symptoms	Pathologic Correlation
R	Small focus of deep soft tissue swelling adjacent to symptomatic metaphysis	1–3 days	Nonsuppurative metaphysitis
S	Focal "cold" lesion	1–3 days	Nonsuppurative metaphysitis, with vascular spasm or vascular thrombosis
S	Focal "hot" lesion	1–3 days	Nonsuppurative metaphysitis, without vascular spasm or thrombosis
S	Focal "hot" lesion	3–5 days or more	Suppurative metaphysitis
S	Focal "cold" lesion	5 days or more	Focal osseous abscess
R	Deep muscular swelling	3–10 days	Suppurative metaphysitis
R	Medullary bone destruction	1–4 weeks	Suppurative metaphysitis
R	New bone formation in medullary cavity	1–4 weeks	Bone reaction adjacent to suppuration or abscess
R	Cortical lucency or endosteal scalloping	1–4 weeks	Cortical suppuration
R	Periosteal "reaction," involucrum	1–4 weeks	Subperiosteal suppuration, with periosteal elevation and new subperiosteal bone formation

*Classic pattern may be modified by antibiotic therapy, host resistance, and virulence of infecting organisms.
†With technetium Tc-99m phosphate agents.

with the expanding intraosseous inflammatory process (compression by purulent material and edema).[63] False-negative bone scintigraphy has particularly been a problem in infants younger than 6 weeks old, but with careful attention to the technical aspects of the examination, it is generally accurate in older infants and children.

Specificity in the diagnosis of infection in bone has increased with the introduction of indium 111– and technetium 99m–tagged WBC studies.[106] The use of technetium 99m hexamethylpropyleneamine (HMPAO)-labeled leukocytes has become popular in children. The radiation burden of technetium 99m–tagged WBCs (lower energy and shorter half-life) is significantly less than that of indium 111–tagged WBCs. Better resolution of the infectious process with technetium 99m–tagged WBCs is permitted by higher counts (approximately 40 times more than indium 111) and, thus, faster imaging times and less patient movement.[72] Imaging with indium 111–tagged WBCs usually requires at least 24 hours. Indium studies are usually reserved for those patients in whom bone scan findings are equivocal or normal and osseous infection is still likely.

Scintigraphy is particularly useful in children in whom the site of infection cannot be localized and for identifying multifocal involvement, which is important in neonatal osteomyelitis and chronic recurrent multifocal osteomyelitis. MRI and CT are usually used when anatomic information is necessary for surgical intervention or for confirmation of disease.

The ease of performing ultrasound, its widespread availability, its speed, and its low cost when compared with cross-sectional imaging, as well as the possibility of ultrasound-guided aspiration, make this technique attractive. Ultrasound can be helpful in detecting fluid collections in the soft tissue and subperiosteal regions and may guide localization for aspiration or drainage.[1,70] Fluid against bone has been called "pathognomonic" for osteomyelitis, and although this is not the case, it is a finding that warrants intervention or additional imaging.

CT is very reliable in detecting cortical destruction, periosteal reaction, soft tissue extension, and gas in soft tissues.[71] It is superior to MRI for the detection of sequestra and the presence of intraosseous gas, an infrequent but reliable sign of osteomyelitis.

MRI provides accurate information on both the soft tissues and bones and is the imaging study of choice for evaluating the local extent of musculoskeletal infections.[117] It is particularly useful in detailing the soft tissue and osseous components of infections involving the axial skeleton (spine and pelvis) or for chronic bone infection.[22] With its sagittal, coronal, and transaxial orientations, it is very sensitive (97%) and specific (92%) in the diagnosis of acute hematogenous infection, because of the greater anatomic detail, the ability to reveal marrow changes, and the superior contrast between bone and soft tissue.

Soon after treatment begins, radiographs may be misleading if increased bone lysis is misinterpreted as progression of infection. In fact, early healing is often characterized by bone resorption, reflecting removal of damaged osseous matrix and associated mineral crystals. Bone scintigrams are also unreliable indicators of the response to antibiotic therapy because of continued hyperemia and increased bone metabolism, which are slow to resolve despite control of the infection and which persist during the healing and remodeling phase.

After a clinical diagnosis of recrudescent or prolonged persistent infection (i.e., chronic osteomyelitis) is established, radiographs can show the location and extent of disease in terms of bony sclerosis, destruction, and sequestration. However, gallium or radiolabeled leukocytes are much more effective indicators of the activity of the disease.

Imaging findings in early acute hematogenous osteomyelitis are listed in Table 20–6. The earliest radiographic evidence of osteomyelitis is a focus of deep soft tissue edema, which may appear within 3 days of the onset of symptoms.[17] This focal soft tissue swelling is due to the hyperemia and edema caused by nonsuppurative medullary metaphysitis. Comparison views are often necessary for confident recognition of the swelling (Fig. 20–29).

Focal osteoporosis or poorly defined focal areas of medullary radiolucency are the earliest bony changes visible radiographically. These findings are caused by extensive medullary infection with trabecular destruction and suppuration. Such findings may be seen as early as 6 days after the onset of symptoms but generally are not apparent until 10 to 14 days. Cortical lucencies and endosteal scalloping reflect spread of suppuration to the cortex. Periosteal elevation and new bone formation result from centrifugal spread of the infection. These cortical and periosteal alterations are initially apparent between 10 and 20 days after the onset of symptoms. Extensive periosteal elevation occurring circumferentially results in a sleeve of periosteal new bone referred to as the *involucrum*. The increased intramedullary pressure associated with the inflammation often results in devitalized bone in the center of the infected region, which becomes visible as an island of sclerotic bone (i.e., a sequestrum). These classic features of osteomyelitis are uncommon with effective antibiotic therapy.

Skeletal scintigraphy is accurate in the early identification of osteomyelitis. High-resolution techniques including pinhole collimator views are essential to resolve small or subtle abnormalities in the areas of intense bone metabolic activity of the growing metaphyses (Figs. 20–30 and 20–31). Long scanning times are required, especially for pinhole collimator images,

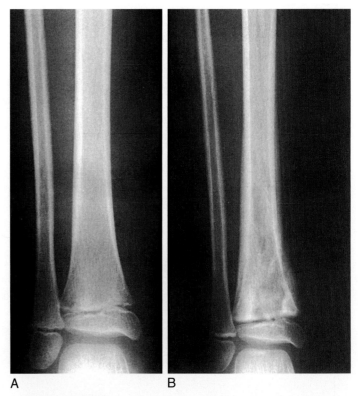

A   B

Figure 20–29
Osteomyelitis. *A,* Anteroposterior radiograph of the right leg of a child who had had pain and was limping for 2 weeks shows radiolucent destructive areas and a central sclerotic region in the medullary space of the distal tibial metaphysis. *B,* Two months later, extensive periosteal new bone has been laid down. Considerably larger areas of destruction and reactive sclerosis are present in the distal half of the tibia. Radiographic findings at this stage of disease do not reliably reflect disease activity.

so sedation is almost always used in children younger than 10 years old. Inadequately sedated children should be remedicated, because even minor amounts of motion can irreparably degrade image quality. Physical restraints such as sandbags or immobilization boards are often desirable, particularly in patients younger than 5 years.

In all patients, the entire skeleton is surveyed with high-resolution collimator or whole-body imaging, because osteomyelitis may affect multiple bones in 5% to 10% of patients, and metastatic neoplasm (especially neuroblastoma and leukemia) may present with a clinical picture that suggests bone or joint infection.

In children with cellulitis, diffusely increased activity in the abnormal region is typically shown on blood-pool images and disappears or becomes less obvious on delayed images. MRI is an excellent modality for distinguishing cellulitis from osteomyelitis.[120]

CT can distinguish cortical and periosteal involvement from medullary involvement by a change in the medullary density numbers. It will demonstrate the cortical destruction,

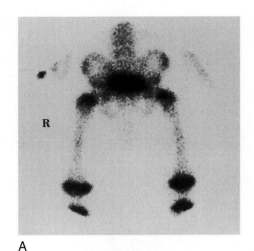

A

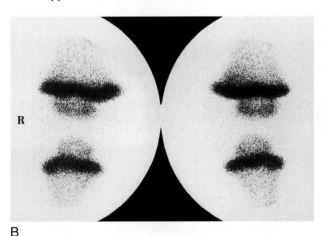

B

Figure 20–30

A, Osteomyelitis. High-resolution collimator image of a Tc-MDP bone scintigram in a 6-month-old infant with fever and irritability. The image shows only very subtle asymmetry of distal femoral activity. *B,* Images obtained with a 3-mm pinhole collimator clearly demonstrates the focus of osteomyelitis in the medial aspect of the left distal femoral metaphysis. Radiographs were normal.

periosteal reaction, and soft tissue extension. MRI shows a localized area of heterogenous signal alteration with a decreased signal on T1-weighted images and increased signal intensity on T2-weighted images. The best predictors of acute osteomyelitis are poorly defined thickened cortex, and a relatively good interface between normal and diseased bone marrow. MRI contrast studies using gadolinium enhance the detection of osteomyelitis and abscess formation (Fig. 20–32).[19,99] Septic arthritis exhibits fluid collections within the joint spaces with signal intensity similar to that of water on the T2-weighted image and less than to slightly greater than that of muscle on the T1-weighted image. Healed osteomyelitis is identified on follow-up examinations by normalization of the marrow and soft tissue signals.[9,120]

In patients with sickle cell anemia, osteomyelitis and bone infarction can present similar clinical pictures. Skeletal scintigraphy with technetium 99m phosphate agents and bone marrow scintigraphy with technetium 99m sulfur colloid can frequently differentiate between these entities. It is important to perform the scintigraphic evaluation within the first week of the illness. With phosphate agents, an infarct appears as a large "cold" area in the medullary space, often in the diaphysis, surrounded by increased activity at the ends of the bone. Later, during the revascularization and healing phases, the infarct may display increased activity throughout the lesion. Bone marrow imaging reveals a lack of activity within the infarct, which persists indefinitely, depending on the type of healing that occurs.[111]

DISKITIS AND VERTEBRAL OSTEOMYELITIS

As with many diseases of obscure etiology, diskitis is known by several names that reflect possible pathogenesis, including spondyloarthritis, nonspecific spondylitis, intervertebral disk-space infection, and benign osteomyelitis of the spine. Diskitis is an inflammatory process that arises in the intervertebral disk space and occurs much more commonly in children than in adults. Diskitis generally affects children younger than 5 years of age and is associated with absent or low-grade fever and an elevated sedimentation rate. It occurs nearly exclusively in the lumbar region, causing refusal to walk or progressive limp. Some 2 to 3 weeks into the illness, radiographs demonstrate narrowing of the disk space with variable degrees of destruction of adjacent vertebral end plates.

Vertebral osteomyelitis typically occurs in older children who are febrile and complain of back pain in the lumbar, thoracic, or cervical regions. Vertebral osteomyelitis in pediatric patients accounts for only 1% to 2% of all children with osteomyelitis. Vertebral osteomyelitis is much rarer in children than in adults. Vertebral osteomyelitis has a peak during adolescence and a more prominent one in patients older than 50 years of age. It is usually more virulent than diskitis with a greater number of positive cultures. The usually isolated organism is *S. aureus.* In contrast, children with vertebral osteomyelitis are more likely to be febrile and ill-appearing at the time of presentation than those with diskitis.

Pathophysiology

The pathophysiology of diskitis and vertebral osteomyelitis remains poorly understood, but differences in blood supply to the intervertebral disk by age have been implicated for both. Diskitis is thought to occur in childhood owing to the presence of vascular channels in the cartilaginous region of the disk space that disappear later in life (up to 20 years) and because of abundant intraosseous arterial anastomoses in childhood that promote clearance of microorganisms or entrapped emboli. Whether the primary nidus is the intervertebral disk extending to involve both end plates or the

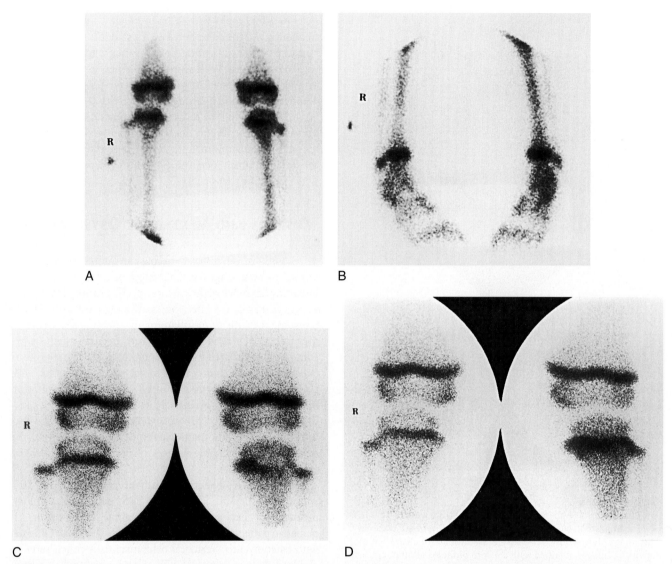

A

B

C

D

Figure 20–31
Osteomyelitis. *A* and *B*, High-resolution collimator images of the lower extremities in a 2-year-old girl with 2 days of fever and refusal to bear weight on the left leg show increased radiotracer activity throughout the distal left lower extremity from the knee down. This type of diffuse increase can be seen in any form of regional hyperperfusion. *C*, Pinhole collimator images of the knees obtained at the same time show a photon-deficient region affecting the lateral two thirds of the left tibial metaphysis. Expanding early osteomyelitis has occluded the blood supply focally to this region. *D*, Pinhole collimator images of the knees obtained 6 days after symptoms began show that the photon-deficient region has filled in, and the entire proximal tibial metaphysis and epiphysis demonstrate increased activity. Radiographs were normal.

vertebral end plate extending across the disk space to involve the other end plate is controversial. Vertebral osteomyelitis, in contrast, is thought to occur when microorganisms lodge in the low-flow, end-organ vasculature adjacent to the subchondral plate region with the infection spreading further into the vertebral body and sometimes involving the adjacent intervertebral disk space. The end plate is a metaphysis-equivalent site because of a similar microvascular anatomy that provides a favorable setting for hematogenous osteomyelitis. Most authors propose an infectious cause for diskitis. No conclusive data are available, however, and the fact that most

cultures are sterile and patients recover without antimicrobial therapy mitigates against this hypothesis. Other mechanisms such as trauma and noninfectious inflammation have been proposed. Infection with *S. aureus* has been documented in a few pediatric patients by blood or disk biopsy culture.[124] Vertebral osteomyelitis, although infrequently encountered, can be an atypical manifestation of *Bartonella henselae* infection. The availability of specific serologic assays allowed the confirmation of this cat-scratch disease organism. In patients who have exposure to cats, this etiology should be considered.[100]

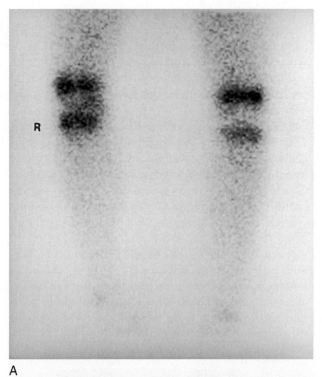

A

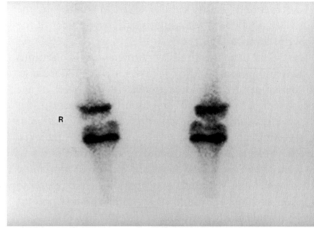

B

C

Figure 20–32

Osteomyelitis of the proximal tibia. This 6-year-old girl presented with pain and swelling of the knee; there was no bone abnormality on plain films. The bone scan blood pool *(A)* and delayed *(B)* images show increased uptake in the joint and symmetrically on each side of the joint, a pattern seen with septic arthritis. However, MRI was positive for osteomyelitis. *C*, Sagittal T1-weighted fat-saturated postgadolinium image shows enhancement of the marrow in the proximal tibial epiphysis and metaphysis. There is fluid in the knee joint with synovial enhancement.

Clinical Presentation

A broad spectrum of severity exists in diskitis and is related to the virulence of the responsible organism and the vigor of host defenses. Diskitis is biphasic, with a higher incidence early in childhood and a less prevalent peak during adolescence. In a recent series, the mean age at presentation was 2.8 years with a range of 7 months to 16 years.[34] Apparently, adults may have essentially the same disease, although vertebral destruction is usually more extensive in adults.[28] In one study, 78% of children with diskitis had involvement of the lumbar or lumbosacral area.[21]

The typical patient with diskitis experiences the insidious or fluctuating onset of low back pain, irritability, malaise, and low-grade fever. Children younger than 3 years of age present with refusal to walk or with a limp, whereas older patients often complain of back pain. The painful portion of the illness usually lasts from 2 to 4 weeks. In some patients, usually toddlers, nerve root irritation may cause hip pain that is more severe than the back pain and results in limping early in the illness. Within days to weeks, the child refuses to walk and later may refuse to sit or stand; these symptoms may be diagnostically confusing.

The majority of children with vertebral osteomyelitis present with back pain. Other presenting symptoms include neck, shoulder, rib, and abdominal pain. Fever is more frequent and usually higher and of longer duration in children with vertebral osteomyelitis. Blood cultures and more invasive procedures, including biopsy, should be strongly considered in patients with suspected vertebral osteomyelitis, for which definition of a causal agent is particularly important in selection of the appropriate antimicrobial therapy and in defining its duration. Tuberculosis and brucellosis should be excluded by skin or serologic testing.

Controversy exists concerning treatment methods for diskitis. Most authorities believe that antibiotic therapy is warranted, particularly when blood culture results are positive. However, with diskitis, blood cultures are infrequently positive. Other clinicians omit antibiotic therapy because they believe there is insufficient evidence showing that such therapy significantly affects outcome. Almost all authorities agree that immobilization (body cast or bed rest) for 3 months is advisable. Pain is usually rapidly relieved by immobilization.

Diagnostic Imaging

Radiographic evidence of diskitis is typically not apparent until 2 to 4 weeks after the onset of symptoms. Skeletal scintigraphy is warranted when radiographs are still normal. The interval between disease onset and the possibility of disease being seen on scintigraphic examination is unknown.

If early radiographic findings of diskitis (disk narrowing or minimal end-plate indistinctness) are equivocally present, scintigraphic examination can be used. MRI can demonstrate altered bone marrow and a disk signal early in the course of osseous infection and can demonstrate the relationship of

soft tissue swelling and suppuration of neural structures. Destructive vertebral lesions, early disk inflammation, and paraspinal soft tissue swelling also can be seen. MRI has been very effective in detailing the processes of diskitis and vertebral osteomyelitis. After diskitis is diagnosed, plain radiographs are used for surveillance and for evaluation of residual deformities.

Initial radiographs of the spine may be normal in both diskitis and vertebral osteomyelitis. The earliest radiographic abnormality of disk space infection is narrowing (loss of height) of the disk space, which may not occur for 2 to 4 weeks after the onset of symptoms (Fig. 20–33). The compromise of the disk from infection may appear in just 10 days in the younger age group, or it may take 2 to 4 weeks in the older age group. Disk space narrowing is not specific for infection and can be found in trauma and Scheuermann's disease. The narrowing is postulated to result from herniation of the nucleus pulposus into the vertebral body through the weakened end plate, although some component of disk destruction also may be involved. Within a few weeks after disk

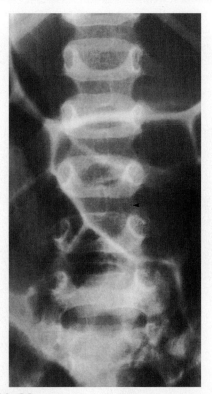

Figure 20–33
Diskitis: AP view of the lumbar spine in a 2-year-old girl who presented with abdominal pain of 2 weeks' duration. The intervertebral disk spaces widen progressively downward to the L3–L4 level (*arrowhead*), which is narrower than the interspace above. Vertebral end-plate indistinctness is not yet present. Note the moderately dilated bowel loops. Close evaluation of the vertebral bodies in the abdominal films of children with unexplained abdominal pain is important.

narrowing occurs, the vertebral end plates usually become indistinct, and there may be widening of the paraspinal lines. The inflammatory process may be completely confined to the disk space or may involve the adjacent vertebrae with obvious destruction. Generally, both adjacent end plates display similar destructive changes, but one is often more severely affected than the other. The earliest radiographic change noted in osteomyelitis is the rarefaction in the superior or interior region of the involved vertebrae adjacent to the cartilaginous plate. Such radiographic changes occur 3 to 6 weeks after the onset of sepsis. Like diskitis, the changes include disk narrowing, demineralization of adjacent vertebral end plates, and widening of the paraspinal lines. At 6 to 10 weeks following the onset of symptoms, frank destruction of the end plates and extension of the lytic process to the central portion of the vertebral body occurs (Fig. 20–34). The body becomes compressed and a paravertebral soft tissue mass may be evident. The presence of a suppurative soft tissue mass (abscess) is more typical of osteomyelitis than of pure diskitis.

In evaluating disk-space narrowing, note that the disk spaces normally become slightly wider at each segment, proceeding from the lower thoracic region caudally to L5. Even a subtle loss of height or lack of the normal increase in height is highly suggestive of diskitis in the proper clinical setting. The L5–S1 disk space is normally narrower than L4–L5; thus, at this level, direct bone changes are more helpful diagnostically than is disk space height. In most patients,

diskitis involves a single disk in the lumbar region, most often L4–L5 or L3–L4. Disk involvement above T9 is very unusual, but cases of diskitis in the cervical spine have been reported.

During healing, areas of sclerosis develop in the affected vertebral bodies. Persistent disk narrowing is the rule after healing, but the degree of residual deformity is extremely variable, with some patients appearing almost normal radiographically and others developing severe kyphosis. Calcification in the disk has been reported as a rare late finding. Following treatment, the osteomyelitis site also develops reactive sclerosis. Bony bridging, vertebral fusion, or both may develop.

Positive findings on bone scintigraphy may predate radiographic changes by weeks. The usual scintigraphic finding of diskitis is increased radiotracer deposition in the vertebral end plates adjacent to the affected disk (Fig. 20–35). Characteristic findings can be seen on blood pool images. With vertebral osteomyelitis, bone scintigraphy usually shows diffuse uptake of the radiopharmaceutical in the involved vertebra on both blood-pool and delayed images. The findings are generally shown clearly on high-resolution collimator images (including posterior oblique views), but pinhole collimator views permit increased confidence in the diagnosis. SPECT imaging can also resolve the distribution of activity in the spine. If the abnormally intense area of activity is not in the end plate but in the pedicle or another posterior element of the vertebral arch, other diagnoses, such as fracture or osteoid osteoma, should be strongly considered. The sensitivity of bone scintigraphy for the detection of osteomyelitis, diskitis, and aseptic spine diseases is high (more than 90%). Bone scans, however, are nonspecific. With indium 111–labeled leukocyte scintigraphy, the specificity is improved, but the sensitivity is rather low (17%).[113] Indium 111–labeled WBCs may be photopenic in the involved segments. Lack of accumulation of the radiotracer may be related to the somewhat chronic nature of vertebral osteomyelitis without much polymorphonuclear response.[96] Because of the high rate of false-negative studies in the presence of infective spondylitis, it may be helpful only in selected patients. Gallium 67 scanning is quite specific for vertebral infection, particularly when combined with bone scintigraphy.[48] A butterfly pattern of uptake on gallium scintigraphy has been described in vertebral osteomyelitis.[15]

CT accurately demonstrates end-plate erosions and paravertebral masses. After administration of intravenous contrast medium, there is enhancement of the intervertebral disk, reflecting inflammatory hyperemia. CT displays anatomic detail well and may be used to guide percutaneous biopsy or drainage and for preoperative planning.

The advantages of multiplanar MRI include the direct demonstration of bone marrow involvement, the assessment of spinal canal involvement and soft tissue abscesses, and the visualization of neural structures. Because of this, MRI has replaced CT in many institutions for evaluation of inflammatory conditions of the spine and is the choice for imaging

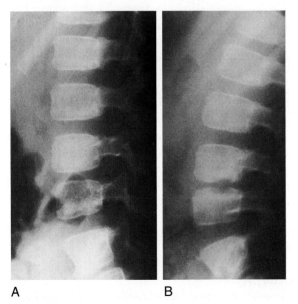

A   B

Figure 20–34
Diskitis: lateral view. *A,* Early diskitis is clearly indicated with narrowing of the L4–L5 disk space but, as yet, no evidence of bony destruction. *B,* Two months later, sclerosis of the end plates is noted with obvious focal destruction of a rounded area at the same portion of each end plate. These lucent regions probably represent herniation of the nucleus pulposus into the vertebral body.

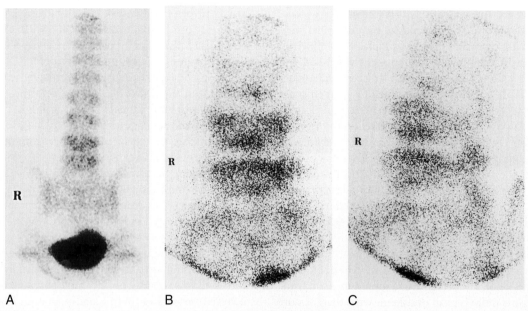

A   B   C

Figure 20–35
Diskitis. *A,* High-resolution collimator images of a 3-year-old girl with L4–L5 diskitis whose radiographs were normal. Increased radiotracer deposition in the L4 and L5 vertebrae is obvious. *B,* A pinhole collimator image in the posterior projection from the same scintigram demonstrates a relative increase in radiotracer deposition in the upper end plate of L5, in addition to generalized increase in uptake throughout the L4 and L5 vertebral bodies. *C,* A left posterior oblique projection utilizing the pinhole collimator separates the right pedicles and right laminae from the vertebral bodies, showing that the predominant areas of abnormality lie anteriorly.

of infections of the spine. MRI is both sensitive and specific for diskitis and vertebral osteomyelitis. MRI examination is sensitive to the change in disk hydration, which takes place early in the course of the disease. Normally, the nucleus has a higher signal intensity than the annulus because of its greater water content. The MRI appearances of disk space infection vary according to the stage of the disease and the age of the patient.[29] In young children, the infected sites display decreased signal on both T1- and T2-weighted images, whereas in older patients the T1-weighted images show low signal in the affected portions of the vertebral bodies but high signal with T2 weighting.[29] The affected disk may also be enhanced following gadolinium chelate administration (Fig. 20–36). The earliest response to vertebral osteomyelitis is the accumulation of water in the extracellular bone marrow. This bone marrow edema is detected by a uniform pattern of signal changes with low signal intensity on T1-weighted images. MRI findings for vertebral osteomyelitis include decreased signal intensity in the disk and adjacent vertebral bodies (as well as loss of end-plate definition on T1-weighted images). Increased signal intensity of the disk, the involved paraspinal, and the epidural tissues is seen on T2-weighted imaging. The adjacent vertebral bodies are enhanced only 50% of the time on T2-weighted imaging. Contrast enhancement of the disk and adjacent vertebral bodies, as well as ring enhancement of paraspinal and epidural abscesses and homogeneous enhancement of phlegmon, occurs in most examples of vertebral osteomyelits.[88] Some radiologists prefer

proton density T2-weighted fat-saturated sequences for appreciation of increased signal intensity in the disk and adjacent vertebral bodies. Because the findings change very little during the healing phase despite a good clinical response, MRI is not useful for monitoring this phase except to discover complications such as neural impingement from the protruding disk or paravertebral abscess.

SLIPPED CAPITAL FEMORAL EPIPHYSIS

Radiographic evidence of a SCFE is essential for diagnosing the condition. Because radiographic manifestations may initially be subtle, imaging examination must be performed with care. In particular, the frog-leg lateral hip view, which is more sensitive to the early changes of slipped epiphysis than the AP view, should be a routine part of the radiographic assessment of an adolescent who presents with a limp and hip or knee pain.

Pathophysiology

Several maturation factors relative to growth and epiphyseal development are deficient in patients with SCFE, including bone age, height and weight, thyroid functions, sex hormone levels, and growth hormone levels. Most patients (71%) weigh more than the 80th percentile. The level of active thyroid hormone (triiodothyronine) was significantly low in 25% of patients with SCFE. Testosterone levels and growth

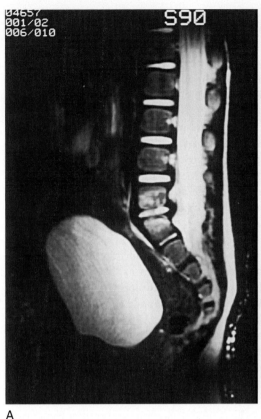
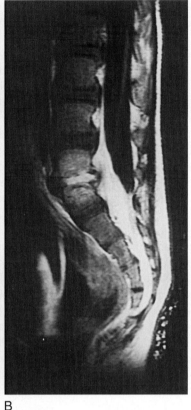

A   B

Figure 20–36
Diskitis: *A,* A T2-weighted (4/108) sagittal image reveals mottling of the intervertebral disk at the L5–S1 disk space and mottling of the marrow signal of the adjacent vertebral bodies. Also note the posterior mass effect and bulging into the spinal canal. *B,* A T1-weighted (0.8/25) image shows that the abnormal disk has a very high signal.

hormone levels were markedly reduced in the majority of patients with SCFE who were tested.[83]

The essential lesion of SCFE is a spontaneous medial and posterior displacement of the capital femoral epiphysis on the femoral neck. A combination of mechanical and hormonal factors probably account for this lesion. In early adolescence, the proximal femoral growth plate rotates from a horizontal to an oblique orientation and, with concomitant rapid growth, becomes more vulnerable to the shearing forces of ordinary weight bearing. The weakest plane in the physis is between the zones of cartilage hypertrophy and provisional calcification. Multiple endocrine factors such as low testosterone and growth hormone levels, along with a tendency toward hypothyroidism, lend support to the biochemical theory of a delicate hormonal imbalance in SCFE. It is of interest that several diseases involving endocrine imbalance are associated with SCFE (Table 20–7).

Clinical Presentation

Males are affected by SCFE up to five times more commonly than females. The peak age range is 13 to 16 years in males and 11 to 14 years in females. The large, obese, sexually underdeveloped adolescent is affected far more commonly than the adolescent who is tall, thin, and rapidly growing. Half of patients exceed the 95th percentile in weight for their height.[69] African-American children are affected more frequently than Caucasian children.[12] Bilateral involvement occurs in 15% to 25% of patients. Patients typically present with groin, thigh, or knee pain and a limp. The limp is most often antalgic, but a Trendelenburg gait may also be seen. There are no systemic symptoms. On physical examination, limitation of abduction, flexion, and internal rotation of the affected hip are evident. Patients with more severe disease display a tendency toward external rotation of the femur as the hip is flexed, and the thigh does not reach the abdomen even with maximal flexion.

TABLE 20-7 CONDITIONS ASSOCIATED WITH SLIPPED CAPITAL FEMORAL EPIPHYSIS
Chronic renal failure
Hypothyroidism
Craniopharyngioma
Primary hyperparathyroidism
Acromegaly
Rickets
Turner's syndrome
Klinefelter's syndrome
Ovarian dysgenesis
Radiotherapy

Prevention of further slipping is the usual objective of therapy, rather than attempts to correct displacement and angulation at the physis when the slip is mild to moderate. Fixation is most often accomplished with surgical pinning, which can be done percutaneously.[91,93] Closed complete reduction of the slip is not often undertaken because vigorous manipulation in such attempts may increase the risk of AVN of the femoral head. Open reduction of severe slips has a significant risk of avascular necrosis (reportedly occurring in about one third of these patients). Chondrolysis, or acute cartilage necrosis of the capital femoral epiphysis, is the most common and important complication and can occur in treated and untreated SCFE. Its exact etiology has not been conclusively determined, and there may be some connection with hardware penetration into the joint and its development. Because chondrolysis can occur in both treated and untreated hips, an immune mechanism has been postulated. Although some evidence of an immune reaction has been confirmed in the joint, no screening test has yet been developed to determine susceptible individuals. The incidence of chondrolysis varies from 1.8% to 55% in patients with SCFE.[43,56] The more severe the slip is and the longer its duration, the more likely is the development of secondary chondrolysis. Prolonged immobilization may induce chondrolysis due to a reduction in production of synovial fluid. The nutritional needs of articular cartilage are supplied mainly by synovial fluid. Restoration of lost joint width can occur, and joint width may return to nearly normal in 3 months to 1 year with aggressive rehabilitation. In a large series of patients with SCFE and chondrolysis who were followed for 7 years, 32% of patients had some evidence of restoration of cartilage.[64] Nonetheless, the prognosis for SCFE is good in three fourths of patients with slips of 40 degrees or less.[64]

Diagnostic Imaging

Radiographs of the pelvis in the anteroposterior neutral and frog-leg position generally are sufficient to make the diagnosis. The frog-leg lateral view is essential for detection of subtle, minimal posterior slippage. Scintigraphic examination may be useful to assess vascularity of the femoral head and the presence of chondrolysis.

In the earliest stage (preslip) before there is any noticeable evidence of shift in the position of the femoral head, the radiograph may reveal only an apparent widening of the physis (epiphyseal plate). With mild slipping (defined as up to 1 cm of displacement), the AP view in neutral position may appear deceptively normal, but careful analysis reveals slight widening of the physis, which has slightly irregular margins, and failure of the lateral corner of the epiphysis to extend lateral to the lateral femoral neck. The medial corner of the metaphysis descends to about the lower margin of the acetabulum (Fig. 20–37). The frog-leg position view makes

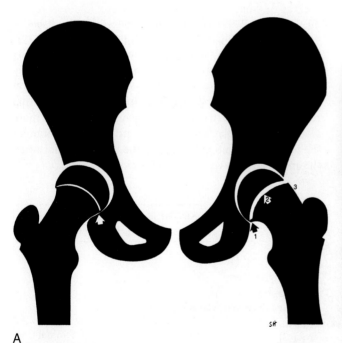 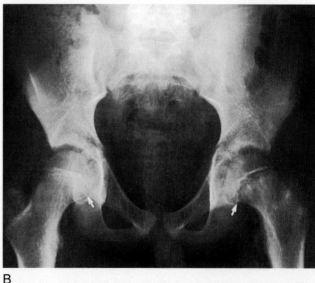

A   B

Figure 20–37

Slipped capital femoral epiphysis. *A,* Diagrammatic representation. Normal right hip and abnormal left hip. An abnormally low location of the proximal medial femoral metaphysis *(black arrow with 1).* Epiphyseal widening is characteristic *(white arrow with 2),* as is the medial location of the lateral margin of the femoral head, such that a line drawn along the lateral femoral neck (3) will not intersect the femoral head. *B,* Radiograph. In this frontal view of the hips (in neutral position) of a 10-year-old boy with a limp and left hip pain for several weeks, apparent widening of the physis of the proximal left femur is evident. The left femoral head does not project lateral to the margin of the femoral neck, and the medial corner of the proximal metaphysis *(arrow)* does not extend as deeply into the acetabulum as on the normal side.

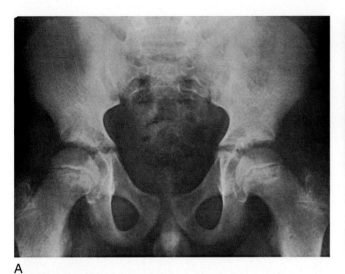

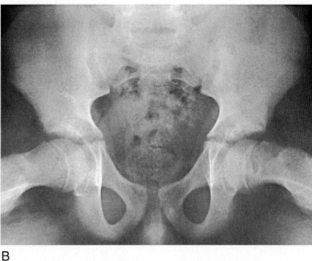

A   B

Figure 20–38

Slipped capital femoral epiphysis. *A,* The anteroposterior view of the pelvis (in neutral position) of a 12-year-old boy with hip pain shows no obvious abnormalities. However, a peculiar elliptical area of increased density runs across each proximal femoral metaphysis. *B,* These findings emphasize that the frog-leg lateral view is much more reliable than the AP view in diagnosing mild slipped capital femoral epiphysis, present in this patient bilaterally.

the findings much easier to detect because the femoral head displacement is perpendicular to the radiographic beam (Fig. 20–38). In a moderate slip, the head is displaced more than 1 cm but less than two thirds the width of the femoral neck. Displacement of greater than two thirds of the width of the femoral neck is described as a severe slip.

SCFE may be acute or chronic. Chronic epiphyseal slip (symptoms lasting longer than 3 weeks) can be confirmed radiographically by the increased cortical bone buttressing the inferior aspect of the femoral neck (Fig. 20–39). The femoral neck bows cephalad to accommodate the slip and, in severe

cases, the lateral position of the femoral neck may actually articulate with a portion of the acetabulum. Femoral shortening occurs due to the bowing phenomenon and sometimes premature fusion of the physis. Determination of the head-neck angle from axial CT is the most accurate and reproducible method for measuring the true posterior angulation and epiphyseal displacement. This method reduces the variability caused by positioning of the patient on the true lateral and frog-leg lateral views. CT could help standardize the assessment of slip severity but is not done routinely.[20] Sequential radiographic examinations can mislead the

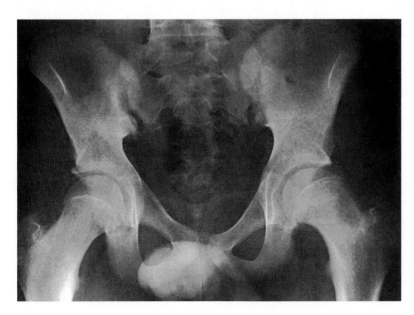

Figure 20–39

Chronic slipped capital femoral epiphysis. This AP pelvis film shows remodeling of the left femoral neck into a distinctive curved shape with thickening of its medial cortex (buttressing). Note that as in acute slippage, the femoral head does not project lateral to the lateral margin of the femoral neck. Also, the medial corner of the proximal lateral metaphysis does not extend as deeply into the acetabulum as on the normal side. This 13-year-old boy presented with chronic left hip pain and a limp.

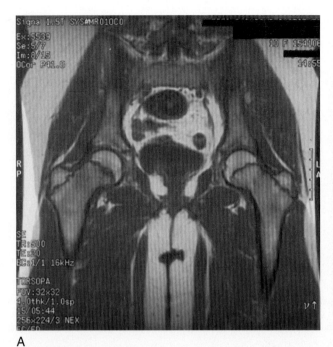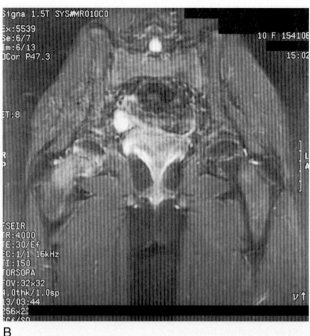

A   B

Figure 20–40
Early right slipped capital femoral epiphysis in a 10-year-old female. *A,* Coronal T1-weighted image shows widening of the right physis and low signal intensity in the femoral neck. *B,* Coronal inversion recovery image shows increased signal intensity in the marrow of the right capital femoral epiphysis adjacent to the growth plate and in the metaphysis of the neck.

observer by different positioning of the patient and placement of the x-ray beam, which results in changing head-neck relationships and positioning of pins.

Bone scintigraphy usually is not needed to make the diagnosis of SCFE. A small percentage of patients may undergo scintigraphy when the radiographic examination is incomplete or incorrectly interpreted and if a complication such as AVN, chondrolysis, or both[77] is suspected. High-resolution (pinhole) magnification anterior views with the hip in neutral and frog-leg lateral positions should be performed. Increased uptake in the physis and in the adjacent proximal femoral metaphysis is the most common finding in SCFE. This pattern reflects the increased metabolic activity at the site of cartilage plate disruption. Almost all scans of SCFE show increased periarticular activity, which represents an associated reactive synovitis. In active chondrolysis, the early-phase soft tissue images show significant increased periarticular activity. On delayed bone scan images, periarticular increased uptake in association with premature closure of the physis of the greater trochanter has been described as being indicative of chondrolysis. Bone scan findings can predict subsequent narrowing of the joint space (seen later on radiographs).[81] The radiographic findings of chondrolysis include persistent juxta-articular osteoporosis, progressive narrowing of the joint space to 50% or less of the normal width, and erosion of the subarticular bony cortex.[43]

Avascular necrosis of the femoral head is uncommon except in moderate or severe slips, particularly after open reduction.

This complication is identified most effectively with skeletal scintigraphy or MRI. The presence of metallic pins in the femoral neck may interfere with MRI evaluation of avascular necrosis. MRI has been accurate in predicting the presence of an acute slip in the contralateral asymptomatic side.[39] It may also be used in patients with symptoms of preslip in whom radiographs are equivocal. Growth plate changes and bone marrow edema confirm the diagnosis (Fig. 20–40).

Long-term sequelae of SCFE include femoral shortening from early growth plate closure, varus deformity (often severe), femoral neck deformity (shortening and broadening), and degenerative arthritis.

UNCOMMON CAUSES OF LIMPING

A variety of uncommon causes of limping occur at different ages, with abnormal gaits appropriate to the area involved. Such causes, listed in Table 20–8, should be considered when the more common etiologies are excluded.

SUMMARY

Diagnostic imaging plays an important role in the evaluation of children whose limp is due to a problem other than minor soft-tissue injury. Knowledge of the age relationship

TABLE 20-8 UNCOMMON CAUSES OF LIMPING (ALL AGES)

Congenital Conditions
Focal femoral deficiency
Hemihypertrophy
Congenital absence or shortening of the tibia
Tibial pseudarthrosis
Tarsal coalition
Accessory navicular bone
Traumatic Causes
Spondylolysis
Spondylolisthesis
Inflammatory Diseases
Juvenile rheumatoid arthritis
Rubella
Rubella vaccination
Caffey's disease
Henoch-Schönlein purpura
Rheumatic fever
Dermatomyositis
Appendicitis
Iliac adenitis
Thrombophlebitis
Neuromuscular Diseases
Hemiatrophy
Muscular dystrophy
Polio
Myositis
Peripheral nerve trauma or pressure
Spinal muscular atrophies
Amyoplasia congenital
Metabolic Diseases
Rickets
Scurvy
Hypervitaminosis A
Glycogen storage disease
Porphyria
Neoplastic Diseases
Leukemia
Osteosarcoma

Ewing's sarcoma
Neuroblastoma
Bone cyst
Osteoid osteoma
Rhabdomyosarcoma
Eosinophilic granuloma
Central nervous system tumors
Hemangioma
Lymphangioma
Lymphoma
Multiple exostoses
Enchondromatosis
Fibrous dysplasia
Giant cell tumor
Systemic Diseases and Syndromes
Hemophilia
Sickle cell anemia
Neurofibromatosis
Gaucher's disease
Larsen's disease
Chondrodysplasias
Mucopolysaccharidoses
Other bone dysplasias
Klippel-Trenaunay-Weber syndrome
Hypertrophic osteoarthropathy
Other Causes
Reflex sympathetic dystrophy
Köhler's bone disease
Freiberg's infarction
Leg-length discrepancy
Chondromalacia of patella
Blount-Barber syndrome
Ischemic contractures
Ingrown toenail
Idiopathic chondrolysis of the hip
Scoliosis
Psychological (mimicry)

and pathophysiology of diseases with acute gait disturbance allows the radiologist to intelligently recommend the most appropriate imaging procedure. Plain films and ultrasound are typically the first steps because they are convenient to obtain. Use of scintigraphy, CT, or MRI is needed as a second step for accurate diagnosis, because early in the course of many diseases, findings are limited to soft tissue and bone marrow. In pediatric patients, failure to diagnose infection has profound consequences and justifies the use of multiple studies to confirm or rule out its presence. Radiologists must accept the fact that there is no universal agreement on what

imaging modality may be best in a given situation. Some institutions and individuals may be more skilled in one modality than another, and this factor should be considered. A correctly performed and thoughtfully interpreted study will often make a difference.

REFERENCES

1. Abiri MM, Kirpekar M, Ablow RC. Osteomyelitis: Detection with US. Radiology 172:509–511, 1989.

2. Adam R, Hendry GM, Moss J, Wild SR, Gillespie I. Arthrosonography of the irritable hip in childhood: A review of 1 year's experience. Br J Radiol 59:205–208, 1986.

3. American Academy of Pediatrics. Clinical practice guideline: Early detection of developmental dysplasia of the hip. Committee on Quality Improvement, Subcommittee on Developmental Dysplasia of the Hip. Pediatrics 105:896–905, 2000.

4. American College of Radiology. American College of Radiology Standards 1999–2000. Reston, VA: American College of Radiology, 2000.

5. Arcomano JP, Stunkle G, Barnett JC, Sackler JP. Muscle group signs and pubic varus as a manifestation of hip disease in children. J Bone Joint Surg 89A:966–969, 1963.

6. Aronson J, Garvin K, Siebert J, Glasier C, Tursky EA. Efficiency of the bone scan for occult limping toddlers. J Pediatr Orthop 12:38–44, 1992.

7. Aronsson DD, Goldberg MJ, Kling TF Jr, Roy DR. Developmental dysplasia of the hip. Pediatrics 94:201–208, 1994.

8. Beaupre A, Carrol IN. The three syndromes of iliac osteomyelitis in children. J Bone Joint Surg 61A:1087–1092, 1979.

9. Beltran J, Noto AM, McGhee RB, Freedy RM, McCalla MS. Infections of the musculoskeletal system: High-field-strength MR imaging. Radiology 164:449–454, 1987.

10. Bennett OM, Namnyak SS. Bone and joint manifestations of sickle cell anaemia. J Bone Joint Surg 72B:494–499, 1990.

11. Bertol P, Macnicol MF, Mitchell GP. Radiographic features of neonatal congenital dislocation of the hip. J Bone Joint Surg 64B:176–179, 1982.

12. Bishop JO, Oley TJ, Stephenson CT, Tullos HS. Slipped capital epiphysis. A study of 50 cases in black children. Clin Orthop 135:93–96, 1978.

13. Blumberg K, Patterson RJ. The toddler's cuboid fracture. Radiology 179:93–94, 1991.

14. Brown I. A study of the "capsular" shadow in disorders of the hip in children. J Bone Joint Surg 57B:175–179, 1975.

15. Bruschwein DA, Brown ML, McLeod RA. Gallium scintigraphy in the evaluation of disk-space infections: Concise communication. J Nucl Med 21:925–927, 1980.

16. Burnett MW, Bass JW, Cook BA. Etiology of osteomyelitis complicating sickle cell disease. Pediatrics 101:296–297, 1998.

17. Capitanio MA, Kirkpatrick JA. Early roentgen observations in acute osteomyelitis. AJR Am J Roentgenol 108:488–496, 1970.

18. Chung SMK. Identifying the cause of acute limp in childhood. Clin Pediatr 13:769–772, 1974.

19. Cohen MD, Cory DA, Kleiman M, Smith JA, Broderick NJ. Magnetic resonance differentiation of acute and chronic osteomyelitis in children. Clin Radiol 41:53–56, 1990.

20. Cohen MS, Gelberman RH, Griffin PP, Kasser JR, Emans JB, Millis MB. Slipped capital femoral epiphysis: Assessment of epiphyseal displacement and angulation. J Pediatr Orthop 6:259–264, 1986.

21. Conway JJ. A scintigraphic classification of Legg-Calvé-Perthes disease. Semin Nucl Med 23:274–295, 1993.

22. Dangman BC, Hoffer FA, Rand FF, O'Rourke EJ. Osteomyelitis in children: Gadolinium-enhanced MR imaging. Radiology 182:743–747, 1992.

23. De Smet AA, Fisher DR, Burnstein MI, Graf BK, Lange RH. Value of MR imaging in staging osteochondral lesions of the talus (osteochondritis dissecans): Results in 14 patients. AJR Am J Roentgenol 155:555–558, 1990.

24. De Smet AA, Fisher DR, Graf BK, Lange RH. Osteochondritis dissecans of the knee: Value of MR imaging determining lesion stability and the presence of articular cartilage defects. AJR Am J Roentgenol 155:549–553, 1990.

25. De Valderrama JAF. The observation hip syndrome and its late sequelae. J Bone Joint Surg 45B:462–470, 1963.

26. Deutsch AL, Resnick D, Campbell G. Computed tomography and bone scintigraphy in the evaluation of tarsal coalition. Radiology 144:137–140, 1982.

27. Dich VQ, Nelson JD, Haltalin KC. Osteomyelitis in infants and children. A review of 163 cases. Am J Dis Child 129:1273–1278, 1975.

28. Digby JM, Kersley JB. Pyogenic non-tuberculous spinal infection. An analysis of thirty cases. J Bone Joint Surg 61B:47–55, 1979.

29. du Lac P, Panuel M, Devred P, et al. MRI of disc space infection in infants and children. Report of 12 cases. Pediatr Radiol 20:175–178, 1990.

30. Dunbar JS, Owen HF, Nogrady MB, McLeese R. Obscure tibial fracture of the infant: The toddler's fracture. J Can Assoc Radiol 15:136–144, 1954.

31. Egund N, Hasegawa Y, Pettersson H, Wingstrand H. Conventional radiography in transient synovitis of the hip in children. Acta Radiol 28:193–197, 1987.

32. Elsig JP, Exner GU, von Schulthess GK, Weitzel M. False-negative magnetic resonance imaging in early stage of Legg-Calvé-Perthes disease. J Pediatr Orthop 9:231–235, 1989.

33. Englaro EE, Gelfand MJ, Paltiel HJ. Bone scintigraphy in preschool children with lower extremity pain of unknown origin. J Nucl Med 33:351–354, 1992.

34. Fernandez M, Carrol CL, Baker CJ. Discitis and vertebral osteomyelitis in children: An 18-year review. Pediatrics 105:1299–1304, 2000.

35. Fink CW, Nelson JD. Septic arthritis and osteomyelitis in children. Clin Rheum Dis 12:423–435, 1986.

36. Fisher RL. An epidemiological study of Legg-Perthes disease. J Bone Joint Surg 54A:769–778, 1972.

37. Fisher RL, Roderique JW, Brown DC, Danigelis JA, Ozonoff MB, Sziklas JJ. The relationship of isotope bone imaging findings to prognosis in Legg-Perthes disease. Clin Orthop 150:23–29, 1980.

38. Fredrickson BE, Baker D, McHolick WJ, Yuen HA, Lubicky JP et al. The natural history of spondylolysis and spondylolisthesis. J Bone Joint Surg 66A:699–707, 1984.

39. Futami T, Suzuki S, Seto Y, Kashiwagi N. Sequential magnetic resonance imaging in slipped capital femoral epiphysis: Assessment of preslip in the contralateral hip. J Pediatr Orthop 10:298–303, 2001.

40. Gershuni DH, Axer A, Hendel D. Arthrographic findings in Legg-Calvé-Perthes disease and transient synovitis of the hip. J Bone Joint Surg 60A:457–464, 1978.

41. Gelfand MJ, Ball WS, Oestreich AE, Crawford AH, Jolson R, Perlmen A. Transient loss of femoral head Tc-99m diphosphonate uptake with prolonged maintenance of femoral head architecture. Clin Nucl Med 8:347–354, 1983.

42. Gilley JS, Gelman MI, Edson M, Metcalf RW. Chondral fractures of the knee. Arthrographic, arthroscopic, and clinical manifestations. Radiology 138:51–54, 1981.

43. Goldman AB, Schneider R, Martel W. Acute chondrolysis complicating slipped capital femoral epiphysis. AJR Am J Roentgenol 130:945–950, 1978.

44. Graf R. Classification of hip joint dysplasia by means of sonography. Arch Orthop Trauma Surg 102:248–255, 1984.

45. Green NE, Beauchamp RD, Griffin PP. Primary subacute epiphyseal osteomyelitis. J Bone Joint Surg 63A:107–114, 1981.

46. Grissom LE, Harcke HT, Kumar SJ, Bassett GS, MacEwen GD. Ultrasound evaluation of hip position in the Pavlik harness. J Ultrasound Med 7:1–6, 1988.

47. Guyer B, Smith DS, Cady RB, Bassano DA, Levinsohn EM. Dosimetry of computerized tomography in the evaluation of hip dysplasia. Skeletal Radiol 12:123–127, 1984.

48. Hadjipavlou AG, Cesani-Vazquez F, Vallaneuva-Meyer J, et al. The effectiveness of gallium citrate Ga 67 radionuclide imaging in vertebral osteomyelitis revisited. Am J Orthop 27:179–183, 1998.

49. Harcke HT, Grissom LE. Performing dynamic sonography of the infant hip. AJR Am J Roentgenol 155:837–844, 1990.

50. Haueisen DC, Weiner DS, Weiner SD. The characterization of "transient synovitis of the hip" in children. J Pediatr Orthop 6:11–17, 1986.

51. Henderson RC, Renner JB, Sturdivant MC, Greene WB. Evaluation of magnetic resonance imaging in Legg-Perthes disease: A prospective, blinded study. J Pediatr Orthop 10:289–297, 1990.

52. Hensinger RN. Congenital dislocation of the hip. Treatment in infancy to walking age. Orthop Clin North Am 18:596–616, 1987.

53. Hoffman EB, de Beer JD, Keys G, Anderson P. Diaphyseal primary subacute osteomyelitis in children. J Pediatr Orthop 10:250–254, 1990.

54. Holder LE, Michael RH. The specific scintigraphic pattern of "shin splints in the lower leg": Concise communication. J Nucl Med 25:865–869, 1984.

55. Howard JB, Highgenboten CL, Nelson JD. Residual effects of septic arthritis in infancy and childhood. JAMA 236:932–935, 1978.

56. Hughes AW. Idiopathic chondrolysis of the hip: A case report and review of the literature. Ann Rheum Dis 44:268–272, 1985.

57. Illingworth CM. 128 limping children with no fracture, sprain, or obvious cause. Seven were found to have Perthes' disease, 76 seemed to have transient synovitis of the hip, and in 45, the cause seemed to be in the ankle or knee. Clin Pediatr 17:139–142, 1978.

58. Illingworth CM. Recurrences of transient synovitis of the hip. Arch Dis Child 58:620–623, 1983.

59. Ippolito E, Tudisco C, Farsetti P. The long-term prognosis of unilateral Perthes' disease. J Bone Joint Surg 69B:243–250, 1987.

60. Johnson GF. Pediatric Lisfranc injury: "Bunk bed fracture." AJR Am J Roentgenol 137:1041–1044, 1981.

61. Johnson ND, Wood BP, Jackman KV. Complex infantile and congenital hip dislocation: Assessment with MR imaging. Radiology 168:151–156, 1988.

62. Jones DA, Powell N. Ultrasound and neonatal hip screening. A prospective study of 'high risk' babies. J Bone Joint Surg 72B: 457–459, 1990.

63. Jones DC, Cady RB. "Cold" bone scans in acute osteomyelitis. J Bone Joint Surg 63B:376–378, 1981.

64. Jones JR, Paterson DC, Hillier TM, Foster BK. Remodelling after pinning for slipped capital femoral epiphysis. J Bone Joint Surg 72B:568–573, 1990.

65. Jones MM, Moore WH, Brewer EJ, Sonnemaker RE, Long SE. Radionuclide bone/joint imaging in children with rheumatic complaints. Skeletal Radiol 17:1–7, 1988.

66. Kallio P, Ryoppy S, Kunnamo I. Transient synovitis and Perthes' disease. Is there an aetiological connection? J Bone Joint Surg 68B:808–811, 1986.

67. Kaye JJ, Winchester PH, Freiberger RH. Neonatal septic "dislocation" of the hip: True dislocation of pathological epiphyseal separation? Radiology 114:671–674, 1975.

68. Keats TE. Atlas of Normal Roentgen Variants That May Stimulate Disease. 3rd ed. Chicago: Year-Book Medical Publishers, 1984.

69. Kelsey JL, Acheson RM, Keggi KJ. The body build of patients with slipped capital femoral epiphysis. Am J Dis Child 124:276–281, 1972.

70. Kothari NA, Pelchovitz DJ, Meyer JS. Imaging of musculoskeletal infections. Radiol Clin North Am 39:653–671, 2001.

71. Kuhn JP, Berger PE. Computed tomographic diagnosis of osteomyelitis. Radiology 130:503–506, 1979.

72. Lantto T, Kaukonen JP, Kokkola A, Laitinen R, Vorne M. Tc99m-HMPAO labeled leukocytes superior to bone scan in detection of osteomyelitis in children. Clin Nucl Med 17:7–10, 1992.

73. Lateur LM, Van Hoe LR, Van Ghillewe KV, Gryspeert SS, Baert AL, Dereymaeker GE. Subtalar coalition: Diagnosis with the C sign on lateral radiographs of the ankle. Radiology 193:847–851, 1994.

74. Laxer RM, Allen RC, Malleson PN, Morrison RT, Petty RE. Technetium 99m-methylene diphosphonate bone scans in children with reflex neurovascular dystrophy. J Pediatr 106:437–440, 1985.

75. Lee SK, Suh KJ, Kim YW, et al. Septic arthritis versus transient synovitis at MR imaging: Preliminary assessment with signal intensity alterations in bone marrow. Radiology 211:459–465, 1999.

76. Leibowitz E, Levin S, Torten J, Meyer R. Interferon system in acute transient synovitis. Arch Dis Child 60:959–962, 1985.

77. Lubicky JP. Chondrolysis and avascular necrosis: Complications of slipped capital femoral epiphysis. J Pediatr Orthop 5:162–167, 1996.

78. MacEwen GD, Bassett GS. Current trends in the management of congenital dislocation of the hip. Int Orthop 8:103–111, 1984.

79. Mandell GA, Harcke HT, Bowen JR, Sharkey CA. Transient photopenia in the femoral head following arthrography. Clin Nucl Med 14:397–403, 1989.

80. Mandell GA, Harcke HT, Hugh J, Kumar SJ, Maas KW. Detection of talocalcaneal coalitions by magnification bone scintigraphy. J Nucl Med 31:1797–1801, 1990.

81. Mandell GA, Keret D, Harcke HT, Bowen JR. Chondrolysis: Detection by bone scintigraphy. J Pediatr Orthop 12:80–85, 1992.

82. Mandell GA, MacKenzie WG, Scott CI Jr, Harke HT, Wills JS, Bassett GS. Identification of avascular necrosis in the dysplastic proximal femoral epiphysis. Skeletal Radiol 18:273–281, 1989.

83. Mann DC, Weddington J, Richton S. Hormonal studies in patients with clipped capital femoral epiphysis without evidence of endocrinopathy. J Pediatr Orthop 8:543–545, 1988.

84. Marchal GJ, Van Holsbeeck MT, Raes M, et al. Transient synovitis of the hip in children: Role of US. Radiology 162:825–828, 1987.

85. Matin P. Bone scintigraphy in the diagnosis and management of traumatic injury. Semin Nucl Med 13:104–122, 1983.

86. McNally EG, Tasker A, Benson MK. MRI after operative reduction for developmental dysplasia of the hip. J Bone Joint Surg 79B:724–726, 1997.

87. Mellick LB, Reesor K, Memers D, Reinker KA. Tibial fractures of young children. Pediatr Emerg Care 4:97–101, 1988.

88. Miaux Y, Dion-Voirin E, Genant HK. Re: MR imaging of vertebral osteomyelitis revisited. AJR Am J Roentgenol 169:1459, 1997.

89. Minikel J, Sty J, Simons G. Sequential radionuclide bone imaging in avascular pediatric hip conditions. Clin Orthop 175:202–208, 1983.

90. Miralles M, Gonzalez G, Pulpeiro JR, et al. Sonography of the painful hip in children. 500 consecutive cases. AJR Am J Roentgenol 152:579–582, 1989.

91. Morrissy RT. Slipped capital femoral epiphysis, technique of percutaneous in situ fixation. J Pediatr Orthop 10:347–350, 1990.

92. Mukamel M, Litmanovitch M, Yosipovich A, Grunebaum M, Varsano I. Legg-Calvé-Perthes disease following transient synovitis. How often? Clin Pediatr 24:629–631, 1985.

93. Nguyen D, Morrissy RT. Slipped capital femoral epiphysis: Rationale for the technique of percutaneous in situ fixation. J Pediatr Orthop 10:341–346, 1990.

94. Nixon GW. Hematogenous osteomyelitis of metaphyseal-equivalent locations. AJR Am J Roentgenol 130:123–129, 1978.

95. Ozonoff M. Pediatric Orthopedic Radiology. Philadelphia, WB Saunders, 1979.

96. Palestro CJ, Kim CK, Swyer AJ, Vallabhajosula S, Goldsmigh SJ. Radionuclide diagnosis of vertebral osteomyelitis: Indium-111-leukocyte and technetium-99m-methylene diphosphonate bone scintigraphy. J Nucl Med 32:1861–1865, 1991.

97. Pay NT, Singer WS, Bartal E. Hip pain in three children accompanied by transient abnormal findings on MR images. Radiology 171:147–149, 1989.

98. Polaneur PA, Harcke HT, Bowen JR. Effective use of ultrasound in the management of congenital dislocation and/or dysplasia of the hip (CDH). Clin Orthop 252:176–181, 1990.

99. Poyhia T, Azouz EM. MR imaging evaluation of subacute and chronic bone abscesses in children. Pediatr Radiol 30:763–768, 2000.

100. Robson JM, Harte GJ, Osborne DR, McCormack JG. Cat-scratch disease with paravertebral mass and osteomyelitis. Clin Infect Dis 28:274–278, 1999.

101. Rosenbaum DM, Blumhagen JD. Acute epiphyseal osteomyelitis in children. Radiology 156:88–92, 1985.

102. Rush BH, Bramson RT, Ogden JA. Legg-Calvé-Perthes disease: Detection of cartilaginous and synovial change with MR imaging. Radiology 167:473–476, 1988.
103. Salter RB, Harris WR. Injuries involving the epiphyseal plate. J Bone Joint Surg 45A:587–622, 1963.
104. Saraste H. Long-term clinical and radiological follow-up of spondylolysis and spondylolisthesis. J Pediatr Orthop 7:631–638, 1987.
105. Schauwecker DS. Osteomyelitis: Diagnosis with In-111-labeled leukocytes. Radiology 171:141–146, 1989.
106. Schauwecker DS, Park HM, Mock BH, et al. Evaluation of complicating osteomyelitis with Tc-99m MDP, In-111 granulocytes, and Ga-67 citrate. J Nucl Med 25:849–853, 1984.
107. Scoles PV, Hilty MD, Sfakianakis GN. Bone scan patterns in acute osteomyelitis. Clin Orthop 153:210–217, 1980.
108. Scotti DM, Sadhu VK, Heimberg F, O'Hara AE. Osgood-Schlatter's disease, an emphasis on soft tissue changes in roentgen diagnosis. Skeletal Radiol 4:21–25, 1979.
109. Sebag G, Ducou Le Pointe H, Klein I, et al. Dynamic gadolinium-enhanced subtraction MR imaging-a simple technique for the early diagnosis of Legg-Calvé-Perthes disease: Preliminary results. Pediatr Radiol 27:216–220, 1997.
110. Sharwood PF. The irritable hip syndrome in children. A long-term follow-up. Acta Orthop Scand 52:633–638, 1981.
111. Skaggs DL, Kim SK, Greene NW, Harris D, Miller JH. Differentiation between bone infarction and acute osteomyelitis in children with sickle cell disease with use of sequential radionuclide bone marrow and bone scans. J Bone Joint Surg 83A:1810–1813, 2001.
112. St. Pierre P, Staheli LT, Smith JB, Green NE. Femoral neck stress fractures in children and adolescents. J Pediatr Orthop 15:470–473, 1995.
113. Stabler A, Reiser MF. Imaging of spinal infection. Radiol Clin North Am 39:115–135, 2001.
114. Starshak RJ, Simons GW, Sty JR. Occult fracture of the calcaneus-another toddler's fracture. Pediatr Radiol 14:37–40, 1984.
115. Sutherland AD, Savage JP, Paterson DC, Foster BK. The nuclide bone-scan in the diagnosis and management of Perthes' disease. J Bone Joint Surg 62B:300–306, 1980.
116. Swischuk LE, John SD, Tschoepe EJ. Upper tibial hyperextension fractures in infants: Another occult toddler's fracture. Pediatr Radiol 29:6–9, 1999.
117. Tang JS, Gold RH, Bassett LW, Seeger LL. Musculoskeletal infection of the extremities: Evaluation with MR imaging. Radiology 166:205–209, 1988.
118. Taylor GR, Clarke NM. Management of irritable hip: A review of hospital admission policy. Arch Dis Child 71:59–63, 1994.
119. Thompson GH, Salter RB. Legg-Calvé-Perthes disease. Current concepts and controversies. Orthop Clin North Am 18:617–635, 1987.
120. Unger E, Moldofsky, Gatenby R, Hartz W, Broder G. Diagnosis of osteomyelitis by MR imaging. AJR Am J Roentgenol 150:605–610, 1988.
121. Vila-Verde VM, da Silva KC. Bone age delay in Perthes disease and transient synovitis of the hip. Clin Orthop 385:118–123, 2001.
122. Volberg FM, Sumner TE, Abramson JS, Winchester PH. Unreliability of radiographic diagnosis of septic hip in children. Pediatrics 74:118–120, 1984.
123. Waldvogel FA, Medoff G, Swartz MN. Osteomyelitis: A review of clinical features, therapeutic considerations and unusual aspects. N Engl J Med 282:198–206, 1970.
124. Wenger DR, Bobechko WP, Gilday DL. The spectrum of intervertebral disc-space infection in children. J Bone Joint Surg 60A:100–108, 1978.
125. Wilson AJ, Murphy WA, Hardy DC, Totty WG. Transient osteoporosis: Transient bone marrow edema? Radiology 167:757–760, 1988.
126. Wingstrand H, Egund N, Carlin NO, Forsberg L, Gustafson R, Sundnen G. Intracapsular pressure in transient synovitis of the hip. Acta Orthop Scand 56:204–210, 1985.
127. Woodhouse CF. Dynamic influences of vascular occlusion affecting the development of avascular necrosis of the femoral head. Clin Orthop 32:119–129, 1964.
128. Yablon IG. Limp in childhood. J Fam Pract 2:291–295, 1975.

ADDITIONAL READING

American Institute of Ultrasound in Medicine. AIUM Practice Guideline for the performance of ultrasound examination for detection of developmental dysplasia of the hip. J Ultrasound Med 2003;22:1131-6.
Carty H, Burnnell F, Stringer DA, et al. Imaging Children, 2nd ed. London: Churchill Livingstone, 2004.
Chau CL, Griffith JF. Musculoskeletal infections: ultrasound appearances. Clin Radiol 2005;60:149-59.
Chung T. Magnetic resonance imaging in acute osteomyelitis in children. Pediatr Infect Dis 2002;21:869-70.
Coffey C, Haley K, Hayes J, Groner JI. The risk of child abuse in infants and toddlers with lower extremity injuries. J Pediatr Surg 2005;40:120-3.
Connolly LP, Connolly SA, Drubach LA, Jaramillo D, Treves ST. Acute hematogenous osteomyelitis of children: assessment of skeletal scintigraphy-based diagnosed in the era of MRI. J Nucl Med 2002;43:1310-6.
Feingold R, Saigal G, Azouz EM, Morales A, Albuquerque PA. Imaging of low back pain in children and adolescents. Semin Ultrasound CT MR 2004;25:490-505.
Futami T, Suzuki S, Seto Y, Kashiwagi N. Sequential magnetic resonance imaging in slipped capital femoral epiphysis: assessment of preslip in the contralateral hip. J Pediatr Orthop 2001;10:298-303.
Lalaji A, Umans H, Schneider R, Mintz D, Liebling MS, Haramati N. Skeletal Radiol 2002;31:362-5.
Ledermann HP, Schweitzer ME, Morrison WB, Carrino JA. MR imaging findings in spinal infections: rules or myths? Radiology 2003;228:506-14.
Marin C, Sanchez-Alegre ML, Gallego C, Ruiz Y, Collado E, Garcia JA, Mardones GG. Magnetic resonance imaging of osteoarticular infections in children. Curr Probl Diagn Radiol 2004;33:43-59.
Newberg AH, Newman JS. Imaging the painful hip. Clin Orthop Relat Res 2003;406:19-28.
Saigal G, Azouz EM, Abdenour G. Imaging of osteomyelitis with special reference to children. Semin Musculoskelet Radiol 2004:8:255-65.
Stanitski CL. Changes in pediatric acute hematogenous osteomyelitis management. J Pediatr Orthop 2004;24:444-5.
Swischuk LE. Pediatric hip pain. Emerg Radiol 2002;9:219-24.
Teo HEL, Peh WCG. Skeletal tuberculosis in children. Pediatr Radiol 43:853–860, 2004.

INDEX

Page numbers in italics refer to illustrations; page numbers followed by t refer to tables.

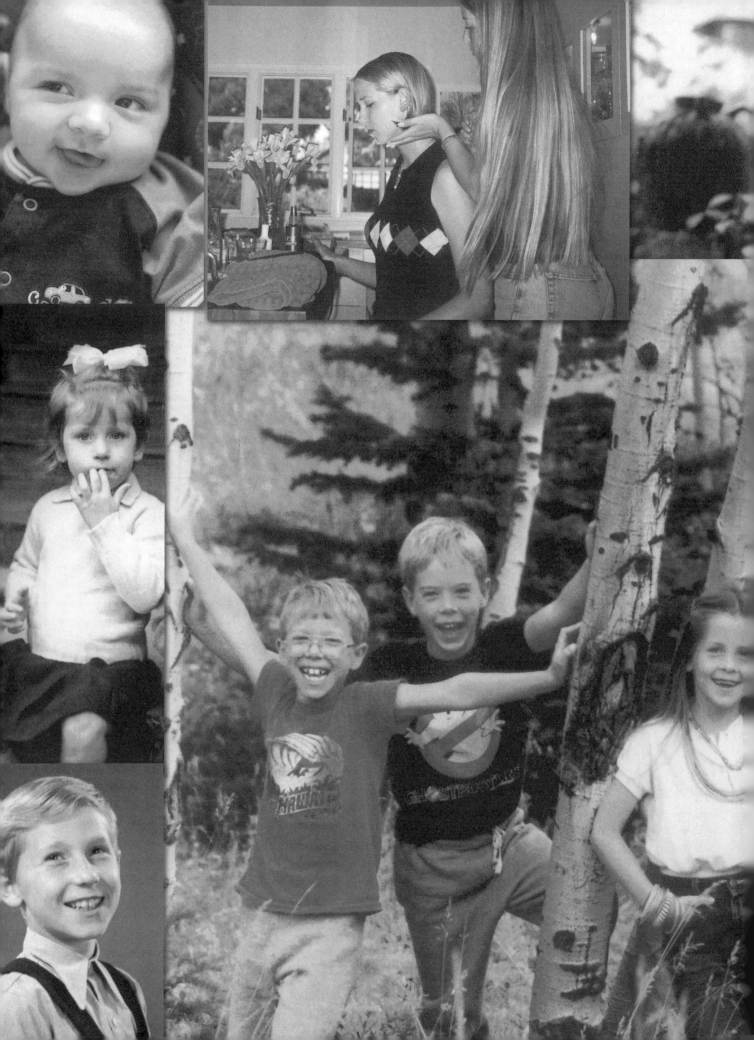